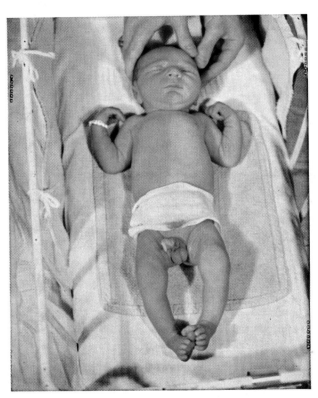

*Harlequin color change. Note the sharp line of demarcation in the midline of the face and trunk separating the reddened right half of the body and the blanched left half. (From M. Birdsong and J. E. Edmunds: Obstet. Gynecol., Vol. 7. Reproduced with permission of the senior author.)*

# *4*th Edition
# DISEASES
# *of the*
# NEWBORN

## ALEXANDER J. SCHAFFER, M.D.

Professor of Pediatrics
University of Maryland School of Medicine;
Associate Professor Emeritus of Pediatrics
The Johns Hopkins University School of Medicine
Baltimore, Maryland

## MARY ELLEN AVERY, M.D.

Thomas Morgan Rotch Professor of Pediatrics
Harvard Medical School;
Physician-in-Chief
The Children's Hospital Medical Center
Boston, Massachusetts

W. B. SAUNDERS COMPANY
Philadelphia, London, Toronto

W. B. Saunders Company: West Washington Square
Philadelphia, PA 19105

1 St. Anne's Road
Eastbourne, East Sussex BN21 3UN, England

1 Goldthorne Avenue
Toronto, Ontario M8Z 5T9, Canada

**Library of Congress Cataloging in Publication Data**

Schaffer, Alexander J

Diseases of the newborn.

Includes bibliographies and index.

1. Infants (Newborn)—Diseases.     I. Avery, Mary Ellen,
   joint author.    II. Title.

RJ254.S3 1977        618.9′201        75–38155

ISBN 0–7216–7947–1

Listed here is the latest translated edition of this
book together with the language of the translation
and the publisher.

Spanish (*3rd Edition*)—Salvat Editores, S.A., Barcelona,
                Spain

Diseases of the Newborn                                    ISBN   0-7216-7947-1

Last digit is the print number:     9    8    7    6    5    4    3    2

# CONTRIBUTORS

JACOB V. ARANDA, M.D., Ph.D.
Assistant Professor of Pharmacology and Therapeutics and Pediatrics, McGill University. Staff Neonatologist, McGill University Teaching Hospitals, Montreal, Quebec.
*Principles of Neonatal Pharmacology*

WILLIAM E. BELL, M.D.
Director, Section of Pediatric Neurology, Department of Pediatrics, The University of Iowa College of Medicine, Iowa City, Iowa.
*Neurologic Assessment of the Newborn Infant; Perinatal Trauma to the Head and to Cranial and Peripheral Nerves; Perinatal Insults to the Brain and Spinal Cord; Abnormalities in Size and Shape of Head; Seizures in the Newborn Infant; Miscellaneous Disorders of the Intracranial Contents; Miscellaneous Disorders of the Spine, Spinal Cord, and Peripheral Nervous System*

T. BERRY BRAZELTON, M.D.
Associate Professor of Pediatrics, Harvard Medical School. Director, Child Development Unit, Children's Hospital Medical Center, Boston, Massachusetts.
*Neonatal Behavior and Its Significance*

MARVIN CORNBLATH, M.D.
Professor and Head, Department of Pediatrics, University of Maryland Hospital, Baltimore, Maryland.
*Disorders of Carbohydrate Metabolism*

NANCY B. ESTERLY, M.D.
Associate Professor, Department of Pediatrics, Pritzker School of Medicine, University of Chicago. Director, Division of Dermatology, Department of Pediatrics, Michael Reese Hospital, Chicago, Illinois.
*Congenital and Hereditary Disorders of the Skin; Infections of the Skin; Nevi and Cutaneous Tumors; Miscellaneous Skin Disorders*

F. CLARKE FRASER, Ph.D., M.D., D.Sc., F.R.S.C.
Professor of Medical Genetics, Department of Biology, and Professor of Pediatrics, McGill University. Director of Medical Genetics, The Montreal Children's Hospital, Montreal, Quebec.
*The First Arch Syndrome, Cleft Lip and Cleft Palate; The Chondrodystrophies; Other Congenital Defects Involving Bones; Congenital Defects Involving Joints; Gross Chromosomal Aberrations; Genetic Counseling; Some Multiple Malformation Syndromes not Caused by Gross Chromosomal Aberrations*

**BERTIL E. GLADER, Ph.D., M.D.**

Assistant Professor of Pediatrics, Harvard Medical School. Associate Hematologist, Children's Hospital Medical Center, Boston, Massachusetts.
*Bleeding Disorders in the Newborn Infant; Neonatal Leukocyte Disorders; Erythrocyte Disorders in Infancy*

**WILLIAM RICHARD GREEN, M.D.**

Associate Professor of Ophthalmology and Pathology, Johns Hopkins University School of Medicine. Ophthalmologist and Pathologist, The Johns Hopkins Hospital, Baltimore, Maryland.
*Tumors of the Eye and Orbit*

**WARREN E. GRUPE, M.D.**

Associate Professor of Pediatrics, Children's Hospital Medical Center, Harvard Medical School. Director, Pediatric Nephrology, Children's Hospital Medical Center, Boston, Massachusetts.
*General Considerations; Disorders of the External Genitals; Major Congenital Malformations of the Genitourinary Tract; Congenital Malformations of the Kidney; Hydronephrosis; Renal Vascular Thrombosis; Hypertension; Differential Diagnosis of Enlarged Kidney; Nephropathies; Disorders of the Female Genitourinary Tract*

**JORGE B. HOWARD, M.D.**

Ayudante, Escuela de Medicina de la Universidad de Chile, Santiago. Formerly Infectious Diseases Fellow, Department of Pediatrics, University of Texas Southwestern Medical School, Dallas, Texas.
*Bacterial and Viral Infections of the Newborn*

**HARVEY L. LEVY, M.D.**

Assistant Professor of Neurology, Harvard Medical School. Assistant in Neurology, Massachusetts General Hospital. Assistant Director of Health Services, Director of the Massachusetts Metabolic Disorders Screening Program, Massachusetts Department of Public Health, Boston, Massachusetts.
*General Considerations; Inborn Errors of Carbohydrate Metabolism; Inborn Errors of Amino Acid Metabolism; Inborn Errors of Organic Acids; Inborn Errors of Lipid Metabolism; Miscellaneous Inborn Errors of Metabolism*

**PETER M. LOUGHNAN, M.B., B.S., M.R.C.P.**

Department of Clinical Pharmacology, Royal Children's Hospital, Melbourne, Australia.
*Principles of Neonatal Pharmacology*

**MILTON MARKOWITZ, M.D.**

Professor and Head, Department of Pediatrics, University of Connecticut School of Medicine, Farmington, Connecticut.
*General Considerations; Congenital Heart Disease; Myocarditis; Cardiac Arrhythmias; Miscellaneous Conditions; Differential Diagnosis of Neonatal Cardiac Problems; Treatment*

**GEORGE H. McCRACKEN, JR., M.D.**

Professor of Pediatrics, University of Texas Southwestern Medical School. Attending Physician, Parkland Memorial Hospital and Children's Medical Center of Dallas, Dallas, Texas.
*Bacterial and Viral Infections of the Newborn*

AUBREY MILUNSKY, MB.B.Ch., M.R.C.P., D.C.H.
Assistant Professor of Pediatrics, Harvard Medical School. Director, Genetics Laboratory, Eunice Kennedy Shriver Center. Assistant Pediatrician, Massachusetts General Hospital, Boston, Massachusetts.
*Antenatal Diagnosis of Genetic Disorders; Causes of Abnormalities in Newborns*

ALLEN H. NEIMS, M.D., Ph.D.
Associate Professor, Department of Pharmacology and Therapeutics and Pediatrics, McGill University. Director, Roche Developmental Pharmacology Unit, and Department of Developmental Biology, Montreal Children's Hospital, Montreal, Quebec.
*Principles of Neonatal Pharmacology*

FRANK ARAM OSKI, M.D.
Professor of Pediatrics, Upstate Medical Center, State University of New York. Chairman, Department of Pediatrics, Upstate Medical Center, State University of New York, Syracuse, New York.
*General Considerations; Physiologic Icterus (Jaundice) of the Newborn; Hemolytic Disease of the Newborn; Kernicterus; Obstructive Jaundice; Prolonged Obstructive Jaundice of Uncertain Etiology (Neonatal Giant-Cell Hepatitis); Jaundice of Other Varieties; Differential Diagnosis of Jaundice*

ROBERTSON PARKMAN, M.D.
Assistant Professor of Pediatrics, Harvard Medical School. Associate in Medicine (Immunology), Children's Hospital Medical Center. Associate in Medicine, Peter Bent Brigham Hospital. Senior Clinical Associate, The Sidney Farber Cancer Center, Boston, Massachusetts.
*Immunology*

JOHN S. PARKS, M.D., Ph.D.
Assistant Professor of Pediatrics, University of Pennsylvania School of Medicine. Associate Physician and Associate Endocrinologist, The Children's Hospital of Philadelphia, Philadelphia, Pennsylvania.
*Disorders of Mineral Metabolism; Disorders of the Adrenal Glands; Disorders of the Thyroid Gland; Abnormalities of Sexual Differentiation*

ARNALL PATZ, M.D.
Professor of Ophthalmology and the Seeing Eye Research Professor, Johns Hopkins University School of Medicine. Director, Retinal Vascular Center, Wilmer Ophthalmological Institute, The Johns Hopkins Hospital, Baltimore, Maryland.
*Disturbances of Motility; Other Neonatal Disorders of the Eyes; Infections Within and About the Eye; Tumors of the Eye and Orbit*

JOHN R. RAYE, M.D.
Associate Professor, Department of Pediatrics, The University of Connecticut Health Center, Farmington, Connecticut.
*Feeding the Normal Newborn; Feeding the Low Birth Weight Infant; Disorders of Vitamins and Trace Minerals*

ALLEN DAVID SCHWARTZ, M.D.
Associate Professor, Department of Pediatrics, University of Maryland School of Medicine. Head, Division of Pediatric Hematology and Oncology, University of Maryland Hospital, Baltimore, Maryland.
*Congenital Malignant Disorders*

ARNOLD L. SMITH, M.D.
>    Associate Professor of Pediatrics, Harvard Medical School. Associate in Infectious Disease, Children's Hospital Medical Center, Boston, Massachusetts.
>    *Fungus Infections*

LAWRENCE M. SOLOMON, M.D.
>    Professor and Head, Department of Dermatology, Abraham Lincoln School of Medicine, University of Illinois, Chicago, Illinois.
>    *Congenital and Hereditary Disorders of the Skin; Infections of the Skin; Nevi and Cutaneous Tumors; Miscellaneous Skin Disorders*

# FOREWORD
# to the Fourth Edition

Some 20 years ago, Dr. Schaffer was persuaded to make available to the general medical public the encyclopedic knowledge he had accumulated in many years of astute observation of healthy and sick newborn infants. He wrote the first edition of Diseases of the Newborn in early morning hours, before starting on the daily duties of his busy life as one of the most respected and beloved private practitioners and teachers of pediatrics in Baltimore. The effort and strain were great, but so also has been the acceptance of the book by those charged with the care of sick newborn infants throughout the world. House officers, medical students and nurses can be seen poring over its contents in copies chained to desks in many nurseries. In this edition, as in the previous one, Dr. Schaffer is joined not only by his long time colleague Dr. Milton Markowitz but also by co-author Dr. Mary Ellen Avery, one of his most illustrious and productive "fellow students." Dr. Avery's continuing contributions to the understanding of pulmonary maturation, her clinical skills, her finely reasoned judgment of research and clinical data and the clarity of her thinking and language ensure the book's continuing usefulness.

During the past two decades a marked increase has occurred in both laboratory and clinical research related to neonatal mortality and morbidity, and to the residua of the latter. The care of sick neonates has passed from relatively passive to active to intensive. Therapeutic procedures remain under continuing study because, beneficial though they are, they may produce new syndromes, as, for example, did the use of both oxygen and chloramphenicol some years ago.

The development of regional centers for "high-risk" infants or infants of "high-risk" mothers, now becoming more popular in this country, permits collection of more adequate evaluative data, both short and long term, even in the absence of a national health plan. Judgments are made difficult not only by multiple perinatal and neonatal circumstances which may affect the central nervous system particularly, but also by specific nutritional factors before and during pregnancy. Furthermore, the separation of infants from their mothers and the deprived environment to which many are discharged require collection of data which must be judged according to principles of nutrition of the soul. Finally, centers need to help develop guidelines for studying the ethical issues raised by new techniques which increase the chances of survival of badly malformed or badly damaged infants.

Neonatology thus cannot be a narrow subspecialty concerned only with the syndromes seen in the intensive care unit. It must remain loyal to its parent, pediatrics, which is oriented toward family, community and healthy as well as high-risk infants. The broad and particular experiences of the authors continue to ensure a comprehensive source of reference.

HARRY H. GORDON, M.D.
*NARC–Grover F. Powers*
*Professor of Pediatrics*
*Albert Einstein College of Medicine*
*Yeshiva University*

# PREFACE
## to the Fourth Edition

Almost incredible is the change in attitude toward the newborn infant, the abundance of information now at hand and the dramatic reduction in mortality and morbidity that have occurred since the first edition of this compilation of Diseases of the Newborn was published in 1960. During the few decades of practice of pediatrics and observation of the problems of newborn infants that preceded the publication of the First Edition, the senior author witnessed a decline in infant mortality from 47 per 1000 live births in 1940 to 26 per 1000 live births in 1960. By 1974 that number was further reduced to 16.5 per 1000 live births, and the contribution of deaths under 28 days of age reached an all-time low of 12.1 per 1000 live births.

What factors have been responsible for the increased interest in the fate of the newly born, and for the remarkable advances in understanding of their problems? Evidence for the interest is abundant in the genesis of neonatal intensive care units, regional programs to make such care widely available, training programs for neonatologists and, we might add, a number of excellent textbooks on the physiology of the newborn infant and disorders of infants. Monographs describing problems of one or another organ system may indeed be replacing more comprehensive textbooks devoted to a description of most disorders, but we hope our readers will continue to find a single text, now requiring a group of authors, however superficial its coverage of certain subjects, to be a welcome starting place for investigating and understanding the problem to be solved.

One of the factors most responsible for the explosion of interest and information has been the national commitment to research, as expressed through support of the National Institutes of Health intra- and extramural programs. Perhaps the junior editor feels the impact of this support most vividly, since the first 10 years of her academic pursuits were funded largely by the National Institutes of Health through personnel support programs and individual project grant support. The public has expressed its interest in improving the care of newborn infants in a variety of other ways as well, and we should note the major role of voluntary health agencies, such as United Cerebral Palsy Association, the Association for Aid to Crippled Children, the Markle Foundation, the National Foundation, the American Lung Association, the American Heart Association, and many others of both national and local scope. Granting agencies provide not only the needed dollars for research and study but also the encouragement to carry on. They are saying, "We believe in what you are trying to achieve," and that vote of confidence may be even more valuable than money in producing an appropriate climate for research and study.

We as a profession would be remiss if we did not also acknowledge our sensitivity to criticism. Occasionally physicians have not fully informed the parents of infant patients of the need for certain kinds of intervention, or of the necessity to evaluate a proposed therapy by a controlled clinical trial. The formation of a national commission to provide guidelines for fetal research is the outgrowth of a concern that the physician-investigator must interact with the public on issues of mutual concern, and we welcome this interaction. Issues of the definition of viability, of the rights of the newborn, of the meaning of informed consent, are of central concern as we move toward even further reductions in mortality and morbidity in the decades ahead.

Understanding of problems in human development has received a major thrust from advances in other disciplines and, perhaps most importantly, from a new technology. We worried about hypoxia and hyperoxia in the 1940's, we measured oxygen concentration in incubators in the 1950's, but we could not measure the most important variable, the oxygen tension in the blood, until the 1960's. When it became possible by microchemical methods to measure not only blood gases but also many other substances, we could practice modern scientific medicine to aid in the diagnosis and treatment of our small patients.

We have also seen the application of some fundamental advances in molecular biology to the management of our fetal and newborn patients. For example, the ability to identify the abnormal globin changes on trace amounts of fetal hemoglobin now permits prenatal diagnosis of sickle cell disease and beta-thalassemia. Indeed most prenatal diagnosis today depends on the application of biochemical detection of enzyme abnormalities, or of chromosome identification, which were outgrowths of support of basic cellular biology.

Those who are engaged in developmental biology today have at their hands tools of unparalleled potential for separating proteins, for establishing amino-acid sequences, for identifying topographical relationships in membranes and for understanding the most fundamental cellular processes. They tell us through tissue culture techniques about the regulation of synthesis and secretion of cell products, and hormonal and neural interactions in these processes. Inevitably the decades ahead will see the application of such sophisticated technology to the solution of the human problems of disordered growth and disease.

We view the Fourth Edition of this book as a statement of the state of the clinical art as we see it in 1976. We hope we are at the beginning of a new era of translation of the excitement of the last decade of monumental laboratory advances to the needs of our newborn infants. We feel the presence of a very large gap between the sophistication of science and the level of care we can bring to our patients. This book describes the ways we currently make a diagnosis, and the care we can offer. We want it to be outdated very soon.

ALEXANDER J. SCHAFFER
MARY ELLEN AVERY

# FOREWORD
## to the First Edition

Although there is controversy about "new" and "old" pediatrics, everyone recognizes the responsibility of physicians—be they obstetricians, pediatricians or general practitioners—to newborn infants. Dr. Ethel C. Durham, a pioneer in this field, posed the problem as follows: One must learn new facts about the newborn; one must spread more widely what is already known; one must make it possible to apply these facts. Dr. Schaffer's book is an important direct step toward these goals. Out of his extensive experience as a critical clinician and teacher he has written a book to help physicians judge the significance of symptoms in newborn infants. Appraisal of the neonate is most difficult, but careful history and careful physical examination are, as in all medicine, the basic modalities with which the physician must deal. The art is to know how to interpret findings, how to know when laboratory assistance is required. Direct experience with large numbers of newborn infants and understanding of their physiology are the bases for expert clinical judgment. Neither is a substitute for the other. During his more than thirty-five years as a leading practitioner of pediatrics in Baltimore, Dr. Schaffer has made careful clinical observations of thousands of newborn infants not only in the nurseries of Johns Hopkins, Sinai and the Women's Hospitals, but also as the infants have grown. He has maintained a continuing interest in the anatomic, biochemical, immunologic, pathologic, physiologic and psychologic peculiarities of the newborn infant, as befits a man who was Dr. John Howland's chief resident, and who became a leading teacher of pediatrics at Johns Hopkins University under Dr. E. A. Park and his successors.

Dr. Schaffer and his associate Dr. Milton Markowitz have for years demonstrated their consummate skill in diagnosis and treatment of newborn infants to those colleagues fortunate enough to work with them on a day-to-day basis. This book extends their influence for the benefit of newborn infants and their parents, wherever they are.

HARRY H. GORDON, M.D.

*Professor of Pediatrics*
*Albert Einstein College of Medicine*
*New York, New York*

# PREFACE
## to the First Edition

This book was intended to be an Atlas of Diseases of the Newborn. It was to consist of a large number of illustrations and a minimum number of words. Justifiably or not, we soon found ourselves changing this plan. The chief reason was that many important topics were simply not amenable to photographic treatment. How does one go about handling galactosemia or phenylketonuria pictorially? Of what use to a student or a practitioner would a book on the newborn be which omitted any discussion of an inborn error of metabolism whose early recognition spells the difference between vision and blindness, intelligence and stupidity, longevity and early death?

The second consideration which changed the structure of this book was the gigantic growth within the past decade of the corpus of knowledge concerning the newborn. Pathologists, physiologists of many varieties, radiologists and clinicians have begun to swarm over the newborn in ever-increasing numbers. Much has been learned, even though much still remains to be discovered. We felt that the time was ripe for this new knowledge to be collected and to be integrated with the old into an omnium gatherum of Diseases of the Newborn. This could not be accomplished with pictures alone.

We were then confronted with the apparently insurmountable obstacle of our own limitation of knowledge. Clearly no one man can hope to know as much about disturbances in bodily chemistry *and* endocrinology *and* congenital heart disease *and* the premature infant as do the various subspecialists in these limited fields. Would not a collection of essays written by eight or ten of these specialists constitute a superior kind of volume to this necessarily less erudite and less detailed one? We ventured to guess that, for the purpose we had in mind, it would not be as useful. For we practitioners of pediatrics are the newborns' first and primary physicians. We are the ones who should be aware of genetic predispositions which may dictate laboratory studies even before our newborn becomes ill. In this connection we call to your attention the proper management of babies born in families which contain known sufferers from congenital galactosemia or phenylpyruvic oligophrenia. We are the ones who should not, indeed must not, allow even the most trifling deviations from normal to escape our attention in our original examination. Overlooking a cornea which is larger than it should be may spell the difference between ultimate good vision and blindness. Not noticing, or attaching no significance to, a tiny red spot over the spine may mean that the baby will suffer one or two bouts of staphylococcal meningitis before his dermal sinus is diagnosed and excised. In these situations the ophthalmologist and the neurologic surgeon are of absolutely no help to us until we have made the all-important original observation. Finally we are the ones called when cyanosis, dyspnea, fever or convulsions appear, and we must make rapid decisions as to immediate treatment and further study. We must categorize the illness accurately and ask help, when needed, of the proper subspecialist. We have quoted in the text the unfortunate story of a newborn with dextrocardia for whom the aid of a cardiologist was sought. Both practitioner and cardiologist stood by while the infant died of untreated pneumothorax.

In actuality the situation of the pediatrician practicing neonatology differs but little qualitatively from his everyday posture with respect to older infants and children. Much of his function consists in screening, expediting and directing his patients to other subspecialists. But quantitative differences exist in the neonatal period. When newborns are sick they are often so terribly sick that one is loath to endanger their lives by performing diagnostic procedures that would be sheerest routine in older infants. At the same time physical examination is less rewarding in them. Finally the clinical entities peculiar to their age group are just beginning to be defined and are far from being neatly classified in any fixed nosologic schema. Thus even the simplest decisions, for instance whether cyanosis is caused by a congenital heart defect or by pulmonary or intracranial disorder, can be far from simple in the neonate. We believe the practitioner needs a reference book which brings these matters up to date and which may permit him to make these important decisions more promptly and more accurately. Detailed information about pathologic physiology, pathology and embryology may be obtained from other sources.

This then, is a book on clinical neonatology, written by a practitioner who is neither pathologist nor physiologist, neither biochemist nor virologist. It will therefore have suffered from lack of detailed knowledge in these fields. It is our hope that it will have gained something by virtue of the author's preoccupation for many busy years with the diagnosis, natural history and treatment of disorders of the sick newborn.

Many acknowledgments are in order, too many to detail in this place. The first must go to my wife, who accepted with extraordinary good grace almost complete withdrawal from social life plus the inconvenience of having been awakened at or before dawn every morning for about five years. The second is directed to Dr. Harry H. Gordon, who stimulated me to begin this work and whose constant interest and affectionate concern were mine throughout its long-drawn-out course. He must not be held responsible for any of its imperfections. Neither must my associate, Dr. Milton Markowitz, who not only wrote the section devoted to cardiac disorders, but also struggled with me over most of the sick infants who formed the basis of such knowledge of neonatology as we may possess. Dr. Anthony Perlman, my former associate, was equally conscientious in the matters of diagnosis and treatment of many of these infants and in the mechanical job of keeping detailed day-by-day records of their progress. Pathologists at three hospitals have cooperated freely at the expense of much of their valuable time. Dr. William J. Lovitt, Dr. Ella Oppenheimer and Dr. Tobias Weinberg of The Hospital for the Women of Maryland, The Johns Hopkins and the Sinai Hospitals of Baltimore, respectively, deserve my thanks. The interpretations placed upon their observations are my own. So do the librarians of the Medical and Chirurgical Faculty of Maryland, chiefly Miss Louise D. C. King and Miss M. Florence Woods, and my own secretary Miss Patricia Lilly. I am obligated deeply to all those physicians and surgeons who have given permission to utilize cases and have supplied me with prints of illustrations which my own files did not contain. In this connection the photographers at the various hospitals must be thanked, especially Mr. Harold A. Thomas at The Sinai Hospital of Baltimore.

I am singularly indebted to three good friends whose financial aid made it possible for me to amass an extensive and expensive collection of prints, lantern slides and color transparencies. They are the Messrs. Alan Wurtzburger, James H. Levi and the late Stuart M. Weiler and their wives. Dr. Markowitz is equally grateful to the Benjamin and Minnie Landsberg Memorial Foundation for their support of his studies in the field of heart disease in infancy and childhood.

I must mention my special feeling of gratitude to my publishers, W. B. Saunders Company. My contacts and correspondence with them were effected largely through the medium of John Dusseau, less often through Robert Rowan. Their help, their encouragement, their sound advice and, not least, their exhilarating senses of humor have carried me over many rough spots.

Finally I must thank the administrators of the aforementioned hospitals, plus those of the Union Memorial, University and Lutheran Hospitals of Baltimore, and the heads of their respective Pediatric and Obstetrical Departments for their permission to utilize their cases to illustrate many of my points.

ALEXANDER J. SCHAFFER
*Baltimore, Maryland*

# CONTENTS

## APPENDICES

# INTRODUCTION

## THE AIMS OF NEONATOLOGY

We trust we have been forgiven for coining the words "neonatology" and "neonatologist." The one designates the art and science of diagnosis and treatment of disorders of the newborn infant, the other the physician whose primary concern lies in this specialty. The words follow logically the stem "neonate," in common usage, and seem to be at least as appropriate as the neologisms "geriatrics" and "geriatrist" or "gerontologist." A new subspecialty has emerged in pediatrics, at least as defined by board certification and fellowship training programs. Such a subdivision has, we suspect, as much merit as does adolescent medicine or even pediatric endocrinology and pediatric cardiology. The period of greatest mortality in life is the first day, and a high mortality rate characterizes the entire first month (Fig. I–1). If we add to these the deaths which take place in the last months of pregnancy and during labor and delivery, the sum total of so-called perinatal deaths adds up to a staggering figure, a figure which has not fallen nearly so rapidly since the dawn of modern medicine as have the mortality rates for any of the other age groups. Table I–1 and Figure I–2 show the main causes of infant deaths in the first year, and Table I–2 the position the United States currently occupies among 25 selected countries. The perinatal period, therefore, represents the last frontier of medicine, territory which has just begun to be cleared of its forests and underbrush in preparation for its eagerly anticipated crops of saved lives. Until such time as a new subspecialty may be established, it behooves the pediatrician and the general practitioner who supervise the growth and development of infants and children to become more adept in diagnosis, therapy and prevention of the disorders of the newborn infant.

That a great deal of progress has been made in the past 15 years is attested to by the graphic representation of the fall in neonatal mortality in various time periods (Fig. I–3 and Table I–3).

## THE ORIGINAL EXAMINATION

The first task is the performance of a thorough physical examination. This does not differ in technique from the one the physician performs upon an older infant, but its orientation is different because of the special problems unique in this age group.

The first examination of a newborn baby should be an exciting event. It is unfortunate that because there are so many babies born and because one so seldom discovers deviations from the normal, the average practitioner or house officer assigned that duty is inclined to look upon it as a chore. In actuality it is a task of the utmost importance which, performed conscientiously, pays large dividends.

It should be routine for the examiner to scan the labor sheet with care before looking at the baby. On this he should be able to find at a glance the mother's age, parity and the outcome of her previous pregnancies, if any, her blood type and that of her husband. Matters of significance are her estimated date of confinement, the total duration of labor and the length of the second stage, and the day and hour her membranes ruptured, so that he may calculate the length of time they had been ruptured prior to delivery. Any instrumental aid to delivery should be known, as well as the presentation of the fetus. Several notations of fetal heart rate should appear on this sheet. The characteristics and quantity of amniotic fluid are of equal importance, as are the drugs which the mother has taken at any time during pregnancy, whether they have been ones directed toward the relief of pain, hypertension or edema, or for control of seizures, fever or arthritic symp-

1

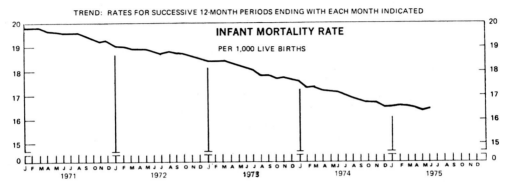

*Figure I–1.* Infant mortality rates for the United States, 1971 to 1975. (From Wegman, M. E.: Pediatrics, 56: 963, 1975.)

**TABLE I–1.** *Infant Mortality Rates by Age and Selected Causes for the United States, 1964 and 1974*

| Age and Cause of Death | 1974 (est.) | 1964 |
|---|---|---|
| *Age* | | |
| Total under 1 year | 16.5 | 24.8 |
| Under 28 days | 12.1 | 17.9 |
| 28 days to 11 months | 4.4 | 6.9 |
| *Causes* | | |
| Certain gastrointestinal diseases | 0.3 | 0.6 |
| Influenza and pneumonia | 0.9 | 3.1 |
| Congenital anomalies | 2.9 | 3.6 |
| Birth injuries | 0.6 | 0.7 |
| Asphyxia of newborn, unspecified | 1.5 | 3.7 |
| Immaturity, unqualified | 1.5 | 3.5 |
| Other diseases of early infancy | 5.3 | 5.8 |
| All other causes | 3.7 | 3.7 |

*Adjusted to compensate for differences between the seventh and eighth revisions of the International List of Causes of Death. (From Wegman, M. E.: Pediatrics 56:960, 1975.)

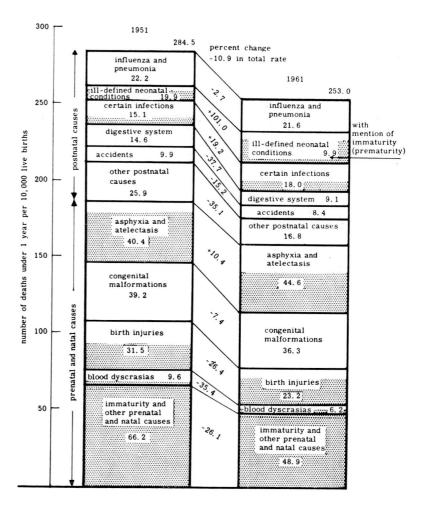

*Figure 1-2.* Infant mortaltiy, United States, 1951 and 1961: main causes by international lists (sixth and seventh revisions). (Department of Health, Education, and Welfare, Welfare Administration, Children's Bureau. Based on data from the Public Health Service, National Vital Statistics Division.)

toms. Every effort will be made to rule in or out the regular use of addictive drugs.

Finally there should appear on this same sheet the obstetrician's or anesthesiologist's estimate of the baby's condition one minute and five minutes after delivery, according to the method of Apgar. All this consumes but a few moments. To the neonatologist these obstetrical data are as significant as a detailed record of the past history of an adult is to the internist. Their significance is discussed later. (See Chapter 5.)

The pediatrician has a special responsibility for knowledge of the action of drugs that may affect the fetus after maternal ingestion, and of those agents available for treatment of the infant. The tragedy of the thalidomide disaster and the rise in neonatal mortality associated with routine use of chloramphenicol in the mid-1950's are perhaps the most spectacular illustrations of the price paid for indiscriminate use of drugs in the absence of knowledge of potential toxicity for the fetus.

These facts ascertained, the examiner turns to the two principal questions under scrutiny: First, have the rigors of pregnancy, labor and delivery rendered the newborn infant ill in any way? Second, has the mother produced a sound baby free of congenital malformations?

A thorough physical examination of a newborn differs from that of a 6 year old only with respect to differences in focus. One's sights must be set on those signs which help to answer the two questions posed above. A rapid survey of the specific data we search for follows. Although the list seems long, the trained examiner can complete such an examination within 10 to 15 minutes.

One begins with an estimation of the gestational age at the moment of birth, using the scoring method of Dubowitz or some similar one. (See Appendix.) Ideally, this estimate should approximate closely the figure calculated from the date of the last menstrual period. Then one takes an over-all look at the baby. Does he appear to be sick or well? Is he normally fashioned or not? More specifically, one examines his color, looking for pallor, the pallid cyanosis of shock, cyanosis and jaundice. If his skin is pale, are his mucous membranes and nail beds also pale? Or is the pallor a grayish sickly color of the skin alone while nail beds and lips are duskily blue? If the latter, the discoloration is more likely to be the result of shock; if the former, of anemia. Cyanosis may be generalized, or it may be localized to the distal parts of the extremities, to the head and face, to one side of the body or to the upper or lower half of the trunk. The significance of these color changes will be discussed later. Does cyanosis disappear in an environment of 30 to 40 per cent oxygen? of 100 per cent oxygen? Is it deepened or does it clear with crying? Jaundice may be intense and obvious, or one may have to bring out the yellow color of the milder forms by thumb pressure blanching of the skin.

Respirations may be irregular, but should number no more than 40 per minute.

**TABLE I–2.** *Infant Mortality Rates for Lowest 25 Countries With Populations Over 2,500,000*

| Country | 1973 | 1974 |
|---|---|---|
| Sweden | 9.6 | 9.2° |
| Finland | 10.0 | |
| Japan | 11.3 | |
| Netherlands | 11.5 | 11.0° |
| Denmark | 11.5 | |
| Norway | 11.8° | |
| Switzerland | 13.2° | |
| France | 15.5° | |
| Canada | 15.6 | |
| German Democratic Republic | 16.0 | |
| New Zealand | 16.2° | |
| Australia | 16.5° | |
| Hong Kong | 16.8° | 17.7° |
| England and Wales | 16.9 | 15.5° |
| Belgium | 17.0° | |
| **United States** | **17.7** | **16.5°** |
| Ireland | 18.0 | |
| Spain† | 20.0 | 18.5 |
| Czechoslovakia | 21.2 | |
| German Federal Republic | 22.7 | |
| Israel | 22.8 | |
| Austria | 23.8 | 23.4° |
| Greece | 24.1 | 24.0° |
| Italy | 25.7 | |
| Poland | 25.8 | 23.5° |

°Provisional data.

†Data from Anuario Estadistico, Madrid, including deaths in the first day of life (omitted in United Nations' figures for Spain).

(From Wegman, M.: Pediatrics 56:960, 1975.)

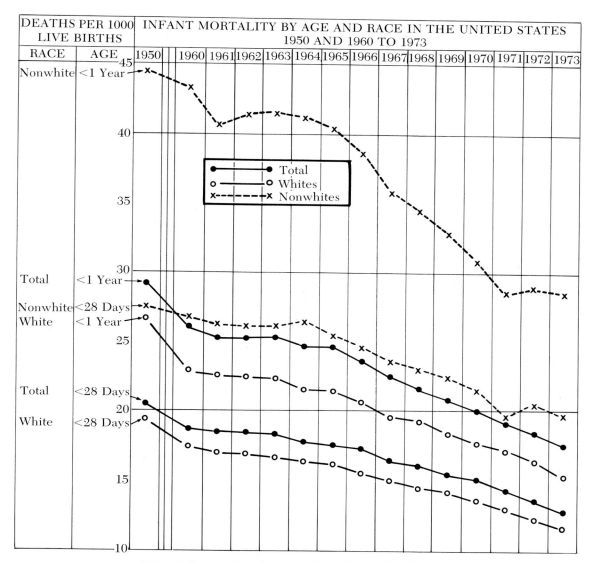

*Figure I–3.*   Data from Wegman, M. Pediatrics 54:677, 1974.

Apnea, bradypnea or tachypnea will be noted, as will unusually irregular, periodic and gasping breathing. Normally fairly shallow, breaths may be abnormally shallow or deep. Obstruction to the airway will be evidenced by retraction of intercostal spaces, suprasternal notch, sternum and lower ribs in ascending order of degree of obstruction. Stridor during inspiration or expiration, or both, is of significance, as is wheezing or grunting expiration.

The cry should be lusty and angrysounding with repetitive bursts after a single stimulus. Weak cry, high-pitched cry, hoarseness and aphonia call for study.

When undisturbed, the infant should lie quietly. If cold or annoyed or hurt, he will cry violently and move his extremities vigorously and jerkily. If he cries constantly when undisturbed or if he cries not at all when disturbed, his behavior is not normal. Similarly, if he is in constant mo-

**TABLE I–3.**  *Infant Mortality by Age and Race for the United States, 1950 and 1960 to 1973*[*][†]

| Year[‡] | Total | | | White | | | All Other | | |
|---|---|---|---|---|---|---|---|---|---|
| | Under 1 Year | Under 28 Days | 28 Days to 11 mo | Under 1 Year | Under 28 Days | 28 Days to 11 mo | Under 1 Year | Under 28 Days | 28 Days to 11 mo |
| 1950 | 29.2 | 20.5 | 8.7 | 26.8 | 19.4 | 7.4 | 44.4 | 27.5 | 19.9 |
| 1960 | 26.0 | 18.7 | 7.3 | 22.9 | 17.2 | 5.7 | 43.2 | 26.9 | 16.4 |
| 1961 | 25.3 | 18.4 | 6.9 | 22.4 | 16.9 | 5.5 | 40.7 | 26.2 | 14.5 |
| 1962 | 25.3 | 18.3 | 7.0 | 22.3 | 16.9 | 5.5 | 41.4 | 26.1 | 15.3 |
| 1963 | 25.2 | 18.2 | 7.0 | 22.2 | 16.7 | 5.5 | 41.5 | 26.1 | 15.4 |
| 1964 | 24.8 | 17.9 | 6.9 | 21.6 | 16.2 | 5.4 | 41.1 | 26.5 | 14.6 |
| 1965 | 24.7 | 17.7 | 7.0 | 21.5 | 16.1 | 5.4 | 40.3 | 25.4 | 14.9 |
| 1966 | 23.7 | 17.2 | 6.5 | 20.6 | 15.6 | 5.0 | 38.8 | 24.8 | 13.9 |
| 1967 | 22.4 | 16.5 | 5.9 | 19.7 | 15.0 | 4.7 | 35.9 | 23.8 | 12.1 |
| 1968 | 21.8 | 16.1 | 5.7 | 19.2 | 14.7 | 4.5 | 34.5 | 23.0 | 11.6 |
| 1969 | 20.9 | 15.6 | 5.3 | 18.4 | 14.2 | 4.2 | 32.9 | 22.5 | 10.4 |
| 1970 | 20.0 | 15.1 | 4.9 | 17.8 | 13.8 | 4.0 | 30.9 | 21.4 | 9.5 |
| 1971 | 19.1 | 14.2 | 4.9 | 17.1 | 13.0 | 4.0 | 28.5 | 19.6 | 8.9 |
| 1972 | 18.5 | 13.7 | 4.8 | 16.3 | 12.3 | 4.0 | 29.0 | 20.6 | 8.5 |
| 1973 | 17.6 | 12.9 | 4.7 | 15.2 | 11.5 | 3.7 | 28.8 | 19.8 | 9.0 |

[*]From Wegman, M.: Pediatrics *54:*677, 1974.
[†]Rates per 1000 live births.
[‡]Data for 1972 and 1973 are estimations based on a 10 per cent sample of deaths; all other years are based on final figures.

tion or is unusually still, one has cause for alarm. Violent, anxious overactivity and stupor or coma are especially disturbing. Muscle tonus is normally a bit exaggerated, but true rigidity and its opposite, flaccidity, are frightening; so are signs of cerebral irritation such as muscle twitching and convulsions.

A few exact measurements are important at all ages, but perhaps more so in the neonatal period. Weight and over-all length must be considered in relation to gestational age, and excesses as well as deficits in the average figures must be noted and explained. It is useful to measure the distances from the top of the head to symphysis and from symphysis to heel and to figure the ratio of the upper to the lower segment. Noting the circumferences of the head and chest is mandatory; noting that of the abdomen as well does no harm. One should pay particular attention, without necessarily measuring them, to the length of extremities in relation to that of the trunk, estimating whether they are unduly long and slender or unusually short and broad. With these base lines fixed at birth, later measurements throughout infancy take on added meaning.

With these general observations behind us we may turn to the examination of specific subdivisions. Variations in color of skin we have mentioned above. At birth the skin is usually covered with white vernix, which is most abundant in premature infants and becomes less prominent toward term. Post-term infants characteristically have no vernix caseosa, and the skin is dry, cracked and wrinkled. Its texture must be investigated with special reference to dryness, scaliness, flakiness, inelasticity or extraordinary elasticity, unusual thinness or thickness. Is edema present or not, and if so, is it generalized or localized? One looks for tumors, mainly hemangiomas, although others may be found, and for urticarial, pustular, vesicular, petechial, ecchymotic, nodular or gangrenous rashes. Lest one forget, one searches at this point for dermal sinuses in the midline of the back from occiput to coccyx and in the pilonidal region and near the ears and in the neck.

The *head* must be the focus of intense scrutiny. Its size is of utmost importance, both largeness and smallness attracting deep interest. Its shape is of equal importance, but molding during descent through the birth canal may obscure significant alterations which will only come to light some days later. At that time excessive height or length, narrowness or broadness or bizarre knobbings and depressions may be noted. Tumors or protrusions of various kinds will be noted. The fontanels and sutures are also often distorted by molding, so that instead of separations one palpates ridges where cranial bones override others. Again after a few days one can estimate better the size of fontanels and their flatness, fullness or tenseness and the width of suture lines. Absent sutural separations are as significant as excessive spreading of the lines, and one should make a practice of running a fingertip from occiput to nasion along the sagittal and metopic sutures, from one temporal region to the other along the coronal suture, and over the occipitoparietal junctures to define the lambdoidal sutures. One should look carefully along the midline for dimples, sinuses, small red spots, hirsute areas or cystic swellings which suggest the presence of congenital cranial dermal sinuses or other defects in the underlying vertebral column.

The features deserve their share of minute observation, especially the eyes. Their recent irritation by silver nitrate will make the task no easier, but they will usually open when the infant is held upright. The color of the conjunctiva and the presence of discharge within its sac may or may not indicate irritative response to the antigonorrheal bactericide recently instilled. The size of the eyeball is significant, as is true of apparent proptosis; so is its tension, and estimation of the tension of all eyeballs is recommended so that increase will be appreciated when encountered. Breadth of cornea is of utmost significance. Haziness or cloudiness of the cornea or lens or media can be quickly noted. Tumors such as small dermoids and hemangiomas are easy to see, but one may need tangential illumination to make out the grayish color of retinoblastoma through the dilated, fixed pupil. Squint or ptosis of the upper lids will be obvious, as will inability to close one or both eyes owing to peripheral facial nerve palsy. Unusual slanting of the lid slit, whether it be upward from within outward as in mongolism, or downward from within outward as in mandibulofacial dysostosis, deserves attention, as does epicanthus. The fundi can usually be seen, fleetingly at least, to provide assurance that a red reflex is present. Flame-shaped and linear hemorrhages in the retina may be seen in approximately one third of all babies born after cephalic deliveries.

Ears can be grossly malformed, uncommonly large or small, angled abnormally or set lower on the head than is usual. Very low placement plus unusual size, floppiness and perpendicularity to the skull suggest renal agenesis or gross chromosomal aberration. The ears often partake in malformations stemming from the first branchial arch, and one must always look carefully for abnormal skin tags, dimples and deep sinuses, especially in front of and below the tragus. The newborn infant should respond to a loud noise or tone. Although not usually routine, otoscopic examination is important if the infant has been in an infected intrauterine environment.

An excess of mucoid secretion in the mouth and pharynx suggests esophageal atresia. Clefts of the lip are obvious. One corner of the lip should not droop, and on crying both corners should move equally well; it may be necessary to apply a painful stimulus to a toe or the sole of the foot in order to demonstrate this. The alveolar ridges must be inspected for tumors (epignathus, epulis) and for clefts, for retention cysts (which resemble unerupted teeth, but are not) and for the elevated plaques of thrush. The tongue may be too large for the mouth and may tend to fall backward to block the pharynx. If possible, one should get a clear view of the pharynx, but the newborn's tongue is exceedingly difficult, at times impossible, to depress. One often does better by forcibly depressing the lower jaw and making the baby cry than by using a tongue depressor. One is looking for nasopharyngeal teratoma, aberrant thyroid and thyroglossal duct cysts, among other items.

The size of the jaw is a matter of great moment. The small, undershot jaw of micrognathia can be the source of great respiratory and feeding difficulty. Otherwise unexplainable bouts of cyanosis may be understood if this observation has been made.

The nose, too, can be the site of airway obstruction productive of dyspnea. One can and should assure oneself at the original examination that the posterior choanae are patent so that the newborn can breathe, as he almost must, through his nose. This can be accomplished by holding the mouth forcibly closed and watching for evidences of respiratory distress, or by listening with the stethoscope to the outrush of air from each naris when the mouth is closed and the other naris is occluded. One will, upon occasion, be rewarded for having got a good view high up within each naris, by seeing a tumor, at times an encephalocele, in the nasal airway.

Rarely the neck is unusually short and poorly mobile, suggesting that the Klippel-Feil syndrome may be present. The neck is the site of important congenital cysts arising from the branchial arches and of dimples and sinuses which are related to them. Sternomastoid tumor, hygroma, thyroglossal duct cyst and enlarged thyroid should be sought for. Stiffness and retraction are important signs. Webbing caused by abnormal folds of skin running from mastoid to acromial area is highly significant. One runs a finger the length of each clavicle to be sure that it has not been fractured.

The *chest* deserves the position of primacy as the site of the majority of troubles, both acquired and inborn, which affect the newborn, and therefore demands more thorough examination than any other part. By observation one notes whether it is overfilled with air, whether it moves adequately with respiration and whether it is symmetrical with respect to both size and motion of either side. One assesses the rate, rhythm and depth of respiration and presence or absence of retraction and of use of accessory muscles to aid breathing. Percussion and auscultation are not nearly so rewarding as they are in older children, but hyperresonance or dullness, diminution of air entry, rales, rhonchi, bowel sounds and wheezes may be heard either generally or locally. Equally important is determination of the heart size and position and of mediastinal shift by these methods of physical examination. The interpretation of these physical signs is based upon the same principles one utilizes in older patients, aided by the foreknowledge of the statistical incidence of various disorders in the neonate. What is of greatest moment is that one examine every newborn by these methods, gaining assurance from year to year in one's ability to distinguish deviations from the normal. Interpretation will follow naturally.

As concerns the heart, its size and position, rate, rhythm and strength of sounds are as important as, if not more than, the presence or absence of murmurs. Extrathoracic signs such as cyanosis, size of the liver and dilatation of superficial veins and palpability of femoral and other distal arterial pulsations are equally significant in arriving at diagnoses in the cardiac field.

In the *abdomen* one looks for unusual flatness or emptiness as an aid in diagnosing diaphragmatic hernia, and for abnormal fullness. If distention is present, one must determine by palpation, percussion and auscultation whether this is due to an excess of air within or outside of the bowel, to excess of fluid which might be clear or chylous exudate, purulent or sanguineous, to an enlarged viscus or viscera or to the presence of a cystic or solid tumor. One determines carefully the size of the liver, the edge of which is normally palpable just below the costal margin, and of the kidneys, whose lower poles one can usually barely feel deep in the flanks. Being able to feel many small hard masses throughout the distended, doughy abdomen is highly significant. One looks also for evidence of venous obstruction in the form of dilated veins over the abdominal wall or, when severe, of cyanosis and edema of genitals and legs. Visible gastric or bowel patterns may be considered an almost unimpeachable mark of obstruction. The umbilicus will be inspected carefully for signs of infection, bleeding, polyp, granuloma or abnormal communication with intra-abdominal viscera.

The *genitals* deserve minute scrutiny. Items one must note in the apparent male include size and formation of the penis, position of the meatus, size of the scrotum and nature of its skin, and descent or nondescent of testes. In the apparent female one notes the size of the clitoris, the nature of the skin of the labia majora, degree of fusion or nonfusion of the labia and, if possible, the position of the vaginal and urethral orifices. One should also palpate carefully over the inguinal canals for possible presence of hernias or gonads.

The perineum will be scrutinized for unusual bulging. One must ascertain that the anus is perforate. Some pediatricians make a practice of performing a digital rectal examination as part of their original examination of a newborn. We have never felt this to be mandatory, preferring to take the first temperature with a rectal thermometer to check on the patency of the anus, and of course to document the time of passage of the first stool.

With the baby prone one examines the posterior portion of the chest by percussion and auscultation. This is the time when one can inspect and feel the occipital region minutely for hemangioma, cephalhematoma, encephalocele and congenital dermal sinuses. With this last possibility in mind one scans the midline of the back, finally spreading the buttocks to ascertain the depth of the pilonidal dimple. The lumbosacral region and buttocks are inspected and probed for possible teratoma or meningocele or lipomeningocele. With the baby still prone one inspects the creases in the two thighs. If these do not match, further observations are in order. With the infant supine again, one attempts to compare the lengths of the two legs and then to abduct the thighs from a position of right-angle flexion laterally and downward to the table top. The significance of these findings is discussed under Congenital Dislocation of the Hip.

A quick assessment of the *extremities* follows naturally. Do all four move well and approximately symmetrically, or is one arm limp or one wrist dropped? Unusual resistance to flexion or extension or its converse, excessive malleability or flaccidity, will be noted. Deep tendon reflexes can be tested in a moment. The distal extremities must be scrutinized for polydactylism or syndactylism, for clubbing, for edema and for unusual creasing of the palms or soles.

A fairly complete neurologic examination will have been performed during the general one, since reaction to stimuli, activity, grasping, and character of the cry are readily noted. See Chapter 77 for details of the neurologic assessment.

### ACCESSORY MODES OF EXAMINATION

Examination of the *blood* is often unrewarding, but there are instances when it can be extremely helpful. The pale, shocked baby immediately after delivery is apt to be labeled as having asphyxia pallida, and the usual resuscitative measures are performed. A determination of hemoglobin content or hematocrit value might demonstrate that he does not fit into that category at all, but is suffering from posthemorrhagic anemia. He needs blood rather than oxygen and probably will die unless he receives blood promptly. Conventional examinations of blood, such as hemoglobin content, white cell count, differential count, sedimentation rate and study of the stained smear may give us valuable information. The discovery of the occasional anemia, of hyperleukocytosis or leukopenia, of platelet deficiency or of abnormally formed red blood cells makes this procedure worthwhile considerably more often than it is performed. Interestingly enough, more complicated studies such as those relative to hemolytic disease of the newborn (Coombs test, antibody titration, determination of blood types, and so on) are made more universally than are the simpler ones. Tests designed to differentiate various kinds of bleeding tendency are similarly being made for clear indication.

Cultures are of immense importance if there was prolonged membrane rupture time or any suggestion of maternal infection, or if the infant had been intubated or was born under unsterile conditions. The external auditory canal and stool should be sterile unless the amniotic fluid was infected. After the first day of life, of course, both sites are likely to be contaminated. Smear and Gram stain of the gastric aspirate are useful in the hours after birth to ascertain organisms that may have been in the amniotic liquid.

The *urine* is not examined as promptly or frequently as it should be. Anorexia, vomiting, failure to gain weight, fever, listlessness, edema, jaundice and diarrhea are among the symptoms which demand at least one urine examination.

Radiographic examinations are of immense value.

We shall never forget our amazement when we looked at the chest films of a one day old who sounded for all the world as though he had asthmatic bronchitis. He did not seem very ill. His chest was emphysematous, and expiration was a bit prolonged and was accompanied by typical musical wheezes, rales and rhonchi. The film showed a heart so large that it practically filled the entire chest! The increased area of cardiac dullness had been obscured to our percussing finger by emphysema.

Without the x-ray film one often cannot differentiate pneumothorax from emphysema, cystic disease of the lung from unilobar emphysema, or mediastinal cysts and tumors from vascular obstruction to the tracheobronchial tree. Nor can one be sure whether one is dealing with amniotic aspiration, pneumonia or lobar atelectasis, inter alia. The list of respiratory diagnoses in which radiologic examination is helpful is very long, indeed. We need not point out that in disorders of the gastrointestinal tract and abdomen, of the genitourinary system and of the central nervous system, as well as of the bony skeleton, radiographic studies are not only helpful, but often, if performed quickly and interpreted accurately, mean the difference between life and death. We often hear the statement that "no x-rays were taken because the baby was too sick." Our comment in response is that "if he was that sick, he should not have been denied the possible benefits of x-ray study."

*Electrocardiograms* yield useful information when one is confronted with diagnostic problems in neonatal cardiology. The value of *electroencephalograms* is more limited and is just beginning to be appreciated. Blood chemical concentrations have the same usefulness as they have at any other period of life, and pertinent ones should be determined on the slightest indication.

A flashlight with a rubber sleeve projecting about $1/4$ inch from its forward end is a useful instrument with which to attempt to transilluminate the skull. Similarly, transillumination of abdominal and scrotal masses can aid in their diagnosis just as it does in the cases of hydranencephaly, subdural hematoma and pneumothorax.

The nasal catheter should be used freely to demonstrate choanal atresia and esophageal stenosis. In some delivery rooms these two diagnoses are proved or eliminated routinely before the infant is transferred to the nursery.

## PREVENTION OF FUTURE TROUBLE

A great part of the pediatrician's task is preventive rather than therapeutic. This is no less true for the newborn than for the older infant.

### BREAST FEEDING

There are compelling reasons why human milk is optimal for the human infant. All mammalian milks have highly specific biochemical compositions. Cow's milk modified to resemble human milk does not succeed in matching it in all respects, such as amino acid and fatty acid composition. For example, human milk contains particularly high levels of lactose, cystine, cholesterol and polyergic fatty acids. In addition, secretory immunoglobulin A, lysozyme, the bifidus factor and lactoferrin are thought to enhance resistance to enteric infection.

The act of suckling promotes pituitary release of prolactin and other hormones which have an anovulatory effect, thus having a contraceptive child-spacing action.

The social, psychological and economic considerations that support the tremendous significance of breast feeding in the underdeveloped world were analyzed by Jelliffe in 1975. The arguments are no less significant for the Western world, since in the United States less than 20 per cent of mothers nurse their infants. (See also pages 840–846.)

## Inborn Errors of Metabolism

We have discussed in great detail later in the text the two inborn errors of metabolism in which early recognition and prompt prophylactic therapy may result in the saving of sight, intellectual capacity and life itself, i.e., congenital galactosemia and congenital phenylketonuria (phenylpyruvic oligophrenia). These disorders stem from a gene defect which in turn deprives the infant of a specific enzyme. If there is a known case of either of these disorders in the family of a newborn, the pediatrician will repeatedly perform the simple tests required to establish the diagnosis until its presence or absolute absence is ascertained. When the family history gives no warning, galactosemia must come to mind automatically at the appearance of any suggestive signs so that it can be ruled in or out with no delay. Other metabolic defects will be signaled by convulsions, lethargy or ketosis, or by a striking odor to the urine or sweat. In the case of phenylketonuria one dare not wait for first symptoms, since hope for future intellectual normality may be gone by the time these appear. We screen every newborn for evidences of this metabolic defect, and the time may be coming when we screen for many others. Thus far our best method of treatment is removal from the diet of the substrate which cannot be properly metabolized. We anticipate that many other single enzyme defects will be uncovered for which preventive treatment will be valuable and that, in due time, we may even be able to supply the missing enzyme.

**MASS SCREENING.** The only disease currently being sought in all newborn infants in most states of this country is phenylketonuria. A sample of blood collected from the heel of an infant at the time of discharge from the hospital (or at least 2 weeks of age in the case of premature infants) is usually sent to a central laboratory for determination of phenylalanine levels by the Guthrie test. A positive test requires confirmation by direct measurement in the blood. (See pages 545 and 546.)

Many centralized facilities for screening of blood or urine samples by chromatography allow a search for multiple abnormalities, including tyrosinemia, histidenemia and branched-chain hyperaminoacidemias such as maple syrup urine disease. Other forms of screening that are increasingly available are for albumin in meconium, indicative of cystic fibrosis, and chromosomes for XYY and other syndromes.

The most important indication for screening is the detection of a disabling disorder for which a treatment is available, as in phenylketonuria. Prenatal screening of the 10 per cent of pregnancies in women over 35 years of age for Down's syndrome could reduce the incidence by one half if abortion were carried out. Early detection of cystic fibrosis can lead to better treatment and genetic counseling.

**PRENATAL DIAGNOSIS.** Prenatal diagnosis is now possible for a large number of metabolic disorders by study of cultivated amniotic fluid cells. Chromosome alterations may also be identified in cells aspirated from amniotic liquid, from which the sex of the fetus can be ascertained. Clearly the way is open to predict, and perhaps treat, some diseases in utero. The next few years should be exciting ones in this area. (See Chapter 2.)

## PREVENTION OF INFECTION

The prevention of infection remains a most important task for those caring for newborn infants. Handwashing on entrance to a nursery, and between examinations of infants, has been documented as most helpful in the control of infection (Mortimer et al.). The wearing of caps, masks and gowns has recently been abandoned in many nurseries except for special procedures such as exchange transfusions. The control of airborne infection is best achieved by adequate ventilation of the nursery (eight to ten air changes per hour), and isolation of an infant is possible in an incubator attached to a tube that brings outside air into its heating system. Any standing pool of water in a nursery is apt to be contaminated with gram-negative "water bugs," such as Pseudomonas and Aerobacter, which can be pathogenic to infants. A useful preventive measure is to eliminate such pools when possible, or change them at least daily. One does not add water to the pan in the incubator unless added oxygen is being administered, since the nursery should be kept at a controlled humidity of 50 to 60 per cent.

Infants are bathed once a day with a bland soap and water, unless they are ill. The use of a soap with 3 per cent hexachlorophene is widely advocated, since it will reduce the colonization of the infant by staphylococci (Farquharson et al.). Its routine use is debatable, however, on the basis of the demonstrated potentiation of colonization with gram-negative organisms after the use of hexachlorophene. More recently, concern about absorption through the skin of solutions with 3 per cent hexachlorophene, with measurable blood levels, raised further doubts about its routine use in low-birth-weight infants. High blood levels can lead to neurotoxicity. The 1972 recommendations are to restrict its routine use to those situations in which staphylococcal disease is present.

Although the history of the care of newborn infants includes attempts to control infection by the routine administration of antibiotics, the havoc wrought by such attempts far outweighs the gain. Not only do resistant organisms emerge, but the toxicity of antibiotics in infants makes such a practice dangerous.

## PREVENTION OF EMOTIONAL DISTURBANCE

Prevention of emotional disturbance in later life clearly merits the leading position in this listing of preventable disorders. The tremendous increment of knowledge and the overwhelming quantity of oral and written communication in this field over the course of the past few decades render detailed examination of this subject as unnecessary as its broad scope makes it unfeasible here. It is now certain that the newborn infant requires a great deal of physical contact with the mother or a mother substitute, and that breast-feeding and rooming-in are valuable in this regard. On the other hand, sheer permissiveness is as unnatural and as unrewarding as stark regulation. The middle-of-the-road course is preferable, in which one regulates within reason, disciplines for good cause while remaining indifferent to minor deviations in behavior from that which in our culture is considered proper, while over all the environment the unobtrusive love and sympathy of the parents is forever almost palpably present. When we chat with new parents, we oversimplify the prescription for successful parenthood in the succinct injunction to "love deeply, but be apparently indifferent." This apparent indifference one demonstrates in the neonatal period by lack of overt concern over failure to drink specified quantities of milk at stated intervals, or over periods of crying or seeming discomfort or over mild constipation, frequency of bowel movement or regurgitation. The practices of feeding and refeeding after short intervals when the baby has eaten little at one mealtime, of overreacting to spells of crying by repeatedly picking up, fondling, dandling, rocking, diaper changing, offering food or water, burping and reburping, inserting suppositories, giving medicines of one kind or another, and the like, inevitably produce the result opposite to the one desired. That is, they increase anorexia and discomfort, and they invite the child to cry in order that he may achieve the constant attention he desires. The manipulation and fondling the infant should receive before, during and for a short time after feedings and diaper changings ought to satisfy his emotional needs.

## REGIONALIZATION OF PERINATAL CARE

Increase in the ability to detect high-risk pregnancies, fetal monitoring and intensive care have demonstrated their value in the reduction of neonatal mortality and morbidity. It is at once obvious that expensive facilities and highly trained personnel cannot be multiplied in every obstetrical service. Consequently, infant transport to appropriately equipped neonatal units is the current compromise when infants are at risk of postnatal problems.

Collaboration between state agencies, third-party payment sources and obstetrical and pediatric groups is necessary to effectively regionalize perinatal care. Regional systems in Wisconsin, Maryland and Arizona are operational, and many other areas are analyzing their own situation.

The Canadian experience in Quebec and Ontario is one of the best documented and shows the reduction in mortality possible with utilization of intensive care.

The most desirable, but sometimes unobtainable, ingredients in perinatal intensive care are a neonatal facility contiguous with the delivery room, both areas equipped with monitoring equipment, adequate space for care of the infant, equipment to maintain optimal temperature, respirators, means of administering phototherapy, x-ray facilities, and appropriately located sinks, electrical outlets, oxygen and compressed air. Of overriding importance are highly trained and motivated physicians and nurses available in sufficient numbers 24 hours a day to make the critical decisions without life-threatening delays.

## REFERENCES

Behrman, R. E. (ed.): Neonatology: Diseases of the Fetus and Infant. St. Louis, The C. V. Mosby Co., 1973.

Clow, C., Scriver, C. R., and Davies, E.: Results of mass screening for hyperaminoacidemias in the newborn infant. Am. J. Dis. Child. *117*:48, 1969.

Davies, P. A., Robinson, R. J., Scopes, J. W., et al.: Medical Care of Newborn Infants. Philadelphia, J. B. Lippincott Co., 1972.

Fantz, R. L.: Pattern vision in newborn infants. Science *140*:296, 1963.

Farquharson, C. D., Penny, S. F., Edwards, H. E., and Barr, E.: The control of staphylococcal skin infections in the nursery. Can. Med. Assoc. J. 67:247, 1952.

Genetic Disorders: Prevention, Treatment, and Rehabilitation. Report of a WHO Scientific Group, Scriver, C. R., Chairman. WHO Technical Report Series No. 497, 1972.

Jelliffe, D. B., and Jelliffe, E. F. P.: Human milk, nutrition, and the World Resource Crisis. Science *188*:557, 1975.

Kopelman, A. E.: Cutaneous absorption of hexachlorophene in low-birth-weight infants. J. Pediatr. 82:972, 1973.

Light, I. J., Sutherland, J. M., Cochran, M. L., et al.: Ecologic relation between Staphylococcus aureus and Pseudomonas in a nursery population. N. Engl. J. Med., 278:1243, 1968.

Lockhart, J. D.: How toxic is hexachlorophene? Pediatrics *50*: 229, 1972.

Lockhart, J. D., and Simmons, H. E.: Hexachlorophene decisions at the FDA. Pediatrics *51*:430, 1973.

Lucey, J. F. (ed.): Problems of Neonatal Intensive Care Units. Fifty-ninth Ross Conference on Pediatric Research. Columbus, Ohio, 1969.

Mortimer, E. A. Lipsitz, P. J., Wolinsky, E., et al.: Transmission of staphylococci between newborns. Am. J. Dis. Child. *104*:113, 1962.

Nadler, H.: Prenatal detection of genetic defects. J. Pediatr., *74*:132, 1969.

Rosenstock, I. M., Childs, B., and Simopoulos, A. P.: Genetic Screening: A Study of the Knowledge and Attitudes of Physicians. Washington, D.C., National Academy of Sciences, 1975.

Segal, S. (ed.): Transport of High-Risk Newborn Infants. Canadian Paediatric Society, 1972.

Sunshine, P. (ed.): Regionalization of Perinatal Care. Report of the 66th Ross Conference on Pediatric Research, 1974.

Swyer, P. R.: The regional organization of special care for the neonate. Pediatr. Clin. N. Amer. 17:761, 1970.

Williams, C. P. S., and Oliver, T. K.: Nursery routines and staphylococcal colonization of the newborn. Pediatrics, *44*:640, 1969.

# I

# The Normal and the Abnormal Newborn

# 1 FETAL GROWTH AND NEONATAL ADAPTATIONS

**FETOLOGY.** Just as neonatology has emerged as a specialty, fetology is an area of increasing interest to obstetricians, physiologists, biochemists and pediatricians alike. The concept of developmental biology includes early embryonic life, later intrauterine life and postnatal growth and maturation. Increasingly investigations on the fetus in utero are being undertaken, sometimes for the sake of learning more of the physiology of labor and birth, sometimes for prenatal diagnosis and now also for treatment before birth. Fetology as a component of perinatology is surely one of the rapidly developing frontiers of pediatric research.

**PRENATAL ASSESSMENT OF FETAL SIZE.** Obstetricians continue to search for reliable estimates of gestational age, fetal size and fetal maturity. When the mother's estimate of dates is uncertain, or the early months of pregnancy are marked by some vaginal bleeding, other means of assessment of the "readiness" for delivery are needed. The increasing availability of reliable predictors of fetal maturity should eliminate the tragedy of elective section of an immature infant, or the prolongation of a pregnancy at the expense of fetal well-being.

Maternal urinary estriol excretion reflects fetal well-being. Since the metabolism of estriol requires participation of the feto-placental unit in its production, estriol excretion by the mother depends on fetal well-being. Although the levels excreted per 24 hours increase with fetal weight, the variability is too great for prediction of fetal size.

Amniotic liquid constituents are useful indicators of fetal functional maturity. Most widely used is the lecithin-sphingomyelin ratio to assess lung maturity. Since lecithin concentrations increase with differentiation of alveolar cells and pulmonary surfactant production, the presence of lecithin in excess of sphingomyelin indicates a degree of lung maturity sufficient to support postnatal respiration. A simple and direct measure of lung surface active materials in amniotic liquid can be made with alcohol extraction of serial dilutions of amniotic liquid. The tubes if shaken will form stable bubbles at the air surface if the pulmonary surfactant is present and will fail to form bubbles if it is absent. The "shake" test requires only test tubes and alcohol and gives an answer within ten minutes.

A major advance in the estimate of fetal size (in contrast to lung maturity or fetal-placental well-being) was the introduction of ultrasound to measure the biparietal diameter. Introduced by Donald et al. in 1958, the technique has been extensively evaluated, and normal values have been established (Fig. 1–1).

This tool has been useful in measuring early fetal growth, with movements of the fetal heart detectable by seven weeks. Crown-rump measurements are possible between 6 and 14 weeks, and are reliable indicators of gestational age in early pregnancy. Serial measurement of length and head size allow determination of intrauterine growth and detection of its retardation, and provide important aid in selecting the optimal time for delivery.

**MONITORING FETUS DURING LABOR.** Extensive studies on fetal electrocardiograms and acid-base balance make it clear that continuous monitoring of selected high-risk pregnancies may permit early intervention by cesarean section (or on the other hand, may section to be deferred) to the advantage of the infant. Technical problems and the need for elaborate instrumentation have prevented the wide application of these procedures at this time. It is nonetheless worth noting a few of the observations that have been made, chiefly by Caldeyro-Barcia and associates in Montevideo, Uruguay. He has emphasized the significance of the transient fall in fetal heart rate that occurs after uterine

16

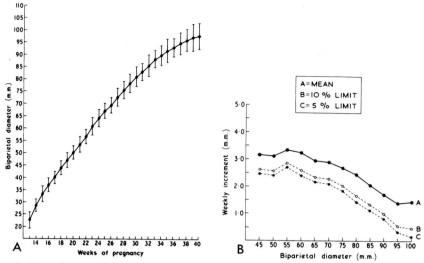

*Figure 1–1.* A, Mean biparietal diameter values (± 2 S.D.) for each week of pregnancy from 13 to 40 weeks menstrual age; 1029 individual readings made during normal pregnancy. This graph is used to assess fetal maturity and size. B, Mean weekly increments in the fetal biparietal diameter with lower tolerance limits according to the size of the biparietal diameter; longitudinal data obtained from normal pregnancies. This graph is used to assess the fetal growth rate. (From Campbell, S.: Clinics in Perinatology. *1*:512, 1974. Reproduced with permission.)

contraction. When the heart rate is slowest, 30 to 60 seconds after the peak contraction (Type II dip), fetal blood shows a significant reduction in oxygen tension and pH. These events, in turn, are correlated with depression of the infant at birth and, perhaps, with later respiratory distress.

*Fetal scalp blood sampling,* first systematically studied by Saling in Berlin, has added another dimension to prenatal diagnosis. Puncture of the fetal scalp with withdrawal of a sample of capillary blood allows measurement of fetal blood gases. When these are done at the same time that maternal blood gases are measured, it is possible to assess the functional capacity of the placenta with respect to gas exchange. James and others have emphasized the poor prognosis when fetal acidosis is present in the absence of maternal acidosis. In general if fetal pH is less than 7.10, the infant will be very depressed at birth.

*Amniocentesis* is now widely used for sampling and study of amniotic fluid. Spectrophotometric examination of bilirubin breakdown products allows prediction of the extent of hemolysis in utero, and is now routinely used in severely Rh sensitized women. Further mention of pigments in amniotic fluid will be found on page 640. Study of cells aspirated from amniotic fluid

for chromosomes or enzymes is also attracting much interest (see p. 32). Analysis of phospholipids in amniotic fluid permits prediction of the presence or absence of the pulmonary surfactant. (See Chapter 13.)

**FETAL GROWTH.** The newborn infant may be born after a shorter than average gestation, in which event he is said to be premature. He may be born of low birth weight for gestational age, either before or at term, in which instance he is undergrown. Such infants are often described as having intrauterine growth retardation, or as being "small for dates." Some babies are the products of a prolonged gestation, and are therefore termed postmature. It is the purpose of this chapter to consider fetal growth, variations in the size of the infant and some of the physiological events at the time of birth.

**SIZE AT TERM.** The length of gestation in the human is variable. "Term" is arbitrarily defined as the duration at which most infants more than 19 inches (48 cm) in length and 6 pounds (2800 gm) in weight are born (Fig. 1–2). Thus 280 to 284 days after the first day of the last menstrual period is the most likely gestational period, although infants born at any time from the beginning of the thirty-eighth week to the forty-third week have similar character-

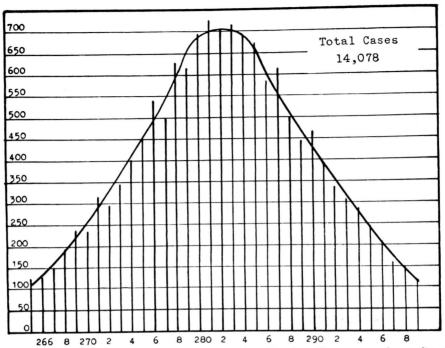

*Figure 1–2.*  Distribution curve of duration of pregnancy (from first day of last menstrual period) in 14,078 cases. The infants were at least 48 cm in length and 2800 gm in weight. Note that the median duration of pregnancy in this series was 282 days. (From Speitkamp.)

istics and a low mortality. The average weight of an infant born at term is approximately 7 pounds 8 ounces (3400 gm) for the white male at sea level, and 7 pounds (3200 gm) for the white female at sea level. Negro infants tend to weigh about 1/2 pound (200 gm) less than white infants at term. Excessive weight is sometimes encountered, presumably as high as 17 pounds (7700 gm), although our own record for weight was 12 pounds 5 ounces (5600 gm). The usual length of a term infant is 20 inches (51 cm), with a range of 18 1/2 to 23 inches (46 to 57 cm). Head circumference is a remarkably constant 13 to 15 inches (33 to 37 cm). The chest is usually nearly the same circumference as the head or a few centimeters smaller. The body segment from crown to symphysis pubis is about 1.7 times the length from pubis to heel.

**PREMATURITY.**    The former definition of prematurity had been birth weight of or under 5 pounds 8 ounces (2500 gm). The definition was based on the ease and accuracy of the measurement of weight and the difficulty of measuring the length of gestation. More accurately, the word pre-

maturity should not be synonymous with low birth weight, since it is widely recognized that many factors can produce low birth weight in infants born at term. It is nonetheless useful for statistical purposes to report mortality by weight groups, usually in 500-gm, but preferably in 250-gm increments.

Infants born before the thirty-seventh week are considered premature, and they are usually of low birth weight. The most common exception is the infant of the diabetic mother, whose size often is large for his gestational age. Perinatal mortality is clearly related to the length of gestation, increasing at either extreme from the lowest mortality of thirty-eight- to forty-two-week pregnancies (Fig. 1–3).

The intrauterine growth charts constructed by Usher and McLean are shown in Figure 1–4. These charts, and others for somewhat different populations, are of great value in assessing the appropriateness of weight for stated gestational age. Some differences exist in the many fetal growth charts that have been constructed in recent years, depending in part on the

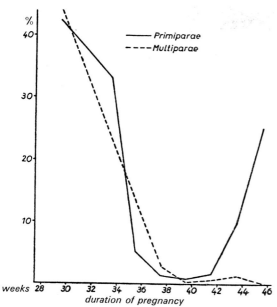

*Figure 1–3.* Perinatal mortality rate in primiparous and multiparous women. (Kloosterman, G. J.: Aspects of Prematurity and Dysmaturity. Nutricia Symposium. Leiden, H. E. Stenfert Kroese, 1968.)

sorts of infants included, and on the region of the world. The Denver data of Lubchenco are representative of infants born at an elevation of approximately 1 mile. Infants born at sea level are slightly heavier at a given gestational age. In a detailed study in England, Thomson and co-workers note the significant effects of sex and birth order, the first-born females being lighter at a given gestational age. (See Appendix for table of gestation length and embryonic and fetal bodily dimensions.)

Increasingly those writing about newborn infants speak of size as "under the tenth percentile" or under two standard deviations from the mean weight for age when identifying undergrown infants. Note that the period of most rapid weight gain is from 32 to 38 weeks, the time in gestation when the fetus stores both fat and carbohydrate. Infants born before then appear wasted.

**LOW BIRTH WEIGHT FOR GESTATIONAL AGE.** Approximately one in three infants under 2500 gm birth weight is undersized for his gestational age. These infants differ in a number of important respects from those of similar size who were born after a gestational interval appropriate for their size. Even the group identified as undergrown is a heterogeneous one, since a variety of different events may predispose to poor intrauterine weight gain.

The identification of the small-for-dates infant depends on collecting the appropriate historic and clinical information. Growth retardation should be suspected if there is a discrepancy in weight and dates, if any of the conditions cited in Table 4–5 are present and if physical signs and neurologic findings are present that indicate maturation inappropriate to the low birth weight. Usher and his colleagues have listed some of the important clinical signs that are indices of physical maturation (see Table 4–7).

Perhaps of most value in assessment of gestational age is a careful examination of the nervous system (see page 687).

**BODY COMPOSITION.** Important changes in body and organ composition take place during fetal and neonatal life. As Widdowson remarked, "In some respects we can regard birth as an incident in chemical development, which pursues the same steady course if all goes well from conception to maturity, and it matters little whether the organism spends the last few weeks of normal gestation inside or outside the uterus." Among the major trends in maturation are a decrease in body water, from 86 to 90 per cent at 28 weeks to 70 to 74 per cent by 6 months of postnatal age (Fig. 1–5). The concentration of nitrogen in fat-free tissues doubles in the last half of pregnancy; in the skin it doubles again by adulthood.

The stores of fat and carbohydrate increase approximately fivefold in the last trimester of pregnancy, and are the food reserves for the newborn infant. Protein stores provide very few calories for the starving newborn, only 4 per cent of the total as compared to 20 per cent in the starving adult. This protein-sparing during starvation is a manifestation of the anabolic tendency of the baby.

Minerals are stored in the body during pregnancy. The average term infant is born with 270 mg of iron, approximately 140 to 170 mg of which is in hemoglobin. During the first week of life, in association with decreased erythropoiesis and red cell destruction, some iron is excreted into the in-

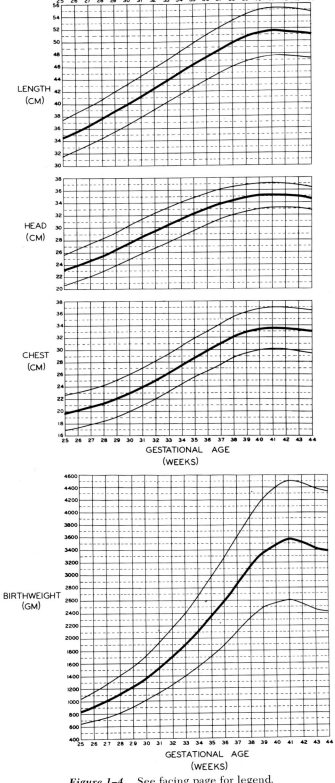

*Figure 1-4.*   See facing page for legend.

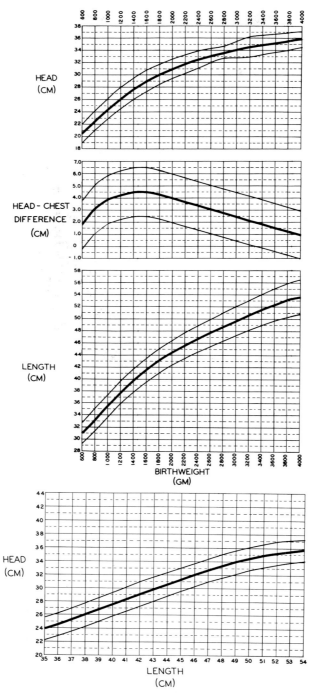

*Figure 1–4.* Smooth curve values of the mean plus or minus two standard deviations (third and ninety-seventh percentiles). Caucasian infants at sea level (Montreal). (Usher, R., and McLean, F.: J. Pediat., *74*:901, 1969.)

**TABLE 1–1.** *Reflexes of Value in Assessing Gestational Age*[*]

| Reflex | Stimulus | Positive Response | Gestation (Weeks) If Reflex Is | |
|---|---|---|---|---|
| | | | Absent | Present |
| Pupil reaction | Light | Pupil contraction | <31 | 29 or more |
| Traction | Pull up by wrists from supine | Flexion of neck or arms | <36 | 33 or more |
| Glabellar tap | Tap on glabella | Blink | <34 | 32 or more |
| Neck-righting | Rotation of head | Trunk follows | <37 | 34 or more |
| Head-turning | Diffuse light from one side | Head-turning to light | Doubtful | 32 or more |

[*]Robinson, R. J.: Arch. Dis. Childhood, *41*:437, 1966.
Note: "29 weeks" means 203 days after the first day of the last menstrual period. If there is a conflict between two results, the reflex placed higher in the table is more likely to give the true gestational age.

testine. The negative iron balance persists for the first few months of life, at which time there is little utilization of dietary iron as well. Serum iron levels at birth are about 160 $\mu$g of iron per 100 ml of serum. The level falls to 50 $\mu$g per 100 ml by 24 hours after birth, and then rises over the next two weeks.

Calcium accumulates in the body approximately linearly from the eighth week to term, when it is about 1.0 gm per 100 gm of fat-free body tissue. The calcium-phosphorus ratio is about 1.75. Magnesium doubles in amount per 100 gm of tissue from the twelfth to the fortieth week of gestation, when it is about 0.2 gm per 100 gm of fat-free tissue (Table 1–2).

Concentrations of sodium tend to fall and those of potassium to rise during fetal life and in the weeks after birth, when intracellular potassium concentrations increase markedly. Despite such marked changes in intracellular and extracellular distribution of ions, their concentrations in blood remain markedly constant. The serum sodium and chloride concentrations are the same in an immature fetus as in an adult.

The full-term infant has three times the copper content per kilogram (4.5 mg per kilogram) of the adult (1.5 mg per kilogram). The concentration in the liver falls after the second month of postnatal life. Surprisingly, the serum copper is lower at birth than at any other time of life—50 $\mu$g per 100 ml, associated with low levels of the copper-protein enzyme, ceruloplasmin.

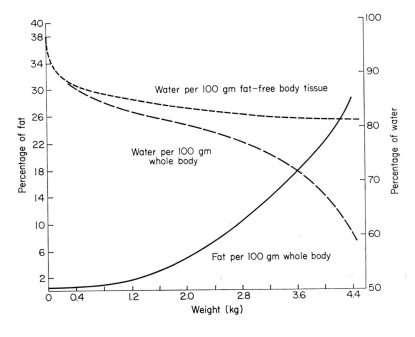

*Figure 1–5.* Percentage of water and fat in the human fetus in relation to body weight. (Widdowson, E., in Assali, N. S. [ed.]: Biology of Gestation. Vol. II. New York, Academic Press, 1968. Reproduced with permission.)

TABLE 1–2.  *Total Amounts of Water, Fat, Nitrogen, and Minerals in the Body of the Developing Fetus*°

| Body Weight (gm) | Approximate Fetal Age (Weeks) | Water (gm) | Fat (gm) | N (gm) | Ca (gm) | P (gm) | Mg (gm) | Na (mEq) | K (mEq) | Cl (mEq) | Fe (mg) | Cu (mg) | Zn (mg) |
|---|---|---|---|---|---|---|---|---|---|---|---|---|---|
| 30 | 13 | 27 | 0.2 | 0.4 | 0.09 | 0.09 | 0.003 | 3.6 | 1.4 | 2.4 | – | – | – |
| 100 | 15 | 89 | 0.5 | 1.0 | 0.3 | 0.2 | 0.01 | 9 | 2.6 | 7 | 5.1 | – | – |
| 200 | 17 | 177 | 1.0 | 2.8 | 0.7 | 0.6 | 0.03 | 20 | 7.9 | 14 | 10 | 0.7 | 2.6 |
| 500 | 23 | 440 | 3.0 | 7.0 | 2.2 | 1.5 | 0.10 | 49 | 22 | 33 | 28 | 2.4 | 9.4 |
| 1000 | 26 | 860 | 10 | 14 | 6.0 | 3.4 | 0.22 | 90 | 41 | 66 | 64 | 3.5 | 16 |
| 1500 | 31 | 1270 | 35 | 25 | 10 | 5.6 | 0.35 | 125 | 60 | 96 | 100 | 5.6 | 25 |
| 2000 | 33 | 1620 | 100 | 37 | 15 | 8.2 | 0.46 | 160 | 84 | 120 | 160 | 8.0 | 35 |
| 2500 | 35 | 1940 | 185 | 49 | 20 | 11 | 0.58 | 200 | 110 | 130 | 220 | 10 | 43 |
| 3000 | 38 | 2180 | 360 | 55 | 25 | 14 | 0.70 | 240 | 130 | 150 | 260 | 12 | 50 |
| 3500 | 40 | 2400 | 560 | 62 | 30 | 17 | 0.78 | 280 | 150 | 160 | 280 | 14 | 53 |

°Widdowson, E.: in Assali, N. S. (ed.): Biology of Gestation. Vol. II. New York, Academic Press, 1968.

It rises during the first week after birth to 150 $\mu$g per 100 ml, and then falls to the adult value of 100 $\mu$g per 100 ml.

**NEONATAL WEIGHT LOSS.** A postnatal weight loss of 5 to 8 per cent of the body weight is a constant feature of the first few days of life. The magnitude of the loss is affected by feeding practices, and to a lesser extent by the humidity in the environment. Some of the weight is lost in the form of meconium, vernix and the remnant of the umbilical cord, but most of the loss is in the form of insensible water and urine.

Redistribution of body fluids occurs in the first days of postnatal life in association with the excretion of water and electrolytes. The changes are most evident in premature infants who seem gelatinous and puffy at birth with their relatively large extracellular fluid accumulations. After several days, they assume a more wizened look. Significant shifts in electrolyte concentrations between intracellular and extracellular tissues occur, as sodium is lost from cells and intracellular potassium concentrations rise.

**TEMPERATURE REGULATION.** A low birth weight infant is at a disadvantage in maintaining body temperature chiefly because of a large surface to volume ratio and relatively little insulating subcutaneous tissue. Frequently soon after birth the infant's skin becomes pale or blue, and the rectal temperature falls, often several degrees below the intrauterine temperature of 37.6°C (99 to 100°F). This phenomenon of a rapid fall in body temperature, most pronounced in very small infants, is such a regular occurrence that the concept that infants are poikilothermic became widely accepted. Studies done mostly in the late 1950's and early 1960's have established that the infant is indeed homeothermic and tries to regulate his body temperature, although often he cannot match heat losses in the minutes or hours after birth. The avenues of heat loss in the infant are evaporation (particularly at birth when he is covered with amniotic liquid), radiation, conduction and convection. The magnitude of the losses depends upon environmental conditions. The sources of heat production are his basal metabolism, muscular activity and chemical thermogenesis mediated through the release of catecholamines. Shivering, an important form of muscular activity that increases heat production 200 to 300 per cent in the adult, is rarely seen in the infant. Chemical thermogenesis appears to be a particularly important mechanism for added heat production in the infant. Skin receptors, presumably concentrated in the face, sense the change in temperature and transmit this information to the central nervous system, which then activates the autonomic nervous system. Sympathetic impulses cause a release of norepinephrine, both from the adrenal and locally at nerve endings in the brown fat. Peripheral vasoconstriction occurs, and the brown fat is activated to break down stores of triglyceride to fatty acids, with the local production of heat. Indeed brown fat—located chiefly in the interscapular area, the nape of the neck and around the heart and kidneys—has greater oxidative capacity per milligram of protein than any other organ, and has led George Cahill to suggest that fat is not only an insulator, but perhaps an electric blanket as well.

Thermographic studies in infants show the increase in skin heat over brown fat after 30 minutes of cold exposure in about 25 per cent of infants in the first postnatal hour, but in all infants between 1 and 14 days of age. This response disappeared by 3 to 6 months of age (Rylander).

The increase in metabolism that is a consequence of cold stress is measured as an increase in oxygen consumption (Fig. 1–6). The magnitude of the effect is apparent from the many reported studies on infants of differing size and postnatal age. A *fall in environmental temperature of only two degrees centigrade, from 33 to 31° C (91.4 to 87.8° F), is a sufficient stimulus to double the oxygen consumption of a term infant* (Hill and Rahimtulla). A change in environmental temperature from 36 to 34° C (96.8 to 93.2° F) will be associated with a similar doubling of oxygen consumption in infants under 1.5 kg (Scopes). The necessity to increase oxygen consumption to maintain body temperature requires approximately the same percentage of increase in ventilation. For the normal term infant, this increase in ventilation is usually reached without difficulty. The low birth weight infant, on the other hand, frequently has some pulmonary insufficiency in the first days of life and may be unable to achieve the appropriate increase in ventilation when chilled. The consequence of increased oxygen needs in the face of pulmonary insufficiency is an oxygen debt, or the accumulation of lactate, leading to metabolic acidosis. Importantly, it has also been shown by at least three independent studies that *the survival rate of low birth weight infants is less when the environmental temperature is several degrees below their thermal neutral environment,* defined as that temperature at which oxygen consumption is minimal (Silverman et al.; Buetow and Klein; Day et al.).

The ability of the infant to increase his oxygen consumption during cold stress is depressed in a low oxygen environment. An arterial oxygen tension of 45 to 55 mm Hg depresses the response, and a $pO_2$ of 30 mm Hg abolishes it. The fall in body temperature in infants with respiratory distress has been used as a rough index of their blood oxygenation.

The difficulties in knowing the optimal thermal environment for a given infant have been discussed by Adamsons and Scopes. Practically, it appears that it is optimal to maintain the skin temperature at 36 to 36.5° C (96.8 to 97.6° F). This can be achieved by servo-incubators or by the use of thermistors to record skin temperature continuously, with judicious adjustment of the incubator to achieve the desired skin temperature. In the absence of servo-incubators, general guidelines for appropriate incubator temperatures were proposed by Hey, as shown in Table 1–3.

**FLUID BALANCE IN THE NEONATE.** The general principles governing fluid balance

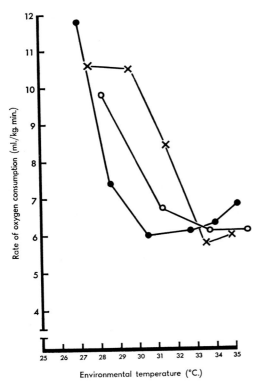

×——× 2,340-g. baby, 35 weeks' gestation, age 4 days
○——○ 2,430-g. baby, 38 weeks' gestation, age 4 days
●——● 3,800-g. baby, 40 weeks' gestation, age 5 days

*Figure 1–6.* Relation of oxygen consumption rate to environmental temperature in three babies. (Scopes, J. W.: Brit. Med. Bull., 22:88, 1966. Reproduced with permission.)

**TABLE 1–3.** *The Mean Temperature Needed to Provide Thermal Neutrality for a Healthy Baby Nursed Naked in Draught-Free Surroundings of Uniform Temperature and Moderate Humidity After Birth*

| Birth-Weight (kg) | Operative Environmental Temperature* | | | |
|---|---|---|---|---|
| | 35°C | 34°C | 33°C | 32°C |
| 1.0 | For 10 days → | After 10 days → | After 3 weeks → | After 5 weeks |
| 1.5 | — | For 10 days → | After 10 days → | After 4 weeks |
| 2.0 | — | For 2 days → | After 2 days → | After 3 weeks |
| >2.5 | — | — | For 2 days → | After 2 days |

*To estimate operative temperature in a single-walled incubator subtract 1°C from incubator air temperature for every 7°C by which this temperature exceeds room temperature.
(From Hey, E.: Brit. Med. Bull. *31*:72, 1975.)

at all ages apply to the newborn infant. Knowledge of daily requirements, assessment of any unusual losses or gains from illness or environmental conditions in the recent past and prediction and measurement on ongoing water losses or gains allows a rational approach to management.

The special conditions that affect the calculation of water requirements in the newborn include differing needs as a function of gestational age, postnatal age, activity and the environment (i.e., incubator humidity, respiration and temperature). We agree with the guidelines stated by Davies et al. for the infant without disease, in about 40 per cent humidity in a thermoneutral environment (Table 1–4).

The changes in body composition with gestational age include an increase in mass, a relative increase in the intracellular compartment with a decrease in the extracellular one, and an increase in the proportion of protein and fat. The clinical relevance of these changes would be that the very immature infant has minimal reserves and the greatest need for growth. Thus prolonged fasting, or deprivation of basal caloric needs would seem to be most serious in the undersized infant.

The changes with postnatal age include the shift of intracellular water to the extracellular space and its excretion, which accounts for the 5–8 per cent weight loss seen in most infants during the first day of postnatal life. Of course, the degree of postnatal weight loss is influenced by fluid intake; the average values cited are for normal infants, offered some 5 per cent dextrose water by mouth, and their nutrients by nursing. The quantity of solutes

excreted is relatively independent of the water intake. Thus, the solutes tend to determine the urine volume rather than urine volume determining solute excretion.

Environmental influences such as temperature and humidity greatly affect insensible water losses. For example O'Brien et al. estimated that at 30–50 per cent relative humidity the average term infant lost 24 ml of water/kg/day, approximately 60 per cent from the lungs and 40 per cent from the skin. These losses are prevented by breath-

**TABLE 1–4.**

| Fluid | Amount |
|---|---|
| Age 0–48 hrs | Pre-term (>1500 gms) 60–70 ml/kg/day |
| 5–10% dextrose in water | Term 50–60 ml/kg/day |
| | Small for dates— up to 90 ml/kg/day |
| | Increase to 100–150 ml/kg/day |

Age over 48 hrs
0.18% NaCl in 4.3% dextrose or 0.2% NaCl in 5% dextrose
(The above regimen averages 3 mEq/kg/day sodium to infants over 48 hrs)

Age over 96 hours
5–10% dextrose does not meet basal caloric needs. If oral feedings cannot be tolerated, proprietary solutions of amino acids and lipids may be used to supplement oral intake, or for total intravenous alimentation if necessary. Potassium up to 3 mEq/kg/day is required.

(Modified from Davies, P. A., et al.: Medical Care of Newborn Babies. Philadelphia, J. B. Lippincott, 1972.)

ing air saturated with water vapor at body temperature and in a similar warm and moist incubator. Fanaroff et al. found weight losses of 60 gm/kg/day in infants under 1250 grams studied nude in single-walled incubators. They reduced these losses with the addition of a plastic heat shield, which presumably altered patterns of air flow over the skin.

Some of the unusual environmental influences need to be considered for sick infants. For example, the influence of continuous distending airway pressure is to impede venous return to the heart. The effect of a decreased central blood volume is to stimulate antidiuretic hormone production, reduce urine volume and promote fluid retention. Salt and water requirements are reduced under these circumstances. The degree of reduction differs as a function of the condition of the individual infant and is best ascertained by measuring urine output and daily weight. An accentuation of postnatal water loss is found in infants under phototherapy, who not infrequently have loose stools, and have increased insensible water loss as well. Oh and Karecki found increased respiratory rates and more skin evaporation in term infants under phototherapy. The oral intake of the infants was about 20 per cent greater when under phototherapy. Since these infants may be on respirators as well, the complexity of writing a prescription for their fluid needs becomes obvious. Only careful clinical observation and weights can guide the therapist.

Of central importance is the recognition that every infant should be given at least his basal caloric needs each 24 hours. The absence of provision of calories forces the utilization of limited stores or tissue breakdown. The extent of the stress of forcing catabolism on an organism geared for growth has not been studied adequately in the human, but logic dictates that it should be avoided if possible. Total caloric needs cannot be met by 10 per cent dextrose in water. For example, a 1 kg infant requires at least 60 cal/24 hours to sustain life. If the infant receives 100 ml of 10 per cent dextrose in water, he is receiving only 40 cal/24 hours. For the first few days of life, glucose alone may be adequate, but the infant must be put in positive nitrogen balance after that time to prevent tissue breakdown.

WATER BALANCE IN THE VERY LOW BIRTH WEIGHT INFANT. When infants under 1500 grams are cared for in an environment of 40–60 per cent humidity, their fluid needs may be significantly greater than those of term infants in a similar environment. Presumably their relatively large surface to volume ratio and perhaps their relatively thin skin promote more insensible losses. Average total combined intake (parenteral and gastrointestinal) is shown in Table 1–6. Of course, individual needs may depart from these guidelines.

ACID-BASE DISTURBANCES. Significant departures from normal hydrogen ion concentrations are common in the neonatal period. Intrauterine asphyxia can result in a severe metabolic acidosis at birth, and postnatal asphyxia adds a respiratory component, so that pH values may be 6.8–7.0 in some asphyxiated infants. Adequate ventilation and oxygenation, increased cardiac output and renal perfusion operate toward rapid correction of the acidemia in the minutes and hours after birth.

**TABLE 1–5.  *Partition of Daily Caloric Expenditure in a Typical Growing Premature Infant***

| Item | Cal/kg/24 hr |
|---|---|
| Resting caloric expenditure | 50 |
| Intermittent activity | 15 |
| Occasional cold stress | 10 |
| Specific dynamic action | 8 |
| Fecal loss | 12 |
| Growth allowance | 25 |
| TOTAL | 120 |

(From Driscoll, J. M., *in* R. E. Behrman, (Ed.): Neonatology. St. Louis, C. V. Mosby Company, 1973.)

**TABLE 1–6.  *Average Total Fluid Intake in ml/kg/day for Infants of Different Birth Weights***

| | Birth Weight | |
|---|---|---|
| | < 1000 grams | 1000–1500 grams |
| Day 1 | 100–120 | 80–100 |
| Day 2 | 140–160 | 110–130 |
| Day 3 | 180–200 | 140–180 |

(Data of Roy, R. N., and Sinclair, J. C.: Clinics in Perinatology 2:393, 1975.)

In profound asphyxia, intravenous infusion of 5 to 10 ml of 25 mEq per 100 ml $NaHCO_3$ in water at a rate of 1 mEq per minute is recommended, concomitant with artificial ventilation to facilitate removal of carbon dioxide. Thereafter maintenance infusion of 5 to 15 mEq $NaHCO_3$ per 100 ml in 5 to 10 per cent glucose is appropriate, as indicated by serial measurements of pH, $Pco_2$, and $HCO_3^-$. If hyponatremia and a hypertonic urine are found, inappropriate ADH secretion is likely, which is an occasional result of severe asphyxia.

The weight of recent evidence supports slow infusions of alkali to correct a metabolic acidosis with a maximum of 6 mEq per kg per 24 hours of $NaHCO_3$. Rapid infusions of hyperosmolar solutions have been associated with hypernatremia and intracranial hemorrhage, according to Simmons and others. In infants requiring intravenous fluids for several days, as in the respiratory distress syndrome, the serum calcium may fall, and supplements are occasionally needed.

The effectiveness of parenteral fluid therapy requires close monitoring of the infant with respect to intake, output, body weight and urine specific gravity or osmolarity, and blood $H^+$ concentration and electrolytes. Urine specific gravity should be 1.005 to 1.012 (unless glucosuria is present) with a volume of 35 to 100 ml per kilogram per 24 hours. Urine osmolality of 75 to 300 mOsm per kg indicates appropriate hydration. Higher or lower values indicate stress on the concentrating or diluting mechanisms.

INTRAVENOUS ALIMENTATION. The provision of nutritional support for infants of very low birth weight, and others with gastrointestinal problems such as necrotizing enterocolitis or surgical problems, has included either total or partial intravenous alimentation. Initially this was achieved through central venous cutdowns that would permit infusion of hyperosmolar solutions such as 5 per cent amino acid hydrolysate in 20–25 per cent glucose. Even with meticulous attention to sterile precautions, and the insertion of millipore filters into the feeding line, infection limited the duration of such nutritional support.

The usual composition of a conventional infusate is 2.5 gm per kilogram per day of amino acids, 25 gm per kilogram per day of glucose, and maintenance electrolytes, minerals and vitamins. The osmolarity of that mixture averages 1800 mOsm per kg $H_2O$, the calories are 110 per kilogram per day and water is 125 ml per kilogram per day.

More recently groups in Europe and Canada have been working with nutritional supplements that include lipids and can be administered by peripheral vein. Cashore et al. in Montreal reported growth rates approximating those that would occur in utero in 23 premature infants of less than 1500 grams at birth. The solutions used contained 10 per cent Intralipid (an intravenous soybean preparation), 4.5 per cent amino acid hydrolysate in 9.5 per cent dextrose and 10 per cent dextrose, in sufficient amounts to deliver 140 ml per kilogram per day after 5 days of age, and 93 calories per kilogram per day. Supplementary calcium and vitamins were added, as well as occasional $NaHCO_2$ when acidemia was present. Partial use of these solutions, with oral milk, allows weaning from total parenteral alimentation. The experience with peripheral intravenous feeding is still preliminary (as of 1976) but surely will become an adjunct to the care of the small infant in the future. (See also pp. 845–857.)

## REFERENCES

Adamsons, K., Jr.: The role of thermal factors in fetal and neonatal life. Pediat. Clin. N. Amer. 13:599, 1966.

Beard, R. W., Morris, E. D., and Clayton, S. C.: pH of foetal capillary blood as an indicator of the condition of the foetus. J. Obst. & Gynaec. Brit. Cwlth. 74:812, 1967.

Bergstrom, W. H.: total body water and normal electrolyte composition. Pediat. Clin. N. Amer. 6:5, 1959.

Bevis, D. C. A.: Antenatal prediction of hemolytic disease of newborn. Lancet, 1:395, 1952.

Brück, K.: Temperature regulation in the newborn infant. Biol. Neonat., 3:65, 1961.

Buetow, K. C., and Klein, S. W.: Effect of maintenance of "normal" skin temperature on survival of infants of low birth weight. Pediatrics 34:163, 1964.

Calcagno, P. L., Rubin, M. I., and Singh, W. S. A.: The influence of surgery on renal function in infancy. Pediatrics, 16:619, 1955.

Cashore, W. J., Sedaghatian, M. R., and Usher, R. H.: Nutritional supplements with intravenously administered lipid, protein hydrolysate and glucose in small premature infants. Pediatrics 56:8, 1975.

Cheek, D. B., Maddison, T. G., Malinek, M., and Coldbeck, J. H.: Further observations on the corrected bromide space of the neonate and investigation of water and electrolyte status in infants born of diabetic mothers. Pediatrics 28:861, 1961.

Christie, A., Martin, M., Williams, E. L., Hudson G., and Lanier, J. C.: The estimation of fetal maturity by roentgen studies of osseous development. Am. J. Obst. & Gynec. 60:133, 1950.

Comline, K. S., Cross, K. W., Dawes, G. S., and Nathanielsz, P. W. (Eds.): Foetal and Neonatal Physiology. Proceedings of The Sir Joseph Barcroft Centenary Symposium. Cambridge University Press, 1973.

Darrow, D. C.: The significance of body size. Am. J. Dis. Child. 98:416, 1959.

Davies, P. A., Robinson, R. J., Scopes, J. W., et al.: Medical Care of Newborn Babies. Philadelphia, J. B. Lippincott Co., 1972.

Davis, J. A., and Dobbing, J. (Eds.): Scientific Foundations of Pediatrics. Philadelphia, W.B. Saunders Company, 1974.

Dawkins, M. J. R., and Hull, D.: The production of heat by fat. Sci. Amer. 213:62, 1965.

Day, R. L., Caliguiri, L., Kamenski, C., and Ehrlich, F.: Body temperature and survival of premature infants. Pediatrics 34:171, 1964.

Diczfalusy, E.: Endocrine functions of the human faeto-placental unit. Fed. Proc. 23:791–798, 1964.

Drescher, A. M., Barnett, H. L., and Troupkou, V.: Water balance in infants during water deprivation. Am. J. Dis. Child. 104:366, 1962.

Dunham, E. C., Jenss, R. M., and Christie, A. U.: A consideration of race and sex in relation to the growth and development of infants. J. Pediat. 14:156, 1939.

Elliott, K., and Knight, J. (Eds.): Size at birth. Ciba Foundation Symposium 27 (New series), Elsevier-Excerpta Med. North-Holland, 1974.

Fanaroff, A. A., Wald, M., Gruber, H. S., and Klaus, M. H.: Insensible water loss in low birth weight infants. Pediatrics 50:236, 1972.

Filler, R. M., and Eraklis, A. J.: Care of the critically ill child. Intravenous alimentation. Pediatrics 46:456, 1970.

Finn, R., Harper, D. T., Stallings, S. A., and Krevans, J. R.: Transplacental hemorrhage. Transfusion 3:114, 1963.

Hey, E.: Thermal Neutrality. Brit. Med. Bull. 31:69-74, 1975.

Hey, E., and Katz, G.: Evaporative water loss in the newborn baby. J. Physiol. 200:605, 1969.

Hey, E. N., and Maurice, N. P.: Effect of humidity on production and loss of heat in the newborn baby. Arch. Dis. Child. 43:166, 1968.

Hill, J. R., and Rahimtulla, K. A.: Heat balance and the metabolic rate of newborn babies in relation to environmental temperature, and the effect of age and weight on basal metabolic rate. J. Physiol. 180:239, 1965.

Hofnagel, D., and Lüders, D.: Pediatric history: Ernst Moro (1874–1951). Pediatrics 29:643, 1962.

Kravath, R., Aharon, A., Abal G., and Finberg, L.: Clinically significant physiologic changes from rapidly administered hypertonic solutions: Acute osmol poisoning, Pediatrics 46:267, 1970.

Liley, A. W.: Liquor amnii analysis in the management of the pregnancy complicated by rhesus sensitization. Am. J. Obst. & Gynec. 82:1359, 1961.

Mendez-Bauer, C., Arnt, I. C., Escarcena, L., and Caldeyro-Barcia, R.: Relationship between blood pH and heart rate in the human fetus during labor. Am. J. Obst. & Gynec. 97:530, 1967.

Mestyan, J., Fekete, M., Bata, O., and Jarai, I.: The basal metabolic rate of premature infants. Biol. Neonat. 7:11, 1964.

Nervez, C. T., Shott, R. J., Bergstrom, W. H., and Williams, M. L.: Prophylaxis against hypocalcemia in low-birth-weight infants requiring bicarbonate infusion. J. Pediat. 87:439, 1975.

O'Brien, D., Hansen, J. D. L., and Smith, C. A.: Effect of supersaturated atmospheres on insensible water loss in the newborn infant. Pediatrics 13:126, 1954.

Oh, W., and Karecki, H.: Phototherapy and insensible water loss in the newborn infant. Am. J. Dis. Child. 124:230, 1972.

O'Neill, E. M.: Normal head growth and prediction of head size in infantile hydrocephalus. Arch. Dis. Child. 36:241, 1961.

Roy, R. N., and Sinclair, J. C.: Hydration of the low birth weight infant. Clinics in Perinatology 2:393, 1975.

Reynolds, D. W., Dweck, H. S., and Cassady, G.: Inappropriate antidiuretic hormone secretion in a neonate with meningitis. Am. J. Dis. Child. 123:251, 1972.

Rylander, E.: Age dependent reactions of rectal and skin temperatures of infants during exposure to cold. Acta Pediat Scand. 61:579, 1972.

Scopes, J. W.: Metabolic rate and temperature control in the human baby. Brit. M. Bull. 22:88, 1966.

Siggaard-Andersen, O.: The Acid-Base Status of the Blood. 3rd ed. Baltimore, Md., The Williams & Wilkins Company, 1965.

Silverman, W. A., Fertig, J. W., and Berger, A. P.: The influence of the thermal environment upon the survival of newly born premature infants. Pediatrics 22:876, 1958.

Silverman, W. A., Sinclair, J. C., and Agate, F. J., Jr.: The oxygen cost of minor changes in heat balance of small newborn infants. Acta Paediat. 55:294, 1966.

Silverman, W., Zamelis, A., Sinclair, J. C., and Agate, F. J. Jr.: Warm nape of the newborn. Pediatrics 33:984, 1964.

Simmons, M. A., Adcock, E. W. III, Bard, H., and Battaglia, F. C.: Hypernatremia and intercranial hemorrhage in infants. New Engl. J. Med. 291:6, 1974.

Sinclair, J. C., Driscoll, J. M. Jr., Heird, W. C., and Winters, R. W.: Supportive management of the sick neonate; parenteral calories, water, and electrolytes. Pediat. Clin. N. Amer. 17:863, 1970.

Thomson, A. M., Billewicz, W. Z., and Hytten, F. E.: The assessment of fetal growth. Brit. Cwlth. 75:903, 1968.

Usher, R., and McLean, F.: Intrauterine growth of live-born Caucasian infants at sea level. Standards obtained from measurements in 7 dimensions of infants born between 25−44 weeks of gestation. J. Pediat. 74:901, 1969.

Winters, R. W.: Total parenteral nutrition in pediatrics: The Borden Award address. Pediatrics 5:17, 1975.

Winters, R. W., Engel, K., and Dell, R. B.: Acid-Base Physiology in Medicine. Westlake, Ohio, The London Company, 1967.

Wood, C., Ferguson, R., Lecton, J., Newman, W., and Walker, A.: Fetal heart rate and acid-base status in the assessment of fetal hypoxia. Am. J. Obst. & Gynec. 98:62, 1968.

World Health Organization Technical Report Series No. 540: Maturation of Fetal Body Systems. Geneva, 1974.

# ANTENATAL DIAGNOSIS OF GENETIC DISORDERS*

2

By Aubrey Milunsky

A new dimension has been added to genetic counseling. Until very recently it was possible to calculate certain risks of recurrence only *after* the birth of a child with a serious genetic disease or congenital malformation. Previously the determination of the carrier state or analysis of the pedigree allowed for fairly accurate predictions of the likelihood for having offspring with inherited diseases. Now, however, with the advent of antenatal genetic diagnosis, an exact prenatal determination of fetal disease can be made. The purpose of this new technology is to provide parents at risk with the opportunity to have unaffected offspring when the risk for having defective children seems unacceptably high. *The emphasis is not on the removal of defective offspring but on the provision of life for children who without antenatal diagnosis might never even be born.* Indeed about 95 per cent of all prenatal studies in the high-risk categories conclude at present with the demonstration that the fetus is unaffected. Parents who have had a defective child or who are known carriers may now elect to have a full family with the assurance that subsequent tragedy can be averted.

The neonatologist faced with a newborn with serious genetic disease or congenital malformation cannot but reflect upon the possibility that the diagnosis might have been made in utero. Parents, too, upon learning that possibilities existed for prevention of such outcomes, will frequently feel anger or frustration. They may even resort to litigation. These early reactions may be followed by unfavorable attitudes relative to the rearing of children with "preventable" genetic defects.

It is a small though important consolation to the parents to know that antenatal diag-

nosis is possible in subsequent pregnancies. Communication of this information is important soon after birth of the affected child. More crucial is the need to inform such parents of the possibly high risk of recurrence of a disorder which is *not* diagnosable antenatally. Not infrequently the next pregnancy is conceived before the couple have really been able to understand the implications of the genetic disorder in question.

Antenatal genetic diagnosis has in fact only been available for a short time. While the feasibility of sex prediction from amniotic fluid cells was demonstrated in 1955, this technique was first applied some 5 years later with the precise goal of preventing sex-linked genetic disease. Necessary technological refinements in human cell cultivation led over the next 5 years to the successful demonstration of normal fetal karyotypes from cultured amniotic fluid cells. Only then were the first abnormal fetal karyotypes determined from such cells, and it took a few years more before prenatal diagnostic studies became more generally available.

## THE APPROACH TO ANTENATAL DIAGNOSIS (Fig. 2–1)

Antenatal genetic study is a diagnostic tool, not a screening one. Because only a small number of cells can usually be grown from an amniotic fluid sample, the aim is to answer a sharply defined question specifying a particular disease entity, including its subtype. Knowledge of the family history is therefore crucial, and the greatest efforts must be made to gather all the information available. In addition to the necessary pedigree analysis, care should be exercised to examine photographs of deceased siblings and relatives and to obtain hospital and autopsy records and even frozen or living tis-

*Supported in part by U.S.P.H.S. grant numbers 1-PO1-HD-05515, 1-RO1-HDO9281-01 and 1-T32-GM-07015-01.

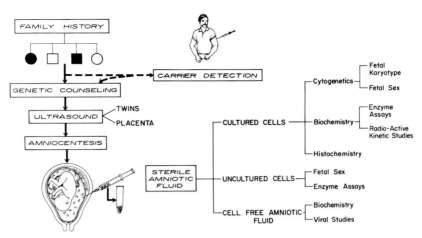

**Figure 2–1.** Schematic approach to the prenatal diagnosis of genetic disorders. (From Milunsky, A.: The Prenatal Diagnosis of Genetic Disorders. Springfield, Ill., Charles C Thomas, 1973.)

sues, such as cultured skin fibroblasts, from allegedly similarly affected individuals.

The mode of inheritance may become evident from the family history. The history may show on the maternal side, for example, a few female newborns who suffered from linearly arranged vesicular lesions with pigmented skin in curious whorls and streaks, perhaps associated with mental retardation and cerebral palsy. The diagnosis of incontinentia pigmenti should come to mind, and with it the realization that the parents can have normal unaffected males in this autosomal dominant sexlinked disorder.

Consideration of antenatal diagnosis ideally should take place prior to planned pregnancy. At this time genetic counseling would be useful to limit the risks, and carrier detection tests, which are becoming available for an increasing number of disorders, could be given. Thus, although both parents may be found to be carriers for an autosomal recessive disorder (e.g., Tay-Sachs disease), they may nevertheless proceed with childbearing with the assurance that antenatal diagnosis will allow them to have unaffected offspring selectively. Questions concerning heterozygosity should be looked into prior to conception rather than during pregnancy, since the activity of certain enzymes such as hexosaminidase, may change during pregnancy thereby providing unreliable results.

When the determination is made that antenatal diagnosis is a clear option, ultrasound studies are routinely recommended prior to amniocentesis. Their use to localize the placenta may diminish the frequency of bloody taps and decrease the chances of fetal loss. Occasionally such studies themselves reveal unsuspected pathology, such as hydrocephaly or anencephaly (Fig. 2–2). They also show the presence of multiple fetuses. Since amniocentesis performed without prior ultrasound will provide fluid from only one amniotic sac, the later discovery of multiple pregnancy may seriously complicate the obstetric and psychological management. The twin studied may be affected by a serious genetic disorder but no information will be available on the other, or vice versa. In this situation, both counselor and parents may be faced with an exceedingly difficult decision.

## AMNIOCENTESIS

The procedure of transabdominal amniocentesis has been performed for at least 45 years, in most cases to obtain fluid during the third trimester of pregnancy for the management of Rh disease. Although amniocentesis for prenatal genetic studies is recommended at 14 to 16 weeks, much experience is still needed to truly assess the real risks and accuracy of this procedure at this stage of pregnancy. Thus far there has been no maternal mortality and only minor maternal morbidity (one patient required a laparotomy to treat retroperitoneal hemor-

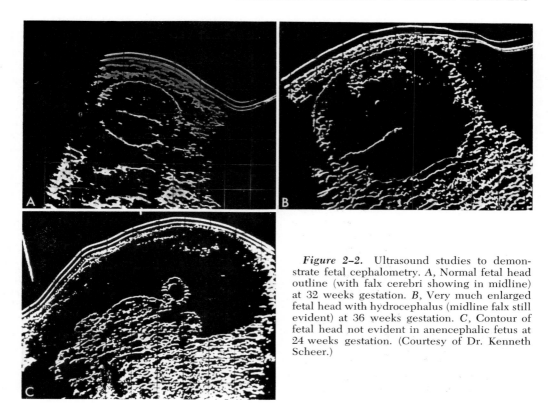

*Figure 2–2.* Ultrasound studies to demonstrate fetal cephalometry. *A*, Normal fetal head outline (with falx cerebri showing in midline) at 32 weeks gestation. *B*, Very much enlarged fetal head with hydrocephalus (midline falx still evident) at 36 weeks gestation. *C*, Contour of fetal head not evident in anencephalic fetus at 24 weeks gestation. (Courtesy of Dr. Kenneth Scheer.)

rhage). Major fetal complications include fetal loss, fetal damage and stillbirth. Detailed studies of over 1000 amniocenteses in the second trimester, together with matched controls, have been done by the Collaborative Amniocentesis Registry Project at the National Institutes of Child Health and Human Development. This study concluded that the risk during the second trimester did not exceed the background risk of fetal loss in pregnancies not complicated by amniocentesis. It would, however, seem safe to assume that the introduction of a needle into the uterus carries at least a marginal risk. This fractional risk must be balanced against the indication for amniocentesis for a disorder with a low risk of occurrence or recurrence.

Failure to aspirate amniotic fluid occurs in 6 to 10 per cent of cases, most often when ultrasound has not been used prior to amniocentesis. Repeat procedures at 1 to 2 week intervals almost always succeed. Grossly bloody samples are obtained in 5 to 10 per cent of attempts, leading to somewhat slower amniotic cell growth and the hazard of maternal cell mixture. Results are obtained from the first sample in about 90 per cent, a second tap being necessary in 6 to 10 per cent. Very occasionally even a third tap is needed. The commonest reason to repeat taps is poor cell growth. Other indications are contaminated cell cultures, admixture with blood, ruined or lost transported samples and verification of diagnosis.

The amniotic fluid, containing cells from amnion, fetal skin and intestinal, respiratory and urinary tracts, is best subjected to tissue culture studies for both chromosomal analysis and biochemical assays. Cultured fibroblasts and amniotic fluid cells retain their enzymatic machinery through successive generations in culture, thereby facilitating the demonstration of diminished or absent enzyme activity or the detection of excess storage material. Uncultured amniotic fluid cells are in various stages of demise and provide an unreliable and inconsistent tissue for diagnosis. They are therefore not recommended for either biochemical or chromosomal analysis. Only rarely is cell-free amniotic fluid useful for antenatal diagnosis. The single best example is alpha-fetoprotein analysis when open neural tube defects in the fetus are suspected (vide infra).

Unfortunately, the new technologies for prenatal genetic diagnosis have not been error free. Recent experience suggests an error rate of approximately seven per 1000 cases studied. This is disturbing, since virtually no opportunity exists for repeat studies until after birth. The commonest error has been in prenatal sex determination. Fortunately, these incorrect results have not been costly, since in no case yet has the error occurred where the risk was for sex-linked disease. Karyotyping errors have also occurred. At least two infants have been born with trisomy 21 in whom the antenatal diagnosis was "normal karyotype." There have also been errors in the antenatal diagnosis of biochemical disorders of metabolism. In one case although a diagnosis of galactosemia was made, the parents opted to continue the pregnancy. The infant when delivered was free of galactosemia. Not so fortunate, however, were other infants born after reassuring prenatal diagnoses had been made. At least three infants with Hurler's syndrome and one with Tay-Sachs disease have been delivered after assurance that these disorders had been excluded.

## INDICATIONS FOR ANTENATAL DIAGNOSIS

### CHROMOSOMAL ABNORMALITIES

Advanced maternal age is the most common reason for antenatal genetic studies. The chance of a prospective mother between 40 and 44 years of age having a child with a chromosomal abnormality is approximately 1 in 40. While the disorder found most often in this group is Down's syndrome, other maternal age dependent abnormalities include trisomy 13, trisomy 18, Klinefelter's syndrome and XXX. Available data for women between 35 and 39 years of age suggest a risk of about 2 per cent for all chromosomal abnormalities. In Massachusetts, amniocentesis is recommended for all women 35 years of age and over.

The second indication for study is when one of the parents is a known translocation carrier. The risks in such cases range between 4 and 20 per cent, depending upon which parent is the carrier and the disorder in question. About 50 per cent of D/G translocations appear to be inherited while most G/G translocations occur sporadically. 21/21 translocation carriers carry a 100 per cent risk of having an affected child.

The third major indication for study is a previous child with trisomy 21. The risk for recurrence for women below 35 years of age is 1 to 2 per cent.

Other miscellaneous indications that exist but arise only occasionally include abnormal parental karyotypes (e.g., mosaicism), possibly maternal hypo or hyperthyroidism, hereditary disorders in which chromosomal breakage may occur (e.g., Bloom's or Fanconi's syndrome), satellite associations seen in the karyotypes of either parent, or finally in situations of habitual abortion. It should be noted that while chromosomal aberrations may occur in the following situations, antenatal studies are not recommended for rubella, toxoplasmosis, cytomegalic inclusion disease, or following maternal irradiation or maternal drug ingestion (e.g., LSD). In all these conditions chromosomal breakage may be seen in cultured amniotic cells, but it is not possible to extrapolate from such observations to the fetal well-being. Further, although congenital rubella and cytomegalic inclusion disease have been diagnosed from isolation of live virus in amniotic cells, failure to grow virus does not exclude these disorders in the fetus. Moreover, cytomegalovirus excretion in an infant at birth does not necessarily imply congenital defect.

Cytogenetic observations from amniotic cell cultures may on occasion present difficulties in interpretation. It is now known that high degrees of polyploidy are compatible with the birth of a karyotypically normal child. Mosaicism may be easily missed. Spontaneous changes such as translocations may occur in cell culture. Variations of the pH of the culture medium have been observed to induce chromosomal errors. Contamination of cultures by mycoplasma may on occasion cause chromosomal abnormalities including unusual mosaicism.

## SEX-LINKED DISORDERS

Accurate prenatal sex determination is crucial to the management of about 150 sex-linked disorders. If the fetus is found to be male there is a 50 per cent risk that the fetus is affected. These disorders are carried by females but generally affect males only (e.g., hemophilia, muscular dystrophy, chronic granulomatous disease). There are at present only three disorders in this category that can specifically be diagnosed in the affected fetus (Hunter's, Lesch-Nyhan's, Fabry's). Progress in making specific antenatal x-linked diagnoses in male fetuses is likely to increase through utilization of fetal blood sampling and fetal skin and muscle biopsy. Ultimately, however, sex selection prior to pregnancy will likely prove to be the most valuable resource in the prevention of sex-linked disease. Technological refinements in separating X from Y-bearing sperm will allow couples to selectively have female offspring, obviating the need for amniocentesis, prenatal genetic studies and therapeutic abortion of male fetuses.

## HEREDITARY BIOCHEMICAL DISORDERS OF METABOLISM

Until very recently antenatal studies were utilized only for those parents who already had an affected child. Now, with the advent of large scale population screening for heterozygotes, an increasing number of couples without history of tragedy are seeking antenatal studies. Approximately 66 biochemical disorders are now diagnosable in utero (Table 2–1). Although accurate carrier detection is possible for some of these, it is not available on a population basis. However, in families where such disorders have occurred it is often possible to do heterozygote studies on a limited basis on all family members.

Great care must be exercised in securing antenatal diagnosis of a biochemical disorder. There are many variables in tissue culture that may affect the activity of the enzyme being measured. These need not be specified in detail in a communication written for the general pediatrician. However, it must be stressed that all assays must be done on control-matched samples handled identically and at the same time.

To complicate matters further, determination of heterozygosity has been compounded in at least three different lysosomal enzyme disorders having direct implications for prenatal diagnosis. In Tay-Sachs disease, Krabbe's disease and metachromatic leukodystrophy, examples have appeared in which apparently healthy though obligate carrier *parents* have been found to have enzyme activities in the homozygous range. These observations have been interpreted as manifestations of heterozygosity in these asymptomatic normal parents. The interpretation has been that each of the deficient enzymes (e.g., hexosaminidase A for Tay-Sachs) possesses polypeptide sub-units which may be subject to mutation in utero as well as after birth. To avoid such possibilities it might be wiser to delineate the heterozygote status of prospective parents, preferably prior to pregnancy.

## MISCELLANEOUS GENETIC DISORDERS

The observation in Edinburgh of an association between neural tube defects (e.g., anencephaly, spina bifida) and elevated amniotic fluid alpha-fetoprotein has provided the most significant advance in the prenatal diagnosis of such disorders. Alpha-fetoprotein is a specific alpha-1-globulin and is synthesized by normal embryonal liver cells, the yolk sac and the gastrointestinal tract of the human conceptus. Its serum concentrations rise from about the sixth week of gestation to a peak between 12 and 14 weeks and then steadily fall toward term. The concentration gradient between fetal serum and amniotic fluid is about 200:1. Unlike other proteins, the major source of amniotic fluid alpha-fetoprotein appears to be fetal urine, in which the concentration is higher than in amniotic fluid.

In this fluid, alpha-fetoprotein concentrations decrease from about the fifteenth week of gestation until delivery, at which time they are similar to those in maternal serum (Fig. 2–3). This steady decrease is evident even when there is an open neural defect. Hence the optimal time for amniocentesis for these studies is between 14 and 16 weeks of gestation. In *open* neural tube defects, alpha-fetoprotein moves from fetal

**TABLE 2–1.** *Inherited Metabolic Disorders Potentially Diagnosable Prenatally*

*Lipidoses*
  Cholesterol ester storage disease
  Fabry's disease
  Farber's disease
  Gaucher's disease
  Generalized gangliosidosis
    (GM₁ gangliosidosis type 1)
  Juvenile GM₁ gangliosidosis
    (GM₁ gangliosidosis type 2)
  Tay–Sachs disease
    (GM₂ gangliosidosis type 1)
  Sandhoff's disease
    (GM₂ gangliosidosis type 2)
  Juvenile GM₂ gangliosidosis (GM₂ gangliosidosis
    type 3)
  GM₃ sphingolipidystrophy
  Krabbe's disease (globoid cell leukodystrophy)
  Metachromatic leukodystrophy
  Niemann-Pick disease type A
  Niemann-Pick disease type B
  Refsum's disease
  Wolman's disease

*Mucopolysaccharidoses*
  MPS I – Hurler
  MPS I – Scheie
  MPS – Hurler/Scheie
  MPS II A – Hunter
  MPS II B – Hunter
  MPS III – Sanfilippo A
       – Sanfilippo B
  MPS IV – Morquio's syndrome
  MPS VI A – Maroteaux-Lamy syndrome
  MPS VI B – Maroteaux-Lamy syndrome
  MPS VII – β-glucuronidase deficiency

*Amino Acid and Related Disorders*
  Argininosuccinic aciduria
  Aspartylglucosaminuria
  Citrullinemia
  Congenital hyperammonemia
  Cystathionine synthase deficiency
    (homocystinuria)
  Cystathioninuria
  Cystinuria
  Hartnup disease
  Histidinemia
  Hypervalinemia
  Iminoglycinuria
  Isoleucine catabolism disorder
  Isovaleric acidemia

Maple syrup urine disease
  Severe infantile
  Intermittent
Methylmalonic aciduria
  Unresponsive to vitamin B₁₂
  Responsive to vitamin B₁₂
Methylenetetrahydrofolate reductase deficiency
Ornithine–α–ketoacid transaminase deficiency
Propionyl CoA carboxylase deficiency
  (ketotic hyperglycinemia)
Succinyl–CoA: 3 ketoacid CoA–transferase
  deficiency
Vitamin B₁₂ metabolic defect

*Disorders of Carbohydrate Metabolism*
  Fucosidosis
  Galactokinase deficiency
  Galactosemia
  Glucose–6–phosphate dehydrogenase
    deficiency
  Glycogen storage disease (type II)
  Glycogen storage disease (type III)
  Glycogen storage disease (type IV)
  Mannosidosis
  Phosphohexose isomerase deficiency
  Pyruvate decarboxylase deficiency
  Pyruvate dehydrogenase deficiency

*Miscellaneous Hereditary Disorders*
  Acatalasemia
  Adenosine deaminase deficiency
  Chediak-Higashi syndrome
  Congenital erythropoietic porphyria
  Cystinosis
  Familial hypercholesterolemia
  Hypophosphatasia
  I–cell disease
  Leigh's encephalopathy
  Lesch-Nyhan syndrome
  Lysosomal acid phosphatase deficiency
  Lysyl-protocollagen hydroxylase deficiency
  Myotonic muscular dystrophy
  Nail-patella syndrome
  Orotic aciduria
  Saccharopinuria
  Sickle cell anemia
  Testicular feminization
  Thalassemia
  Xeroderma pigmentosum

serum to cerebrospinal fluid, then egresses through the open lesion into the surrounding amniotic fluid. Hence, assay of this protein is useful only in open neural tube defects and not in the 10 per cent in which the defects are covered by skin.

The alpha-fetoprotein diagnostic test is non-specific, there being other conditions in which marked elevations may occur (Table 2–2). These studies may be particu-

larly complicated by the presence of fetal blood in the sample. Measurements of other protein markers have been attempted for the same purpose, and have included beta-trace protein, the neuronal specific S-100 protein, alpha 2-macroglobulin and, most recently, fibrin-fibrinogen degradation products. The alpha-fetoprotein assay remains the test of choice.

Observations in England have indicated

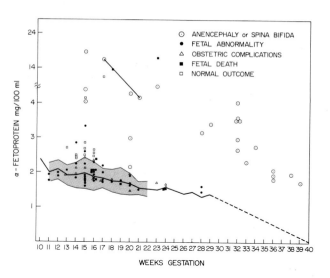

*Figure 2-3.* Alpha-fetoprotein (AFP) concentrations (± 2 S.D. shaded area) in normal amniotic fluid (918 cases), anencephaly or spina bifida (27 cases), various fetal abnormalities (38 cases), fetal death (10 cases), obstetric complications (15 cases) and normal outcomes (12 cases). Note the striking fall in AFP concentration (16.5 to 4.55 mg/100 ml) between weeks 16 and 21 in one case of anencephaly. Elevated AFP values in pregnancies with normal outcomes mostly reflect fetal blood contamination of the amniotic fluid sample.

that maternal serum alpha-fetoprotein may be elevated in pregnancy when the fetus is afflicted with an open neural tube defect. Initial estimates, which may be optimistic, suggest that about 80 per cent of anencephalic fetuses and almost 60 per cent of those with spina bifida are detectable by such studies during the second trimester. Should the prospective studies now underway in both the United Kingdom and the

United States show even some proximity to these first estimates (based on very few cases) a major screening tool will find its way into routine obstetric practice. Current studies are offered only to parents who have already had a child with a neural defect and to the few parents who themselves have suffered one.

Human fetal reticulocytes have been shown to synthesize hemoglobin A as early as the ninth week of gestation. The beta chain of hemoglobin S is synthesized as early as the fifteenth week. These facts, plus the recognition that mixed maternal-fetal blood obtained from the placenta contains adequate numbers of fetal reticulocytes, have set the stage for the prenatal diagnosis of hemoglobinopathies, especially sickle cell anemia and beta-thalassemia. But placental aspiration for mixed fetal-maternal samples is, unfortunately, not often successful. Morever, roughly 50 per cent of mothers have a posterior placenta and are therefore not approachable by the blind technique. The development of the small caliber fiberoptic fetoscope has allowed fetal blood sampling under direct vision. While this technique must still be regarded as experimental, it is already apparent from tiny fetal blood samples (measured in lambdas) that it is possible to make the prenatal diagnosis of hemoglobinopathies. However, instruments currently available do not allow for fetal blood sampling under direct vision when the placenta is anteriorly situated. Further tech-

**TABLE 2-2.  *Conditions with Associated Elevated Amniotic Fluid AFP***

|                              | < 24 wks | > 24 wks |
| ---------------------------- | -------- | -------- |
| Anencephaly                  | +        | +a       |
| Myelomeningocele             | +a       | +a       |
| Encephalocele                | +a       | +a       |
| Omphalocele                  | +a       | ?        |
| Esophageal atresia           | ?        | +        |
| Duodenal atresia             | +        | ?        |
| Hydrocephalus                | +a       | +a       |
| Congenital nephrosis         | +        | +        |
| Meckel's syndrome            | +        | ?        |
| Turner's syndrome            | +        | ?        |
| Cystic hygroma               | +        | ?        |
| Fetal death                  | +        | +        |
| Fetal blood contamination    | +        | ?        |
| Twins                        | +a       | ?        |
| Rh disease                   | +        | +        |
| Spontaneous abortion         | +a       | +        |
| Sacrococcygeal teratoma      | ?        | +        |
| Congenital skin defects      | ?        | +        |
| Tetralogy of Fallot          | ?        | +        |
| Respiratory distress syndrome | ?       | +        |

*a = AFP level known to be *not* invariably elevated.

nical modifications are required on the fetoscopes available, after which tests of their safety will be required. Through direct visualization of the phenotype of the fetus, the antenatal diagnosis of at least 60 hereditary congenital malformation syndromes associated with mental retardation may also become possible.

## REFERENCES

Atkins, L., Milunsky, A., and Shahood, J. M.: Prenatal diagnosis: Detailed chromosomal analysis in 500 cases. Clin. Genet. 6:317, 1974.

Bloom, A. D., Schmickel, R., Barr, M., et al.: Prenatal detection of autosomal mosaicism. J. Pediatr. 84:732, 1974.

Brock, D. J. H., Bolton, A. E., and Monaghan, J. M.: Prenatal diagnosis of anencephaly through maternal serum alpha-fetoprotein measurement. Lancet 2:923, 1973.

Brock, D. J. H., and Scrimgeour, J. B.: Early prenatal diagnosis of anencephaly. Lancet 2:1252, 1972.

Brock, D. J. H., and Sutcliffe, R. G.: Alpha-fetoprotein in the antenatal diagnosis of anencephaly and spina bifida. Lancet 2:197, 1972.

Burton, B. K., Gerbie, A. B., and Nadler, H. L.: Present status of intrauterine diagnosis of genetic defects. Am. J. Obstet. Gynecol. 118:718, 1974.

Campbell, S.: The assessment of fetal development by diagnostic ultrasound. In Milunsky, A. (Ed.): Clinics in Perinatology. Symposium on Management of the High-Risk Pregnancy. Vol. 1. Philadelphia, W. B. Saunders Company, 1974, p. 507.

Cox, D. M., Niewczas-Late, V., Riffell, I., et al.: Chromosomal mosaicism in diagnostic amniotic fluid cell cultures. Pediatr. Res. 8:679, 1974.

Doran, T. A., Rudd, N. L., Gardner, H. A., et al.: The antenatal diagnosis of genetic disease. Am. J. Obstet. Gynecol. 118:310, 1974.

Ellis, J. R.: Spontaneous translocation in a cell culture. Ann. Hum. Genet. 26:287, 1963.

Frigoletto, F. D., and Griscom, N. T.: Amniography for the detection of myelomeningocele. Obstet. Gynecol. 44:286, 1974.

Galjaard, H., Hoogeveen, A., Keijzer, W., et al.: The use of quantitative cytochemical analyses in rapid prenatal detection and somatic cell genetic studies of metabolic diseases. Histochem. J. 6:491, 1974.

Galjaard, H., Mekes, R., De Josselin De Jong, J. E., et al.: A method for rapid prenatal diagnosis of glycogenosis II (Pompe's disease). Clin. Chim. Acta 49:361, 1973.

Gerbie, A. B., Nadler, H. L., and Gerbie, M. V.: Amniocentesis in genetic counseling. Am. J. Obstet. Gynecol. 109:765, 1971.

Hilton, B., Callahan, D., Harris, M., Condliffe, P., and Berkley, B. (Eds.): Ethical Issues in Human Genetics. Genetic Counseling and the Use of Genetic Knowledge. New York, Plenum Press, 1973.

Hobbins, J. C., Mahoney, M. J., and Goldstein, L. A.: New method of intrauterine evaluation by the combined use of fetoscopy and ultrasound. Am. J. Obstet. Gynecol. 118:1069, 1974.

Hollenberg, M. D., Kaback, M. M., and Kazazian, H. H., Jr.: Adult hemoglobin synthesis by reticulocytes from the human fetus at midtrimester. Science 174:698, 1971.

Hsu, Y. F., Dubin, E. C., Kerenyi, T., et al.: Results and pitfalls in prenatal cytogenetic diagnosis. J. Med. Genet. 10:112, 1973.

Huijing, F., Warren, R. J., and McLeod, A. G. W.: Elevated activity of lysosomal enzymes in amniotic fluid of a fetus with mucolipidosis II (I-cell disease). Clin. Chim. Acta 44:453, 1973.

Kajii, T.: Pseudomosaicism in cultured amniotic fluid cells. Lancet 2:1037, 1971.

Kan, Y. W., Dozy, A. M., Alter, B. P., et al.: Detection of the sickle gene in the human fetus. Potential for intrauterine diagnosis of sickle cell anemia. New Engl. J. Med. 287:1, 1972.

Kan, Y. W., Dozy, A. M., Alter, B. P., et al.: Intrauterine diagnosis of thalassemia. Ann. N.Y. Acad. Sci. 232:145, 1974.

Kan, Y. W., Golbus, M. S., Klein, P., et al.: Successful application of prenatal diagnosis in a pregnancy at risk for homozygous β-thalassemia. New Engl. J. Med. 292:1096, 1975.

Kardon, N. B., Chernay, P. R., Hsu, L. Y., et al.: Pitfalls in prenatal diagnosis resulting from chromosomal mosaicism. J. Pediatr. 80:297, 1972.

Leck, A. E., Ruoss, C. F., Kitaw, M. J., et al.: Raised α-fetoprotein in maternal serum with anencephalic pregnancy. Lancet 2:385, 1973.

Lorber, J., Stewart, C. R., and Ward, A. M.: Alpha-fetoprotein in antenatal diagnosis of anencephaly and spina bifida. Lancet 1:1187, 1973.

Macri, J. N., Weiss, R. R., and Joshi, M. S.: Beta trace protein and neural tube defects. Lancet 1:1109, 1974.

Macri, J. N., Weiss, R. R., Joshi, M. S., et al.: Antenatal diagnosis of neural tube defects using cerebrospinal fluid proteins. Lancet 1:14, 1974.

Milunsky, A.: The Prenatal Diagnosis of Hereditary Disorders. Springfield, Charles C Thomas, Publisher, 1973.

Milunsky, A. (Ed.): The Prevention of Mental Retardation and Genetic Disease. Philadelphia, W. B. Saunders Company, 1975.

Milunsky, A., and Alpert, E.: The value of alpha-fetoprotein in the prenatal diagnosis of neural tube defects. J. Pediatr. 84:889, 1974.

Milunsky, A., Alpert, E., and Charles, D.: Amniotic fluid alpha-fetoprotein in anencephaly. Obstet. Gynecol. 43:592, 1974.

Milunsky, A., and Annas, G. J. (Eds.): Genetics and the Law. Proceedings of a National Symposium, Boston, Plenum Press, 1975.

Milunsky, A., and Atkins, L.: Prenatal diagnosis of genetic disorders. An analysis of experience with 600 cases. J.A.M.A. 230:232, 1974.

Milunsky, A., Atkins, L., and Littlefield, J. W.: Amniocentesis for prenatal genetic studies. Obstet. Gynecol. 40:104, 1972.

Milunsky, A., Littlefield, J. W., Kanfer, J. N., et al.: Prenatal genetic diagnosis. New Engl. J. Med. 283:1370, 1441, 1498, 1970.

Milunsky, A., Macri, J. N., Weiss, R. R., et al.: Prenatal

detection of neural tube defects. Comparative studies between alpha-fetoprotein and β-trace protein. Am. J. Obstet. Gynecol. *122*:313, 1975.

Milunsky, A., and Reilly, P.: Medico-legal issues in the prenatal diagnosis of hereditary disorders. Am. J. Law Med. *1*:71, 1975.

Nadler, H. L., and Gerbie, A. B.: Role of amniocentesis in the intrauterine detection of genetic disorders. New Engl. J. Med. *282*:596, 1970.

Patrick, J. E., Perry, T. B., and Kinch, R. A. H.: Fetoscopy and fetal blood sampling: A percutaneous approach. Am. J. Obstet. Gynecol. *119*:539, 1974.

Philip, J., Bang, J., Hahnemann, N., et al.: Chromosome analysis of fetuses in risk pregnancies. Acta Obstet. Gynecol. Scand. 53:9, 1974.

Purves, L. R., and Purves, M.: Serum alpha-fetoprotein. VI. The radioimmunoassay evidence for the presence of AFP in the serum of normal people and during pregnancy. S. Afr. Med. J. *46*:1290, 1972.

Robinson, A., Bowes, W., Droegemueller, W., et al.: Intrauterine diagnosis: Potential complications. Am. J. Obstet. Gynecol. *116*:937, 1973.

Schneider, E. L., Stanbridge, E. J., Epstein, C. J., et al.: Mycoplasma contamination of cultured amniotic fluid cells: Potential hazard to prenatal chromosomal diagnosis. Science *184*:477, 1974.

Scrimgeour, J. B.: Other techniques for antenatal diagnosis. *In* Emery, A. E. H. (Ed.): Antenatal Diagnosis of Genetic Disease. Baltimore, The Williams & Wilkins Company, 1973, p. 40.

Seppälä, M.: Increased alpha-fetoprotein in amniotic fluid associated with a congenital esophageal atresia of the fetus. Obstet. Gynecol. 42:613, 1973.

Seppälä, M.: Alpha-fetoprotein in the management of high-risk pregnancies. *In* Milunsky, A. (Ed.): Clinics in Perinatology. Symposium on Management of the High-Risk Pregnancy. Vol. 1. Philadelphia, W. B. Saunders Company, 1974, p. 293.

Seppälä, M., and Ruoslahti, E.: Radioimmunoassay of maternal serum alpha-fetoprotein during pregnancy and delivery. Am. J. Obstet. Gynecol. *112*: 208, 1972.

Seppälä, M., and Unnerus, H.-A.: Elevated amniotic fluid alpha-fetoprotein in fetal hydrocephaly. Am. J. Obstet. Gynecol. *119*:270, 1974.

Shapiro, S., Levine, H. S., and Abramowicz, M.: Factors associated with early and late fetal loss. Excerpta Med. Int. Congr. Ser. 224:45, 1970.

Spranger, J. W., and Wiedemann, H. R.: The genetic mucolipidoses. Humangenetik 9:113, 1970.

Toop, J., and Emery, A. E. H.: Muscle histology in fetuses at risk for Duchenne muscular dystrophy. Clin. Genet. 5:230, 1974.

Valenti, C.: Endoamnioscopy and fetal biopsy. A new technique. Am. J. Obstet. Gynecol. *114*:561, 1972.

Valenti, C.: Antenatal detection of hemoglobinopathies. A preliminary report. Am. J. Obstet. Gynecol. *115*:851, 1973.

Warburton, D., and Fraser, F. C.: Spontaneous abortion risks in man: Data from reproductive histories collected in a medical genetics unit. Am. J. Hum. Genet. *16*:1, 1964.

# NEONATAL BEHAVIOR AND ITS SIGNIFICANCE

3

*By T. Berry Brazelton*

The newborn infant has been thought of as neurologically insufficient (Flechsig), subcortical in his behavior (Lorenz), a blank slate to be written upon by his environment, his world a blooming, buzzing confusion (James). None of these descriptions fits the kind of predictable, directed responses one sees in a neonate when he is in a social interaction with a nurturing adult or as he responds to an attractive auditory or visual stimulus. For, when positive rather than intrusive stimuli are utilized, the neonate has marvelous capacities for alerting and attention, for suppressing interfering reflex responses in order to attend. With very predictable behaviors, he responds to and interacts with his environ-

ment from birth. But this predictability requires a knowledge of his ongoing state of consciousness.* When "state" is accounted for, most of his reactions are predictable—both to negative and to positive stimuli, from internal as well as external sources. State becomes a matrix for under-

---

*State of consciousness or "state" of the infant becomes a most important matrix for interpretation of neonatal behavior. His reactions to all stimuli—internal and external—are dependent on his ongoing state of consciousness. Using "state" as a matrix, behavioral responses become quite predictable. "State" depends on physiological variables such as hunger, nutrition, degree of hydration, and the timing within the wake-sleep cycle of the infant. Our criteria for state throughout this chapter are based on the descriptions of Prechtl and Beintema (see p. 47).

standing his reactions. It qualifies stimulation as appropriate or inappropriate to his ongoing organization.

The classical pediatric neurological assessment of the neonate is based on his responses to painful or intrusive stimuli, and, as such, the resulting reflex behavior is, indeed, mediated by the midbrain. A standard neurological evaluation simply evaluates the integrity of the brain stem as it "copes" with these stimuli. But such an examination neglects the available organized behavior which the infant can demonstrate as he suppresses reflexive behavior in order to attend to more "interesting" stimuli—such as the human face or voice, a soft rattle or a light caress:

> As a newborn lies undressed and uncovered in the nursery, his color begins to change, with mottled uneven acrocyanosis of his extremities, as he attempts to control loss of body heat. He begins to shiver, then to cry and flail his limbs in jerky thrusting movements in an effort to raise his own temperature. In the face of such enormous demands, as one speaks gently and insistently into one ear, his movements become smoother, slower, and he gradually quiets completely. His face softens then brightens, his eyes move smoothly to the side from which the voice is coming. His head follows with a sudden smooth turn toward the voice, and he searches for the face of the speaker. He fixes on the eyes of the examiner and listens intently for several minutes. If the examiner moves his face slowly to the baby's midline and then across to the other side, the newborn will track him, his head and eyes smoothly turning in an 180° arc.

This complex interaction of visual, auditory and motor behavior to respond to a human stimulus is managed by the neonate despite the enormous physiological demands of being undressed and unrestrained in a cold, overstimulating nursery. If one ignores the importance of this capacity as he evaluates the neurological and physiological integrity of the neonate, he misses the implication of the powerful effect of the cortex on the autonomic and physiological systems in the neonatal period. As pediatricians, we must be aware of the interactions between physiological and psychological mechanisms, as they represent integrity in the neonate and predict the individual differences in developmental outcome.

A pediatrician has tools for assessing the central nervous system of a neonate. A neonate may pass him by unless he pays attention to the baby's capacity to quiet down when spoken to, to alert when picked up and handled and to lock onto and follow the examiner's face when the eyes are open.

## INTRAUTERINE INFLUENCES

The neonate's behavioral responses have already been powerfully influenced by intrauterine events and experiences. The extent of intrauterine shaping of behavior can only be guessed. Intrauterine nutrition and infection would be expected to be powerful in determining the DNA and RNA complements of the central nervous system and other organs, such as adrenals and thyroids, which underly neonatal behavior.

Winick suggests that as much as 40 per cent of the expectable DNA content of a neonate's brain may be reduced by prolonged, severe intrauterine malnutrition. We have examined a group of neonates from protein-caloric deprived Guatemalan women in a nutritional study by Incap (Brazelton et al., 1975). We have found that caloric intake during pregnancy correlates with the behavior of the neonate. Infants with higher birth weight were more vigorous and motorically mature as well as more able to attend to visual and auditory stimuli than were low birth weight infants. These infants were the offspring of better nourished mothers.

In addition to the physiological effects of intrauterine depletion from under-nutrition and infection, we have been impressed with other intrauterine influences—for example, the influence of maternal experience on the behavior of the offspring. Animal work by Thompson and Keeley has indicated that severe behavioral and physiological stress to rats and mice during pregnancy (conditioned anxiety, crowding, epinephrine injection) produced permanent changes in the behavior of their offspring. Open field activity and maze learning of the newborn pups were severely impaired. Lieberman produced the same kinds of changes in mice offspring by injection during pregnancy of stress-syndrome hormones (hydrocortisone and norepinephrine). When these hormones were injected into chick eggs the resultant offspring showed delays in pecking and in seeking contact for protection. On the other hand, epinephrine injections given to the mouse mother just prior to delivery and into chick eggs produced more vigorous, rapidly responsive offspring.

Sontag first suggested that in utero conditioning of human fetal behavioral responses might represent a kind of "learning" which would contribute to individual differences seen in neonatal behavior. When the fetal heart rate was monitored by a cardiotachometer placed on the mother's abdomen, the fetal heart responded to auditory stimuli, cigarette smoking and emotional shocks administered to the mother. As these stimuli were repeated, the fetal heart rate response became diminished and its latency prolonged. The infant was "learning" not to respond to such stimuli. In another study Ando and Hattori (1969) demonstrated that infants near an airfield in Okinawa who had been exposed to high noise levels during the first four months of gestation were significantly less reactive to loud sounds after birth. Thus, one can expect that all kinds of information and stimulation—both that directly received by the fetus and that received via the neurological and chemical responses of the mother—might shape infant behavior. But effects may not be seen as linear in the outcome behavior of the neonate. For example, the fetus may respond to anxiety in the mother by becoming more active and reactive (more anxious); or he may "learn" to cope with the stress induced by her anxiety and become quieter—having learned to shut down on his own responses to her signals. At birth, the baby may be intensely driving, overreactive, or he may be quietly able to handle stimulation *or* he may demonstrate a mixture of both these mechanisms.

Unfortunately there has been little documentation so far of sensorimotor behavior in the premature infant. We can now see that even 34 week premature infants do fix on and track a visual object. They can attend to and even turn their heads toward a human voice or soft rattle, although their response often seems more obligatory and rigid than they are in full term infants (Als, work in progress). There seems to be a kind of organized state control available, although states in the premature are less well defined than those of the full term infants. Their state controls are more fragile, and the impinging demands of physiological adjustments become major sources of interference with these responses. We can begin to credit the premature infant with a capacity to attend to and organize cues from his environment. When he will attend to the human voice, fix on and follow the face or a shiny moving object, we can be sure that his capacity to master the demands of an immature physiology allows him to begin to organize around important environmental input. We can predict that he is a "better" premature than one who is still at the mercy of obligatory respiratory or cardiac demands or of a poorly organized central nervous system. In other words, a pediatrician should be aware of and responsive to the premature's sensorimotor behavioral responses in much the same way as he is to that of a mature neonate.

## ORGANIZATION OF MOTOR BEHAVIOR

The organization and quality of the newborn's motor behavior can provide much information on the current state of the newborn. But one must be constantly aware of the conditions that will influence his performance in a period of observation. These include 1) his state of arousal; 2) environmental factors such as temperature, lighting and sound levels which influence his arousal state; 3) chemical imbalance such as hypoglycemia or hypercalcemia; 4) state of hydration; 5) state of wellbeing—e.g., illness or other stress; and 6) degree of recovery from perinatal and other stresses. Effective hand to mouth activity may be important not only because it signifies the baby's capacity to perform a complex motor feat but also because he may use it for quieting himself in order to attend to his environment or keep himself under control. Then it becomes a significant observation in the neonatal nursery.

Complex behavioral patterns available to

the neonate become a way of measuring his integrity. Spontaneous hand to mouth efforts as he becomes upset and tries to keep himself under control, or hand to mouth response as his cheek is stroked, or his palm is touched, become a way of seeing his capacity for motor organization. This complex behavioral arc of hand to mouth was first described and named by Babkin.

Defensive reactions are structured motor patterns, and the infant's effectiveness in approaching and removing an obtrusive stimulus becomes a way of testing for motor pathways and their organization. For example, covering the baby's face with a cloth elicits a series of motor maneuvers. First he roots, then twists his head from side to side, stretches his neck backward in active arching, and finally brings each arm up to swipe at the offending cloth. Many newborns effectively push the cloth off the face. These responses (hand to mouth, defensive movements or other sequential motor acts) may be of equal value to elicited reflexes as the examiner assesses the upper extremities for neurological adequacy.

Motor activity may be observed for other than its value as an assessment of neurologic integrity and maturation. There have been reports in the literature which seem to point to differences in genetic endowment. Geber first described a kind of motor precocity in African neonates which seemed to place them 4 to 6 weeks ahead of a control group of European neonates. Her methodology and findings are under dispute (Warren), but Super has found that East African mothers stimulate their babies in a way that fosters early motor development. This raises the question as to whether mothers are sensing a kind of motor "excitement" in their babies which they foster in subsequent interactive behavior which leads to precocity. This is supported by findings of extremely balanced motor tone and well organized, smooth movements of Gusii newborns in Kenya (Keefer).

To assign genetic differences in precocity of motor behavior without seeing this neonatal behavior as an interaction between genetic endowment and intrauterine experience would be naive, for we are becoming more aware of nutritional and chemical effects on motor development in utero. Hence, the reports of genetic differences must be evaluated with intrauterine shaping in mind.

There is little question that the neonate's motor potential and his kind of motor activity react powerfully on the environment around him. For example, an intensely driving motoric neonate can be predicted to be fussy, "colicky." This kind of infant is easily aroused to intense, driving motor activity. His response to almost any stimulus is a startle, followed by an intense crying state. He thrusts his arms and legs in violent activity. This reaction sets off startles which continue to upset him. Each startle produces more activity and crying. He tends to perpetuate this cyclical, disturbed crying activity for long periods. A parent's upset reaction to this crying contributes more tension, and one sees the anlage for "colic" in the neonatal period. When one assesses such a neonate and finds this hyperreactivity to stimuli not suppressed by him or by reasonable, calming maneuvers, one can predict a "colicky" infant and a period of stress for the parents. With such a prediction the physican can begin to intervene in the neonatal period; and his or her role becomes supportive to the neonate's parents: 1) relieving them of their inevitable upset in having fostered his disturbed behavior, and in being unable to find a "magical" solution which will soothe him and suppress his hyperactive, hypersensitive behavior; and 2) predicting for them that a consistent, low-keyed environment will lead to relief from the baby's "colicky" behavior after a few months and eventually, in all likelihood, to a well-organized, rather exciting baby. As a result, careful observation and assessment of the way an infant moves and how he uses his motor capacities may be extremely important as a predictor of his CNS integrity, of his genetic and intrauterine experience, of his perinatal recovery, of his individual temperamental endowment, and of his potential influence on the environment around him.

## SENSORY CAPACITIES

The newborn is equipped with the capacity for processing complex visual stimulation and showing organized visuomotor behavior. When a bright light is flashed into a neonate's eyes, his pupils constrict, he blinks, his eyelids and whole face contract, he withdraws his head by arching his whole body, often setting off a complete startle as he withdraws, his heart rate and respirations increase and there is an evoked response registered on his visual occipital EEG. Repeated stimulation of this nature will induce diminishing responses. For example, in a series of 20 bright-light stimuli presented at 1 minute intervals, we found that the infant rapidly "habituated" out the behavioral responses, and by the tenth stimulus, not only had his observable motor responses decreased but his cardiac and respiratory responses had also begun to decrease markedly. The latency to evoked responses as measured by EEG tracings was increasing, and by the fifteenth stimulus his EEG reflected the induction of a quiet, unresponsive state similar to that seen in sleep (Brazelton). His capacity to shut out repetitious disturbing visual stimuli protects him from having to respond to visual stimulation and at the same time frees him to save his energy to meet his physiological demands. The capacity to habituate to visual stimuli is decreased, although it is present, in immature infants (Hrbek), and is depressed by medication such as barbituates given to mothers as premedication at the time of delivery. This has led Brazier to postulate that the primary focus for this mechanism is in the reticular formation and midbrain. However, the cortical control over this mechanism seems apparent as one observes a neonate who is initially in irregular, light sleep become drowsier with repeated stimulation. He then becomes deeply asleep, with tightened flexed extremities, little movement except jerky startles, no eyeblinks, deep, regular respirations and rapid, regular heart rate. This state seems to resemble a defense against the assaults of the environment, and upon cessation of the stimulation the infant almost immediately goes back to his initial state or an even more alert state. One can often see neonates in noisy, brightly lighted neonatal nurseries in this "defensive" sleep state.

Just as he is equipped with the capacity to shut out certain stimuli, he also demonstrates the capacity to alert to, and to turn his eyes and head to follow and fix upon a stimulus which appeals to him. Fantz first pointed out neonatal preference for complex visual stimuli. More recently, Goren (1975) showed that immediately after delivery, a human neonate would not only fix upon a drawing that resembled a human face, but would follow it in 180 degree arcs, with eyes and head turning to follow. A scrambled face did not demand the same kind of attention, nor did the infant follow the distorted face with his eyes and head for the same degree of lateral following.

Extremes of brightness and noise in the environment have been found to interfere with the neonate's capacity to respond. In a noisy, overlighted nursery, the neonate tends to shut down on his capacity to attend, but in a semidarkened room, a normal neonate in an alert state can be brought to respond to the human face as well as to a red or shiny object. For example, the following description indicates the behaviors of which the infant is capable:

> The neonate is held or propped up at a 30° angle. Vestibular responses enhance eye opening and tend to bring him to a more alert state (Korner). His eyes begin to scan the environment with a dull look, wide pupils and

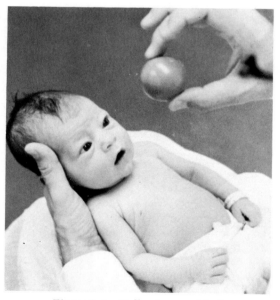

*Figure 3–1.*  Following a red ball.

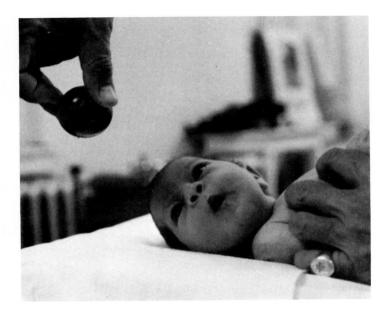

*Figure 3–2.* Head turning to follow.

saccadic lateral movements of both eyes.

As a bright red ball is brought into his line of vision and is moved slowly up and down to attract his attention, his pupils contract slightly. As the ball is moved slowly from side to side, his face begins to brighten, his eyes widen, his limbs still, and he stares fixedly at the object, beginning slowly to track the ball from side to side. He maintains the stilled posture in order to attend to the ball. His eyes first track in small arcs that take him off the target, but as he becomes more invested, the eye movements become smoother. As his eyes move laterally, his head begins to turn, and he moves his head from side to side in order to facilitate the tracking of the object. He is able to follow it for as much as 120°, to right and left, and will even make eye and head movements to follow it 30° up or down. Meanwhile, interfering body movement or startles seem to be actively suppressed. He can maintain this intense visual involvement for several minutes before he startles, becomes upset or dull, and loses the alert state necessary to this kind of visual behavior.

Tronick and Clanton have experimentally demonstrated that these complex patterns of coordination of head and eye movements appear to be very organized, and they suggested that the infant has a cortically controlled visual system at birth that coordinates head and eye for the extraction of information from the environment.

Adamson has demonstrated the importance of vision to the neonate by covering an alert baby's eyes with both an opaque and a clear plastic shield. He swipes at and attempts vigorously to remove the opaque shield, building up to frantic activity to do so and quieting suddenly when it is removed. When the clear shield is substituted, he becomes calm enough to look interestedly through it.

Bower and Tronick have demonstrated that neonates will actively defend themselves from looming visual targets with a defensive reaction to an approaching object. This defense includes head turning and directed arm movements.

Salapatek and Haith have found that the highest points of concentration of fixation in the neonatal period are on the contrasting edges of an object. In the neonate, the eyes or sides of the head seem to be the most compelling features of the face. Thus, the neonate seems to be highly programed for visual learning from birth. The visual stimuli which are "appropriate" or appealing, such as the human face and eyes, or a moving object, seem to be adapted to capture his attention very early. This allows for very early learning about his human caretakers and the world around him. If his physiological systems are not overwhelmed with demands of too much

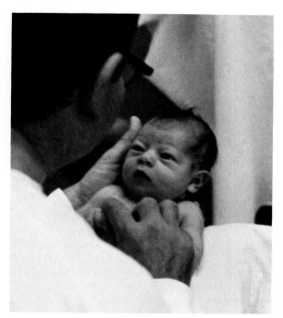

***Figure 3-3.*** Fixation and intense interest in the human face.

information or too prolonged a period of attention, he will attend for long alert periods.

When an examiner can produce graded visual and motor responses in a neonate, he can be encouraged to predict to a normal, well-integrated nervous system.

### AUDITORY

The neonate's auditory responses are specific and well organized. But often assessments are not sensitive to the complexity of newborn behavior. For example, the loud clackers used in the Collaborative Project of NINDB for early detection of central nervous system defects were ineffective in loud, noisy nurseries. A large percentage of neonates tested with such a routine were unresponsive and appeared to have shut out or habituated to auditory stimuli. Another approach in these conditions would have been to use a soft rattle. This stimulus would have been more appropriate to the habituated state of these neonates. Hence a routine test for hearing should include several stimuli — animate as well as inanimate — with careful pairing of the stimulus so that it will break through

the neonate's present state of consciousness; for example, a rattle in light sleep, a voice in awake states and a clap in deep sleep. Respirations and eyeblinks, as well as more obvious behavioral responses, should be monitored for reactions to auditory stimuli.

A pediatrician can test this in the nursery. By speaking softly in a high-pitched voice to one side of the baby's head, he should be able to see the infant become quiet and alert-looking and gradually turn his head toward the voice. As the doctor continues to talk, the infant begins to search for the source of the voice with his eyes, his face intent. This train of behavior is found in intact, normal infants and is a good sign of central nervous system integrity.

Kearsley has demonstrated the importance of rise time on the neonate's behavioral responses. Sounds with prolonged onset times and low frequencies produced eye opening and cardiac deceleration, while sounds with rapid onset and high frequency produced eye closing, cardiac acceleration and increased head movements. Thus, different quality sounds produced an alerting or a defensive reaction.

In sum then, as one defines the neonate's behavioral response to an appropriate sound, one sees a series of regular steps. As the sound is localized (Leventhal and Lipsitt), cardiac rate first increases (Steinschneider) and may be accompanied by a mild startle. If the auditory stimulus is attractive to the infant, his face will brighten, his heart rate will decelerate, his breathing will slow and he will alert and search with his eyes until the source of the sound is localized and in the "en face" midline of the baby. This train of behavior, which occurs as a response to an attractive auditory stimulus such as the human voice, becomes a measure of the neonate's capacity to organize his central nervous system.

### OLFACTORY

Engen et al. have demonstrated differentiated responses to acetic acid, anise, asafetida and alcohol in the neonatal period. More recently, MacFarlane has shown that 7-day-old neonates can reliably distinguish their own mothers' breast pads from those of other mothers. They turn their heads toward their own mothers' breast pads with 80 per cent reliability, after controls for laterality are imposed. We have seen that breastfeeding infants at 3 weeks may refuse to accept a formula from their mothers. This refusal seems to be related to the infants' ability to choose the available breast by smell. Yet fathers are successful in giving a bottle to these same babies. Thus, it seems that the neonate does have the capacity to make choices from olfactory stimuli, and that this information too can be used as part of the attachment process.

## TASTE

The newborn has fine differential responses to taste. Nelson (Jensen) observed differentiated sucking responses to sugar, salt, quinine water and citric acid solutions, with increased sucking to sugar and decreased sucking to the others. More recently, it has been reported that a newborn's differentiation is expressed in an even more complex fashion. When an infant is fed different fluids through a monitored nipple, his sucking pattern is recorded. With a cow's milk formula he will suck in a rather continuous fashion, pausing at irregular intervals. If breast milk is fed to him in this paradigm, he will register his recognition of the change after a short latency, then suck in bursts, with frequent pauses at regular intervals. The pauses seem to be directly related to breast milk as if he were programed for other kinds of stimuli (such as social communication) in the pauses.

## TACTILE

The sensitivity of the infant to handling and to touch is quite apparent. A mother's first response to an upset baby is to contain him—to shut down on his disturbing motor activity by touching or holding him. Swaddling has been used in many cultures to replace the important constraints offered first by the uterus and then by mothers and caretakers. As a restraining influence on the overreactions of hyperreactive neonates, the supportive control which is offered by a steady hand on a baby's abdomen or by holding his arms so that he cannot startle reproduces the swaddling effects of holding or wrapping a neonate. This added control of disturbing motor responses allows the neonate to attend to and interact with his environment.

First used for containment, tactile stimuli can be used to rouse or sooth the neonate. A patting motion of 3 times per minute seems to be soothing, whereas at 5 or 6 times a minute he becomes more excited and alerted for other kinds of stimuli.

A test of the baby's responsiveness may be to place a hand firmly on his belly when he is beginning to become upset. If he can utilize this tactile pressure to calm himself down, the examiner can feel better about him. Holding onto the arm or arms of a crying, flailing baby will usually break through the cycle of startling and crying to comfort him.

This is a maneuver to use when the infant is undressed and beginning to become upset, in order to auscultate the heart and lungs.

## SUCKING

The awake, hungry newborn exhibits rapid searching movements in response to tactile stimulation in the region around the mouth, and even as far out on the face as the cheek and sides of the jaw and head (Peiper, Blauvelt). This is called the rooting reflex and is present in the premature even before sucking itself is effective (Prechtl).

The infant sucks in a more or less regular pattern of bursts and pauses. During nonnutritive sucking, his rate varies around two sucks a second (Wolff). Bursts seem to occur in packages of 5 to 24 sucks per burst (Kaye). The pause between bursts has been considered to be a rest and recovery period as well as a period during which cognitive information is being processed by the neonate (Halverson, Bruner). Kaye found that the pauses were important ethologically, since they are used by mothers as signals to stimulate the infant to return to sucking. However, the mother's jiggling actually prolongs the pause as the infant responds to the information given to him by his mother.

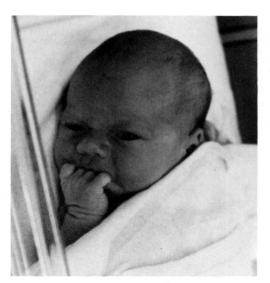

*Figure 3–4.*   Sucking.

Finger sucking is common in the neo-natal period, and there is evidence that the insertion of parts of the hand in the mouth occurs commonly in the uterus. The impor-tance of sucking as a regulatory response can be seen in a newborn as he begins to build up from a quiet state to crying. His own attempts to achieve hand to mouth contact in order to keep his activity under control are fulfilled when he is able to in-sert a finger into his mouth, suck on it and quiet himself. The sense of satisfaction and of gratification at having achieved this self-regulation are apparent. His face softens and alerts as he begins to concentrate on maintaining this kind of self-regulation. A pacifier can achieve this same kind of quieting in an upset baby, but may not serve the self-regulatory feedback system as richly as the baby's own maneuver.

The newborn sucks most when highly aroused and is, in general, soothed through the sucking act. Piaget asserts that the first changes in sucking which come about as part of his learning about the world are "the beginning of the infant's psychology."

We should add to our neonatal examina-tion a test for CNS integration: 1) Insert a gloved finger into the baby's mouth to pro-duce a sucking response; 2) as soon as he is sucking well, test his hearing and his vi-sion by observing his sucking response to a light and a rattle or a voice; 3) if he re-sponds by a brief cessation of sucking, as he should, repeat the auditory or visual stimulus several times at short intervals. He should gradually lose interest in the stimulus and continue his sucking pattern without interruption. This simple set of maneuvers demonstrates auditory, and vi-sual integrity as well as his capacity for complex interactions between systems, and, most important, his ability to shut out repeated nonsignificant information.

## HEART RATE AS A MEASURE OF ATTENTION AND HABITUATION

The neonate's capacity to attend to exter-nal stimuli is coupled with the capacity to habituate or tune them out. In states of alert inactivity, he can be brought to a state of alert attention by many kinds of stimuli. His capacity to discriminate between stim-uli, to attend to or to shut out stimuli, is complex and highly organized.

The Law of Initial Values (Lacey) plays an important role in any assessment of car-diac responses. Bridger and Reiser, and Lipton et al. have demonstrated that the prestimulus heart rate is likely to be in-versely correlated with the response as well as the magnitude of heart rate response. Most infants have a reliable resting heart rate toward which their post-stimulus rate will trend in a cyclic homeostatic curve. If the infant's prestimulus rate is high, a re-sponse will bring about relative decelera-tion; if his prestimulus rate is low, his response will be toward acceleration. Nega-tive or disturbing stimuli produce little or no deceleration; soothing stimuli produce a mild decrease in base rate and a stable low-grade homeostatic response; whereas an at-tractive or interesting stimulus may bring about marked, brief acceleration followed by a period of observable deceleration.

Habituation to repeated stimuli can be monitored by this technique (Bartoshuk, Bridger). Since habituation is generally thought to reflect cortical storage of infor-mation about a stimulus, the decrease in heart rate response over repeated trials with a stimulus might reflect the infant's cortical functioning. With an intrusive stim-ulus, one sees a gradual, diminishing shut-down on the degree of acceleratory cardiac responses to the repetitious stimulus. With an interesting stimulus, the acceleratory component may decrease slightly, but the deceleratory phase is markedly affected with repeated presentations. This, then, becomes a measure of cortical function. Dishabituation (or recovery of the total response) when the stimulus is changed can be seen in the neonatal period and can be used as a further measure of cortical and subcortical function in the neonatal period (Brackbill, Eisenberg).

Since these measures are dependent on the integrity of the central nervous system as well as upon the demands on the cardiac system, it is not surprising that stressed infants do not demonstrate this complex behavior. Lester demonstrated a substantial orienting response followed by rapid habituation to auditory signals with dishabituation to changes in tonal frequency in well nourished infants. But infants who had been undernourished showed an attenuation or complete absence of the orienting response and no dishabituation to changes in tonal frequency. The decrease in these responses seemed highly correlated with the degree of malnutrition to which the infants had been exposed. This lack of orienting in attentional mechanisms suggests itself as a precursor for disabilities in learning later on.

The use of heart rate responses to auditory, visual, tactile and kinesthetic stimuli has been underutilized in assessing the cognitive and physiological status of stressed neonates. We have utilized both negative (bright light, bell) and positive stimuli (soft rattle, touch, human voice) in assessing immature infants and have monitored changes in skin color as we presented the stimuli. One can observe clinically an initial change in skin color, followed by recovery to good color when the infant can either habituate to disturbing stimuli or attend to interesting stimuli. When he cannot habituate or attend, his poor color increases and he can be stimulated until he is in cardiovascular collapse (as was observed with repeated visual responses in an anencephalic baby [Brazelton, Scholl and Robey]).

## STATE

The matrix of state as a concept for organization in the neonate has become of importance since its use as a background for neurological behavior in Prechtl's assessment. Within the context of optimal state of alertness, he demonstrated that the newborn's midbrain reflexive behavior improved, and the neurologic exam became a better diagnostic measure.

Sleep states have been recognized and defined since 1937 by Wagner. She described some of the behaviors seen in deep or regular sleep—jerky startles and relative unresponsiveness to external stimuli, and more regulated smooth movements accompanied by responsiveness to stimuli in lighter sleep. Wolff added his observations of deep sleep—regular, deep respirations with sudden spontaneous motor patterns such as sobs, mouthing and sucking, and erections which occurred at fairly regular intervals in an otherwise inactive baby. He observed that babies were more responsive to stimuli in light sleep. Aserinsky and Kleitman described cycles of quiet, regular sleep followed by active periods of body movements and rapid eye movements (REMs) under closed lids. Hence, light sleep has come to be designated as REM sleep. At term, active sleep (REM) occupies 45 to 50 per cent of total sleep time, indeterminate sleep occupies 10 per cent and quiet sleep 35 to 45 per cent. The predominance of active sleep has led to the hypothesis that REM sleep mechanisms stimulate the growth of the neural systems by cyclic excitation, and it is in REM sleep that much of the differentiation of neuronal structures and neurophysiological discharge patterns occurs (Anders and Roffworg). Quiet sleep seems to serve the purpose of inhibiting CNS activity and is truly an habituated state of rest.

The length of sleep cycles (REM active and quiet sleep) changes with age. At term they occur in a periodicity of 45 to 50 minutes, but immature babies have even shorter, less well defined cycles. Newborn infants have as much active REM in the first half of the deep period as in the second half. Initial brief, individual sleep and wake patterns coalesce as the environment presses the neonate to develop diurnal patterns of daytime wakefulness and night sleep. Appropriate feeding patterns, diet, absence of excessive anxiety, sufficient nurturing stimulation and a fussing period prior to a long sleep have all been implicated as reinforcing to the CNS maturation necessary to the development of diurnal cycling of sleep and wakefulness. Sleep polygrams, as determined by both EEG and activity monitoring, are proving to be sensitive indicators of neurological maturation and integrity in the neonatal period. Steinschneider has analyzed the occurrence of apnea episodes during sleep as part of a study on the sudden infant death syndrome (SIDS). He found that these episodes are more likely to occur during REM sleep, and has suggested that prolonged apnea, a concomittant of sleep, is part of a final physiological pathway culminating in SIDS.

In our behavioral assessment of neonates, we have utilized the two states of deep, regular and active REM sleep described by Wolff and Prechtl. These states can be reliably determined by observation and without any instrumentation.

1. Deep sleep: regular breathing, eyes closed, spontaneous activity confined to startles and jerky movements at quite regular intervals. Responses to external stimuli are partially inhibited and any response is likely to be delayed. No eye movements, and state changes are less likely after stimuli or startles than in other states.
2. Active REM sleep: irregular breathing, sucking movements, eyes closed but rapid eye movements can be detected underneath the closed lids, low activity level, irregular smooth organized movements of extremities and trunk. Startles or startle equivalents as response to external stimuli occur with change of state.

Alert states have been separated into four states for our behavioral assessment:

1. Drowsy: semidozing, eyes may be open or closed, eyelids often fluttering, activity level variable, with interspersed mild startles and slow, smoothly monitored movements of extremities at periodic intervals; reactive to sensory stimuli but with some delay, state change frequently after stimulation.
2. Wide awake: alert bright look; focuses attention on sources of auditory or visual stimuli; motor activity suppressed

in order to attend to stimuli. Impinging stimuli break through with a delayed response.
3. Active awake: eyes open, considerable motor activity, thrusting movements of extremities, occasional startles set off by activity. Reactive to external stimulation with an increase in startles or motor activity, discrete reactions difficult to distinguish because of general high activity level.
4. Crying: intense crying, jerky motor movements, difficult to break through with stimulation.

The waking states are easily influenced by fatigue, hunger, or other organic needs, and may last for variable amounts of time. However, in the neonatal period, they are at the mercy of the sleep cycles, and surround them in a fairly regular fashion. Waking states are infrequently observed in noisy, overlighted neonatal nurseries, but in a rooming-in situation or at home, they become a large part of each four hour cycle, and the neonate lies in his crib looking around for as much as 20 to 30 minutes at a time. Appropriate stimulation can bring him up to a responsive state 2. Rocking, gently jiggling, crooning, stroking, setting off vestibular responses by bringing him upright or by rotating him all serve to open his eyes. Then his interest in visual and auditory stimuli helps him to maintain a quiet alert state. In this state his respirations are regular at a rate of 50 to 60 a minute, his cardiac rate, too, is regular and fairly slow (around 100 to 120/min.), his eyes are wide, shiny, and capable of conjugate movements to scan and to follow with head turning to appropriate objects; his limbs, trunk and face are relaxed and inactive; the skin is pink and uniform in color. Alert inactive states occur in the first 30 to 60 minutes after delivery but then are likely to decrease in duration and occurrence over the next 48 hours as the infant recovers, but they return after the first 2 days, and make up as much as 8 to 16 per cent of total observation time in the first month (Wolff).

Kleitman talks of wakefulness of "necessity" and of "choice." Wakefulness of necessity is brought about by stimuli such as hunger, cold and bowel movements, or by external stimuli which disturb sleep cycles. Sleep recurs as soon as the response to the disturbing stimuli is completed. Wakefulness of choice is related to neocortical activity and is a late acquisition coinciding with the emergence of voluntary motor actions and a mature capacity to achieve and maintain full consciousness. Absence of hunger and fatigue, bowel and bladder activity and gross motor activity are necessary to this state. After a few weeks this state can accompany gross motor activity as long as the infant is not too active. Pursuit movements of his extremities accompany visual fixation and following as early as 2 to 3 weeks (Brazelton, 1974). The occurrence and duration of these quiet inactive states may be highly correlated with intactness and mature organization of the neonate's central nervous system.

A pediatrician can obtain a sense of the infant's state organization from the mother by asking her how long and deeply he sleeps, and how much time he spends in wideawake alertness. When he is easily disorganized or thrown from either of these states by minor stimuli, one can suspect a hypersensitive central nervous system. Such an infant is difficult for parents, and they will need advice as to maneuvers which will help the infant to control his reactions; e.g., advice as to swaddling, pacifiers, rocking in order to help him to quiet down to sleep, and so on. This hypersensitivity can be observed in the nursery or the pediatrician's office as well.

Crying serves many purposes in the neonate—not the least of which is to shut out painful or disturbing stimuli. Hunger and pain are also responded to with crying which brings the caretaker to him. And there is a kind of fussy crying which occurs periodically throughout the day—usually in a cyclic fashion—which seems to act as a discharge of energy, and an organizer of the states which ensue (Brazelton). After a period of such fussy crying, the neonate may be more alert or he may sleep more deeply.

As a behavior for organizing his day and for reducing disturbance within his CNS, crying seems to be of real importance in the neonatal period. Most parents can distinguish cries of pain, hunger and fussiness by 2 to 3 weeks, and learn quickly to respond appropriately (Wolff). So the cry is of ethological significance to elicit appropriate caretaking for the infant.

Parents need to be reassured that there is a certain amount of normal crying to be expected—usually at a regular time, at the end of the day. This crying period is predictable and is not a sign of "colic" or internal stress, as it is likely to be interpreted by parents. They feel that they should and must find the right solution to it and it will stop. As their efforts to quiet the baby increase, the crying period can increase from 1 1/2 hours to as much as 6 to 8 hours a day, as the infant begins to reflect the anxiety and unpredictable handling of the frantic parents. By warning new parents in advance that a certain amount of fussiness is normal, and by assuring them that there are no magical cures they are missing, a pediatrician can often nip this disturbance in their relationship in the bud, and prevent the more severe colic (Brazelton, 1962).

The neonate's cry has been analyzed by Lind (Wasz-Hockert et al., 1968), Wolff (1969) and others for diagnostic purposes. It is a complex, serially organized acoustical pattern that is directly regulated by the CNS. Wolff (1969) found that there were three distinct acoustical patterns of cries in normal infants: hunger, anger and pain. Lind (Wasz-Hockert et al., 1968) found four patterns: birth, hunger, pain and pleasure.

We have found differences in newborns in their use of states. The difficulty in rousing certain infants from sleep states to alert or crying with disturbing stimuli versus the rapidity with which others go from sleep to crying and down again, or the lability which certain newborns demonstrate as they move rapidly from one state to another, or others who are consoled easily from crying, and the self-quieting efforts on the part of other infants in order to maintain alert or quiet states, are all differentiating characteristics that will help to predict in neonates their future individualities. Certainly these differences will affect the kind of nurturing they will receive from their environments. We reported an infant whose rapidly labile movement from crying to deep sleep left no opportunity for his mother to reach him. She found him such a difficult infant that we correctly predicted profound difficulties in their relationship. Since we had found this difficult state of lability and unreachability in the neonatal period, we were able to support the mother with extra advice, along with a preventive approach to her anxiety. We supported her in maintaining their relationship until the baby could begin to develop more adequate state controls. As his threshold for sensory input became more adequate, his state behavior became smoother, and he became more reachable by those around him. In this case, neonatal observations served to prevent a serious breakdown in the mother-infant interaction, as we could assure the mother that his lability was not due to her handling of the infant.

## EVALUATION OF THE NEONATE

As the potential for early intervention increases, it becomes more important to identify at-risk infants as early as possible. The Apgar score is the most universal criterion for assessing the newborn's well-being in the delivery room. But since it is a measure of the infant's capacity to cope with stress in the first 15 minutes after delivery only, it does not tap in on the depth of depression which inevitably follows this stress reaction (James). Subtler effects are overlooked by this score, as it necessitates a substantial insult to impair the Apgar scores. As his physiologic demands take precedence and his habituation mechanisms begin to function to shut out his reactions to stimuli and thus add to the depressed autonomic and central reactions, the baby may end up in a rather frightening behavioral slump after initially good Apgars.

Repeated evaluations in the neonatal nursery are necessary in order to record the depth and duration of postdelivery depression. Scanlon has developed an assessment technique which has high reliability among observers and serves to record the depth of the newborn's depression. It seems to be sensitive to the effects of maternal medication and anesthesia, as well as to hypoxic events in the immediate paranatal period. This test includes two categories of responses: 1) neuromuscular—body tone,

arm recoil, truncal tone, head control, Moro response, root and suck—and 2) adaptive—observations of alertness to auditory and visual stimuli and capacity to shut out such stimuli, including pinprick, Moro, bright light and loud noises. He follows babies hourly over the first 6 hours with this 5 minute test and can predict to recovery and postdict to the effects of paranatal variables on this recovery curve.

Graham was the first to use behavioral measures as part of a predictive neurological exam. Her techniques included qualitative assessments of tension and motor response measures, tactile responses, irritability ratings, ease of quieting and visual and auditory responsiveness. She evaluated these measures within the context of state of arousal. Rosenblith established the validity of her assessment as a predictor as well as its day to day test-retest reliability, finding correlations between many of the newborn measures and their outcome at 4, 8 and 12 months and at 2 years in the Collaborative Perinatal Research Project.

In order to record and evaluate some of the integrative processes evidenced in neonatal behavior we have developed a behavioral evaluation scale (Brazelton) which tests and documents the infant's use of state behavior (state of consciousness) and the response to various kinds of stimulation.

Since the infant's reactions to all stimuli are dependent on his ongoing "state," any interpretation of them must be made with this in mind. His use of state to maintain control of his reactions to environmental and internal stimuli is an important mechanism and reflects his potential for organization. State no longer need be treated as an error variable but serves to set a dynamic pattern to allow for the full behavioral repertoire of the infant. Specifically, our examination tracks the lability and direction of state changes over the course of the examination. The variability of state points to the infant's capacities for self-organization. His ability to quiet himself as well as his need for stimulation also measure this adequacy.

The behavior examination tests for neurological adequacy with 20 reflex measures and for 26 behavioral responses to environmental stimuli, including the kind of interpersonal stimuli which mothers use in their handling of the infant as they attempt to help him adapt to the new world. In the examination, there is a graded series of procedures—talking, hand on belly, restraint, holding and rocking—designed to soothe and alert the infant. His responsiveness to animate stimuli, such as voice and face, and to inanimate stimuli, such as rattle, bell, red ball, white light and temperature change, is assessed. Estimates of vigor and attentional excitement are measured; and motor activity and tone are assessed, as is autonomic responsiveness, as he changes state. With this examination given on successive days we have been able to outline 1) the initial period of alertness immediately after delivery, presumably the result of stimulation from labor and the new environment after delivery; 2) the period of depression and disorganization which follows and lasts for 24 to 48 hours in infants with uncomplicated deliveries and no medication effects, but which lasts for periods of 3 to 4 days if they have been compromised by medication given their mothers during labor; and 3) the curve of recovery to "optimal" function after several days. This third period may be the best single predictor of individual potential function, and it seems to correlate well with the neonate's retest ability at 30 days. The shape of the curve made by several examinations may be the most important assessment of the basic CNS intactness, of the neonate's ability to integrate CNS and other physiological recovery mechanisms, and of the strength of his compensatory capacities when there have been compromising insults to him during labor and delivery. Test-retest reliability is greater than .8, and interscorer reliability of 90 per cent can be achieved with training, and maintained for at least a year. The examination takes 20 minutes to perform and 10 minutes to score reliably.

This neonatal behavioral examination has been used in cross-cultural studies to outline genetic differences, with prematures to predict their outcome successfully, to document behavioral correlates of intrauterine protein depletion, to determine the effects of uteri depleted by rapidly repeated pregnancies, and to assess the influence of heavy medication given the mother during labor, as well as maternal addiction to heroin and methadone.

The behavioral items are as follows:

Response decrement to repeated visual stimuli

Response decrement to repeated auditory stimuli

Response decrement to pinprick

Orienting responses to inanimate visual and auditory stimuli

Orienting responses to the examiner's face and voice

Quality and duration of alert periods

General muscle tone—in resting and in response to being handled (passive and active)

Motor maturity

Traction responses as he is pulled to sit

Responses to being cuddled by the examiner

Defensive reactions to a cloth over his face

Consolability with intervention by examiner

Attempts to console self and control state behavior

Rapidity of build up to crying state

Peak of excitement and capacity to control himself

Irritability during the examination

General assessment of kind and degree of activity

Tremulousness

Amount of startling

Lability of skin color (measuring autonomic lability)

Lability of states during entire examination

Hand-to-mouth activity

In addition to 26 items of behavior, assessed on a 9-point scale, there are 20 reflex responses which are also assessed.

We feel that the behavioral items are tapping in on more important evidences of cortical control and responsiveness, even in the neonatal period. The neonate's capacity to manage and overcome the physiological demands of this adjustment period in order to attend to, to differentiate and to habituate to the complex stimuli of an examiner's maneuvers may be an important predictor of his future central nervous system organization. Certainly, the curve of recovery of these responses over the first neonatal week must be of more significance than the midbrain responses detectable in routine neurological examinations.

It is not necessary to perform behavioral evaluation in order to get a feeling for the neonate's integrity, but it is important to test for and record a certain number of sensory and motor responses. In addition, his capacity to quiet himself, to use the examiner in order to control himself, and then to attend to and respond to the examiner's maneuvers in any pediatric examination can be an excellent way of assessing his CNS integrity and his temperamental style of cementing his parents to him. When the infant is difficult or aberrant, a pediatrician can begin an alert and interventive approach to help the parents adjust to him. Then, instead of compounding his difficulties by their anxiety over his not responding to their nurturing as they expect, parents can see their role more clearly as that of gradually but surely teaching him how to achieve an integrated response system to important environmental cues. This is an important preventive role for the pediatrician or caring professional.

## THE NEONATE AS A SOCIAL BEING

The newborn infant is obviously not prepared to exist outside of a matrix of social supports from a responsive care giver. But he is also *not* passive within this matrix. On the contrary, the behavior patterns and sensory capabilities discussed elsewhere in this chapter shape the caretaker's behavior. Moreover, the "feelings of efficacy" which are engendered in the infant and his caretakers by the mutuality which is established becomes a source of energy to each participant (White).

Moss and Goldberg point to the trigger-like value in setting off mothering activities of the newborn's small size, helpless appearance and distress cries. Klaus and Kennell have described the kinds of initial contacts mothers make with their newborn infants and the distortions in this behavior when the mother is depressed by abnormalities in the baby, such as prematurity, illness in the neonatal period, etc. Eye-to-eye contact, touching, handling and nursing behavior on the part of the mother may be assessed and judged to predict her ability to relate to the new baby. Changes in these behaviors over time are stressed as indicators of recovery or nonrecovery of maternal capacity to attach to the baby by mothers who have been depressed and unable to function optimally by having produced an infant at risk.

The ability of the baby to precipitate and encourage the mother's attachment and care taking behavior must be considered. With an unresponsive neonate, the feedback mechanisms necessary to fuel mothering behavior are severely impaired. The possibility of creating or compounding the problems of infants at risk by a distortion of the environment's reactions to them is too important, and our tools for predicting this should be sharpened in the lying-in period. The opportunity for observing the pair together is never again as available, and surely we are missing valuable predictive information when we do not make regular, repeated observations of interactive situations, such as feeding periods, bathing and "play" periods after feeding.

In the normally competent dyad, there are preadapted complementary behaviors that guarantee a high level of mutually produced contingency experience (Goldberg). A competent infant is one who roots and sucks efficiently, alerts to stimulation selectively, modulates states of arousal, cries loudly when uncomfortable and quiets when comforted. Lorenz pointed out that certain features make up a "kewpie doll" face which elicits parenting responses—the short vertical axis and puffed cheeks of the face, the relatively large head to body size, the uncoordinated body movements, the soft fuzzy skin and hair. The fact that the infant prefers and quiets down to human stimuli such as the voice and face are critical to maternal attachment. Fathers report that they begin to develop strong affectional ties only after the infant has begun to look at and smile at them, and many mothers do not feel attachment until the second or third month, when eye-to-eye contact and rhythmic reactive behaviors are firmly established (Robson and Moss).

In stressed neonates, the responsive behavior which normally exists to feed back to the mother may not be present or satisfying and the relationship may flounder. If the eliciting stimuli the normal baby presents to care-givers are not forthcoming or are distorted, parental behavior in turn becomes distorted. Prechtl reports the high incidence of brain-damaged infants who appear normal externally but elicit anger and rejection from their parents, even before an official diagnosis of damage has been made. Klein and Stern report an unexpectedly large number of battered children from a premature population. Klaus and Kennell attribute this in part to the effects on the parents of early separation from their prematures. We would add the effects of maternal depression after the delivery of a sick neonate. And the syndrome of failure to thrive seems to be a sequel to many infants who are small for gestational age at birth. Many SGA infants are later given up for adoption (Miller and Hassanian).

We are interested in determining the role of aberrant behavior in the premature or SGA infant that might lend itself to an already adversely influenced maternal attachment. Als et al. are also trying to define the aberrant releasors in the behavior of the neonate, using the Brazelton Neonatal Assessment. We have found that premature and SGA babies are poorer in interactive behaviors, in alerting responses and in selecting for the female voice, for the human face in auditory and visual responses, in state modulation and in producing satisfactory motor behavior. Throughout the first year of life these SGA babies evidence a high incidence of hyperactivity and temperamental and organizational instability. These difficulties are bound to and do result in parental frustrations (Als).

It is, thus, apparent that in addition to the physiological and neurological problems at-risk newborns have to cope with, they generate by their distorted behavior deficient parenting patterns which, in turn, exacerbate an already compromised start on life. The interactive cyclical nature of this process cannot be overstressed and must be taken into account whenever one deals with other than healthy normal newborns.

We have seen that the infant in the first few weeks requires that the mother adapt her behavior to a cyclic attentional cycle which comes from the infant and which is dependent on the homeostatic requirements of the infant's immature physiological systems. When an infant attends to and becomes intensely involved with a familiar adult, he attends to her with a cyclical pattern of attention—withdrawal and recovery—which resembles a homeostatic curve, at a rate of four cycles per minute in a period of intense interaction. A mother or father who is sensitive to the baby's needs reflects this self-regulatory mechanism and regulates her/his affective and cognitive information to the infant's requirements. An insensitive parent overloads the neonate, and their interaction becomes stressed.

In an optimal interaction, the reciprocity that is established on these cycles of attention and recovery becomes the base for affective development, and fuel for learning about his environment. This interdependency of rhythms seems to be at the root of their attachment, as well as of their communication (Brazelton, Chapple). From this interdependency, the infant learns rules about his environment and about himself. Thus, the quality of the interaction becomes more important in assessing an at-risk pair than does an evaluation of either participant alone. Prevention of future difficulties for the child may well hinge on early identification of failure in this interaction.

A pediatrician can observe and record a lack of synchrony or "fit" between a mother and her baby. When they are unable to achieve a rhythmic period of playing looking or vocal games with each other, he should be alerted to an interaction which may well be at risk for future stress or failure.

## SUMMARY

An assessment of the neonate's behavioral responses should be a part of every pediatric examination. Integration of his central and autonomic nervous systems is necessary for him to overcome the physiological demands of recovery in the immediate period after delivery. This very fact makes such an assessment a valuable opportunity to see and quantitate his stage of well-being. That behavioral responses are dependent on his capacity to regulate his states of consciousness is of primary importance in such an assessment. For his state behavior marks both his capacity to alert to an interesting or appropriate stimulus and his capacity to shut out a disturbing or inappropriate one. This potential signifies his viability as well as his capacity to adapt to his environment with a potential for learning the information necessary to his future progress. It is also involved in his capacity to respond to his care-giver in a way that will hook her or him to the infant in a mutual feedback system which will provide the nurturing necessary to his future affective and cognitive growth.

The pattern of recovery of the infant's potential for behavior becomes the most important way of predicting not only his immediate coping capacity but also his future reactions to stress. Thus, several assessments in the perinatal period become of significance.

The wealth of data about neonatal responses has accumulated to such a degree that it behooves us as pediatricians to be aware of the behavioral richness of the neonate for assessment and prediction of his future integrity.

## REFERENCES

Adamson, L.: Infants response to visual and tactile occlusions. Ph.D. Dissertation, University of California at Berkeley, in preparation, 1976.

Als, H., Tronick, E., Adamson, L., and Brazelton, T. B.: Revisions of the Brazelton Neonatal Behavioral Assessment Scales with premature and other at risk newborns. Personal commun., 1975.

Anders, T. F., and Roffwarg, H.: The effects of selective interruption and total sleep deprivation in the human newborn, Develop. Psychobiol. 6:77–89, 1973.

Anders, T. F., and Weinstein, P.: Sleep and its disorders in infants and children: A review. Pediatrics 50:312, 1972.

Ando, Y., and Hattori, H.: Effects of intense noise during fetal life upon postnatal adaptability. J. Acoust. Soc. Am. 47:(4) 1128, 1970.

Apgar, V. A.: A proposal for a new method of evaluation of the newborn infant. Curr. Res. Anesth. Analg. 32:260, 1960.

Aserinsky, E., and Kleitman, N.: A motility cycle in sleeping infants as manifested by ocular and gross motor activity. J. Appl. Physiol. 8:11, 1955.

Babkin, P. S.: The establishment of reflex activity in early postnatal life. In Central Nervous System and Behavior, 3rd Conference, Princeton, N.J., U. S. Dept. HEW (OTS 62-43772), 24-31, 1960.

Ball, W., and Tronick, E.: Infant response to impending collision: optical and real. Science 171:818-820, 1971.

Bartoshuk, A. K., and Tennant, J. M.: Human neonatal correlates of sleep wakefulness and neural maturation. J. Psychiat. Res. 2:73, 1964.

Brigman, T., Haith, M. M., and Mann, L.: Development of eye contact and facial scanning in infants. Paper presented at Soc. Res. Child Devel., Minneapolis, April 1974.

Blauvelt, H., and McKenna, J.: Mother neonate interaction: Capacity of the human newborn for orientation. In B. M. Foss (Ed.): Determinants of Infant Behavior, New York, John Wiley & Sons, 1961.

Bower, T. G. R.: The determinants of perceptual unity in infancy. Psychon. Sci., 3:323, 1965.

Bowlby, J.: Attachment and Loss, Vol. I: Attachment. New York, Basic Books, 1969.

Brackbill, Y.: Continuous stimulation and arousal level in infants: Additive effects. Proc. 78th Annual Convention. Am. Psychol. Assn. 5:271, 1970; and in Stone, L. V., Smith, H. T. and Murphy, L. B. (Eds.): The Competent Infant. New York, Basic Books, 1973, p. 300.

Brazelton, T. B.: Sucking in infancy. Pediatrics, 17:400, 1956.

Brazelton, T. B.: Psychophysiologic reactions in the neonate. J. Pediatr. 58:513, 1961.

Brazelton, T. B.: Observations of the neonate. J. Acad. Ch. Psych. 1:38, 1962.

Brazelton, T. B.: Infants and Mothers: Differences in Development. New York, Delacorte Press, 1969.

Brazelton, T. B.: Effect of prenatal drugs on the behavior of the neonate. Am. J. Psychiat. 126:95, 1970.

Brazelton, T. B.: Assessment of the infant at risk. Clin. Obstet. Gynec. 16:361, 1973.

Brazelton, T. B.: Influence of perinatal drugs on the behavior of the neonate. In Hellmuth, J. (Ed.): Exceptional Infant. Vol. 2, New York, Bruner Mazel, 1971, p. 419.

Brazelton, T. B., Koslowski, B., and Main, M.: Origins of reciprocity, In Lewis, M., and Rosenblum, L. (Eds.): Mother Infant Interaction. New York, Wiley, 1974, pp. 49–76.

Brazelton, T. B., Koslowski, B., and Tronick, E.: Study of neonatal behavior in Zambian and American neonates. Am. Acad. Child Psychiat. 15:97, 1976.

Brazelton, T. B., Robey, J. S., and Collier, G. A.: Infant development in the Zinacantec Indians of Southern Mexico. Pediatrics 44:274, 1969.

Brazelton, T. B., Scholl, M. L., and Robey, J. S.: Visual responses in the newborn. Pediatrics 37:284, 1966.

Brazelton, T. B., Tronick, E., Lechtig, A., and Lasky, R.: Biomedical variables and neonatal performance of Guatemalan infants. Paper presented at American Academy Cerebral Palsy, New Orleans, 1975.

Brazelton, T. B., Tronick, E., Wise, S., Als, H., Adamson, L., and Scanlon, J: The effects of regional obstetric anesthesia on newborn behavior over the first ten days of life, Pediatrics (in press) 1976.

Brazier, M. A. B. (Ed.): The central nervous system and behavior. Trans. 2nd Conf., Josiah Macy Fdn., 1959.

Bruner, J. S.: Eye, hand and mind. *In* D. Elkind and J. H. Flavell (Eds.): Studies in Cognitive Development. New York, Oxford University Press, 1969, p. 223.

Bridger, W. H.: Sensory habituation and discrimination in the human neonate. Am. J. Psychiat. *117*:991, 1961.

Bridger, W. H., and Reiser, M. F.: Psychophysiologic studies of the neonate: An approach toward the methodological and theoretical problems involved. Psychosom. Med. *21*:265–276, 1959.

Chapple, E.: Experimental production of transients in human interaction. Nature *228*:630, 1970.

Clifton, R. K.: Cardiac conditioning and orienting in the human infant. *In* Obrist, P., Black, A. H., Brener, J., and DiCara, L. (Eds.): Cardiovascular Physiology. Chicago, Aldine Press, 1974, p. 479.

Dayton, G. O. Jr., Jones, M. H., Aiu, P., Rawson, R. A., Steele, B., and Rose, M.: Developmental study of coordinated eye movements in the human infant. Arch. Ophthalmol. *71*:865, 1964.

Drage, J. S., Kennedy, C., and Berendes, H.: The 5 minute Apgar scores and 4 year psychological performance. Devel. Med. Child Neurol. *8*:141, 1966.

Dreyfus-Brisac, C., Flescher, J., and Plessart, E.: C'électroencephalogramme: critère d'âge conceptionnel du nouveau-né a terme et prématuré, Biol. Neonatol. *4*:154–173, 1962.

Dreyfus-Brisac, C.: The bioelectrical development of the central nervous system during early life. *In* Falkner, J. (Ed.): Human Development. Philadelphia, W. B. Saunders Co., pp. 286–305, 1966.

Dubowitz, L.: Personal communication, 1975.

Dubowitz, L., and Dubowitz, V.: Clinical assessment of gestational age in the newborn infant. J. Pediatr. *77*:1, 1970.

Dubowitz, V., Whittaker, G. F., Brown, B. H., and Robinson, A.: Nerve conduction velocity: An index of neurological maturity of the newborn infant. Developm. Med. Child Neurol. *10*:741, 1968.

Eisenberg, R. B.: Auditory behavior in the human neonate: Methodologic problems. J. Audio. Res. *5*:159, 1965.

Ellingson, R. V.: Cortical electrical responses to visual stimulation in the human infant. Electroenceph. Clin. Neurophysiol. *12*:663, 1960.

Engen, T., Lipsett, L. P., and Kaye, H.: Olfactory responses and adaptation in the human neonate. J. Comp. Physiol. Psychol. *56*:73, 1963.

Fantz, R. L.: Visual perception from birth as shown by pattern selectivity. Ann. N.Y. Acad. Sci. *118*:793, 1965.

Farr, V., Mitchell, R. G., Nelligan, G. A., and Parkin, V. M.: The definition of some external characteristics used in the assessment of gestational age in the newborn infant. Developm. Med. Child Neurol. *8*:507, 1966.

Flechsig, P. E.: Anatomie des menschlichen Geherns und Ruckenmarks auf myelogenetischer Grundlage. Leipsiz, G. Thieme, 1920.

Firestone, J., Lesser, K., Strauss, M. E., Starr, R. H., and Ostrea, E. M.: Behavioral characteristics of methadone addicted neonates. Technical Report, 02–74, Mimeo, 1974.

Fisichelli, V., and Karelitz, S.: The cry latencies of normal infants and those with brain damage. Pediatr. *62*:724–734, 1963.

Freedman, D. C., and Freedman, N.: Behavioral differences between Chinese American and American newborns. Nature *224*:227, 1969.

Geber, M., and Dean, R. F. A.: The state of development of newborn African children. Lancet *272*:1216, 1957.

Gesell, A.: The Embryology of Behavior. New York: Harper, 1945.

Goldberg, S.: Competence reconsidered: A model of parent infant interaction. Personal communication, Brandeis University, 1975.

Goren, C., Sarty, M., and Wu, P.: Visual following and pattern discrimination of face-like stimuli by newborn infants. Pediatrics *56*:544, 1975.

Gorman, J. J., Cogan, D. G., and Gillis, S. S.: An apparatus for grading the visual acuity of infants on the basis of opticokinetic nystagmus. Pediatrics *19*:1088, 1957.

Graham, F. K., Matarazzo, R. G., and Caldwell, B. M.: Behavioral differences between normal and traumatized newborns. Psychol. Mono. *70*:427, 1956.

Graham, F. K., and Clifton, R. K.: Heart rate change as a component of the orienting response. Psychol. Bull. *65*:305–320, 1966.

Graziano, L. J., Weitzman, E. D., and Velasco, M. S. A.: Neurologic maturation and auditory evoked responses in low birth weight infants. Pediatrics *41*:483, 1968.

Gryboski, J. D.: The swallowing mechanism of the neonate: esophageal and gastric motility. Pediatrics *35*:445, 1965.

Haith, M. M., Kessen, W., and Collins, D.: Response of the human infant to level of complexity of intermittent visual movement. J. Exp. Child Psychol. *7*:52, 1969.

Halverson, H. M.: Mechanisms of early feeding. J. Genet. Psychol. *64*:185, 1944.

Haynes, H., White, B. L., and Held, R.: Visual accommodation in human infants. Science *148*:528, 1965.

Hershenson, M.: Visual discrimination in the human newborn. J. Comp. Physiol. Psychol. *58*:270, 1964.

Hooker, D.: The Prenatal Origin of Behavior. 3rd edition. New York, Hafner Publishing Co., 1969.

Horowitz, F. D., Self, P. A., Paden, L. N., Culp, R., Laub, K., Boyd, E., and Mann, M. E.: Newborn and four week retest on a normative population using the Brazelton Newborn Assessment Procedure. Paper presented at Soc. Res. Child Devel. Meetings, Minneapolis, 1971.

Hrbek, A., and Mares, P.: Cortical evoked responses to visual stimulation in full term and premature infants. EEG Clin. Neurophysiol. *16*:575, 1964.

Humphry, J.: Postnatal repetition of human prenatal activity sequences with some suggestions of their neuro-anatomical basin. *In* R. J. Robinson (Ed.): Brain and Early Behavior. London, Academic Press, 43–84, 1969.

Hutt, C., and Ounsted, C.: The biological significance of gaze aversion with particular reference to the syndrome of infantile autism. Behavioral Science *11*:346–356, 1966.

Illingsworth, R.: Crying in infants and children. Br. Med. J. *1*:75, 1955.

James, L. S.: The effect of pain relief for labor and delivery of the fetus and newborn. Anesthesiology *21*:405, 1960.

James, W.: The principles of psychology. New York, Henry Holt, 1890, p. 488.

Jensen, K.: Differential reactions to taste and temperature stimuli in newborn infants. Genet. Psychol. Monogr. *12*:361, 1932.

Kaplan, S. L., et al.: Correlations between scores on the Brazelton Neonatal Assessment Scale, measures of newborn sucking behavior, and birthweight in infants born to narcotic addicted mothers, *In* Ellis, N. R. (Ed.): Aberrant Development in Infancy. Hillsdale, N.J., Lawrence Erlbaum Assoc., 1975.

Karelitz, S., and Fischelli, V.: The cry thresholds of normal infants and those with brain damage. J. Pediatr. *61*:679–685, 1962.

Kaye, H.: Infant sucking and its modification. *In* L. P. Lipsitt and C. C. Spiker (Eds.): Advances in Child Development and Behavior. Vol III, New York: Academic Press, 1967, p.1.

Kaye, K., and Brazelton, T. B.: The orthological significance of the burst-pause pattern in infant sucking. Paper given at Soc. for Res. in Child Devel., Minneapolis, April, 1971.

Keefer, C.: Neonatal assessment in Gusii infants in Kenya. work in progress, Harvard University, 1976.

Keefer, C., Tronick, E., Levine, R., and Brazelton, T. B.: Motor development in Gusii infants, manuscript of work in progress, Harvard University, 1976.

Keeley, K.: Prenatal influence on the behavior of offspring of crowded mice. Science *135*:44, 1962.

Kessen, W., Haith, M. M., and Salapatek, P. H.: Human infancy: A bibliography and guide. *In* Mussen, P. (Ed.): Carmichael's Manual of Child Psychology. Vol 1, New York, Wiley and Sons, 1970, p. 287.

Klaus, M. H., and Kennell, J. H.: Mothers separated from their newborn infants. Ped. Clin. N. Am. *17*:1015, 1970.

Klein, M., and Stern, L.: Low birthweight and the battered child syndrome, Am. J. Dis. Child. *122*:15, 1971.

Korner, A. F., and Thoman, E. B.: Visual alertness in neonates as evoked by maternal care. J. Exp. Child Psychol. *10*:67, 1970.

Kron, R. E., Stein, M., and Goddard, K. E.: A method of measuring sucking behavior of newborn infants. Psychosom. Med. *25*:181, 1963.

Lester, B. M.: Cardiac habituation of the orienting response to an auditory signal in infants of varying nutritional status. Developm. Psychol. *11*:432, 1975.

Lewis, M., Bartels, B., Campbell, H. and Goldberg, S.: Individual differences in attention, Am. J. Dis. Child. *112*:461, 1967.

Lind, J., Wasz-Hockert, O., Vuorenkoski, F., Partanen, T., Theorell, K., and Valanne, E.: Vocal responses to painful stimuli in newborn and young infants. Ann. Paediatr. Fenn. *12*:55–63, 1966.

Lipsitt, L. P.: Learning in the human infant. *In* H. W. Stevenson, M. D. Rheingold and E. Hess (Eds.) Early Behavior: Comparative and Behavioral Approaches. New York, Wiley, 1967, 225–247.

Lipton E. L., Steinschneider, A., and Richmond, J.: Auditory sensitivity in the infant: Effect of intensity on cardiac and motor responsivity. Child Dev. *37*:233–252, 1966.

Lipton, E. L., Steinschneider, A., and Richmond, J.: Swaddling—a child care practice: Historical, cultural and experimental observations. Monogr. Pediatr. *35*:521–67, 1965.

Lorenz, K.: Die angeborenen Formen möglicher Erfahrung. *In* J. Nash (Ed.): Developmental Psychology: A Psychobiological Approach. Englewood, N. J., Prentice-Hall, 1970.

Lubchenco, L. O., Bard, H., Goldman, A. L., Coyer, W. E., McIntyre, C., and Smith, D.: Newborn intensive care and long-term prognosis, Dev. Med. Child Neurol. *16*:421–431, 1974.

Lubchenco, L. O., Hansman, C., Dressler, M., and Boyd, E.: Intrauterine growth estimated from liveborn, birthweight data at 24 to 42 weeks of gestation. Pediatrics *32*:793, 1963.

Lieberman, M. W.: Early developmental stress and later behavior. Science *141*:824–825, 1963.

MacFarlane, A.: Olfaction in the development of preferences in the human neonate. *In* Parent-Infant Evaluation. Ciba Foundation Symposium 33. American Elsevier, N. Y., 1975, 103–119.

Michaelis, R., Parmelee, A., Stern, E., and Haber, A.: Activity states in premature and term infants. Dev. Psychobiol. 6:209, 1973.

Michaelis, R., Schulte, F. J., and Nolte, R.: Motor behavior of small for gestational age newborn infants. J. Pediatr. 76:208, 1970.

Miller, H. and Hassanein, K.: Fetal malnutrition in white newborn infants: Maternal factors. Pediatrics 52:504, 1973.

Minde, K., Ford, M. A., Cellhofer, E., and Boukydis, C.: Mothers of premature infants. Dept. of Psychiatry, Hospital for Sick Children, Toronto, 1975.

Moss, H. A.: Methodological issues in studying mother-infant interaction. Am. J. Orthopsych. 35:482, 1965.

Osofsky, J. and Danzger, B.: Relationships between neonatal characteristics and mother-infant interaction, Dev. Psychol. 10:124, 1974.

Parmelee, A.: Infant crying and neurologic diagnosis. J. Pediatr. *61*:801, 1962.

Parmelee, A. H., and Michaelis, R.: Neurologic examination of the newborn. *In* J. Hellmuth (Ed.): Exceptional Infant. Vol. II, New York, Bruner Mazel, 1971. pp. 3–24.

Parmelee, A. H., Jr., Schulte, F. J., Akiyama, Y., Wenner, W. H., Schultz, M. A. and Stern, E.: Maturation of EEG activity during sleep in premature infants. Electroenceph. Clin. Neurophysiol. 24:319, 1968.

Partanen, J., Wasz-Hockert, O., Vuroenkoski, V., Theorell, K., Valann, E., and Lind, J.: Auditory identification of pain cry signals of young infants in pathological conditions and its spectrographic basis. Ann. Paediatr. Fenn. 13:56, 1967.

Peiper, A.: Cerebral Function in Infancy and Childhood. New York, Consultants Bureau, 1963.

Piaget, J.: The Construction of Reality in the Child. New York, Basic Books, 1954.

Porzes, S. W.: Indices of newborn attentional responsivity. Merrill Palmer Quart. 20:231, 1974.

Pratt, K. C.: The effects of repeated visual stimulation upon the activity of newborn infants. J. Genet. Psychol. 44:117, 1934.

Prechtl, H. F. R.: The directed head turning response and allied movements of the human baby. Behavior 13:212, 1956.

Prechtl, H., and Beintema, D.: The neurological examination of the full term newborn infant. Clin. Devel. Med., National Spastics Monograph No 12. London: W. M. Heinemann and Sons, 1964.

Preyer, W.: The Mind of the Child. New York, Appleton, 1888.

Ray, W. S.: A preliminary study of fetal conditioning. Child Devel. 3:173, 1932.

Robinson, R. J.: Assessment of gestational age by neurological examination. Arch. Dis. Child. *41*:437, 1966.

Robson, K. S., and Moss, H. A.: Patterns and determinants of maternal attachment. J. Pediatr. 77:976, 1970.

Rosenblith, J. F.: Prognostic value of behavioral assessment of neonates. Biol. Neonatol. 6:76, 1964.

Saint-Anne Dargassies, S.: La maturation neurologique des prématures. Etudes Neonat. *4*:71, 1955.

Saint-Anne Dargassies, S.: Neurological maturation of the premature infant of 28 to 41 weeks gestational age. *In* F. Falkner (Ed.): Human Development. Philadelphia, W. B. Saunders Co., 1966.

Salapatek, P. H., and Kessen, W.: Visual scanning of triangles by the human newborn, J. Exp. Child Psychol. 3:155, 1966.

Sameroff, A. J.: The components of sucking in the human newborn, J. Exp. Child Psychol. 6:607, 1968.

Scanlon, J. W., Brown, W. V., Weiss, J. B., and Alper, N. H.: Neurobehavioral responses of newborns after maternal epidural anesthesia. Anesthesiology *40*:121, 1974.

Scarr, S., and Williams, M.: The effects of early stimulation on low birthweight infants. Child Dev. *44*:94, 1973.

Schulte, F. J., Michaelis, R., Linke, I., and Nolte, R.: Motor nerve conduction velocity in term, preterm, and small for dates newborn infants. Dev. Psychobiol. *1*:41, 1968.

Sontag, L. W., and Richardo, T. W.: Studies in fetal behavior: Fetal heart rate as a behavioral indicator. Monogr. Soc. Res. Child Devel. 3:(4), 1938.

Soule, A. B., Standley, K., Copans, S. A., and Davis, M.: Clinical uses of the Brazelton Neonatal Scale. Pediatrics *54*:583, 1974.

Stechler, G., and Latz, E.: Some observations on attention and arousal in the human infant. J. Acad. Child Psych. 5:517, 1966.

Strauss, M. E.: Early development of narcotic addicted infants. Progress Report, 1973.

Super, C.: Motor Performance in Kenyan infants. Colloquium, University of Nairobi, February, 1975.

Truby, H. M., Bosma, J. F., and Lind, J.: Newborn infant cry. Acta Pediatr. Scand. Suppl. *163*, 1965.

Wagner, I. F.: The establishment of a criterion of depth of sleep in the newborn infant. J. Genet. Psychol., *51*:17, 1937.

Warkany, J., Monroe, B., and Sutherland, B.: Intrauterine growth retardation. Am. J. Dis. Child. *102*:127, 1961.

Warren, N.: Reevaluation of motor precocity in African children. Personal communication, 1972.

Wasz-Hockert, O., Lind, J., Vuorenkoski, V., Partanen, T., and Valanne, E.: The infant cry. Clin. Dev. Med. *29*, 1968.

Weitzman, E. D., Fishbein, W., and Graziani, D.: Auditory evoked responses obtained from the scalp EEG of the full term infant during sleep. Pediatrics 35:458, 1965.

White, R. W.: Motivation reconsidered: The concept of competence. Psychol. Rev. 66:297, 1959.

Windle, W.: Reflexes of mammalian embryos and fetuses. *In* P. Weiss (Ed.): Genetic Neurology, Chicago, University of Chicago Press, 1950, pp. 214–222.

Winick, M.: Malnutrition and brain development, J. Pediatr. *74*:667, 1969.

Winick, M.: Nucleic acid and protein content during growth of human brain. Pediatr. Res. 2:352, 1968.

Wolff, P.: The causes, controls, and organization of behavior in the neonate. Psychol. Monogr. 5: (no. 17) 1966.

Wolff, P.: The natural history of crying and other vocalizations in early infancy. *In* B. W. Foss (Ed.): Determinants of infant behavior. IV, London, Methuen & Co., 1969. p. 81.

# 4

# THE UNDERSIZED INFANT

## TRUE PREMATURITY

The primary statistical criterion of prematurity used to be a birth weight of 5½ pounds (2500 gm) or less. By this standard a good many infants of more than 37 weeks' gestational age are undoubtedly included. Both race and sex affect the expected weight for gestational age. A white male infant at term would average 300 grams heavier than a black female infant. The effect of race appears to reverse between 34 and 36 weeks, in that black infants are relatively heavier at a given gestational age below 34 weeks (Hoffman et al.).

**INCIDENCE.** The proportion of infants born earlier than 37 weeks varies widely from country to country, or even from city to city, largely reflecting socioeconomic factors. Usher, in Montreal, reports that borderline premature infants, of 37 to 38 weeks, with weights of 2500 to 3250 grams, make up 16 per cent of all live births; infants of 31 to 36 weeks make up 16 per cent; while those of

**TABLE 4–1.** *Events Associated with Prematurity*

| |
|---|
| Female infants more often than male |
| Maternal age less than 16 years, or over 35 years |
| History of previous premature birth |
| History of previous fetal death |
| Illegitimate pregnancy |
| Short intervals between pregnancies |
| Asymptomatic bacteriuria |
| Lower socioeconomic status |
| Maternal cyanotic heart disease |
| Elective induction of labor |

24 to 30 weeks (extremely premature infants) make up only about 1 per cent. This latter group contributes significantly to neonatal deaths and to later handicapped infants.

**ETIOLOGY.** The reasons for low birth weight are legion, although more often than not obscure in a given patient (Table 4–1). The highest prematurity rates are among individuals in low socioeconomic classes. Which of the many conditions associated with poverty are the critical ones remains to be established. Maternal nutrition has been thought crucial by some, and was supported by the findings of Antonov that the prematurity rate at the Leningrad State Pediatric Institute was 49 per cent in the first half of 1942 during the siege. In many studies in this country and in Europe the prematurity rate has been shown to be 15 per cent or more in the poorer classes, and 5 to 7 per cent in the upper classes. In a municipal hospital in Bombay it was 36.3 per cent in 1956.

**PHYSICAL FINDINGS.** Infants of different gestational ages differ from each other in many respects just as infants of one and two months' postnatal age are dissimilar. An infant born with a weight of 4 pounds (1800 gm) bears little resemblance to one who weighs 1800 grams at 2 months of age. Not only are appearances different, but maturation of function, risks of certain disorders and metabolic needs are dissimilar in infants of different birth weights and gestational ages.

The smallest viable premature infants give one the impression of having suffered from profound malnutrition, since they lack any significant fat stores and muscle mass. After their postnatal water losses, the impression of malnutrition is all the stronger as one sees skin stretched like parchment over the skeleton. The head is relatively large, the fontanels wide, the chest wall very compliant, the abdomen often distended and the genitalia very immature with undescended testicles and a poorly developed scrotum. Pigmentation is usually absent at birth.

The premature infant often has a gelatinous feel, and is usually coated with white vernix caseosa at birth. The skin over the hands and soles is smooth, lacking most of the creases seen at term. Over the next few days, he loses his vernix, and the skin becomes dry and often scaly. The ruddy look of the first days of life fades to a paler hue as the hematocrit falls. Commonly some physiological jaundice is present; it may peak at 5 to 7 days, or somewhat later than in the term infant. When the bilirubin is rising, a yellow hue is noted first in the face, descending then to involve the feet last. The color is usually yellow-orange on the third or fourth day, turning a paler yellow after the first week.

## FUNCTIONAL IMMATURITY

One generally thinks of the prematurely born infant as handicapped in contrast to the term infant, and no one would maintain that our present methods of care are as satisfactory as the normal intrauterine environment. Yet it is impressive that so many infants delivered after only two thirds of the normal gestational period can make a good adjustment to the extrauterine milieu. It is worthy of emphasis that over 70 per cent of infants born in the weight range of 1000 to 1500 grams survive, and the majority of them have normal neuromuscular and mental function. Such a positive approach is not stated to ignore the significant mortality and morbidity that remains, but to suggest that some of the difficulties encountered by some premature infants may not be attributed solely to immaturity but to postnatal aberrations that might be remediable.

Perhaps the most striking of the evidences of physiologic immaturity is the occurrence of jaundice late in the first week of life. The breakdown of hemoglobin and reduced capacity of the liver to conjugate and excrete bilirubin contribute to the degree of hyperbilirubinemia (see pp. 641–645). Ultimately activity catches up with need, and jaundice disappears (Chap. 70). Blood glucose levels often lower than those of mature infants also stem in all probability from immaturity of hepatic function, as do hypoproteinemia and hypoprothrombinemia.

The kidneys of premature infants function less efficiently than do those of full-term babies. Glomeruli and their nephrons are still developing at a rapid rate in the normal kidney until term and later. Birth before the thirty-seventh week implies possession of less than the full complement of functioning nephrons, and this deprivation varies inversely with the age of the fetus. It results in a diminution in functional capacity, including glomerular filtration rate and tubular functions. Premature infants can concentrate urine, but not to the same degree as can more mature infants, and their capacity for osmotic diuresis is limited. Clearance of urea, chloride, potassium and phosphorus are diminished. The kidneys are therefore limited in their capacity to handle emergency work loads, with the result that infection, vomiting, diarrhea or heat stress leads quickly to acidosis or alkalosis.

The commonest form of respiratory irregularity in the premature infant is so-called periodic respiration. Thirty to 40 per cent of all prematures are subject to it, breathing periods of 10 to 15 seconds alternating with apneic periods of 6 to 7 seconds. Similar breathing irregularity does not affect the full-term newborn at sea level, although it frequently does at high altitudes. Its cause is not fully understood.

The digestive powers of the premature infant appear to approximate those of the mature one with one notable exception. It has been demonstrated beyond doubt that the premature infant handles fat less well than does the mature infant. When he is fed the full complement of fat in cow's milk (4 per cent), a great deal may be excreted in the stool. Considerably less is lost when the intake is reduced by half. Some artificial formulas with added vegetable oils bind calcium in the intestinal tract with resulting negative calcium balance in the first few weeks of life. Although the amounts lost are probably not very significant, early introduction of vitamin D will improve the situation in infants fed on cow's milk formulas. The ability of the premature infant to absorb and metabolize proteins and carbohydrates seems unimpaired (see Chap. 93).

The total caloric requirement of the premature infant approximates that of the mature one. A somewhat increased basal need, perhaps due to increased ratio of surface area to weight, plus an increased requirement for more rapid growth and increased fecal loss on diets of unskimmed milk is counterbalanced by a lesser caloric need for muscular activity. An average intake of 120 calories per kilogram is adequate for steady gain in weight. Higher caloric intakes may possibly increase the speed of gain and shorten hospital stay without injury to the infant (see Chap. 93).

Low birth weight infants are well known to be predisposed to intracranial and pulmonary hemorrhage. Bleeding has been associated with hypoxia, traumatic deliveries, hypoglycemia and the respiratory distress syndrome. Very few systematic correlations between clinical hemorrhage and hemostatic functions have been reported. Low birth weight infants as a group have lower levels of factor II, V, VII and X activity, a defect in serum thromboplastic activity and reduced numbers of platelets (see Chap. 64).

The final disability of the premature infant consequent upon immaturity, the one which accounts for much mortality and morbidity, is his extraordinary susceptibility to infection. We shall discuss later (Chap. 84) some of the factors which play some part in this lack of resistance. Bacteriostatic and bactericidal activity of the blood serum is less vigorous than in mature infants and older persons. Their white blood corpuscles phagocytize bacteria less efficiently than do those of the mature infant. They have been deprived of some maternal antibodies that would normally cross the placenta in the last trimester. The premature infant also does not manufacture antibody in response to injection of antigen to the same degree as does the mature infant. The sum total of these humoral deficiencies may be significant, but many believe that there must be factors of resistance inherent in the tissues themselves which are not well developed and which contribute heavily toward the unusual susceptibility to infection.

SUSCEPTIBILITY TO MATERNAL ANESTHETICS AND ANALGESICS. Prematurity carries with it susceptibility to the deleterious effects of maternal anesthetics and analgesics. Oversedation adds the hazard of depression of respiratory center responsiveness, with the result that the tiny infant does not make the continuous respiratory effort requisite for survival. An additional hazard, we believe, is loss of sensitivity in the mechanism which defends against tracheal aspiration of oropharyngeal secretions and food. The resultant aspiration pneumonitis is rapidly fatal.

VITAMIN REQUIREMENTS. A fortuitous combination of circumstances renders the premature infant much more liable to rickets than is his mature counterpart. Virtually every one of them who dies after having survived a few weeks shows the pathologic changes of rickets at the ends of the long bones. If bone x-ray films are taken routinely, many will reveal rachitic alterations ranging from barely recognizable to florid ones. The blood calcium or phosphorus levels in the more severe cases will be diminished. The circumstances responsible are an increased need for vitamin D and calcium because of the uncommon rapidity of bone growth in premature infants and the excessive fecal loss of ingested vitamin D because of inefficiency in the absorption of fat from the intestine.

This latter factor is operative in the case of vitamin A, another fat-soluble vitamin. In addition, the premature infant is often fed low-fat milk, and milk fat is the natural source of vitamin A. Add to these the fact that the store of this vitamin in the liver of the premature infant is considerably smaller than that in the mature baby's liver, and one has the perfect setup for the development of vitamin A deficiency. Unless adequate amounts of the water-miscible form of the vitamin are added to the diet early,

subclinical avitaminosis A supervenes not uncommonly, although the full-blown deficiency disease rarely makes its appearance (p. 859).

The other two fat-soluble vitamins may be in short supply for similar reasons. Deficiency in vitamin K superimposed upon hypoprothrombinemia and vascular fragility so often encountered in prematurity can only aggravate the tendency to excessive bleeding. Laboratory evidence of vitamin E deficiency is routinely met in premature infants, and this lack occasionally causes anemia and edema (p. 573).

Premature infants who are not given supplementary vitamin C may acquire scurvy with unusual rapidity. They also require additional ascorbic acid for the complete metabolism of certain amino acids (p. 865).

ANEMIA. We discuss in detail the physiologic anemia to which premature infants are subject and point out that it is not preventable or permanently cured by iron or transfusions (Chap. 66). Supplemental iron, starting at 4 to 8 weeks of age, is recommended, however, because rapid growth will quickly deplete iron stores.

HYPERBILIRUBINEMIA. The premature infant is more prone to hyperbilirubinemia than is the mature one. If there is a pathologic basis for jaundice, such as hemolytic disease or sepsis, the jaundice which results is likely to be more severe in the premature. Even without a reason such as one of these, the premature is prone to hyperbilirubinemia because of immaturity in respect to the elaboration of glucuronyl transferase in his liver. Until this enzyme is formed in sufficient quantity, bilirubin cannot be conjugated into the glucuronated form (direct-reacting) and therefore cannot be excreted (see Chap. 70).

HYPOGLYCEMIA. Blood sugar determinations made in the first 12 hours or more of life show that the original fall in blood sugar concentration is more profound in many premature infants than in mature ones. Fifty per cent of prematures versus 15 per cent of matures experience a drop to hypoglycemic levels (see Chap. 57).

RETROLENTAL FIBROPLASIA (see also page 985). The eye of the infant is not fully vascularized until several weeks after term birth. When oxygen tension in the arterial blood is elevated, retinal vasospasm may develop, leading to ischemic injury to the retina. Later fibrous tissue forms and retinal detachment may occur. The condition, once the leading cause of blindness in the United States, was virtually eliminated with severe restriction of oxygen therapy to premature infants. More recently, as it has become evident that some infants with severe lung disease may need high concentrations of inspired oxygen to maintain life, oxygen has been used more liberally. On occasion it has been used longer than needed, or in excess concentration, and arterial oxygen tensions have reached toxic levels. A substantial increase in the numbers of infants with retrolental fibroplasia has been noted in this country in recent years.

The only safeguard for the infant who needs some added oxygen, but in whom too much may cause visual impairment or blindness, is to measure arterial oxygen tensions several times daily whenever inspired concentrations of greater than 40 per cent are indicated. In our hands umbilical arterial oxygen tensions of over 40 mm Hg and under 80 to 100 mm Hg have not led to retrolental fibroplasia. It would be ideal to measure oxygen tensions in samples of temporal or radial artery blood, but it is difficult to obtain serial samples from these sites in a tiny premature infant.

**FEEDING THE PREMATURE INFANT.** The time at which feedings should be instituted for the premature infant has been the subject of some debate in past years. Partisans of late feeding base their argument largely upon the valid reason that swallowing is imperfect in the immature, and that reflux, with its danger of aspiration pneumonitis, is extremely hazardous. Proponents of early feeding have proved beyond reasonable doubt that this regimen minimizes the dangers of hypoglycemia, hyperbilirubinemia and excess catabolism of the small neonate. They point out that the hazard of aspiration may be virtually eliminated by intravenous feeding in those infants who are so immature that they may be prone to gastroesophageal reflux and subsequent aspiration. Thus, early feeding, begun within four to eight hours after birth, is appropriate and such early feeding is

often best accomplished by intravenous rather than oral or nasogastric tube feeding.

One error to be avoided is feeding too large quantities. All sorts of schedules have been devised, but fixed schemes are to be avoided, since much depends upon the hunger and the capacity of the individual baby. The alert vigorous one may be offered 4 ml to begin with and the quantity increased by 2 ml whenever the previous amount has been taken well. The maximum increment in any one day on this regimen will be 1/2 ounce (16 ml). Most will reach satiety at an intake of approximately 120 calories per kilogram, but some will demand as much as 160 to 180 calories. There seems to be no valid reason why they should not have this much.

The low birth weight baby soon demonstrates whether or not he can take in by his own efforts sufficient food upon which to gain weight. Inability to do so or the appearance of cyanosis during early attempts at feeding calls for the institution of gavage. Intermittent gavage is to be preferred for larger premature infants, in whom the procedure will probably be necessary for only a few days. It may be performed every 3 or 4 hours, preferably the latter, until trials with nipple or medicine dropper indicate readiness to resume oral feeding. An indwelling polyethylene catheter is to be preferred in those infants who are so small that gavage feeding will be needed for many days or weeks or are in such delicate respiratory balance that the act of passing the gavage tube induces apnea and cyanosis. Small feedings can then be introduced every three hours through a No. 5 or No. 8 French nasogastric tube. It should be withdrawn and replaced through the other nostril periodically, approximately every two days, since esophageal and gastric erosion and hemorrhage have been known to follow prolonged use of indwelling catheters. Gastrostomy has been advocated as a way to feed small premature infants, but controlled studies comparing gastrostomy with gavage favored the latter. Peritonitis, sepsis and central nervous system hemorrhage were significantly greater in the gastrostomy group (Raffensperger et al.).

Nasojejunal feedings are useful in some infants in whom regurgitation is a problem.

The position of the tube can be ascertained by testing the aspirate with litmus. When a pH of 5 to 7 is found, abdominal films are indicated to place the end of the tube beyond the ligament of Treitz. Infusions by slow drip of infusion pump are tolerated well by most infants. Great care must be taken not to overload the intestine (see page 853).

Volumes have been written about the relative merits of human milk versus cow's milk, of whole milk versus skimmed milk mixtures and of simulated human milk products versus the less complex cow's milk or evaporated milk formulas. It is apparent that many low birth weight infants have done well when raised on breast milk, and in many parts of the world that is the only safe, sterile form of milk available. When infants are too feeble to suck, breast milk may be expressed and fed the infants by gavage. The low solute load and optimal calcium-phosphorus ratios of breast milk may be mimicked by suitable processing of cow's milk, although the benefit of protection from enteric infection cannot be duplicated by cow's milk.

In this country, the current trend is to give low birth weight infants cow's milk, modified to reduce the fat content and electrolyte load, and with adjustments in protein composition to reach a level of 4 gm per kilogram per day, or somewhat greater than that found in breast milk. The demands of growth require added protein to maintain a positive nitrogen balance. High protein intake (6 gm per kilogram per day) such as is found in half-skimmed milk has been shown to result in significant elevations of plasma phenylalanine and tyrosine in some infants, and is not currently recommended, since some adverse effects of such changes in serum amino acids have been reported (Momunes et al.).

Our current practice with very small infants is to give the water requirements of 60 to 80 ml per kilogram per day intravenously for the first few days. As soon as peristalsis begins, we give 1 to 2 ml of formula at a concentration of 0.8 calories per milliliter every two to three hours. As the infant demonstrates he can tolerate larger volumes of formula, we discontinue intravenous feedings and give formula at a concentration of 0.8 calories per milliliter, working up to 150 ml per kilogram per day by the end of the first week to 10 days. We feed premature infants arbitrarily at 3-hour intervals until such time as their capacity permits sufficient intake per feeding for the number to be reduced to 6 per day. This is usually possible when a body weight of 4 pounds 8 ounces or 4 pounds 12 ounces (2000 or 2100 gm) has been reached. At this point we ordinarily change the feeding to an iron- and vitamin-enriched prepared formula and the schedule to an every-four-hour one in preparation for the infant's discharge after having reached a weight of 5 pounds (2250 gm) (see Appendix II).

Neither breast milk nor commercial formulas without added iron meet the relatively high requirements of the pre-term infant for iron, vitamin E and folate. Iron deficiency may not be manifest until several months of age; low levels of vitamin E and folate are detectable in the first weeks of life. Recommendations for pre-term infants are 2 mg/kg of iron starting within 4 to 8 weeks of birth, 5 to 25 I.U./day of alpha-tocopherol acetate starting in the first week of life, and 50 $\mu$g per day of folic acid. Folate and vitamin E can be combined in a single oral preparation.

Pre-term infants also require relatively higher doses of vitamin C to maintain normal tyrosine levels, and doses of 75 mg/day are recommended. Vitamin D requirements are 400 units per day, and administration should begin by mouth, if possible not later than 2 weeks of age.

Low birth weight infants frequently have low serum calcium levels, with or without symptoms. Since proprietary formulas do not provide the amount of calcium such an infant would normally acquire in utero, supplement in the form of oral calcium is recommended. When serum concentrations of calcium are less than 7.5 mg per 100 ml, Fomon recommends oral calcium gluconate 0.5 to 1.0 gm per kilogram per day for several days (see Chaps. 92 and 93).

**PREVENTION OF INFECTION IN PREMATURE INFANTS.** Low birth weight infants, as well as those at high risk, should be in an intensive care nursery. Their nurses and nurses' aides must never be permitted to care for, indeed to come in contact with,

*TABLE 4–2.* *Mortality of Premature Infants*

| Birth Weight | No. Infants | Mortality (%) | No. Infants | Mortality (%) |
|---|---|---|---|---|
| < 1 kg. | 759 | 87 | 182 | 82 |
| 1–1.25 kg. | 834 | 58.5 | } 192 | 35 |
| 1.25–1.5 kg. | 1410 | 36.3 | | |
| 1.5–2 kg. | 3549 | 17.3 | 480 | 8.9 |
| 2–2.5 kg. | 2470 | 9.3 | 1671 | 2.6 |
| All | 9022 | 27.4% | 2525 | 12% |
| | 1922–1952 | | 1967–1968 | |
| | (Hess, *Pediatrics*, 11:425, 1953) | | (Baltimore City Health Department) | |

parents or adult patients. It would be better if they had no contact with full-term infants either, but considerations of expense may render this specialization unfeasible. The care of premature infants should not be entrusted to student nurses except under direct supervision of experienced graduate nurses.

The most scrupulous isolation technique is mandatory in an intensive care nursery. Hands must be washed before entering the nursery, and rewashed before examination of each baby. Gowns need to be worn only

if an infant is to be handled. We no longer advise the use of masks. Personnel with respiratory infection may not be allowed to rely upon masks as sufficient protection against transmitting infection. They must be assigned other duties until free from disease. Personnel with cutaneous infection are as unclean as were lepers in biblical days. They must be excluded from any contact with premature infants until clinical cure has been verified by three successive negative cultures.

We no longer insist on isolation of in-

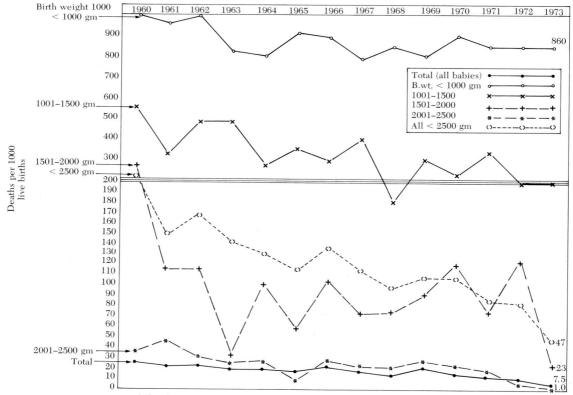

*Figure 4–1.* Neonatal death rates per 1000 single live births, the Johns Hopkins Hospital (1960–1973).

fected infants in nurseries where ventilation is good and hand-washing scrupulous.

**PROGNOSIS.** A steady decline in mortality of premature infants has followed almost universal adoption of the practices outlined in the preceding paragraphs. Table 4–2 demonstrates some of the trends over the years. Prematurity is still the primary cause of death in more than half of the newborns who succumb for all reasons, even though their mortality rate decreased from 1940 to 1950 by 23 per cent (Dunham). Figure 4–1 is characteristic of the more recent decline in many hospitals throughout the world. Table 4–3 illustrates the fall in weight-specific mortality in New York City from 1962 through 1971. The outlook for survival of very small infants remains poor but is improving (Fig. 4–2).

The principal causes of death in the first days of life have changed in relative incidence in recent years. In the 1940's and 1950's trauma, asphyxia and isoimmunization were more frequent than in the 1960's. Even malformations are less common in the 1970's compared to the 1950's. The data in Table 4–4 come from consecutive autopsies at Babies' Hospital, New York, 1960–68.

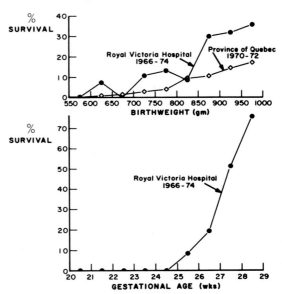

**SURVIVAL RATES AT THE BORDERLINE OF VIABILITY**

*Figure 4–2.* Survival rates at the borderline of viability. (Courtesy of Dr. Robert Usher, Royal Victoria Hospital, Montreal, Quebec, Canada.)

*1962–1971*

**TABLE 4–3.** *Neonatal Survival Rate in New York City by Weight at Birth and Race (Per Cent Live Births)*

| Weight at Birth in Grams | 1962 | 1963 | 1964 | 1965 | 1966 | 1967 | 1968 | 1969 | 1970 | 1971 |
|---|---|---|---|---|---|---|---|---|---|---|
| Under 1000 | 12.5 | 12.9 | 11.6 | 12.1 | 13.6 | 15.1 | 17.5 | 14 | 20 | 21 |
| White | 8.5 | 11.6 | 6.7 | 8.2 | 9.9 | 11.4 | 11.7 | 5 | 18.7 | 12.7 |
| Nonwhite | 16.4 | 14.2 | 16.1 | 15.5 | 16.7 | 17.9 | 22.6 | 21.2 | 21.2 | 28.2 |
| | | | | | | | | | | |
| 1001–1500 | 55 | 55.7 | 56.2 | 59.2 | 63.4 | 64.1 | 65.5 | 61 | 66.6 | 66.2 |
| White | 49.5 | 50.2 | 47.4 | 52 | 59.1 | 56.8 | 61.1 | 52.5 | 61.6 | 57.2 |
| Nonwhite | 61.7 | 62.1 | 65.8 | 66.7 | 68.2 | 71.4 | 70.5 | 70.1 | 71.5 | 75.2 |
| | | | | | | | | | | |
| 1501–2000 | 85.6 | 87.9 | 87.1 | 88.5 | 89 | 89 | 88.8 | 89.2 | 90 | 90.8 |
| White | 82.6 | 85.3 | 84 | 86 | 86.9 | 86.6 | 86.8 | 87.2 | 86.9 | 87.1 |
| Nonwhite | 90.1 | 91.4 | 91.1 | 91.6 | 91.8 | 92.3 | 91.6 | 91.6 | 93.7 | 94.2 |
| | | | | | | | | | | |
| 2001–2500 | 96.8 | 97.2 | 97.2 | 97.4 | 97.6 | 97.8 | 97.7 | 97.4 | 97.7 | 97.5 |
| White | 96.5 | 96.8 | 96.9 | 96.9 | 97.2 | 97.5 | 97.1 | 97.1 | 97.3 | 96.8 |
| Nonwhite | 97.4 | 98 | 97.7 | 98.1 | 98.2 | 98.4 | 98.7 | 97.9 | 98.3 | 98.4 |
| | | | | | | | | | | |
| Under 2501 | 85.2 | 86 | 85.4 | 86.1 | 87.2 | 87.2 | 87.5 | 86.7 | 88.5 | 89.1 |
| White | 85.7 | 86.4 | 85.5 | 86.6 | 87.7 | 87.9 | 87.6 | 86.7 | 88.5 | 88.2 |
| Nonwhite | 84.3 | 85.4 | 85.1 | 85.3 | 86.5 | 86.2 | 87.3 | 86.7 | 88.4 | 90.2 |

(Courtesy of Behrman, R. E., and Rosen, T. S.: Report to The National Commission for The Protection of Human Subjects. 1975.)

*TABLE 4–4. Incidence at Autopsy of Common Fetal, Neonatal and Maternal Conditions*°

| | Gestational Age in Weeks | |
| --- | --- | --- |
| | 28–33 | 34–37 |
| Amniotic fluid infection syndrome | 29% | 11% |
| Hyaline membrane disease | 88% | 48% |
| Pulmonary hemorrhage | 18% | 9% |
| Intraventricular and/or subarachnoid hemorrhage | 61% | 15% |
| Antenatal hypoxia | 13% | 21% |
| Congenital anomalies | 6% | 73% |
| Toxemia of pregnancy | 8% | 22% |
| Polyhydramnios | 3% | 22% |
| Number of cases | 201 | 93 |

°(Data of Naeye, R. L., and Blanc, W. A. *In* Milunsky, A. (Ed.): Clinics in Perinatology, Philadelphia, W. B. Saunders Company, September, 1974.)

As recently as the 1960's, the prevailing experience with the follow-up of low birth weight infants was dismal. In general, the lower the birth weight, the worse the prognosis (Drillien). Among 91 infants with birth weights under 1500 grams, Lubchenco et al. found 50 per cent to have moderate to severe handicaps a decade later. In contrast, infants born in the 1970's, and cared for in neonatal intensive care units, are doing much better. In the series of Rawlings at University College Hospital, London, 90 per cent are normal. Davies and Tizard found 10.3 per cent of their infants under 1500 grams birth weight born during 1961–1964 had spastic diplegia. None born after that date had that lesion. The improvement in outcome was concurrent with closer attention to keeping infants warm and with earlier feeding, as well as other aspects of neonatal intensive care.

Although in general mortality and morbidity are greatly improved, among infants of less than 32 weeks' gestational age referred to a neonatal intensive care unit, Fitzhardinge found some major problems. Gross central nervous system defects (hydrocephaly and microcephaly) were found in 22.5 per cent of 40 boys in her series, and in none of the 27 girls. The mean postconceptional developmental quotients were 110 for the girls and 108 for the boys. Careful follow-up of survivors of neonatal intensive care is clearly of great importance.

# CONSIDERATIONS ON THE DEFINITION OF VIABILITY

Two relatively recent events in American society have prompted a consideration of the definition of viability of the human fetus. One event is the liberalization of indications for abortion, and the inevitability of an occasional error in calculation of gestational age. Although the error is reduced by use of ultrasound to measure fetal head diameter, and by careful clinical assessment, nonetheless infants of 600 to 700 gm are sometimes the product of an elective abortion. The other event is the application of intensive care and technical advances permitting the occasional survival of a 700 gm infant, and the increasingly frequent intact survival of infants weighing more than 800 gm. These events bring into focus the question of when to treat "the product of conception" as any piece of tissue removed at operation, or when to mobilize the facilities of a neonatal intensive-care unit to promote a small possibility of survival.

Any attempt to answer this question must be in the context of the environment in which one lives. For example, neonatal intensive care is not available to all infants born everywhere on earth, so that this issue is not particularly relevant in all societies. Furthermore, any answer has to be based on a judgment of where one is willing to draw the line of probability of a successful outcome. If the chance of survival is one in a million, should intensive care be mobilized, at an estimated cost of $500 per day, with the possible consequence being a denial of such care to situations of greater expectancy of a positive yield? Finally, any modus operandi that might be agreed upon in 1975 may need revision in 1976 if major medical advances permit a better outlook for even smaller infants.

Of first importance would seem to be an analysis of existing experience with infants of very low birth weight. A review of the literature will unearth the case reports of some very small infants, although the reports are usually unsupported by photographs or evidence of careful documentation not only of weight but also of size and gestational age. Surely one of the smallest documented infants was reported by Lelek et al. in 1973. An infant weighing 450 gm at birth fell to a low weight of 360 gm, with a length of 27 cm at 27 weeks, and was alive and doing well at three months of age. A study of populations of infants is difficult since traditional reporting assigns them to a category of less than 1000 gm, and thereby blurs the important differences between infants of 500 gm and those of 900 gm.

In the Quebec perinatal mortality survey, survival by weight group of 50-gm increments for a total population was recorded (Usher RH: Personal communication). No infant of less than a 600-gm birth weight was discharged home. Of 999 infants with weights between 501 and 1000 gm, 56 lived to go home, and 41 of these weighed more than 850 gm at birth. Seen from another perspective, these data indicate that of all infants born over a 3-year period in Quebec, 277,445 births from 1970 through 1972, only four were discharged home after being born with weights from 601 to 700 gm. Thus, the issues concern only a minute fraction of live births. The poignancy of the problem, however, revolves around the circumstances that sometimes a 600-gm fetus is much desired by a couple with a bad reproductive history, and sometimes it is the product of a planned abortion. At present, the view of most obstetric and pediatric personnel seems reasonable: that the wishes of the parents of a 600-gm infant be respected, and the choice for or against intensive supportive care be on that basis.

**RULES FOR CARE OF PREMATURE INFANTS.** The American Academy of Pediatrics has issued a schedule of rules and regulations covering the proper management and feeding of newborn infants. The reader is referred to this invaluable pamphlet, *Standards and Recommendations for Hospital Care of Newborn Infants, Full-Term and Premature* (see also Appendix I).

## INTRAUTERINE GROWTH RETARDATION

Increasing recognition of the heterogeneity of the population of low birth weight infants has led to separation of undergrown infants from true prematures. The usual operational definition of such an infant is that his weight is under two standard deviations of that expected for his gestational age, on the basis of one of the several charts of fetal growth now available. Accurate assessment of gestational age is often difficult. Skeptics would assert that only in the event of twins of unequal size could one be certain that the smaller was "small for dates," and even then some would question whether the larger was "large for dates." Obstetricians and pediatricians, however, are convinced that many fetuses fail to thrive *in utero,* with resulting small size for gestational age. They constitute 1.5 to 2 per cent of all births and their overall neonatal mortality is between 3 and 4 per cent.

**ETIOLOGY.** Many adverse conditions can impair intrauterine growth. Some of them are listed in Table 4–5 and Figure 4–3. It is at once obvious that the causes of fetal growth failure are multiple, and the conclusion is inescapable that studies of body composition, diseases and prognosis that are based on the fact of intrauterine growth retardation alone, without regard to etiology, are likely to give variable and conflicting results. For example, some cite the improved chances for survival in infants of over 37 weeks' gestation but undersized, compared to infants of similar and appropriate size but under 37 weeks' gestation. Statistics may support such a conclu-

**TABLE 4–5.   *Some Findings Associated with Intrauterine Growth Retardation***

Maternal factors
   Infections such as rubella, cytomegalovirus, toxoplasmosis, syphilis
   Toxemia
   Heart disease
   Short stature
   Primiparity
   Severe malnutrition
   Cigarette smoking
   Narcotic usage
   Low maternal age
Environmental factors
   Residence at high altitude
   Radiation
   Exposure to teratogens
Placental factors
   Infarcts
   Thrombosis of fetal vessels
   Single umbilical artery
   Premature partial separation
Fetal factors
   Twins
   Chromosomal abnormalities
   Other congenital malformations

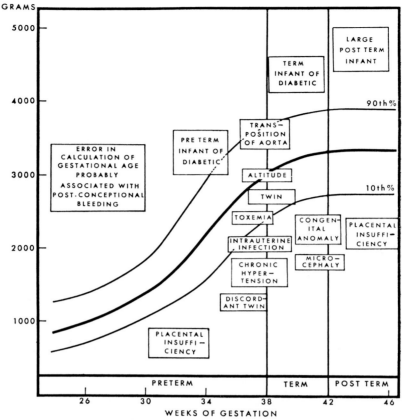

*Figure 4–3.*  Graphic representation of conditions associated with deviations of intrauterine growth. The boxes symbolize the approximate birth weight and gestational age at which the condition is likely to occur. (Lubchenco, L. D., et al.: Factors influencing fetal growth. *In* Jonxis, J. H. P., Visser, H. K. A., and Troelstra, J. A. [Eds.]:Aspects of Praematurity and Dysmaturity. Leiden, H. G. Stenfert Kroese, 1968.)

sion during one study if the cause of fetal growth retardation is maternal toxemia or cigarette smoking. If, on the other hand, a rubella epidemic had occurred, the small-for-dates infants would have a higher mortality than true prematures of comparable birth weight.

**PATHOLOGY.**  The findings at autopsy of undersized infants have been described in detail by Gruenwald and are summarized in Table 4–6. Organ maturation proceeds even though the expected increase in body size does not occur. The small size of the thymus and adrenal has been cited as evidence of chronic intrauterine stress.

**PHYSICAL FINDINGS.**  Small-for-dates infants may be distinguished by a neurologic performance more compatible with that of an older infant (see p. 687) and by

certain characteristics of the physical examination. Table 4–7 lists some of the clinical markers of gestational age tabulated by Usher et al. Discrepancies may be found within an individual with respect to the presence or absence of findings characteristic of a given gestational age. On the whole, however, a careful clinical and neurologic assessment will allow a useful evaluation of the degree of maturity of the infant.

Other laboratory aids in assessing the length of gestation have some usefulness in a statistical sense but little or no predictive value for the individual, since the scatter of findings is so great. For example, fetal hemoglobin concentrations tend to fall with advancing gestational age; the distal femoral epiphysis usually appears at 36

**TABLE 4–6.** *Pathologic Findings in Intrauterine Growth Retardation*

Placenta: Findings are variable. Occasionally the placenta is small; microinfarcts and occlusion of vessels in small villous systems may be present
Organs that tend to be heavier than expected for weight:
  Brain
  Heart
  Spleen
Organs that tend to be lighter than expected for weight:
  Lungs
  Liver
  Thymus
  Adrenals
Gross findings: More convolutions in brain than expected for weight
  Greater glomerular development than expected
  Alveolar development appropriate for gestational age rather than weight
  Scant extramedullary erythropoiesis

weeks; thigh girth and skin thickness increase with age; but individual variation in all these indices is great.

COURSE. The likelihood of some post-natal problems such as the respiratory distress syndrome and hyperbilirubinemia is reduced with increasing gestational age. In low birth weight infants, the risk of hypoglycemia and pulmonary hemorrhage is substantially increased. The possibility of fetal infection, chromosomal abnormalities and other congenital malformations is greater in such infants, since those events are etiological in the production of growth retardation.

MANAGEMENT. Recognition of the significant risk of symptomatic hypoglycemia makes serial measurements of blood glucose advisable (see pp. 519–525). We attempt to determine blood glucose by the glucose oxidase method on capillary blood by 4 hours of age, and again at twelve and 24 hours. Prevention of hypoglycemia seems warranted and is achieved by the early institution of oral feedings if the infant is vigorous or by the intravenous route if depressed. We aim to give glucose and water in some form to undersized infants

**TABLE 4–7.** *Clinical Criteria for Classification of Low Birth Weight Infants (Premature vs. Dysmature ["Small for Dates"])*[*]

| Criteria | 36 Weeks (Premature) | 37–38 Weeks (Borderline Premature) | 39 Weeks (Full Term) |
|---|---|---|---|
| Creases on sole of foot | One or two transverse creases running anteriorly, smooth posterior 3/4 of foot | More creases appear anteriorly, heel remains smooth | Creases extend throughout soles, prominent deep clefts |
| Size of breast nodule (large nodules, full term; but small ones may be premature or small for dates) | Not palpable before 33 wks.; rarely exceeds 3 mm. by 36 weeks | Average is 4 mm. | Average is 7 mm., sizable mass, readily seen |
| Hair on head | Cotton wool quality, difficult to distinguish one strand from another | Same, with some progression toward 38 weeks characteristic | Silky texture because of thickening of hair; can distinguish each strand of hair |
| Cartilaginous development of earlobe | Shapeless, pliable with little cartilaginous support | | Rigid earlobe, stiffened with cartilage; folds of helix and anthelix prominent (distinct ridges) |
| Testicular descent and scrotal changes | Small scrotum with rugae on its inferior aspect limited to a small area; testes at junction of inguinal canal and superior aspect of scrotum not completely descended | Gradual descent with scrotal enlargement | Enlarged scrotum with fully descended testes, pendulous in appearance; inferior surface of scrotum completely covered with rugae |

[*]Modified from Usher, R., et al.: *Pediat. Clin. N. Amer.*, 13:835, 1966.

no later than 4 hours of postnatal age and often earlier.

Undersized infants have been shown by Sinclair, Scopes and Silverman to have a greater oxygen consumption per kilogram of body weight than true premature infants. This evidence of "hypermetabolism" probably relates to the percentage of body weight contributed by visceral organs with relatively large oxygen consumptions per unit size. The practical point to emerge from measurements of metabolism is that fluid and caloric needs of undersized infants are somewhat increased when calculated per kilogram of body weight. We try to individualize the requirements of each infant. Some, who seem hungry, may reach full oral feedings by 3 days of age; others tolerate only those amounts that would be accepted by the true premature. When offered formula early, the infants show less postnatal weight loss than true premature infants, and may gain weight more rapidly.

Screening for occult intrauterine infection with cord IgM levels would seem appropriate in these undersized infants.

**PROGNOSIS.** The longterm outcome of intrauterine growth retardation of unknown etiology remains under active study. The reports of Fitzhardinge and Steven suggest that some remain undersized, others show complete catch-up growth. The best predictor of later growth is the growth rate in the first 12 months of life. Cerebral palsy was rare among these infants, but minimal cerebral dysfunction was present in 25 per

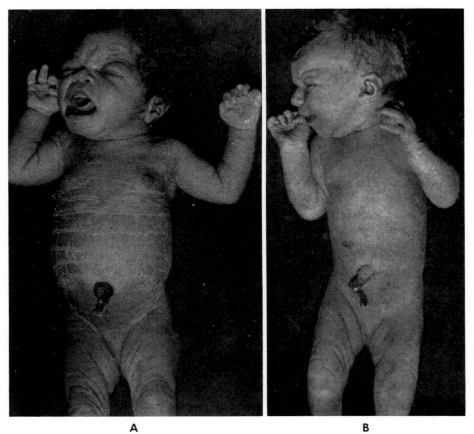

**A**                                          **B**

*Figure 4–4.*   *A,* First stage of postmaturity (placental dysfunction syndrome). Gestational age, 310 days; birth weight, 6 pounds 12 ounces. Relatively long and thin. Dry, cracking, collodionlike skin. No staining. Notable loss of subcutaneous tissue. *B,* Third stage of postmaturity (placental dysfunction). Gestational age, 290 days. Yellow-stained skin and green-yellow cord and membranes. Generalized desquamation. Long, thin, wasted muscles and subcutaneous tissue. (Clifford, S. H.: J. Pediat. *44:*1, 1954.)

cent. Speech problems were noted in one third of the boys and in one fourth of the girls. Poor performance in school was a common problem, present in half of the boys and more than one-third of the girls.

## PROLONGED GESTATION (POSTMATURITY)

Some infants are born appearing normal after a gestation of 300 days or longer; others appear to have suffered intrauterine weight loss, have macerated and wrinkled skins and may die in the first days of life. This latter group of infants may be designated as "postmature."

INCIDENCE. Kunstadter and Schnitz found that 247 of 2877 infants had gestational ages of 42 weeks or over; 132 of these were over 43 weeks. This incidence of 4.59 per cent is lower than Sjöstedt's 9.5 per cent, but agrees with the findings of Clifford and most other observers.

ETIOLOGY. Until the mechanisms of the initiation of normal labor are more clearly understood, it seems unlikely that the etiology of prolonged gestation will be evident. The observations of Liggins on pregnant ewes suggest that the fetal pituitary-adrenal axis may be central to the initiation of labor. Whether or not this is true in the human remains to be established.

DIAGNOSIS. The salient features of the infant are the apparent recent weight loss, an appearance of unusual alertness or a wide-eyed look, absence of vernix caseosa, dry skin, and often a greenish color of the umbilical cord and skin (Fig. 4–4). The skull is well calcified and feels harder than normal. Resuscitative efforts will often have been required in the delivery room. Aspiration of meconium and squames is common, and pulmonary hemorrhage has been noted in this group of infants. Hypoglycemia may be more common among these infants.

TREATMENT. Many postmature infants require no special treatment. If they seem hungry, it is our practice to feed them full-strength formula as early as 4 hours. If they are depressed, intravenous fluids with 10 per cent dextrose are indicated prophylaxis for hypoglycemia. Increasingly obstetri-cians are inducing delivery in women with prolonged gestation. The increase in mortality in pregnancies of over 42 weeks supports this approach, now that induction with oxytocic agents can be monitored carefully. Neonatal mortality in postmature infants is much greater if the interval since the preceding pregnancy has been of the order of ten years.

## REFERENCES

Alexander, H. E.: Seminar on premature and newborn infants, coordinated by R. L. Day, and W. A. Silverman. Pediatrics 20:143, 1957.

Antonov, A. N.: Children born during the siege of Leningrad in 1942. J. Pediat. 30:250, 1947.

Avery, M. E.: Considerations on the definition of viability. New Engl. J. Med. 292:206–207, 1975.

Babson, S. G., Kangas, J., Young, N., and Bramhall, J. I.: Growth and development of twins of dissimilar size at birth. Pediatrics 33:327, 1964.

Battaglia, F. C., Frazier, T., and Hellegers, A. E.: Obstetric and pediatric complications of juvenile pregnancy. Pediatrics 32:902, 1963.

Beard, A. G., Panos, T. C., Marasigan, B. V., Eminians, J., Kennedy, H. F., and Lamb, J.: Perinatal stress and the premature neonate. II. Effect of fluid and calorie deprivation on blood glucose. J. Pediatr. 68:329, 1966.

Brockway, G. E., Reilly, E. T., and Rice, M. M.: Premature mortality: An analysis of 518 cases of prematurity with a comparison of Negro and White races. J. Pediatr. 37:362, 1950.

Calcagno, P. L., and Rubin, M. I.: Effect of added carbohydrate on growth, nitrogen retention, and renal water excretion in premature infants. Pediatrics 13:193, 1954.

Chernick, V., Heldrich, F., and Avery, M. E.: Periodic breathing of premature infants. J. Pediatr. 64:330, 1964.

Clifford, S. H.: Postmaturity—with placental dysfunction; clinical syndrome and pathologic findings. J. Pediatr. 44:1, 1954.

Dallman, P. R.: Iron, vitamin E and folate in the preterm infant. J. Pediatr. 85:742–752, 1974.

Davidson, M., Levine, S. Z., Bauer, C. H., and Dann, M.: Feeding studies in low-birth-weight infants. J. Pediatr. 70:695, 1967.

Davies, P. A., and Stewart, A. L.: Low-birth-weight infants: Neurological sequelae and later intelligence. Brit. Med. Bull. 31:85–91, 1975.

Davies, P., and Tizard, J. P. M.: Very low birth weight and subsequent neurological defect. Devel. Med. Child Neurol. 17:3, 1975.

Drillien, C. M.: Growth and development in a group of children of very low birth weight. Arch. Dis. Child. 33:10, 1958.

Dunham, E. C.: Septicemia in the newborn. Am. J. Dis. Child. 45:229, 1933.

Dunham, E. C.: Quoted by H. Reardon, J. L. Wilson, and B. Graham (see below).

Eastman, N. J.: Williams Obstetrics. 11th ed. New York, Appleton-Century-Crofts, Inc., 1956.

Fitzhardinge, P. M.: Early growth and development in low-birth-weight infants following treatment in an intensive care nursery. Pediatrics 56:162, 1975.

Fitzhardinge, P. M., and Steven, E. M.: The small-for-date infant. I. Later growth patterns. Pediatrics 49:671, 1972.

Fitzhardinge, P. and Steven, E.: The small-for-date infant: II. Neurological and intellectual sequelae. Pediatrics 50:50, 1972.

Flax, L., Levert, E. L., and Strong, R. A.: A study of premature mortality. J. Pediatr. 21:717, 1942.

Fomon, S. J.: Infant Nutrition. 2nd ed. Philadelphia, W. B. Saunders Co., 1974.

Frazier, T. M., Davis, G. H., Goldstein, H., and Goldberg, I. D.: Cigarette smoking and prematurity: A prospective study. Am. J. Obstet. Gynecol. 81:988, 1961.

Gordon, H. H., and Levine, S. Z.: The metabolic basis for the individualized feeding of infants, premature and full-term. J. Pediatr. 25:464, 1944.

Gordon, H. H., Levine, S. Z., and McNamara, W.: The feeding of premature infants, a comparison of human and cow's milk. Am. J. Dis. Child. 73:442, 1947.

Gruenwald, P.: Abnormalities of placental vascularity in relation to intrauterine deprivation and retardation of fetal growth: Significance of avascular chorionic villi. New York State J. Med. 61:1508, 1961.

Gruenwald, P.: Chronic fetal distress and placental insufficiency. Biol. Neonat. 5:215, 1963.

Gruenwald, P., and Minh, H. N.: Evaluation of body and organ weights in perinatal pathology. Am. J. Obstet. Gynecol. 82:312, 1961.

Harper, P. A., Fischer, L., and Rider, R.: Neurological and intellectual status of prematures at three to five years of age. J. Pediatr. 55:679, 1959.

Hodes, H. L.: Antibiotic prophylaxis. Pediatrics 24:126, 1959.

Johnson, L., Schaffer, D., and Boggs, T. R.: The premature infant, vitamin E deficiency and retrolental fibroplasia. Am. J. Clin. Nutr. 27:1158, 1974.

Jonsen, A. R., Phibbs, R. H., Tooley, W. H. and Garland, M. J.: Critical issues in newborn intensive care: A conference report and policy proposal. Pediat. 55:756, 1975.

Jonxis, J. H. P., Visser, H. K. A., and Troelstra, J. A. (eds.): Aspects of Praematurity and Dysmaturity. Nutricia Symposium. Leiden. H. E. Stenfert Kroese. 1968.

Knobloch, H., Rider, R., Harper, P., and Pasamanick, B.: Neuropsychiatric sequelae of prematurity. J.A.M.A. 161:581, 1956.

Kunstadter, R. H., and Bartelme, P. F.: Infants surviving a low weight of less than 1,000 grams. In J. H. Hess, G. J. Mohr, and P. F. Bartelme: The Physical and Mental Growth of Prematurely Born Children. Chicago, University of Chicago Press, 1934, Part III, Chap. 13, pp. 221–239.

Kunstadter, R. H., and Schnitz, S. E.: Postmaturity and the placental dysfunction syndrome. J.A.M.A. 161:151, 1956.

Liggins, G. C.: Premature delivery of fetal lambs infused with glucocorticoids. J. Endocrinol. 45:515, 1969.

Lubchenco, L., Deliveria-Papadopoulos, M., and gestational age on sequelae. J. Pediatr. 80:509–512, 1972.

Lubchenco, L. O., Bard, H., Goldman, A. L., Coyer, W. E., McIntyre, C., and Smith, D. M.: Newborn intensive care and long-term prognosis. Devel. Med. Child. Neurol. 16:421–431, 1974.

Lubchenco, L. O., Hansman, C., Dressler, M., and Boyd, E.: Intrauterine growth as estimated from liveborn birth-weight data at 24 to 42 weeks of gestation. Pediatrics 32:793, 1963.

Mamunes, P., et al.: Intellectual deficits after transient tyrosinemia in the term neonate. Pediatrics 57:675, 1976.

Neims, A. H., Warner, M., et al.: Relative deficiency in the elimination of hexachlorophene by neonatal rodents. In Marselli, P. L., et al. (Eds.): Basic and Therapeutic Aspects of Perinatal Pharmacology. New York, Raven Press, 1975.

Nyhan, W. L., and Fousek, M. D.: Septicemia of the newborn. Pediatrics 22:268, 1958.

Peterson, H. G., Jr., and Pendleton, M. E.: Contrasting roentgenographic pulmonary patterns of the hyaline membrane and fetal aspiration syndromes. Am. J. Roentgenol. 74:800, 1955.

Pincus, J. B., Gittleman, Z. F., Saito, M., and Sobel, A. E.: A study of plasma values of sodium, potassium, chloride, carbon dioxide, carbon dioxide tension, sugar, urea and the protein base-binding power, pH and hematocrit in prematures on the first day of life. Pediatrics 18:39, 1956.

Potter, E. L.: Quoted by H. Reardon, J. L. Wilson, and B. Graham (see below).

Potter, E. L.: Pathology of the Fetus and the Newborn. Chicago, Year Book Publishers, Inc., 1952.

Radde, I. C., et al.: Growth and mineral metabolism in very low birth weight infants. I. Comparison of two modes of $NaHCO_3$ treatment of late metabolic acidosis. Ped. Res. 9:564, 1975.

Raffensperger, J. G., Shakunthala, V., Pildes, R. S., Strohl, E. L., and Cornblath, M.: Feeding gastrostomy in premature infants. Arch. Surg. 97:190, 1968.

Rawlings, G., Reynolds, E. O. R., Stewart, A., and Strang, L. B.: Changing prognosis for infants of very low birth weight. Lancet 1:516, 1971.

Reardon, H., Wilson, J. L., and Graham, B.: Physiological deviations of the premature infant, with summary of principles of care. A.M.A. Am. J. Dis. Child. 81:99, 138, 1951.

Schlesinger, E. R.: Neonatal intensive care: Planning for services and outcomes following care. J. Pediatr. 82:916–920, 1973.

Scott, K. E., and Usher, R.: Fetal malnutrition. Its incidence, causes and effects. Am. J. Obstet. Gynecol. 94:951, 1966.

Silverman, W. A.: Commentary: Low birth weight. Pediatrics 32:791, 1963.

Silverman, W. A., and Sinclair, J. C.: Evaluation of precautions before entering a neonatal unit. Pediatrics 40:900, 1967.

Sinclair, J. C., Scopes, J. M., and Silverman, W. A.: Metabolic reference standards for the neonate. Pediatrics 39:724, 1967.

Sjöstedt, S., Engleson, G., and Rooth, G.: Dysmaturity. Arch. Dis. Child. 33:123, 1958.

Smith, C. A.: Prenatal and neonatal nutrition. Borden Award Address. Pediatrics 30:145, 1962.

Stiehm, E. R.: Fetal defense mechanisms. Am. J. Dis. Child. 129:438, 1975.

Taylor, W. C., James, J. A., and Henderson, J. L.: The

significance of yellow vernix in the newborn. Arch. Dis. Child. 27:442, 1952.

Terris, M.: The epidemiology of prematurity: Studies of specific etiologic factors. *In* S. Chipman, et al.: Research Methodology and Needs in Perinatal Studies, Springfield, Ill., Charles C Thomas, 1966.

Thomson, A. M., Billewicz, W. Z., and Hytten, F. E.: The assessment of fetal growth. J. Obstet. Gynaecol. Br. Commonw. 75:903, 1968.

Usher, R., McLean, F., and Scott, K. E.: Judgment of fetal age. II. Clinical significance of gestational age and an objective method of its assessment. Pediat. Clin. N. Amer. 13:835, 1966.

Van den Berg, B. J., and Yerushalmy, J.: The relationship of the rate of intrauterine growth of infants of low birth weight to mortality, morbidity, and congenital anomalies. J. Pediatr. 69:531, 1966.

Wagner, E. A., Jones, D. V., Koch, C. A., and Smith, G. D.: Polyethylene tube feeding in premature infants.

J. Pediatr. *41*:79, 1952.

Wennberg, R. P., Schwartz, R., and Sweet, A. Y.: Early versus delayed feeding of low birth weight infants: Effects on physiologic jaundice. J. Pediatr. 68:860, 1966.

Widdowson, E. M.: Changes in the composition of the body at birth and their bearing on function and food requirements. *In* J. H. P. Jonxis, H. K. A. Visser and J. A. Troelstra (Eds.): The Adaptation of the Newborn Infant to Extra-uterine Life. Leiden, H. E. Stenfert Kroese, 1964.

Widdowson, E. M.: The relation between the nature of the fat in the diet of young babies and their absorption of calcium. Biol. Neonatol. 9:279, 1966.

Wu, P. Y. K., Teilman, P., Gabler, M., Vaughan, M., and Metcoff, J.: "Early" versus "late" feeding of low birth weight neonates: Effect on serum bilirubin, blood sugar, and responses to glucagon and epinephrine tolerance tests. Pediatrics 39:733, 1967.

# CAUSES OF ABNORMALITIES IN NEWBORNS

# 5

*Revised by Aubrey Milunsky*

## CONGENITAL MALFORMATIONS

Congenital anomalies, defects and malformations are responsible for approximately one tenth of the deaths in the first month of life. The deaths represent but a small fraction of the total disability which they cause. McIntosh et al. found that 3.6 per cent of consecutive newborns in a large series manifested at least one *major* congenital anomaly, defined by Marden et al. as one which has an adverse effect upon either function or social acceptability. When these babies were followed closely, the percentage of anomalies which must have dated from birth rose to 7.5 per cent by the age of 5 years. Marden and his collaborators found one or more *minor* anomalies in 14.7 per cent of more than 5000 consecutive liveborns. Polani, in England, estimates that 6 per cent or more of all persons "suffer from developmental disorders manifest at birth or in early life ranging from mild to severe, from curable through irremediable to untreatable or even lethal." In this volume congenital malformations will be treated as

the highly important segments of the disorders of each special system which they are, and they will therefore be found scattered through the entire book. Multiple congenital defects and disorders not readily classifiable in any one system have been assigned a section of their own (Chapter 102) (Table 5–1).

**ETIOLOGY.** Congenital malformations and defects are caused by a variety of diverse pathogenetic agents. These fall into the following main categories.

**GROSS CHROMOSOMAL ABERRATIONS.** The pathogenesis of gross chromosomal aberrations and the descriptions of the syndromes which are clearly associated with them are given in detail in Chapter 100.

**DEFECTIVE GENES.** The malformations and malfunctions in this group are by definition familial and hereditary. Some are transmitted as dominants, some as recessives; some may be sex-linked. Examples include classic achondroplasia, often transmitted as a dominant, and hemophilia A, a sex-linked defect.

The occurrence of major genetic disease

**TABLE 5–1.**   *Etiology of Serious Malformations in 18,555 Newborns at Boston Hospital for Women, 1972–1974*[*]

|  | Total Malformations | Per Cent of Total Newborns |
|---|---|---|
| I. Multifactorial inheritance | 127 | 0.7 |
| II. Single mutant gene with Mendelian inheritance | 67 | 0.4 |
| III. Chromosome abnormalities[**] | 28 | 0.2 |
| IV. Other (includes possible teratogens and unknowns) | 95 | 0.5 |
|  | 317 | 1.8 |

[*]Courtesy of Dr. Lewis B. Holmes.
[**]Only infants with malformations were karyotyped.

in a newborn without a family history usually implies an autosomal recessive disorder or a mutational event. That the latter is not an unusual occurrence is exemplified by the knowledge that approximately one third of all sex-linked hereditary disorders occur as a consequence of mutation. Significant mutation rates also occur in the dominant genetic disorders; for example, approximately 50 per cent of infant tuberosclerosis, retinoblastoma and many other dominant disorders are due to sporadic mutations.

Congenital malformations caused by sex-linked inheritance may be particularly important since, potentially, prenatal sex determination may assist in their subsequent prevention. Hydrocephalus in some forms, imperforate anus, microphthalmia, anhidrotic ectodermal dysplasia and certain biochemical disorders represent only a few of the more than 30 syndromes noted in this category.

Multifactorial (polygenic) inheritance re-

**TABLE 5–2.** *Incidence and Sex Ratio of the Commoner Malformations in England and Wales*[*]

|  | Incidence per 1000 Live Births | Sex Ratio, Male / Female |
|---|---|---|
| Anencephaly | 2 | 0.4 |
| Spina bifida | 2.5 | 0.8 |
| Down's syndrome | 2 | 1.0 |
| Pyloric stenosis | 3 | 5.0 |
| Cleft lip | 1 | 1.8 |
| Talipes equinovarus | 1 | 2.0 |
| Congenital hip dislocation | 1 | 0.15 |
| Congenital heart malformations | 4 | 1.0 |

[*]Carter, C. O.: Proc. Roy. Soc. Med. *61*:991, 1968.

flects the additive effects of several minor gene abnormalities and environmental factors. Neural tube defects (anencephaly, spina bifida) are perhaps the commonest examples in this group, which also includes pyloric stenosis, dislocation of the hips, cleft lip and palate and many others. Genetic factors (increased frequency in people of Irish extraction) in the neural tube defects mix with recognizable environmental components which include low socioeconomic classes, more frequent winter and fall births and changing frequency with variable geographic location.

X-IRRADIATION OF THE FETUS. Exposure of the developing human fetus to radiant energy has been known to affect it deleteriously. Until recently reports of this kind of injury were confined to single cases in which the mother's pelvis had been irradiated vigorously for a medical reason. Microcephaly was the usual outcome. Dropping the atomic bomb afforded an unwelcome opportunity to study the wholesale effects of overexposure to radiant energy. Plummer found that 11 pregnant women had been within 1200 meters of the hypocenter at the moment of explosion at Hiroshima. Seven of their babies born thereafter were microcephalic. The other four had been fortuitously shielded by thick concrete walls. No pregnant women farther than 1200 meters from the hypocenter bore microcephalic infants. The incidence of congenital malformations other than microcephaly was no greater in the exposed group, no matter how close to the hypocenter, than in the control unexposed population. Too little time has elapsed to determine the incidence of genetic mutation in the irradiated segment.

**TABLE 5–3.** *Drugs with Teratogenic Potential*

| Drugs | Effect on Fetus |
|---|---|
| A. *Drugs with known teratogenic effects* | |
| Amphetamines | Congenital heart disease, transposition of great vessels |
| Aminopterin (methotrexate) | Abortion, multiple malformations |
| Methyltestosterone | |
| 17-alpha-Ethanyl-19-nor-testosterone (Norlutin) | Masculinization of female fetus |
| Progesterone | |
| 17-alpha-Ethanyl-testerone (Progestoral) | |
| Diethylstilbestrol | Masculinization of female fetus, vaginal adenocarcinoma in adolescence |
| Thalidomide | Phocomelia and other malformations |
| Trimethadione and paramethadione | Abortion, multiple malformations, mental retardation |
| Warfarin | Hypoplasia of nasal structures, optic atrophy and mental retardation |
| B. *Drugs with suspected teratogenic potential* | |
| Busulfan (Myleran) | Stunted growth, corneal opacities, cleft palate, hypoplasia of ovaries, thyroid and parathyroids |
| Chlorobiphenyls | Cola-colored newborns, intrauterine growth retardation and exophthalmos |
| Chlorpropamide | Abortion |
| Cyclophosphamide | Multiple malformations |
| Diphenylhydantoin | Facial clefts and cardiovascular defects |
| 6-Mercaptopurine | Multiple malformations |
| Phenobarbitone | Facial clefts and cardiovascular defects |
| Tolbutamide | Multiple malformations |

CHEMICAL AGENTS. The principles of drug-induced teratogenesis are now well defined in experimental animals. The severe malformations produced in human embryos by small maternal doses of thalidomide emphasized that these principles apply also to man. The probability that a woman's exposure to a drug will produce a malformation in her baby depends on the dose, route of administration, stage of gestation and genotype of mother and embryo. Drugs at non-teratogenic levels can become highly teratogenic in the presence of other drugs or environmental variables such as specific nutritional deficiency, hypoxia or food and water restriction. Each drug has its own "critical period," the gestational age at which it is most teratogenic; these differ for different teratogens, and may anticipate, by varying lengths of time, the developmental event that they interrupt.

Until recently, only teratogens with major effects, and a high probability of producing malformations at the observed doses, have been recognized in man. These include radiation in large amounts, thalidomide, certain antimetabolites used in cancer therapy and certain androgens and synthetic progestational agents. With more intensive search, and larger bodies of data becoming available, the list is being extended to a number of other drugs with a lower, but appreciable, risk of producing malformations. These include certain estrogen/progestogen preparations used as pregnancy tests or to treat threatened abortion, several anti-epileptic drugs and ethyl alcohol. In fact, Dilantin and maternal alcoholism are now known to produce specific phenotypes in a portion of exposed embryos. Still others, such as the phenothiazines and Valium, are under suspicion. In our present state of knowledge it is best to assume that any drug has some risk of producing a malformation if presented to a genetically susceptible embryo at a susceptible stage, in the presence of potentiating environmental factors (Wilson).

The best known human teratogen is thalidomide, which, paradoxically, might not have been detected by screening methods in pregnant animals, since the time of its action on limb buds is so sharply circumscribed.

The teratogenic effects of antimetabolites and folic acid antagonists have been well recognized. One infant reported by the author eight years ago was born after the failed abortifacient use of methotrexate.

Other infants similarly exposed had comparable phenotypic abnormalities. This child, now over 8 years of age, remains with incompletely ossified skull defects, an I.Q. within the normal range, and an extremely small stature.

Maternal ingestion of steroid hormones with androgenic activity may lead to masculinization of female infants. Recently a suspected association between multiple congenital anomalies and the ingestion in early pregnancy of a progestogen/estrogen compound or a progestogen alone has been reported. While the large study in progress to make a more accurate determination of this association is continuing, prudence would dictate the verification of the absence of pregnancy prior to initiating oral contraception, as well as discontinuing hormonal agents as tests for pregnancy.

Hydantoin anticonvulsants during pregnancy have been associated with craniofacial anomalies, nail and digital hypoplasia, prenatal onset of growth deficiency and mental deficiency. The incidence and relationship of these malformations to the use of hydantoin has not been firmly established. The frequency and severity of maternal seizures may dictate continued use of these agents in some pregnancies, even though the "fetal hydantoin syndrome" is a possibility (Hanson and Smith).

The number of drugs proved to be teratogenic in the human is very small, compared with the large number of such agents in animals. Nonetheless, caution in drug administration during pregnancy is to be advised.

The only clearly demonstrated harm of smoking in pregnancy is the tendency to smaller babies with a higher mortality. We have detected the presence of nicotine and cotinine in the amniotic fluid of smoking mothers as early as 14 weeks' gestation. It might still be premature to conclude on the basis of statistical surveys that smoking has indeed no relationship to congenital malformations.

DELAYED EFFECTS OF MATERNAL DRUG INGESTION. The most recent and perhaps most worrisome sequel to maternal drug ingestion during pregnancy has been the occurrence of adenocarcinoma of the female genital tract following *intrauterine exposure to stilbestrol*. This observation in 1971 pointed to the remarkable occurrence of vaginal adenocarcinoma occurring at an average of 17.5 years with 90 per cent of cases occurring after 12 years. While many of these cases have been clearly associated with maternal hormone exposure, there are well documented numbers of cases where no such exposure occurred. The total dosages of stilbestrol ingested during pregnancies by these mothers with affected daughters has varied enormously. In all cases, however, therapy began prior to the 18th week of pregnancy.

A propensity toward the development of malignancy also exists in association with certain well-defined genetic disorders (e.g., Bloom's syndrome, Fanconi's syndrome and ataxia-telangiectasia). What environmental or other genetic influences exert their effects on the early developing embryo, with manifestations of congenital malformation or genetic disorder at birth and the development of malignancy many years later, are still essentially unknown.

VITAMIN DEFICIENCY OR EXCESS. Warkany and his co-workers have explored this aspect of the problem most fully. There is no doubt that the deficiency of vitamin A in the diet of pregnant rats leads to an excess of various malformations in their offspring. It is probable that dietary deficiencies in riboflavin, pantothenic acid and folic acid produce similar results. Whether human offspring are damaged in the same manner by maternal dietary deficiencies is a moot question. Clement Smith's study of the offspring of mothers who were forced to live on a starvation diet during the German occupation of The Netherlands uncovered no excess of congenitally malformed newborns. Interestingly enough, Cohlan presented evidence indicating that an excess of vitamin A given to pregnant rats produces congenital defects very like those caused by its deficiency!

MATERNAL INFECTION. Infection during pregnancy is not an insignificant cause of subsequent congenital defect. Approximately 8 to 10 per cent of women in the child-bearing age are susceptible to rubella. In one study, about 2 to 3 per cent of cases of mental deficiency were related to rubella and toxoplasmosis infection during pregnancy. Cytomegalovirus infection was associated with 10 per cent of cases with microcephaly and mental retardation. An important problem in discerning the cause of congenital malformations due to maternal infection is the not infrequent occurrence of subclinical or inapparent infection with unrecognized maternal disease. Inapparent maternal infection by rubella, toxoplasmosis or cytomegalovirus, for example, may still be related causally to malformations. While rubella reinfection after natural disease may be an unusual event, this is not the case following immunization. Some protective mechanisms are operative, since many mothers with proved rubella infection in the first trimes-

ter of pregnancy may have totally unaffected offspring (Table 5–4).

Cytomegalovirus infection may occur in as many as 6 per cent of pregnancies, but cytomegalovirus excretion is found in only 0.5 to 2.0 per cent of newborns, of whom only about 1 in 3000 develops the classical syndrome of cytomegalic inclusion disease.

The incidence of toxoplasmosis in pregnancy has been estimated to be as high as 4 to 6 per 1000, with congenital toxoplasmosis occurring as frequently as 1 per 1000 births. Thorough neonatal examinations, including examination of the ocular fundi, may reveal no abnormal typical signs of rubella, toxoplasmosis or cytomegalic in-

**TABLE 5–4.** *Pregnancy Outcomes of Patients Who Experienced Clinical Rubella With Antibody Response**

| Time of Rubella | No. of Patients | Race | | | Elevated Cord IgM† | Outcome |
|---|---|---|---|---|---|---|
| | | White | Negro | Puerto Rican | | |
| Preconception (0 to 28 days before conception) | 7 | 3 | 4 | 0 | 0/5‡ | 1 Congenital rubella (21 days before conception)<br>1 Abortion<br>1 Stillbirth<br>1 Multiple infections in first year<br>3 Normal |
| First trimester (0 to 12 weeks after conception) | 42 | 16 | 25 | 1 | 9/27 | 7 Congenital rubella<br>1 Stillbirth (rubella)<br>7 Therapeutic abortions (rubella)<br>4 Suspect congenital rubella<br>5 Lost to follow-up<br>18 Normal |
| Second trimester (13 to 26 weeks after conception) | 58 | 21 | 31 | 6 | 9/50 | 6 Congenital rubella<br>1 Stillbirth (rubella)<br>1 Stillbirth<br>1 Therapeutic abortion (rubella)<br>4 Suspect congenital rubella<br>2 Lost to follow-up<br>43 Normal |
| Third trimester (≧ 26 weeks after conception) | 21 | 7 | 14 | 0 | 2/19 | 3 Lost to follow-up<br>18 Normal |
| Total | 128 | 47 | 74 | 7 | 20/101 | 14 Congenital rubella<br>2 Stillbirths (rubella)<br>2 Stillbirths<br>1 Abortion<br>8 Therapeutic abortions (rubella)<br>8 Suspect congenital rubella<br>1 Multiple infections in first year<br>10 Lost to follow-up<br>82 Normal |

*Sever, J. L., Hardy, J. B., Nelson, K. B., and Gilkeson, M. I.: Am. J. Dis. Child. *118*:125, 1969.
†IgM indicates immune globulin. >25 mg. per 100 ml.
‡Number elevated per number available and tested.

clusion disease. Months or years may pass before any abnormality is detected. Perceptive deafness, for example, diagnosed years after birth may be the only manifestation of congenital rubella. Recent disturbing reports suggest that maternal rubella infection *after* 14 weeks' gestation may lead to communication defects and developmental retardation observed months to years later (see Chapter 87).

Other maternal viral infections may be associated with congenital malformations in the offspring. Viruses suspected of possibly being teratogenic have included coxsackie A and B, influenza A, varicella, and herpes simplex.

The important questions as to whether abortion should be advised when a pregnant woman develops rubella, or whether and when gamma globulin should be administered if she has been exposed to rubella, are discussed in Chapter 87 (see pp. 807–809). So is the still somewhat moot question concerning the usefulness of determining Toxoplasma antibody titers of mothers during pregnancy, and the indication for treating her or her newborn or both (Chap. 89).

MATERNAL INGESTION OF POISONS. A 17 per cent mortality rate has been reported in the offspring of women with chronic alcoholism. In addition, 44 per cent of 23 offspring reported were found to have borderline to moderate mental retardation, while 32 per cent had sufficiently abnormal physical features to suggest a "fetal alcohol syndrome." The relationship of the dysmorphogenic features to maternal alcoholism still requires better proof. The profound detrimental effects of the disorganized problem family on the psychological and intellectual development of children may possibly prove to be the "cause" of the developmental retardation rather than the alcoholism itself.

Both increased frequency of stillbirth and congenital malformations were noted in infants of mothers with high lead exposure toward the latter part of the 19th century. More recently, attention has focused on neurologic damage in asymptomatic children who have been subjected to an increased lead burden. Studies of lead-associated hyperactivity in mice and the

demonstration of slow learning in sheep with borderline blood-lead levels raise worrisome questions in these suggestive animal models of human disease. Since it is known that lead affects rapidly growing tissues, the observation that increased cord blood lead in infants of mothers in high lead exposure areas (e.g., near expressways) cannot be ignored.

Maternal ingestion of methylmercury occurred in an epidemic in Japan, resulting in microcephaly and cerebral palsy. The cause of these abnormalities was felt to be fish contaminated with methylmercury.

FAULTY NUTRITION OF THE OVUM. Malformed embryos often develop when implantation of the ovum takes place in an unusual site, such as the fallopian tube or the peritoneal surface. It is certain that nutrition is not optimal in these abnormal loci. The same explanation has been advanced for the excessive number of congenitally malformed infants born to women in the more advanced childbearing age as well as for those born to women for whom conception has been difficult as evidenced by a long period of involuntary sterility preceding conception. It appears likely now that many of these are caused by nondisjunction during meiosis. No one knows whether diabetic mothers produce more abnormal fetuses and infants because of placental insufficiency, hence faulty nutrition, or because of the teratogenic influence of excessive or abnormal hormones.

MECHANICAL FACTORS WITHIN THE UTERUS. Denis Browne listed three possible mechanical faults which could be responsible for fetal malformation. These are malposition—that is, the fetus is folded up improperly—increased mechanical pressure and increased hydraulic pressure within the uterine cavity. Normally, he argued, the hips, knees and elbows are flexed, the soles of the feet pressed against the uterine wall. Should the soles of the feet be apposed, metatarsal varus would result, whereas growth with the sides of the feet applied to the uterine wall would result in varus deformity. Dislocation of the hip can be explained by abnormal mechanical pressure upon the knee forcing the femoral head downward and backward. Arthrogryposis can be understood to be the outcome of increased hydraulic pressure, equally distributed, which interferes with venous return from the limbs. This mechanical theory has the merits of simplicity and plausibility and doubtless supplies the proper explanation for some congenital deformities.

HORMONAL DEPRIVATION OR EXCESS. Deprivation of thyroid hormones during fetal life, by absence of iodine in the available drinking water, by maternal ingestion of iodides or antithyroid drugs of the thiouracil family or for other reasons, may lead to the birth of a cretinous child (see Chapter 55). Female pseudohermaphroditism may be caused by the mother's ingestion of testosterone or closely related chemicals (see page 513).

## TRANSPLACENTALLY TRANSMITTED DISORDERS

Many infections pass from mother to fetus by way of the placenta. The list of infective agents capable of traversing the placental barrier includes bacteria, viruses and protozoa. One would suppose that the tinier viruses might be able to wander across tissue separating the two circulations without necessarily causing placentitis, but that this lesion must be set up in order to permit passage of the larger infective agents. On the other hand, it is possible that connections between the circulations, demonstrated by Kline in some placentas, may serve as a direct route for transmigration. Pneumococcus and the Salmonella of typhoid fever were the first known bacterial invaders historically, but many others have since been shown to be capable of passage. *Treponema pallidum* causes congenital syphilis in this way. The viruses of practically all the exanthems have been observed to set up their own patterns of disease in the fetus or newborn following the usual incubation period after having affected the mother, and many of the less common viruses, such as those of encephalitis, cytomegalic inclusion disease and members of the Coxsackie group, often behave in similar fashion. The prime example of a protozoal infection which crosses over is the toxoplasma, and it, like the cytomegalic inclusion virus, may initiate a severe disease in the fetus without having affected the mother at all. Examples of transplacentally transmitted infectious diseases will be discovered scattered through the sections devoted to respiratory disorders and infections.

But living organisms are not the only offenders which pass the barrier to cause trouble for the fetus. The unidentified agents, possibly autoimmune antibodies, responsible for two such widely different disorders as thrombocytopenic purpura and myasthenia gravis at times do the same to set up disease in the newborn similar to that of the mother. Mothers with lupus erythematosus often transmit the L.E. factor, which enables their infants to manufacture L.E. cells for 6 or 7 weeks. Rarely, malignant tumor cells metastasize from mother to fetus. Poisons, such as morphine and quinine, ingested by the mother may be responsible for bizarre disease in the newborn. This important route of pathogenesis, unique to the newborn, must receive much credit for the high morbidity and mortality rates characteristic of this period of life.

## PLACENTAL ACCIDENTS

The intact placenta serves as lungs and kidneys to the fetus, and any interference with anatomic connection or with its functional capacity is a source of great danger. Acute separations, such as abruptio placentae, premature separation, placenta praevia and marginal sinus rupture, give rise to sudden withdrawal of oxygen and glucose from the fetus and permit accumulation in the tissues of carbon dioxide and other metabolites. The ensuing asphyxiation causes widespread physiopathologic alterations which are described elsewhere. The principal signs of disease occur in the brain with its sudden anoxia, and the lungs, which may have become filled with amniotic sac contents as a result of fetal gasping.

Ordinarily the placenta tears away from the uterus by cleavage through its maternal side, and all the blood lost comes from the mother's blood supply, but on rare occasions the fetal pathways are disrupted and blood loss is fetal. Posthemorrhagic anemia of fetus or newborn results.

Placental insufficiency is believed by many observers to be responsible for the increased morbidity and mortality of postmaturity. Maternal toxemia, hypertension and diabetes may operate in the same manner. In these situations the disabilities consequent upon inefficient placental exchange develop slowly and progressively rather than explosively, and fetal disease which results is not apt to be catastrophic.

## UMBILICAL CORD ACCIDENTS

The umbilical cord, whose constant continuity is an absolute must for survival of the fetus, is subject to a variety of accidents. Some cords are malformed, their ends inserting into the placenta after subdivision into numerous branches (velamentous insertion) instead of as a solid rope. Traction exerted by the fetus descending during delivery can tear such delicate vessels. Some cords become knotted in the course of their shiftings and turnings within the amniotic sac, and these knots can be tightened during descent (true knots). It is possible for an excessively short cord to be avulsed from either fetal or placental attachment during descent. Finally the cord may be delivered before the infant, and this prolapsed cord is in danger of being compressed between the descending fetus and a bony prominence. The net result of these accidents is to cause fetal bleeding or asphyxia. Anemia follows bleeding, and cerebral and pulmonary effects result from sudden fetal asphyxia. These seem similar to the effects of placental accidents described above.

## ABNORMAL PRESENTATIONS

Breech presentations and deliveries by the breech are more hazardous than are cephalic ones. Local congestion of the presenting part leads to cyanosis and edema of buttocks and genitals in all ways analogous to caput succedaneum, and need cause no concern. The greatest source of danger appears to be the frequency with which the umbilical cord prolapses and becomes compressed. Even without prolapse the hazard of cord compression is increased, since the abdomen and cord enter the narrow confines of the birth canal relatively earlier than they do in cephalic deliveries, and are subject to abnormal pressures through the entire period when chest, shoulders and head must be delivered. In addition, the placenta may begin to separate when the uterus starts to empty, and in breech deliveries such emptying and placental separation may begin when the head still has the length of the birth canal to traverse. Both situations make it much more probable that the breech baby will be born more deeply asphyxiated than one who presents by the vertex. Manual extraction by vigorous traction upon the feet adds the possibility of tearing the spinal dura or cord, and traction with the body at an angle to the head in the attempt to deliver this aftercoming part carries with it the hazard of brachial plexus injury.

Shoulder dystocia and transverse and face presentations prolong total labor and especially its second stage. To the asphyxial effect of prolongation of labor the operator may have to add the traumatic ones of vigorous manual or instrumental manipulation. Asphyxia neonatorum with cerebral anoxia or massive aspiration of amniotic sac contents or trauma, either intracranial or peripheral, may follow.

Congenital malformations occur nearly twice as often in breech deliveries. Anencephalus is regularly associated with spontaneous face or brow presentations.

## PRECIPITOUS LABOR

Excessively rapid deliveries appear to be as hazardous as prolonged ones. The factor chiefly responsible for trouble in this situation may be quick compression of the skull by its sudden entrance into and passage through the birth canal. Having no time in which to mold gently to conform with the contours of the snugly fitting canal, the head lengthens abruptly in the *anteroposterior* direction, thereby causing sudden broadening of the bitemporal diameter, which stretches and may tear one or both leaves of the tentorium. Subdural hemorrhage follows, which may be supratentorial, infratentorial or both. In some instances the cranial bones override instantaneously and catch bridging veins to the superior longitudinal sinus between them. Other factors, not fully understood, may be operative.

## INSTRUMENTAL DELIVERY

Consummation of delivery by low or outlet forceps is an innocuous procedure. The use of midforceps or high forceps, on the other hand, is associated with an increase in neonatal morbidity and mortality. We use the word "associated" advisedly in order to intimate that not all the trouble which follows necessarily stems from the use of forceps, since they are not applied unless delivery has already been impeded. Tightly applied forceps can fracture the skull. Rarely are these fractures depressed. Excessive compression of the skull may lead to intracranial bleeding. Traction on the head so applied as to pull it to one side stretches and can tear the spinal roots of the brachial plexus of the opposite side.

## PROLONGED RUPTURE OF MEMBRANES

Organisms from the vagina attempt to invade the amniotic interior as soon as the membranes rupture. They succeed in contaminating the fluid in a certain percentage of cases, but not in others. Shubeck has surveyed some 30,000 successive deliveries from the point of view of outcome in relation to length of membrane rupture interval prior to delivery. After 72 hours of rupture, amnionitis was demonstrable in about 50 per cent, funisitis in 25 per cent and infection of the fetus or newborn in 8 per cent. One factor which promotes invasion is the process of active labor, so that 100 per cent of amniotic fluids are infected if membranes have been ruptured and labor has been active for twelve hours or more. If labor has not commenced, some sacs become infected, but many remain sterile for several days or weeks. Perhaps a small tear and a constant outward flow serve as a

physical barrier to the ascent of organisms. Perhaps other factors are operative. If amniotic sac contents have become contaminated, fetal swallowing or aspiration may induce sepsis, intrauterine pneumonia, otitis media, meningitis or other neonatal infections. This matter is discussed in detail in the section on disorders of respiration (Chap. 14).

## LATE OR EARLY PRIMIPARITY

The ideal years for childbearing are from about 16 to the early 30s. As mothers exceed 35 years in age, perinatal mortality more than doubles. In the British Perinatal Study of 1958, the perinatal mortality rate was 51.0 per 1000 for primiparae, and 59.2 per 1000 for mothers of parity 4 after age 35 years. These figures stand in contrast to the lowest rate of 19.8 found in mothers of parity 1 between 25 and 29 years of age.

A sharp increase in perinatal mortality occurs in women under 19 years of age. Pregnancy in adolescence is increasing in the United States at a worrisome rate, so that nearly one in five births is to a mother 18 years or younger.

At least two totally different factors seem to be responsible for the troubles of infants born to elderly primiparae. They give birth to more congenitally malformed fetuses than do younger mothers. The risk of Down's syndrome in pregnancies of women over 40 years of age is 2.6 per cent, compared with an overall incidence of 0.15 per cent. The reason for this proclivity is the greater tendency toward nondisjunction during meiosis exhibited by the germ cells of older than of younger women. In the second place, elderly primiparae contribute more than their statistical share to the traumatic intracranial hemorrhage group. This is understandable in view of the diminished elasticity of their outlets, so that the fetal head must undergo an undue amount of compression and molding while battering its way through the rigid canal. This is especially true if the baby happens to be a larger one.

## OVERSEDATION

By oversedation we mean either the use of excessive anesthetic or analgesic drugs for the purpose of alleviating labor pains or the use of those drugs in acceptable dosage, but too near the moment of the infant's birth. No one can say exactly what the safe interval between medication and delivery should be, but one finds reports indicating superiority in neonatal morbidity and mortality when drugs have been given no closer than 4 hours to birth.

From the pediatrician's point of view the ideal newborn is one who cries lustily within 5 seconds after emergence and establishes spontaneous respirations immediately after the first cry, after which no secondary episode of apnea or bradypnea follows. This is what one encounters when deliveries have been neither too long nor too short, when no instruments have been used and when no drugs at all have been given the mother. When the mother has been anesthetized or oversedated, a sizeable percentage of the newborns will delay their first cry or will fail to breathe easily and regularly after their initial gasps. After resuscitative measures their respiratory rate is likely to be unusually rapid and their color a bit dusky for a variable number of hours.

The cause commonly assigned to this form of respiratory difficulty is depression of the fetal respiratory center by direct action of the drug or by the indirect depressing action of drug-induced maternal hypoxia. We are inclined to believe that a third important source of difficulty resides in the drug-induced loss of laryngeal and pharyngeal reflexes which in the normal state prevent aspiration. Inhalation of vaginal or oropharyngeal secretions leads then to the massive aspiration syndrome (Chap. 10). These various depressant actions affect premature infants to a greater degree than they do those born at full term.

## MATERNAL DIABETES

It has been evident for a long time that mothers with diabetes are not ideal dams. Many of their offspring are stillborn, a higher than expected number of their liveborn babies show lethal and nonlethal congenital abnormalities, and even among those not congenitally malformed, neonatal mortality is high.

**INCIDENCE OF FETAL MORTALITY AND MORBIDITY.** The higher perinatal mortality among offspring of diabetic mothers is compounded of excessive fetal wastage in the last trimester of pregnancy and increased neonatal mortality. In the pre-insulin era perinatal mortality was about 50 per cent, and consisted largely of stillbirths. Neonatal mortality among the survivors was notably low. More recently the outlook has greatly improved. Much of the improvement relates to more careful regulation of maternal blood sugar, and selection of the time for delivery, with urinary estriol determinations, (HPL) levels, and amniocentesis to assess fetal lung maturity with lecithin-sphingomyelin ratios or the foam stability test. The reported perinatal mortality from any center will depend on the degree of severity of maternal disease in the population studied.

**MATERNAL FACTORS.** Perinatal mortality is clearly related to the severity of maternal disease, and to the gestational age of the infant at the time of delivery. The prognosis for the infant is best in the fetal age group of 36 to 38 weeks and in the weight group of $7\frac{1}{2}$ to $8\frac{1}{2}$ pounds (3500 to 3950 gm), according to Brandstrup, Osler and Pedersen. A modified White classification is widely used to characterize maternal disease (Table 5–5).

Gestational diabetes, defined as an abnormality of glucose tolerance demonstrable during pregnancy but reverting to normal within 6 weeks of delivery, has been shown to be associated with a fourfold increase in mortality compared with control pregnancies. (O'Sullivan et al.). Women overweight and over 25 years of age are at greatest risk. Recognition and treatment of this group may significantly reduce the number of oversized infants.

Perinatal mortality reported by Pedersen in relation to White's classification is A, 4.8 per cent; B, 10.4 per cent; C, 25.0 per cent; D, 18.0 per cent; E and F, 47.8 per cent. The overall perinatal mortality in that series published in 1965 was 17.9 per cent. In the period 1970–1972 he found perinatal mortality reduced to 7.4 per cent.

Although maternal acidosis and ketosis appear to have an adverse effect on the fetus, neither maternal hyperinsulinism nor maternal hypoglycemic shock, although

**TABLE 5–5.** *Modified White Classification of Diabetes and Pregnancy**

Class A—High fetal survival, no insulin, minimal dietary regulation
1. Gestational diabetes—abnormal glucose tolerance test during pregnancy which reverts to normal within a few weeks after delivery
2. Prediabetes—normal glucose tolerance test, but family history of diabetes, previous large infants or unexplained stillbirths

Class B—Onset of diabetes in adult life after age 20 years, duration less than 10 years, no vascular disease

Class C—Diabetes of long duration (10–19 years) with onset during adolescence (over 10 years) with minimal vascular disease

Class D—Diabetes of 20 years or more duration, onset before age 10 years, evidence of vascular disease (i.e., retinitis, albuminuria, hypertension)

Class E—Patients with D plus nephritis

* Cornblath, M., Personal communication.

teratogenic early in gestation in some animals, has been reported as harmful to the human fetus. Maternal toxemia increases the likelihood of fetal loss in utero. Hydramnios is frequently found; this may or may not contribute to increased fetal mortality.

**PATHOLOGIC CHANGES IN THE FETUS AND THE NEWBORN.** Some, but by no means all, of the offspring of diabetic mothers demonstrate some or all of the following abnormalities. Macrosomia is fairly frequent, developing apparently from the twenty-eighth week on. Given et al. report that the average weight of newborns at the New York Hospital is 7 pounds 2 ounces (3250 gm). Thirty and six-tenths per cent of the infants of diabetic mothers delivered there weighed more than 8 pounds 15 ounces (4000 gm).

Visceromegaly is usually striking, with increase in weight of the heart and liver. Kidneys are usually of normal weight. The thymus may be undersized, and the brain is regularly of less than expected weight in relation to total body weight. Extramedullary erythropoiesis is common. In the pancreas, the islets of Langerhans are prominent. The beta cells are hyperplastic, and extractable insulin is increased. Interstitial cellular infiltrates consisting mainly of eosinophils are common around the hypertrophied islets. Venous thrombosis, especially in the renal vein, is found with increased frequency in infants of diabetic mothers. If the infant dies after some hours of postnatal life, atelectasis with hyaline membranes is common; this condition accounted for 52 per cent of the deaths in the series of Driscoll et al. Table 5–6 lists the primary causes of neonatal death in the combined series from Boston and Copenhagen, representing 858 infants.

Congenital malformations that may involve any organ system occur more frequently in infants of diabetic mothers than in others of like gestational age. The incidence of malformations depends upon the definitions used, which in turn contribute to the conflicting reports in the literature on this subject. Major malformations occur in about 5 per cent of the infants; in the presence of maternal vascular complications the frequency increases to about 10 per cent. Lenz and Maier called attention to the association of malformations of the spine and maternal diabetes in 1964, and Passarge and Lenz added overwhelming evidence for the association when they accumulated 43 cases of agenesis of the sacrum and coccyx and/or malformations of the lower extremities, all of them in infants of diabetic mothers. The syndrome is fortunately rare, estimated to occur in about 1 per cent of diabetic pregnancies (Fig. 5–1). The mother of the infant shown in Figure 5–1 had an abnormal glucose tolerance test but no overt diabetes. The only other malformation that is overrepresented in association with maternal diabetes is ventricular septal defect (Driscoll et al.).

The pathology of the placenta is notable for the presence of endarteritis and thrombosis, occasionally with calcification of the vessels. Increased erythropoiesis is often

**TABLE 5–6.** *Primary Causes of Neonatal Death in Infants of Diabetic Mothers*

| | |
|---|---|
| Hyaline membrane disease | 45% |
| Other respiratory disorders | 11% |
| Congenital malformations | 28% |
| Infection | 9% |
| Extreme prematurity | 3% |
| Other | 4% |
| | 100% |

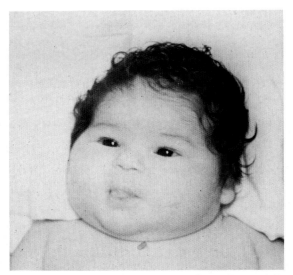

*Figure 5–1.* Photograph showing the puffy rounded contour suggesting the "cushingoid syndrome," characteristic of some infants of diabetic mothers.

evident. No lesions specific for diabetes have been demonstrated by either light or electron microscopy.

**CLINICAL FINDINGS.** Infants of diabetic mothers bear such a resemblance to one another that the experienced pediatrician rarely has any difficulty in spotting one on entry into a nursery. They are usually large, appear puffy and fat, are often of a ruddy color and are frequently limp with legs flexed and abducted. The umbilical cord may be twice normal size. They may have prominent fat pads over their upper backs reminiscent of those seen in Cushing's disease. Indeed their cushingoid appearance has led a number of investigators to study adrenal function, but investigations to date have failed to demonstrate elevated cortisol levels in maternal blood or cord venous blood.

Striking differences exist in body composition between infants of diabetic mothers and others of like gestational age. Briefly they are fat and dry. Subcutaneous fat thickness averages 11 mm compared to 7.5 mm, and total body water is 70 per cent of weight instead of 80 per cent. Glycogen stores in heart and liver are found to be increased.

The infants behave more appropriately for gestational age than weight. Thus they can be thought of as oversized premature infants, or large-for-dates neonates. They are frequently jittery, even when blood glucose and calcium levels are normal. Preliminary reports suggest that ionized calcium may correlate better than total serum calcium with symptoms. They lose water and electrolytes in the first days of life in excess of infants of like weight, and this despite their originally low body water content. Thus depletion of body water is a problem which must be anticipated by early feeding. Like premature infants, paradoxically they may show pitting edema from 24 to 48 hours of age.

Insulin levels are elevated in infants of diabetic mothers. Hypoglycemia is a common complication. At birth, the cord blood sugar is usually a little lower than the maternal. In the next hour, it falls precipitously and may remain depressed over the next 24 hours (see pages 520 and 521).

Hypocalcemia is recognized in these infants, but rarely are the symptoms alleviated by immediate infusions of 5 to 10 ml of a 10 per cent solution of calcium gluconate. Continuous infusions of a balanced salt solution with glucose and calcium are indicated in infants who do not tolerate oral feedings.

Hyperbilirubinemia is more of a problem in infants of diabetic mothers than in infants of nondiabetic mothers, and probably reflects their immaturity. Whether any other factors operate to promote hyperbilirubinemia is not clear. The peak of the jaundice is usually between the fifth and seventh days, somewhat later than that found in term infants.

The major problem and principal cause of death is the respiratory distress syndrome. The disease in infants of diabetic mothers is identical to that found in premature infants.

The combined factors of prematurity and delivery by cesarean section account for excessive frequency of respiratory distress, but when these factors are controlled, the fact of maternal diabetes per se puts the infant at nearly six times the risk of respiratory distress compared with other infants of similar gestation. Smith et al. have suggested that the antagonism of insulin and cortisol inhibits the normal enzyme inductive effects of cortisol on lung maturation. Thus the hyperinsulinemia of the fetus of the diabetic mother may retard lung development with respect to surfactant synthesis, thus predisposing to hyaline membrane disease.

**TREATMENT.** The management of these infants is based on awareness that they are prone to hypoglycemia, hypocalcemia, respiratory distress, hyperbilirubinemia and venous thrombosis. It should be noted, however, that half of them have an uneventful neonatal course.

A pediatrician should be present at the delivery of such an infant because it is a "high risk" baby. Knowledge of the state of the maternal diabetes as well as of the fluid therapy and glucose and insulin the mother has received is important, as are baseline measurements of glucose and calcium on umbilical cord blood. If significant hydramnios is present, a tube should be inserted into the stomach to test the patency of the esophagus, and to withdraw excessive amounts of swallowed fluid which might be vomited and aspirated later. Resuscitation follows the same guidelines as for any infant. On admission to the nursery, glucose and hematocrit are measured on capillary blood. If the infant is jittery, a venous sample should be drawn for a calcium determination. If the infant has any respiratory distress, an umbilical artery catheter is inserted to permit serial sampling of blood for $PO_2$, $PCO_2$, pH and $HCO_3$. Intravenous fluids and oxygen are to be given as indicated by the appropriate measurements. If the blood sugar is 30 mg per 100 ml or lower, one infuses 10 per cent glucose for the first 24 hours, with no or up to 15 mEq. $NaHCO_3$ depending on the pH, at a volume of 60 to 80 ml per kilogram per 24 hours. Oral feedings of formula are offered whenever the infant seems hungry and peristalsis is present. The use of intravenous fluids, preferably via a scalp or antecubital vein, is indicated to correct metabolic acidosis and to forestall high degrees of hyperbilirubinemia. Although some debate the need to give glucose to these infants, who characteristically are not symptomatic when it is low, we elect to try to raise depressed glucose value. In addition to intravenous glucose or early oral feedings, glucagon may be of value. In the first hours of life, 300 micrograms per kilogram—intravenously or intramuscularly—can elevate the blood sugar for two to three hours.

It should be noted that no agreement exists on optimal management of these infants. If the infant is vigorous and looks well, we do not use intravenous fluids, but rather offer formula at about twelve hours of age. Pedersen prefers to withhold all feedings until 24 hours of age. If his infants are jittery, he gives small doses of phenobarbital rather than calcium. Urinalyses are appropriate on the first and fourth or fifth days of life to search for red cells suggestive of renal vein thrombosis.

**PROGNOSIS.** If infants of diabetic mothers survive the hazards of the perinatal period, the prognosis for life is excellent. Detailed psychologic and neurologic examinations fail to reveal any significant abnormalities. The major problem of these infants is their greater risk of having diabetes mellitus. According to White, 7 per cent of them will have diabetes by age 20 years. Farquhar estimates their risk of diabetes to be approximately 20 times that of infants of mothers without diabetes.

## CESAREAN SECTION

**FETAL AND INFANT MORTALITY.** Operative delivery of the fetus by cesarean section saves the lives of many mothers. It also saves many babies. Yet the fetal and infant mortality which follows sections, even those performed by the most skillful surgeons in our leading clinics, remains two to three times as great as that which follows vaginal delivery.

Figures from all our larger hospitals bear this out. Almost at random we pick a table of Landesman, which summarizes the experience at the New York Hospital over three successive 5-year periods, in order to illustrate this and a few other items (Table 5–7). Infant mortality following both cesarean section and vaginal deliveries declined in each of the succeeding periods, but total clinic infant deaths fell a bit faster than did cesarean ones. The ratio of cesarean to clinic deaths was 2.4:1 in the first period, 2.6:1 in the second and 2.8:1 in the

**TABLE 5–7.   *Clinic and Section Mortality (1933–1949) in Percentages*[*]**

|  | 1933–1938 | 1939–1943 | 1944–1949 |
|---|---|---|---|
| Total clinic | 3.9 | 3.2 | 2.2 |
| Total sections | 9.5 | 8.3 | 6.3 |
| Premature sections | 50.0 | 40.0 | 22.1 |
| Full-term sections | 6.5 | 5.5 | 4.4 |

[*]Landesman, R.: Am. J. Obstet. Gynecol., *61*:557, 1951.

last. When only full-term babies were considered, the cesarean mortality was still twice as great as the general clinic infant mortality. Deaths of premature infants delivered by cesarean sections were five or more times as great as of mature ones. Better fetal monitoring and more liberal criteria for section have been associated with a sharp reduction in fetal and neonatal mortality so the more recent figures are less heavily weighted against section.

One other sharp dichotomy can be drawn, and that is the different order of magnitude of infant mortality following emergency section from that following elective section. The emergency procedure is reserved for premature separation, abruptio placentae, severe toxemia, rupture of the uterus, placenta praevia, prolonged labor and other conditions which lead to fetal distress. In many instances the fetus is dead or moribund by the time the operator delivers it. Elective sections, on the other hand, are performed because of a previous section, for cephalopelvic disproportion, in elderly primiparae and for cardiac disease of the mother, inter alia. In these situations the fetus should not have been subjected to distress before delivery. As expected, the infant mortality in the elective group, as derived from Landesman's table, amounted to twenty of 1068, or 2 per cent, while that in the emergency group adds up to 106 of 564, or approximately 19 per cent. There are differences within the latter composite group also, premature separations treated by cesarean section eventuating in a 50 per cent fetal or infant loss, while the same figure for prolonged labors was 10 per cent. The difference between the two great groups is even more striking in King, King and Pitt's statistics from the Touro Infirma-

ry. Gross uncorrected perinatal mortality in their elective group was only 1.4 per cent, while that for their emergency group was 25 per cent. One can conclude that elective cesarean section is as safe for the infant, if not a bit safer than, vaginal delivery.

The sections reported in the British Perinatal Study of 1958 were classified on the basis of the presence of labor. Those sections performed after the onset of labor led to a significantly lower perinatal mortality than those done before labor. The adverse weighting of those not in labor was attributed to immaturity in association with toxemia, placenta praevia and errors in estimation of fetal age. It seems probable that labor is associated with increased fetal blood cortisol levels, and this prenatal glucocorticoid surge sets the stage for normal postnatal respiratory adaptations (see Chapter 13).

**PATHOLOGY AND PATHOGENESIS.** The chief cause of fetal death associated with emergency section is asphyxia from placental separation. The principal disorder of infants born by elective section is the respiratory distress syndrome. When Usher et al. reviewed the outcome of sections by consideration of gestational age, it was evident that the combination of prematurity and section was related to the occurrence of respiratory distress, but that among infants over thirty-eight weeks of gestational age, the route of delivery did not influence the incidence of disease. Similar results were found in the British Perinatal Study.

The question of which aspect of birth by cesarean section predisposes a premature infant to hyaline membrane disease is unanswered. One of the most widely discussed possibilities concerns the time of clamping of the umbilical cord. Several observers have suggested that early clamping, before the first breath, deprives the infant of the blood in the placenta and umbilical cord. It has been shown that as much as one third of the infant's total blood volume can be in the placenta at the moment of birth, and that with delayed clamping of the cord and with the aid of gravity, this "placental transfusion" can be given to the infant. The physiological effects of giving the infant the placental blood have been beautifully documented in a series of papers by Lind, Oh and colleagues. Late clamping is associated with higher hematocrits, higher systemic and pulmonary artery blood pressures, higher right atrial and portal pressures, longer interval until the first breath, higher respiratory rates and reduced lung compliance. Perhaps the most perceptive comment on this problem was made by Clement Smith in an editorial in *Pediatrics* in 1967, when he wrote in answer to the question "When should one ligate the umbilical cord?" posed in 1875, that "92 years and at least 90 published papers later, the question is still unanswered." It seems probable that at times it can be good to give the infant the placental blood, at times it can be bad and, as in most matters of concern in the care of the newborn infant, individual judgment is needed.

Russ and Strong thought that aspiration and aspiration pneumonia were important factors. They advised routine intratracheal catheterization, averring that 3 to 7 cc of mucoid material can be aspirated from these infants as opposed to 1 to 2 cc from babies born vaginally. Gellis et al. thought that the stomachs of these infants contained more secretion and that regurgitation-aspiration constituted a special hazard. They advocated, therefore, routine gastric emptying immediately after delivery. Although this procedure is widely practiced, it has not affected the incidence of hyaline membrane disease. It would seem that the only justifications for the insertion of a catheter into the stomach of a newborn infant are to rule out choanal and esophageal atresia and to remove excesses of swallowed blood, meconium or gastric contents for bacteriological study. None of these conditions relate to the route of delivery; therefore section per se should not be the reason for gastric aspiration.

**TREATMENT.** The sick cesarean-delivered newborn is treated according to the needs of his particular manifestations. Asphyxia, cerebral anoxic damage, massive aspiration and intracranial hemorrhage are managed in the not quite satisfactory ways we manage them in all other newborns. The same statement applies to the hyaline membrane disease.

## HYDRAMNIOS AS A SIGNAL OF CONGENITAL MALFORMATION

When pregnancy nears its termination, the amniotic sac contains approximately 600 to 1500 cc of fluid. Hydramnios exists if more than 2000 cc has accumulated. This happens rather infrequently, once in 1000 deliveries in DeYoung's experience, once in every 232 deliveries in that of Lloyd and Clatworthy.

The dynamics of the circulation of amniotic fluid has been clarified by a number of students of the problem. An essential element of the process appears to be the in-

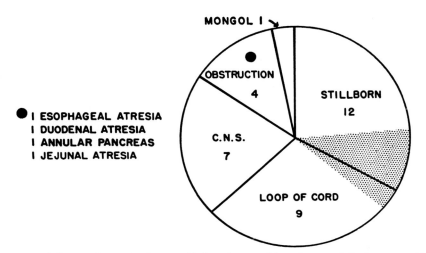

*Figure 5–2.* Type of abnormality in 33 abnormal babies born to 76 mothers with hydramnios. (Lloyd, J. R., and Clatworthy, H. W., Jr.: Pediatrics, *21*:903, 1958.)

termittent swallowing by the fetus of gulps of fluid which is then absorbed from fetal intestine into its circulation and transferred to the maternal blood stream across the placenta. Recent observations by Nichols and Schrepfer suggest strongly that ability or inability to swallow may have been overemphasized as determining factors in hydramnios. Hydramnios was associated with the birth of an anencephalic who *could* swallow, and was absent in the birth of one who *could not* swallow. "Hydramnios is a complicated phenomenon," they conclude. Duffy has recently reported an extraordinary association of hydramnios with fetal renal disease and retroperitoneal fibrosis of undetermined origin. He suggests that the hydramnios may have resulted from fetal proteinuria, which in turn increased the protein concentration of the amniotic fluid.

Hydramnios results from several maternal obstetrical diseases and from any disorder which precludes fetal swallowing. Death of the fetus *in utero,* tight wrapping of the cord about the neck, anencephaly and high obstructions of the gastrointestinal tract are the main responsible causes (Fig. 5–2). For the pediatrician it is this last group which lends importance to the phenomenon. Although high intestinal obstructions and anencephalus are the most common malformations associated with hydramnios, it occurs in nearly one third of the mothers of mongols even in the absence of intestinal obstruction. In the British Perinatal Study, over a quarter of all deaths with malformations followed a pregnancy complicated by hydramnios. When hydramnios has been noted by the obstetrician, the pediatrician must be on the qui vive for the earliest indications of esophageal or high intestinal obstruction if the infant is born alive and is free of any major cranial malformation.

For an excellent overview of many aspects of human malformations the reader is referred to Berry, C. L.: Brit. Med. Bull. 32:1–94, 1976.

# REFERENCES

Adams, J. M., Heath, H. D., Imagawa, D. T., Jones, M. H., and Shear, H. H.: Viral infections in the embryo. A.M.A. Am. J. Dis. Child. 92:109, 1956.

Avery, M. E., Oppenheimer, E. H., and Gordon, H. H.: Renal-vein thrombosis in newborn infants of diabetic mothers. N. Engl. J. Med. 265:1134, 1957.

Baker, J. B. E.: The effects of drugs on the foetus. Pharmacol. Rev. 12:37, 1960.

Benirschke, K., and Kim, C. K.: Multiple pregnancy. New Engl. J. Med. 288:1276, 1973.

Berry, C. L. (Ed.): Human malformations. Brit. Med. Bull. 32:1–94, 1976.

Boston Collaborative Drug Surveillance Program: Diethylstilbestrol in pregnancy. Frequency of exposure and usage patterns. Cancer 31:573, 1973.

Brandstrup, E., Osler, M., and Pedersen, J.: Perinatal mortality in diabetic pregnancy. Acta Endocrinol. 37:434, 1961.

Browne, D.: Congenital deformities of mechanical origin. Arch. Dis. Child. 30:37, 1955.

Butler, N. R., and Alberman, E. D.: Perinatal Problems. The Second Report of the 1958 British Perinatal Mortality Survey. London, E. & S. Livingstone, Ltd., 1969.

Butler, N. R., and Bonham, D. G.: Perinatal Mortality. The First Report of the 1968 Perinatal Mortality Survey. London, E. & S. Livingstone, Ltd., 1963.

Carter, C. O.: The genetics of congenital malformations. Proc. Roy. Soc. Med. 61:991, 1968.

Cohlan, S. Q.: Congenital anomalies in the rat produced by excessive intake of vitamin A during pregnancy. Pediatrics, 13:556, 1954.

Cornblath, M., Levin, E., and Marquetti, E.: Studies of carbohydrate metabolism in the newborn: Effect of glucagon on the concentration of sugar in capillary blood of the newborn infant. Pediatrics 21:885, 1958.

Cornblath, M., and Schwartz, R.: Disorders of Carbohydrate Metabolism in Infancy. Philadelphia, W. B. Saunders Company, 1966, pp. 57–81.

Craig, W. J.: Clinical signs of neonatal tetany: With especial reference to their occurrence in newborn babies of diabetic mothers. Pediatrics 22:297, 1958.

Dekaban, A. S.: Abnormalities in children exposed to x-radiation during various stages of gestation: Tentative timetable of radiation injury to the human fetus, Part I. J. Nucl. Med. 9:471, 1968.

Desmonts, G., and Couvreur, J.: Congenital toxoplasmosis. A prospective study of 378 pregnancies. New Engl. J. Med. 290:1110, 1974.

DeYoung, V. R.: Hydramnios as a signal to the physician responsible for newborn infants. J. Pediatr. 53:277, 1958.

Driscoll, S. G., Benirschke, K., and Curtis, G. W.: Neonatal deaths among infants of diabetic mothers. Am. J. Dis. Child. 100:818, 1960.

Duffy, J.: Fetal retroperitoneal fibrosis associated with hydramnios. J.A.M.A. 198:993, 1966.

Ekelund, H., Kullander, S., and Kallen, B.: Major and minor malformations in newborns and infants up to one year of age. Acta Paediat. Scand. 59:297, 1970.

Farquhar, J. W.: Prognosis for babies born to diabetic mothers in Edinburgh. Arch. Dis. Child. 44:36, 1969.

Fields, G. A., Schwarz, R. H., Dickens, H. O., and Tunnessen, W.: Sacral agenesis in the infant of a gestational diabetic. J. Obstet. Gynecol. 32:778, 1968.

Fraser, F. C., and Sainstat, T. D.: Production of congenital defects in the offspring of pregnant mice treated with cortisone; Progress report. Pediatrics 8:527, 1951.

Fraumeni, J. F., Jr.: Chemicals in human teratogenesis and transplacental carcinogenesis. Pediatrics 53:807, 1974.

Fuccillo, D. A., and Sever, J. L.: Viral teratology. Bacteriol. Rev. 37:19, 1973.

Gellis, S. S. and Hsia, D. Y.-Y.: The infant of the diabetic mother. A.M.A. J. Dis. Child. 97:1, 1959.

Gregg, N. M.: Congenital cataract following German measles in mother. Tr. Ophth. Soc. Australia (1941) 3:35, 1942.

Holmes, L. B.: Inborn errors of morphogenesis—a review of localized hereditary malformations. New Eng. J. Med. 291:763, 1974.

Holowach, J., Thurston, D. L., and Becker, B.: Congenital defects in infants following mumps during pregnancy; a review of the literature and a report of chorioretinitis due to fetal infection. J. Pediatr. 50:689, 1957.

Hsia, Y. E., Bratu, M., and Herbordt, A.: Genetics of the Meckel syndrome (dysencephalia splanchnocystica). Pediatrics 48:237, 1971.

Jones, K. L., Smith, D. W., Streissguth, A. P., et al.: Outcome in offspring of chronic alcoholic women. Lancet 1:1076, 1974.

Jones, K. L., Smith, D. W., Ulleland, C. N., et al.: Pattern of malformation in offspring of chronic alcoholic mothers. Lancet 1:7815, 1973.

King, J. A., King, E. L., and Pitt, McB.: A study of fetal mortality in cesarean section. South. M. J., 46:491, 1953.

Kline, B. S.: Microscopic observation of development of human placenta. Am. J. Obstet. Gynecol. 61:1065, 1951.

Krugman, S.: The clinical use of gamma globulin. New Engl. J. Med. 269:195, 1963.

Krugman, S. (Ed.): International Conference on Rubella Immunization. Am. J. Dis. Child. 118:1, 155, 1969.

Lapinleimu, K., Koskimies, O., Cantell, K., et al.: Association between maternal herpesvirus infections and congenital malformations. Lancet 1:1127, 1974.

Leck, I., and Record, R. G.: Seasonal incidence of anencephalus. Br. J. Prev. Soc. Med. 20:67, 1966.

Lenz, W., and Maier, W.: Congenital malformations and maternal diabetes. Lancet 2:1124, 1964.

Levine, P.: Serological factors as possible causes of spontaneous abortions. J. Hered. 34:71, 1943.

Lloyd, J. R., and Clatworthy, H. W., Jr.: Hydramnios as an aid to the early diagnosis of congenital obstruction of the alimentary tract: A study of the maternal and fetal factors. Pediatrics 21:903, 1958.

Lubs, H. A., and Ruddle, F. H.: Chromosomal abnormalities in the human population: Estimation of rates based on New Haven newborn study. Science 1969:495, 1970.

Marden, P. M., Smith, D. W., and McDonald, M. J.: Congenital anomalies in the newborn infant, including minor variations. J. Pediatr. 64:357, 1964.

McIntosh, R., Merritt, K. K., Richards, M. R., Samuels, M. H., and Bellows, M. T.: The incidence of congenital malformations: A study of 5964 pregnancies. Pediatrics 14:505, 1954.

Meltzer, H. J.: Congenital anomalies due to attempted abortion with 4-aminopteroglutamic acid. J.A.M.A. 161:1253, 1956.

Mikamo, K.: Anatomic and chromosomal anomalies in spontaneous abortions. Am. J. Obstet. Gynecol. 106:243, 1970.

Miller, H. C.: Cardiac hypertrophy and extramedullary erythropoiesis in newborn infants of prediabetic mothers. Am. J. M. Sc. 209:447, 1945.

Miller, L. H., Reifsnyder, D. N. and Martinez, S. A.: Late onset of disease in congenital toxoplasmosis. Clin. Pediat. 10:78, 1971.

Miller, R. W.: Relation between cancer and congenital defects in man. New Engl. J. Med. 275:87, 1966.

Milunsky, A. (Ed.): Clinics in Perinatology. Vol. II., Philadelphia, W. B. Saunders Company, 1974.

Milunsky, A. (Ed.): The Prevention of Mental Retardation and Genetic Disease. Philadelphia, W. B. Saunders Company, 1975.

Milunsky, A., Graef, J., and Gaynor, M.: Methotrexate-induced congenital malformations, with a review of the literature. J. Pediatr. 72:790, 1968.

Monson, R. R., Rosenberg, L., Hartz, S. C., et al.: Diphenylhydantoin and selected congenital malformations. New Engl. J. Med. 289:1049, 1973.

Neel, J. V.: A study of major congenital defects in Japanese infants. Am. J. Hum. Genet. 10:398, 1958.

Nichols, J., and Schrepfer, R.: Polyhydramnios in anencephaly. J.A.M.A. 197:549, 1966.

Oh, W., Wallgren, G., Hanson, J. S., and Lind, J.: The effects of placental transfusion on respiratory mechanics of normal term newborn infants. Pediatrics 40:7, 1967.

Oppenheimer, E. H., and Esterly, J. H.: Thrombosis in the newborn: comparison between infants of diabetic and nondiabetic mothers. J. Pediatr. 67:549, 1965.

Osler, M., and Pedersen, J.: The body composition of newborn infants of diabetic mothers. Pediatrics 26:985, 1960.

O'Sullivan, J. B., Mahan, C. M., Charles, D. and Dandrow, R. V.: Medical treatment of the gestational diabetic. Obstet. Gynec. 43:817, 1974.

Passarge, E., and Lenz, W.: Syndrome of caudal regression in infants of diabetic mothers. Observations of Further Cases. Pediatrics, 37:672, 1966.

Pedersen, J.: The Pregnant Diabetic and Her Newborn. Problems and Management. Baltimore, Williams and Wilkins Company, 1967.

Pedersen, J., Mølsted-Pedersen, L. and Andersen, B.: Assessors of fetal-perinatal mortality in diabetic pregnancy. Diabetes 23:302, 1974.

Penrose, L. S., and Svith, G. F.: Down's Anomaly. Boston, Little, Brown and Company, 1966.

Pildes, R. S.: Infants of diabetic mothers. N. Engl. J. Med. 289:902, 1973.

Plummer, G.: Anomalies occurring in children exposed in utero to the atomic bomb in Hiroshima. Pediatrics, 10:687, 1952.

Polani, P. E.: Incidence of developmental and other genetic abnormalities. Proc. R. Soc. Med. 66:1118, 1973.

Pritchard, J. A.: Fetal swallowing and amniotic fluid. Obst. Gynecol. 28:606, 1966.

Reardon, H. S., et al.: Treatment of acute respiratory distress in newborn infants of diabetic and "prediabetic" mothers. Tr. Soc. Ped. Res., 1957.

Rothman, K. J., and Fyler, D. C.: Seasonal occurrence of complex ventricular septal defect. Lancet 2:193, 1974.

Rowland, T. W., Hubbell, J. P., and Nadas, A. S.: Congenital heart disease in infants of diabetic mothers. J. Pediatr. 83:815, 1973.

Rubin, A. and Murphy, D. P.: Studies in human

reproduction. III. The frequency of congenital malformations in the offspring of nondiabetic and diabetic individuals. J. Pediatr. 53:579, 1958.

Rugh, R.: X-irradiation effects on the human fetus. J. Pediatr. 52:531, 1958.

Rusnak, S. L., and Driscoll, S. G.: Congenital spinal anomalies in infants of diabetic mothers. Pediatrics 35:989, 1965.

Schaffer, A. J.: The pathogenesis of intrauterine pneumonia: A critical review of the evidence concerning intrauterine respiratory-like movements. Pediatrics 17:747, 1956.

Sever, J., and White, L. R.: Intrauterine viral infections. Ann. Rev. Med. 19:471, 1968.

Shubeck, F.: Spontaneous rupture of membranes. Feb, 2, 1965. Collaborative Perinatal Project No. 64–002–2.

Shepard, T. H.: Catalog of Teratogenic Agents. Baltimore, Johns Hopkins University Press, 1973.

Siegel, M.: Congenital malformations following chickenpox, measles, mumps, and hepatitis. Results of a cohort study. J.A.M.A. 226:1521, 1973.

Siegel, M., and Greenberg, M.: Fetal death, malformation and prematurity after maternal rubella. New Engl. J. Med. 262:389, 1960.

Smith, B. T., Giroud, C. J. P., Robert, M., and Avery, M. E.: Insulin antagonism of cortisol action on lecithin synthesis by cultured fetal lung cells. J. Pediatr. 87:953, 1975.

Smith, C. A.: Effects of maternal undernutrition upon the newborn infant in Holland (1944–1945). J. Pediatr. 30:229, 1947.

Smith, C. A.: When should one ligate the umbilical cord? Editorial. Pediatrics 40:5, 1967.

Speidel, B. D., and Meadow, S. R.: Maternal epilepsy and abnormalities of the fetus and newborn. Lancet 2:839, 1972.

Stevenson, A. C.: The association of hydramnios with congenital malformations. In Wolstenholm, G. E. W., and O'Conner, C. M. (Eds.): Ciba Foundation Symposium on Congenital Malformations. Boston, Little, Brown & Company, 1960, p. 241.

Takeuchi, A., and Benirschke, K.: Renal vein thrombosis of the newborn and its relation to maternal diabetes. Biol. Neonatol. 3:237, 1961.

Usher, R., McLean, F., and Maughan, G. B.: Respiratory distress syndrome in infants delivered by cesarean section. Am. J. Obstet. Gynecol. 88:806, 1964.

Usher, R., Shephard, M., and Lind, J.: The blood volume of the newborn infant and the placental transfusion. Acta Paediat. Scand. 52:497, 1963.

Van Vunakis, H., Langone, J. J., and Milunsky, A.: Nicotine and Cotinine in the amniotic fluid of smokers in the early period of gestation. Am. J. Obstet. Gynecol. 120:64, 1974.

Wallace, H. M., Hoenig, L., and Rich, H.: Newborn infants with congenital malformations or birth injuries. A.M.A. J. Dis. Child. 91:529, 1956.

Warkany, J.: Etiology of congenital malformations. Advances in Pediatrics. New York, Interscience Publishers, Inc., 1947, Vol. 2.

Warkany, J.: Congenital Malformations. Notes and Comments. Chicago, Year Book Medical Publishers, Inc., 1971.

White, P.: Diabetes mellitus in pregnancy. Clinics in Perinatology. 1st ed., Philadelphia, W. B. Saunders, 1974, p. 331.

White, P.: Pregnancy and diabetes, medical aspects. Med. Clin. N. Amer. 49:1015, 1965.

Wilson, J. G.: Present status of drugs as teratogens in man. Teratology 7:3, 1973.

# II

# Disorders of the
# Respiratory System

An understanding of the disorders of respiration in the neonatal period demands a fairly clear understanding of the physiology of respiration in the fetus and in the neonate, and of the alterations which accompany the precipitous changeover from the aquatic state to the air-breathing state. Within a matter of seconds after the placenta has separated, the newborn must be transformed, as it were, from larva to adult, from tadpole to frog. Little wonder that mortality is higher at this moment than at any other period of life! Unfortunately our knowledge of the physiologic processes accompanying this changeover is far from complete.

## THE FETAL LUNG

The fetal lung does not function as an organ of gas exchange, but it must develop in such a way that it can assume this role as soon as the placental circulation is interrupted at birth. In fetal life, only 4 per cent of the cardiac output perfuses the pulmonary vascular bed; after birth the whole of the cardiac output must go through the lung. The vascular bed must develop the capacity to accept this enormous increase in perfusion. Similarly, the airways and terminal air spaces are distended with liquid in fetal life; after birth they must adapt to a gaseous environment and remain inflated at end-expiration. Rapid, irregular respiratory movements are present some of the time in utero; after birth the central respiratory regulatory apparatus not only must initiate the forceful respirations needed to inflate the airless lung but also must sustain rhythmic breathing. Such major physiological adjustments in the circulatory, respiratory and central nervous systems are not required at any other time of life. Little wonder that they sometimes fail to function perfectly. The remarkable fact is that they so often succeed so perfectly, and that cardiorespiratory function is nearly normal within hours of the moment of birth.

The fetal lung contains liquid that in the normal state is the product of the lung itself. Its volume, estimated on the basis of studies in animals, is about 40 to 60 ml; its composition differs from amniotic liquid in being somewhat more acid (pH 6.43, compared to 7.07 of amniotic liquid), with a $CO_2$ level of 4.4 mEq per liter compared to 18.4 mEq per liter of amniotic liquid. Fetal lung liquid contains acid mucopolysaccharides, mucoproteins and surface-active lipoproteins, and has a variable total protein content averaging 300 mg per cent. Occasionally there is admixture of the fetal lung liquid with amniotic liquid, presumably from gasping in utero. Squamous epithelial cells from the infants' skin have been identified in lungs of some infants who died weeks after birth from nonpulmonary causes. They are not regularly present in the lungs of all infants, however, and the weight of the evidence at hand is that the fetal lung, as well as the kidney, is the normal source of amniotic liquid rather than that the amniotic liquid is aspirated and distends the fetal lung. In the lamb over 100 ml per day of lung liquid is produced. Fetal swallowing also occurs, on the average of 100 ml/kg/day.

The gaseous environment of the fetus is maintained by the placenta. Studies in monkeys with catheters placed in fetal vessels reveal the arterial oxygen saturation to be between 80 and 95 per cent, $pO_2$ between 30 and 40 mm of mercury, pH 7.37 to 7.40 and $pCO_2$ approximately 35 to 40 mm of mercury.

Measurements of capillary blood from the human fetal scalp during labor show a pH of approximately 7.30, standard bicarbonate of 19 mEq per liter, $pCO_2$ of 44 mm of mercury and $pO_2$ of approximately 20 to 25 mm of mercury. It can be safely assumed that fetal arterial blood before labor would have a slightly higher pH and $pO_2$ and a lower $pCO_2$. Sampling of fetal scalp blood, plus comparison with maternal capillary blood, has become a useful tool in the detection of stress in the fetus.

## THE FIRST BREATH OF AIR

The introduction of air into the airless lung requires higher pressure than those needed at any other time of life. Actual measurements of the forces applied by the infant range from 10 to 70 cm of water for intervals lasting 0.5 to 1.0 second. The first expiration is usually associated with a positive pressure of 20 to 30 cm of water. These pressures should be interpreted in the context of the 4 cm of water required on the average for normal breathing in the infant after the first few breaths, as in the adult.

The reason higher pressures are required at birth is the necessity to overcome the opposing forces of the viscosity of liquid in the airways (some 100 times that of air) and of surface tension, whose effect is maximal in the airways of smallest caliber. Associated with the introduction of the 50 or so milliliters of air that is usual with the first breath is the necessity that some of it, usually 20 to 30 ml, remain behind to establish the functional residual capacity. At the same time, the liquid that was in the air spaces must be removed. Some of it is aspirated from the oropharynx or expelled

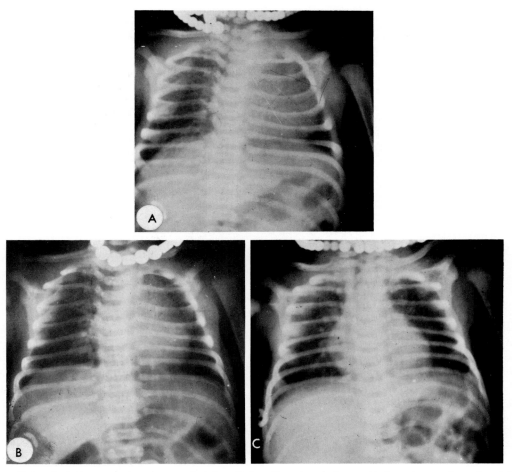

*Figure 6–1.* A, Anteroposterior view on first day. Not well centered, it nevertheless shows a large heart, broad mediastinum, coarse mottling of the right lung, the left being hidden by the heart, and a faint but definite line between the right upper and middle lobes. B, Film taken on the second day, showing diminution in heart size and mediastinal breadth. The lung mottling is less coarse and less well defined. C, Film taken on the fifth day. The heart and mediastinum appear to be in perfect proportion to chest width now. Root shadows are still prominent, but the peripheral portions of the lungs are clear. (These films were lent us by Dr. Charles Weymuller. They are one series in his early studies on chest radiography in the newborn, made in 1928, and thus are of historical interest. They appeared in *Am. J. Dis. Child.*, 35:837, 1928.)

by the infant; most of it is removed by the pulmonary circulation, which increases manyfold at birth. The proteins in the lung liquid, and as much as one third of the total volume, are removed through the rich lymphatic network of the lung.

The stimuli to the initiation of breathing at birth are multiple. Uncertainty still persists as to their relative importance. The changes in blood gases after interruption of the placental circulation are predictable, namely, a fall in oxygen tension and pH and a rise in $pCO_2$. These changes at first stimulate respiration, although they can quickly become so profound as to depress it. Very low oxygen tensions suppress the responsiveness of the central nervous system, just as high $CO_2$ tensions can be narcotizing. Nonchemical stimuli, such as a change in temperature and tactile input, enhance "neuronal traffic" through the medulla and increase the discharge of the central respiratory neurons. It seems possible that added neural stimuli are associated with changes in the distribution of fetal blood flow after the umbilical cord is clamped. In the exteriorized fetal animal, the most reliable stimulus to the initiation of breathing is clamping the cord. In the human, the first breath may precede clamping the cord, although interruption of the umbilical circulation in the course of delivery may have the same physiological consequences.

## BREATHING PATTERNS

Irregularities in respiratory patterns occur in all newborn infants, increasingly so in the more premature ones. When the pattern is characterized by a ventilatory burst, then an apneic pause of 5 to 15 seconds, repetitively, it is called periodic breathing. More sporadic and prolonged apneic intervals are called "apneic spells." Breathing patterns are influenced greatly by state of consciousness; deep sleep is associated with reasonably regular patterns, rapid eye movement (REM) sleep by periodic breathing and wakefulness by grossly irregular breathing associated with muscle movement, sucking and crying. Inspiratory gasps are frequent, occasionally characterized by a second inspiration imposed on the first to achieve a doubling or more of tidal volume.

## Periodic Breathing

Some of the characteristics of periodic breathing may be summarized as follows:

1. Periods of apnea of 5 to 10 seconds
   Periods of ventilation of 10 to 15 seconds
   Average rate 30 to 40 per minute
   Rate during ventilatory interval 50 to 60 per minute
2. Periodic breathing is most common in most premature infants, but is rarely seen in first few days of life
3. It is more common during REM sleep
4. Period breathing persists intermittently until infants are about 36 weeks of gestational age, regardless of time of birth
5. It is more common at altitude than at sea level
6. It can be abolished with increased inspired oxygen and increased carbon dioxide
7. The net effect of periodic breathing is slight hyperventilation
8. An increase in lung volume tends to reduce the amount of periodic breathing
9. No significant changes in heart rate occur during the apneic interval
10. No prognostic significance is associated with periodic breathing

## Apneic Spells

In contrast with periodic breathing, apneic spells are associated with other illnesses, such as sepsis, pneumonia, meningitis, hypoglycemia and intracranial hemorrhage. They may also occur in very premature infants in the absence of recognized pathology. Much recent study has been directed toward understanding the etiology and evaluating the therapy of apneic spells, in part because they are known to carry a poor prognosis and sometimes, if unrecognized, can be fatal. The overrepresentation of low birth weight among infants who die suddenly and unexpectedly at several months of age further stimulates interest and study of apneic spells as observed in the nursery.

Infants prone to have apneic spells may be moderately depressed from other causes. Unlike most of those with periodic breathing, they can have some carbon dioxide retention, with $PA_{CO_2}$ of 40–60 cm Hg. Occasionally periodic breathing may precede a series of apneic spells, and the same infants can, and often do, display both types of respiratory patterns.

Among the means to lessen the frequency of apneic spells have been gentle stimulation, achieved through rocking incubators or water beds. Maintenance of an abdominal wall temperature of 36° instead of 36.5° C has been an adequate thermal stimulus to respiration to reduce the incidence of apneic spells. Humidity of 50 to 60 per cent in incubators permits a lower ambient temperature and likewise has been found to reduce the number of apneic spells.

Pharmacologic stimulation as well, such as theophylline in a dose of 2 to 3 mg per kilogram orally every 6 hours, with maintenance of blood levels of 6 to 12 $\mu$g per ml has been found effective in the reduction of incidence of apneic spells (Shannon et al.).

Studies on the etiology of apnea have demonstrated a number of associated events. Minimal upper respiratory infection, but perhaps enough to produce nasal obstruction, has been found in infants who die suddenly. Airway occlusion, deliberately with a mask or inadvertently by position of the neck may not be associated with gasping in some infants, particularly if in deep sleep. Regurgitation of gastric contents, with spillover into the airway, may be a way in which airway obstruction can occur in those infants whose reflexes for coughing and gagging are suppressed or immature.

We most need ways to detect infants at special risk of failure to respond to the usual ventilatory stimuli after airway occlusion from whatever cause. Given such information, prophylaxis with physical or pharmacologic stimuli, and appropriate use of apnea monitors may lessen the tragic occurrence of sudden infant death syndrome.

## EVALUATION OF THE NEWBORN

Until relatively recently the condition of newborns had been summarily described as good, fair or poor. Apgar attempted, in the early 1950's to evaluate their conditions upon more objective grounds, so that one might compare infants born in different hospitals and under diverse conditions of anesthesia and delivery, or of health, with greater precision. She assigned a figure of 0, 1 or 2 to five objective signs determined 1 minute after delivery, the sum constituting

**TABLE 6–1.   Causes of Respiratory Distress**

I. Obstruction of the airway
   A. Choanal atresia
   B. Congenital stridors
   C. Tracheal stenosis
   D. Bronchial stenosis
II. Lung parenchymal disease
   A. Aspiration syndromes
   B. Atelectasis
   C. Hyperinflation
   D. Pneumomediastinum and pneumothorax
   E. Idiopathic lobar emphysema
   F. Congenital pulmonary lymphangiectasis
   G. Wilson-Mikity syndrome
   H. Hyaline membrane disease
   I. Pneumonia
   J. Retained lung liquid (transient tachypnea of the newborn)
III. Nonpulmonary causes
   A. Heart failure
   B. Intracranial lesions
   C. Salicylism
   D. Metabolic acidosis
IV. Miscellaneous
   A. Pulmonary agenesis
   B. Disorders of the diaphragm and chest wall
   C. Tracheoesophageal fistula
   D. Pulmonary cysts
   E. Intrathoracic tumors and cysts
   F. Pulmonary sequestration
   G. Pleural effusions
   H. Pulmonary hemorrhage

the infants' score. Thus (1) a heart rate of 100 to 140 rates a figure of 2, no heart beat, of 0, less than 100, of 1; (2) respiratory effort is rated 2 if the infant breathes promptly and cries lustily, 0 if apneic or if only one or two gasps are made, and 1 for anything in between; (3) reflex irritability is rated 2 if good, 0 if there is no response to stimulation, 1 for anything between; (4) muscle tone is assigned 0 for flaccidity, 2 for good tone, 1 for intermediate tone or for hypertonus; and (5) color is rated 2 if the entire body is pink, 0 if all blue, 1 if anything between. In Apgar's own series, scores of 0, 1 or 2 presaged a 14 per cent mortality, of 3, 4, 5, 6 or 7, 1.1 per cent, and of 8, 9 and 10, 0.13 per cent. Apgar scoring has been universally accepted as a useful procedure. The correlation with mortality in the first 28 days is greater with the 5-minute score than at 1 minute, and scoring at both times seems appropriate.

A great variety of disorders cause the neonate to breathe with excessive effort. Some are listed in Table 6–1.

TABLE 6–2.   *Clues to Diagnosis of Types of Respiratory Distress*

| Information from Maternal History | Most Likely Condition in Infant |
|---|---|
| Prematurity | Hyaline membrane disease |
| Diabetes | Hyaline membrane disease |
| Hemorrhage in the days before premature delivery | Hyaline membrane disease |
| Infection | Pneumonia |
| Premature rupture of membranes | Pneumonia |
| Prolonged labor | Pneumonia |
| Meconium-stained amniotic fluid | Meconium aspiration |
| Hydramnios | Tracheoesophageal fistula |
| Excessive medications | Central nervous system depression |
| Reserpine | Stuffy nose |
| Traumatic or breech delivery | Central nervous system hemorrhage |
|  | Phrenic nerve paralysis |
| Fetal tachycardia or bradycardia | Asphyxia |
| Prolapsed cord or cord entanglements | Asphyxia |
| Postmaturity | Aspiration |

| Signs in the Baby | Most Likely Associated Condition |
|---|---|
| Single umbilical artery | Congenital anomalies |
| Other congenital anomalies | Associated cardiopulmonary anomalies |
| Scaphoid abdomen | Diaphragmatic hernia |
| Erb's palsy | Phrenic nerve palsy |
| Cannot breathe with mouth closed | Choanal atresia |
|  | Stuffy nose |
| Gasping with little air exchange | Upper airway obstruction |
| Overdistention of lungs | Aspiration, lobar emphysema, or pneumothorax |
| Shift of apical pulse | Pneumothorax |
|  | Chylothorax |
|  | Hypoplastic lung |
| Fever, or rise in temperature in a constant temperature environment | Pneumonia |
| Shrill cry, hypertonia, or flaccidity | Central nervous system disorder |
| Atonia | Trauma, myasthenia, poliomyelitis, amyotonia |
| Frothy blood from larynx | Pulmonary hemorrhage |
| Head extended in the absence of neurologic findings | Laryngeal obstruction or vascular rings |
| Choking after feedings | Tracheoesophageal fistula or pharyngeal incoordination |

*From Avery, M. E., and Fletcher, B. D.: *The Lung and Its Disorders in the Newborn Infant.* 3rd. ed.

## FREQUENCY OF DISORDERS OF RESPIRATION

The frequency of any given cause of respiratory distress will depend on the gestational age of the infant under consideration, the condition of the mother, and the environment. Table 6–1 lists some causes of respiratory distress.

The differential diagnosis of the many causes of dyspnea in the newborn infant appears throughout the text. Some useful clues to diagnosis are included in Table 6–2.

## REFERENCES

Adams, F. H.: Functional development of the fetal lung. J. Pediatr. 68:794, 1966.

Apgar, V.: A proposal for a new method of evaluation of the newborn infant. Anesth. Analg. 32:260, 1953.

Apgar, V., Holaday, D. A., James, L. S., et al.: Evaluation of the newborn infant—Second report. J.A.M.A. 168:1985, 1958.

Avery, M. E., and Fletcher, B. D.: The Lung and Its Disorders in the Newborn Infant. 3rd ed. Philadelphia, W. B. Saunders Company, 1974.

Barcroft, J.: Fetal circulation and respiration. Physiol. Rev. 16:103, 1936.

Barcroft, J., and Barron, D. H.: The genesis of respiratory movements in the foetus of the sheep. Physiology 88:56, 1936-7.

Bundesen, H. N., Potter, E. L., Fishbein, W. I., et al.: Progress in the reduction of needless neonatal deaths. J.A.M.A. *148*:907, 1952.

Burns, B. D.: The central control of respiratory movements. Br. Med. Bull. *19*:7, 1963.

Chernick, V., Heldrich, F., and Avery, M. E.: Periodic breathing of premature infants. J. Pediatr. *64*:330, 1964.

Daily, W. J. R., Klaus, M., and Meyer, H. B.: Apnea in premature infants. Monitoring incidence, heart rate changes, and an effect of environmental temperature. Pediatrics *43*:510, 1969.

Davis, M. E., and Potter, E. L.: Intrauterine respiration of the human fetus. J.A.M.A. *131*:1194, 1946.

Dawes, G. S., Fox, H. E., Leduc, B. M., et al.: Respiratory movements and rapid eye movement sleep in the foetal lamb. J. Physiol. *220*:119, 1972.

DeReuck, A. V. S., and Porter, R. (eds): Development of the Lung. Ciba Foundation Symposium. London, J. & A. Churchill, Ltd., 1967.

Drage, J. S., Kennedy, C., and Schwarz, B. K.: The Apgar Score as an index of neonatal mortality. A report from the Collaborative Study of Cerebral Palsy. Obstet. Gynecol. *24*:222, 1964.

Eastman, N. J., Geiling, E. M. K., and DeLawder, A. M.: Fetal blood studies: IV. The $O_2$ and $CO_2$ dissociation curves of foetal blood. Bull. Johns Hopkins Hosp. *53*:246, 1933.

Farber, S., and Sweet, L. K.: Amniotic sac contents in lungs of infants. Am. J. Dis. Child. *42*:1372, 1931.

Farber, S., and Wilson, J. L.: Atelectasis of the newborn: A study and critical review. Am. J. Dis. Child. *46*:572, 1933.

Fenner, A., Schalk, U., Hoenicke, H., et al.: Periodic breathing in premature and neonatal babies. Pediat. Res. 7:174, 1973.

Gabriel, M., Albani, M., and Schulte, F. J.: Apneic spells and sleep states in preterm infants. Pediatrics 57:142, 1976.

Karlberg, P.: The adaptive changes in the immediate postnatal period, with particular reference to respiration. J. Pediatr. *56*:585, 1960.

Klemperer, H. H.: Experimentelle Studien zur Physiologie der ersten Atemzuges. Arch. Gynäkol. *154*:108, 1933.

Miller, H. C., and Conklin, E. V.: Clinical evaluation of respiratory insufficiency in newborn infants. Pediatrics *16*:427, 1955.

Miller, H. C., Behrle, F. C., and Snull, N. W.: Apnea and irregular respiratory rhythms among premature infants. Pediatrics 23:676, 1959.

Noback, C. J.: A contribution to the topographic anatomy of the thymus gland, with particular reference to its changes at birth and in the period of the newborn. Am. J. Dis. Child. 22:120, 1921.

Oliver, T. K. (ed.): Neonatal Respiratory Adaptation. Bethesda, Md., U.S. Department of Health, Education, and Welfare, 1964.

Perlstein, P. H., Edwards, N. K., and Sutherland, J. M.: Apnea in premature infants and incubator-air-temperature changes. N. Engl. J. Med. 282:461, 1970.

Rigatto, H., and Brady, J. P.: Periodic breathing and apnea in preterm infant. I. Evidence for hypoventilation possibly due to central respiratory depression. Pediatrics 50:202, 1972.

Rigatto, H., Verdazco, R., and Cates, D. B.: Effects of $O_2$ on the ventilatory response to $CO_2$ in preterm infants. J. Appl. Physiol. 39:896, 1975.

Runge, M.: Die Ursache der Lungenathmung des Neugeborenen. Arch. Gynäkol. *46*:512, 1894.

Scarpelli, E. M., and Auld, P. A. M.: Pulmonary Physiology of the Fetus, Newborn, and Child. Philadelphia, Lea and Febiger, 1975.

Shannon, D. C., Gotay, F., Stein, I. M., et al.: Prevention of apnea and bradycardia in low-birth-weight infants. Pediatrics, 55:589, 1975.

Smith, C. A., and Nelson, N. M.: Physiology of the Newborn Infant. 4th ed. Springfield, Ill., Charles C Thomas, 1976.

Strang, L. B.: The lungs at birth. Arch. Dis. Child. *40*:575, 1965.

Thibeault, D. W., Wong, M. M., and Auld, P. A. M.: Thoracic gas volume changes in premature infants. Pediatrics *40*:403, 1967.

# ATRESIA OF THE POSTERIOR CHOANAE

## 7

A rare congenital defect is obstruction at the junction of the posterior terminus of the nasal airway and the nasopharynx, the so-called posterior naris or choana. The obstructing element is most commonly a bony plate 1/8 to 1/4 inch in thickness, but it may be a thin membrane. Obstruction may be unilateral and partial, or bilateral and complete. Symptomatology varies considerably in these two varieties. Associated congenital defects include Treacher Collins syndrome, palatal abnormalities, colobomas, tracheoesophageal fistula and congenital heart disease, according to the series of Flake and Ferguson. The abnormality is twice as frequent on the right side as on the left, and twice as frequent in girls as in boys. The estimated frequency of 1 in every 8000 births may be low, since unilateral lesions may be unrecognized.

**ETIOLOGY AND PATHOGENESIS.** The familial tendency to choanal atresia is evident from most large series reported, including McGovern's cases as well as those of Phelps.

The mouth and nares develop from invaginations which deepen caudad in the embryonic head, while the primitive foregut and its offshoot, the trachea, grow cephalad. Normally these canals meet in the region of the pharynx and fuse into the widely patent foodway and airway. Rarely the embryologic septum separating nares from foregut fails to disappear, leaving the foodway intact but the airway obstructed. The septum may remain membranous, but commonly it becomes converted into bone.

**DIAGNOSIS**

BILATERAL CHOANAL OBSTRUCTION. Symptoms may or may not be manifest immediately after birth. Two of our four infants cried and breathed within seconds after delivery, but one was described as "limp and cyanotic at birth," while another did not breathe immediately or well and was said to have become "full of mucus" very shortly. All had breathing difficulty within a few hours. In some this was episodic and associated with attempts to feed; in others it was constant.

The diagnosis is suspected when an infant has marked retractions and is mouth-breathing. If the nostrils are occluded, no adverse effect is noted; if the mouth is occluded, the infant may struggle and become cyanotic and limp. The inability to pass a feeding tube through the nostril suggests the diagnosis. It may be confirmed by the instillation of a few drops of methylene blue dye into the nostril; if the nares are patent, the dye can be seen in the pharynx. Radiographic studies with contrast media may confirm the diagnosis, but are not essential (Fig. 7–1).

UNILATERAL CHOANAL ATRESIA. When congenital obstruction is limited to one side, which is the case in about 20 per cent of infants, the diagnosis is seldom made in

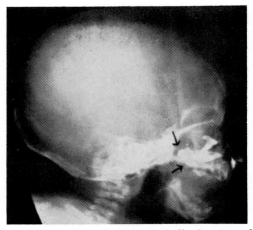

*Figure 7–1.* Lateral view of skull after Lipiodol had been instilled into the nares. The dye can be seen pooled in the nose and nasopharynx, but none has entered the oropharynx.

the neonatal period. In four cases with which we are acquainted it was not arrived at until the ages of 3, 6, 10 and 38 years. In all these the retrospective story was that of inability to breathe through one side of the nose since birth, unilateral nasal discharge and often-repeated upper respiratory tract infections.

**TREATMENT.** If the obstruction is membranous, an attempt to perforate it may be made as soon as the diagnosis is made. A polyethylene or rubber catheter may then be threaded through and left in place for a few days. Dilatation may have to be repeated from time to time. When the obstruction is bony, as it almost always is, definitive operative repair should not be undertaken until the child is 12 to 18 months old at the earliest. In the interim, and especially in the first month or two of life, much ingenuity is required to keep the infant alive and gaining. Usually a preliminary period of gavage feeding is indicated. Subsequently the infant learns to feed, first from a dropper, then from a bottle, without becoming too distressed. Feedings must be slow and interrupted and, in order to spare the baby undue exhaustion, should be frequent and small. Gradually this task becomes easier and less fraught with danger. Trouble is often encountered even between feedings, cyanotic spells developing because the tongue drops backward into close apposition with the soft palate. Some observers believe, and we are inclined to agree, that this difficulty is due less to the choanal atresia than to associated micrognathia (q.v.). Whatever the cause, serious spells of choking and cyanosis may necessitate immobilization of the tongue by stitching its lower surface to the lower jaw.

Erickson et al. have pointed out that these infants can be managed easily and successfully by introducing an oral airway and feeding by gavage for the first week or so. Over the next 2 or 3 weeks they can be weaned from the airway and taught to eat and breathe through the mouth intermittently. From then on feeding goes smoothly, if a bit slowly, and definitive operation may be postponed for 4 years or more, at which time it is easier and more likely to eventuate in successful cure.

The operation of choice at present consists in formation of bony windows through a transpalatal approach and covering the raw edges with split-thickness grafts.

CASE 7-1

A white female infant whose family history was unimportant and whose mother's pregnancy, labor and delivery were not unusual was limp and cyanotic at birth. She was resuscitated with positive pressure oxygen and placed in a warmed incubator. Birth weight was 7 pounds 5 ounces (3315 gm), but during the first 11 days of life she lost 2 pounds. Feeding had been extremely difficult because throughout all attempted bottle feedings spells of severe cyanosis occurred. Between feedings the baby lay limp and inactive. She had been offered Olac, 1/2 ounce every 3 hours, and had been given 5 per cent glucose subcutaneously, as well as penicillin intramuscularly, and had been kept in humid oxygen. She was transferred to the Sinai Hospital of Baltimore on the eleventh day of life with the probable diagnosis of congenital heart disease.

Physical examination at age 11 days showed weight 5 pounds 6 ounces (2440 gm). She was a small, well developed, well nourished infant receiving oxygen. Her color was good; there was no distress. The nose was full of thick mucus, and its mucous membranes were reddened. The mouth was held constantly open. The head was held retracted in a position of opisthotonos, but this was apparently voluntary, since no difficulty was experienced in flexing the neck. When she was first seen, breathing was easy and quiet, but slight sternal retraction was noted. Breath sounds were audible everywhere.

When she was moved or when bottle feedings were attempted, the infant became highly excited. Retraction increased with deepening of respiration, and she became slightly cyanotic. On these occasions the percussion note became

hyperresonant, but breath sounds were poorly heard. After suctioning the nares and pharynx, breath sounds reappeared. The rest of the examination was negative in all respects.

She was kept in humid oxygen and fed by gavage. Shortly after admission deep cyanosis developed and persisted, and nasal suction was attempted. The catheter encountered a firm obstruction after being introduced into each naris and passed only a few centimeters. It could not be forced into the oropharynx through either the right or the left nostril. Lipiodol was then instilled into the nose, and x-ray films revealed bilateral choanal atresia (Fig. 5-1).

X-ray study of the chest showed questionable generalized overinflation. A barium swallow esophagram revealed no esophageal anomaly. Blood was normal except for anemia (hemoglobin 12.5 gm). Urine was normal.

**COMMENT.** In this example the infant was in trouble from birth, being limp and cyanotic, and there had been no antecedent obstetrical difficulty to account for this. After this initial period she seemed not too ill unless stimulated, especially by attempts to feed. These produced agitation, increased respiratory difficulty and cyanosis. Only after transfer to a different hospital at 11 days was this intermittent dyspnea correlated with the complete nasal obstruction of bilateral choanal atresia. The diagnosis was suggested by inability to force a catheter through the nares into the pharynx and was verified by x-ray film after instillation of Lipiodol.

## REFERENCES

Cohen, H. J., and Witchell, I. S.: Bilateral congenital choanal atresia in newborn. A.M.A. Am. J. Dis. Child. 83:328, 1952.

Erickson, D. J., Lodge, J. L., and Tomsovic, E. J.: Medical management of bilateral choanal atresia. J. Pediatr. 63:561, 1963.

Fearon, B., and Dickson, J.: Bilateral choanal atresia in the newborn. Plan of action. Laryngoscope 9:1487, 1968.

Ferguson, C. F., and Kendig, E. L.: Pediatric Otolaryngology. 2nd ed. Philadelphia, W. B. Saunders Co. 1972, pp. 1002-1112.

Flake, C. G., and Ferguson, C. E.: Congenital choanal atresia in infants and children. Ann. Otol. Rhinol. Laryngol. 73:458, 1964.

Grahne, B., and Kaltiokallio, K.: Congenital choanal atresia and its heredity. Acta Otolaryngol., 62:193, 1966.

McGovern, F. H.: Congenital choanal atresia. Laryngoscope 60:815, 1950.

Phelps, K. A.: Congenital occlusion of choanae. Ann. Otol. Rhinol. Laryngol. 35:143, 1926.

Strome, M.: Differential Diagnosis in Pediatric Otolaryngology. Boston, Little, Brown and Co., 1975.

The term "congenital stridors" is used to include all cases in which a stridulous or crowing noise is made from birth or begins within a few weeks after birth. Stridor is produced when the glottis or trachea is narrowed or deformed, when neighboring structures intrude upon the glottic opening or trachea or when the vocal cords move abnormally. The primary cause may lie within or near the larynx, within the chest or within the central nervous system. A suggested system of classification follows:

    I. Simple congenital laryngeal stridor
   II. Congenital anomalies of larynx or trachea
      A. Laryngeal webs
      B. Laryngeal stenosis
      C. Tracheal stenosis
        1. Congenital hypoplasia
        2. Compression by neighboring structures
  III. Cysts and neoplasms of larynx
  IV. "Neurogenic" stridor
   V. Vocal cord paralysis
  VI. Acquired laryngeal lesions (inflammation, foreign body, trauma, edema)

## SIMPLE CONGENITAL LARYNGEAL STRIDOR

This term we use to designate those instances of stridor in which, because of various clinical characteristics, no serious laryngeal or extralaryngeal lesions are suspected, or in which, if studies are performed, only minor alterations in laryngeal structure or function are discovered.

**INCIDENCE.** The condition is common. Holinger and associates were able to report upon 305 cases gathered in a period of seven years. Every pediatrician encounters one every few months in the course of a practice of average size.

**ETIOLOGY.** There is no complete unanimity of opinion as to the cause of simple congenital stridor. Laryngoscopy generally reveals a larynx that is softer than usual,

which collapses abnormally with inspiration. At times the epiglottis seems at fault, being overlong, curved, even tube-shaped, and drawn into the glottic opening with the indrawn breath. At other times the arytenoids may be loose and flabby or the aryepiglottic folds redundant, and these tissues may sag into the glottis with inspiration. For these reasons the disorder has been also called laryngomalacia, congenital flaccid larynx and inspiratory laryngeal collapse.

A few cases have been associated with micrognathia and a few with pectus excavatum. Innumerable infants with stridor have been diagnosed as having an enlarged thymus and have been treated by irradiation. In practically all these instances the diagnosis was incorrect and the treatment unwarranted.

**DIAGNOSIS.** The onset of noisy respiration is commonly stated to be noted at birth or shortly thereafter. In our experience stridor is rarely heard in the newborn nursery, and when it is heard that early in life, it is more likely to be one of the more serious varieties of the disorder. Simple stridor is usually brought to the attention of the pediatrician at the first monthly checkup, not too infrequently at the second and occasionally as late as four months. The noise is unlike the pharyngeal moist snore. It may at times have the quality of a dry, high-pitched crowing inspiration, though more often it is lower pitched and vibratory or fluttering. The noise is generally confined to the inspiratory phase, but rarely, in severe examples, expiration may also be noisy.

These points are of importance in distinguishing simple stridor from the more serious varieties. Phonation is unimpaired; voice and cry are strong. It is commonly intermittent rather than constant, increasing with excitement and physical activity, diminishing and often disappearing when the infant is at complete rest. It is altered by change of position, being intensified when the infant is supine, ameliorated when prone. Most important of all, although the parents are greatly disturbed by the extraordinarily noisy breathing, the infant himself seems not bothered by it at all. His color remains good, his appetite unimpaired, and his weight curve rises steadily. This is true in spite of the observation that during the periods when stridor is at its height there is usually retraction with inspiration of the suprasternal notch and intercostal spaces and even of the sternum itself. This type of stridor has been convincingly demonstrated radiographically by Dunbar. With the infant in the supine position, horizontal beam lateral views of the neck are made with high speed cine-recording. When stridor is present, antero-inferior dispalcement and vibration of the aryepiglottic folds can be seen on inspiration.

**PROGNOSIS.** Simple congenital stridor usually disappears between 6 months and 1 year of life. It may last longer. We have in our practice two children who became stridulous when excited, one until she was 6 years old, the other until he was 8. The disorder does not carry with it any strong predilection for either upper or lower respiratory tract infections.

**TREATMENT.** No specific treatment is required or indicated. The appearance of stridor within the first month or so demands a leisurely detailed discussion of the problem with the parents. It must be explained that most of these infants suffer from no great abnormality, but that a few of them do. If the child fails to feed properly, if weight does not rise satisfactorily, if his color becomes poor either constantly or in attacks, if his voice does not remain strong or if he appears restless or unhappy, studies should then be made to rule out more serious causes of stridor. Some parents will prefer that such studies be made immediately, and to this there appears to be no valid contraindication. Direct laryngoscopy, and x-ray pictures of the neck to show the larynx and trachea, and of the chest should be sufficient for a start. If the physician is truly suspicious that the stridor is not of the simple kind, he must add to these procedures esophagram, tracheogram, perhaps cine-esophagram, bronchoscopy and bronchogram and, in certain instances, angiocardiogram.

## CONGENITAL LARYNGEAL AND TRACHEAL STENOSES

Under this all-inclusive term are grouped the various anatomic lesions which produce narrowing of the laryngeal airway, including the trachea just beneath the larynx, which may produce stridor at or shortly after birth. They are thrown into this heterogeneous group because the pediatrician cannot hope to differentiate one from the other by simple physical examination owing to the similarity of their symptoms and signs. Differentiation and therapy lie in the domain of the otolaryngologist. The pediatrician should, however, be aware of the various possibilities.

Nabarro has reported a remarkable instance of stridor from birth in which there was extensive calcification of laryngeal and tracheal cartilages.

### LARYNGEAL WEBS

Webs are usually glottic in location; i.e., they obstruct at the level of the true vocal cords, but they may be supraglottic or subglottic. They may be small, connecting only the anterior ends of the cords, or they may cover the entire glottic chink. In the first instance symptoms may be lacking; in the second, respiratory difficulty is great.

**ETIOLOGY.** Webs arise in the seventh to tenth week of gestation. At this time the larynx is developing from the floor of the pharynx and from outgrowths of the third, fourth and fifth branchial arches, around the stem of the trachea. Like many other embryologic lumens, the stoma which originally opens from the floor of the pharynx into the trachea becomes fused by epithelial ingrowth. After a few weeks this obliteration is dissolved and the lumen is re-established. Incomplete recanalization of the primitive laryngeal airway results in web formation.

**INCIDENCE.** Although laryngeal webs are well recognized, and Holinger has reported 32 in a series of 866 patients with laryngeal abnormalities, his experience is that of a laryngologist to whom those patients were referred. A pediatrician rarely sees one, since they occur approximately once in 10,000 births.

**DIAGNOSIS.** Symptoms are usually

present at birth, and the degree of symptomatology depends upon the extent of the web. If it is complete, a few gasps may occur before death. If it is partial, in addition to the stridor the cry will be weak or hoarse, and respirations labored. Definitive diagnosis depends on direct laryngoscopy.

**TREATMENT.** Perforation of an obstructing web may be lifesaving. Partial webs may be incised or dilated; tracheostomy may be needed during these procedures until dilatation is adequate.

### CONGENITAL ATRESIA OF THE LARYNX

A few cases of complete obstruction to the airway at birth have been reported. In Holinger's case the entire glottis was encased in a thick fibrous sheet, almost cartilaginous in consistency.

These are of importance only because someone in the delivery room — obstetrician, anesthetist or nurse — must recognize immediately that violent inspiratory effort without resultant air entry distinguishes them from the run-of-the-mill asphyxias of the newborn. Unless an airway can be established immediately, either by producing an aperture in the membrane or by tracheotomy, death in a few minutes is inevitable.

### CONGENITAL SUBGLOTTIC STENOSIS

This group also is rare. Pathologically this condition is extremely variable and difficult to evaluate, consisting as it does of nonspecific thickening of any of the structures beneath the glottis. Obstruction is usually maximal 2 to 3 mm beneath the glottic chink and is almost never inflammatory. In two of Holinger's cases the cricoid cartilage itself seemed deformed, its anteroposterior measurement increased so that it protruded into the airway.

There is stridor from birth unless the stenosis is minimal. In this instance stridor may only follow respiratory infection, the children having repeated attacks of "croup," often with superimposed laryngotracheobronchitis. Since the narrowing is subglottic, the voice is unaffected.

Tracheotomy is often required for severer degrees of stenosis or during inflammatory episodes in the milder ones.

Growth of the larynx with advancing age ameliorates the condition when narrowing is slight, but more advanced stenosis demands repeated dilatations.

### TRACHEAL STENOSIS

Narrowing of the trachea may be either intrinsic or extrinsic. A few cases are on record of extreme *congenital hypoplastic narrowing of the trachea.* They are suspected because of persistent inspiratory difficulty with stridor, present from birth until death. Laryngeal stenosis can be differentiated by the fact that the voice is unimpaired. Diagnosis can be made only by bronchoscopy or tracheography and bronchography. Both because of its extreme rarity and because no definitive treatment is available for this lethal congenital defect, we shall not describe it in detail.

### Tracheal Compression by Neighboring Structures

Both the larynx and the trachea may be narrowed by extrinsic masses. These include tumors of the neck and mediastinal cysts and tumors, which are discussed elsewhere (Chap. 19). Perhaps the most common form of compression of the airway is that produced by a blood vessel which pursues an abnormal course through the mediastinum. Because these are not exceedingly rare and because diagnosis can now be arrived at fairly early in life and definitive treatment may be lifesaving, these are considered in some detail in the following pages.

## ANOMALIES OF THE GREAT VESSELS

Maldevelopment of the aortic arch and malposition of one or more of the great vessels arising from the arch produce important and recognizable clinical syndromes in the infant. Early recognition is of considerable importance, since early surgical correction saves lives and eliminates much serious morbidity. Many minor deviations from the normal in origin and course of intrathoracic arteries go unnoticed because in their anomalous locations they do not impinge upon either the trachea or the esophagus. Neuhauser classified the group as follows:

I. Right aortic arch
    A. With situs inversus viscerum
    B. Without inversion

      1. Anterior type
      2. Posterior type
II. Double aortic arch
III. Anomalous right subclavian artery
IV. Patent ductus arteriosus
V. Coarctation of the aorta

Patent ductus arteriosus and coarctation of the aorta are described in Chapter 23.

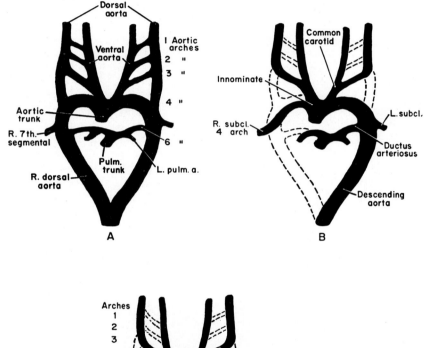

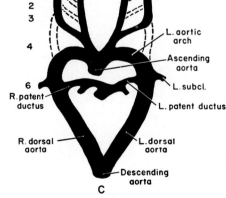

*Figure 8–1.* Normal development of the aortic-arch system includes progressive development as well as regression. Asymmetry is still another characteristic of this normal development. Not all the aortic arches are present simultaneously.

*A*, Primitive pattern consisting of a double aortic arch, right and left patent ductus arteriosus and a midline descending aorta. *B*, The final asymmetrical pattern representing the normal aortic-arch system. A left aortic arch and left patent ductus arteriosus are present. *C*, Failure of regression of either fourth arch, resulting in a persistent double aortic arch. Usually either right or left ductus arteriosus regresses, the aorta descending on either the right or left. In most instances the posterior arch is the larger of the two. A localized area of constriction often represents minimal regressive developmental change. (Blumenthal, S., and Ravitch, M. M.: Pediatrics, *20:*896, 1957.)

The first two conditions listed are discussed here because the symptom-complex they induce is more closely identified with the respiratory and gastrointestinal systems than with the cardiovascular system. Rarer anomalies such as left-sided right subclavian artery, anomalous left common carotid artery, anomalous innominate artery and aberrant or right-sided patent ductus will not be discussed individually.

In addition to the obstructive disorders which arise from anomalies of the aortic arch or one of its branches, one encounters occasional instances in which similar trouble is engendered by aberrant pulmonary arteries.

**ETIOLOGY.** The development of the aortic arch is effected by a complicated series of evolutions of the primitive paired aortic arches. These are clearly illustrated in Figure 8-1.

**INCIDENCE.** The total number of anomalies in this category is large, but only a minority produce symptoms. In the symptomatic group double aortic arch is the commonest malformation. Wolman, in his stimulating report in 1939, was able to find six cases in the literature. One might safely guess that hundreds of cases have come to operation in this country alone since that time. Right aortic arch is also not at all uncommon, but an even larger proportion of these produce no symptoms. They are symptomatic only when a ductus arteriosus or ligamentum arteriosum and another anomalously placed vessel complete the encircling ring.

**DIAGNOSIS.** The symptoms and signs produced depend upon the location of the aberrant vessel or vessels and the degree to which they compromise the esophagus and airway. A combination of respiratory and digestive signs is to be expected in double aortic arch, although respiratory symptoms are distinctly the more prominent. Dyspnea is present from birth or appears within several weeks. Respirations are stridulous in the majority, although in many expiratory wheezing rather than inspiratory stridor is heard. Stridor often persists during sleep and is increased by crying. Cyanosis may be constant or episodic. Feeding is likely to initiate or accentuate stridor and to produce or deepen dyspnea and cyan-

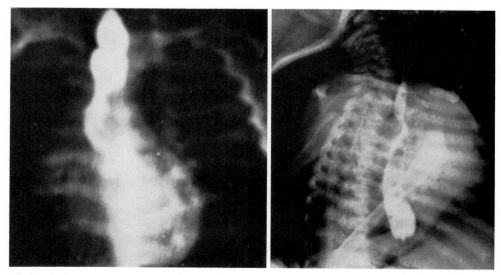

*Figure 8-2.* A, Anteroposterior view of chest with esophagus filled with barium. Smooth indentations can be seen on either side, the deeper one being on the left. B, Lateral view. The esophagus is displaced anteriorly, and there is a deep, smooth indentation of the posterior wall. The combination of A and B is diagnostic of double aortic arch. This infant was dyspneic immediately after spontaneous respiration was established, and vomited; episodes of cyanosis and stridor followed. Wheezes were heard constantly. Stridor became constant after the tenth day. The diagnosis was finally made after two months; operation was performed, and after a stormy postoperative course she recovered completely.

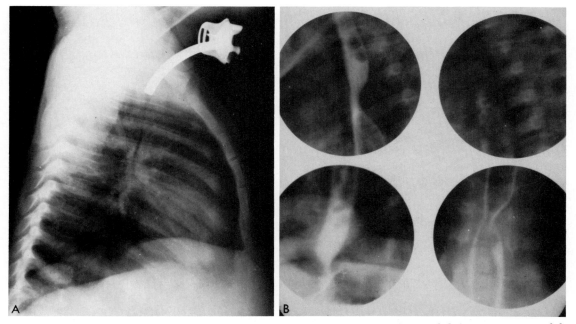

*Figure 8–3.* *A*, Plain lateral view of chest shows a tracheotomy tube in place and definite narrowing of the trachea beneath the lower end of the tube. *B*, Four spot films with barium filling the esophagus show the deep indentation of the posterior margin (upper left) and the compression patterns of the right and left borders, the one on the left being deeper than that on the right.

This case history is not abstracted in the text. Stridor was present from birth, feedings were taken poorly and often vomited, and feeding usually increased stridor. Repeatedly respiratory infections produced croupy dyspnea diagnosed as laryngotracheobronchitis. In one of these attacks the patient had to be tracheotomized. At operation a double aortic arch was found, as expected, and one limb was resected. Unfortunately the patient died within the immediate postoperative period.

osis. Food offered by nipple is often taken poorly and may be regurgitated. Vomitus may contain fresh or altered blood. Feeding may also stimulate paroxysmal cough. All signs are aggravated by the respiratory infections which repeatedly plague these infants. During these infections breathing may be exceedingly difficult and "croupy," suggesting that caused by acute laryngotracheobronchitis. *Severely affected babies prefer to lie with the head sharply retracted, and flexion of the neck exaggerates dyspnea.* The cough is characteristically brassy or bitonal.

Right aortic arch per se produces no or few symptoms. Rarely, as it turns to the right instead of the left, it may impinge upon the trachea or it may compress the bronchi to any of the right lung lobes. Compression then results in either atelectasis or emphysema or a combination of these. Trouble most often arises when it forms one limb of a complete vascular ring,

the others comprised of a patent ductus arteriosus or ligamentum arteriosum and a pulmonary artery or an anomalous left carotid or left subclavian artery. When a constricting vascular ring is present, it is clinically indistinguishable from double aortic arch.

The most common anomaly in the course of a single vessel involves the left subclavian, which arises from the right side of the arch and crosses to the left. Usually it courses behind the esophagus, infrequently between the esophagus and the trachea or, rarely indeed, in front of the trachea. Symptoms, if present, are apt to be restricted to dysphagia, but if one of the two less usual courses is followed, respiration may also be involved.

Respiratory symptoms in the absence of esophageal symptoms should suggest compression of the trachea by an anomalous innominate artery. Signs and symptoms may not be present at birth, but may become more severe in the first months of life and subside thereafter. Episodic apnea, limpness and cyanosis may occur in this condition, as in other forms of tracheal compression from aberrant vessels.

**RADIOGRAPHIC DIAGNOSIS.** Localized atelectasis or emphysema in the newborn, if persistent, should make one consider vascular compression of a major bronchus as a possible cause. Visualization of the trachea in plain posteroanterior and lateral films at times reveals narrowing above the carina plus displacement in either the sagittal or horizontal plane. The most fruitful diagnostic procedure is the barium swallow cineradiographic examination, which demonstrates abnormalities in esophageal contour. High kilovoltage films will improve the contrast between air and soft tissues and aid in identification of tracheal compression.

Neuhauser summarized his vast experience in this field in 1946. He pointed out that right aortic arch might be suspected in the plain anteroposterior film if the aortic arch was observed to lie to the right, if the "knob" on the left was absent, and if the trachea was deviated to the left. Esophagram reveals a rounded indentation into the right border of the esophagus, but none on the left or on the anterior or posterior face. Double aortic arch is characterized by narrowing and anterior displacement of the trachea, seen in the plain lateral film. When the esophagus is filled with barium, it is seen to be displaced forward by a rounded, pulsating mass. Spot films show constriction from both sides and, in the lateral view, deep indentation both in front and in back. An anomalous right subclavian artery taking its usual course from left to right produces an oblique defect in the posterior aspect of the esophagus about 0.5 cm wide and 3 to 4 cm long.

Contrast tracheograms and angiograms are indicated in those instances in which plain films and esophagrams have not sufficed to establish the suspected diagnosis. They are also useful to the surgeon by indicating whether the anterior or the posterior arch is the smaller one, hence the one he will wish to ligate. His choice of incision may be determined by this information.

**PROGNOSIS.** The outlook varies with the degree of tracheal obstruction, the nature of the anomaly and the treatment given. Infants symptomatic early must be observed carefully, since tightness of the ring often increases with growth. Sudden death may occur. Lower respiratory tract infections are common, some pneumonic, most resembling severe laryngotracheobronchitis. After operative correction one expects stridor to persist for many months even though dyspnea has been relieved promptly.

**TREATMENT.** Successful surgical correction, pioneered by Gross, has been accomplished in all types of vascular ring anomalies. Operative risk is still not inconsiderable, especially for double aortic arch. In selecting the proper time for operation this risk must be balanced against the degree of respiratory difficulty. If this is severe from the start, surgery is indicated in the neonatal period. If one can wait, one does, but each respiratory infection must be treated with antimicrobial agents both early and vigorously.

The most common problem in the postoperative period is the persistence of respiratory distress after division of the obstructing vessel. The failure of the trachea to resume normal dimensions may result from hypoplastic segments of trachea, and these may require further operative intervention. Vasko and Ahn have reported the use of autologous rib as a tracheal splint for symptomatic tracheomalacia. Tracheostomy may be necessary in some situations.

## CASE HISTORIES

### CASE 8–1

A white male infant weighing 8 pounds 4 ounces (3745 gm) was born to a primiparous mother after an uneventful pregnancy and labor. The baby breathed promptly and seemed quite well. At 8 hours a nurse noted that he was breathing with a little difficulty and that his color was dusky. Examined at 15 hours, his chest was emphysematous, and inspiration was accompanied by stridor and retraction and expiration by audible wheezes. The note was hyperresonant throughout, breath sounds were somewhat diminished, and inspiratory rales and expiratory wheezes and rhonchi were heard everywhere. The heart seemed normal in size and sound. Though he was placed in humidified ox-

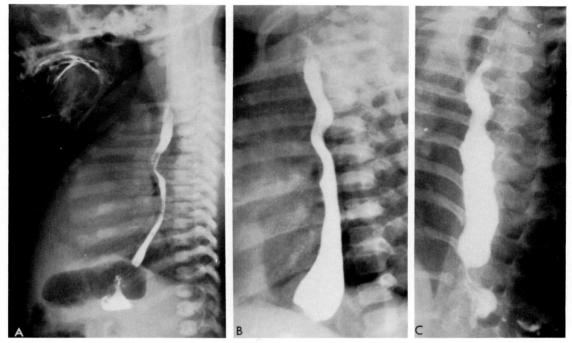

*Figure 8–4.* *A,* Lateral view of chest taken after a barium swallow had filled the esophagus. At the junction of the upper and middle thirds the esophagus is displaced anteriorly, and its lumen is narrowed. *B,* Spot film of same patient taken in an oblique position. A deeper posterior and shallower and longer anterior compression can be distinguished. *C,* Another spot film taken in a more nearly anteroposterior projection. Now the compressions can be seen on both sides, deeper on the left than on the right, produced by a right aortic arch and a fibrous band.

ygen and given Achromycin by mouth, his condition worsened over the next 12 hours, and he was transferred to the Harriet Lane Home. Here an x-ray film showed a huge heart almost filling the entire chest. The sounds were fairly strong, the rate rapid but regular, and no murmurs were heard. Soon the liver edge descended, and dyspnea and wheezing increased. His head was held retracted. He was digitalized over the next 12 hours and kept in humidified oxygen. Much to our surprise he came out of his heart failure, and over the next 10 days his heart rapidly returned to normal size. Inspiratory stridor, expiratory wheeze and head retraction persisted. An esophagram done because of persistence of these signs showed unmistakable evidence of a constricting vascular ring (Fig. 8–4).

He was discharged from hospital on the eleventh day on maintenance oral doses of digitalis. At home he did well except that inspiratory stridor, expiratory wheeze and head retraction persisted. These were all accentuated during an upper respiratory tract infection at 6 months. At 7 months he was readmitted for operation, which was performed by Dr. Henry Bahnson. A vascular ring was found, composed of a right aortic arch, a fibrous band running

from the origin of the left subclavian artery to the posterior portion of the right arch and an obliterated ductus arteriosus pulling the pulmonary artery backward. These two were divided. The constriction was obviously relieved. One month later stridor and wheeze were diminished, head retraction was gone. By the age of 10½ months nothing abnormal was noted except a hint of hoarseness on crying.

**COMMENT.** This extraordinary infant had cardiac asthma about 8 hours after birth. After heart failure had been overcome, persistent stridor, wheezing and head retraction suggested vascular ring. This was demonstrated by esophagram, and the constriction was relieved at 7 months of age. Stridor and wheezing persisted about 5 weeks, then rapidly diminished.

CASE 8–2

A white female infant was said to have been born after normal pregnancy and labor, to have breathed and cried promptly and to have been quite well until 3 weeks of age. At this time cyanosis of the face was noted when she cried; then respirations became labored, and paroxysmal cough appeared, accompanied by low fever. Symptomatic treatment was ineffective, and at 7 weeks of age she was admitted to a local hospital. There findings' led to diagnoses of atelectasis of the left upper lobe, pneumonitis, and congenital heart disease, a long, loud, blowing systolic murmur having been heard over the entire precordium. In spite of vigorous antibiotic therapy two episodes of high fever with generalized crackling rales punctuated this admission.

She was transferred to the Harriet Lane Home

at the age of 7 months. She was small and poorly nourished, decidedly tachypneic, with suprasternal, supraclavicular and subcostal retraction. Temperature was 40° C, pulse 140, respirations 100 per minute. Percussion note was dull in the left axilla and back, breath sounds were diminished throughout the left lung field, and many fine rales were audible over the left upper lobe. A soft apical systolic murmur was heard; the second pulmonary sound was accentuated and split. The rest of the examination was negative. Hemoglobin was 15.5 gm, white blood cell count 19,000, with 57 per cent polymorphonu-

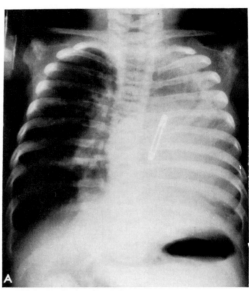

*Figure 8–5.* A, Anteroposterior view of chest showing (1) emphysema of the right lung, (2) herniation of the right upper lobe into the left upper hemithorax, (3) dislocation of heart and mediastinal contents far to the left, and (4) contraction and virtual absence of air-containing lung in the left hemi-thorax. This picture strongly suggests left pulmonary agenesis. B, Two weeks later the picture has changed considerably. Emphysema of the right lung has diminished, and the herniation has disappeared. The heart has moved a little closer to the midline, although still dislocated to the left, and there is air-containing lung clearly visible along the left lateral chest wall. C, Bronchogram shows almost complete obstruction of the left major bronchus. An anomalous pulmonary artery and patent ductus arteriosus were found to be responsible for the obstruction and atelectasis.

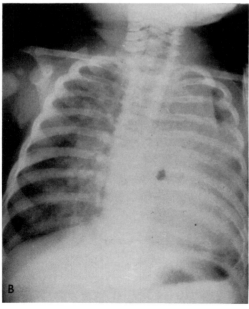

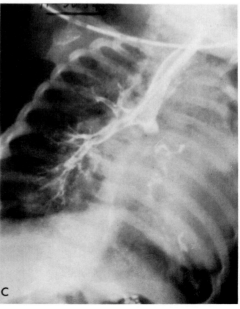

clears, platelets numerous. Tuberculin test result was negative. Electrocardiogram showed a balanced axis, right ventricular hypertrophy and a T wave abnormality.

The original anteroposterior film of the chest showed opacification of the left hemithorax, emphysema of the right lung with herniation into the left upper hemithorax and displacement of the heart and mediastinum to the left (Fig. 8–5A). It was highly suggestive of left pulmonary agenesis. After vigorous treatment with tetracycline the temperature became normal.

Further studies were made. Stool enzymes were normal. Cardiac catheterization revealed right ventricular and pulmonary artery hypertension, but it was not certain that this was not secondary to pulmonary disease. Angiocardiogram was interpreted as showing atrial septal defect. A repeat x-ray examination 2 weeks after the first ruled out pulmonary agenesis (Fig. 8–5B). The emphysema of the right lung had diminished, herniation being no longer seen; the heart and mediastinum had shifted back toward the right, although not reaching their normal position, and the left lung was seen to be air-containing. Bronchograms were then taken which showed almost complete obstruction to the left main bronchus (Fig. 8–5C).

Operation was performed by Dr. Alfred Blalock. The left lung was almost completely atelectatic and contained much boggy secretion. The pulmonary artery was large, and there was a large patent ductus arteriosus. The left pulmonary artery was small and ran an anomalous course. The left main bronchus was constricted 1 cm beyond the carina between the patent ductus and the aberrant left pulmonary artery. Left pneumonectomy and ligations of the ductus were carried out.

Postoperative course was uneventful.

COMMENT. This fascinating case puzzled us in the first instance by its striking resemblance to left pulmonary agenesis. Even now, as we look at the original film, we find it difficult to avoid this diagnosis. Probably the suggestion of air-containing lung visible at the left costophrenic angle should have warned us that complete agenesis could not have been present. The change in the appearance of the lungs 2 weeks later clarified this point. We were also disinclined to credit the story of a loud, long systolic murmur having been heard 5 months before in another hospital, since we never heard more than a soft, low-pitched, short apical blow. We ourselves were never convinced until the broncho-gram was made that an abnormal vessel was responsible for the atelectasis of the left lung. Once we had seen the bronchogram, of course, no further doubt could be entertained. No stridor was heard in this example because obstruction was not to the trachea, but to a major bronchus.

Welsh and Munro encountered congenital stridor caused by an aberrant pulmonary artery which coursed between the trachea and esophagus.

## CYSTS AND NEOPLASMS OF THE LARYNX

*Cysts* arise either from one of the three branchial arches concerned in the development of the larynx or, as retention cysts, from its lining mucous membrane. Laryngoceles may simulate true cysts in both appearance and symptomatology, but these are encountered only rarely in infancy.

The presenting signs of cyst are hoarseness, muffled voice or aphonia plus stridor. Onset is usually at birth, but may be delayed weeks or months. Severity of dyspnea depends upon the size of the cyst. Diagnosis rests upon laryngoscopy.

Treatment is carried out through the laryngoscope and consists in either aspiration or resection. Tracheotomy is indicated for some patients until respiratory obstruction can be controlled. External operative approach is seldom required.

A limited variety of *tumors* has been discovered to involve the larynx. The angioma group, including hemangioma, lymphangioma and hemangioendothelioma, has supplied the greatest number. Some of the hemangiomas have been limited to the larynx, but in others laryngeal tumor was part of a widespread angiomatous involvement of the face, neck and pharynx. Fibrosarcomas of the larynx and trachea have been reported, as has a neurofibroma which at autopsy proved to be but one of many such new growths scattered throughout the body.

Tumors of neighboring structures such as cystic hygroma of the neck, thyroglossal duct cyst or aberrant thyroid at the base of the tongue, and congenital goiter often produce dyspnea, but seldom cause stridor.

Treatment of laryngeal tumor depends

upon its histologic characteristics. Remarkable regression in cutaneous hemangiomas occurs after 1 to 2 weeks of steroid therapy, in the dose range of prednisone, 2 to 3 mg per kilogram per day. Laryngeal hemangiomas sometimes respond to oral corticosteroid therapy within a few days, and usually by 10 days. Tracheostomy may be necessary for control of dyspnea until these definitive measures are undertaken.

## NEUROGENIC STRIDOR

It has been suspected for a long time that certain examples of stridor might be initiated by some aberration in nervous control of the larynx. Thus Schwartz wrote of an "overzealous reflex of laryngeal closure during the threatening experience of regurgitation." Allen, Towsley and Wilson elaborated on this problem in a beautifully comprehensive study of the literature plus a careful investigation of four instructive case histories of their own. They came to the conclusion, impossible to gainsay from the evidence presented, that episodes of stridor coupled with apnea and cyanosis, often hazardous to life, may be precipitated by a neurogenic mechanism. This differs from idiopathic epilepsy by the fact that the stimulus is an identifiable, localizable trigger mechanism, such as nipple feeding, regurgitation or tactile stimulation of the esophagus or larynx. In one of their cases carotid sinus pressure induced heart block. This child was greatly improved by administration of atropine. In their first patient, in whom attacks of stridor, apnea and cyanosis precipitated by bottle feeding were at times followed by convulsion, the electroencephalogram was distinctly abnormal. Anticonvulsant therapy (phenytoin and phenobarbital) not only put an end to attacks, but also quickly improved the electroencephalographic tracing.

This syndrome is particularly frequent following repair of tracheo-esophageal stricture. We have ourselves encountered one infant in whom bougienage for stricture subsequent to this operation induced complete heart stoppage. The two mechanisms must not be dissimilar.

Allen and coworkers conclude that avoidance of esophageal stimulation at the one end (gavage rather than nipple feeding), depression of the cerebrum at the other (anticonvulsive therapy) or breaking the reflex arc at the level of the vagus nerve (atropine) are effective methods of combatting attacks of neurogenic stridor.

## PARALYSIS OF VOCAL CORDS

**INCIDENCE.** The literature abounds with reports of vocal cord paralysis in adults, but few cases have been reported in the newborn. That it is not an extreme rarity is attested to by the fact that we saw two such cases within 2 years.

**ETIOLOGY.** Paralysis may be bilateral or unilateral. When bilateral, it is almost invariably central in origin and nature, producing spastic palsy. In the newborn, birth trauma involving the brain stem seems to be the only important etiological factor.

Unilateral palsies are peripheral and flaccid and are almost always left-sided, although a few right-sided ones are met. The left-sided variety predominates for two reasons: (1) because the recurrent laryngeal nerve on that side arises lower in the neck and its course is therefore longer, and (2) because it loops around the aorta from front to back before ascending alongside the trachea. It is thus susceptible to injury by dilatation of the aorta or by this vessel's displacement by enlargement of the conus or of nearby chambers of the heart. A few cases are caused by pressure upon the nerves by mediastinal tumors.

**DIAGNOSIS.** Hoarseness or aphonia is present, depending upon the type and degree of paralysis. Stridor almost invariably is heard, inspiratory in time, and often associated with deep thoracic retraction. Laryngoscopic inspection is required in order to differentiate the stridor of vocal cord paralysis from that due to laryngeal stenosis. Concomitant signs of congenital heart disease or mediastinal tumor may or may not be elicited.

**PROGNOSIS.** The outcome depends entirely upon the basic disorder. Central paralyses commonly disappear with the subsidence of edema or absorption of blood within the cranial cavity. Palsies caused by pressure will persist until pressure is relieved.

**TREATMENT.** This is directed toward discovery and, if possible, relief of the basic disorder. The finding of unilateral vocal cord paralysis calls for careful study of the mediastinal contents and includes fluoroscopy, x-ray films, barium swallow films and often angiocardiography.

# REFERENCES

Allen, R. J., Towsley, H. A., and Wilson, J. L.: Neurogenic stridor in infancy. A.M.A. Am. J. Dis. Child. 87:179, 1954.

Ardran, G. M., and Kemp, F. H.: The mechanism of changes in form of the cervical airway in infancy. Med. Radiogr. Photogr., 44:26, 1968.

Baker, D. C., Jr.: Congenital disorders of the larynx. N.Y. J. Med., 54:2458, 1954.

Berdan, W. E., Baker, D. H., et al.: Innominate artery compression of the trachea in infants with stridor and apnea. Radiology 92:272, 1969.

Blumenthal, S., and Ravitch, M. M.: Seminar on aortic vascular rings and other anomalies of the aortic arch. Pediatrics 20:896, 1957.

Bradham, R. R., Sealy, W. C., and Young, W. G.: Respiratory distress associated with anomalies of the aortic arch. Surg. Gynecol. Obstet. 126:9, 1968.

Butz, R. O.: Length and cross-section growth patterns in the human trachea. Pediatrics 42:336, 1968.

Campbell, J. S., Wiglesworth, F. W., Latorroca, R., et al.: Congenital subglottic hemangiomas of larynx and trachea. Pediatrics 22:727, 1958.

Clerf, L. H.: Unilateral vocal cord paralysis. J.A.M.A. 151:900, 1953.

Dunbar, J. S.: Upper respiratory tract obstruction in infants and children. Am. J. Roentgenol. 109:227, 1970.

Fearon, B., and Shortreed, R.: Tracheobronchial compression by congenital cardiovascular anomalies in children. Syndrome of apnea. Ann. Otol. Rhinol. Laryngol. 72:949, 1963.

Ferguson, C. F.: Congenital abnormalities of the infant larynx. Otol. Clin. N. Am., 3:185, 1970.

Fost, N. C., and Esterly, N.: Successful treatment of juvenile hemangiomas with prednisone. J. Pediatr. 72:351, 1968.

Glaser, J., Landau, D. B., and Heatly, C. A.: Subglottic laryngeal stenosis in infancy. Am. J. Dis. Child. 50:1203, 1935.

Gross, R. E., and Neuhauser, E. B. D.: Compression of the trachea or esophagus by vascular anomalies: Surgical therapy in 40 cases. Pediatrics 7:69, 1951.

Holinger, P. H., Johnston, K. C., and Schiller, F.: Congenital anomalies of the larynx. Ann. Otol. Rhinol. Laryngol. 63:581, 1954.

Holinger, P. H., Johnston, K. C., and Zoss, A. R.: Tracheal and bronchial obstruction due to congenital cardiovascular anomalies. Ann. Otol. Rhinol. Laryngol. 57:808, 1948.

Holinger, P. H., Schild, J. A. and Weprin, L.: Pediatric laryngology. Otol. Clin. N. Am., 3:625, 1970.

Holinger, P. H., Slaughter, D. P., and Novak, F. J., III: Unusual tumors obstructing the lower respiratory tract of infants and children. Trans. Am. Acad. Ophthal. 54:223, 1949-50.

Hudson, P.: Congenital web of larynx. A.M.A. Am. J. Dis. Child. 81:545, 1951.

Keleman, G.: Congenital laryngeal stridor. A.M.A. Arch. Otolaryngol., 58:245, 1953.

Loeb, W. J., and Smith, E. E.: Airway obstruction in a newborn by pedunculated pharyngeal dermoid. Pediatrics 40:20, 1967.

Mercer, R. D.: Laryngeal stridor with temporary cardiac and respiratory arrest. Am. J. Dis. Child. 70:336, 1945.

Morrison, L. F.: Recurrent laryngeal nerve paralysis; A revised conception based on the dissection of one hundred cadavers. Ann. Otol. Rhinol. Laryngol. 61:567, 1952.

Nabarro, S.: Calcification of the laryngeal and tracheal cartilages associated with congenital stridor in an infant. Arch. Dis. Child. 27:185, 1952.

Neuhauser, E. B. D.: The roentgen diagnosis of double aortic arch and other anomalies of the great vessels. Am. J. Roentgenol. 56:1, 1946.

Sayre, J. W., and Hall, E. G.: Anomalies of larynx associated with tracheo-esophageal fistula. Pediatrics 13:150, 1954.

Schwartz, A. B.: Functional disorders of the larynx in early infancy. J. Pediatr. 42:457, 1953.

Suchs, O. W., and Powell, D. B.: Congenital cysts of the larynx in infants. Laryngoscope 77:654, 1967.

Vasko, J. S., and Ahn, C.: Surgical management of secondary tracheomalacia. Ann. Thorac. Surg. 6:269, 1968.

Welsh, T. M., and Munro, J. B.: Congenital stridor caused by aberrant pulmonary artery. Arch. Dis. Child. 29:101, 1954.

Wilson, T. G.: Some observations on the anatomy of the infantile larynx. Acta Otolaryngol. 43:95, 1953.

Wolman, I. J.: Syndrome of constricting double aortic arch in infancy; Report of a case. J. Pediatr. 14:527, 1939.

# TRACHEOESOPHAGEAL FISTULA
# AND
# ESOPHAGEAL ATRESIA

Both esophageal atresia and tracheoesophageal fistula are encountered as separate congenital defects. Each alone is exceedingly rare. More commonly one finds the two associated in a compound defect. The possible varieties are (1) esophageal atresia alone, (2) tracheoesophageal fistula alone, and (3) esophageal atresia with (*a*) upper fistula, (*b*) lower fistula or (*c*) double fistula. Diagrammatically, the principal types are shown in Figure 9–1.

## TRACHEOESOPHAGEAL FISTULA
## WITH ESOPHAGEAL ATRESIA

**INCIDENCE.** Esophageal atresia with tracheoesophageal fistula is by no means rare. There are probably local differences in its frequency depending upon the varying genetic constitution of populations, but these are not likely to be as great as incidences of one to 500 in the Boston area versus one to 10,000 in the Philadelphia area that have been reported. An overall incidence of one in 2500 deliveries is generally accepted. In a recent series of 103 cases, 63 were males, 40 females.

Approximately 85 per cent of the reported cases consist of esophageal atresia with a fistulous connection between the lower esophageal pouch and the trachea. Reflux of gastric contents into the trachea is responsible for the severe pulmonary symptoms.

Although premature births account for 8 per cent of children born in the United States, 34 per cent of infants with esophageal atresia weigh less than 2.5 kg. The proportion of low birth weight infants with esophageal atresia who are undersize for gestational age is not certain.

**ETIOLOGY.** The disorder is due to an error in ontogenetic development which occurs before the eighth week of gestation. It results from the embryologic fact that the trachea develops as an outgrowth from the foregut, and from that portion of the foregut which is destined to become the esophagus. During this complex series of evolutions incomplete separation of the primitive tubes and imperfect recanalization of the esophageal column may occur.

**DIAGNOSIS.** In most cases the newborn infant cries immediately, breathes spontaneously and acquires a healthy pink color. After minutes or a few hours it is noted that inordinate quantities of mucus are accumulating in the pharynx, and these may overflow from the nose and mouth onto bed linen or may be regurgitated. Sooner or later, and in all gradations of severity, respiratory difficulty becomes associated with this embarrassing accumulation of mucus. There may be only mild duskiness with rasping inspiration or expiration, or deep cyanosis may supervene with labored inspiration or expiration. Pharyngeal suction commonly ameliorates this situation for a

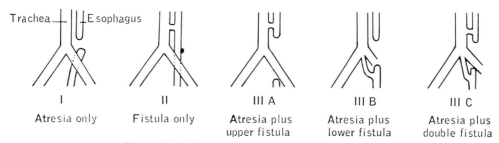

| I | II | III A | III B | III C |
|---|---|---|---|---|
| Atresia only | Fistula only | Atresia plus upper fistula | Atresia plus lower fistula | Atresia plus double fistula |

*Figure 9–1.* Types of tracheoesophageal fistulas.

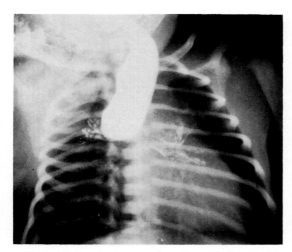

*Figure 9–2.* Anteroposterior view of chest made on the second day of life, after a Lipiodol swallow. A large, dilated upper esophageal pouch ending blindly in midchest can be seen. There is no air in the abdomen, a fact suggesting either that there is no fistula or that, if one is present, it is an upper one. Some Lipiodol has seeped into the lungs, and one can actually see the outlines of a broad fistulous tract coursing to the left of the lower end of the pouch.

time. Attempted feeding causes an exacerbation of respiratory difficulty and is followed by prompt regurgitation of the ingested fluid mixed with much thick mucus. After feedings a previously clear chest may become full of coarse rales and rhonchi.

As one listens to the lungs of some of these infants great variations in air entry may be heard. First one major bronchus and then another becomes plugged, and breath sounds diminish and vanish over large areas for shorter or longer periods. Vigorous pharyngeal or endotracheal suction may reopen the airways. Atelectasis, of the right upper lobe especially, may develop and persist.

This combination of signs, consisting of (1) excessive accumulation of mucus, (2) respiratory difficulty, either persistent or in spells, and (3) regurgitation of all ingested fluids, is pathognomonic of esophageal atresia.

If the abdomen remains flat and airless, one can be certain that no fistula connects the trachea with the lower esophageal pouch. There may be no fistula at all, or the fistula may run from the upper pouch to the trachea. In the latter instance respiratory

difficulty and cough, especially after attempts to feed, are apt to be considerably greater.

If, on the other hand, the abdomen rapidly becomes distended and the intestine fills with air promptly, one can be certain that the defect is the usual one, i.e., esophageal atresia with a fistula connecting the trachea and lower esophageal pouch.

Diagnosis can be confirmed in several ways. A catheter may be passed into the esophagus, where it will meet obstruction a few inches from the mouth. Rarely one may be misled by its easy passage far enough to have reached the stomach, when actually it is coiling in the blind upper pouch. Simultaneous fluoroscopy clarifies this point.

Further confirmation by x-ray film is advisable. A plain roentgenogram may demonstrate clearly the air-filled upper pouch. Instillation of 0.5 cubic centimeters of contrast medium demarcates the pouch more sharply, and may reveal the fistula itself.

The degree of dyspnea varies from case to case. It may be almost nonexistent, perhaps associated with attempts to feed, or it may be severe enough to require tracheostomy.

**TREATMENT.** Treatment should begin with suction to the upper pouch, followed

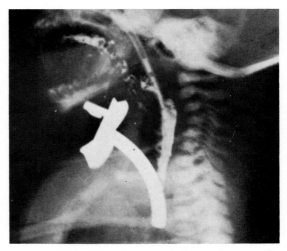

*Figure 9–3.* Lateral view of chest taken on the fourth day of life after Iodochloral had been instilled by nasal catheter into the esophagus. A tracheostomy tube is in place because of unusually severe dyspnea. Dye fills an upper segment which ends blindly about the level of the carina.

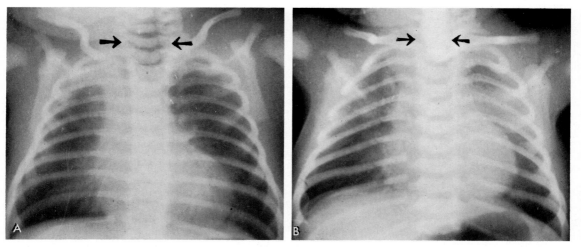

*Figure 9–4.* *A*, Anteroposterior view of chest taken on the first day of life. One can see clearly the blind upper esophageal pouch sharply outlined by its air content. Air within the abdomen bespeaks lower tracheoesophageal fistula. *B*, After instillation of Lipiodol the upper esophageal pouch stands out clearly.

This case is not abstracted in the text. It is included only to point out again that diagnosis may often be made on the basis of plain films alone, without Lipiodol instillation.

by gastrostomy to prevent further reflux of gastric contents into the lung. Repair of the fistula and esophagus should be undertaken whenever the infant's general condition permits it. Pneumonia is inevitable, but is minimal and reversible when the period of gross infection is brief. Pneumonia was found in all nine of the infants who did not survive operation in the series of Grow and Neerken.

The operation of choice is division of the fistula and end-to-end anastomosis of the esophageal ends, successfully performed first by Cameron Haight. When this procedure cannot be carried out because of excessive distance between the upper and lower pouches, various alternatives remain. One of these is transplantation of a portion of colon to form a continuous tube between the upper and lower segments. An alternative approach is elongation of the proximal pouch by periodic bougienage over a period of 1 to 3 months. Sometimes a tube can be fashioned from the greater curvature of the stomach. Replacement procedures are usually deferred until 6 months to 1 year of age.

Postoperative care consists in adequate antibiotic treatment directed toward the pulmonary infection and careful protection of the anastomotic site. This means that nothing is to be taken by mouth for approx-

imately 7 to 10 days. Hydration, proper electrolyte balance and caloric intake can be maintained by gastrostomy feedings, supplemented at first by intravenous fluids. Most authorities agree that it is safer to err a little on the side of underhydration rather than of overhydration. A daily total quota of 75 ml. per kilogram of body weight of intravenous fluids should suffice.

**PROGNOSIS.** Prognosis depends upon several factors. Prematures do less well than large, mature infants. Babies diagnosed and operated upon early do better than those who come to surgery late. This difference results from the better state of hydration and blood chemical balance of the younger infant as well as from the fact that pulmonary infection is less deeply seated. There is little excuse in our present state of knowledge for gastrostomy to be

*TABLE 9–1.* **Anatomical Incidence and Survival Rate**

| Anomaly | Number of Patients | Number of Survivors |
|---|---|---|
| Esophageal atresia without TEF | 82 | 46 (56%) |
| Esophageal atresia with proximal TEF | 9 | 5 (56%) |
| Esophageal atresia with proximal and distal TGF | 7 | 5 (71%) |
| Esophageal atresia with distal TEF | 916 | 559 (61%) |
| TEF without atresia | 44 | 30 (68%) |

**TABLE 9–2.** *Associated Anomalies*

| Type of Anomaly | Number of Patients | Number of Survivors |
|---|---|---|
| None | 478 | 373 (78%) |
| Congenital heart disease | 171 | 37 (22%) |
| Imperforate anus | 88 | 38 (43%) |
| Genitourinary malformations | 98 | 22 (22%) |
| Intestinal atresia | 30 | 4 (13%) |

Data of Holder et al. Pediatrics 34:542, 1964.

delayed beyond the second day of life. Emergency gastrostomy is a vital first step; definitive repair can be delayed until the infant's condition improves. The third variable factor is the skill of the operator and of the teams supplying preoperative and postoperative care. These differences are reflected in various reports. Haight, the originator of direct anastomosis, and Leven, who was able to report 68 personal cases of primary closure, achieved survival rates slightly in excess of 60 per cent. In a sur-

vey of experience from many pediatric centers 1958–1962, Holder et al. confirmed a similar overall survival rate (Table 9–1). A major determinant of outcome is the presence of associated anomalies. Holder et al. surveyed their own experiences and that of their colleagues with the results shown in Table 9–2.

Almost all the infants who die have widespread bronchial pneumonia. Leakage from the anastomotic site is responsible for mediastinitis and a stormy postoperative course in a high percentage of the unsuccessful cases. Most of these problems can be managed by prolonged tube drainage of the thorax, and nutritional support with intravenous alimentation. By far the most common complication is the development of stricture at the operative site. When this is severe, one may be forced to resort to bougienage, but there is general agreement that the hazards of instrumental dilatation warrant great care with this procedure.

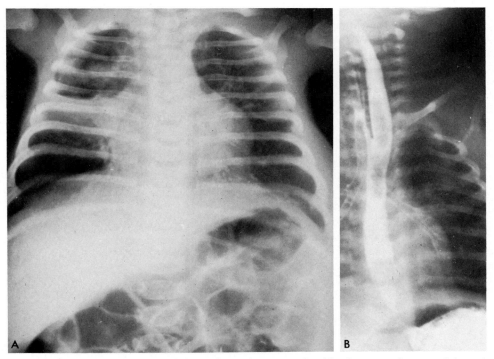

**Figure 9–5.** *A*, Anteroposterior view of chest of an infant 6 months old. There is atelectasis of the right middle lobe, hyperinflation of the right lower lobe and some patchy opacification elsewhere. *B*, Spot film taken after barium swallow outlines the esophagus and a fistula of large caliber coursing from it upward toward the trachea. A faint bronchogram is visible. There is no atresia or stenosis of the esophagus.

A tracheoesophageal fistula without esophageal atresia was found at autopsy. (The films were obtained for us by Dr. Thomas D. Michael of Baltimore.).

## TRACHEOESOPHAGEAL FISTULA WITHOUT ESOPHAGEAL ATRESIA

The defect of single or multiple fistulas alone is rare indeed. Only 1 to 3 per cent of fistulas are unassociated with esophageal atresia. Gross found the compound defect to be 60 times, Haight 30 times, as frequent as the solitary one. Although most of the fistulas are somewhere near the carina, a few have been reported in the neck. Multiple fistulas without atresia are very rare, but have been reported by Rehbein in 1964 and by Eckstein and Somasundaram in 1966.

**DIAGNOSIS.** In 1951 Helmsworth and Pryles felt that the clinical picture was so conclusive that surgical treatment could be undertaken without x-ray confirmation. As slightly modified by Herweg and Ogura, the criteria include (1) coughing, choking and cyanosis immediately after ingesting fluids, (2) no difficulty in swallowing, the distress occurring a few seconds later, (3) clear lung fields becoming full of coarse rales and rhonchi after swallowing, (4) absence of symptoms after gavage feeding, and (5) gastric distention after crying, straining and coughing.

We insist on confirmation of the diagnosis by cineradiographic studies or endoscopy before surgery is undertaken. The contrast material should be injected through a feeding tube inserted into the esophagus at different levels to permit filling of a small fistula, which often attaches to the trachea cephalad to its level in the esophagus.

**TREATMENT.** Once the diagnosis has been made, surgery offers the only possibility of cure. The operation is comparatively simple, exposure and ligation of the fistulous tract being all that is required. The approach is usually through the neck; thoracotomy is rarely indicated.

## TRACHEOESOPHAGEAL FISTULA WITH A LARGE ESOPHAGEAL DIVERTICULUM

Sir Douglas Robb described an interesting variant of the previously described congenital developmental defects involving the trachea and esophagus together. In his

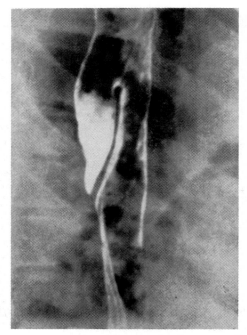

*Figure 9–6.* Roentgenogram after barium swallow, showing diverticulum before operation. The fistula is not demonstrated. (Robb, D.: Austr. N. Zeal. J. Surg. 22:120, 1952.)

case there was a fistulous connection between foodway and airway, and instead of an atretic esophagus, there was a large diverticulum at the same level. An abstract of his case follows.

### CASE 9–1

"This 11 year old boy had had attacks of choking from birth. After a meal he would cough, choke, become blue, having to be watched day and night. Sitting him up and patting his back helped. Attacks became less frequent and less severe with advancing age, and he learned to manage them himself. He developed and gained satisfactorily.

"At the age of 5 years the diverticulum was visualized by x-ray and a fistulous connection was suspected. The diverticulum was demonstrated again on this admission but on neither occasion was the fistula seen (Fig. 9–6). At operation a bulky esophagus was seen and a line of demarcation could be recognized dividing the main lumen from the pouch. This measured 3.5 cm in length. About 1 cm. above the junction of esophagus and pouch a dimple was seen through which a probe could be passed upward for 3 or 4 cm. This fistula was divided and ligated and the pouch was excised. Convalescence was uneventful and a barium swallow film taken 3 weeks later showed a normal esophagus."

**COMMENT.** This case report is included even though the child was 11 years old by the time definitive treatment was carried out. The defect was clearly a congenital one and might have been repaired when the lad was much younger.

## LARYNGOTRACHEOESOPHAGEAL CLEFT

A midline communication between the posterior laryngeal wall and the esophagus presents with the same symptoms as an H-type tracheoesophageal fistula. This rare congenital defect may be very difficult to diagnose either by direct vision or radiographically, but careful endoscopy and repeated contrast studies may reveal the cleft. According to Burroughs and Leape, 34 such infants had been described in the literature by 1974, with nine survivors, all of whom had had operative repair with tracheostomy. Our patient with a cleft survived without operation, requiring nasogastric tube feedings to prevent aspiration for the first three months of life. Thereafter he had no difficulty with swallowing, aspiration or phonation. A more severe form of this rare anomaly is a persistent esophagotrachea, such as described by Griscom, which is not compatible with life.

## REFERENCES

Avery, M. E., and Fletcher, B. D.: The Lung and Its Disorders in the Newborn Infant. Philadelphia, W. B. Saunders Co., 1974.

Bond-Taylor, W., Starer, F., and Atwell, J. D.: Vertebral anomalies associated with esophageal atresia and tracheoesophageal fistula with reference to the initial operative mortality. J. Pediatr. Surg. 8:9, 1973.

Burroughs, N., and Leape, L. L.: Laryngotracheoesophageal cleft: Report of a case successfully treated and review of the literature. Pediatrics 53:516, 1974.

Clatworthy, H. W., Jr.: Esophageal atresia; importance of early diagnosis and adequate treatment illustrated by a series of patients. Pediatrics 16:122, 1955.

Colten, D. H., Middleton, B. W., and Fletcher, J.: Gastric tube esophagoplasty. J. Pediat. Surg. 9:451, 1974.

Eckstein, H. B., and Somasundaram, K.: Multiple tracheoesophageal fistulas without atresia. Report of a case. J. Pediat. Surg. 1:381, 1966.

Ferguson, C. C.: Replacement of the esophagus by colon in infants and children. Can. J. Surg. 13:396, 1970.

Griscom, N. T.: Persistent esophagotrachea: The most severe form of laryngotracheoesophageal cleft. Am. J. Roentgen. 97:211, 1966.

Gross, R. E., and Firestone, F. N.: Colonic reconstruction of the esophagus in infants and children. Surgery 61:995, 1967.

Grow, J. B., and Neerken, A. J.: Esophageal atresia and tracheoesophageal fistula. J.A.M.A. 152:1614, 1953.

Haight, C.: In Leven et al., pp. 717–18.

Helmsworth, J. A., and Pryles, C. V.: Congenital tracheoesophageal fistula without esophageal atresia. J. Pediatr. 38:610, 1951.

Herweg, J. C., and Ogura, J. H.: Congenital tracheoesophageal fistula without esophageal atresia; endoscopic diagnostic technique. J. Pediatr. 47:293, 1955.

Hodge, G. B., and Johnson, G. D.: Congenital esophageal atresia with tracheoesophageal fistula. Am. Surgeon 19:569, 1953.

Holder, T. M., and Ashcraft, K. W.: Esophageal atresia and tracheosophageal fistula. (Collective review). Ann. Thorac. Surg. 9:445, 467, 1970.

Holder, T. M., Cloud, D. T., Lewis, J. E. Jr., et al.: Esophageal atresia and tracheoesophageal fistula. Pediatrics 34:542, 1964.

Kappelman, W. M., Dorst, J., Haller, A., et al.: H-Type tracheoesophageal fistula. Am. J. Dis. Child. 118:568, 1969.

Kraus, M., and White, H.: Congenital tracheo-esophageal fistula in the neck without atresia. J. Pediatr. 51:580, 1957.

Leven, N. L., Varco, R. L., Lannin, B. G., and Tongen, L. A.: The surgical management of congenital atresia of the esophagus and tracheoesophageal fistula. Ann. Surg. 136:701, 1952.

Mahour, G. H., Woolley, M. M., and Gwinn, J. L.: Elongation of the upper pouch and delayed anatomic reconstruction in esophageal atresia. J. Pediatr. Surg. 9:373, 1974.

Rehbein, F.: Esophageal atresia with double tracheoesophageal fistula. Arch. Dis. Child. 39:138, 1964.

Robb, D.: Congenital tracheo-esophageal fistula without atresia but with a large esophageal diverticulum. Aust. N.Z. J. Surg. 22:120, 1952.

Ware, G. W., and Cross, L. L.: Congenital tracheoesophageal fistula without atresia of the esophagus. Pediatrics 14:254, 1954.

Waterston, D. J., Bonham Carter, R. E., and Aberdeen, E.: Congenital tracheo-esophageal fistula in association with oesophageal atresia. Lancet, 2:55, 1963.

By both clinical and pathological evidence, aspiration is one of the most common accidents that affect the lungs of newborn infants. If aspiration occurs before birth, amniotic debris, including squamous epithelial cells, may be found in lungs studied post mortem. If it occurs after premature separation of the placenta, the lungs may be full of maternal blood. Aspiration of infected amniotic sac contents or cervical mucus is a cause of postnatal pneumonia. In infants born after term or after fetal distress for any reason it is not unusual to find meconium-stained amniotic liquid aspirated.

Postnatal aspiration of gastric contents, milk and vitamins is well recognized, and constitutes a danger in depressed infants in particular.

**INCIDENCE.** Considering the many possible times that aspiration may occur, it is not surprising that it remains among the most common causes of respiratory distress in infants. The radiographic features of aspiration were noted by Peterson and Pendleton to occur in 34 infants during the same period in which they discovered 104 infants with the radiographic features of hyaline membrane disease. Meconium was seen in the trachea of 0.5 per cent of infants examined prospectively by Gregory et al.; 20 per cent of their group of meconium-stained infants had pulmonary disease.

**PATHOLOGY.** The lungs of fetuses or infants who have aspirated before or during delivery are firm and poorly aerated and sink in the fixing solution. The bronchi contain fluid or thin mucus. Cut surfaces exude fluid. Under the microscope (Fig. 10–1) many alveoli are collapsed, but others are overexpanded, filled with fluid and, in some instances, squamae and other recognizable amniotic debris. In many, congestion, edema and hemorrhage are prominent. Segments or patches of atelectasis or areas of emphysema, or both, are seen. In a number of the lungs simple emphysema has progressed to one of its more advanced stages. Pleural fluid is found on occasion.

Intracranial hemorrhage, cerebral venous congestion or cerebral edema often coexists. So do petechial hemorrhages and ecchymoses in many other sites.

In many lungs overfilling and distention of pulmonary capillaries are visible, and in a few this finding is striking. Dilatation of the right side of the heart may be obvious.

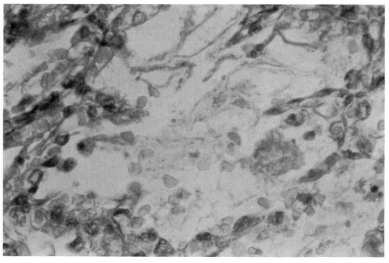

*Figure 10–1.* Section of lung of a 7 pound 8 ounce (3400 gm) full-term infant who died fifteen minutes after birth after having gasped only a few times. Prolonged labor, uterine inertia, stimulation of labor by a Pitocin drip, and finally midforceps extraction characterized his delivery. The microscopic section shows much fluid, debris and many squamae within dilated terminal air spaces. Virtually every section from both lungs looked like this one.

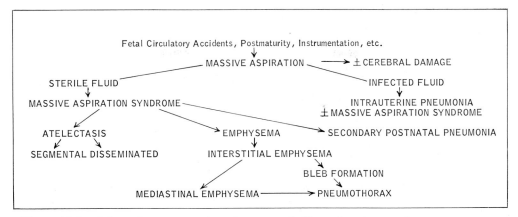

**Figure 10–2.** Schematic representation of causes and effects of aspiration of amniotic contents.

**PATHOGENESIS.** Our tentative concept of the causes and effects of prenatal or perinatal aspiration is schematized in Figure 10–2.

It is generally agreed that conditions tending to produce fetal asphyxia cause the fetus to make deepened respiratory-like movements, or to gasp, in the uterus or birth canal. Such movements have been attributed to anoxia or hypoxia. The vague term "asphyxia" seems to be more desirable in this connection. Accidents responsible include abruptio placentae, premature separation, marginal sinus rupture, sudden maternal hypotension, uterine tetany, cord prolapse, entanglements or tears, indeed any mishap which compromises the circulation of the placenta or of the fetus itself. A second excitant of prenatal gasping may be vigorous manual or instrumental manipulation of the fetus.

Peterson and Pendleton concluded that postmaturity was the most frequent cause of fetal aspiration. We agree completely that it plays an important role. In our own experience postmaturity, or placental insufficiency, as indicated by low birth weight in relation to gestational age, or by the clinical signs detailed in Section I (p. 00), accounts for a large proportion of the cases,

**Figure 10–3.** Anteroposterior view of chest made at ten hours of age in an 8 pound, 8 ounce (3855 gm) male infant, born ten days after his E.D.C. and an uncomplicated labor and delivery. He was covered with thick meconium at birth. He was tachypneic and dyspneic for two days, better on the third day, and well on the fourth day.

Note the intense patchy opacification almost filling the right hemithorax, maximal about the heart shadow, but extending to the periphery in the right middle zone. Some, but much less, is seen on the left side.

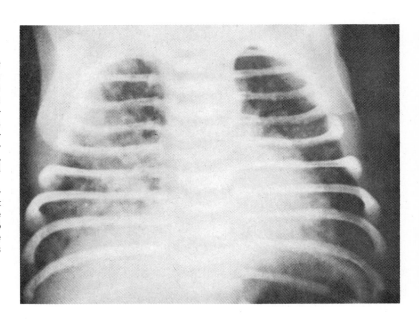

but term infants also suffer from massive aspiration, and premature infants are far from immune to it. Assuming placental insufficiency to be the seat of the trouble in postmature infants, the effect upon the fetus would be that of slow asphyxia rather than the explosive form engendered by circulatory accidents.

When aspiration has occurred in utero, it often follows a period of fetal distress marked by the passage of meconium. Other infants demonstrate clinical features of massive aspiration without having suffered fetal distress. In some of them we have noted that large doses of analgesics have been given the mothers within 2 hours of delivery, and speculate on the possibility of drug-induced loss of mechanisms to prevent aspiration. Second-born twins, infants delivered by the breech and those born after a prolonged second stage of labor are predisposed to aspiration of amniotic and cervical contents.

Postnatal aspiration may occur in depressed infants after gavage feeding, after overfeeding, sometimes in association with swallowing excessive amounts of air and with intestinal obstruction. Infants of low gestational age and birth weight seem particularly prone to aspiration after feedings, and that has been the principal argument for a delay in their first feeding. The benefits to them of adequate fluid and caloric intake probably outweigh the risks of aspiration if care is taken to give feedings frequently in small quantities.

In the event of recurrent aspiration, or whenever coughing or choking occurs with feedings, the possibility of an anatomic defect should be considered. The most common of these is tracheoesophageal fistula, but posterior laryngeal clefts can produce similar symptoms.

A functional cause of recurrent aspiration was described by DeCarlo and others in 1952 and was later labelled "pharyngeal incoordination of infancy." Apparently 10 to 15 per cent of all infants aspirate somewhat during the first days of life, but rarely thereafter. The diagnosis is made by the demonstration of oily contrast medium entering the trachea as well as the esophagus. When pharyngeal incoordination persists, the diagnosis of dysautonomia should be entertained.

**DIAGNOSIS.** Infants who have aspirated in utero may have blood or meconium in the oropharynx and deserve immediate suctioning of pharynx and trachea. They may be profoundly asphyxiated and require intubation, further suction and positive pressure applied to the tube to inflate the lungs. In a series of 20 liveborn infants with aspiration of amniotic sac contents, Schaffer noted that 12 were severely asphyxiated at birth. The physical signs are exceedingly variable, dependent in part on the vigor of the infant and the extent of aspiration. Significant hyperinflation of the chest is usual, with a prominent anterior sternal bulge and depressed diaphragms. Tachypnea is regularly present. Retraction is not uncommon. Dullness to percussion is sometimes present. Coarse rales and rhonchi are usual but not invariable. Continuous production of mucus, occasionally bloody or meconium-stained, is usual.

The course of the illness is also variable. It is most prolonged when the aspirated material contains meconium or is contaminated. The rare death from uninfected aspirate takes place within 24 hours; recovery is usually evident by several days, but in a few instances radiographic changes and tachypnea persist for weeks. Pneumothorax is a recognized complication of meconium aspiration.

**RADIOGRAPHIC FEATURES.** Coarse, irregular densities usually follow the distribution of the bronchial tree. Focal areas of hyperinflation are common, and occasionally the domes of the diaphragm are flattened. Some clearing is usually evident by 24 hours. The lesion is not pathognomonic for aspiration and is indistinguishable from pneumonia and hemorrhage. Persistent air trapping and even pneumatocele formation may be evident for several months.

In the following pages we cite brief case reports, one of a stillborn infant whose lungs contained inordinate amounts of aspirated amniotic debris in order to indicate pathogenetic mechanisms, another of an infant who died after some hours with massive aspiration to point out some aspects of their symptomatology, and, finally, the clinical courses and radiographic appearance of the lungs of infants who seem to fit in the same category, but who survived.

## CASE HISTORIES

### CASE 10–1

A white 25 year old primipara began to bleed slightly 6 days after her estimated due date. Labor began the following day with rupture of the membranes. The fluid was meconium-stained. The mother's urine on admission showed 2-plus albumin. She became fully dilated after 8 hours of labor, after which time the fetal heart sounds became slow and disappeared. Delivery was hastened with forceps and was accomplished 50 minutes after fetal distress had been noted, 6 minutes after fetal heart sounds were last heard. Pregnancy was estimated at 287 days.

The stillborn infant weighed 7 pounds 1 ounce (3215 gm). Her lungs were not air-containing, the pleural surfaces contained scattered focal hemorrhages, and the alveoli were greatly distended with amniotic fluid, debris and squamae. The placenta showed considerable calcification, with hyaline degeneration of the decidual plate.

**COMMENT.** The history of this stillborn infant from the files of the Johns Hopkins Hospital has been selected as illustrative of the problem of stillbirth in general. In this one the fetus was postmature, and placental insufficiency may have been the pathogenetic factor. Others could have been chosen to demonstrate the same pulmonary lesion following cord prolapse, placental separation, prolonged labor due to shoulder dystocia or to difficult instrumental delivery necessitated by macrosomia and other asphyxia-producing accidents. Second, the aspirate which distends terminal air spaces need not contain meconium. Just how much trouble, if any, excess fluid without debris might cause a liveborn infant we cannot say. We know that under normal conditions large quantities of fluid are taken up into the circulation with great rapidity. Nor can we say what the appearance of such a waterlogged lung might be by x-ray examination.

### CASE 10–2

A primiparous 21 year old black girl went into labor on the two hundred ninety-seventh day of her gestation. Her blood pressure rose to 150/100 after the onset of labor and remained high until delivery. The membranes ruptured 1½ hours before delivery, the amniotic fluid being meconium-stained. The fetal heart remained strong and of good rate throughout. The first stage lasted 6 hours, 45 minutes, the second stage 1 hour, 30 minutes.

Birth weight was 7 pounds 12 ounces (3540 gm). The infant was covered with thick meconium. She was pale and limp and made no effort to breathe. The heart rate was 60 per minute. After pharyngeal suction and positive pressure resuscitation the color improved and the heart speeded up. After 10 minutes, when spontaneous respirations were established, she breathed about 40 times a minute, with some retraction. Air entry was fair throughout, and innumerable coarse and fine rales were heard over the entire chest. At 2 hours she was still flaccid, responded but poorly to stimuli and her color was good. Respirations were still shallow, had become more rapid, and an inspiratory wheeze was heard as well as numerous rales. The respiratory rate gradually increased, reaching 120 per minute, but short periods of apnea appeared. Late in the first day she became responsive, then rigid, and then twitchings of the arms and hands were noted. By 12 hours her pulse rate was 132, her respiration rate 115 per minute, her color was gray, her muscle tone generally increased, her head retracted. She died, after her condition had remained essentially unchanged except for repeated generalized convulsions, on the third day.

The placenta showed numerous infarcts. The lungs were the site of massive aspiration of meconium and amniotic debris and of focal hemorrhages. The brain was grossly edematous, with tonsillar herniation and obliteration of the lateral and third ventricles and the aqueduct of Sylvius.

**COMMENT.** This case demonstrates the dual effect upon this fetus of placental insufficiency and prolonged second stage of labor. The brain became intensely edematous to the point of herniation into the foramen magnum. The lungs were the site of massive aspiration. Brain damage led successively to flaccidity and apnea, rigidity, twitching, generalized convulsions. Massive aspiration caused tachypnea, retraction, wheezing. We say this as a statement of fact because less severe cases demonstrate that respiratory signs may be present without cerebral ones.

### CASE 10–3

A 33-week, 2350-gm baby was born to a 35 year old primipara. Presentation was by the breech, and during labor the cord prolapsed. Delivery was accomplished by manual extraction. The amniotic fluid was not meconium-stained, nor was any fetal distress noted. The first breath was taken after 3 minutes. Upon arrival at the nursery her color was good, but she was grunting a bit. She was covered with thick vernix. At 1 hour she was deeply cyanotic and tachypneic and grunted with each expiration. Treated with oxygen, humidity, penicillin and streptomycin, she was better the second day, practically well the third day.

X-ray film taken 4 hours of age showed patchy opacification about the heart and extending outward (Fig. 10–4).

**COMMENT.** This baby was premature by date and weight; she was covered with thick vernix. Prolapsed cord and manual extraction of a breech presentation are more than adequate reasons for massive aspiration. It is well to be reminded that respiratory distress in the premature infant may be caused by several disorders other than hyaline membrane syndrome. It is also clear that meconium is not needed to produce the full-blown massive aspiration syndrome.

### CASE 10–4

A white male infant was born on the expected date of confinement at the Sinai Hospital. The family history was unimportant, pregnancy uneventful, labor short, without apparent difficulty. The mother had been given Demerol, 100 mg, and scopolamine, 0.6 mg, intravenously 56 minutes before delivery. Birth weigh was 7 pounds 2 ounces (3230 gm). The amniotic fluid was not meconium-stained. He breathed and cried immediately and was said to have been quite well for the first 12 hours. At that time grunting respirations were noted.

On physical examination at 12 hours respirations were 40 per minute, with moderate sternal retractions. Breath sounds were diminished generally, but more so over the right lung. Color and activity were good. He was placed in an Isolette. Penicillin and streptomycin were started (50,000 units and 40 mg every 6 hours intramuscularly). At 17 hours he looked fairly well when out of oxygen. Color was good, Moro reflex active. Respirations numbered 60 to 70 per minute with slight retraction. The superior portion of the chest was prominent. The percussion note was resonant throughout, but breath sounds were diminished over the posterior aspect of both lungs and over the right upper lobe in front. No rales or rhonchi were heard.

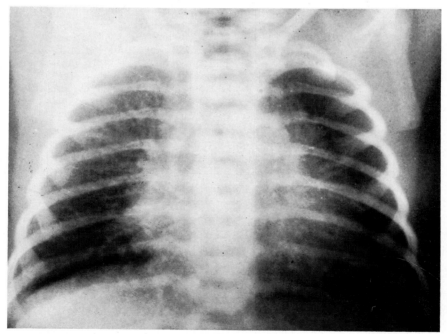

*Figure 10–4.* There is intense infiltration, some patchy, some linear, surrounding the heart and obliterating its normally sharp silhouette. The opacification extends outward and downward a short distance on the left side and toward the right base, but it involves the entire right upper lobe heavily.

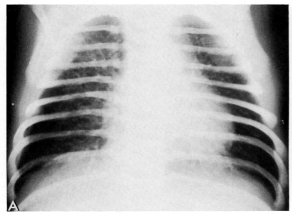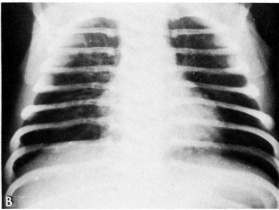

*Figure 10–5.* A, Anteroposterior view of the chest taken on the first day of life. Noteworthy are the heavy patchy infiltration of both lungs, more intense in the upper lung fields, and the overaeration of the lower lobes. The opacification appears soft, not granular. Note, too, the blurring of the normally sharp cardiac silhouette. B, Taken on the third day. There has been some clearing of the opacification, although a moderate amount is still visible, especially in the right upper lobe and hugging the heart shadow. The emphysema appears to have increased somewhat.

The lungs showed patchy infiltration of both upper lobes and of the right middle lobe, whereas both bases were emphysematous. The infiltrate was soft and coarse and was denser at the hili and about the cardiac contour (Fig. 10–5).

On the third day the respirations were still 60 to 70 per minute, but retraction was less, and only at times was expiratory grunting heard. Color was good. Breath sounds were distinctly improved in strength. By the fourth day breathing rate was normal, there was no retraction, and breath sounds came through well everywhere. He was discharged on the sixth day apparently quite well.

**COMMENT.** This child demonstrated the characteristic clinical course and x-ray findings of massive aspiration. It is interesting that he was full-term, neither premature nor postmature, and had suffered no untoward obstetrical accidents. His mother, however, had been given large doses of two analgesic drugs less than an hour before delivery. He was quite well at birth, and breathed and cried immediately, as befits an infant who had suffered no cerebral anoxic damage. But, as we see it, his defenses were down because of the too recent sedation, and he aspirated his own pharyngeal secretions. Within 12 hours the accumulation was great enough, or enough had been gradually sucked into the terminal air spaces, so that obstructive difficulty

developed. The characteristic pattern of atelectasis mixed with emphysema does not require that meconium be part of the aspirate.

For another example in which oversedation seems to have been the cause of massive aspiration leading to obstructive emphysema, see Case 12–1 (p. 128).

**TREATMENT.** Aspiration of clear amniotic sac contents requires only suctioning and the provision of adequate oxygen for a few days. When meconium was part of the aspirate, Gregory et al. achieved remarkably good results by suctioning the trachea dry immediately after birth, and a chest x-ray taken. If there was evidence of meconium aspiration, the baby breathed an ultrasonic mist of NaCl and water and the pharynx was suctioned and the chest percussed and vibrated every $\frac{1}{2}$ hour for four times, then every hour for six times more. Meantime, $O_2$ was supplied to keep the $PA_{O_2}$ above 50 mm Hg.

**PROGNOSIS.** As the illustrative case histories demonstrate, most infants who have aspirated amniotic or vaginal contents do well. They recover clinically after 2 or 3 days, radiologically after 5 to 7 days.

A few die quickly of massive aspiration, usually associated with obvious evidences of cerebral anoxia. A few more develop pneumomediastinum and/or pneumothorax as a result of progressing hyperinflation.

Others develop pneumonitis either because the aspirated amniotic fluid has been contaminated from the start, or secondary to the irritation of aspirated meconium. Total mortality for all these reasons should not exceed 10 to 15 per cent.

## REFERENCES

Baghdassarian, O. H., and Gatewood, W. M.: Barium swallow in evaluation of chronic or recurrent pneumonias in infancy and childhood. Md. State Med. J. *14*:51, 1965.

Bryan, C. S.: Enhancement of bacterial infection by meconium. Johns Hopkins Med. J. *121*:9, 1967.

Case Records of Massachusetts General Hospital. N. Engl. J. Med. *227*:516, 1942.

DeCarlo, J., Tramer, A., and Startzman, H. H.: Iodized oil aspiration in the newborn. Am. J. Dis. Child. *84*:442, 1952.

Farber, S., and Wilson, J. L.: Atelectasis of the newborn: A study and critical review. Am. J. Dis. Child. *46*:572, 1933.

Fletcher, B. D., Outerbridge, E. W., and Dunbar, J. S.: Pulmonary interstitial emphysema in the newborn. J. Can. Assoc. Radiol. *21*:273, 1970.

Green, H., and Apley, J.: Study of cardiac enlargement in infancy, with case reports of reversible enlargement. Pediatrics 5:249, 1950.

Gregory, G. A., Gooding, C. A., Phibbs, R. H., et al.: Meconium aspiration in infant—A prospective study. J. Pediat. 85:848, 1974.

Martin, J. F., and Friedell, H. L.: The roentgen findings in atelectasis of the newborn, with special reference to changes in the cardiac silhouette. Am. J. Roentgenol. 67:905, 1952.

Peace, R. J.: Cor pulmonale in newborn infants. A.M.A. Am. J. Dis. Child. 89:567, 1955.

Peterson, H. G., Jr., and Pendleton, M. E.: Contrasting roentgenographic pulmonary patterns of the hyaline membrane and fetal aspiration syndromes. Am. J. Roentgen. 74:800, 1955.

# 11

# ATELECTASIS

Atelectasis means incomplete expansion of a lung or a portion of lung.

**CLASSIFICATION.** Atelectasis falls naturally into two main categories: initial or primary atelectasis signifies failure of alveolar expansion ab origine, while obstructive, resorption or secondary atelectasis denotes initial filling, but subsequent collapse because further entrance of air has been prevented, or because increased surface forces prevent air from remaining in the alveoli. A simple schema follows.

I. Primary or initial atelectasis
   A. Pulmonary immaturity
   B. Inadequacy of respiratory effort, due to:
      1. Weakness of muscles concerned with breathing
      2. Softness of thoracic cage
      3. Oversedation
      4. Severe illness
      5. Damage to respiratory center
II. Secondary atelectasis
   A. Inhalation of amniotic debris or mucus plugs
   B. Deficiency of the pulmonary surfactant

   C. Congenital anomalies obstructing airway
   D. Abnormal external pressure upon lung

**PATHOGENESIS.** The alveoli of the mature lung at the moment of birth, before the first breath has been taken, are not collapsed and empty. They contain a quantity of liquid which normally is formed in the lung rather than aspirated.

If one judges by the radiographic appearance of the lungs alone, the first few breaths taken by a vigorous newborn produce complete expansion of all parts of the lungs. No dramatic changes in the shape of the thorax or the position of the diaphragm occur, which suggests that the lung liquid that was expelled or absorbed is quickly replaced by an equal volume of air.

A minimal degree of primary atelectasis is probably physiological in the first days of life, since lung function studies show progressive improvement over the first 72 to 96 hours. If for any reason the newborn makes inadequate respiratory efforts, complete expansion may be delayed for days or weeks. Feeble respiration may result from a variety of disorders, infectious, hemolytic and others, which have made the infant ill by the time he is born. It may result from oversedation of the infant by sedatives given the mother in too large quantities or too close to the time of delivery. We make a distinction in this situation between the atelectasis without dyspnea associated with central nervous system depression and that with dyspnea which we think is due to obstructive aspirate. Damage to the respiratory center may result from intracranial hemorrhage or a prior episode of cerebral anoxia.

In the very small premature the respiratory effort may be feeble indeed. The muscles concerned with respiration are small and poorly developed. Their pull is exerted upon a thoracic cage which is softer and more compliant than that of the mature newborn. Much of the negative pressure achieved by breathing effort is therefore wasted, since, instead of inflating the lungs, it sucks the suprasternal notch, intercostal spaces, ribs and sternum inward.

In addition to this mechanical factor, a developmental one of even greater importance may increase atelectasis. The outgrowth of alveoli from respiratory bronchioles and their transformation into their ultimate functioning form go on up to, and for some time after, delivery. From the 28th week on, the lungs of prematures contain progressively fewer and fewer thick-walled airways lined with high columnar epithelium and more and more which are thin, lined with flattened epithelium, and are thoroughly efficient in their function of gas exchange. Not only may the tiny premature, therefore, have difficulty in insufflating adequate amounts of air, but also such air as is inhaled may be wasted in expanding bronchioles, alveolar ducts and thick-walled alveoli.

Fetal lung may fail to expand because abnormal intrathoracic contents literally leave it insufficient room for expansion. Atelectasis is inevitable in lung segments adjacent to an enlarged, congenitally malformed heart, a large diaphragmatic hernia, air-filled or fluid-filled cysts and tumors of any magnitude which might be present at birth. By the same token, a previously expanded segment may collapse if certain abnormal intrathoracic conditions develop after birth. Examples are enlargement of an initially normal heart, distention with air of a congenitally misplaced loop of bowel, sudden onset of pleural effusion, pneumothorax or unilobar emphysema, or the rapid enlargement of an air-filled cyst. Atelectasis in these circumstances is self-explanatory.

Of a different order from these varieties is that type of atelectasis which develops from obstruction to the airway from within, after the lung has expanded fully. Inhalation of particulate amniotic debris or of plugs of mucus may produce blockage to further ingress of air. When this happens, the air already contained is absorbed, and portions of the lung collapse. Depending upon the site of obstruction, collapse may involve an entire lung, a lobe or segment, or if multiple, scattered small areas of both lungs. Regardless of their size or number, these are all examples of so-called resorption atelectasis. Such a mechanism presumably is operative in the presence of severe infections.

Infants who have been intubated and maintained on respirators are particularly prone to develop atelectasis. If the tube occludes a major bronchus, total lung collapse can occur. If secretions puddle in the airways, segmental or lobar collapse occurs. Widespread atelectasis and compensatory overdistention of parts of the lung commonly lead to changing clinical signs and need for oxygen, as well as changing roentgenographic findings. The scarcity of intra-alveolar pores of Kohn in the lung of the newborn infant limits his capacity for collateral ventilation and increases the likelihood of alveolar collapse distal to an obstruction. Frequent change of position and suctioning may be helpful. Physiotherapy applied to the chest is widely advocated, but its efficacy is not documented.

One situation in which massive atelectasis may occur with prompt reversal after a few deep breaths is in apnea after oxygen breathing. The pulmonary circulation quickly takes up the oxygen, which is utilized, so that venous oxygen tensions remain low, and oxygen is rapidly resorbed from the alveoli under these circumstances. Fletcher and Avery demonstrated this phenomenon of reversible gas freeing of lung within minutes in a puppy.

Di Sant'Agnese pointed out another infrequent cause of atelectasis in the newborn or somewhat older infant. Atelectasis of the right upper lobe chiefly, occasionally of other lobes, may precede pulmonary infection in cystic fibrosis of the pancreas. This is doubtless due to the accumulation in a bronchus of the viscid secretion characteristic of mucoviscidosis (Fig. 11–1).

Secondary atelectasis can result from a deficiency of the pulmonary surfactant, either on the basis of extreme immaturity, or from interference with its production, as in hyaline membrane disease. (See Chapter 13.) Deficiency of the surfactant permits the tiny, sharply curved terminal air spaces to collapse at end-expiration from the forces of surface tension. The surfactant, when present, reduces surface tension and thus stabilizes the terminal air spaces; it operates as an anti-atelectasis factor. The time of appearance of the surfactant in the human is variable, but usually it is detectable at 26 or 27 weeks, or when the fetus weighs 700 to 800 gm. It can be found ear-lier in some, and may be lacking later in others.

**DIAGNOSIS.** When atelectasis is secondary to disease elsewhere in the thorax, it may contribute little or nothing to the total clinical picture. The presence of a collapsed lobe or segment alters very little the signs and symptoms produced by diaphragmatic hernia, pneumothorax or a large failing heart. Under these circumstances, therefore, it behaves as a coincidental finding of little importance.

*Primary atelectasis* is suggested by persistent cyanosis associated with feeble respiratory effort, or by intermittent cyanosis associated with irregular respiration and periods of apnea.

In *obstructive atelectasis,* on the other hand, the infant makes vigorous efforts to breathe. The baby may show initial apnea neonatorum or may be normal at birth, crying immediately and breathing spontaneously and well for some hours.

At some point within the first 24 hours dyspnea and cyanosis appear. Examination reveals an infant in respiratory distress, cyanotic when out of oxygen, breathing rapidly and deeply, with visible inspiratory retraction and at times audible expiratory grunt. One hemithorax may move less well

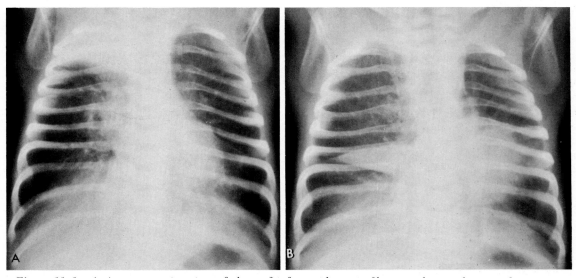

*Figure 11–1.* A, Anteroposterior view of chest of infant with cystic fibrosis, taken at the age of twenty-one days. Segmental atelectasis of the right upper lobe and moderate emphysema of the left lower and possibly of the right lower lobe can be seen. B, At the age of twenty-nine days. Atelectasis is confined to the right middle lobe. (Prints supplied by and reprinted with the kind permission of Dr. Paul A. di Sant'Agnese.)

than the other, and an area of dullness is discovered over which fine tissue-paper rales are audible at the end of inspiration. The heart is dislocated toward the involved side, and the diaphragm is elevated. This combination of signs indicates *lobar* or *segmental obstructive atelectasis*.

The clinical picture of the patchy or lobular atelectasis so characteristic of massive aspiration has been described (p. 118).

**RADIOGRAPHIC CHANGES.** *Primary atelectasis* is manifest on the x-ray film as a diffuse clouding of both entire lungs.

*Lobar* or *segmental atelectasis* produces a homogeneous, sharply outlined shadow resembling that of lobar pneumonia. In addition, the involved hemithorax appears smaller than the opposite one, the ribs are more closely approximated, and the diaphragm is elevated on that side. If the atelectatic area is moderately large, the heart and mediastinum are shifted toward the consolidation (Fig. 11–2).

*Lobular* or *patchy atelectasis* of massive aspiration has been amply illustrated in the preceding chapter.

CASE 11–1

A white male infant whose birth weight was 5 pounds 9 ounces (2525 gm) was born after nor-

mal pregnancy and labor. He breathed and cried immediately, but there was excessive mucus in his pharynx and airway. After vigorous suctioning he was sent to the nursery in excellent condition. One-half hour later rapid respirations and cyanosis were noted by the nursery attendant. Examination at 8 hours revealed an infant whose extremities were cyanotic even while he was receiving oxygen. His respirations numbered 80 to 100 per minute, and there was decided sternal retraction with inspiration. His cry was good, his vigor unabated. Resonance was unimpaired anywhere, air exchange was generally poor, and a few inspiratory rales were heard over the upper lobe of the right lung anteriorly. By 20 hours there was distinct dullness to percussion over the right lung, and numerous fine rales were heard in this area, both front and back. No cardiac shift could be made out by percussion. Fluoroscopy, however, revealed density of the right lung field and shift of the heart to that side. X-ray film verified this (Fig. 11–2). The infant was given penicillin intramuscularly and kept in an atmosphere of humidified oxygen. He gradually improved over the following 3 days, and the lungs were completely normal by the seventh day.

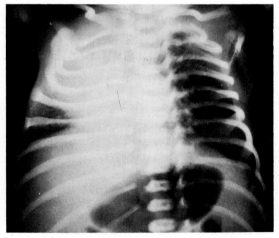

*Figure 11–2.* Anteroposterior view of chest. Almost the entire right lung is solidly radiopaque. The heart and mediastinal contents are shifted far to the right. The right hemithorax is contracted, its intercostal spaces narrower and its diaphragm higher than normal. The left lung is emphysematous, its upper lobe bulging slightly into the mediastinum. Its intercostal spaces are widened, and its diaphragm is low and flattened.

**COMMENT.** This is an example of segmental atelectasis which involved the right upper lobe and probably the right middle lobe also. It cannot be doubted that excessive mucoid secretion was drawn into the bronchi of these lobes, where it acted as a stop-valve which permitted resorption of all air within them. Emphysema of the left lung is compensatory.

**TREATMENT.** In the event of segmental or lobar atelectasis, removal of the cause of the obstruction is of first importance. The repositioning of an endotracheal tube or careful suctioning with sterile technique may be appropriate. Persistent atelectasis may respond to positioning the infant so that the collapsed segment is in the least dependent position. Gentle percussion of the chest wall to dislodge secretions, followed by suctioning, may be useful.

Since tracheal suctioning may be stressful to the infant, it should be done with free-flowing oxygen at hand, and only with sterile catheter and rubber glove technique. An endotracheal tube will impede mucociliary clearance, predispose to pooling of secretions and set the stage for the introduction of infection unless suctioning is done with great care. We find 4-hour intervals are appropriate, but would change the intervals depending on the returns.

## REFERENCES

Avery, M. E., and Said, S.: Surface phemonena in lungs in health and disease. Medicine *44*:503, 1965.

Day, R., Goodfellow, A. M., Apgar, V., et al.: Pressure-time relations in the safe correction of atelectasis in animal lungs. Pediatrics *10*:593, 1952.

di Sant'Agnese, P. A.: Bronchial obstruction with lobar atelectasis and emphysema in cystic fibrosis of the pancreas. Pediatrics *12*:178, 1953.

Donald, I.: Atelectasis neonatorum. J. Obstet Gynaecol. Br. Emp. *61*:725, 1954.

Donald, I: Radiology in neonatal respiratory disorders. Br. J. Radiol. 27:500, 1954.

Farber, S., and Wilson, J. J.: Atelectasis of the newborn. Am. J. Dis. Child. *46*:572, 1933.

Fletcher, B. D., and Avery, M. E.: The effects of airway occlusion after oxygen breathing on the lungs of newborn infants. Radiology *109*:655, 1973.

Lind, J., Tähti, E., and Hirvensalo, M.: Roentgenographic studies of the size of the lungs of the newborn baby before and after aeration. Ann. Paediatr. Fenn. *12*:20, 1966.

Martin, J. F., and Friedell, H. L.: The roentgen findings in atelectasis of the newborn. Am. J. Roentgenol. 67:905, 1952.

Scarpelli, E.: The Surfactant Systems of the Lung. Philadelphia, Lea & Febiger, 1968.

Spear, O. S., Vaeusorn, O., Avery, M. E., et al.: Inclusions in terminal air spaces of fetal and neonatal human lung. Biol. Neonat. *14*:344, 1969.

Wilson, J. L., and Farber, S.: Pathogenesis of atelectasis of the newborn. Am. J. Dis. Child. *46*:590, 1933.

# 12    HYPERINFLATED LUNG; LOBAR EMPHYSEMA; PNEUMOTHORAX; PNEUMOMEDIASTINUM

The lung of the newborn infant becomes hyperaerated with great frequency. Both lungs in their entirety may be so affected, or one lung or a lobe or a segment of a lung. *Simple hyperaeration* (overdistention of terminal air spaces) may progress to *interstitial emphysema,* in which septa are broken and air escapes into interstitial tissue. Collection of this air into bullae or blebs may permit rupture into the pleural space, either directly or after being carried down the sheaths of blood and lymph vessels to the mediastinum.

**PATHOGENESIS.** The only basic causes of hyperinflation are (1) some obstructive process that permits ingress of air into the terminal air spaces but impedes egress, or (2) expansion of a segment of lung by the normally negative intrathoracic pressure to compensate for loss of volume in another lobe.

Some immediate causes of hyperinflation are:

1. Intrinsic partial obstruction by:
   a. Mucus
   b. Meconium or squamous cells
   c. Inflammatory exudate
2. Extrinsic compression by:
   a. Bronchogenic cyst
   b. Aberrant vessel
3. Idiopathic unilobar emphysema
4. Compensatory hyperinflation in presence of:
   a. Atelectasis
   b. Pulmonary agenesis or hyperplasia
5. Iatrogenic

**DIAGNOSIS.** Many of the infants suffering from emphysema will have been born after some abnormality of pregnancy or labor. Postmaturity, toxemia, placental bleeding, cord accidents, maternal hypotension, vigorous instrumental extraction, breech delivery and other problems figure prominently in the histories. Many will have been ill at birth, with breathing and crying time delayed, and positive pressure insufflation will have been attempted. Within a few minutes or hours after spontaneous respiration has become established the signs of emphysema become noticeable. These may begin and remain relatively mild. They may progress over the course of 12 to 48 hours to severer forms or they may strike catastrophically with the first few breaths.

When obstructive emphysema is fully developed, the diagnosis can be made by physical examination with relative ease. The chest is visibly hyperinflated. Respirations are rapid and shallow, with some retraction, and the chest fails to deflate completely upon expiration. Percussion reveals hyperresonance, depressed diaphragm and contracted area of cardiac dullness. Breath sounds are diminished in intensity. Rales are not usually heard. A wheeze may be heard during expiration. Lesser degrees of emphysema and the emphysema which coexists with patchy atelectasis may not produce such characteristic signs and may be diagnosable only by x-ray film.

*Interstitial emphysema* cannot be differentiated by physical examination from the simple form. It may be assumed to be present when emphysema is definite and cyanosis is present, and when the chest remains overinflated at the end of expiration. Infants suffering from interstitial emphysema ordinarily seem quite ill. Blebs and bullae cannot be localized by the percussing finger and the stethoscope.

*Mediastinal emphysema* may also not be recognizable by its signs. When there is great accumulation of air in the mediastinum, the sternum is thrust forward, the percussion note over it and for a short distance to either side is strikingly hyperresonant and, rarely, a clicking or crunching noise may be heard synchronous with the heart beat. Heart sounds may appear to be distant. These infants, too, are extremely ill, and cyanosis may become intense.

## PNEUMOTHORAX

The most common cause of increased intrathoracic tension is pneumothorax, with or without associated pneumomediastinum and interstitial emphysema. Spontaneous pneumothorax is more common in the first days of life than at any other time of childhood.

**INCIDENCE.** When radiographs have been taken on consecutive infants, small asymptomatic pneumothoraces have been detected in about 1 or 2 per cent of them. Symptomatic pneumothoraces are rarer, occurring about once in a thousand live births. A higher incidence than that would suggest overzealous resuscitative efforts in the delivery room.

**PATHOGENESIS.** Clearly the lung can be ruptured by the application of excessive pressure during resuscitation. Equally clearly, pneumothorax can occur in the absence of artificial ventilation. It is associated with postmaturity and meconium staining, suggesting that aspirated materials may partially obstruct portions of the lung and allow excessive pressure to be

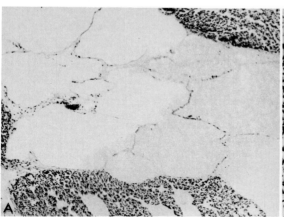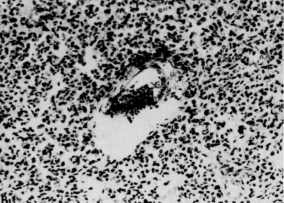

*Figure 12-1.* A, Photomicrograph of lung of an infant who died of emphysema and bilateral pneumothorax. The group of alveoli in the center shows much distention, their septa thinned. Some of the septa have ruptured. In the periphery the lung is atelectatic. B, Higher-power view to show a blood vessel in cross section. The vessel is compressed by a surrounding collar of air which has filled and ballooned the perivascular space.

applied to the previously aerated alveoli by the descent of the diaphragm. This hypothesis to explain the reasons for the predisposition to pneumothorax in the first hours of life was proposed by Chernick and Avery in 1963 after studies on the mechanism of inflation of the airless lung. The serial opening of the terminal ventilatory units would allow shearing forces to be applied to those that are open when others are obstructed. There seems to be no need to consider congenital defects in these lungs, since recurrences after an episode in infancy have not been reported.

Pneumothorax has been described by Lubchenco in premature infants, occurring in the first weeks of life. We also have seen it under those circumstances and have noted it in a number of infants with hyaline membrane disease. Nevertheless, it seems to be overwhelmingly a problem of the mature or postmature infant. Indeed, Adler and Wyszogrodski have demonstrated that the more mature lung ruptures at lower transpulmonary pressures than the less mature lung.

**SYMPTOMS.** Infants with significant accumulation of air in the pleural space are usually tachypneic, often cyanotic, and may have asymmetric chests. Hyperresonance is often evident, but the expected decrease in breath sounds on the affected side may be absent, since breath sounds are so widely transmitted in infants. Irritability is usually prominent. The cardiac impulses may be shifted; indeed, careful following of the point of maximal impulse is a useful guide to the possibility of increase or decrease in the pneumothorax.

**DIAGNOSIS AND TREATMENT.** If the infant is critically ill and the chest is found to be hyperresonant, a needle should be inserted immediately, preferably attached via a three-way stopcock to a syringe. The removal of air under tension should give prompt relief. When the situation is less critical, a chest film is indicated. Kuhns and colleagues have used fiberoptic transillumination to identify and follow pneumothoraces, and we have found this technique very useful. The decision to remove the air by needle aspiration, closed-suction drainage or oxygen breathing depends on the clinical state. If the child is not severely ill, close observation over the

subsequent hours should reveal whether he is getting better or worse. Often, complete resolution occurs without any intervention. Occasionally, removal of the air by a simple aspiration is satisfactory. In the absence of continuing leak, administration of 40 to 50 per cent oxygen will greatly facilitate removal of the loculated air on the basis of nitrogen washout, as demonstrated by Chernick and Avery. If air continues to accumulate, water-seal drainage for a few days may be indicated.

The presence of significant amounts of mediastinal air is indicated by elevation of the thymus as seen on the anteroposterior and lateral chest films (Fig. 12–3). Air in that location and subcutaneous and interstitial air are, of course, difficult to aspirate. Oxygen breathing (even 100 per cent oxygen for a few hours) will hasten removal of air from those locations. High oxygen mixtures should not be given unless symptoms are severe, and then should be withdrawn as soon as the infant has improved.

## CASE HISTORIES

### CASE 12–1

A white male infant whose mother's pregnancy was uncomplicated except by severe nausea and vomiting in the first 4 months was born 2 weeks before the expected date of confinement. Amniotomy was performed at 6 P.M., labor began at 8 P.M. Demerol (100 mg) and scopolamine (0.6 mg) were given 1 hour, and Seconal (100 mg) 2½ hours before delivery, which took place at 1:15 A.M. Birth weight was 6 pounds 13 ounces (3090 gm). He cried and breathed spontaneously, but at 15 minutes was noted to be cyanotic about the face and head. At 3 A.M. respirations were 42 per minute, and color was poor. There was a grunt with each expiration. At 6 A.M. mask oxygen was started.

Physical examination was made at 10 A.M. (age 9 hours). Color was fair when he was in oxygen, but cyanotic when he was out of the incubator. The cry was weak, but respirations now were slow, shallow, regular. Lungs were clear to percussion and auscultation. The impression was oversedation. He was ordered penicillin and streptomycin, oxygen and nothing by mouth.

During the rest of the first day there was little change. Removal from oxygen produced cyanosis. During the night, respirations again became rapid and grunting, and some sternal retraction was noted.

At age 33 hours no improvement was apparent. Respiration varied from 80 to 100 per minute, with some retraction. The chest was symmetrical. Percussion note was dull over most of the right hemithorax, with poor air exchange on this side, very resonant over the sternum, and the heart sounds were a little distant.

On x-ray the left hemithorax was seen to be hyperinflated, the ribs widely separated, the diaphragm low, the left upper lobe herniating slightly into the upper mediastinum. The heart and thymic shadow were displaced to the right. There was soft patchy infiltration into the right lung, denser at the hilus (Fig. 12–2).

By 3 days of age he was definitely improved. Respirations were still rapid, 70 per minute, but no longer labored. Color was good while he was in oxygen, fair out. From then on he made rapid improvement both clinically and by x-ray until by the seventh day he seemed perfectly normal.

**COMMENT.** This infant was well at birth, but became dyspneic and cyanotic within 15 minutes after delivery. Physical signs were never sufficiently characteristic to suggest the correct diagnosis, but x-ray film told the entire story. There was hyperinflation of the entire left lung and patchy atelectasis of the right lung. The sequence of events may have been (1) aspiration of oronasopharyngeal secretions due to oversedation, (2) stop-valve closure of many small bronchi of the right lung, and (3) check-valve closure of the left main bronchus. He improved by the third day and was well by the seventh day of life.

CASE 12–2

A white male infant was born at the Hospital for the Women of Maryland after 43 weeks of

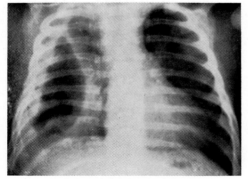

*Figure 12–2.* Anteroposterior view of the chest taken at thirty-three hours of age. Emphysema of the left lung predominates, with ribs widely spread and slight herniation of the upper lobe into the mediastinum. In the right lung there is patchy atelectasis. The mass in the right upper section is almost surely the thymus, slightly dislocated to the right.

gestation to a 25 year old primipara who had suffered from toxemia with hypertension and albuminuria. Delivery was spontaneous, but amniotic fluid was meconium-stained. Birth weight was 6 pounds 3 ounces (2807 gm), Apgar score 6, with first breath and cry delayed. On arrival at the nursery he was cyanotic, with rapid respirations. Color improved in oxygen. The chest was hyperinflated, and there was resonance over the sternum. Rales were heard throughout both lungs. An x-ray film showed mediastinal emphysema (Fig. 12–3). After 2½ days he was able to be removed from the oxygen tent. He remained jittery and tense for 2 more days and thereafter was well.

**COMMENT.** This case illustrates beautifully the sequence of events in many cases of emphysema: postmaturity, meconium-staining of amniotic fluid, massive aspiration, neonatal asphyxia, followed by tachypnea, dyspnea and cyanosis. Hyperinflation and hyperresonance over the sternum signaled the advance of simple emphysema to mediastinal emphysema.

CASE 12–3

A 36 year old para 4 bled briskly at 33 weeks, went into labor at 40 weeks, and delivered spontaneously a 3487-gm baby boy. Amniotic fluid was meconium-stained. The baby was scored 8 on the Apgar scale, but respiratory onset was delayed and respirations were gasping from the start. No positive pressure was used in resuscitation.

On arrival at the nursery he was covered with thick yellow vernix, and respirations were accompanied by retracting and flaring of the alae and by expiratory grunting. In humidified oxygen breathing was easier by 10 hours. By the second day he was much better, and by the third week he seemed well. X-ray film on the first day showed right-sided pneumothorax (Fig. 12–4).

CASE 12–4

A white male infant was born after normal pregnancy and delivery at the Women's Hospital of Maryland. He breathed and cried spontaneously. Within a few minutes, however, he was in great respiratory distress and cyanotic. Birth weight was 6 pounds 4 ounces (2835 gm).

On physical examination his respirations were rapid and labored. Disproportion between the hemithoraces was noted, the left side being much more prominent than the right. Percussion note was hyperresonant on the left, front and back, but dull over the right side. The heart could not be located by percussion, but the

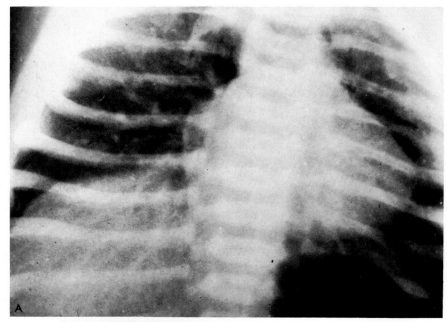

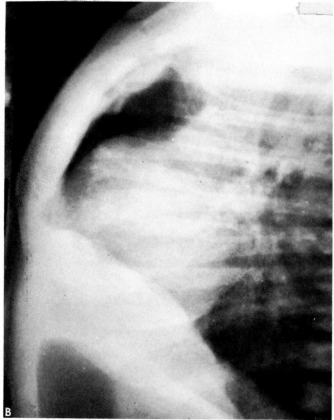

*Figure 12–3.*   *A*, One can see two large bubbles of air in the right upper mediastinum. One of them appears to be lifting the thymus outward and upward. *B*, Lateral view to show the large collection of air in the anterior mediastinum.

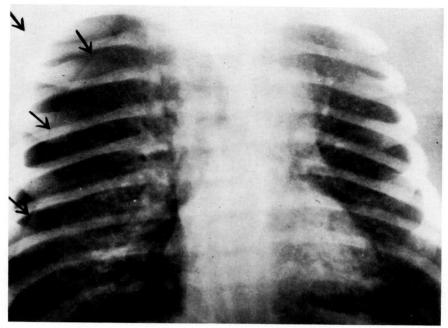

*Figure 12–4.*   Marked pneumothorax is visible on the right.

sounds were maximal to the right of the sternum. Breath sounds were diminished everywhere, and no rales were audible. Fluoroscopy
and x-ray study revealed a high degree of pneu-

mothorax on the left and of atelectasis on the
right with mediastinal dislocation toward the
right (Fig. 12–5).

Thirty-five cubic centimeters of air were re-

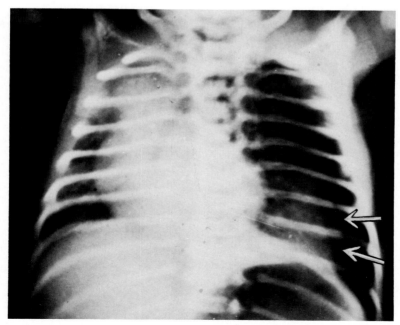

*Figure 12–5.*   Anteroposterior view of chest of infant three hours old. Respiratory distress began, for no known
reason, a few minutes after birth, shortly after the original cry. One sees left pneumothorax, the collapsed left
lung, shift of the heart and mediastinum to the right, and atelectasis of the right upper lobe.

moved by thoracentesis, with improvement. During the course of the day dyspnea again increased, and 15 cc more of air were withdrawn. Moderate respiratory distress continued for 48 hours, but the pneumothorax gradually diminished, while the right-sided atelectasis resolved even more slowly. By the fourth day the clinical condition and x-ray appearance were normal.

**COMMENT.** These two infants suffered pneumothorax within the first hour of life without having been subjected to positive pressure insufflation. Both responded well, one to simple needle-syringe aspiration and the other to nothing more than oxygen.

## LOBAR EMPHYSEMA

This syndrome has also been called congenital lobar emphysema, unilobar obstructive emphysema, localized hypertrophic emphysema and infantile lobar emphysema. In our present confused state of knowledge about causation it would appear to be wise to use the simplest descriptive term without qualifying adjectives which may be apposite for some, but not for all. The syndrome is characterized by emphysematous expansion of one lobe. Dyspnea and cyanosis are produced, and these progress slowly or rapidly until serious respiratory difficulty develops.

**INCIDENCE.** The syndrome has been recognized only in the past 40 years. Up to 1960 about 30 cases had been reported. It is therefore rare, but the rate at which reports have been accruing in the past few years makes the supposition reasonable that it is not the extreme rarity it was once thought to be. Leape and Longino, for example, reported 21 additional cases in 1964, and Lincoln et al. added 28 in 1971.

**PATHOLOGY AND PATHOGENESIS.** At operation or autopsy one lobe (usually an upper, less often the right middle, rarely a lower) is ballooned to many times its normal size. It is usually pink and spongy in appearance, resembling, according to one author, a pink soufflé. When excised, it retains its overinflated appearance. Under the microscope most of the alveoli are distended, many have coalesced because of rupture of the septa, and subpleural blebs may have been formed. Careful postmortem studies by Reid and her colleagues have illuminated the variety of findings in this condition. In some infants, the tissue is normal with respect to alveolar and airway numbers, but simply overdistended, as by a mucous plug. In others, the numbers of airways and alveoli are reduced (a hypoplastic overdistended lobe). Radiographically they are unusually translucent but not overdistended. Rarely, a lobe may show normal airways, but an excess of alveoli, the so-called polyalveolar lobe. Finally, atresia of a bronchus can permit overdistention of some segments, but poor egress of air, leading to radiolucency of segments of lung.

In many lungs lesions have been alleged to have been found to account for the progressive hyperinflation. Bronchial alter-

**TABLE 12–1.    *Types of Childhood Lobar Emphysema***

| Type | No. of Airways | Alveoli | |
|---|---|---|---|
| Polyalveolar lobe | Normal | *Number:* | Increased |
| | | *Size:* | May or may not be increased (i.e. emphysema) |
| Overinflation | Normal | *Number:* | Normal* |
| | | *Size:* | Increased |
| Hypoplastic emphysema | Decreased | *Number:* | Decreased |
| | | *Size:* | Increased |
| Atresia of bronchus | Probably normal | *Number:* | Probably normal* |
| | | *Size:* | Increased |
| Compensatory emphysema | Normal | *Number:* | Normal* |
| | | *Size:* | Increased |

*As alveolar multiplication after birth is so rapid, these two types described as having a normal alveolar number at birth may rapidly come to have too few alveoli for age if the postnatal alveolar multiplication is impaired. (Courtesy of Dr. Lynne Reid)

ations have been described: viz., mucosal folds, diminution, absence or flaccidity of bronchial cartilage, and stenoses due to inflammation, cysts or mucous plugs. Deficient cartilage was found in 22 of 28 resected lobes in the series reported by Lincoln et al. in 1971. Extrabronchial compression by aberrant blood vessels, chiefly the ductus arteriosus or its residual fibrous cord, has been found in a few. A pathological classification of lobar emphysema has been proposed by Dr. Lynne Reid (Table 12–1).

**DIAGNOSIS.** First symptoms are noted at birth in a few cases, during the first week in a few more, between 1 week and 1 month in the majority. In a scattered minority the original signs of illness make their appearance between 1 and 6 months of age. It is therefore by and large a neonatal disease.

Spells of dyspnea with cyanosis ordinarily usher in the disorder, and these signs soon become persistent and severe. Wheezing expiration is noted not too infrequently. Vomiting and cough are encountered rarely.

On examination, dyspnea, with labored inspiration accompanied by retraction of variable degree, and grunting or prolonged wheezing expiration are the rule. An area of hyperresonance involving one upper lobe or one entire lung is discovered, and over this area air entry is diminished. The heart and mediastinum are dislocated away from the hyperresonant side.

**RADIOGRAPHIC FINDINGS.** One lobe, usually the right or left upper or the right middle, is voluminous and radiolucent. It often can be seen crossing the midline anterior to the heart. Adjacent lobes are atelectatic. The heart is shifted to the side opposite the overexpanded lobe and can usually be seen to be pressed posteriorly by the herniated lung.

**TREATMENT.** If the infant is in severe respiratory distress, immediate intervention is indicated. After a chest film, we prefer to invite a pediatric surgeon and an otolaryngologist to work with us, the latter to perform endoscopy on the operating table, with the surgeon prepared to do an immediate thoracotomy if necessary. Occasionally an obstructing mucous plug may be removed by suction, and thoracotomy will not be required. If immediate relief is not forthcoming, thoracotomy is in order. The operative mortality in recent years has been very low. It was zero in 21 cases reported by Leape and Longino in 1964. During the same time interval, 3 infants died who were symptomatic in the newborn period and not operated upon.

In asymptomatic infants in whom lobar overdistention is discovered incidentally, bronchoscopy is indicated. We have elected to follow some such infants without operation and they have remained asymptomatic. Occasionally the overdistended lobe returns to normal volume, as noted by Roghair in 1972.

**PROGNOSIS.** The outlook after operation is usually excellent. Few functional evaluations have been made, but DeMuth and Sloan in 1966 did note some persistent reduction in midexpiratory flow rates in two children, suggesting that the disease is not always limited to the most obviously involved lobes.

## REFERENCES

Adler, S. M., and Wyszogrodski, I.: Pneumothorax as a function of gestational age: Clinical and experimental studies. J. Pediatr. 87:771, 1975.

Aranda, J. V., Stern, L., and Dunbar, J. S.: Pneumothorax with pneumoperitoneum in a newborn infant. Am J. Dis. Child 123:163, 1972.

Boland, R. B., Schneider, A. F., and Boggs, J. D.: Infantile lobar emphysema; Etiological concept. A.M.A. Arch Pathol. 61:289, 1956.

Campbell, P. E.: Congenital lobar emphysema: Etiologic studies. Aust. Paediatr. J. 5:226, 1969.

Chernick, V., and Avery, M. E.: Spontaneous alveolar rupture in newborn infants. Pediatrics 32:816, 1963.

Day, R., Goodfellow, A. M., Apgar, V., et al.: Pressure-time relation in the safe correction of atelectasis in animal lungs. Pediatrics 10:593, 1952.

DeMuth, G. R., and Sloan, H.: Congenital lobar emphysema: Long-term effects and sequelae in treated cases. Surgery 59:601, 1966.

Donahoe, P. K., et al.: Pneumoperitoneum secondary to pulmonary air leak. J. Pediatr. 81:797, 1972.

Emery, J. L.: Interstitial emphysema, pneumothorax and "air-block" in the newborn. Lancet 1:405, 1956.

Fischer, H. W., Potts, W. J., and Holinger, P. H.: Lobar emphysema in infants and children. J. Pediatr. 41:403, 1952.

Hislop, A., and Reid, L.: Growth and development of the respiratory system—Anatomical development. In Davis, J. A., and Dobbing, J. (eds.): Scientific

Foundations of Paediatrics. Philadelphia, W. B. Saunders Co., 1974.

Holzel, A., Bennett, E., and Vaughan, B. F.: Congenital lobar emphysema. Arch. Dis. Child. *31*:216, 1956.

Kuhns, L. R., Bednarek, F. J., Wyman, M. L., et al.: Diagnosis of pneumothorax or pneumomediastinum in the neonate by transillumination. Pediatrics *56*:355, 1975.

Leape, L. L., and Longino, L. A.: Infantile lobar emphysema. Pediatrics *34*:246, 1964.

Lincoln, J. C. R., Stark, J., Subramanian, S., et al: Congenital lobar emphysema. Ann Surg. *173*:55, 1971.

Lubchenco, L. O.: Recognition of spontaneous pneumothorax in premature infants. Pediatrics *24*:996, 1959.

Nelson, T.: Tension emphysema in infants. Arch. Dis. Child. *32*:38, 1957.

Patterson, W. H., and Fawcitt, J.: Non-traumatic mediastinal emphysema in childhood. Arch. Dis. Child. *29*:451, 1954.

Roghair, G. D.: Non-operative management of lobar emphysema. Long-term follow-up. Radiology *102*:125, 1972.

Shaw, R. R.: Localized hypertrophic emphysema. Pediatrics *9*:220, 1952.

Strunge, P.: Infantile lobar emphysema with lobar agenesis and congenital heart disease. Acta Paediatr. Scand. *61*:209, 1972.

Thompson, J., and Forfar, J. O.: Regional obstructive emphysema in infancy. Arch. Dis. Child. *33*:97, 1958.

# 13 HYALINE MEMBRANE DISEASE

Hyaline membrane disease, sometimes referred to as respiratory distress syndrome, surfactant deficiency syndrome or neonatal atelectasis, is the result of ventilation of a lung with inadequate stores of surfactant or the incapability of its continued production.

**EPIDEMIOLOGY.** Although there is no universal agreement on clinical or pathological diagnostic criteria, the almost complete accord between investigators allows assessment of incidence and mortality rates. Described in all populations of the world, it appears to be somewhat more common in prematurely born white compared to black infants, nearly twice as common in males as females, with a familial likelihood of recurrence in a subsequent prematurely born infant. The disorder accounts for about 10,000 deaths per year in the United States, with a mortality rate of about 28 per cent of those afflicted. Age at death is nearly always 72 hours or less, except in some infants who die of complications of the disease or its treatment later in the first few weeks of life.

Infants at special risk are those delivered prematurely, with a rising incidence with greater prematurity. Delivery by section in the absence of previous labor poses an added risk if birth occurs before 37 weeks' gestation. Precipitous delivery after maternal hemorrhage, asphyxia or maternal diabetes is associated with a greater likelihood of hyaline membrane disease. The second-born twin is at greater risk than the first-born. Some maternal conditions are thought to have a sparing effect, namely, conditions associated with chronic intrauterine distress that lead to undersized infants, maternal steroid ingestion and, in some instances, prolonged labor following rupture of the membranes (Table 13–1).

**PATHOLOGY.** On gross examination the lungs are voluminous and liver-like, and generally sink in water or formalin. Under the microscope much of the lung appears solid, owing to the tight apposition of most of the alveolar walls. Scattered throughout are dilated air spaces, respiratory bronchioles, alveolar ducts and a few alveoli, some of whose walls are lined with pink-staining "hyaline" material containing fibrin and cellular debris. The capillaries are strikingly congested, and there may be pulmonary edema and lymphatic distention (Figs. 13–1 and 13–2).

Epithelial necrosis in the terminal bronchioles at sites underlying the membrane suggests that a reaction to injury has taken place. Hypersecretion is evident, and reparative phenomena such as a proliferation

**TABLE 13-1.** *Categorization of Observations in Hyaline Membrane Disease*[*][†]

| Established | Probable | Possible |
|---|---|---|
| **Epidemiology** | | |
| Worldwide | Secondborn twin at greater risk | Maternal diabetes predisposes |
| Prematurity predisposes | PROM spares | Maternal hemorrhage predisposes |
| C-section w/o labor predisposes | IUGR spares | Familial predisposition |
| Perinatal asphyxia predisposes | Maternal toxemia spares | Prenatal corticoids spare |
| Male mortality >female | | Maternal heroin addiction spares |
| | | Late pulmonary sequelae |
| **Clinical signs** | | |
| Onset near the time of birth | Fine inspiratory rales | Pulmonary edema |
| Retractions and tachypnea | Hypothermia | PDA murmur |
| Expiratory grunt | Peripheral edema | |
| Cyanosis | | |
| Systematic hypotension | | |
| Characteristic chest x-ray | | |
| Course to death or recovery lasts 3 to 5 days | | |
| **Pathophysiology** | | |
| Reduced lung compliance | Poor peripheral perfusion | Myocardial malconduction |
| Reduced FRC | Poor renal perfusion | |
| Poor lung distensibility | | |
| Poor alveolar stability | | |
| Right-to-left shunts | | |
| Reduced effective pulmonary blood flow | | |
| **Pathobiochemistry** | | |
| Respiratory acidosis | Hyperbilirubinemia | Hyperkalemia |
| Metabolic acidosis | Decreased total serum proteins | Pepsinogen in lung |
| Decreased saturated P-lipids | Decreased fibrinolysins | |
| Preceded by low AF L/S ratio | | |
| Preceded by low AF surfactant titer | | |
| **Pathology** | | |
| Atelectasis | Osmiophilic lamellar bodies decreased early, increased later | Small adrenal glands |
| Injury to epithelial cells | | Intracranial hemorrhage |
| Membrane contains fibrin and cellular products | | |
| **Etiology** | | |
| Surfactant deficiency during disease | Primary surfactant deficiency (in utero) | Absent corticoid stimulus (in utero) |
| | | DPL synthesis impaired and/or destruction increased |
| | | Autonomic dysfunction |
| | | Primary pulmonary hypoperfusion |
| | | Hypovolemia |

[*]From Farrell, P., and Avery, M. E.: Am. Rev. Resp. Dis., *111*:657, 1975.
[†]The following abbreviations are used in this table: PROM—prolonged rupture of membranes (>16 hours); IUGR—intrauterine growth retardation; PDA—patent ductus arteriosus; FRC—functional residual capacity; AF—amniotic fluid; L/S—lecithin/sphingomyelin ratio; DPL—dipalmitoyl lecithin.

of type II cells are evident in infants who die in the second or third day of life.

**PATHOGENESIS.** Although numerous suggestions as to pathogenesis have been proposed since the first clinical description of this condition in 1949, the weight of evidence supports the central role of immaturity of the lung with respect to surfactant synthesis, or suppression of synthesis adequate to meet postnatal demands, as, for example, by asphyxia. The observations in support of a surfactant deficiency syndrome include: (1) the epidemiological finding of a higher incidence in more immature infants; (2) the postmortem biochemical observations on lungs of infants who die with the disorder; (3) the high order of predictability of this disease in the presence of low lecithin levels in amniotic liquid; (4) the reduced likelihood of the disease after events that accelerate lung maturation, such as intrauterine stress in association with intrauterine growth retardation, maternal heroin addiction or prenatal glucocorticoid therapy; and (5) the increased likelihood of the disease in the presence of maternal diabetes in which fetal insulin production can oppose the lung-maturation effect of corticoid. The 3-day course of mild to moderate hyaline membrane disease is also consistent with postnatal induction of enzyme activity with respect to surfactant synthesis.

Surfactant deficiency interferes with lung function by preventing the formation of a functional residual capacity of air by failing

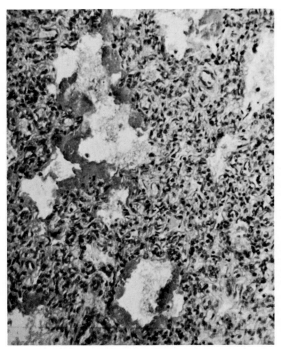

**Figure 13–2.** Photomicrograph of section of lung of a premature infant weighing 5 pounds (2270 gm) at birth, whose dyspnea was first noticed at eight hours and who died after steadily increasing respiratory difficulty at 27 hours. The appearance of the section of lung is in all respects similar to that in Figure 13–1.

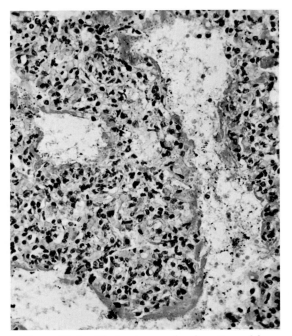

**Figure 13–1.** Photomicrograph of section of lung of a 3 pound 10 ounce (1640 gm) infant born in the thirty-second week of gestation. He seemed well for one hour; then dyspnea appeared and gradually increased with deepening sternal and costal retraction. He died at 22 hours of age. One sees unexpanded lung, with dilated air spaces lined with thick, homogeneously staining membrane.

to stabilize small air spaces at end-expiration. Each new inspiration requires the application of sufficient transpulmonary pressure to reinflate atelectatic air spaces. High frequencies and large applied pressures are employed to maintain alveolar ventilation. Uneven distribution of inspired air and perfusion of atelectatic air spaces result in poor gas exchange, characterized chiefly by hypoxemia. The infant grunts in an attempt to prolong inspiration, a pattern of breathing which can be shown experimentally to improve alveolar ventilation.

Pulmonary vascular resistance is raised by vasoconstriction aggravated by hypoxia, increasing right-to-left shunts through the persistent fetal vascular pathways, ductus arteriosus and foramen ovale. Some blood perfuses airless parts of lung, further contributing to the hypoxemia. As much as 80 per cent of the cardiac output may be shunted past airless lung.

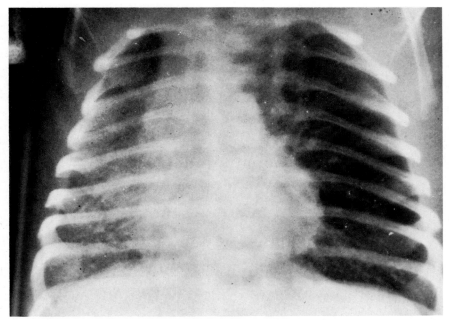

***Figure 13–3.*** Anteroposterior view of chest of a premature infant with typical "hyaline membrane syndrome" on the second day of life. Fine reticulogranular markings can still be seen at the left base. They have disappeared from view in the remainder of the left lung, which has become markedly emphysematous. They have become coarser and more crowded in the right lung as it has become more atelectatic.

Wasted ventilation and perfusion initiate a train of events which accounts for most of the findings in hyaline membrane disease. For example, reduced oxygenation to the heart impairs cardiac output, which in turn means reduced perfusion of organs such as the kidney, whose ability to maintain acid-base homeostasis is compromised. Poor perfusion of peripheral tissues contributes to lactic acidemia and a profound metabolic acidosis. The association of intraventricular hemorrhage with hyaline membrane disease may be related to cerebral hypoxia and ischemia or to intravascular coagulation, which is seen in some seriously ill infants.

**DIAGNOSIS.** The onset of symptoms is within minutes of birth, but often they are not recognized as significant for some hours. Duskiness, tachypnea, grunting and significant retractions are characteristic. Increasing cyanosis, often relatively unresponsive to increased inspired oxygen concentrations, is a necessary feature of the disease. Air exchange may be reduced; rales may or may not be present, and dullness to percussion may be evident, particularly at the lung bases. Sometimes the upper sternum seems prominent as the lower sternum is sucked in with each inspiratory effort.

Death is most likely to occur in the first 24 hours, but may be much later with use of respirators and other life-support interventions.

**RADIOGRAPHIC FINDINGS.** The earliest findings are a fine miliary mottling of the lungs, with consolidation centrally. The air-filled tracheobronchial tree stands out in relief against the opacified hila, which often obscure the cardiothymic silhouette. The radiographic appearance may change minute to minute, depending on the recent lung volume history. For example, a good cry can aerate both lungs, and a deep inspiratory effort may show minimal disease. Expiration, particularly after oxygen breathing, can lead to gas-freeing of lungs and a virtual "white-out" of the thorax.

The miliary reticulogranularity of the lung parenchyma is usually present within minutes of birth. Occasionally the changes are more prominent in the right than in the left hemithorax, and sometimes more evident in lower lobes than in upper lobes.

During the course of the disease, the

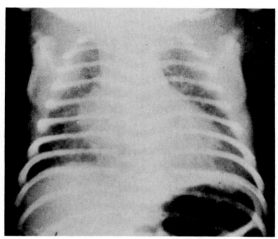

**Figure 13–4.** Anteroposterior view of thorax taken on the second day of life. Note the universal symmetrical, finely reticulogranular appearance of both lung fields.

radiogram may show a number of changes, including interstitial emphysema, pneumomediastinum and pneumothorax. In some infants, recovery is slow, and complex radiologic changes occur over ensuing months. (See pages 180 to 182.)

**PROGNOSIS.** Hyaline membrane disease remains a serious disorder. Approximately 20 to 30 per cent of those in whom we make the diagnosis succumb. Some of the deaths are from pulmonary failure; others are associated with, and perhaps caused by, intraventricular hemorrhage. The smallest infants usually succumb within 24 hours; larger ones may live longer, and some of these die from intercurrent infection. Most deaths occur within 72 hours of birth, unless artificial respiration is employed. Occasionally death occurs much later in those who receive ventilatory assistance. The survivors usually recover completely. Rarely, recurrent pulmonary infection and fibrosis have followed the illness. The outlook for mental and neurological status was reported from infants in a collaborative project by Fisch et al., who found significant impairment at 1 year of age, but no persisting deficits at 4 years of age when compared with infants of like birth weight without hyaline membrane disease.

Stahlman et al. have found no increase in disability among their infants with the disease treated by vigorous intensive care, compared to infants of like weight without the disease.

The many reports on mental and physical development of low-birth-weight infants with and without hyaline membrane disease agree that maintenance of homeostasis with respect to oxygen, acid-base balance, glucose, general nutritional support and careful temperature regulation have virtually eliminated spastic diplegia and have insured a greatly improved outlook with respect to later neuromuscular function.

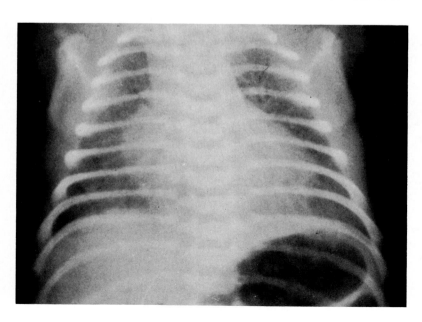

**Figure 13–5.** Anteroposterior view of chest of a prematurely born twin. Tachypnea began immediately after birth and was followed by increasing dyspnea. One sees the fine reticulogranular opacities scattered homogeneously throughout both lungs.

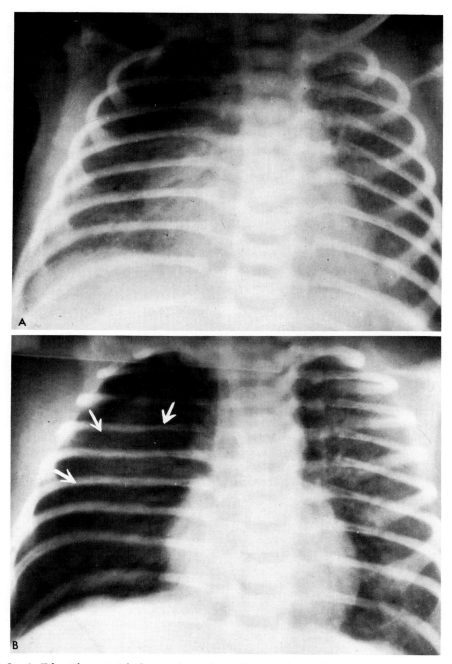

*Figure 13–6.* *A,* Film taken at eight hours of age shows the reticulogranular pattern in the left lung and right base, while the right upper lobe is distinctly hyperinflated. *B,* Six hours later. Now rupture has occurred on the right side, and a large pneumothorax can be seen surrounding the collapsed right lung.

**TREATMENT.** Advocates of one or another approach to treatment of hyaline membrane disease have in the past usually based their recommendations on assumptions derived from postulated pathogenesis rather than clinical, controlled trials. For example, nothing by mouth for 3 days arose from fears of further aspiration; digitalis and diuretics were advocated on the assumption that left heart failure was the primary defect; glucose and bicarbonate were prescribed to correct the metabolic acidosis; and mist with or without enzymes was at one time advocated to dissolve the membrane.

In the light of such a record of trial and error, it may be presumptuous to set forth an approach to treatment in 1976 without the qualifying comment that everything is subject to change.

At least now we have some carefully documented approaches to treatment that deserve emphasis. Of primary importance is the need to oxygenate the infant with whatever inspired mixture is needed to keep arterial tensions at 50 to 70 mm Hg. The goal can be achieved with modest inspired mixtures if continuous distending airway pressure is achieved either by positive pressure at the mouth, or negative pressure around the thorax by cuirass or body tank-type respiration. Alternately, prolonged inspiratory/expiratory ratios can do for the infant what he does with his own larynx in the act of grunting respiration.

One of the major problems faced by the therapist is to know the arterial oxygen tension during the course of a rapidly changing disease state as well as in response to therapeutic interventions. Clearly, continuous recording of transcutaneous $PO_2$ would be ideal, and some approaches have been made in this direction. Intermittent blood sampling is currently available. Some advocate arteriolar blood from finger sticks, others prefer the radial artery, and currently most place a catheter in the umbilical artery so as not to disturb the infant as frequently as gas samples are required. Hazards of umbilical artery catheterization have been detailed in numerous articles and include embolization to vital organs, loss of limbs, sepsis and mesenteric thrombosis. The risks versus benefits must be weighed for each infant, based on severity of illness, amounts of oxygen anticipated, risks of hyperoxygenation, such as retrolental fibroplasia, and risks of underoxygenation, which could lead to death.

RESPIRATORS. The use of continuous distending airway pressure to give the infant the functional residual capacity his unstable alveoli cannot assure him, can be achieved with or without respirators. If oxygenation cannot be maintained with continuous distending airway pressure up to 8 to 10 cm $H_2O$, or if apneic spells intervene, artificial ventilation is indicated. A variety of respirators are available that fulfill the requirements of delivering small gas volumes with either pressure-limited or volume-limited devices. The ability to vary inspiratory-expiratory ratios is helpful, since often 2:1 ratios improve gas exchange and lessen the peak pressures required.

Negative pressure respirators have the advantage of obviating the necessity for endotracheal tubes. On the other hand, they are not always effective in very sick infants with very stiff lungs. Tight-fitting face masks covering nose and mouth, nasal prongs and nasotracheal and endotracheal tubes all have their advocates. Loose-fitting tubes have the advantage of lessening dead space. A new sterile polyvinyl chloride tube is preferred, usually of 2.5 mm internal diameter for infants less than 2000 gm, and 3 mm internal diameter for larger infants. A rule of thumb, proposed by Sinclair, for the distance for insertion (from nares to mid-trachea) is 21 per cent of the baby's crown-heel length. The tube is fixed in position by passing silk sutures through the wall and anchoring them with tape to the skin. Absolute immobility of the tube in relation to the patient is desirable. Suctioning should be with strict sterile technique, including disposable gloves. It can be brief, but should be repeated every 30 to 60 minutes if secretions accumulate. The instillation of a few milliliters of sterile water is useful before suctioning if sticky secretions are present. The tube is changed only if obstructed.

*Complications of Respirator Therapy.* Increasingly infants are found to have interstitial emphysema and pneumothorax during the course of respirator therapy. Alertness as to the possibility of these complications, usually indicated by an abrupt clinical deterioration, can lead to lifesaving intervention. Of central importance is the awareness that the lungs themselves are changing during the course of the disease, so that the 10 cm $H_2O$ distending pressure found to be effective during the early phases of the disease may tamponade the pulmonary circulation during the recovery phase, leading to worsening of hypoxemia and stronger respiratory efforts, with lung rupture and loculated air.

Infants who survive the first week or so of illness may become respirator- and oxygen-dependent. Typically they undergo a series of changes in their lungs characterized by air-trapping, atelectasis, fibrosis, cyst formation and basilar emphysema. Originally described by Northway and Resan in 1967 under the name of bronchopulmonary dysplasia, this condition is now well known to everyone caring for premature infants. The course is chronic, sometimes months or years, with complete recovery a possibility, but death from intercurrent illness a continuing threat. At autopsy the lungs are heavy, hypercellular and fibrotic, with squamous metaplasia of even smaller airways. Since the cilia are gone, it is not surprising that secretions pool; either atelectasis or lobular emphysema is common.

Bronchopulmonary dysplasia is less common when the duration of high concentrations of inspired oxygen is reduced by continuous distending airway pressure or prolonged inspiratory-expiratory ratios. The similarity of the lesion to that of chronic oxygen toxicity is striking, and it may be related to oxygen alone. The contribution of high applied airway pressures to the pathogenesis of the lesion remains a possibility, supported by Reynolds et al., who report a sharp diminution in the lesion since they have limited airway pressures to less than 25 cm $H_2O$ (see page 180).

OTHER METHODS OF IMPROVING OXYGENATION. Increasing blood volume and increasing oxygen delivery by substitution of adult hemoglobin for fetal hemoglobin have much to commend them in the management of sick infants. The maintenance of normal arterial and central venous pressures ensures better distribution of the cardiac output. In at least one controlled trial by Delivoria-Papadopoulos and colleagues, a significant improvement in survival was demonstrated by a two-volume exchange transfusion with fresh blood within 8 hours of birth. We have preferred small transfusions with fresh blood to increase circulating blood volume.

OTHER SUPPORTIVE MEASURES. Nutritional support of the sick low-birth-weight infant is essential for recovery from disease as well as growth. Experience teaches us that aspiration is more likely with high respiratory rates and respiratory distress. For this reason, intravenous fluids are begun early in the course of the disease. On the first day of life 5 per cent glucose with $NaHCO_3$ 5–15 mEq per 100 ml solution depending on the degree of metabolic acidosis, seems appropriate in a volume of 60 to 80 ml/kg body weight. If the infant is breathing air saturated with water vapor, and in a fully saturated environment, water needs may be closer to 50 ml/kg; in a dry environment and with high respiratory rates off a respirator, approximately 100 ml/kg or more may be more appropriate. Over ensuing days it seems important to keep the infants in positive balance with respect to calories, nitrogen and glucose. The addition of amino acid mixtures and lipid emulsions to intravenous therapy seems to be a major advance in management. Although many details remain to be evaluated, it now appears that there is little excuse to superimpose starvation upon sick premature infants.

TEMPERATURE REGULATION. Maintenance of a thermal-neutral environment (defined as that thermal environment in which oxygen consumption is at a minimum) seems to improve survival of sick low-birth-weight infants. Even a few degrees can change oxygen consumption and, hence, metabolic demands, and in turn ventilatory requirements. In practice, maintaining the environmental temperature at 36° to 36.5° C seems best. Peripheral vasoconstriction is a sign of an adverse thermal environment and can be used as an indicator of the appropriateness, or lack thereof, of incubator temperatures.

## PERSISTENT PATENT DUCTUS ARTERIOSUS

With increasing survival of low birth weight infants, we are seeing more and more infants with symptomatic patent ductus arteriosus, sometimes requiring surgical closure. Many are convalescing from their respiratory distress when a systolic or continuous murmur becomes evident, respiratory effort increases, a bounding pulse may appear and the heart enlarges. Digitalis and diuretics prove helpful in most such infants, but a few are in intractable failure and require surgical closure of the ductus.

Edmunds *et al.* reported 21 infants who required operation at ages 16 to 44 days (mean 29 days) in the absence of previous RDS, and 5 to 35 days (mean 15 days) for those who had had RDS. Most infants improve promptly after ligation of the ductus, although some show persistent pulmonary changes similar to those described in bronchopulmonary dysplasia.

Our indications for operation are the demonstration of a left-to-right shunt by scanning or by aortography, and failure of medical management to improve the heart failure.

Closure of the ductus with a prostaglandin inhibitor, indomethacin, was reported by Friedman et al. and appears to be a promising approach.

**PRENATAL DIAGNOSIS AND PREVENTION.** Recognition that a deficiency of alveolar surfactant was an essential aspect of hyaline membrane disease, and knowledge that lung liquids contributed to amniotic liquid, led to a search for components of the surfactant in amniotic liquid. Gluck et

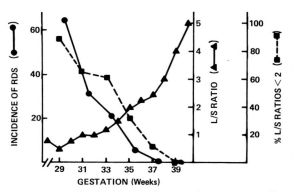

*Figure 13–8.* Comparison of incidence figures for RDS with average values of lecithin/sphingomyelin in amniotic liquid. Each value is plotted as a function of gestational age. (From Farrell, P. M., and Avery, M. E.: Am. Rev. Resp. Dis. *111*:657, 1975)

al. first established the relationship between a low lecithin-sphingomyelin ratio and clinical respiratory distress, establishing the ability to predict with a greater than 90 per cent accuracy which infant was at risk (Fig. 13–7).

Subsequently other approaches to prenatal diagnosis, such as the foam stability test of Clements, have found wide use among obstetricians. It seems inevitable that the next few years will be characterized by improvements in the approach to prenatal estimation of lung maturity.

The possibility of prevention of hyaline membrane disease is at hand with the demonstration that glucocorticoids are the timers of lung cell differentiation. Normally the fetal adrenal produces glucocorticoids toward the end of pregnancy, or earlier given some kinds of intrauterine stress. Amniotic liquid levels of cortisol reflect this activity by increasing after 35 weeks of gestation. Thus, premature birth deprives the infant of the physiologic surge in glucocorticoid activity which presumably is necessary for alveolar cell differentiation with respect to surfactant synthesis. Liggins and Howie first demonstrated that betamethasone given to the mother 24 hours before delivery could reduce deaths from hyaline membrane disease in infants under 32 weeks. It seems probable that this form of intervention, or prenatal treatment, will be indicated whenever delivery can be postponed 24 hours in the presence of a low lecithin/sphingomyelin ratio. More controlled trials and long-term follow-ups are under way.

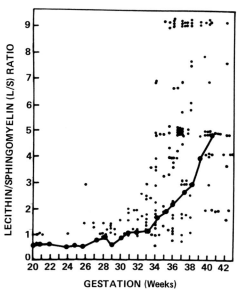

*Figure 13–7.* Note the wide variation among individuals of the same gestational age. The lecithin-sphingomyelin ratio is a better index of lung "maturity" than is gestational age. (Data of L. Gluck et al.) (From Farrell, P. M., and Avery, M. E.: Am. Rev. Resp. Dis. *111*:657, 1975)

# REFERENCES

Ablow, R. C., and Orzalesi, M. M.: Localized roentgenographic pattern of hyaline membrane disease. Evidence that the upper lobes of human lung mature earlier than the lower lobes. Am. J. Roentgenol. *112*:23, 1971.

Auld, P. A. M., Bhangananda, P., and Mehta, S.: The influence of an early caloric intake with I-V glucose on catabolism of premature infants. Pediatrics *37*: 592, 1966.

Avery, M. E.: Pharmacological approaches to acceleration of fetal lung maturation. Br. Med. Bull. *31*:131, 1975.

Avery, M. E., and Fletcher, B. D.: The Lung and Its Disorders in the Newborn Infant. 3rd ed. Philadelphia, W. B. Saunders Company, 1974.

Avery, M. E., and Mead, J.: Surface properties in relation to atelectasis and hyaline membrane disease. Am. J. Dis. Child. *97*:517, 1959.

Bancalari, E., Garcia, O. L., and Jesse, M. J.: Effects of continuous negative pressure on lung mechanisms in idiopathic respiratory distress syndrome. Pediatrics *51*:485, 1973.

Blystad, W., Landing, B. H., and Smith, C. A.: Pulmonary hyaline membranes in newborn infants. Pediatrics *8*:5, 1951.

Bozic, C.: Pulmonary hyaline membranes and vascular anomalies of the lung. Description of a case. Pediatrics *32*:1094, 1963.

Brumley, G. W., Hodson, W. A., and Avery, M. E.: Lung phospholipids and surface tension correlations in infants with and without hyaline membrane disease and in adults. Pediatrics *40*:13, 1967.

Chu, J., Clements, J. A., Cotton, E. K., et al.: Neonatal pulmonary ischemia. Pediatrics *40*:709, 1970.

Clements, J. A., Platzker, A. C. G., Tierney, D. F., et al.: Assessment of the risk of the respiratory distress syndrome by a rapid test for surfactant in amniotic fluid. N. Engl. J. Med., *286*:1077, 1972.

Davies, P. A., Robinson, R. J., Scopes, J. W., et al.: Medical Care of Newborn Babies. Philadelphia, J. B. Lippincott Co., 1972.

DeLemos, R. A., Shermata, D. W., Knelson, J. H., et al.: Acceleration of appearance of pulmonary surfactant in the fetal lamb by administration of corticosteroids. Am. Rev. Resp. Dis. *102*:459, 1970.

Delivoria-Papadapoulos, M., et al.: Effect of exchange transfusion on pulmonary function of infants with severe respiratory distress syndrome. (Abstract.) Pediat. Res. *8*:445, 1974.

DeReuck, A. V. S., and Porter, R. (eds.): Ciba Foundation Symposium: Development of the Lung. London, J. & A. Churchill Ltd., 1967.

Edmunds, L. H., Gregory, G. A., Heymann, M. A., et al.: Surgical closure of ductus arteriosus in premature infants. Circulation *48*:856, 1973.

Evans, J. J.: Prediction of respiratory distress syndrome by shake test on newborn gastric aspirate. N. Engl. J. Med. *292*:1113, 1975.

Farrell, P. M., and Avery, M. E.: Hyaline membrane disease. State of the art. Am. Rev. Resp. Dis. *111*: 657, 1975.

Fanaroff, A. A., Cha, C. C., Sosa, R., et al.: A controlled trial of continuous negative external pressure in the treatment of severe respiratory distress syndrome. J. Pediatr. *82*:921, 1973.

Fencl, M., and Tulchinsky, D.: Total cortisol in amniotic fluid and fetal lung maturation. N. Engl. J. Med. *292*:133, 1975.

Fisch, R. O., Gravem, H. J., and Engle, R. R.: Neurological status of survivors of neonatal respiratory distress syndrome. J. Pediatr. *73*:395, 1968.

Friedman, W. F., et al.: Pharmacologic closure of patent ductus arteriosus in the premature infant. N. Engl. J. Med. *295*:526, 1976.

Gandy, G., Jacobson, W., and Gairdner, D.: Hyaline membrane disease. I. Cellular changes. Arch. Dis. Child. *45*:289, 1970.

Gitlin, D., and Craig, J. M.: The nature of hyaline membrane in asphyxia of the newborn. Pediatrics *17*:64, 1956.

Gluck, L., Kulovich, M. V., Borer, R. C., et al.: Diagnosis of the respiratory distress syndrome by amniocentesis. Used in "A pediatrician's view of hyaline membrane disease." Am. J. Obstet. Gynec. *109*:440, 1971.

Graven, S. N., and Misenheimer, H. R.: Respiratory distress syndrome and the high risk mother. Am. J. Dis. Child. *109*:489, 1965.

Gregory, G. A., Kitterman, J. A., Phibbs, R. H., et al.: Treatment of idiopathic respiratory distress syndrome with continuous positive airway pressure. N. Engl. J. Med. *284*:1333, 1971.

Harrison, V. C., Heese, H. de V., and Klein, M.: The significance of grunting in hyaline membrane disease. Used in "A pediatrician's view of hyaline membrane disease." Pediatrics *41*:549, 1968.

Heymann, M. A., Rudolph, A. M., and Silverman, N. H.: Closure of the ductus arteriosus in premature infants by inhibition of prostaglandin synthesis. N. Engl. J. Med. *295*:530, 1976.

Huch, R., Lübbers, D., and Huch, A.: Reliability of transcutaneous monitoring of arterial $PO_2$ in newborn infants. Arch. Dis. Child. *49*:213, 1974.

James, L. S.: The onset of breathing and resuscitation. Pediatr. Clin. N. Am. *13*:621, 1966.

Klaus, M. H., and Fanaroff, A. A.: Care of the High-Risk Neonate. Philadelphia, W. B. Saunders Company, 1973.

Knelson, J. H., and Avery, M. E.: Site of blood sampling. Letter to editor. Pediatrics *43*:638, 1969.

Knelson, J. H., Howatt, W. F., and DeMuth, G. R.: The physiologic significance of grunting respiration. Pediatrics *44*:393, 1969.

Krouskop, R. W., Brown, E. G., and Sweet, A. Y.: The early use of continuous positive airway pressure in the treatment of idiopathic respiratory distress syndrome. J. Pediatr. *87*:263, 1975.

Landing, B. H.: Pulmonary lesions of newborn infants: A statistical study. Pediatrics *19*:217, 1957.

Lendrum, F. C.: The pulmonary hyaline membrane as a manifestation of heart failure in the newborn infant. J. Pediatr. *47*:149, 1955.

Lewis, S.: A follow up study of the respiratory distress syndrome. Proc. Soc. Med *61*:771, 1968.

Liggins, G. C., and Howie, R. N.: A controlled trial of antepartum glucocorticoid treatment for prevention of the respiratory distress syndrome in premature infants. Pediatrics *50*:515, 1972.

Miller, H. C., and Hamilton, T. R.: The pathogenesis of the "vernix membrane": Relation to aspiration pneumonia in stillborn and newborn infants. Pediatrics *3*:735, 1949.

Mockrin, L. D., and Bancalari, E. H.: Early versus delayed initiation of continuous negative pressure in infants with hyaline membrane disease. J. Pediatr. *87*:596, 1975.

Moss, A. J., Duffie, E. R., Jr., and Fagan, L. M.: Respiratory distress syndrome in newborn: Study on association of cord clamping and pathogenesis of distress, J.A.M.A., *184*:48, 1963.

Nicolopoulos, D. A., and Smith, C. A.: Metabolic aspects of idiopathic respiratory distress (hyaline membrane syndrome) in newborn infants. Pediatrics *28*:206, 1961.

Northway, W. H., and Rosan, R. C.: Radiographic features of pulmonary oxygen toxicity in the newborn: Bronchopulmonary dysplasia. Radiology *91*:49, 1968.

Peterson, H. G., Jr., and Pendleton, M. E.: Contrasting roentgenographic pulmonary patterns of the hyaline membrane and fetal aspiration syndromes. Am. J. Roentgenol. *74*:800, 1955.

Reynolds, E. O. R.: Management of hyaline membrane disease. Br. Med. Bull. *31*:18, 1975.

Rhodes, P. G., Hall, R. T., and Leonidas, J. C.: Chronic pulmonary disease in neonates with assisted ventilation. Pediatrics *55*:788, 1975.

Robert, M. F., Neff, R. K., Hubbell, J. P., Taeusch, H. W., and Avery, M. E.: Association between maternal diabetes and the respiratory distress syndrome in the newborn. N. Engl. J. Med. *294*:357, 1976.

Roberton, N. R. C., Hallidie-Smith, K. A., and Davis, J. A.: Severe respiratory distress syndrome mimicking cyanotic heart-disease in term babies. Lancet *2*:1108, 1967.

Robertson, B., Tunell, R., and Rudhe, U.: Late stages of pulmonary hyaline membranes of the newborn. Acta Paediatr. *53*:433, 1964.

Rokos, J., Vaeusorn, O., Nachman, R., et al.: Hyaline membrane disease in twins. Pediatrics *42*:204, 1968.

Scarpelli, E.: Respiratory distress syndrome of the newborn. Ann. Rev. Med. *19*:153, 1968.

Stahlman, M. T.: In Lucey, J. F. (ed.): Problems of Neonatal Intensive Care Units. Fifty-Ninth Ross Conference on Pediatric Research. Columbus, Ohio, 1969.

Stahlman, M. T., Battersby, E. J., Shepard, F. M., et al.: Prognosis in hyaline membrane disease. N. Engl. J. Med. *276*:303, 1967.

Taghizadeh, A., and Reynolds, E. O. R.: Pathogenesis of bronchopulmonary dysplasia following hyaline membrane disease. Am. J. Pathol. *82*:241, 1976.

Tchou, C.-S., Fletcher, B. D., Branke, P., et al.: Asymmetric distribution of the roentgen pattern in hyaline membrane disease. J. Can. Assoc. Radiol. *23*: 85, 1972.

Thibeault, D. W., Emmanouilides, G. C., Nelson, R. J., et al.: Patent ductus arteriosus complicating the respiratory distress syndrome in preterm infants. J. Pediatr. *86*:120, 1975.

Tran Dinh De and Anderson, G. W.: The experimental production of pulmonary hyaline-like membranes with atelectasis. Am. J. Obstet. Gynecol. *68*:1557, 1954.

Usher, R.: The respiratory distress syndrome of prematurity. Pediatric Clin. N. Am. *8*:525, 1961.

Warley, M. A., and Gairdner, D.: Respiratory distress syndrome of the newborn: Principles in treatment. Arch. Dis. Child. *37*:455, 1962.

# 14                                                        PNEUMONIA

Pneumonia is one of the important causes of perinatal death. It is the sole pathologic lesion discoverable in many stillborn fetuses as well as in many infants who die during the first month of life. In addition, it is a complicating factor in the deaths of many more.

**INCIDENCE.** In consecutive autopsies on stillborns and newborns the percentage of pneumonitis discovered has always been high. In the 1920's and 1930's most figures ranged from 20 to 30 per cent, but Helwig reported 41.5 per cent, and Hook and Katz's result was as high as 51 per cent. In the 1950's the percentages were lower, such as Penner and McInnis's 11.7 per cent and Potter and Adair's 6 per cent. In a review published in 1955 we found evidence of pneumonia in 35 per cent of 76 autopsies, but believed pneumonia to be the sole cause of death in 8 per cent of these newborns.

Autopsy percentages do not tell the entire story. Neonatal pneumonia is not always fatal, and it is an important cause of tachypnea and dyspnea in the first month of life. In 1974, we diagnosed pneumonia in 24 infants among 4000 births, and 9 of the 24 died.

In the differential diagnosis of respiratory difficulty in this age group pneumonia must always be given serious consideration.

**CLASSIFICATION.** Pneumonia may be acquired (1) before the beginning of labor, i.e., in utero, (2) in the course of labor, (3) at the moment of delivery, or (4) after birth. Many attempts have been made to clas-

sify neonatal pneumonias into smaller subgroups in order to clarify some of the confusion which inheres of necessity in a
disease group of such variable etiology, pathology and pathogenesis. We shall base
our discussion upon a schema, in part temporal, in part pathologic and in part pathogenetic.

  I. Intrauterine pneumonia
    A. Ascending infections
    B. Transplacental infections
 II. Paranatally and postnatally acquired pneu-
    monias
    A. Due to aspiration of maternal fecal mat-
       ter
    B. Due to aspiration of food or gastric con-
       tents
    C. Secondary to septicemia
    D. Airborne or contact infections
      1. Bacterial
      2. Viral
      3. Protozoal and fungal
    E. *Pneumocystis carinii* pneumonia

## INTRAUTERINE PNEUMONIA

Intrauterine pneumonia may produce
death of the fetus in utero, or live infants
may be born with fully developed pneumonia which originated within the uterus.
Many of these die within the first 2 or 3
days. The pathologic picture of intrauterine
pneumonia differs considerably from that
of the postnatally acquired disease. The
clinical picture is no less different. The
prognosis is poor but not hopeless.

**PATHOLOGY.** Gross examination of the
lungs is unrewarding. There are no distinct
areas of consolidation or pleurisy, no abscess formation and little or no exudate in
the bronchi. Characteristic is the diffuse-
ness of the involvement on microscopic
examination, practically all the alveoli
in all portions of the lungs being affected.
These are filled with exudate in which
are found polymorphonuclear cells, some
mononuclears, and often red blood cells.
Fibrin is striking by its absence. In some
lungs amniotic debris is virtually absent
(Fig. 14–1); in some, large amounts are
present in distended alveoli (Fig. 14–2).
One assumes that in the latter instance
intrauterine aspiration caused pneumonitis,
whereas the former appearance suggests

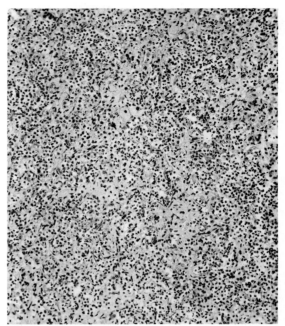

**Figure 14–1.** Microscopic section of lung (× 150)
of an 8 pound 5 ounce (3770 gm) stillborn infant. The
mother's membranes had ruptured 48 hours before
delivery. No treatment had been given. Note the
diffuse pneumonitis, with fluid and inflammatory
cells, mostly polymorphonuclears, homogeneously
and heavily infiltrating interstitial tissue as well as the
potential air spaces. A little amniotic debris is visible.

that pneumonitis was hematogenous in origin.

**INCIDENCE.** Johnson and Meyer found
pneumonia in 19 per cent of 500 consecutive autopsies on stillborns and newborns.
In 13 per cent the evidence indicated that
the infection had been acquired in utero.
MacGregor found this figure to be about 15
per cent. In a series of 1044 consecutive
autopsies of stillborn and newborn infants
from Babies Hospital, New York, Naeye et
al. found congenital pneumonia in 23 per
cent.

In live births intrauterine pneumonia is
uncommon, as contrasted with massive aspiration without infection and with hyaline
membrane disease. We believe that we
make this diagnosis justifiably in five to ten
infants a year on a nursery service of 3000
deliveries each year.

**ETIOLOGY.** The organisms found include, singly or in combination, those
which commonly inhabit the maternal genital tract. These are Group B streptococci,

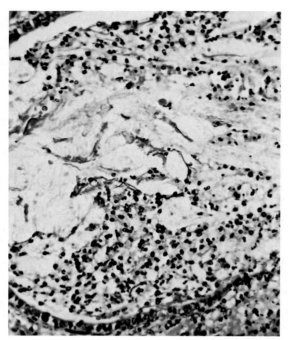

*Figure 14–2.* Microscopic section of lung (× 300) of a full-term infant who lived for two days. The membranes had ruptured 26 hours before delivery, and the cord was wrapped tightly about the baby's neck. Resuscitated with difficulty, she had tachypnea and low-grade fever throughout life. Note the large amount of amniotic aspirate overfilling alveoli in the center, while the surrounding areas are the sites of intense inflammation, most of the cells being polymorphonuclears.

various staphylococci, *Escherichia coli* and other gram-negative bacilli.

**PATHOGENESIS.** From studies of stillborns whose sole cause of death was pneumonia, determined by postmortem examination, and of newborns who lived only a few hours or days and in whom no other cause of death was discovered at autopsy, one concludes that intrauterine pneumonia develops under two different circumstances.

1. Pneumonia may follow prolonged membrane rupture. Amniotic fluids become contaminated by ascending vaginal organisms in increasing numbers the longer the membranes remain ruptured before delivery. If labor is active while membranes are ruptured, such contamination proceeds more rapidly, so that 100 per cent of fluids are infected by the end of 24 hours. Since all fetuses continually swallow amniotic fluid, the oropharynx and the gastrointestinal tract are the most common portals of entry for fetal infection. But since the fetus is induced to gasp as a result of any asphyxial insult, massive aspiration of contaminated amniotic fluid undoubtedly plays a role in pathogenesis.

Kjessler and Pryles et al. have confirmed the importance of prolonged membrane rupture time in the causation of pneumonitis and sepsis, while Blanc described in detail the possible routes of ascending fetal infection under the title "amniotic infection syndrome." Less commonly, infection may ascend through intact, unruptured membrane.

Shubeck has reported the results of a prospective study of more than 30,000 infants born consecutively and included in the Collaborative Perinatal Mortality Study. As membrane rupture time increased from 0 to 72 hours, amnionitis increased in linear fashion to about 50 per cent, funisitis to about 25 per cent, and documented infection of the fetus or the newborn infant to about 8 per cent.

2. Fetal pneumonia may result from transmission of bacteria across the placental barrier to the fetal circulation and thence to the lungs. These organisms may be carried to the placenta by maternal blood. A number of cases of intrauterine pneumococcal pneumonia have developed while the mother suffered from pneumococcal septicemia. That other organisms, including viruses, may cross the placenta in similar fashion appears certain. Placental transmission of viruses is well documented, although usually the impact of fetal viremia is more devastating to the central nervous system, liver and spleen than it is to the lung (Fig. 14–3). Cytomegalovirus, rubella and herpes are all capable of producing fetal pneumonia. Phelan and Campbell described seven infants with interstitial pneumonia caused by rubella, six of whom died of their pneumonia.

**DIAGNOSIS.** A history of precedent obstetrical difficulty is usually obtained. Prolonged ruptured membrane time, especially when this interval has exceeded 12 hours, is highly suggestive. So is maternal antepartum or intrapartum fever or urinary

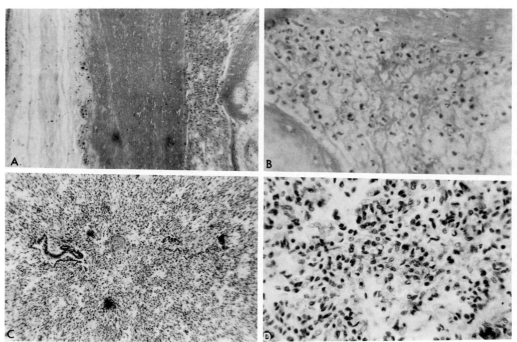

*Figure 14–3.* *A*, Microscopic section of placenta to show ascending fetal infection leading to intrauterine pneumonia. *B*, High-power view of the subchorionic region. *C*, Low-power view of section of lung to show dense homogeneous exudation and leukocytic infiltration. No amniotic debris is visible. *D*, Higher-power view of same.

This case was presented by Dr. Peter Gruenwald at a Johns Hopkins Fetal Mortality Clinic. The photographs are reprinted with his kind permission. The infant was one whose mother's labor was induced, because of Rh incompatibility, two weeks before term. Manual stripping of the membranes did not succeed on one day and was repeated the following day. The infant was promptly exchange-transfused, but died, for unknown reasons, in the midst of the procedure. The findings of placentitis and pneumonitis were unexpected.

tract infection (Fig. 14–4). Obstetrical accidents or prolonged labor leading to fetal asphyxia and vigorous manipulation during delivery, if coupled with prolonged membrane rupture, makes the possibility of intrauterine pneumonia a strong probability.

The infant may be ill at birth with asphyxia of either the livid or pallid variety. The first cry is delayed 2 to 10 minutes or longer, and spontaneous respirations are not established quickly. These infants will have required resuscitative efforts immediately after birth. A falling Apgar score should suggest the possibility of pneumonia.

When respirations become established, they are rapid. Tachypnea may be accompanied by slight or moderate, never severe, retraction. Expiration is often grunting. Fever is present at times in the full-term infant. Often this is low in degree, but on occasion it may reach 104°F or more. Premature infants with pneumonia do not ordinarily become febrile, but they often manifest wide fluctuations of temperature below the normal line. There is no cough.

Physical signs are variable. Occasionally, localized dullness and rales may be heard over several areas of the lung fields on the first examination. Usually the appearance of these signs is delayed for 12 to 48 hours, and at times they can never be elicited through the entire course of the disease. Breath sounds may be diminished over one or more areas or may be generally reduced in intensity, or in places they may be unduly harsh. Seldom does one hear classic tubular breathing.

The white blood cell count in some cases has been in the neighborhood of 30,000, with 75 per cent or more polymorphonuclears, while in a few the count is definitely leukopenic, 4000 per cu ml or less. In the majority the white cell count is within normal limits for the newborn, 5000 to 25,000 and the polymorphonuclear per-

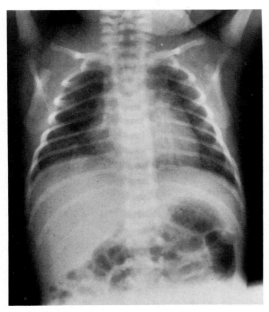

*Figure 14–4.* Film of an infant, age 4 hours, with moderate tachypnea, born of a mother with Group B streptococcal urinary tract infection. Although the infiltrates appear only moderate, the infant died of septicemia and pneumonia at 20 hours of age.

fants become hypertonic, even rigid. Some have muscular twitchings, some frank convulsions. These phenomena are encountered when the disease is severe, and these infants usually do poorly. At autopsy no gross intracranial lesion may be discovered.

Several of our infants with extensive early neonatal pneumonia have had heart failure, signalized by cardiac enlargement, poor, rapid heart sounds and sudden increase in size of the liver.

**RADIOGRAPHIC FINDINGS.** Radiograms supply the supporting evidence for the diagnosis of pneumonia of the newborn. They yield positive evidence in almost all cases in which the clinical picture fits the pattern described above. Pneumonia was not often diagnosed by x-ray study in the past. There are several reasons for this. One is that films taken on the first day of life at times appear normal, and no further ones are taken. In our experience patches of consolidation may not become obvious

centage is not high. In our experience blood cultures have been only rarely positive, and cultures from the throat and nasopharynx have revealed a mixture of the usual vaginal flora. Gastric aspirate obtained in the first hours of life may contain polymorphonuclear cells and bacteria visible with Gram stain (Fig. 14–5). If the pneumonia, progresses, and no organism has been demonstrated from the placenta or gastric aspirate, needle aspirate of the lung may be indicated. The quick insertion and withdrawal of a #23 needle attached to a syringe with about 0.5 ml saline, can contaminate the needle with the offending organism, which may then be cultured. The saline allows the contents of the needle to be flushed into the culture medium.

Virus isolation, demonstration of rising titers of specific antibody, and serum IgM and IgA levels are increasingly available and of essential help in diagnosis of viral infections.

Neurologic abnormalities appear in the course of the disease with unexpected frequency. The infant who was flaccid at birth may remain flaccid for days. Other in-

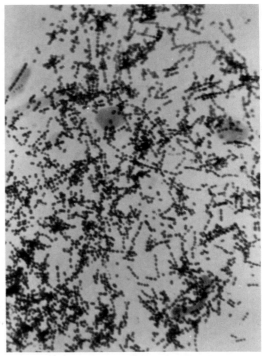

*Figure 14–5.* Gram-stain of gastric aspirate of infant described in legend of Fig. 14–4. Note the myriads of streptococci evident on this smear. (Courtesy of Dr. William Cochran, Boston Hospital for Women.)

until the second or even the third day. This is analogous to the situation in older patients, in whom pneumonic areas may not become radiopaque for a number of days after the onset. Therefore, in doubtful cases x-ray films should be made daily for the first 3 days at least. The second reason is that areas of radiopacity, when seen, are assumed to represent atelectasis. Although this is true at times, at other times they surely are pneumonic patches.

We feel that there are several radiographic patterns of congenital pneumonia. The first is one of bilateral homogeneous opacification involving the major portions of both lungs (Figs. 14–6 and 14–7). This pattern is rarely seen and must be confined to those cases in which pneumonia developed in the fetus many days before delivery. The second pattern is similar to diffuse bronchopneumonia at any age. It consists in coarse irregular opacities heavily clustered about the hilus and extending fanwise in diminishing amounts toward the periphery on both sides. Often it is ill defined on the first day of life, becoming more opaque as well as more extensive on the second and third days. In a few examples we have seen recently there is linear hard-looking opacification extending fanwise from the hilus on one side, while on the other there is an area or several areas of soft-appearing homogeneous density. Peribronchial thickening as a part of the bronchopneumonic process will appear as tiny ring-like densities in the perihilar areas when the bronchi are seen on end. Air bronchograms may also be present as the air-filled bronchi are contrasted against the airless alveoli.

Almost impossible to differentiate from pneumonia is the picture of massive aspiration as described by Peterson and Pendleton, in which opacities assume a "coarse, irregular pattern," and are distributed in exactly the same fashion as we have described for the bronchopneumonic type of congenital pneumonia. There is, however,

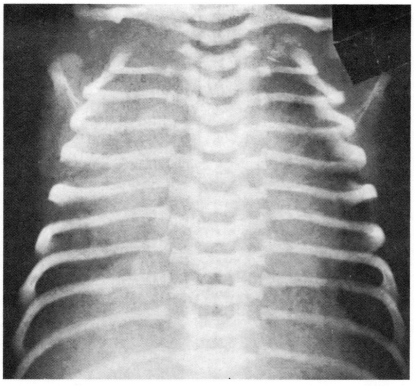

*Figure 14–6.* Anteroposterior view of chest taken at 16 hours of age. The lungs appear to be almost completely consolidated, the periphery of the left lung and the extreme right base alone containing air. The opacification is homogeneous and dense.

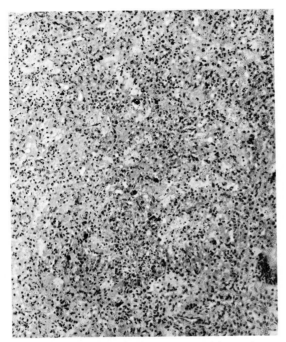

*Figure 14–7.* Microscopic section of lung shows widespread homogenous exudation and leukocytic infiltration. Alveoli, bronchi, and interstitial tissue are all equally involved.

one difference. In pneumonia the radiographic changes may be ill defined on the first day and become more definite within the next few days, whereas in massive aspiration the alterations are maximal early and disappear rapidly in the course of the next few days. If areas of opacification appear soft and homogeneous rather than hard and linear, pneumonia is the more likely diagnosis (Fig. 14–9).

**PROGNOSIS.** It is not true that intrauterine pneumonia is necessarily fatal. This belief arose because until recently the diagnosis was made only post mortem, and because clinicians have not recognized less severe forms. We have now seen many patients who have recovered. It is true, however, that the more seriously ill infants are apt to die in utero or within the first day or two of life regardless of the excellence of treatment. They may die from widespread encroachment of the pneumonic process upon functioning lung tissue alone, or "cerebral deaths" with rigidity and convulsions, or from associated heart failure. It is also a fact that prognosis is bad for the

premature infant with pneumonitis but very good for the term infant. In the course of an unpublished study of one of us (A.J.S.), of approximately 9000 consecutive births at one hospital, four deaths from pneumonia were encountered. All four were infants who weighed less than 2000 gm at birth.

**TREATMENT.** When the diagnosis of intrauterine pneumonia can be made with a fair degree of certainty, treatment must be prompt and vigorous. When pneumonia is suspected antibiotics should be ordered as soon as blood and oropharyngeal cultures and gastric aspirate are collected. The choice of antibiotic depends on knowledge of the organisms in the environment. If the mother was infected and cultures had been taken, we would use antibiotics appropriate to cover her organisms. If the organism is unknown, we use aqueous penicillin, 100,000 units per kilogram per day in two divided doses for the first few days of life, and then in four divided doses. Kanamycin sulfate, 15 mg/kg/day in two divided doses, is also given since it is bacteriocidal against many gram-negative bacilli. Gentamicin, 5 mg/kg/day in the first week and 7.5 mg/kg/day thereafter in divided doses is useful if organisms in the clinic are resistant to Kanamycin. If the cultured organism is not sensitive to those agents, one must use other antibiotics as indicated by sensitivity tests, such as methicillin, ampicillin, streptomycin or colistin. Rarely is chloramphenicol indicated, but if it is used the dosage should be restricted to 25 mg/kg/day and blood levels followed.

Adequate fluids must be supplied, parenterally if necessary. The infants will be kept in a humid environment, with oxygen at a concentration high enough to abolish cyanosis. A sharp lookout must be kept for serious complications, particularly pneumothorax.

**PREVENTION.** Opinion is still divided as to the efficacy of maternal therapy prior to delivery in preventing fetal infection when the membranes have ruptured prematurely. No one any longer advocates treating a mother with full doses of antibiotics for weeks or months. But since concomitant labor seems to hasten upward spread of infection from vagina to fetus, one might logically attempt to prevent as-

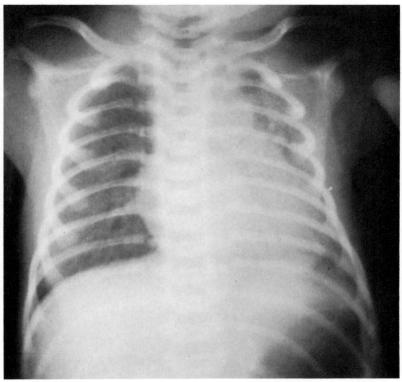

*Figure 14–8.* There is soft linear infiltration spreading outward fanwise from the right hilus. The left lung is almost entirely opacified by confluent areas of homogeneous density. This 4 pound 5 ounce (1956 gm) infant was born after membranes had been ruptured 11½ hours; a second stage of 2½ hours was terminated by mid-forceps extraction. Amniotic fluid was meconium stained; Apgar score was 2 at one minute. Tachypnea and dyspnea were followed by apneic spells and then convulsions; he died at 25 hours of age.

cent by treatment during this critical period. This might be accomplished by beginning vigorous antibiotic therapy a few weeks before the expected date of confinement, continuing it for 2 or 3 days, and then inducing labor. In any event one might give the mother antibiotics from the moment labor begins. Penicillin alone has not been successful in lowering fetal mortality when given to mothers with premature rupture of the membranes (Eastman), and considering the organisms which are usually responsible for intrauterine pneumonia, it would not be expected to be effective. A broad spectrum antibacterial agent such as ampicillin must be used.

The next question is whether one should treat babies routinely who have been born after prolonged membrane rupture time or after asphyxia-producing obstetrical accidents which predispose to neonatal pneumonia. No controlled studies to date have shown that babies so treated suffer less

mortality or morbidity than those from whom treatment is withheld until indicated by appropriate signs or symptoms. But these infants must be monitored assiduously, and vigorous treatment must be instituted at the first sign of respiratory trouble.

## CASE HISTORIES

### CASE 14–1

A full-term 9-pound (4082 gm) female infant was born to a 30 year old primipara. Pregnancy had been uneventful except that the mother had had a hemorrhoidectomy 2 weeks before term. The membranes ruptured 4 hours before delivery. Total labor lasted five hours, the second stage two hours. The infant cried and breathed spontaneously after birth, but the color looked pale and gray. Two hours after birth, respirations were noted to be grunting, and this increased over the next ten hours. At 16 hours the color was gray and she was cyanotic, temperature was 101.6°F, and respirations were rapid and shallow with slight sternal retraction. Per-

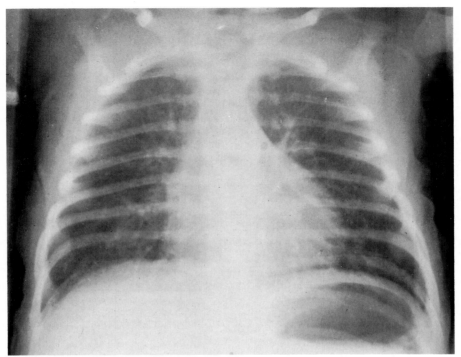

*Figure 14–9.* Anteroposterior view of chest of an infant whose history is not abstracted in the text, who was born 36 hours after membrane rupture and demonstrated fever and tachypnea with mild retraction for five days. He undoubtedly had intrauterine pneumonia.

cussion note was dull everywhere, and many fine rales were heard throughout. Air exchange was poor. Heart sounds were poor, and the liver edge descended to two fingerbreadths below the costal margin. Despite antibiotics, temperature rose to 102.2°F. X-ray film showed very little aerated lung, limited to the periphery (Fig. 14–6). Autopsy showed widespread pneumonia (Fig. 14–7).

**COMMENT.** In this example the pneumonia is diffuse and homogeneous, and neither the radiographic nor the pathologic appearance suggests aspiration. It seems probable that hemorrhoidectomy performed two weeks before term led to maternal bacteremia; bacteria then crossed the placenta and caused fetal septicemia and pneumonia. The clinical course, including tachypnea, mild dyspnea and fever, is characteristic of congenital pneumonia.

CASE 14–2

A white female infant was born at term 4 days after the membranes had ruptured spontaneously. For 3 days the mother had been given penicillin and streptomycin intramuscularly and on the fourth day oxytetracycline by mouth. Labor was finally induced by Pitocin administered intravenously and lasted only 3 hours. At birth the infant was cyanotic and flaccid. Penicillin and streptomycin were given immediately and continued every 6 hours, and she was placed in an incubator with high humidity and oxygen. Physical examination (8 hours) showed that the infant was mildly cyanotic and sluggish, her respirations 40 to 60 per minute, with mild retraction. The lungs were clear to percussion and auscultation. By 33 hours respirations were 100 per minute; her color was dusky when she was out of oxygen. Now air entry into the right base was considerably diminished, but no rales were heard. Twenty-four hours later there was no change. X-ray film at this time (57 hours) showed heavy infiltration in both hili and about the cardiac silhouette, spreading fanwise toward the periphery and concentrating heavily at the right base (Fig. 14–10). Tetracycline was added. On the fourth day she was improved slightly, on the fifth definitely, and she appeared quite well by the ninth day. X-ray study now showed the lungs to be essentially clear. Throughout the first five days of life temperature ranged from 100° to 101.5°F. White blood cell count was 15,150 per cu ml, with 52 per cent polymor-

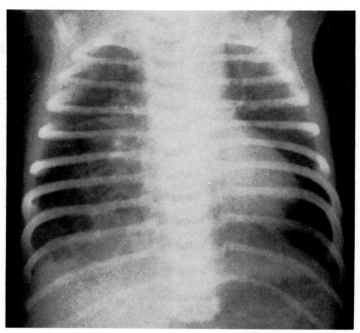

*Figure 14–10.* Anteroposterior view of chest taken on the third day of life. There is heavy infiltration in both root regions extending outward a short distance toward the periphery, but involving the bases, especially the right base, more intensely.

phonuclears on the second day. Nasopharyngeal culture grew out a *Staphylococcus albus;* blood culture was sterile. The placenta showed acute inflammation of amniotic membranes with spread to the decidual layer.

**COMMENT.** In this infant prolonged membrane rupture time, respiratory difficulty from birth with tachypnea and mild dyspnea and persistent fever point strongly toward intrauterine pneumonia. The prolonged course and presence of fever, as well as the unduly long membrane rupture time, argue against simple aspiration. It is possible that treatment of the mother before delivery and of the infant from the moment of birth on was responsible for the favorable outcome. We would no longer use tetracyclines since more effective antibiotics such as ampicillin and gentamicin are available. If the organism had been identified as staphylococcus, we would recommend oxacillin 100 mg/kg/day.

CASE 14–3

A white female infant was born to an elderly secundipara. Pregnancy, labor and delivery were in all respects normal; the membranes had been ruptured only 1 hour before delivery. Birth weight was 6 pounds (2720 gm). The baby did not breathe or cry spontaneously and was resuscitated with difficulty. At one hour of age her

color was fair, respirations were rapid and shallow, and nothing abnormal was noted in the lung fields. She was placed in an incubator, and given streptomycin and penicillin. At 12 hours respirations were rapid and grunting, without retraction. She was tense and jittery. Twitching began and became constant, color deteriorated, and respirations became labored. She died at 60 hours of age.

Autopsy showed generalized areas of consolidation and infiltration of both lungs with inflammatory cells, predominantly polymorphonuclear. Practically no fibrin was seen. Many of the zones of inflammation were confluent. The bronchial tree was filled with similar exudate. No amniotic debris was seen (Fig. 14–12).

**COMMENT.** This example is abstracted briefly for one reason only. Our clinical impression was that the entire trouble stemmed from the neonatal asphyxia and that cerebral anoxia accounted for all the symptoms and signs. The postmortem finding of widespread pneumonia came as a distinct shock. In retrospect we incline to the belief that pneumonia was present before birth, since tachypnea was noted as soon as spontaneous respirations were established. We wonder now whether the cerebral signs were not due entirely to intrauterine pneumonia. Both the history and pathologic appearance suggest that its origin was transplacental.

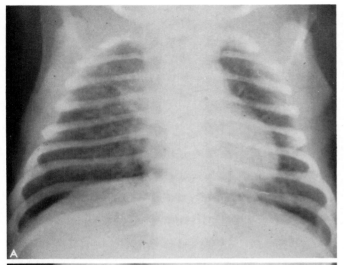
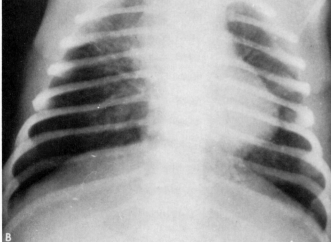

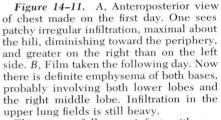

**Figure 14-11.** *A*, Anteroposterior view of chest made on the first day. One sees patchy irregular infiltration, maximal about the hili, diminishing toward the periphery, and greater on the right than on the left side. *B*, Film taken the following day. Now there is definite emphysema of both bases, probably involving both lower lobes and the right middle lobe. Infiltration in the upper lung fields is still heavy.

This was a full term infant with meconium-stained foul-smelling amniotic fluid but no other obstetrical abnormalities. She was dyspneic for 8 days and febrile for most of that time; she then made a perfect recovery, treated with penicillin, streptomycin, and erythromycin. An alpha streptococcus and a hemolytic staphylococcus were grown from the nasopharynx.

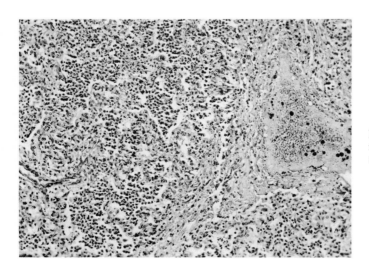

**Figure 14-12.** Microscopic section of lung. Widespread homogeneous pneumonitis with little or no amniotic aspirate is seen.

# PNEUMONIA IN THE PREMATURE INFANT

The premature infant is particularly vulnerable to pneumonia. As in the full-term infant, the disease may be acquired in utero, paranatally or postnatally. The assumption that pneumonia which causes death within the first 3 days is of intra-uterine origin, though true for the term baby, is for the premature probably incorrect. This conclusion is based upon the difference in incidence exemplified in Table 14–1.

Aspiration may contribute to pneumonia acquired by premature infants in the first days of life. The first test feeding should be water, since if aspirated it is less irritating to lung than 5 per cent glucose or milk, as shown by Olson in rabbits.

One frequently discovers pneumonia in the small premature infant in association with either subarachnoid or intraventricular hemorrhage or with hyaline membrane formation, or both. Under these circumstances it is difficult to determine the exact source of the signs displayed.

**PATHOLOGY.** Potter pointed out that the pneumonia of 1½- to 2½-pound (800 to 1200 gm) infants dying within the early neonatal period is usually characteristic in microscopic appearance. The lungs are immature. Only a fraction of the normal complement of alveoli are fully developed. The lumens of the air spaces are filled with leukocytes, and the entire pulmonary tree distal to the bronchioles often is lined by a single layer of macrophages.

**DIAGNOSIS.** In some premature infants the diagnostic signs described on page 147 are discoverable. In others, especially the very small ones, death may occur within 8 to 24 hours after birth with no indication that pulmonary infection is present and progressive. Temperature is normal or subnormal, usually subnormal. The color is dusky or cyanotic, but this may be no more than one expects in so immature an infant. Tachypnea and dyspnea may be absent. Commonly there is great irregularity of respiration with periods of alarming apnea and cyanosis. If one hears generalized dullness, diminished breath sounds and fine crackling rales, these signs may be indistinguishable from those anticipated in immature atelectatic lungs. In brief, pneumonia of the small premature in the first day or two of life may be undiagnosable by physical examination.

X-ray study may or may not reveal the characteristic changes described for intra-uterine pneumonia.

**PROGNOSIS.** Pneumonia is extremely serious in the small premature. Not all, but a very high percentage, die.

**TREATMENT.** The principles of treatment are the same as noted for term infants.

## CASE HISTORIES

### CASE 14–4

A black male infant was born at a gestational age of approximately 28 weeks. Labor was spontaneous and rapid, with no preceding obstetrical complications and short membrane rupture time. Birth weight was 1040 gm (2 pounds 5 ounces), length 35.5 cm (14.2 inches). The infant was born at home and cried immediately, but his color shortly became poor. Admitted to hospital at 3 hours of age, he was cold and moderately cyanotic, respirations were irregular, and there were intermittent short periods of intercostal and subcostal retraction. Air exchange was described as fair throughout, and a few coarse rhonchi were heard. He did not improve in the incubator with high environmental oxygen, and died at 8 hours of age.

Cerebrospinal fluid and blood cultures were negative. Autopsy showed widespread fresh pneumonia, "evidently due to aspiration as the esophagus shows an area of ulcerative inflammation" (Fig. 14–13). There was no hyaline membrane formation or gross intracranial hemorrhage.

**COMMENT.** This tiny premature infant died with extensive pneumonia at 8 hours of age. In a mature baby, death within 2, even 3, days means that the infection was

**TABLE 14–1.** *Incidence of Prematurity among Stillborns with Pneumonia versus Liveborns Who Died of Pneumonia in the First Three Days*

|  | No. | Prematures | Full Term | % Prematures |
|---|---|---|---|---|
| Stillborns | 28 | 4 | 24 | 14 |
| Liveborns | 23 | 14 | 9 | 60 |

acquired prenatally. In this and similar cases we feel fairly sure that it began during or after birth and proceeded rapidly to death. Temperatures remained subnormal throughout, and there were virtually none of the usual signs of pneumonia.

CASE 14–5

A white infant whose birth weight was 920 gm (2 pounds 1 ounce), length 35 cm (14 inches), and approximate gestational age of 28 weeks, was born at home. Pregnancy had been uneventful, labor short and uncomplicated. He cried immediately, and spontaneous respirations were established within a minute, but his color remained dusky. Admitted to hospital at 10 hours of age, he was cyanotic, retracting with each inspiration, but the lungs were clear to percussion and auscultation. He began to cry and grunt with each expiration, and this continued until death at 22 hours. Temperature was subnormal throughout life. Autopsy showed unexpansion, as well as aspiration pneumonia. The alveoli contained amorphous debris, throughout which were scattered many polymorphonuclears.

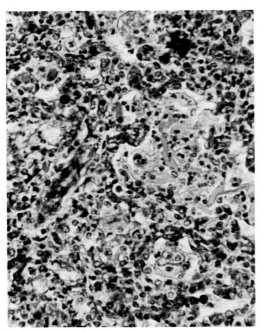

*Figure 14–13.* Microscopic section of lung (× 300) of patient reported in Case 14–4. Note the areas of poor staining interspersed throughout unexpanded lung in which the alveoli are lined by cuboidal epithelium. Throughout are myriads of inflammatory cells, mostly polymorphonuclear cells. The lighter-stained areas seem to be made up of necrotic cells plus aspirate.

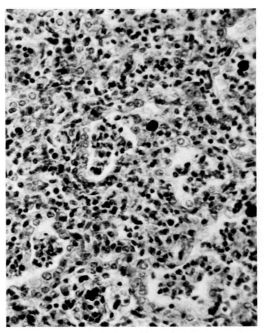

*Figure 14–14.* Microscopic section of lung of a premature infant whose history is not abstracted. Here no aspirate or necrotic cells are seen, but the whole is a mass of unexpanded lung, the alveoli composed of cuboidal cells, all infiltrated by inflammatory blood cells.

**COMMENT.** In this example the clinical picture was highly suggestive of hyaline membrane disease. We cite it only to make the point that differentiation between this disorder and pneumonia is impossible on clinical grounds alone. No radiographs were made.

## PNEUMONIA DUE TO ASPIRATION OF MATERNAL FECAL MATTER

Upon occasion an infant is born in bed unattended and is allowed to lie in the mother's feces. At other times the passage of stool occurs simultaneously with the delivery of the head, and the infant's mouth and nose become soiled by this material. These accidents may incite grave pneumonia, often complicated by septicemia. We have seen this sequence of events twice. Signs of illness appeared in one infant as early as 1 hour after birth, in the other as late as 24 hours. The signs relative to the pneumonia were unmistakable, consisting of tachypnea, slight retraction, grunting expiration, and areas of dullness and rales. Fever was absent in one, present in the other. White blood cell counts were low or normal (4700 and 9100). Blood cultures were positive for *E. coli*. Chest radiographs showed patchy bronchopneumonia. In both infants there was moderate jaundice.

## CASE HISTORIES

### CASE 14–6

A 6 pound 4 ounce (2840 gm) male infant was born at term after an uneventful pregnancy, 6 hours of spontaneous labor, membrane rupture time of 2 hours. The mother had been given an enema during labor, but only a little of fluid was expelled at that time. With the delivery of the head much of the enema fluid was expelled, contaminating the baby's face with fecal matter. He breathed and cried immediately and spontaneously. One hour after birth he discharged mucus from the mouth, and this was repeated at intervals. At 3 hours he was noted to be "feeble." The following day respirations were grunting, but color and tone were good. By that evening he appeared worse and was placed in a heated crib with oxygen. On the third day a pediatrician was consulted.

Examination at this time showed a mildly icteric, lethargic, flaccid infant. Temperature was 96.4° F. There was sclerema of the lower part of the abdomen and buttocks. Respirations were 45 per minute, but were neither labored nor accompanied by retraction. There was dullness at the right base in back with diminished air entry and a few fine rales over this area.

The white blood cell count was 9100, with polymorphonuclears 65 per cent, lymphocytes 24 per cent, monocytes 8 per cent, and eosinophils 4 per cent. The urine showed a trace of albumin and of sugar. Blood culture grew *E. coli*. Nasopharyngeal culture revealed *Aerobacter aerogenes* and *E. coli*.

X-ray film of the chest showed patchy opacities throughout both lung fields (Fig. 14–15). He was given penicillin (25,000 units) and streptomycin (25 mg) intramuscularly every six hours, and chlortetracycline (40 mg) by mouth every six hours.

There was no essential change for 5 days, after which icterus faded, activity and vigor improved, and the sclerema resolved. He was discharged well on the ninth day.

**COMMENT.** This infant surely inhaled and/or swallowed maternal fecal material. He became ill within 1 hour with *E. coli* septicemia and pneumonitis. Subnormal temperature and mild icterus characterized the course. He began to improve after the fifth day and made a good recovery. Our current choice of antibiotics would have been penicillin and gentamicin or kanamycin.

### CASE 14–7

A white female infant was born approximately 2 weeks before term. Pregnancy had been uncomplicated, labor spontaneous and short. The

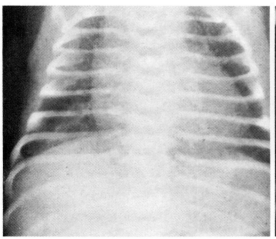 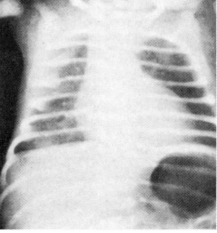

| **A** | **B** |

*Figure 14–15.*  A, Anteroposterior view of chest made on the third day of life. Patchy infiltration of both lungs is seen, somewhat greater at the right base. B, Four days later. The infiltration is more extensive, and the individual patches seem somewhat larger. The left lower lobe may be a trifle hyperinflated.

membranes ruptured 1 hour before delivery. The baby was delivered in bed while no attendants were present and was discovered lying within a pool of semiliquid fecal material. She breathed spontaneously and immediately.

At 24 hours grunting respirations were noted. Temperature was 101.6° F. There was slight jaundice. At 48 hours examination showed severe jaundice, hypertonus, rapid and grunting respirations, generalized dullness to percussion, but no rales and no alteration in breath sounds. Crying was continuous. Voided urine contained gross blood. White blood cells numbered 7400 per cu ml. Blood and urine cultures revealed *E. Coli.*

On the third day, in spite of penicillin, streptomycin and tetracycline therapy, the condition deteriorated. Repeated convulsions occurred. The infant died at 72 hours. Autopsy showed extensive pneumonia, purulent pleurisy and peritonitis, fibrinous meningitis, adrenal abscesses and hemorrhagic medullary renal necrosis.

**COMMENT.** This infant who had pneumonitis, septicemia and pyelonephritis after aspirating maternal fecal material died. Severe jaundice, fever and hematuria appeared and were followed by the signs of meningitis. Pathologically the nature of the pneumonitis plus the purulent pleurisy was totally unlike the picture produced by intrauterine pneumonia. Treatment may not have been ideally chosen or sufficiently vigorous.

## PNEUMONIA DUE TO ASPIRATION OF GASTRIC CONTENTS

One of the commoner forms of neonatal pneumonia is that due to aspiration of food, gastric contents or oronasopharyngeal secretions. Predisposing causes are obstructive lesions anywhere in the gastrointestinal tract such as esophageal atresia, with or without tracheoesophageal fistula, intestinal atresia and imperforate anus, inter alia. Aspiration pneumonia does occur, however, in the absence of organic obstruction, especially in premature or feeble infants, who are prone to regurgitate ingested liquids. It also jeopardizes those infants who experience difficulty in swallowing for various other reasons, such as autonomic dysfunction and thrush esophagitis. Its potential hazard is so great that the order "nothing by mouth" has correctly become

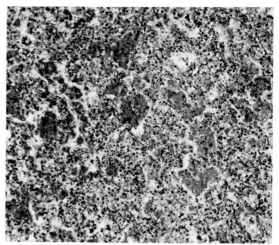

*Figure 14–16.* Photomicrograph of lung. Many large necrotic areas are seen which swarm with gram-negative bacilli when bacterial staining techniques are applied. The alveoli are filled with coagulum, and the whole is infiltrated with polymorphonuclear leukocytes, mononuclear cells and large macrophages.

This 5 pound 8 ounce (2500 gm) infant was born with multiple congenital defects, one of which was an imperforate anus. This was repaired on the third day of life. Feedings begun on the fifth day of life were taken well but occasionally vomited. Two days later he suddenly stopped breathing and rales and rhonchi were heard throughout his chest after sectioning and artificial respiration. A few hours later bloody discharge appeared from the mouth, he became gray and dusky, and soon died. Temperature was subnormal throughout.

one of the commonest and most important prescriptions in neonatal therapeutics.

Whenever an infant is tachypneic or has gastric or abdominal distention, oral feeding should be discontinued. The infant should receive fluid requirements intravenously. If the need to withhold feedings persists more than 24 hours, intravenous alimentation should be considered.

Some infants whose problem is regurgitation or swallowing dysfunction may be fed by a slow infusion into a catheter inserted from nose to jejunum (see page 853).

**PATHOLOGY.** The distribution of aspiration pneumonia is similar to that of other bronchopneumonias. Its cellular reaction differs in that macrophages, often fat-filled if milk has been fed, are present in large numbers. In addition, mononuclear cells and polymorphonuclears are usually found. Scattered patches may be actually necrotic, possibly because of aspiration of gastric digestive juices. These areas often swarm with bacteria of all varieties.

Associated ulcerative lesions of the lower esophagus are not rare.

## STAPHYLOCOCCAL PNEUMONIA

INCIDENCE. Staphylococcal infections of all varieties are a distressing problem in newborn nurseries. They occur sporadically and in epidemics. They were rare until the mid-1940's and became much more frequent in the succeeding 10 or 15 years, but now appear to have declined in numbers throughout most of the United States. Guthrie and Montgomery reported from Glasgow that in the decade 1926–1935 they discovered three primary staphylococcal pneumonias in 2300 consecutive autopsies on babies, whereas in the succeeding decade they found 55 in 2877 autopsies.

It is easy to underestimate the frequency of serious staphylococcal complication, especially in large communities where more than one hospital cares for sick babies. Infants discharged from nurseries with skin or conjunctival infection apparently cured are apt to turn up at another hospital when osteomyelitis, lung abscess or pneumonia supervenes days or weeks later. True incidence can be determined only by painstaking followup study.

In the 1960's, when hexachlorophene-containing soaps were widely used in nurseries, staphylococcal epidemics were rare. When it became known that even 3 per cent solutions of hexachlorophene would give measurable blood levels, and some white matter lesions could be found associated with hexachlorophene toxicity, routine use of such soaps was abandoned, with the consequence of several outbreaks of staphylococcal infection. A reasonable approach would seem to be to recognize the efficacy of hexachlorophene-containing soaps in the face of a high prevalence of staphylococci but to avoid routine bathing of all infants with a potentially toxic substance. Occasional bathing of infected infants, and use by adults for handwashing, should break the chain of spread of staphylococci in nurseries.

ETIOLOGY. The offending organism is usually one of the strains of hemolytic *Staphylococcus aureus*. By and large the pathogenic strains are coagulase-positive. No single strain, as determined by antibiotic resistance pattern or by bacteriophage testing, is totally responsible for an epidemic, although one strain usually outnumbers all others.

Numerous studies have been reported indicating that pari passu with the free use of antimicrobial agents staphylococci have developed resistance in steadily increasing percentages. In the 1930's many became sulfonamide-resistant; in the early 1940's penicillin resistance rapidly increased. Since then they have learned to adapt themselves successively to tetracyclines and erythromycin. Chloramphenicol has remained an effective destroyer of most strains of staphylococcus, and this is possibly because chloramphenicol has been used infrequently in view of its widely publicized hazardous side effects. If it is used in the nursery, the dose should not exceed 25 mg/kg/day, and blood levels should be followed.

Penicillinase-resistant variants of penicillin include methicillin, oxacillin, and others. These agents have proved to be exceedingly valuable in the control of nursery infections, although to date a few resistant strains have emerged.

CONTROL OF AN EPIDEMIC. It is useful to culture the anterior nares of all infants at the time of discharge from the nursery in order to monitor the frequency of colonization and the phage types of the organisms. A colonization rate of about 4 per cent is usual; up to 10 per cent may not be alarming. Any sudden change in the patterns of colonization or the types of organisms should lead to a search for the source and improvement in techniques.

When an epidemic develops, it may be useful to adopt the method of purposeful staph colonization advocated by Shinefield, Eichenwald and others, with a relatively avirulent strain such as 502A. Heavy colonization at birth with 502A interferes with subsequent colonization by more virulent strains. Unfortunately, 502A is not always harmless, so this approach to the control of an epidemic should not be the first one employed.

PATHOGENESIS. Staphylococcal pneumonias fall into two groups: The primary (bronchogenic) form originates in the infant's nasopharynx and spreads downward. The secondary (septic) variety originates in skin or umbilical cord stump, possibly also in the conjunctiva or nasopharynx, and spreads to lung, bone, meninges or other viscera via the blood stream.

The infecting agent may be recovered in the course of a nursery epidemic from the surfaces of the walls, floors and cribs, and from bed linens and infants' clothing. It may also be recovered from the nares and skin of a significant number of the adults comprising the working personnel of the nursery, physicians, nurses and nurses' aides. From all these sources a pool of pathogenic staphylococci is built up in each nursery. Newborn infants admitted to such nurseries become contaminated first externally, i.e., on the skin and umbilical cord stump, and from here the organisms are carried to effect nasal colonization. Staphylococcal disease may or may not follow colonization, depending upon variables such as dosage, degree of pathogenicity and individual immunologic states.

One of the outstanding virtues of "rooming-in" is the comparative freedom of these relatively isolated babies from staphylococcal infections.

Staphylococcal pulmonary infection complicates sooner or later almost all cases of cystic fibrosis of the pancreas. Neonates are not immune to this complication, although in this age group it is rare. The discovery of staphylococcal infection of the lung demands thorough investigation of the infant's enzyme output and studies of the chemical composition of his sweat.

**PATHOLOGY.**    A few cases are fulminating and cause death in 1 or 2 days. In these the lungs are massively consolidated, and with the intense, predominantly polymorphonuclear infiltration one finds equally intense hemorrhagic alteration.

Most cases are less explosive in onset and, if fatal, are less rapidly so. These show patchy infiltration, with clusters of abscesses about the smaller bronchi, especially in the periphery. Pleurisy and empyema are common, as is pyopneumothorax produced by rupture of superficial abscesses into the pleural cavity. Interstitial emphysema, mediastinal emphysema and

pneumothorax are frequently discovered, resulting from extravasation of air into perivascular sheaths and its progression along the blood vessels to the mediastinum. (See Emphysema, p. 126.) Subpleural blebs, or pneumatoceles, are a hallmark of the disease.

**DIAGNOSIS.**    The onset is apt to be mild, with low-grade fever, irritability and usually upper respiratory tract symptoms. These are not invariably present, and not too infrequently vomiting and diarrhea usher in the disease. At times the onset is catastrophic, owing either to the fact that the disease is of the fulminating variety or, as is more likely, to the development of an unheralded pneumothorax. We might point out here that pneumothorax which appears in the first few days of life is apt to be the result of obstructive emphysema, while that which develops in the second week or later is almost always the result of staphylococcal disease.

After 1 to 4 days of mild prodromata, fever rises and respirations become rapid, often labored and accompanied by expiratory grunt. At this stage, areas of dullness and fine crepitant rales may be discovered. Later the signs of pleural effusion, pneumothorax or hydropneumothorax frequently supervene. Distention is often distressing and intractable. Fever may be absent or low-grade, or high and sustained throughout. Scattered pustules may be discovered over the trunk or extremities.

The *course* is variable, from 1 to 8 weeks, depending upon the severity of the infection, the sensitivity of the infecting organism and the accessibility of the abscesses which may form within the thorax or elsewhere.

**LABORATORY FINDINGS.**    By far the majority of these babies show a polymorphonuclear leukocytosis. A few show a normal or leukopenic count, but the widespread notion that leukopenia is characteristic of staphylococcal infection is undoubtedly incorrect. Kanof et al. found granulocytosis in 38 of their 41 reported cases.

Staphylococcus can be grown regularly and readily from pleural exudate and abscess contents. It is almost invariably the predominant organism in throat and nasopharyngeal cultures. In a large percentage of cases it can be cultivated from the blood.

Phage typing and sensitivities will usually demonstrate that the organism belongs to one of several phage types which seem to be particularly pathogenic and that it is insensitive to penicillin and many other antibiotics.

A moderate to severe anemia develops in the course of the disease.

**RADIOGRAPHIC FINDINGS.** Kanof et al. found infiltrations indistinguishable from other forms of bronchopneumonia in all their patients. In addition, empyema was noted in 57 per cent, multiple abscesses in 48 per cent, pneumothorax in 38 per cent and pleural blebs or pneumatoceles in 25 per cent.

**PROGNOSIS.** Before the antibiotic era nearly all neonates died. Since the advent of various antimicrobial agents there has been a succession of periods of favorable and unfavorable prognosis corresponding to the times when staphylococci were sensitive, then insensitive, to each new drug. But with the great variety of drugs now available, one can usually be found which will control the infection. Bloomer et al. were able to report absolutely no mortality in 11 patients 1½ to 16 weeks old, three of whom were less than 1 month of age, treated in the years 1944 to 1955. This result is unusually good. The advent of penicillinase-resistant penicillins has improved our chances of overcoming these infections. All the young babies in the series of Klein et al. who were treated with oxacillin recovered.

The prognosis depends only in part upon control of the pneumonitis; in part it depends also upon the location of metastatic infections secondary to septicemia. Meningitis, pericarditis, peritonitis, renal abscess, brain abscess and osteomyelitis are some of the complications to be expected, and the presence of one or more of these may reduce chances for recovery.

**TREATMENT.** Oxacillin (Prostaphlin) and methicillin (Staphcillin) are the drugs of choice for staphylococcal pneumonitis. They should be used at first in the high dosage of 200 mg/kg/day intramuscularly or intravenously. After defervescence this may be reduced to 100 to 200 mg/kg/day; then oral administration may be substituted for the parenteral route. Parenteral therapy should be continued for a minimum of 10, preferably for 14 days, and should be followed by 14 more days of oral therapy if all has gone well. The changeover to oral medication should not be made until all the clinical, laboratory and radiologic signs have virtually reverted to normal.

*In staphylococcal infections one may not rely upon antibiotics alone. Repeated or constant drainage of pus is imperative, preferably constant.* In the series of Bloomer, thoracentesis was performed one to 23 times in all but two cases of the 11. Closed suction drainage was finally resorted to in eight of the 11, in half of these because of tension pneumothorax, in the other half in order to facilitate drainage.

Fibrinolytic agents such as streptokinase and streptodornase or Tryptar have, in our own experience, been disappointing.

Supportive measures include parenteral fluid therapy, transfusion, gavage feeding, oxygen, high humidity. Others will be resorted to as needed.

### CASE HISTORIES

#### CASE 14–8

A white male infant born in the 35th week of gestation was delivered by cesarean section after a severe vaginal hemorrhage. His birth weight was 5 pounds 6 ounces (2440 gm). He cried immediately and breathed spontaneously, seemed well and was placed in an incubator as a routine procedure. His course in the hospital was uneventful. He was discharged when 14 days old. At home he did well until two days later, when he refused his two morning feedings and seemed irritable. At noon he suddenly became blue and had difficulty in breathing. He was rushed to the hospital and immediately admitted.

On physical examination his temperature was 100° F, pulse 166, respirations 46. He was acutely ill, his color dusky, muscle tone poor. Respirations were slow, shallow and irregular. Only the left side of the chest moved. There was hyperresonance over the entire right hemithorax and dullness with innumerable fine rales over the entire left hemithorax. Blood studies showed a hematocrit level of 46, white blood cell count 27,650, neutrophils 60 per cent, lymphocytes 26 per cent, monocytes 14 per cent; adequate platelets, blood urea nitrogen 57 mg/100 ml, carbon dioxide 16 mEq/liter. X-ray film revealed right tension pneumothorax and left-sided pneumonitis (Fig. 14–17).

Thoracentesis yielded 40 cc of air and 10 cc of sanguineous pus. Immediate apnea followed, but respirations were re-established by positive

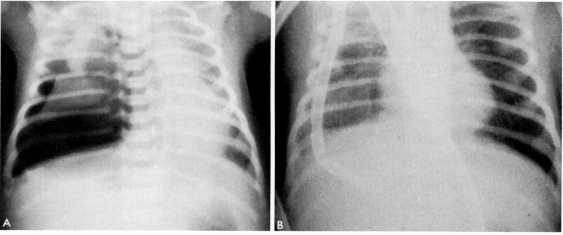

*Figure 14–17.*  *A,* Anteroposterior view of chest made on the first day of the illness, about eight hours after the first symptom had been noted. A great deal of air under tension can be seen to collapse the right lung, flatten the diaphragm and displace the heart and mediastinum far to the left. *B,* Film taken twenty-four hours later, after air and pus had been suctioned continuously from the pleural cavity. The right lung has re-expanded, the left may be a trifle overaerated. Diffuse patchy infiltration can be seen in both lungs now.

pressure oxygen insufflation. A rubber catheter was inserted into the pleural cavity. Smear and culture revealed *Staphylococcus pyogenes.* Some improvement in respiration and general condition followed. He was given chloramphenicol (100 mg) and erythromycin (75 mg) every 8 hours intravenously, and penicillin, 600,000 units every 8 hours intramuscularly, as well as 50 ml of citrated blood and a slow intravenous drip of glucose solution. During the night his condition remained critical, the temperature rising to 102.2° F. He died the following morning.

Autopsy showed right pneumothorax, bronchopneumonia with abscess formation, empyema, right purulent mediastinitis, left lower lobe atelectasis. The portal of entry was not determined.

**COMMENT.** This infant demonstrates well the catastrophic variety of staphylococcal pneumonia in which pyopneumothorax strikes shortly after the onset of the illness. He had been mildly ill for only a few hours, irritable, and not hungry for two successive feedings. He survived little more than 24 hours after his first symptom. Clearly one cannot hope to salvage all neonates with such rapidly advancing disease. We can think of no important differences in treatment which might have altered the outcome, although now we would have given him methicillin in maximum

dosage instead of chloramphenicol and erythromycin.

CASE 14–9

A more recent example was not quite so overwhelming. A 4 week old infant was sick at home for 3 days beore having to be admitted to hospital, and pyopneumothorax did not develop for 2 more days. Constant catheter suction improved him, but dyspnea and fever lasted at least a week after thoracotomy. A huge pneumatocele then developed, covering almost the entire right lung and compressing it sufficiently to cause dyspnea (Fig. 14–18). This refilled as soon

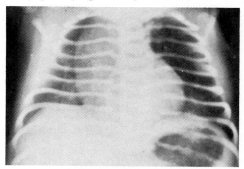

*Figure 14–18.*  Anteroposterior view of chest. A huge pneumatocele fills three quarters of the right hemithorax. There is a broad swath of pleural thickening running the length of the right axillary wall. The right lower and middle lobes appear to be compressed or consolidated. The pleural opacification helps distinguish this pneumatocele from cystic disease of the lung.

as it was emptied by needle and syringe, and it was not disturbed after one such trial. It did not disappear spontaneously in 8 weeks. The organism in this case was not at all or only slightly sensitive to all the usual array of antibiotics tested. Nevertheless, infection responded, albeit slowly, to 2.4 million units of penicillin and 400 mg of chloramphenicol daily, plus closed drainage of the chest cavity with gentle suction.

CASE 14–10

A white male infant was born after an uneventful pregnancy and labor and was discharged from the nursery in good condition on the fifth day. On the tenth day cough and low-grade fever developed. Nothing except nasal congestion and discharge were discovered, but be-

cause of his extreme youth, Aureomycin, 30 mg/kg/day, was begun promptly. By the fourteenth day there had been no improvement, and rales were heard at the right upper lobe anteriorly. He was then admitted to the Harriet Lane Home. The first x-ray film, not reproduced here, showed minimal infiltration of both lung fields, most noted at the right upper lobe, and a small amount of fluid at the right base. *Staphylococcus aureus* hemolyticus was grown from the nasopharyngeal swab. On antibiotics his temperature gradually returned to normal within 3 weeks. Serial x-ray film of the chest showed a constantly changing pattern of pneumatoceles (Fig. 14–19). These finally cleared in 4 months. His subsequent course was entirely without incident.

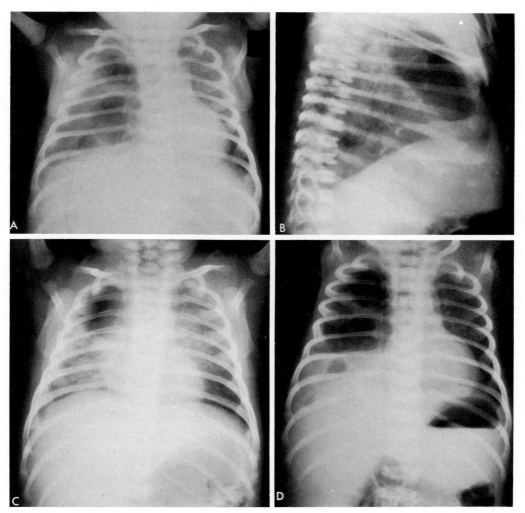

*Figure 14–19.* A, C and D, Anteroposterior projections made at various times throughout the patient's long course. B, Lateral view taken at the same time as A. They show differing degrees of infiltration, pleural thickening and pneumatocele formation.

**COMMENT.** This example of staphylococcal pneumonitis differs from the preceding ones in its relative benignity. The infant was never very ill, his temperature remained low throughout the course, while appetite and vigor were hardly affected at all. Perhaps because of this we entertained the notion that this represented cystic disease of the lung, and for a time we contemplated right pneumonectomy. The subsequent kaleidoscopic changes in the patterns of the translucent areas indicated that they were pneumatoceles rather than congenital cysts.

## KLEBSIELLA-AEROBACTER PNEUMONIA (see p. 794)

It has become customary to regard *Klebsiella pneumoniae* and *Aerobacter aerogenes* as members of the same group in which a great number (77 at last count) of strains are distinguishable on the basis of specific capsular antigens. Within the last decade Klebsiella has become a not uncommon infecting pathogenic organism in the newborn period.

### FRIEDLÄNDER'S BACILLUS (KLEBSIELLA PNEUMONIAE) PNEUMONIA

Pneumonia due to *K. pneumoniae*, formerly called *B. mucosus* capsulatus or Friedländer's bacillus, is moderately rare in infancy and childhood. Several nursery outbreaks have been reported in recent years. We give it brief mention here in order to re-emphasize the point that almost any disorder which involves older persons may attack the newborn. In addition, certain characteristics of its clinicopathologic course are unique.

*Klebsiella pneumoniae* gives rise to two forms of illness: A lobar form is indistinguishable on clinical and radiologic grounds from pneumococcal pneumonia. A chronic type is characterized by an insidious onset, or may follow partial subsidence of the acute form. Progression is marked by pulmonary necrosis, abscess formation, sloughing and cavitation, and, if healing sets in, by fibrosis. Before the antibiotic era the mortality rate was greater than 80 per cent.

CASE 14–11

(Abstracted with the permission of Miller, Orris and Taus.)

A white male infant was born after low forceps delivery with the cord wrapped tightly about the neck. Apneic at birth, he required 9 minutes of artificial respiration. His birth weight was 5 pounds 8 ounces (2500 gm). By the fourth day his weight had dropped to 4 pounds 14 ounces (2210 gm); he was dehydrated, flaccid and cyanotic, even in oxygen. Much yellow mucoid discharge from his nose and mouth necessitated frequent suction. He improved somewhat, but never seemed completely well. On the twentieth day fine moist rales were heard everywhere. Penicillin and sulfadiazine were given. X-ray film showed irregular clouding of both upper lobes and dense round areas in the right middle and left lower lobes (Fig. 14–20). White blood cell count was 16,000, 42 per cent polymorphonuclears. Lumbar puncture yielded normal cerebrospinal fluid.

On the twenty-third day his temperature rose for the first time, to 100.4° F. Ten days later it was down to normal, the physical signs of pneumonia were gone, and therapy was discontinued.

X-ray film taken on the twenty-fourth day showed an increase in size of the round shadows. At the age of 1 month the temperature began to rise again, reaching 104° within 3 days. At this time the left lung was massively consolidated. White blood cell count was 18,200, polymorphonuclears 62 per cent.

Penicillin and sulfadiazine were started again.

At 5 weeks he appeared moribund. Now nasopharyngeal and throat cultures revealed *K. pneumoniae*. Streptomycin was begun, and continued for 10 days. Improvement was immediate, temperature falling to normal after 4 days. Thereafter he seemed quite well.

Three weeks later, at the age of 2 months, repeat x-ray films showed cystic changes in the right upper and left lower lobes. Ten days later these were more pronounced. At the age of 2 months and 3 weeks he was discharged, although cavities were still present, though smaller. His weight was now 8 pounds 4 ounces (3740 gm).

**COMMENT.** This baby was born asphyxiated because of cord entanglement. Pneumonia supervened upon massive aspiration, improved and then exacerbated. At the time of exacerbation *K. pneumoniae* was cultured from the nose and throat. We cannot tell when this organism entered the picture, but it was probably a secondary invader after the first week. By the twentieth day the

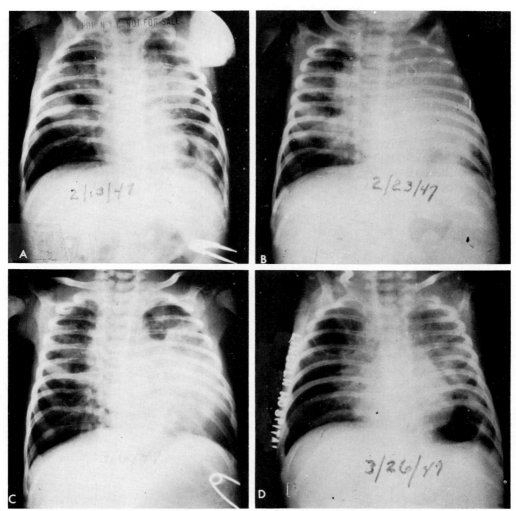

**Figure 14–20.** Friedländer's pneumonia. *A* (2/13/1947), Rounded areas of pneumonic consolidation in both lung fields, which are larger than in typical pneumonia. *B* (2/23/1947), Pneumonic consolidation of entire left lung field (pseudolobar consolidation) due to coalescence of smaller areas of consolidation, blotchy areas of consolidation, throughout the right lung field. *C* (3/6/1947), Moderate clearing of pneumonic consolidation in the left lung field, with an area of decreased density due to cavity formation in the left upper lung field, and clearing of consolidation in the right lung field, with appearance of cavity formation in the upper portion of the lung. *D* (3/26/1947), Coalescence of several cavities at the left base to form one large, thin-walled cavity. The cavity in the right upper lung field is now larger than on previous examination. (Miller, B. W., Orris, H. W., and Taus, H. H.: J. Pediat. *31*:521, 1947.)

characteristic round lesions had appeared, and these areas later excavitated. The cavities had not healed by the age of nearly 3 months, but were becoming smaller then. Fortunately the organism was sensitive to streptomycin.

Thaler reviewed this subject in 1962. He points out that this group of organisms is seldom sensitive to penicillin and, indeed, that it appears as a secondary invader commonly during or after the termination of a course of penicillin therapy. He further stresses the fact that chloramphenicol and streptomycin are the antibiotics of choice against Klebsiella-Aerobacter bacilli, and that, when used together, they should influence the course of disease favorably in 93 per cent of the cases.

## GROUP B STREPTOCOCCAL INFECTIONS

Increasingly Group B streptococcal infections are recognized as a significant cause of pneumonia and suppurative meningitis. Some infants have respiratory distress at the time of delivery, others are considered normal at birth and suddenly deteriorate in the first day or two of life. Clinically they may be indistinguishable from infants with hyaline membrane disease, although the chest radiographs often differ. Streaky infiltrates are more consistent with pneumonia, and a diffuse granular pattern more consistent with hyaline membrane disease.

The early onset of fulminant forms may be fatal, even with prompt and appropriate antibiotic therapy.

Another group of infants has a later onset of illness, characterized by irritability, feeding problems and fever. The onset may be several days or even a week after delivery, and is usually leptomeningeal infection rather than pneumonia.

One of the problems in recognition of this illness is that hospital laboratories may not report Group B hemolytic streptococci by that name, since grouping by the precipitin method is not always available. They can be suspected by colony morphology and type of hemolysis, and may be bacitracin-resistant. Apparently most beta-hemolytic streptococci isolated from the vagina will be Group B.

Prevention is achievable by culture of the vagina, and of the husband's urethra if streptococci are recovered from the vagina. Franciosi et al. recommend 1.2 M units parenteral benzanthine penicillin be given to the parents. (See page 148.)

## PSEUDOMONAS (B. PYOCYANEUS) PNEUMONIA

**INCIDENCE.** The pseudomonas group of bacilli, like staphylococci and some fungi, have benefited by the widespread use of antibiotics. In the last 25 years their importance as pathogens has increased. This increase in morbidity and mortality is most notable in nurseries and infants' wards.

**ETIOLOGY.** Pseudomonas is a group of organisms of low pathogenicity. It is, in fact, practically nonpathogenic for a mature, healthy person unless ingested or inoculated in overwhelming dosage or unless its growth potential is artificially increased by the destruction of its normal antagonists, the gram-positive cocci. This effect is successfully achieved by the prolonged use of penicillin.

The organism is variable in its sensitivity to various antibiotics. Dilute acetic acid inhibits its growth and is useful in water chambers of incubators or humidifiers (6 ml of 2 per cent acetic acid per liter).

**PATHOLOGY.** Pseudomonas is almost unique in that it calls forth no inflammatory response in invaded tissues. Infected areas of lung or intestine are killed by its toxin, but few polymorphonuclear or mononuclear cells wander into the devastated areas. The resultant lesions have been called necrobiotic. In addition, it stimulates no leukocytosis of the peripheral blood. In many instances, indeed, it appears to suppress leukocytes, causing profound leukopenia and granulocytopenia, as well as platelet production. Suppression of platelet production is responsible for intractable bleeding which may complicate the late stages of the disease and which, at times, may constitute the presenting sign at its onset.

**PATHOGENESIS.** An occasional infant becomes infected by the ingestion of large quantities of contaminated water, which can be traced to a shallow well or cistern. This source is becoming more and more infrequent. Most infections are acquired in the hospital, either in the premature or full-term nurseries or in the wards for sick infants. As is the case with the staphylococcus, pseudomonas pneumonia may be primary, i.e., a direct result of infection of the upper respiratory tract by extension downward, or secondary, as a metastatic infection from generalized septicemia. These originate in some instances from a primary focus in the gastrointestinal tract, in others from an accidental or operative wound in either skin or mucous membrane.

Once having gained a foothold in a nursery or ward, pseudomonas is difficult to eradicate. It can be cultivated from walls and floors, furniture and linens, and even from basins of many conventional antiseptic solutions. This ubiquity renders it a constant potential hazard, not to the healthy newborn so much as to the premature infant or the one enfeebled by other disease. It is particularly prone to gain entrance to the blood stream by invading operative wounds. Prolonged use of penicillin in any child, in prophylactic or therapeutic dosage, makes him more liable to pseudomonas infection, and its continued use is apt to make that infection more hazardous. In a series of eight cases reported from the Brooke General Hospital, including gangrenous infections of the skin, gastroenteritis and respiratory infections, and ranging in patient age from 5 days to 9 years, penicillin had been given for various reasons and varying periods to every child.

**DIAGNOSIS.** The rare case of primary pneumonia due to *Pseudomonas aeruginosa* differs in no recognizable way, clinically or radiologically, from pneumonia of the newborn caused by many other organisms. Diagnosis depends entirely upon recovery of the organism from the nose or throat. The diagnosis of secondary pseudomonas pneumonia may be made more easily if other signs, particularly characteristic skin lesions, are present. These will be discussed fully in the section on infections of the newborn (pp. 794 and 795).

**TREATMENT.** As indicated earlier, there is no regularity of response of various strains of Pseudomonas to the antimicrobial agents. Most are killed in vitro by polymyxin B, but the clinical response to this drug is not so striking as its performance in vitro. A combination of polymyxin B in small dosage (1.0 mg/kg/day) with streptomycin (20-40 mg/kg/day) or colistin (2 to 5 mg/kg/day) is often effective. Polymyxin B and colistin have a similar spectrum of activity, and both can be toxic to the kidneys. Daily urinalyses are indicated. Gentamicin 5 mg/kg/day or carbenicillin is useful.

The usual supportive measures will be utilized. Multiple small transfusions may be required if granulopenia and thrombocytopenia ensue, but the appearance of these hematologic complications makes the prognosis exceedingly grave.

**PREVENTION.** The ubiquitous "water bugs," as they have been labeled, depend on moist surfaces for growth. Prevention depends on meticulous cleansing and drying of incubators and inhalation therapy equipment. A 0.25 per cent solution of acetic acid in incubators or nebulizers has been shown by Edmondson and others to reduce contamination. A regimen of gas sterilization or autoclaving of all nebulizers and suction equipment every 48 hours is recommended.

## VIRUS PNEUMONIA

Adams described several epidemics of a type of pneumonia which attacks newborns in nurseries and differs from intrauterine and other forms of bacterial pneumonia in several particulars. Although its occurrence is usually epidemic, sporadic cases may be encountered. In these one or both parents have a respiratory infection. From pharyngeal scrapings of both parent and infant numerous epithelial cells are seen to contain eosinophilic inclusion bodies. They represent the pathognomonic sign of the disease.

Neonates in the first week of life are affected in largest numbers, although one as old as 32 weeks was discovered. Premature infants are most highly susceptible, and in them the mortality rate is high.

The *clinical picture* includes an acute onset, with sneezing, coughing, fever of 100 to 103° F, dyspnea and cyanosis. The upper respiratory tract alone may be involved, or rales and x-ray shadows resembling those of bronchopneumonia may indicate spread to the lower respiratory tract. In severe cases extreme dyspnea with deep retraction and cyanosis, either persistent or in bouts, develops. Exudate in the pharynx is abundant, whitish, thick and tenacious. The white blood cell count is normal or slightly elevated, with increased percentage of lymphocytes.

The *course* of the nonfatal cases is usually short, from 3 to 10 days. Mortality rate in the first epidemic Adams observed was 20 per cent, deaths being confined almost entirely to premature infants.

In *treatment* drugs are of no use, oxygen is beneficial, and adult human serum or gamma globulin is useful "in prophylaxis."

An outbreak of pneumonitis in term infants in Sendai, Japan, was attributed to parainfluenza I. Ten of 17 afflicted infants died of the disease, notable for a leukocytosis of 15,000 to 40,000 cells, 60 to 80 per cent of which were polymorphonuclear.

Our only comment about this disease entity is that it should be easy to diagnose in the very young newborn because of the prominence of cough. Coughing is one of the rarest sounds heard in the newborn nursery. Stridor, grunting and wheezing are commonplace, but cough accompanies no other form of pneumonia and is associated with few syndromes.

For the sake of completeness it should be added that Ludlam doubts the specificity of the finding of inclusion bodies in the pharyngeal epithelium. He maintains that they occur as often in well as in sick babies, and in adults unrelated to the latter as often as in their parents.

## PLASMA CELL PNEUMONIA (PNEUMOCYSTIS CARINII PNEUMONIA)

*Pneumocystis carinii* pneumonia is exceedingly rare in newborn nurseries in this country, although it has been noted in epidemics in Europe. It occurs most commonly in infants of several months or years of age with other debilitating disease, such as immune deficiency states and malignancies.

**INCIDENCE.** In Germany, Poland, Czechoslovakia, Switzerland and Scandinavia, indeed in all of Central Europe, it is common in the form of epidemics involving newborns and especially premature infants. Elsewhere in the world it is a rare and sporadic disorder which strikes, with few exceptions, infants and children debilitated by some severe underlying disease.

**ETIOLOGY AND PATHOLOGY.** The offending organism, the *Pneumocystis carinii*, has not been classified with certainty. It is believed to belong to the family of protozoa by most, of fungi by some. The organism is widely distributed among animals, including rats, mice, dogs, cats, sheep and goats, and has been identified in all parts of the world. It is found, often with difficulty, in Giemsa-stained sections of involved lungs. These are voluminous, emphysematous, inelastic and firm, and under the microscope heavy interstitial fibrous proliferation and cellular infiltration are seen. In the European form most of

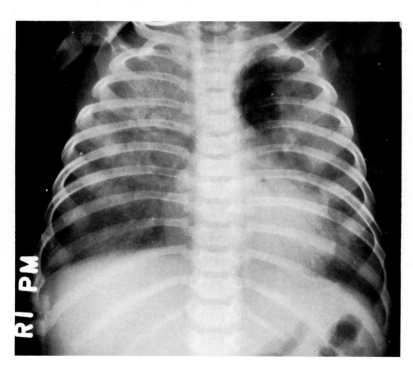

*Figure 14–21.* Chest film of a white male infant, six months of age, who had a cough and some cyanosis, with severe respiratory distress. No rales were heard, despite the extensive homogeneous infiltrates on the film. He had no measurable gamma globulins. *Pneumocystis carinii* was seen on smear of a lung aspirate.

these cells are plasma cells, whereas elsewhere in the world, when hypogammaglobulinemia is the underlying predisposing disorder, as it often is, lymphocytes and macrophages make up the infiltrate. The alveoli are distended with foamy, lacy, honeycombed exudate in which the cysts may be found.

**DIAGNOSIS.** In its epidemic form the disease begins within the second month of life or a bit later. A short period of loss of appetite and failure to gain is followed by duskiness and tachypnea. Cyanosis deepens gradually, and mild to severe dyspnea may appear. The lungs seem normal to percussion and auscultation, but radiographs characteristically show bilateral ground-glass hazing extending outward from the hilar regions. There is little or no fever and usually no cough. The white blood count may be normal or elevated.

The diagnosis depends on seeing the organism. Occasionally it can be recovered from tracheal aspirates. More commonly, a lung aspirate is required. Smear of the aspirated cells, and Giemsa stain, may reveal the encysted organism.

In its sporadic form, as seen in the United States, the disease strikes later, usually from 4 months to 2 years, and involves almost only infants or children who have impaired immunologic responses. A few others debilitated by advanced malignancy, or after prolonged steroid therapy, have been reported. In the case of Kramer et al. a hypogammaglobulinemic infant died with heavy infection with both Pneumocystis and cytomegalic inclusion virus. Since reduction of gamma globulin is associated with sparsity or absence of plasma cells, it is understandable that these cells are not found in the pneumonitis of these children. In other respects the sporadic disease is similar to the epidemic form.

**TREATMENT.** Definite clinical improvement has been noted in some infants with the use of pentamidine isethionate, 4 mg/kg/day intramuscularly. Gamma globulin injections are indicated if the blood levels are low. Steroids are contraindicated since they may further depress host resistance.

## REFERENCES

Adams, J. M.: Congenital pneumonitis in newborn infants. Am. J. Dis. Child. 75:544, 1948.

Adams, J. M.: Primary pneumonitis in infancy. J.A.M.A. 138:1142, 1948.

Alford, C. A., Stagno, S., and Reynolds, D. W.: Diagnosis of chronic perinatal infections. Am. J. Dis. Child. 129:455, 1975.

Baker, C. J., Barrett, F. F., Gordon, R. C., et al.: Suppurative meningitis due to streptococci of Lancefield group B: A study of 33 infants. J. Pediatr. 82:724, 1973.

Blanc, W. A.: Amniotic infection syndrome: Pathogenesis, morphology and significance in circumnatal mortality. Clin. Obstet. Gynecol. 2:705, 1959.

Bloomer, W. E., Giammona, S., Lindskog, G. E., et al.: Staphylococcal pneumonia and empyema in infancy. J. Thorac. Surg. 30:265, 1955.

Browne, F. J.: Pneumonia neonatorum. Br. Med. J. 1:469, 1922.

Calkins, L. A.: Premature spontaneous rupture of the membranes. Am. J. Obstet. Gynecol. 64:871, 1952.

Ceruti, E., Contreras, J., and Neira, M.: Staphylococcal pneumonia in childhood. Am. J. Dis. Child. 122:386, 1971.

Ciba Foundation Symposium 10 (new series): Intrauterine Infections. Elsevier, Excerpta Medica, North Holland, 1973.

Davies, P. A., and Aherne, W.: Congenital pneumonia. Arch. Dis. Child. 38:598, 1963.

Edmondson, E. B., Reinarz, J. A., Pierce, A. K., et al.: Nebulization equipment: A potential source of infection in gram-negative pneumonias. Am. J. Dis. Child. 111:357, 1966.

Erchul, J. W., Williams, L. P., and Meighan, P. B.: Pneumocystis carinii in hypopharyngeal material. N. Engl. J. Med. 267:926, 1962.

Franciosi, R. A., Knostman, J. D., and Zimmerman, R. A.: Group B streptococcal infections, J. Pediatr. 82:707, 1973.

Gajdusek, D. C.: Pneumocystis carinii — Etiologic agent of plasma cell pneumonia of premature and young infants. Pediatrics. 19:543, 1957.

Geppert, L. J., Baker, H. J., Copple, B. I., et al.: Pseudomonas infections in infants and children. J. Pediatr. 4:555, 1952.

Gordon, A. S., and Lederer, M.: Intrauterine lobar pneumonia and pneumococcemia. Am. J. Dis. Child. 36:764, 1928.

Guthrie, K. J., and Montgomery, G. L.: Staphylococcal pneumonia in childhood. Lancet 2:752, 1947.

Harnaes, K., and Torp, K. H.: Congenital pneumonia in the neonatal period. Arch. Dis. Child. 30:99, 1955.

Helwig, F. C.: Congenital aspiration pneumonia in stillborn and newborn infants. Am. J. Obstet. Gynecol. 26:849, 1933.

Hess Thaysen, T. E.: Die akuten nichtspezifischen Pneumonien der ersten Lebenstag. Jahrb. Kinderh. 79:140, 1914.

Hook, H., and Katz, K.: Über angeborene nichtspezifische Pneumonie und Pneumonie der ersten Lebenstage nach Aspiration innerhalb der Geburts-wege. Virchow's Arch. Pathol. Anat. *267*:571, 1928.

Johnson, W. C., and Meyer, J. R.: A study of pneumo-nia in the stillborn and newborn. Am. J. Obstet. Gynecol. *9*:151, 1925.

Kanof, A., Epstein, B. S., Kramer, B., et al.: Staphylo-coccal pneumonia and empyema. Pediatrics *11*:385, 1953.

Kjessler, A.: The time factor in rupture of the mem-branes and its influence on perinatal mortality. Acta Obstet. Gynecol. *35*:495, 1956.

Kramer, R. I., Cirone, V. C., and Moore, H.: Intersti-tial pneumonia due to Pneumocystis carinii, cyto-megalic inclusion disease and hypogammaglobulin-emia simultaneously in an infant. Pediatrics *29*:816, 1962.

Light, I., Sutherland, J. M., and Schott, J. E.: Control of a staphylococcal outbreak in a nursery: Use of bacterial interference. J.A.M.A. *193*:699, 1965.

Ludlam, G. B.: The incidence and probable signifi-cance of pharyngeal inclusion bodies, with special reference to their presence in newborn infants. J. Pathol. Bacteriol. *63*:687, 1951.

MacGregor, A. R.: Pneumonia in the newborn. Arch. Dis. Child. *14*:323, 1939.

Miller, B. W., Orris, H. W., and Taus, H. H.: Fried-länder's pneumonia in infancy. J. Pediatr. *31*:521, 1947.

Moran, T. S.: Milk aspiration pneumonia in human and animal subject. Arch. Pathol. *55*:286, 1953.

Naeye, R. L., Dellinger, W. S., and Blanc, W. A.: Fetal and maternal features of antenatal bacterial infec-tions, J. Pediatr. *69*:733, 1971.

Neter, E., and Weintraub, D. H.: An epidemiologic study of Pseudomonas aeruginosa (B. Pyocyanes) in premature infants in the presence and absence of infection. J. Pediatr. *46*:280, 1955.

Olsen, M.: The benign effects on rabbits' lungs of the aspiration of water compared with 5% glucose and milk. Pediatrics *46*:538, 1970.

Overall, J., and Glasgow, L.: Virus infections of the fetus and newborn infant. J. Pediatr. *77*:315, 1970.

Penner, D. W., and McInnis, A. C.: Intrauterine and neonatal pneumonia. Am. J. Obstet. Gynecol. *69*:147, 1955.

Peterson, H. G., and Pendleton, M. E.: Contrasting roentgenographic pulmonary patterns of the hyaline membrane and fetal aspiration syndromes. Am. J. Roentgenol. *74*:800, 1955.

Phelan, P., and Campbell, P.: Pulmonary complica-tions of rubella embryopathy. J. Pediatr. *75*:202, 1969.

Potter, E. L.: Pathology of the Fetus and Newborn. Chicago, Year Book Medical Publishers, Inc., 1952.

Potter, E. L., and Adair, F. L.: Fetal and Neonatal Death. 2nd ed. Chicago, University of Chicago Press, 1949.

Pryles, C. V., Steg, N. L., Nair, S., et al.: A controlled study of the incidence of prolonged premature rup-ture of the amniotic membranes. Pediatrics *31*:608, 1963.

Rackow, F.: Staphylococcal pyothorax in infants. Br. Med. J. *1*:11, 1953.

Robbins, J. B.: Pneumocystis carinii pneumonitis: A review. Pediatr. Res. *1*:131, 1967.

Sano, T., Niitsu, I., and Nakagawa, I.: Newborn virus pneumonitis (Type Sendai). I. Report: Clinical ob-servation of a new virus pneumonitis of the new-born. Yokohama Med. Bull. *4*:199, 1953.

Schaffer, A. J., Markowitz, M., and Perlman, A.: Pneu-monia of newborn infants. J.A.M.A. *159*:663, 1955.

Shinefield, H. R., Wilsey, J. D., Kibble, J. C., et al.: In-teractions of staphylococcal colonization. Am. J. Dis. Child. *111*:11, 1966.

Shubeck, F., Benson, R. C., Clark, W. W., et al.: Fetal hazard after rupture of the membranes. A report from the collaborative project. Pediatrics *37*:672, 1966.

Slemons, J. M.: Placental bacteremia. J.A.M.A. *65*:1265, 1915.

Smith, J. A. M., Jennison, R. F., and Langley, F. A.: Perinatal infection and perinatal death; Clinical aspects. Lancet *2*:903, 1956.

Snyder, F. F.: Obstetric Analgesia and Anesthesia. Philadelphia, W. B. Saunders Company, 1949.

Thaler, M. M.: Klebsiella-Aerobacter pneumonia in infants: A review of the literature and report of a case. Pediatrics *30*:206, 1962.

Warren, W. S., and Stool, S.: Otitis media in low-birth-weight infants. J. Pediatr. *79*:740, 1971.

# MISCELLANEOUS PULMONARY DISORDERS

15

## TRANSIENT TACHYPNEA OF THE NEWBORN*

First described as a syndrome in 1966 on the basis of eight infants with very similar

*This section reproduced from Avery, M. E., and Fletcher, B. D.: The Lung and Its Disorders in the Newborn, Philadelphia, W. B. Saunders Co., 1974.

signs and clinical course, the pathogenesis is unknown and the diagnosis is one of exclusion of other known causes of respira-tory distress (Avery et al.). "Transient res-piratory distress of the newborn" or "wet-lung disease" have been offered as alterna-tive names for this syndrome; a number of these babies, however, had birth asphyxia.

The infants are usually born at term, with

no specific antenatal events in common. In the first hours of life they exhibit elevated respiratory rates, up to 120/min, in the absence of significant retractions or rales. They may be minimally cyanotic, but alveolar ventilation is normal as measured by blood pH and $PCO_2$. No cardiovascular abnormalities have been found. Sundell et al. reported 36 infants with problems similar to those described by Avery et al. They used the name "type II respiratory distress" to designate their infants, most of whom were born prematurely, although late in gestation. Mild depression at birth was common in the series described by Sundell. Prompt increase in oxygenation on administration of oxygen distinguished these infants from those with hyaline mem-

brane disease. A benign course was emphasized by both groups reporting on this disorder.

The chest radiographs show prominent, ill defined vascular markings, edematous interlobar septa and pleural effusions in the costophrenic angles and interlobar fissures, typical of interstitial edema. On occasion, alveolar edema may be present. The lungs tend to be slightly hyperaerated. Clearing of the lungs is usually evident the next day, although complete clearing may require 3 to 7 days (Fig. 15–1).

One suggested mechanism for the tachypnea is a delay in resorption of fetal lung liquid. The prominent perihilar streaking may represent engorgement of the periarterial lymphatics, which have

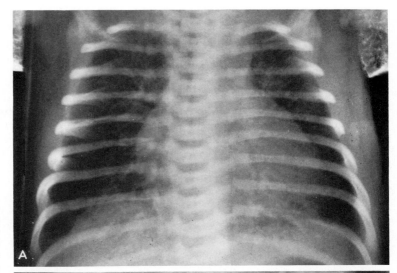

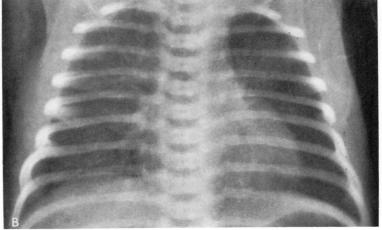

*Figure 15–1.* The large cardiovascular silhouette, air bronchogram and streaky lung fields were seen at 2 hours of age (*A*), but had cleared by 24 hours of age (*B*), typical of transient tachypnea of the newborn or delayed clearance of lung liquid via the lymphatics after birth.

been shown to participate in clearance of alveolar liquid with the initiation of air breathing. Fletcher et al. tested the possibility that delayed clearance of lung liquid could account for the findings by sequential chest films in newborn lambs. When lung water content was elevated, and radiographic abnormalities were present, the respiratory rates were increased.

Sequential films in asymptomatic newborn infants sometimes show vascular engorgement in the first 2 hours of life. Northway et al. and Steele and Copeland pointed out that the vascular engorgement was not always associated with tachypnea.

The process is self-limited, and infants followed as long as 1 year had no recurrence of tachypnea or other evidence of pulmonary dysfunction.

## PERSISTENT LIQUID-FILLED LUNG

Animal experiments involving fetal tracheal ligation established the fetal lung as a secretory organ in which liquid could accumulate (Jost and Policard; Lanman et al.). It is hardly surprising, then, that bronchial occlusion in utero can promote liquid accumulation in the affected lobe. Griscom et al. reported two infants in whom bronchial obstruction was present with a space-occupying radiopaque mass noted on roentgenogram. At operation liquid-filled lung distal to the obstruction was noted. With removal of the obstruction, aeration occurred in one; in the other, normal lung was resected.

## RESPIRATORY DISTRESS FROM PULMONARY VASCULAR DISORDERS (PERSISTENT PULMONARY HYPERTENSION)

Both pulmonary arterial and veno-occlusive disease have been described in the lungs of infants. Wagenvoort et al. added the twelfth patient to the literature with intimal thickening of the pulmonary veins in association with a chronic interstitial pneumonia and subacute myocarditis. Their infant was symptomatic from birth, with cyanosis and cough. The chest film showed a reticular pattern, but the heart was normal size. On cardiac catheterization pulmonary artery pressure was 110/45, and left atrial pressure was 3. Wedge pressure was 15. The infant died at 8 weeks of age. The only hint as to pathogenesis was a respiratory infection in the mother during the last weeks of pregnancy.

A less severe and perhaps more common problem was described by Siassi et al. in a group of five full-term infants who presented with cyanosis and tachypnea at birth, persisting for 5 to 7 days. On cardiac catheterization pulmonary artery pressures were elevated, with the mean between 48 and 68 mm Hg. Four of them had right-to-left ductal shunts. One infant died at 3 days of age and, on histologic examination of the lung, thickening of the media of the arterioles was noted. No inflammation was noted. The authors considered intrauterine hypoxia or hypervolemia as perhaps etiologic in the persistent pulmonary hypertension.

Progressive and fatal pulmonary hypertension in two infants born at term who died in the third month of life was described by Burnell et al. No associated cardiac or respiratory disease was present. Mean pulmonary artery pressures persisted at fetal levels of 66 mm Hg in one infant and 42 mm Hg in the other. Pressures fell to normal on breathing oxygen in one infant, but not in the other. At autopsy the pulmonary vessels showed an abnormal pattern of branching, with thickening of the walls of the preacinar arteries. Intimal thickening was described in some vessels (see p. 303).

## PULMONARY AGENESIS

All gradations of underdevelopment of the lung are encountered, ranging from hypoplasia of one segment or lobe to complete absence of both lungs. Schneider, in Schwalbe's monumental treatise on congenital malformations, classified all cases into three categories: *agenesis* (complete absence of lung and bronchus), *aplasia* (rudimentary bronchus, but no alveolar tissue), and *hypoplasia* (underdeveloped alveolar tissue).

INCIDENCE.    The condition is extremely rare. Olcott and Dooley reported the first case found at autopsy in the New York

Hospital in more than 10,000 postmortem examinations. Théremin found but two in 30,000 autopsies. In 1953 Oyamada, Gasul and Holinger were able to find, in an exhaustive survey of the world literature, 109 reported cases of all varieties. Fifty of these were right-sided defects, 59 left-sided.

**ETIOLOGY.** Agenesis, aplasia and hypoplasia are all congenital defects. They represent failure of development of the primitive lung bud in slightly different stages of ontogeny. Although Warkany was able to demonstrate an increased number of offspring with this defect from rat mothers fed a grossly deficient diet, this mechanism has not been proved to be of importance in the production of agenesis in the human being.

**DIAGNOSIS.** The time of onset of symptoms is remarkably variable. Some infants are in great difficulty at birth and survive only one or two gasping respirations. Levy's 49 year old patient, on the other hand, complained of only occasional slight dyspnea, while the 40 year old woman reported by Nesbit et al. stated merely that she never had had the reserve strength of her associates, her activity having been limited somewhat by dyspnea.

The presenting symptom is at times tachypnea without cyanosis, or with cyanosis only upon undue exertion. More often the presenting complaint has been repeated attacks of lower respiratory tract infection, described as bronchitis, asthmatic bronchitis or pneumonia. A few infants have been noted to have had "stertorous breathing" or to have made "gurgling sounds" from birth. Wheezing respirations, either in attacks or present constantly, have been reported.

Physical examination reveals characteristic signs. The affected hemithorax may be a trifle flattened, but usually little difference can be made out in the size of the two sides. One side, however, moves less well than the other. On this side the percussion note is flat from top to bottom, front and back, at first, but later some resonance appears over the upper part of the chest in front where the emphysematous normal lung has herniated across the midline. Breath sounds follow the same pattern, completely absent over one lung at first, later present but diminished over the upper lobe in front. The heart and medias-

tinum are found, by percussion and auscultation and by observation and palpation of the apex beat, to have shifted far to the affected side. The note on the good side is resonant or hyperresonant, the breath sounds are stronger, and no adventitious sounds are heard.

**DIFFERENTIAL DIAGNOSIS.** Clinically, there is no possible method of differentiating complete agenesis from massive atelectasis involving one entire lung. Atelectasis of this degree is much less frequently encountered than is agenesis, rare as the latter is. On only one occasion has almost complete collapse of one lung, caused by anomalous vascular compression of the main bronchus, confused us in this fashion. The case has been described (Case 8–2, Fig. 8–5). It is at times difficult to be certain that there is no lesion on one side which dislocates the heart and mediastinal contents in the opposite direction, but the complete normality of physical signs on that side is usually distinction enough. Solid tumor or fluid-filled cyst or pleural effusion should be appreciated easily by percussion changes. Air-filled cyst and pneumothorax should produce hyperresonance bordering upon tympany, and in all these conditions breath sounds are commonly diminished to a considerable degree.

**RADIOGRAPHIC FINDINGS.** Anteroposterior films show almost complete opacity of the affected side. If the agenesis is of the left lung, the right border of the heart and mediastinum is seen as a sharp perpendicular line at or within the left border of the sternum. The left border, when agenesis is right-sided, is found well to the right of the sternum, the entire cardiac shadow often being continuous with that of the liver. The trachea deviates toward the affected side. As the infant grows older the good lung can be seen to overexpand across the midline until a sizable amount of aerated lung lies within the opposite upper hemithorax. In the lateral film this herniated lung can be seen just beneath the sternum, pressing the heart and great vessels posteriorly. If aerated lung is visible anywhere, either far laterally or toward the base, the disorder is not complete agenesis; it is either incomplete atelectasis or hypoplasia of one lung.

**BRONCHOSCOPY.** Through the bronchoscope often no carina is seen. The single main bronchus appears continuous with the trachea. In aplasia a narrow bronchus may be seen which terminates completely after a course of a few centimeters, or the bronchus may be represented only by a dimple in the tracheal wall. The remaining normal bronchus turns sharply toward the side which contains normal lung.

**BRONCHOGRAPHY.** Bronchogram shows the absent or rudimentary main bronchus. Films of the well developed lung are usually normal, with the exception of deviation of the bronchial tree toward the opposite side and the demonstration of herniated lung in the anterior mediastinum and the upper portion of the opposite hemithorax.

**PROGNOSIS.** Half of all the reported patients die either at birth or within the first 5 years of life. Some die as a result of concomitant congenital malformations. The majority die in the course of one of their repeated lower respiratory tract infections. Three children died during bronchoscopy while attempts were being made to remove a foreign body from the single main bronchus after having been asymptomatic until that moment.

Persons with agenesis of the left lung have a longer life expectancy than do those with agenesis of the right lung (Fig. 15–2).

This statement is based upon an analysis of the cases compiled by Oyamada, Gasul and Holinger. Beginning with 50 right-sided and 59 left-sided instances of agenesis, it was found that only 16 of the former versus 35 of the latter patients survived the first year of life, while the figures for 5 years were 9 versus 32, for 10 years 8 versus 26, and for 20 years 7 versus 20. No significant difference was found in the percentage of associated congenital malformations. We are forced to assume, therefore, that right-sided agenesis is more hazardous than left-sided agenesis. The only reason for this discrepancy which comes to mind is that the shift of mediastinal contents is greater when agenesis is right-sided. Thus, there is more lateral deviation of great vessels and large bronchi, and these may actually become kinked or compressed in the process. The prominence of lower respiratory tract disease in the histories of the patients suggests that malposition of the larger bronchi is the fact of greater importance.

**TREATMENT.** No definitive treatment has been attempted. Each successive respiratory infection has been managed in the conventional fashion. In those who have frequent repetitions of lower respiratory tract infection, prophylactic antimicrobial therapy might be considered.

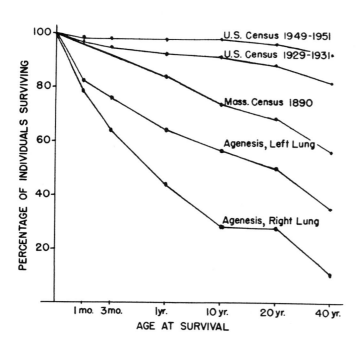

*Figure 15–2.* Comparative survival curves of patients with agenesis of a lung are contrasted with those of total population 25 years (topmost curve) and 45 years ago (second from top), and of the state of Massachusetts at the end of the nineteenth century. It is clear that survival with agenesis of either lung is poorer than that of the general population, and that survival with agenesis of the right lung is significantly worse than when the left lung is missing from birth. (Schaffer, A. J., and Rider, R. V.: Tr. Am. Climatol. Assn. 68:25, 1956.)

## CASE HISTORIES

### CASE 15–1

A black female infant whose birth weight was 5 pounds 1 ounce (2300 gm) was born spontaneously after a long first stage but short second stage of labor. Pregnancy had been complicated by laparotomy at the second month of gestation for abdominal pain, when nothing abnormal was found, and an episode of pyuria in the sixth month. She cried spontaneously, but soon became cyanotic, making regular but not vigorous respiratory efforts. On examination shortly after birth the right hemithorax was flat to percussion, the left dull. Heart sounds were loudest to the right of the sternum. With positive pressure oxygen followed by high environmental oxygen there was improvement. The second day her

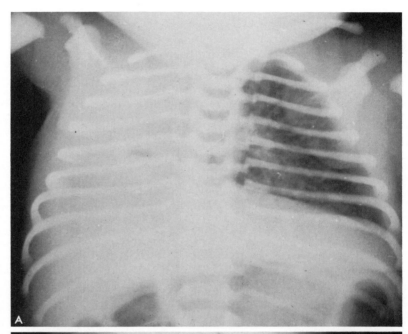

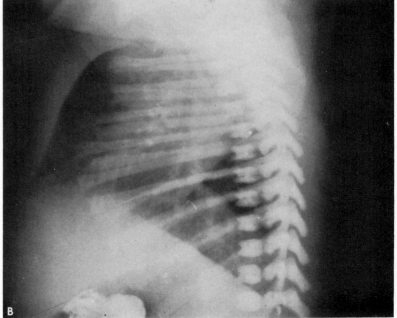

*Figure 15–3.* A, Anteroposterior view of chest made on the second day of life. There is complete opacity of the right hemithorax except for a small bubble of air in midchest. The heart and mediastinal contents are displaced entirely into the right side. The left lung is somewhat emphysematous, the ribs on that side are more widely spread, and the diaphragm is flattened. B, Lateral view. The anterior mediastinum is deep, and there is a broad band of translucency between sternum and heart. This indicates herniation of the left upper lobe toward the right.

color in oxygen was good except for cyanosis of the hands and feet. Breath sounds were now loud over the left hemithorax, inaudible over the right. Fluoroscopy and x-ray study revealed a homogeneously dense right hemithorax (Fig. 15–3). There was slow improvement, but feeding remained difficult, and cyanosis reappeared when she was removed from the incubator.

Bronchoscopy on the fifth day of life showed no excess mucus in the airway. The rest of this examination was unsatisfactory.

For the next 3 weeks the infant ate better and gained slowly. At 4 weeks the temperature began to rise, reaching 105° F a few days later. Death occurred on the thirty-fifth day.

At autopsy the right lung was represented by a fleshy mass 3 by 3 by 1 cm in size. This lay posteriorly and was connected to the mediastinum by a tiny bronchus and a small artery. The right ventricle was large and dilated, the ductus arteriosus was patent, and no right pulmonary artery was seen. Under the microscope the hypoplastic lung was almost completely atelectatic, but did contain a little air in some sections, while the left lung was patchily consolidated, with mononuclear infiltration and edema.

**COMMENT.** In this case cyanosis was prominent, dyspnea not great, almost immediately after birth. Signs suggested complete absence of the right lung, with me-diastinal shift to that side. Bronchoscopy was not helpful, as it frequently is not in such small infants. X-ray film showed virtual absence of the right lung and emphysema of the left, the lateral view in particular revealing herniation of lung into the anterior mediastinum. At autopsy the right lung was represented by a small hypoplastic mass. Death was due to pneumonia of the remaining lung.

CASE 14–2

A white female was born prematurely after an otherwise uneventful pregnancy, a short labor and a spontaneous delivery. She seemed well until the twelfth day, when tachypnea and mild dyspnea were noted. Cyanosis with feedings appeared 2 days later, and a heart murmur was heard. Respiratory difficulty increased over the next few days. Several prior examinations were said to have been normal, but on the seventeenth day a pediatric consultant found hyper-resonance of the entire right hemithorax and over the sternum, dullness over the left hemithorax and shift of the heart to the left. The systolic murmur was rough and loud. X-ray film showed emphysema of the right lung, with herniation of its upper lobe far over into the left upper hemithorax, heart dislocated to the left and downward and, probably, a small segment of aerated lung at the left costophrenic angle (Fig. 15–4). Bronchoscopy revealed no main left

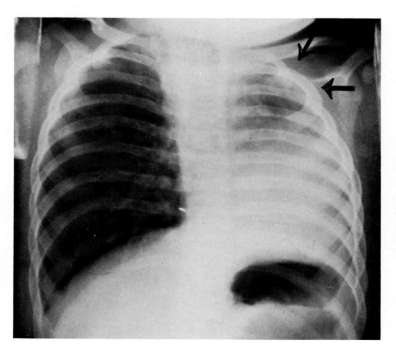

*Figure 15–4.* Anteroposterior view of chest made when patient was 3 weeks old. The right hemithorax is expanded, the left contracted. The right lung is emphysematous, and its upper lobe has herniated across the midline to fill almost completely the left upper hemithorax. The heart is displaced far to the left and downward. There may be a small segment of aerated lung tissue in the left costophrenic angle.

bronchus, but the operator was not too sure of his findings. Mild tachypnea persisted, but the child ate well, and her color remained good. She was discharged from hospital at 5 weeks of age.

We saw her fairly frequently in the 5 years after her birth. She is prone to upper respiratory tract infections, but vigorous antibiotic therapy from the onset of each one has prevented lower respiratory tract trouble. Throughout one winter she was kept on antibiotic medication. The murmur is still present, but is now soft and not impressive.

COMMENT. Even at this late date it is hard to be certain of the proper diagnosis in this child. The films strongly suggest almost complete agenesis of the left lung with, possibly, a small hypoplastic segment its only remnant. On the other hand, the history of normal examinations prior to appearance of symptoms and of the heart murmur makes one keep in mind the possibility of vascular bronchial compression and atelectasis. We could not prevail upon the mother to permit bronchography and angiocardiography, both of which were surely indicated.

## HYPOPLASTIC LUNGS

Hypoplastic lungs are most often associated with other congenital malformation, such as anomalous vertebrae and especially diaphragmatic hernia.

INCIDENCE. Roe and Stephens described 10 instances in a series of 24 infants with diaphragmatic hernia. The degree of hypoplasia presumably relates to the time of abdominal visceral migration into the hemithorax, as well as to the extent of it. The lung may be normal histologically and reduced in weight, or there may be retardation in pulmonary differentiation and a reduction in the number of bronchial branches.

PROGRESS. Impaired lung function is the most common cause of death in association with diaphragmatic hernia. Recognition of the likelihood of pneumothorax on either side is the best preventive of fatal tension phenomena with mediastinal shift.

An unusual type of hypoplastic lung with systemic arterial supply and venous drainage into the inferior vena cava, the "scimi-

tar syndrome," was reported in a father and daughter by Neill et al. The father was asymptomatic, but the daughter had dextroposition of the heart and pulmonary hypertension, and died after a pneumonectomy.

Hypoplastic lungs are regularly found with renal agenesis (Potter's syndrome). (See page 430.)

## CONGENITAL PULMONARY LYMPHANGIECTASIS

Congenital pulmonary lymphangiectasis, a rare disorder first described over 100 years ago by Virchow, has been reported in only about 25 infants. It is usually lethal in infancy, and diagnosed only on postmortem examination; sometimes, however, it is compatible with longer life, and may even be asymptomatic.

CLINICAL MANIFESTATIONS. In the majority of infants reported, respiratory distress was noted at birth, and cyanosis was marked and persistent. The duration of life in such infants has ranged from 30 minutes to 30 days. Very rarely, symptoms abate and survivals up to 4 years are known in infants who were symptomatic in infancy. Those children with asymptomatic pulmonary lymphangiectasis have usually had associated malformations of the lymphatic system such as lymphangiomas of the extremities or intestinal lymphangiectasis. The pulmonary lesion has on occasion been recognized only after a routine chest film was taken. The condition has been reported twice as commonly in males as in females, and usually after term birth. Other congenital malformations, particularly of the cardiovascular system, have been noted in over half the cases coming to autopsy.

RADIOGRAPHIC FEATURES. The lungs are usually diffusely involved with a reticular pattern, and sometimes the fissures are prominent. Hyperaeration is regularly noted, and helps to distinguish the condition from hyaline membrane disease, with which it may be confused.

PATHOLOGY. Grossly the lungs show thin-walled vesicles on their surfaces, and thickened, interlobular septa; they tend to be heavy and airless. The cut surface reveals a honeycomb pattern of irregularly

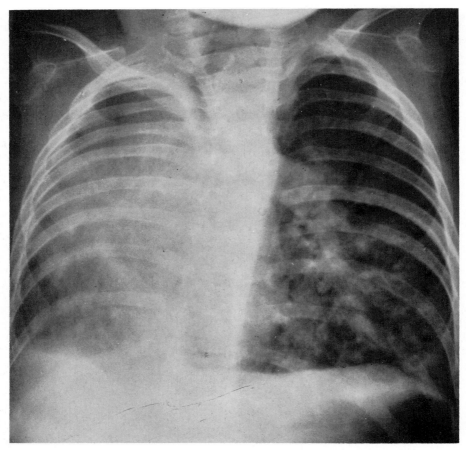

*Figure 15–5.* Anteroposterior view of chest shows heart shifted far to right, trachea also dislocated to right, moderate emphysema of left lung, and diminution in size of the right hemithorax. Much increase of vascular shadows on the left.

This case history is not abstracted in the text. The infant was well at birth, but respirations were rapid from the start, and a loud systolic murmur was heard on the original examination. He improved, but suffered numerous respiratory infections throughout infancy.

His mother and brother have hypoplastic right lungs, eventration of the right diaphragm and anomalous venous return. This infant almost surely has the same defects without the eventration. (We are indebted to Dr. Olga M. Baghdassarian for this film.)

shaped, fluid-filled cysts, which on microscopic examination are dilated lymphatic vessels lined by a thin layer of elongated epithelial cells. The surrounding connective tissue is loose and embryonal, and the pulmonary parenchyma airless and underdeveloped.

**PATHOGENESIS.** This congenital malformation presumably results from persistence of wide fetal lymph trunks in the connective tissue septa of the lung. The reason for this developmental defect and the commonly associated cardiovascular and other lymphatic anomalies remains obscure. The disorder is not known to be familial.

## WILSON-MIKITY SYNDROME

As more attention has been focused on premature infants, and more chest films obtained, it is not surprising that new syndromes have been identified. One of these was first reported in 1960 by Wilson and Mikity, and in recent years has borne their names.

**INCIDENCE.** The disorder has been reported in widely separated centers in Europe and North America. Mikity et al. estimate the incidence at 1:450 live births of premature infants. Apparently the condition is restricted to infants of less than 36 weeks' gestational age and appears to be more frequent in those of very low birth weight. It has been noted in black and white infants of both sexes.

**CLINICAL FINDINGS.** No consistent abnormalities of pregnancy have been noted. The infants may have some respiratory distress at birth, occasionally severe and thought to be hyaline membrane disease. Others may have no respiratory symptoms and receive no added oxygen, but some weeks later have the insidious onset of cyanosis and a rapid respiratory rate. Even those with early respiratory distress usually improve for a week or more before cyanosis and retractions reappear. On the whole, the symptoms increase over a 2- to 6-week interval and may persist for several months. The infants characteristically appear in good general condition, gain weight and are active. Their symptomatology is restricted to the lung and is characterized by a striking oxygen dependency. Fine rales and sometimes wheezing have been noted, but more commonly breath sounds have a grating, sandpaper quality to them.

An associated finding of interest in several reported series is a fractured rib. The etiology of the rib fracture has not been determined, and fractures in other bones have not been reported.

**LABORATORY FINDINGS.** Exhaustive attempts to define an etiologic agent by laboratory studies during life and examination of the lungs post mortem have failed to unearth a causative organism. The association of ECHO type 19 virus was noted in one infant, but has not been found in others. Serologic studies for respiratory viruses, routine blood studies, and sweat chloride determinations have all been negative. Definite abnormalities of pulmonary function have been documented, mostly by Swyer et al., who report $CO_2$ retention, substantial right-to-left shunts, a reduction in lung compliance and an increase in airway resistance. Cardiovascular function is usually normal, except very late in the illness when cor pulmonale may occur.

**RADIOGRAPHIC FINDINGS.** In the first weeks of life, the chest film is usually normal. Early abnormalities are a bilateral, coarse, streaky infiltrate, and, later, cystic lesions in both lungs. The walls of the cysts average 0.5 to 1 mm in thickness, and the cysts themselves 1 to 4 mm in diameter. Later the cysts enlarge and coalesce, and

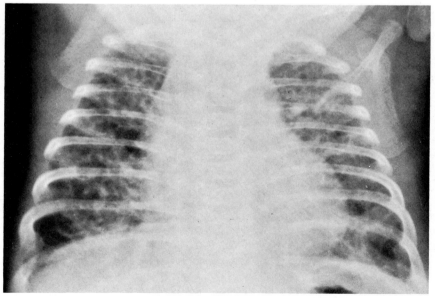

*Figure 15–6.* Posteroanterior view of chest shows a lacy network of linear opacifications throughout both lungs. Many round dark areas are seen. (Baghdassarian, O., Avery, M. E., and Neuhauser, E. B.: Am. J. Roentgenol. 89:1020, 1963.)

overexpanded hyperlucent lungs are seen. Resolution of these changes lags behind clinical improvement; complete radiographic clearing may not occur until two years of age (Mikity et al.) (Fig. 15–6).

PATHOLOGIC FINDINGS. A similarity to interstitial fibrosis was noted by Wilson and Mikity in their original article, but since then major differences have become apparent. The excised lung, inflated, has a characteristic hobnail appearance on the surface, as if terminal air spaces were overdistended and restricting fibrous septa were prominent. The lung contains more air per gram of tissue than would be expected, unlike interstitial fibrosis. Histologically, there are no pathognomonic features. Some of the alveolar septa appear thick; however, no increase in fibrotic tissue is found.

Electron microscopic studies have not uncovered any characteristic lesion (Swyer et al.). It is felt that an arrest in lung development may have occurred, with an inadequate alveolar-capillary interface to support gas exchange in the growing infant.

TREATMENT. Only supportive measures can be recommended at this time. It is of critical importance to use only as much added oxygen as needed to overcome cyanosis or to keep the arterial blood tensions in a safe range, presumably 60 to 80 mm Hg. Attempts to alter the course of the disease by digitalization, use of steroids and antibiotics have been fruitless.

## BRONCHOPULMONARY DYSPLASIA

Low birth weight infants who require high concentrations of oxygen and ventilatory support may show persisting, chronic pulmonary dysfunction, named by Northway et al. "bronchopulmonary dysplasia."

INCIDENCE. This problem occurs only in neonatal intensive care centers among infants who have required vigorous therapy to sustain life. It normally follows hyaline membrane disease, and occurs in only a few per cent of such infants. The chronicity of the illness (often months) and the continued dependency on oxygen and respirators makes the problem seem common, since most active centers have one or more such infants under care at any time.

DIAGNOSIS. Persistent pulmonary insufficiency after seeming improvement from the respiratory distress syndrome raises the possibility of bronchopulmonary dysplasia. In the first week or two of life, a persistent patent ductus arteriosus can produce similar symptoms. Radiographic changes are non-specific but nonetheless helpful. The lung markings are prominent, and areas of radiolucency may appear. Lobular or even lobar atelectasis can occur, alternating with hyperinflation. The infants often fail to grow, remain hyperemic in room air, may have apneic spells, and often require continuous or intermittent artificial ventilation.

PATHOGENESIS. The disorder may represent the result of lung injury from hyaline membrane disease, oxygen toxicity, or stresses from mechanical ventilation. DeLemos et al. produced similar lung changes in newborn lambs breathing 95+ per cent oxygen with or without a respirator, and Robinson et al. documented chronic proliferative pulmonary lesions, with squamous metaplasia in adult monkey lungs on prolonged exposure to high oxygen. On the other hand, in a review of the experience at University College Hospital, London, Reynolds found the form of mechanical ventilation to be more critical than the amount of oxygen. When he changed the ventilatory pattern to a rate of 30 cycles/minute and a 2–3:1 inspiratory-expiratory ratio (with a peak pressure no higher than 25 cm $H_2O$), he greatly reduced the problem in his nursery.

TREATMENT. Optimal nutrition, oxygenation and general supportive care to encourage growth and development is all we have to offer. Although glucocorticoids have been tried, no documented success has been recorded, and the hazards of reducing host defenses against infection and growth suppression would seem to contraindicate them. Antibiotics are appropriate for intercurrent infections. Chest physical therapy may help if atelectasis is present. Diuretics or fluid restriction should be considered if rales are prominent and pulmonary edema thought to be present. Increased inspired oxygen sufficient to keep the arterial level at about 60 mm/Hg and maintenance of a hematocrit of over 30 to 35 to provide adequate oxygen-carrying capacity would seem appropriate.

### CASE 15–3

The female infant was delivered of a 21 year old mother after the spontaneous onset of labor at a presumed gestational age of 37 weeks with a weight of 1600 grams. On physical examina-

tion the infant had characteristics more consistent with 33 weeks of development. Immediately after birth there was grunting respiration with tachypnea and retractions (Fig. 15–7A and B). The infant required 60–80 per cent of oxygen for the first 3 days of life but gradually was able to tolerate 40–50 per cent over the next several days. During this first week of life the infant was ventilated with positive pressure and con-

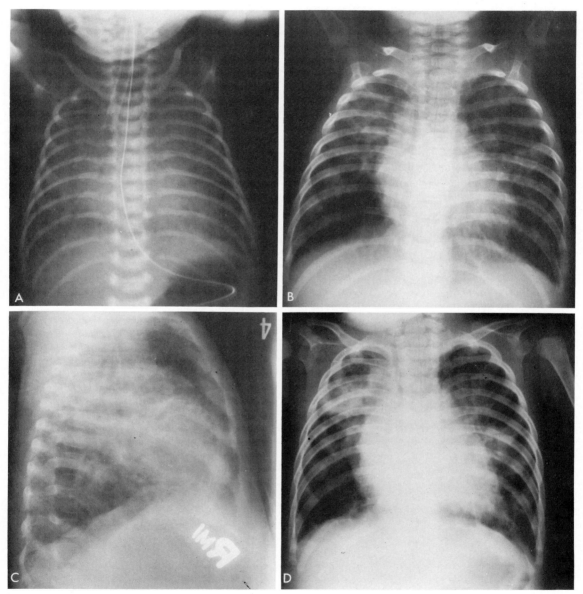

*Figure 15–7.*   A, Film on first day of life, 1600 gram infant, with respiratory distress. A feeding tube and an endotracheal tube are in place. A diffuse reticulogranular pattern is present in both lungs. B and C, The same infant, age 5 months, with areas of infiltration and hyperaeration. D, Age 11 months, the infant continued to need intermittent artificial respiration and 25 to 30 per cent oxygen. The heart is enlarged, with ECG evidence of right ventricular enlargement.

tinuous end-expiratory pressure through an endotracheal tube. Dependence on the respirator persisted through the first month of life, but the baby was successfully extubated at one month of age. However, shortly thereafter there was evidence of increasing respiratory difficulty in association with a large patent ductus arteriosus. This was managed medically with digitalis and there was subsequent improvement; however, there were continued failure to gain weight, apneic episodes and intermittent dependence on a respirator. By 5 months of age the infant had grown to a weight of 2900 grams and was discharged home briefly. There were several subsequent admissions, however, for increasing cyanosis and labored respirations, usually associated with new pulmonary infiltrates, sometimes thought to be pneumonic, sometimes thought to be atelectatic. The chest film never cleared completely and by 8 months of age showed persistent scarring in the right upper lobe and the left lower lobe (Fig. 15–7C). By 11 months of age the infant had been readmitted to the hospital requiring intubation, artificial ventilation and 40–50 per cent oxygen. Because she seemed too weak to suck well she had failed to gain weight sufficiently so that at 1 year of age she weighed only 4.1 kilo. For this reason a gastrostomy was inserted for nutritional support with slow, subsequent weight gain. However, during this period there was an increase in cardiomegaly persistent right heart failure refractory to oxygen and diuretics (Fig. 15–7D). The infant died of respiratory failure at 13 months of age.

# REFERENCES

Areechon, W., and Reid, L.: Hypoplasia of lung with congenital diaphragmatic hernia. Br. Med. J. *1*:230, 1963.

Baghdassarian, O., Avery, M. E., and Neuhauser, E. B. B.: A form of pulmonary insufficiency in premature infants: Pulmonary dysmaturity? Am. J. Roentgenol. 89:1020, 1963.

Dahms, B. B., Krauss, A. W., and Auld, P. A. M.: Pulmonary function in dysmature infants. J. Pediatr. *84*:434, 1974.

deLemos, R., et al.: Lung injury from oxygen in lambs: The role of artificial ventilation. Anesthesiology *30*:609, 1969.

deLormier, A. A., Tierney, D. F., and Parker, H. R.: Hypoplastic lungs in fetal lambs with surgically produced congenital diaphragmatic hernia. Surgery *62*:12, 1967.

De Weese, E. R., and Howard, J. C., Jr.: Congenital absence of a lung diagnosed before death. Radiology *42*:389, 1944.

Field, C. E.: Pulmonary agenesis and hypoplasia. Arch. Dis. Child. *21*:61, 1946.

Giammalvo, J. T.: Congenital lymphangiectasis of the lung: A form of cystic disease. Lab. Invest. *4*:450, 1955.

Hodgman, J. E., Mikity, V. G., Tatter, O., et al.: Chronic respiratory distress in the premature infant. Wilson-Mikity syndrome. Pediatrics *44*:179, 1969.

Javett, S. N., Webster, I., and Braudo, J. L.: Congenital dilatation of the pulmonary lymphatics. Pediatrics *31*:416, 1963.

Klein, Z. L.: An accessory lobe of lung in a newborn. Pediatrics *45*:118, 1970.

Laurence, K. M.: Congenital pulmonary cystic lymphangiectasis. J. Pathol. *70*:325, 1955.

Levy, C. S.: Congenital absence of one lung. Am. J. Med. Sci. *159*:237, 1920.

Mikity, V., Hodgman, J. E., and Tatter, D.: The radiological findings in delayed pulmonary maturation in premature infants. Progr. Pediatr. Radiol. *1*:149, 1967.

Neill, C. A., Ferencz, C., Sabiston, D. C., and Sheldon, H.: The familial occurrence of hypoplastic right lung with systemic arterial supply and venous drainage "Scimitar Syndrome" Bull. Johns Hopkins Hosp. *107*:1, 1960.

Nesbit, W. M., Paul, K. W., and Middleton, W. S.: Congenital aplasia of the lung: A case report. Am. J. Roentgenol. *57*:446, 1947.

Northway, W. H., Jr., and Rosan, R. C.: Radiographic features of pulmonary oxygen toxicity in the newborn. Radiology *91*:49, 1968.

Northway, W. H., Jr., Rosan, R. C., and Porter, D. Y.: Pulmonary disease following respirator therapy. N. Engl. J. Med. *276*:357, 1967.

Olcott, C. T., and Dooley, S. W.: Agenesis of lung in an infant. Am. J. Dis. Child. *65*:777, 1943.

Oyamada, A., Gasul, B. M., and Holinger, P. H.: Agenesis of the lung. Am. J. Dis. Child. *85*:182, 1953.

Pearl, M.: Sequestration of the lung. Am. J. Dis. Child. *124*:706, 1972.

Reynolds, E. O. R., and Taghizadeh, A.: Improved prognosis of infants mechanically ventilated for hyaline membrane disease. Arch. Dis. Child. *49*:505, 1974.

Rhodes, P. G., Hall, R. T., and Leonidas, J. C.: Chronic pulmonary disease in neonates with assisted ventilation. Pediatrics 55:788, 1975.

Robinson, R. F., Harper, D. T., Thomas, A. S., et al.: Proliferative pulmonary lesions in monkeys exposed to high concentrations of oxygen. Aerospace Med. 38:481, 1967.

Roe, B. B., and Stephens, J. B.: Congenital diaphragmatic hernia and hypoplastic lung. J. Thorac. Surg. *32*:279, 1956.

Schaffer, A. J., and Rider, R. V.: A note on the prognosis of pulmonary agenesis and hypoplasia according to the side affected. Trans. Am. Clin. & Climat. Assoc. 68:25, 1956.

Swyer, P. R., Delivoria-Papadopoulos, M., Levison, H., et al.: The pulmonary syndrome of Wilson and Mikity. Pediatrics 36:374, 1965.

Thomas, L. B., and Boyden, E. A.: Agenesis of the right lung; Report of 3 cases. Surgery *31*:429, 1952.

Thurlbeck, W. M.: Postnatal growth and development of the lung. Am. Rev. Resp. Dis. *111*:803, 1975.

Tsang, R. C., Chen, I., Hayes, W., et al.: Neonatal hypocalcemia in infants with birth asphyxia. J. Pediatr. *84*:428, 1974.

Valle, A. R., and Graham, E. A.: Agenesis of the lung. J. Thorac. Surg. *13*:345, 1944.

Wexels, P.: Agenesis of the lung. Thorax *6*:171, 1951.

Wilson, M. G., and Mikity, V. G.: A new form of respiratory disease in premature infants. Am. J. Dis. Child. 99:489, 1960.

# DISORDERS OF THE DIAPHRAGM

# 16

## CONGENITAL DIAPHRAGMATIC HERNIA

Congenital diaphragmatic hernia is characterized by the presence of abdominal viscera in the thoracic cavity, above one or both diaphragms. Usually the abnormally placed viscera are the hollow ones, stomach, small or large bowel, but spleen and liver may also be present. Herniation ordinarily occurs through the left diaphragm. The proportion of left-sided to right-sided hernias varies in reported series from four to one to eight to one. They are rarely bilateral.

**INCIDENCE.** It is difficult to assign a firm figure for the frequency of diaphragmatic hernia. Estimates range from as many as one in 1196 deliveries to as few as one in 10,000. In the British Perinatal Survey of March 1958, diaphragmatic hernias were found in 1.4 per cent of all postmortems, and once in every 2200 total births.

In our experience it ranks fairly high among the causes of respiratory distress in the neonatal period.

**ETIOLOGY.** In older persons diaphragmatic hernia may be produced by trauma. In the newborn it invariably results from congenital defect, from "absence of one or more of the embryological components of the diaphragm or from a failure of two or more of these components to fuse" (Zimmerman and Anson). The most common abnormality is incomplete closure of the pleuroperitoneal sinus (foramen of Bochdalek), situated in the posterolateral aspect of the diaphragm. Less common are herniations through the substernal sinus (of Morgagni or Larrey) and through the esophageal hiatus. Thoracic stomach with short esophagus is a different type of defect which will be discussed with diseases of the gastrointestinal tract (p. 330).

The hernias are usually "false;" that is, not covered by a peritoneal sac. Rarely a sac is present, indicating that migration of abdominal contents took place a little later in embryologic life, after rather than before the peritoneal lining was completed. It is of no clinical importance except that the sac may confuse diagnosis because it simulates diaphragm, as it did on one occasion in our own experience.

**DIAGNOSIS.** The diagnostic criteria of congenital diaphragmatic hernia vary with the volume of viscera herniated and, perhaps because of this, with the time of onset of symptoms. Infants may be seriously ill at the moment of birth; others may become ill at any time during infancy, childhood or even adult life. Indeed, some hernias remain completely asymptomatic and are discovered only in the course of routine x-ray examination of the chest.

If the volume of intrathoracic abdominal viscera is great, symptoms are apt to appear immediately after birth. The symptoms are entirely respiratory at this stage The commonly repeated dictum that the diagnosis of diaphragmatic hernia is suggested by a combination of respiratory and gastrointestinal symptoms is true only for those which manifest themselves later. Usually the baby, born after normal pregnancy and labor, breathes or gasps once and is then seen to be in great trouble. He may make no further respiratory effort until resuscitative measures have been taken. Cyanosis develops. When spontaneous respirations are established, they are deep and labored, often gasping and irregular, and associated with deep sternal and costal retraction. Cyanosis may or may not clear in high concentrations of oxygen.

In other instances difficulty does not become manifest until some hours or days after birth. Tachypnea may be the first sign, followed by a variable degree of retraction. Attempts at feeding may initiate vomiting, but this is not common. Rarely the first intimation that hernia is present is supplied

**183**

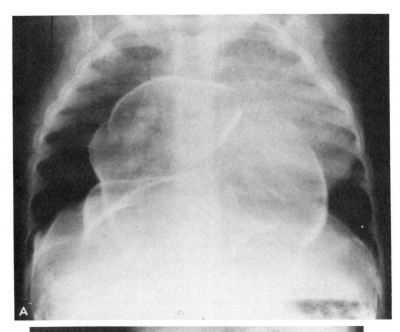

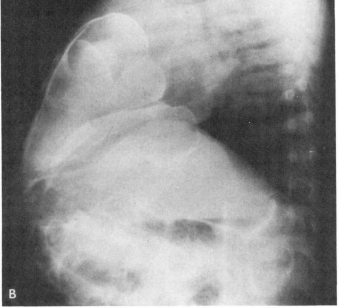

*Figure 16–1.* Hernias of the foramen of Morgagni frequently present as a mass, contiguous with the right heart margin. Water soluble contrast medium injected into the peritoneal cavity outlines the mass.

(*A*, From Oh, K. S., et al.: Radiology *108*:647, 1973.)

by the signs of intestinal obstruction produced by strangulation of intrathoracic bowel.

Physical signs are variable, depending not only upon the quantity of displaced viscera but also upon their consistency. Observation may yield the valuable information that the chest, especially the left hemithorax, is overfilled, while the abdomen is flat or scaphoid. Air-filled bowel produces a tympanitic note upon percussion, but over empty bowel, liver and spleen the note is flat. In our experience with large hernias the combination of flatness over one portion of the hemithorax and tympany over another was almost always discovered. Tinkling peristaltic sounds are heard after air has penetrated thoracic bowel. The heart is displaced to the side opposite the lesion, usually to the right. Part of the adjacent and opposite lung is invariably atelectatic; therefore over these areas the percussion note is dull, and fine crackling rales may be heard. Rarely one hears bronchial breath sounds over such collapsed areas.

Differential diagnosis is not too difficult. In lobar atelectasis difficult respiration begins some hours after birth. The heart is shifted toward the affected side, and the lung of the side opposite the shift appears normal or emphysematous. Physical examination alone may not be sufficient to differentiate from hernia all the other lesions which dislocate the heart and mediastinal structures toward the opposite side. Tympany could signify pneumothorax, lobar emphysema or air-containing cyst as well as air-filled hollow viscus. Dullness or flatness might indicate tumor, fluid-filled cyst or pleural effusion as well as solid abdominal viscus. A combination of tympany over one portion of the affected hemithorax and flatness over another, such as was encountered in two of our abstracted cases, is strongly suggestive of diaphragmatic hernia. An overfilled chest and concave abdomen constitute strong evidence for this diagnosis. Pathognomonic are tinkling peristaltic sounds heard in the chest.

Plain x-ray films, anteroposterior and lateral, should resolve any residual doubt. It is unwise to rely entirely upon fluoroscopy. The variety of pictures produced by congenital diaphragmatic hernia is consistent with the variation in quantity and type of abdominal viscera which may be displaced. Rather than describe all possible combinations and permutations, a number of examples are reproduced. If any doubt exists that the air-containing shadows in the chest are stomach or bowel, a barium meal x-ray series may be made.

**TREATMENT.** *Once the diagnosis is suspected, a feeding tube should be inserted into the stomach and, with continuous suction, air and gastric contents aspirated.* The only treatment available is replacement of the displaced viscera into the abdominal cavity and surgical correction of the congenital defect. It is imperative that this be effected immediately, as soon, that is, as the diagnosis is established and proper preoperative preparation has been completed. The hazards of delay are sudden death, probably owing to dislocation of mediastinal contents, and the supervention of pneumonia. The newborn within the first day or two of life tolerates protracted procedures as well as or better than he does later. Nothing is gained and much may be lost by waiting.

The choice of surgical approach, whether thoracic, abdominal, or both, is a moot question which the pediatrician fortunately does not have to answer. The abdominal approach would appear to be superior for several reasons. It is likely, however, that prognosis depends less upon the approach than upon the skill of the surgeon. He will no doubt get the best results by utilizing the method in which he has become adept. Meeker and Snyder make a strong case for gastrostomy as a useful device for minimizing distention and improving postoperative respiratory exchange.

**PROGNOSIS.** That some patients survive is demonstrated by our first illustrative case. The percentage of cure varies directly with (1) the promptness with which diagnosis is made and operation is performed, (2) the experience and skill of the operator, (3) the excellence of preoperative and postoperative care and (4) the degree of hypoplasia of the compressed lung.

In a review of 142 patients, McNamara et al. report that only 56 per cent of critically ill infants presenting within 24 hours of birth survived, whereas 94 per cent of those over 1 day survived. Presumably the infants with herniations of less severity or shorter duration could survive the first day of life and were thus excellent candidates for successful repair. Postoperatively pneumothorax is common. Gentle catheter suction of the ipsilateral thorax is appropriate, and concern for rupture of the contralateral lung is important.

The prognosis may depend as well on the presence of other anomalies. In nearly half the infants in the British Perinatal Study, other major anomalies were present and severe enough to account for death. These included anencephalus, Arnold-Chiari malformation, hydrocephalus and iniencephalus. Congenital heart disease and urogenital anomalies may also coexist with diaphragmatic hernias.

## CASE HISTORIES

### CASE 16–1

An infant whose family history was unimportant and whose mother's pregnancy and labor were not remarkable cried and breathed immediately after birth and seemed perfectly normal. At 14 hours glucose solution feedings were

begun and taken well. He voided early and passed a meconium stool at 30 hours. At 36 hours rapid respiration was noted by the nurse, and 1 hour later he was examined by a pediatrician.

He was a well-developed, vigorous full-term infant, slightly icteric, not cyanotic. Respirations were 45 per minute and were accompanied by moderate subcostal retraction. The entire chest seemed full, but the left side bulged more than the right. The percussion note was hyperresonant over the left front, but dull to flat over the entire left back. Heart sounds were faint over the left lower hemithorax, maximal near the nipple line in the right lower hemithorax. Breath

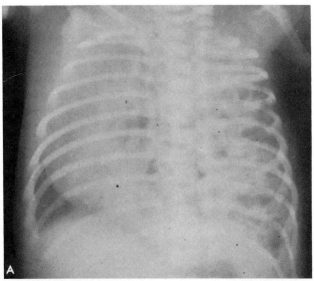
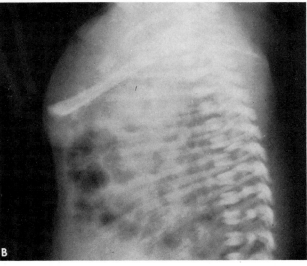

*Figure 16–2. A,* Anteroposterior view of chest made on the second day of life. The heart is displaced far to the right. The left hemithorax is filled with irregular translucent areas which bulge across the midline to occupy part of the right side of the chest. *B,* Lateral view made simultaneously. Here the pattern can be seen more clearly to be that of small bowel for the most part. Note the dilated loops between sternum and cardiac border which press the heart backward.

sounds were diminished over the entire left lung field except at the base posteriorly, where they were bronchial. In this area tinkling sounds were often audible. Breath sounds were somewhat diminished also over the entire right lung, but here no rales were heard.

X-ray film of the chest showed the heart and mediastinum shifted to the right. Irregular translucent areas suggestive of bowel were seen throughout the left hemithorax (Fig. 16–2).

Operation was performed immediately. An opening 1 inch in diameter was found in the left posterior leaf of the diaphragm in the region of the pleuroperitoneal foramen. The entire small and large bowel had escaped into the left hemithorax, the liver, spleen and stomach remaining within the abdomen. The bowel was replaced without much difficulty and the defect repaired. The left lung expanded promptly. Postoperative course was complicated by left pneumothorax which was successfully treated by constant low-pressure catheter suction.

Feedings were begun the third day after operation, and the infant was discharged 7 days later. At 13 months of age, he was in excellent physical condition.

**COMMENT.** This infant did not present symptoms until the second day of life, presumably until air entered the stomach and bowel and produced increased pressure upon the thoracic contents. Physical signs and x-ray study were characteristic, operation was simple, and the result was perfect.

## DIAPHRAGMATIC PARALYSIS

Unilateral paralysis of the diaphragm is encountered rarely in the newborn. Approximately three quarters of the cases are associated with Erb's palsy of the arm of the same side. Most are right-sided.

**INCIDENCE.** France was able to discover only 39 reported cases up to 1954, when he added another of his own. By 1957, Richard et al. identified 64 cases, and added 10 new ones. Paralysis was on the right in 58 cases, and on the left in only 16. It is probable that many mild instances of the disorder have been overlooked because of failure to perform fluoroscopic examination on all dyspneic newborns.

**ETIOLOGY.** Most cases follow difficult breech deliveries. Lateral hyperextension of the neck causes overstretching of the nerves of the brachial plexus and avulsion of the anterior roots supplying the phrenic nerve. In France's case there was complete avulsion of the anterior roots of C 3, C 4 and C 5.

**DIAGNOSIS.** How frequently the diagnosis of diaphragmatic paralysis is missed is exemplified by Schifrin's experience, reported in 1952. He described in detail the histories of four infants. In none of these was the diagnosis made before the age of 6 weeks. Three had been discharged

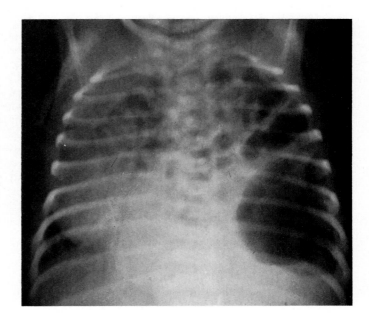

*Figure 16–3.* Anteroposterior view of chest taken on the second day of life. The chest is overexpanded and barrel-shaped. Round translucencies of varying size fill the left hemithorax and part of the right. The heart occupies the lower lateral corner of the right hemithorax. Both diaphragms are depressed, the left more than the right. The translucency in the left lower hemithorax resembles stomach, one or two above it look like large bowel, while the remainder appear to be loops of small bowel.

from the nursery at the end of the first week in spite of the fact that all were tachypneic. Two had had x-ray examination, none fluoroscopy. The fourth infant remained in the hospital with tachypnea and bouts of cyanosis, as well as two episodes of pneumonia, but he was 3 months old before the right diaphragm was noted to be elevated. Many x-ray films had been made prior to this one, but there is no report of his having been studied by fluoroscopy.

Many of the infants are flaccid and make poor respiratory effort immediately after birth. This initial difficulty may be ascribed to the prolonged and difficult labor and instrumental delivery rather than to the diaphragmatic palsy. After resuscitation, if needed, and the establishment of spontaneous respiration the infants are tachypneic or dyspneic. Dyspnea may subside within a few days to be followed by persistent tachypnea. Episodes of transient cyanosis may occur. The situation may deteriorate and terminate in death within the first few months, or improvement may begin as early as the second week or as late as the fifth month and total recovery ensue.

Physical examination shows diminished respiratory excursion on the affected side, which after several weeks may appear flattened. There are dullness and diminished breath sounds over the affected base and often signs of atelectasis over the lung above. Later these findings may be confused by the signs of complicating pneumonia. The heart may or may not be shifted toward the side opposite the lesion. Diaphragmatic movement or its absence can at times be appreciated by deep palpation of the upper part of the abdomen just beneath the ribs.

**RADIOGRAPHIC FINDINGS AND FLUOROSCOPY.** Within the first few days only slight elevation of the affected diaphragm may be seen by x-ray film, and this may be so minor that its significance is overlooked. Later the diaphragm rises higher, the heart and mediastinal contents are displaced and areas of atelectasis may be seen to abut the elevated diaphragm as well as the displaced heart.

The only certain way to clinch the diagnosis early in the course of the disorder is by fluoroscopy. *Under the fluoroscope characteristic paradoxical movement can be seen, the paralyzed diaphragm rising with inspiration and descending with expiration, while its normal mate moves simultaneously in the opposite direction.*

**PROGNOSIS.** France's compilation of 40 reported cases revealed an overall mortality rate of 22.5 per cent (nine deaths). He pointed out, however, that prognosis was much better if there was no associated Erb's palsy (one of 11, or 9 per cent) than if brachial palsy was also present (eight of 29, or 27.6 per cent). Death occurred in 15 of the 74 cases reviewed by Richard et al., usually from infection of the atelectatic lung.

Recovery is often accomplished by gradual restoration of power and movement to the affected diaphragm. This occurred early in our first abstracted case, being complete by the age of 6 weeks, but was not complete in Schifrin's case IV even at the age of 17 months. It is likely that some patients recover clinically, though their diaphragms never regain movement. These may account for cases diagnosed later as eventration of the diaphragm (q.v.).

**TREATMENT.** Placing the infant in an environment with increased oxygen concentration usually suffices to tide him over the first hazardous days. Whether movement of the diaphragm will return depends upon the degree of avulsion of the roots and the possibility of reestablishment of continuity of the torn tissue. It is unlikely that measures such as faradic stimulation will have any effect on the ultimate outcome, although this has been attempted. Faradic stimulation may be used, however, as a prognostic test, since absence of any response indicates complete phrenic nerve degeneration. If after 3 or 4 months electrical stimulation produces no diaphragmatic movement, and if serious symptoms persist or increase, one might consider operative intervention. The operation of choice is plication of the paralyzed diaphragm. (See Eventration of the Diaphragm.)

**CASE 16–2**

A white male infant was born at the Hospital for the Women of Maryland. Labor was complicated by uterine inertia, lasted 30 hours and was finally terminated by manual breech delivery. Great difficulty was experienced in delivering the right shoulder. Birth weight was 10 pounds 2 ounces (4590 gm). The infant cried and breathed spontaneously, but respirations were shallow and rapid. He appeared depressed and generally flaccid. The next day's examination showed tachypnea, mild dyspnea with slight sternal retraction and intermittent cyanosis. There was limitation of motion of the right arm and obvious pain on passive motion of the right shoulder. Crepitus could be felt over the right clavicle. There was no neurologic defect. The chest was described as entirely clear.

X-ray examination revealed elevation of the right diaphragm and a fractured right clavicle. Fluoroscopy revealed paradoxical movement of the right diaphragm.

The infant was kept in hospital for 2 weeks, at first in humidified oxygen. Breathing gradually improved, all dyspnea and cyanosis disappeared, but mild tachypnea persisted until the day of discharge. He was seen regularly thereafter, and by the age of 6 weeks breathing was completely normal.

COMMENT. This story is characteristic in many respects. The infant was large and presented by the breech. Extraction was difficult, and much force was used to free the right shoulder. In the process the right clavicle was broken and the brachial plexus injured. Tachypnea, mild dyspnea and cyanosis were replaced by simple tachypnea, and all difficulty disappeared by the age of 6 weeks.

## EVENTRATION OF THE DIAPHRAGM

Laxdal, McDougall and Mellin defined this condition aptly and succinctly: "One leaf of the diaphragm balloons abnormally high in the chest and yet retains its continuity and normal attachments to the costal margins."

INCIDENCE. The disorder has been discovered in mass x-ray surveys of adults approximately once in 10,000 films. Only within the past 20 years has it been realized that it may cause serious trouble in young infants, including the newborn.

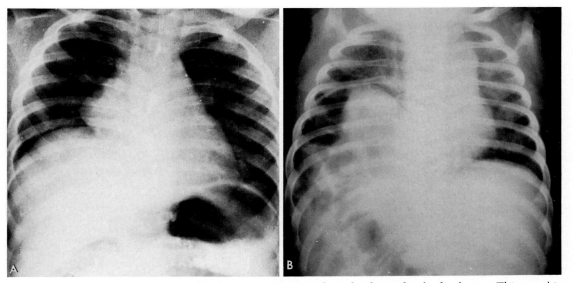

*Figure 16-4.* A, Anteroposterior view of chest to show a moderately elevated right diaphragm. This case history is not summarized in the text because the infant was completely asymptomatic, the x-ray picture having been taken because a sibling had tuberculosis. There had been no difficulty in labor and no respiratory trouble in the neonate. The probable diagnosis is eventration of the diaphragm. B, Anteroposterior view of chest taken at 6 weeks of age. The right diaphragm takes off from the axillary wall a bit lower than usual, rises fairly steeply toward midthorax, after which it becomes cone-shaped or tented in its medial half. Translucent areas which resemble bowel can be seen high in the right hemithorax beneath the elevated diaphragmatic leaf. This case history is not abstracted in the text.

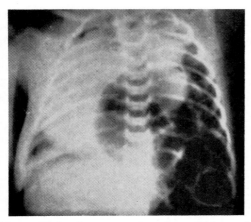

*Figure 16–5.* Anteroposterior view of chest of a newborn with a huge left-sided diaphragmatic hernia. Hollow viscera fill the left hemithorax except the extreme upper portion, where atelectatic lung is seen, and protrude far into the right hemithorax. The heart is pushed to the axillary wall on the right, and little aerated lung can be seen anywhere. This case history is not summarized in the text.

Thus far only a few cases have been reported in this age group.

**ETIOLOGY.** Most cases of eventration appear to be due to congenital insufficiency of muscle. A few follow phrenic nerve paralysis.

**DIAGNOSIS.** Many of the adults in whom eventration was discovered by routine x-ray examination had been completely symptom-free. In the newborn the symptoms and signs may duplicate those of congenital diaphragmatic hernia. After prompt initial respiration, tachypnea, dyspnea and intermittent cyanosis appear. Dullness and absent breath sounds over the lower half or two thirds of one hemithorax are the only consistent abnormal physical findings. The heart may be displaced toward the opposite side.

Anteroposterior and lateral films show the greatly elevated diaphragm and the displaced heart and mediastinum. Under the fluoroscope the excursion of the elevated diaphragm is at first diminished, but in the proper direction; later it may become paradoxical.

**PROGNOSIS.** Some of the reported patients have died. Judging from the comparatively large number of cases discovered in adults, it is evident that many patients survive the neonatal period. We cannot be sure that all these were symptom-free as newborns.

**TREATMENT.** Undoubtedly many patients recover with the aid of simple sup-

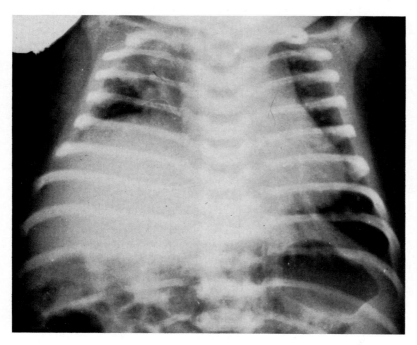

*Figure 16–6.* Anteroposterior view of chest made when patient was 3 weeks old.

Labor had been difficult and prolonged because of shoulder dystocia; delivery was completed by forceps extraction. Right-sided Erb's palsy, tachypnea, and dyspnea were noted, and there was one severe bout of pneumonitis at 4 weeks. All finally cleared at 2½ months of age.

The right diaphragm is elevated to the level of the fourth rib. The right lung contains patches of increased density. The heart is displaced a little toward the left. The left lung is moderately emphysematous, its diaphragm flattened and depressed.

portive measures. When, in spite of these, dyspnea persists and serious episodes of cyanosis do not diminish, or increase in frequency and severity, surgical intervention is indicated. There is on record one operative success in a 9 day old infant (Leahy and Butsch), two in 6 week olds (Bisgard and Robertson) and one in a 7 week old (Laxdal et al.). Operation consists of plication of the elevated leaf of the diaphragm.

CASE 16–3

A black male infant was born after a normal pregnancy and delivery, his birth weight 7 pounds (3175 gm.). He was kept in an incubator because of "weakness" for 3 days, but was sent home at the usual time. He was said to have had a "cold" continuously since birth. Feeding was well supervised, and milk, pablum and egg yolk, and adequate amounts of vitamins A, C and D had been taken. When he was 3 months old, his "cold" became worse and wheezing was noted. He was irritable, ran a low-grade fever, and was treated with penicillin. A few days later he was diagnosed as having left-sided pneumonia. He was then hospitalized locally, and a diagnosis of eventration of the left diaphragm was made. He was referred to the Johns Hopkins Hospital. Neither cyanosis nor dyspnea had ever been noted.

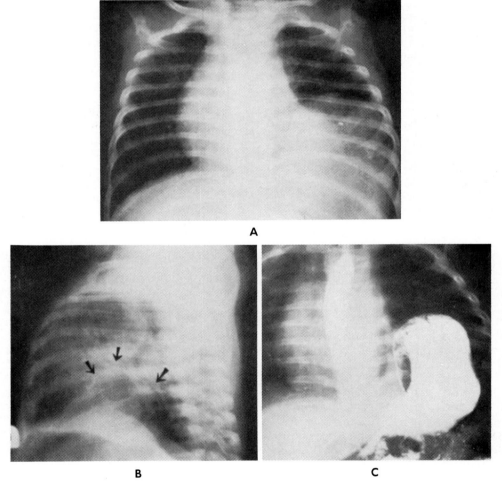

**A**

**B**                    **C**

*Figure 16–7.* *A*, Anteroposterior view of chest made at 3½ months of age. The left diaphragm is elevated to the level of the fourth rib. The heart is displaced a little to the right. *B*, Lateral view on same date. The left diaphragm can be seen considerably higher in the chest than the right. Arrows point to the domed diaphragm. *C*, With barium in the esophagus and stomach the stomach can be seen to lie largely within the thorax. It is inverted. The esophagus is displaced toward the right.

Admission examination (age 3½ months) showed a temperature of 37.4° C., pulse 144, respirations 52, weight 6.24 kg. (13 pounds 12 ounces). Nutrition was fair. His abdomen appeared small. The heart was slightly displaced to the right. Percussion note over the left hemithorax was flat, and over this area no breath sounds were heard. X-ray film shows elevation of the left diaphragm. Gas-filled structures are seen within the thorax beneath it. The heart is displaced to the right (Fig. 16–7). Fluoroscopy on the same day revealed good motion of both leaves of the diaphragm. Operation was performed. The stomach, duodenum, left lobe of the liver and the spleen lay within the left hemithorax beneath a saccular structure which terminated in lateral ridges of muscle. The sac was later found to contain a few muscle fibers. It was removed, and the ridges of muscle were sewn tightly together. The central portion of this diaphragm was a sac almost devoid of muscle. Whether this was a congenital defect or the late result of diaphragmatic paralysis one cannot say.

**COMMENT.** The birth of this infant was said to have been easy, and he was not unusually large. There is little evidence to make one suspect paralysis of the diaphragm due to brachial plexus trauma. He was neither tachypneic nor dyspneic. Nor was paradoxical movement ever demonstrated. The likelihood, then, is that the weak, elevated diaphragm containing very little muscle tissue represents a congenital defect, or a true eventration. Operation successfully restored the proper anatomic relationships.

## ACCESSORY DIAPHRAGM

This extremely rare anomaly consists of a supernumerary membranous and muscular structure which divides the hemithorax into two compartments. Four cases have been reported in the past three or four decades. Hashida and Sherman, who described the most recent example, state that "pressure at the hiatus and disturbed mechanics due to . . . interference with function, especially of the contents of the inferior compartment" are responsible for the signs and symptoms. Anomalies of vascular supply and of lobulation may coexist. Their own infant was mildy cyanotic from birth,

became more deeply so steadily and developed grunting and x-ray evidence of pneumothorax. The left hemithorax moved poorly, and breath sounds over it were absent. He died at 5 hours of age.

The left hemithorax was divided into two unequal compartments by an accessory diaphragm. A semicircular orifice through which bronchi and vessels passed divided the upper from the lower compartment.

## REFERENCES

Allen, M. S., and Thomson, S. A.: Congenital diaphragmatic hernia in children under one year of age: a 24 year review. J. Pediat. Surg., 1:157–161, 1966.

Arnheim, E. E.: Congenital hernia of the diaphragm, with special reference to right-sided hernia of the liver and intestines. Surg. Gynec. & Obstet. 95:293, 1952.

Baran, E. M., Houston, H. E., Lynn, H. B., et al.: Foramen of Morgagni hernias in children. Surgery 62:1076, 1967.

Bisgard, J. D., and Robertson, G. E.: Congenital eventration of the diaphragm; surgical management. Am. J. Surg. 70:95, 1945.

Bishop, H. C., and Koop, C. E.: Acquired eventration of the diaphragm in infancy. Pediatrics 22:1088, 1958.

Bowers, V. M., Jr., McElin, T. W., and Dorsey, J. M.: Diaphragmatic hernia in the newborn; diagnostic responsibility of the obstetrician. Obstet. & Gynecol. 6:262, 1955.

Butler, N., and Claireaux, A. E.: Congenital diaphragmatic hernia as a cause of perinatal mortality. Lancet 1:659, 1962.

Comer, T. P., and Clagett, O. T.: Surgical treatment of hernia of the foramen of Morgagni. J. Thoracic Cardiovasc. Surg. 52:461, 1966.

France, N. E.: Unilateral diaphragmatic paralysis and Erb's palsy in the newborn. Arch. Dis. Childh. 29:357, 1954.

Hashida, Y., and Sherman, F. E.: Accessory diaphragm associated with neonatal respiratory distress. J. Pediatr. 59:529, 1961.

Johnson, D. G., Deaner, R. M., and Koop, C. E.: Diaphragmatic hernia in infancy: factors affecting the mortality rate. Surgery 62:1082, 1967.

Laxdal, O. E., McDougall, H. A., and Mellin, G. W.: Congenital eventration of the diaphragm. N. Engl. J. Med. 250:401, 1954.

Leahy, L. S., and Butsch, W. L.: Surgical management of respiratory emergencies during the first few weeks of life. Arch. Surg. 59:466, 1949.

Levy, J. L. Jr., Guynes, W. A. Jr., Louis, J. E., et al.: Bilateral congenital diaphragmatic hernias through the foramina of Bochdalek. J. Pediat. Surg. 4:557, 1969.

Longino, L. A., and Jewett, T. C.: Congenital bifid sternum. Surgery 38:610, 1955.

McNamara, J. J., Eraklis, A. J., and Gross, R. E.: Congenital posterolateral diaphragmatic hernia in the newborn. J. Thorac. Cardiovasc. Surg. 55:55–59, 1968.

Perinatal Mortality: The First Report of the British Perinatal Mortality Survey. Edinburgh and London, E. & S. Livingstone, Ltd., 1963.

Philipp, E. E., and Skelton, M. O.: Congenital diaphragmatic hernia in siblings. Br. Med. J. 1:1283, 1952.

Richard, J., et al.: Diaphragmatic obstetric paralysis. Report of 10 cases. Arch. Franç. Pediat. 14:563, 1957.

Rickham, P. P.: Strangulated diaphragmatic hernia in the neonatal period. Thorax 10:104, 1955.

Schifrin, N.: Unilateral paralysis of the diaphragm in the newborn infant due to phrenic nerve injury, with and without associated brachial palsy. Pediatrics 9:69, 1952.

Smith, B. T.: Isolated phrenic nerve palsy in the newborn. Pediatrics 49:449, 1972.

Tolins, S. H.: Congenital diaphragmatic hernia in the newborn. Ann. Surg. 137:276, 1953.

Zimmerman, L. M., and Anson, B. J.: The Anatomy and Surgery of Hernia. Baltimore, Williams & Wilkins Company, 1953.

# DISORDERS OF THE CHEST WALL

# 17

Abnormalities of bone and muscle of the chest wall may occur and be a mechanical hindrance to ventilation. Although bony abnormalities are rare, they may be recognized immediately and are sometimes amenable to operative correction.

Defects in the fusion of the sternum are uncommon, but numerous instances have been described since 1947, when Burton reported two cases in which successful operative repair was accomplished. *Complete separation of the sternum* allows protrusion of cardiovascular structures (ectopia cordis). Lethal malformations of the heart are commonly associated with that condition. *Upper sternal clefts* are more common. Early operation is advised in order to shield the underlying structures from injury and because of the greater ease of approximating the separated parts in the first days of life than later.

The most common of the sternal defects is *pectus excavatum*, sometimes associated with the Pierre Robin syndrome and Marfan's syndrome. A similar deformity is commonly seen in premature infants with respiratory distress which commonly resolves in time. Rarely is it a fixed or severe deformity until several months of postnatal age. Although the lesion may be sporadic in occurrence, it is often familial. The indications for operative correction are debatable. In our opinion, correction should not be undertaken until several years of age and then only in those few children in whom the deformity appears to be progressing.

A rare deformity of the thoracic cage, *asphyxiating thoracic dystrophy of the newborn*, was described by Jeune et al. in 1954. It is thought to be a manifestation of a generalized chondrodystrophy. The relatively small and immobile thorax results from short hypoplastic ribs. Death has occurred in the first year of life in most of the reported cases.

Other causes of thoracic dysfunction are diseases of the muscles, including myasthenia gravis, poliomyelitis, amyotonia congenita, muscular dystrophy, glycogen storage disease and spinal cord injury or tumor. Such conditions are usually recognized in the context of the associated systemic muscular weakness or paralysis.

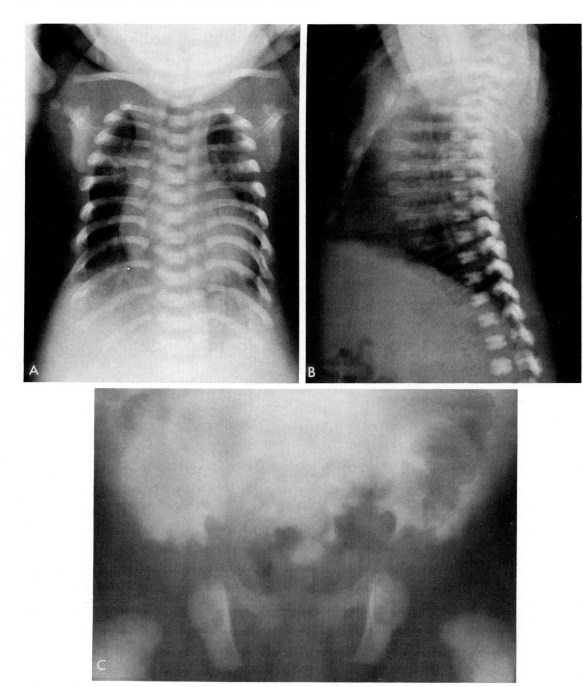

***Figure 17–1.*** *A,* Anteroposterior film of infant with asphyxiating thoracic dystrophy. The thoracic circumference is reduced as compared with the abdominal circumference, and the liver and spleen are displayed downward.

*B,* Lateral projection of the same infant demonstrates further the reduced thoracic volume. (*A* and *B* courtesy of Dr. John Kirkpatrick).

*C,* The film of the pelvis shows flaring of the iliac crest and irregular calcification of the triradiate cartilage with typical bony protrusions. (*C* From Avery, M. E., and Fletcher, B. D.: The Lung and Its Diseases in the Newborn Infant. 3rd ed. Philadelphia, W. B. Saunders Co., 1974.)

They should be suspected in any infant in whom hypoventilation is present when the chest film shows normal heart and lungs.

## REFERENCES

Jeune, N., Carron, R., Berand, C., et al.: Polychondro-dystrophie avec blocage thoracique d'évolution fatale. Pédiatrie 9:390, 1954.

Kohler, E., and Babbitt, D. P.: Dystrophic thoraces and infantile asphyxia. Radiology 94:55, 1970.

Maier, H. C., and Bortone, F.: Complete failure of sternal fusion with herniation of pericardium. J. Thorac. Surg. 18:851, 1949.

Sabiston, D. C.: The surgical management of congenital bifid sternum with partial ectopia cordis. J. Thorac. Surg. 35:118, 1958.

# PULMONARY CYSTS

# 18

Air-containing cysts within the lung are not encountered frequently, but cysts are present in such a variety of forms that they constitute an interesting diagnostic and therapeutic problem in the neonatal period. They may be single or multiple, unilateral or bilateral, filled with air or fluid, or both. They may be infected or clean, and the air within them may or may not be under tension. They may be congenital or acquired. At times conservative measures of treatment are proper, but upon occasion immediate surgical intervention is required.

**INCIDENCE.** By 1933 Anspach and Wolman were able to find 150 cases in the medical literature, and the number has surely doubled since then. Cooke and Blades stated that one asymptomatic case per 20,000 was found in mass surveys, and that one admission to the Walter Reed Hospital in every 2400 was for pulmonary cyst. In spite of these low figures they concluded that the disease was "relatively common." Few of the total make their presence known during the first month of life.

**CLASSIFICATION.** Cooke and Blades proposed the following simple classification:

I. Congenital pulmonary cysts
   A. Bronchogenic cell type
      1. Solitary
      2. Multiple (synonyms: congenital or fetal bronchiectasis)
   B. Alveolar cell type
      1. Solitary (synonyms: balloon cyst, pneumatocele)
      2. Multiple
   C. Combination of A and B
II. Acquired pulmonary cysts
   A. Bullous emphysema
   B. Subpleural blebs

**PATHOLOGY AND PATHOGENESIS.** Congenital cysts form when there is a developmental error in the ontogeny of the lung in the region of the medium-sized bronchi (*bronchogenic* cell type) or just proximal to the alveoli (*alveolar* cell type). These defects may be single or multiple. If multiple, they usually involve several segments of one lobe, more rarely of two or three contiguous lobes, but fortunately they are almost never bilateral. Characteristics of the congenital variety are said to be a wall containing smooth muscle and bits of cartilage. Being lined by epithelium is no proof of congenital origin, since epithelial cells have been found to grow over and line a resected surface. In the bronchogenic cell type the lining cells are cuboidal or columnar and ciliated; in the alveolar type they are squamous. Caffey doubts the specificity of these pathologic alterations, maintaining that acquired cysts may present the same picture.

Congenital cysts usually have a connection with the bronchial tree. Often this is a minute tortuous passage to a small bronchiole. Acquired cysts, on the other hand, connect freely with adjacent bronchioles in many places.

The circumstance of their being in free communication with the tracheobronchial tree is responsible for almost all the trouble lung cysts cause. Infection spreads readily from bronchi into the interior of cysts, where, once established, it may be difficult to eradicate. Besides this, free egress of inspired air may be impeded by check-valve action at the communicating channel, resulting in increased tension. Without infection or tension most pulmonary cysts go unnoticed only to be discovered by x-ray films taken for some other reason.

Emphysematous bullae and subpleural blebs are produced by either obstruction or infection (see Hyperinflated Lung, p. 126).

A rare form of congenital cystic disease is characterized by a mass of cysts lined by proliferating bronchial or cuboidal epithelium. To date 47 instances of this condition, called *cystic adenomatoid malformation of the lung*, have been described. The disorder has been noted in all lobes of the lung. Gottschalk and Abramson in 1957 described its association with placental edema and fetal hydrops, presumably on the basis of obstruction to venous return. Merenstein found hydramnios associated with 8 and anasarca with 14 of the 47 cases reported.

**DIAGNOSIS.** Newborns who become ill with cystic disease of the lungs usually suffer from the effects of rapid expansion of the cysts. Tachypnea or dyspnea may begin at birth or at any time thereafter. Dyspnea may progress rapidly or slowly. In the first instance the infant's condition can become critical within hours; in the latter it may remain almost static for weeks or months.

A minority of neonates demonstrate the effects of infection rather than of increased tension. In these, persistent or repeated exacerbations of pneumonitis are the presenting symptom. When this is so, it is often difficult to decide whether infection came first and produced emphysematous bullae and subpleural blebs, or whether the cystic areas were true congenital cysts which became secondarily infected.

When cysts are solitary and large, they are discoverable by flatness of the percussion note if pus filled, or hyperresonance or tympany if, as is more commonly the case, they are air filled. Breath sounds are diminished to absent over them. The heart is shifted away from the affected side unless a cyst lying adjacent to a bronchus has completely occluded it and has produced atelectasis of the distal segment of lung. Rales may be heard, owing to compression of contiguous lobes. Even when multiple cysts are present, the physical signs may be exactly the same, since the condition of the largest of the cysts dominates the clinical picture.

**RADIOGRAPHIC FINDINGS.** Large balloon cysts filled with air under tension are often mistaken for tension pneumothorax. One hemithorax is overfilled, the diaphragm flattened or even concave, the mediastinum and heart pushed to or beyond the midline. Points which may distinguish balloon cysts from pneumothorax are (1) a delicate linear pattern within the translucent area denoting their fine trabeculation, (2) the presence of compressed lung at the apex and at the costophrenic and cardiohepatic angles, often demarcated from the cyst by a curving line visible in one or another projection, and (3) the absence of all hilar shadows. In pneumothorax the collapsed lung is often visible as a dense shadow projecting from the hilar region or upward from the diaphragm.

Multiple cysts are visualized as a collection of round or oval translucent areas within the hemithorax. If similar shadows are present in both sides of the chest, they are more likely to represent emphysematous bullae or blebs, but unilaterality does not rule out the latter possibility.

The round or oval areas of translucency produced by intrathoracic bowel may offer difficulty at times. When one is in doubt about the possibility of diaphragmatic hernia, a barium meal gastrointestinal series must be performed.

Large cysts containing both air and fluid are hard to differentiate from hydropneumothorax or pyopneumothorax. Here again visualization of a curved concave border between the cyst and compressed lung at the apex or base is the important differentiating feature.

**PROGNOSIS.** Since many cystic lesions of the lung are completely asymptomatic and are discovered accidentally on chest films, it is safe to assume that a good many of those which might be discovered in this way in the neonatal period will never cause trouble. Once symptoms have developed, whether of increasing tension or of infection, the outlook becomes more serious. It is nevertheless true that most cystic-appearing lung lesions disappear with no surgical treatment. Whether one agrees with Caffey that this proves that most of them are not congenital lesions, or with Blades that even congenital cysts may disappear spontaneously, is of little moment.

TREATMENT. The absolute indication for immediate surgical treatment is increasing air tension within the cyst. This indication is unequivocal, and, what is more, radical intervention is called for. Repeated aspirations of air by needle and syringe or constant suction through an introduced catheter gives no more than temporary relief. They should be used, if at all, only for that reason, to tide the infant over a critical period until definitive operative measures can be taken. Operation should then consist in removal of as small a portion of the lung as is necessary, either a segment of a lobe or one or two lobes or the entire lung.

Infection within the cyst cavity constitutes the second indication for lobectomy or pneumonectomy. When there is pus, with or without air, within the cyst cavity, operation may be delayed until antibiotic and supportive therapy has improved the infant's general condition.

The therapeutic approach to acquired cysts should be conservative, since in Caffey's experience eight of 13 cases cleared completely. Cystic lesions subsequent upon obstruction or infection are seldom lethal in themselves, and only treatment directed toward the underlying condition is indicated. If, after a waiting period of months, improvement has not occurred or if growth and development are retarded by persistent or repeated respiratory infection, lobectomy or pneumonectomy may have to be undertaken.

## CASE HISTORIES

### CASE 18–1

(Case of Fischer, Tropea and Bailey, Hahnemann Hospital of Philadelphia, abstracted, and prints reproduced, with kind permission of Dr. Fischer.)

A white female infant, birth weight 5 pounds 12 ounces (2600 gm), pregnancy and labor uncomplicated, breathed with some difficulty from birth, but thrived for 2 weeks. She then failed to gain for the next 2 weeks. Physical examination (1 month) revealed dyspnea, and the chest was partially fixed in expansion with infracostal and suprasternal retraction. Percussion note was hyperresonant over the entire right hemithorax and left upper anterior hemithorax. The heart was displaced into the left axilla. A few crepitant rales were heard over the right back. X-ray film showed large air-containing cysts in the upper and middle thirds of the right hemithorax (Fig. 18–1). Needling produced air under pressure which displaced the plunger of the syringe to the 40-cc mark, with moderate relief. She seemed worse the next day, and subcutaneous emphysema of the chest wall had appeared. She was operated upon, and multiple air-containing cysts were found in the right upper and middle lobes. These two lobes were removed. Convalescence was uneventful. Sections showed many cysts of various sizes, all air-containing, their walls composed of bronchial epithelium superimposed upon hyperplastic muscularis. There was no inflammation.

COMMENT. Multiple cysts commonly involve only one lobe or two contiguous lobes. In this example the right upper and middle lobes were filled with cysts of various sizes, some under tension, none infected, while the right lower lobe was intact. Symptoms and signs were those of dyspnea due to encroachment of the distending cysts upon normal lung plus displacement of the heart and mediastinal structures far to the opposite side. This was probably the first newborn to be lobectomized for cystic disease of the lung. The diagnosis, if made now, would surely have been cystic adenomatoid malformation.

### CASE 18–2

(Case of Dr. Lee Forrest Hill, presented at a conference at the Raymond Blank Hospital for Children, Des Moines, Iowa. Abstracted and prints reproduced with kind permission of Dr. Hill.)

A white male infant aged 8 weeks was admitted because of paroxysmal cough since 1 week of age. Birth weight was 7 pounds 8 ounces (3400 gm); pregnancy and labor had been normal. At times tachypnea had been noted, but never cyanosis or dyspnea. He was alert, in no

*Text continued on page 201*

A

B

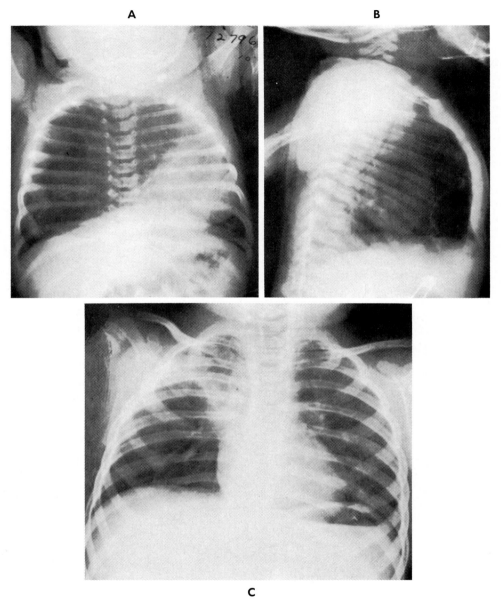

C

*Figure 18–1.* *A*, Anteroposterior film of chest taken at 1 month of age. A number of cystic shadows can be made out within the right lung field. The right lung herniates across the midline to half fill the left upper part of the chest. The heart is displaced far to the left. *B*, Lateral view, same time. The sternum is thrust forward, the heart dislocated posteriorly by herniated lung in the anterior mediastinum. Rounded cystic shadows can again be seen. *C*, Two years after operation. Aside from pleural thickening at the right upper lobe and overaeration of the right lower lobe, the lungs appear quite normal. (Fischer, C. C., Tropea, F., Jr., and Bailey, C. P.: J. Pediatr. 23:219, 1943.)

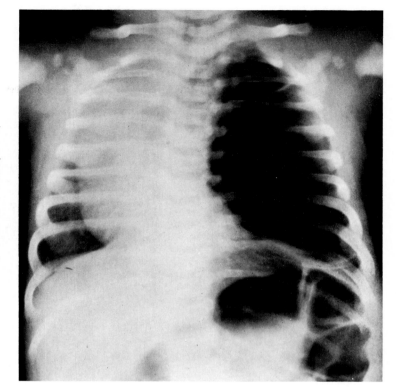

*Figure 18–2.* Anteroposterior film of chest made at 8 weeks of age. Note the shift of heart and mediastinum far to the right, herniation of left lung into right hemithorax and deviation of trachea to the right. The overfilled, overaerated left hemithorax suggests the appearance of tension cyst rather than pneumothorax, because the left hilus is empty and the lower border is curved. No collapsed lung can be seen. (Hill, L. F., J. Pediatr. 38:511, 1951.)

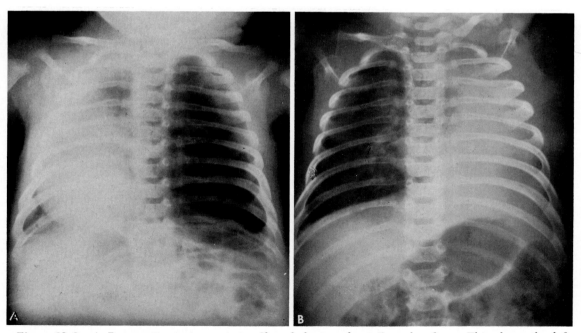

*Figure 18–3.* A, Preoperative anteroposterior film of chest made at 7 weeks of age. This shows the left hemithorax overexpanded by a huge translucent mass. Pneumothorax can be ruled out because the lower border is rounded, there is no shadow of collapsed lung, and fine trabecular markings are visible throughout most of the translucent area. The left upper lobe is herniated into the right upper hemithorax, and the heart and mediastinum are dislocated far to the right. B, Postoperative film shows the heart now displaced to the left, homogeneous opacification of the entire left hemithorax, probably due to thickened pleura, and compensatory emphysema of the right lung. (Leahy, L. J., and Butsch, W. L.: Arch. Surg. 59:466, 1949.)

**199**

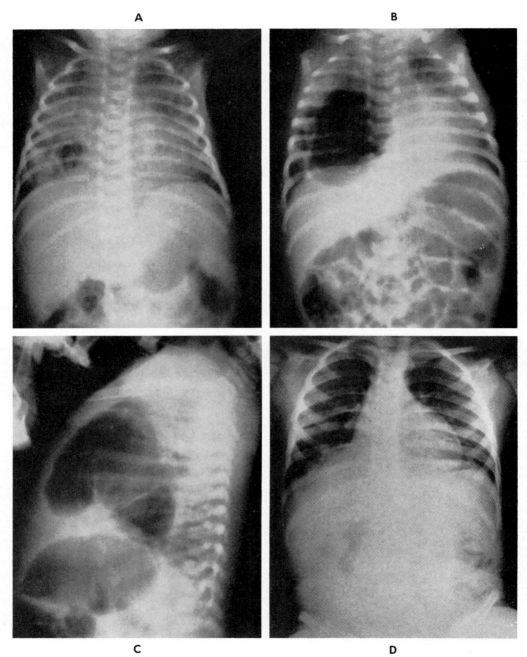

A                                                    B

C                                                    D

*Figure 18–4.*   A, Anteroposterior view of chest taken on the twenty-first day of life. An air-filled cyst can be seen in the right lower part of the chest. *B* and *C*, Thirty days later, showing great increase in size of cyst and dislocation of heart toward the left axilla. *D*, Anteroposterior view at the age of 3 years. The lungs appear essentially normal. (Swan, H., and Aragon, G. E.: Pediatrics *14*:651, 1954.)

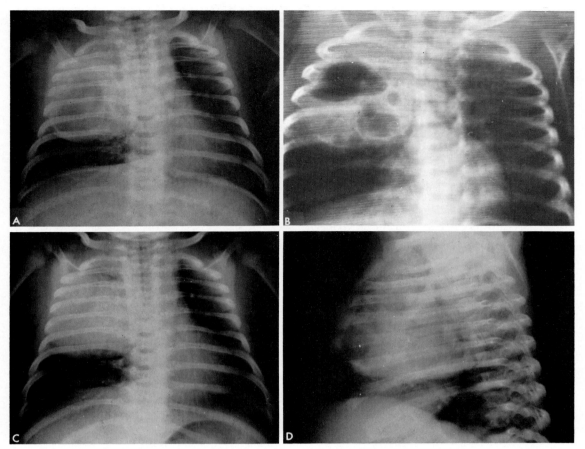

***Figure 18–5.*** *A, B* and *C*, Anteroposterior views of chest of an infant at different times to show the great variability in appearance of the same cystic lung. Differences in appearance depend upon whether one or all of the component cysts are air-filled or fluid-filled at that particular time. *D*, Lateral view made on the same day that *C* was taken. This complicated case history is not abstracted in the text.

distress. There was hyperresonance over the entire left hemithorax; the heart and trachea were shifted to the right. Breath sounds were absent on the left. Hemoglobin was 10.0 gm, red blood cell count 3,000,000, white blood cell count 10,150, with 69 per cent lymphocytes. X-ray film showed a large air-containing cyst, filling the left hemithorax and herniating into the right (Fig. 18–2).

At operation a solitary cyst was found within the left lower lobe. The entire lobe was removed.

The pathologist reported a cyst with surrounding atelectatic lung. No communication with a bronchus could be discovered. The wall consisted of bronchial epithelium, and contained bits of cartilage.

**COMMENT.** This solitary cyst was filled with air under sufficient tension to shift the heart and trachea toward the opposite side, but not enough to produce serious dyspnea. Although no connection with the tracheobronchial tree could be found, one must have been present.

CASE 18–3

(Case 3 of L. J. Leahy and W. L. Butsch, abstracted with permission of the authors.)

A white male infant was born after normal pregnancy and delivery. There was some dyspnea at first, but this improved. The infant seemed to become exhausted easily, however, and he became cyanotic after crying. No physical findings are recorded. X-ray film taken at 7 weeks showed what was interpreted to represent emphysema of the left lung with large bleb formation, shift of the heart and mediastinum to the right and atelectasis of the right lung (Fig.

18–3). Operation revealed numerous cysts in the entire left lung, the upper lobe, particularly involved, having been replaced completely by cysts. Pneumonectomy was performed. The cysts were lined with high columnar epithelium resting upon a thin mesenchymal membrane attached to a thin layer of smooth muscle. Postoperative course was uneventful.

**COMMENT.** This example is almost identical with that of Dr. Hill. Nevertheless at operation, instead of a large solitary cyst, numerous cysts involving the entire lung were discovered. This demonstrates the virtual impossibility of distinguishing single from multiple cysts in many cases.

CASE 18–4

(Case 2 of H. Swan and G. E. Aragon, abstracted with kind permission of Dr. Swan.)

An infant was admitted to the premature nursery on the sixteenth day of life because of attacks of cyanosis and hyperpnea. Weight on admission was 2 pounds 15 ounces (1340 gm). Shallow and irregular respirations were associated with intermittent episodes of cyanosis. She was treated with Terramycin. On the twenty-first day an x-ray film of the chest showed a small air-filled cyst in the lower right lung (Fig. 18–4, *A*). Respiratory difficulty increased steadily, and serial x-ray films show rapid increase in size of the cyst (Fig. 18–4, *B*, *C*). By 30 days after admission dyspnea was severe and cyanosis constant and deep. Operation was performed then, at 6 weeks, and the cyst-containing middle lobe was removed. Weight at the time was 4 pounds 3 ounces (1900 gm). Three years later she was a perfectly normal child, and her chest film appeared normal.

**COMMENT.** This case demonstrates the first great hazard of pulmonary air-containing cysts, that of increasing tension. At times ballooning is explosive, at times steady but slow, as in this instance.

## REFERENCES

Anspach, W. E., and Wolman, I. J.: Large pulmonary air cysts of infancy, with special reference to pathogenesis and diagnosis. Surg., Gynec. Obstet. 56:634, 1933.

Buntain, W. L., Isaacs, H., Payne, V. C., et al.: Lobar emphysema, cystic adenomatoid malformation, pulmonary sequestration and bronchogenic cyst in infancy and childhood: A clinical group. J. Pediatr. Surg. 9:85, 1974.

Burnett, W. E., and Caswell, H. T.: Lobectomy for pulmonary cysts in a fifteen-day-old infant with recovery. Surgery 23:84, 1948.

Caffey, J.: On the natural regression of pulmonary cysts during early infancy. Pediatrics 11:48, 1953.

Clark, N. S., Nairn, R. C., and Gowar, F. J. S.: Cystic disease of the lung in the newborn treated by pneumonectomy. Arch. Dis. Child. 31:358, 1956.

Cooke, F. N., and Blades, B. B.: Cystic disease of the lungs. J. Thorac. Surg. 23:546, 1952.

Fischer, C. C., Tropea, F., Jr., and Bailey, C. P.: Congenital pulmonary cysts; report of an infant treated by lobectomy with recovery. J. Pediatr. 23:219, 1943.

Gottschalk, W., and Abramson, D.: Placental edema and fetal hydrops. Obstet. Gynecol. 10:626, 1957.

Gross, R. E.: Congenital cystic lung: Successful pneumonectomy in a three-week-old baby. Ann. Surg. 123:229, 1946.

Hill, L. F.: Conference at Raymond Blank Memorial Hospital for Children, Des Moines, Iowa. J. Pediatr. 38:511, 1951.

Holder, T. M., and Christy, M. G.: Cystic adenomatoid malformation of the lung. J. Thorac. Cardiovasc. Surg. 47:590, 1964.

Kwittken, J., and Reiner, L.: Congenital cystic adenomatoid malformation of the lung. Pediatrics 30:759, 1962.

Leahy, L. J., and Butsch, W. L.: Surgical management of respiratory emergencies during the first few weeks of life. Arch. Surg. 59:466, 1949.

Merenstein, G. B.: Congenital cystic adenomatoid malformation of the lung. Am. J. Dis. Child. 118:772, 1969.

Swan, H., and Aragon, G. E.: Surgical treatment of pulmonary cysts in infancy. Pediatrics 14:651, 1954.

# 19  INTRATHORACIC TUMORS AND FLUID-FILLED CYSTS

A large variety of solid tumors and fluid-filled cysts, in addition to the air-filled cysts just described, are encountered in the thoraces of adults. Many of these have already been observed in newborns, and we have no doubt that others will be recorded. Those which result from congenital maldevelopment, such as intrathoracic cysts of gastrointestinal origin, and dermoid cysts or teratomatous tumors, are more common in the neonatal period than are neoplasms and lymphomas. This last group, so common in adults as to comprise up to 40 per cent of most series of mediastinal tumors, is of small numerical importance in the young infant. Too few neonatal cases have accumulated up to the present to warrant detailed classification.

Hope and Koop believe that intrathoracic mass lesions are best subdivided into those which arise in the posterior, middle and anterior mediastinal spaces. A few others arise within the substance of the lung itself. In the posterior space neurogenic tumors, duplications of the foregut, and neurenteric and bronchogenic cysts are most commonly encountered in the neonate. The middle mediastinum is the site al-

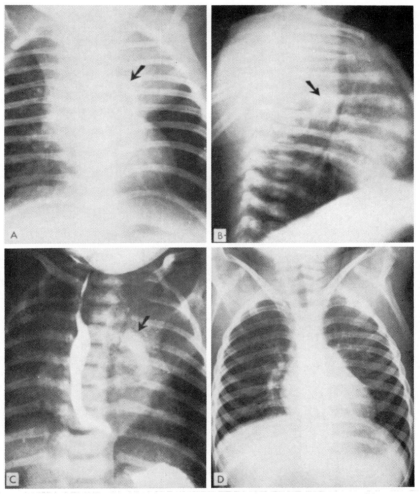

*Figure 19–1.* A 7-week-old male infant entered the hospital for repair of an inguinal hernia and was found to have a lymph node in the left cervical region. This finding resulted in a roentgen examination of the chest. *A*, Anteroposterior roentgenogram showing a large area of density in the left upper hemithorax. Within the homogeneous density a curvilinear calcification is present (arrow). *B*, Lateral roentgenogram showing the mass lesion to be in the posterior mediastinum with some anterior deviation of the trachea. The calcification appears to be in the shape of a horseshoe (arrow). *C*, Anteroposterior view of barium-filled esophagus which shows the large size of the mass lesion more graphically. The calcification is more clearly visualized (arrow). At operation the lesion proved to be a neuroblastoma. It was entirely excised. *D*, Posteroanterior roentgenogram 5 years later showing a normal chest. (Hope, J. W., and Koop, C. E.: Pediatr. Clin. N. Amer. 6:379, 1959.)

most exclusively of vascular lesions, while enlarged thymus and teratomas are masses most often seen in the anterior mediastinal space.

## MEDIASTINAL NEUROBLASTOMA

Neuroblastoma, the most common solid tumor in the mediastinum of infants, arises from neural tissue, either intercostal or sympathetic nerves for the most part. It lies typically in the thoracic gutter, therefore is almost always posterior in location, and may involve superior, mid- or inferior mediastinum. From here it may extend to either side and invade one or both lungs.

**DIAGNOSIS** is suggested by the discovery of an intrathoracic mass. It may follow roentgenography of the chest because of lower respiratory tract infection. Such infections afflict these infants more commonly than others because the growing tumor compresses bronchi. Or x-ray films may be taken because of increasing dyspnea coupled with the physical signs of a solid intrathoracic mass.

Differentiation from other posterior mediastinal masses may be impossible before exploration. Neuroblastoma is not likely to be so sharply demarcated or to have so smooth and round a lower border as does a mediastinal cyst. Invasion of neighboring lung parenchyma argues strongly in favor of neuroblastoma.

**TREATMENT.** Exploration is indicated for any intrathoracic mass. If the tumor proves to be neuroblastoma, as much of it should be excised as is feasible surgically. Excision should be followed by irradiation and, if necessary, by one or another of the chemotherapeutic agents effective against neuroblastoma (see p. 1012).

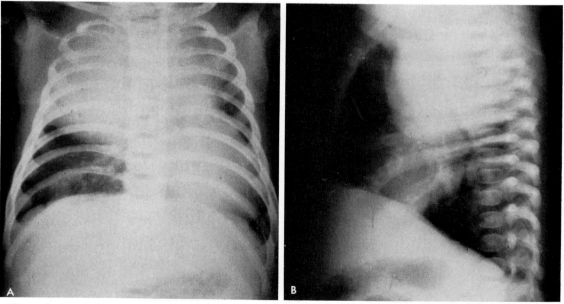

*Figure 19–2.* *A*, Anteroposterior view of chest of a 7-week-old infant admitted because of a severe respiratory infection. An opacity is seen filling the upper half of the right hemithorax and extending beyond the midline halfway to the left axilla. Its lower and left borders are rounded. The heart is displaced to the left and downward. It gives the appearance of a solid tumor. *B*, Lateral view. The opaque mass juts forward from the posterior chest wall, from clavicle halfway down the chest to abut on the heart. Its outline is round.

At operation a tumor was seen in the mediastinum which invaded all adjacent structures, including the left upper lobe. Biopsy revealed neuroblastoma. No excision was attempted. Radiotherapy was ineffective. Aminopterin was begun 2 months later and was followed by rapid improvement. Two years later she appeared perfectly well, and no tumor was visualized on x-ray films. (Case 7 of Dr. Gladys Boyd, abstracted with her kind permission.)

**PROGNOSIS.** The outlook in neuroblastoma, here as in other locations, is surprisingly good. One may look forward to cure in approximately 50 per cent of the cases.

## BRONCHOGENIC CYSTS

Fluid-filled cysts of tracheobronchogenous origin are distinguished with difficulty from those of gastroenterogenous origin.

**INCIDENCE.** In several series of cases of neoplasms and cysts of the mediastinum among patients of all ages reported from various clinics, bronchogenic cysts outnumber those of gastric or enteric derivation. Most observers comment upon the fact that the distribution differs in young infants and children, so that gastroenterogenous and enterogenous ones outnumber the bronchogenic. In a 20 year experience and review of the literature deParedes et al. found 68 cases and added 12 of their own. In the neonate bronchogenic cysts are encountered infrequently.

**PATHOLOGY.** Bronchogenic cysts seldom attain large size. They contain clear fluid and are lined with columnar, cuboidal or pseudostratified epithelium, and their walls generally contain smooth muscle and cartilage. They may, but do not always, communicate with the tracheobronchial tree. They tend to lie in the posterior mediastinum, but some have been found in the anterior space.

**DIAGNOSIS.** Lying as they do, near the carina, these cysts commonly produce signs of respiratory embarrassment from birth or soon after. Generally their size is not such that they can be discovered by percussion or auscultation, but physical signs are likely to reveal their secondary effects, emphysema or atelectasis, rather than the tumor itself. Opsahl and Berman reported a case which showed emphysema on the left, followed by clearing, then equally notable emphysema on the right.

X-ray examination often shows a mass projecting forward from the superior mediastinal shadow, not large, and not necessarily rounded.

Barium swallow may reveal indentation of the esophagus from an anterior direction.

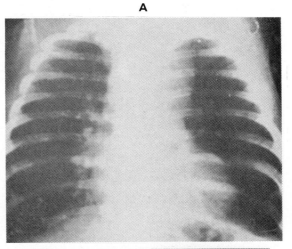

**A**

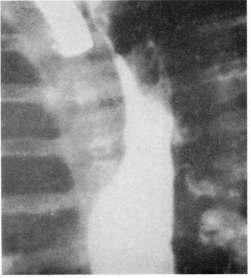

**B**

*Figure 19–3.* Four-month-old female infant with cough and stridor from birth. Both lungs were hyperresonant. *A*, Mass in left mediastinum with trachea pressed to right. *B*, With barium swallow there is a large defect in left side of the esophagus. At operation, a large cyst, not attached to either the trachea or esophagus, was removed. The infant died 2 days later. The specimen was lined by ciliated columnar epithelium, and was diagnosed as bronchogenic cyst. (Kraus, M.: Case Reports Children's Memorial Hosp. *15*:4061, 1957.)

Bronchoscopy reveals compression of the trachea and often of one major bronchus.

**TREATMENT.** Immediate excision should be performed.

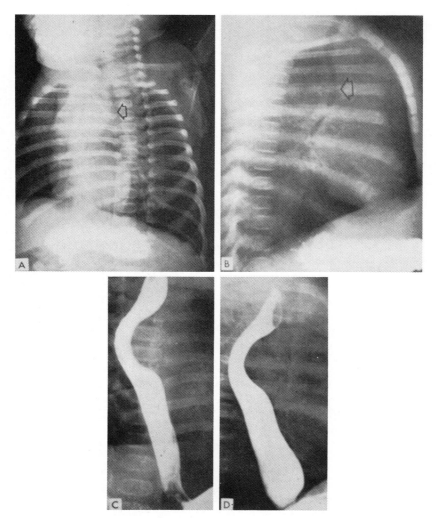

**Figure 19–4.** A 10-week-old male infant with dyspnea since birth. *A*, Left anterior oblique roentgenogram showing a mass lesion just below the carina (arrow). *B*, Lateral roentgenogram showing anterior deviation of the trachea (arrow). *C*, Anteroposterior view of barium-filled esophagus showing extreme deviation of the esophagus to the right just above the level of the carina. *D*, Lateral view of barium-filled esophagus showing posterior deviation of the esophagus just above the level of the carina. At operation a bronchogenic cyst was removed. (Hope, J. W., and Koop, C. E.: Pediatr. Clin. N. Amer. 6:379, 1959.)

## ESOPHAGEAL, GASTROGENIC AND ENTEROGENOUS CYSTS

These three varieties of intrathoracic fluid-filled cysts are discussed together since they are indistinguishable on clinical grounds.

**INCIDENCE.** Together they comprise a large group of mediastinal masses in the neonatal period. Although they are not encountered frequently, they are far from uncommon.

**PATHOLOGY AND ETIOLOGY.** These cysts are duplicated segments of gut which have become partially or completely detached from the parent viscus. They lie in or near the posterior mediastinum, but with increasing size may project far into one or the other hemithorax. Their walls are composed of a mucosal layer characteristic of that of their site of origin, and of one or more muscular layers. They contain fluid which is also similar to the secretion normally manufactured in their parent locus.

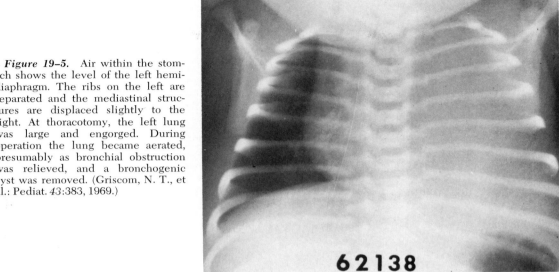

*Figure 19–5.* Air within the stomach shows the level of the left hemidiaphragm. The ribs on the left are separated and the mediastinal structures are displaced slightly to the right. At thoracotomy, the left lung was large and engorged. During operation the lung became aerated, presumably as bronchial obstruction was relieved, and a bronchogenic cyst was removed. (Griscom, N. T., et al.: Pediat. 43:383, 1969.)

The material within gastrogenic cysts contains pepsin and protein and inorganic salts in roughly the same concentrations as are present in gastric juice.

The foregut becomes duplicated in the course of embryonic development by failure of complete resorption of occluding epithelium, resulting in the formation of a supernumerary wall. The high percentage of vertebral malformations coincident with gastroenterogenous cysts led Veeneklaas to suggest that the primary embryonic defect lies in abnormal persistence of the primitive adherence of notochord to foregut. When foregut descends from its early position in the region of the neck, this adhesion causes anomalies in vertebral bodies derived from notochord, and pinches off a portion of the foregut and prevents its descent.

**DIAGNOSIS.** Symptoms depend upon the size and location of the cyst. Since the cysts are all posterior and lie close to the trachea, esophagus and great vessels, they are seldom symptomless. Cyanosis, tachypnea and dyspnea are often present from birth. Swallowing difficulty and vomiting are less frequent. Recurrent lower respiratory tract infections characterize a few. Hemorrhage, from either the mouth or nose, from lungs or stomach, or in the form of melena, is not at all uncommon. In most instances hemorrhage indicates that the cyst is of gastrogenic origin, since the fluid within these cysts contains pepsin and is capable of eroding through the cyst wall to break down adjacent blood vessels.

X-ray films of the chest show abnormal shadows which are often difficult to distinguish from unusual cardiac contours. Lateral and oblique films may be needed in order to make the differentiation with certainty. In one or another projection the rounded border of the cyst contiguous to the heart should be able to be visualized. Barium swallow commonly shows displacement of the esophagus.

Bronchoscopy and esophagoscopy are not ordinarily required in order to clinch the diagnosis. When performed, they may show compression of one or both structures from without.

Cyst puncture need not be performed, but it does add information which aids differential diagnosis. Mediastinal meningocele contains fluid whose specific gravity is considerably lower and whose calcium content is about half that found in gastroenterogenous cysts. Proteolytic ferments are present in cysts, not in meningoceles. In actual practice one does not perform cyst puncture in the newborn.

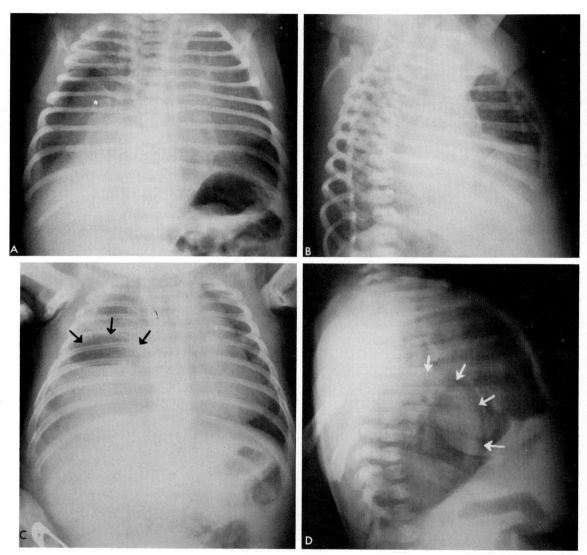

*Figure 19–6.* *A,* Anteroposterior view of chest taken within the first week of life, interpreted as showing atelectasis of right upper and lower lobes. The left border of the heart almost touches the left axillary wall, while its right border appears to be almost as far in the right hemithorax. It is difficult to tell whether this shadow is that of a hugely enlarged heart or whether it is composed of more than one element. *B,* Lateral view. In this view the opacity filling the lower half of the chest is also difficult to diagnose, but it almost surely is not all heart. *C,* Anteroposterior view taken 4 weeks later. In the interim, fluid had been withdrawn six times, and in the process air had been introduced into the right hemithorax. Now one can see a mass in the right middle and lower hemithorax containing a bubble of air which delineates its rounded upper border. Removal of fluid has permitted the heart to return to a position more nearly normal. *D,* Lateral view, same day. Here the rounded margin of almost the entire cyst can be visualized. (Leahy, L. J., and Butsch, W. L.: Arch. Surg., 59:466, 1949.)

**TREATMENT.** Operation is indicated as soon as the diagnosis of mediastinal mass is made. It is neither necessary nor wise to delay exploration until a specific diagnosis has been made.

### CASE 19–1

(Case 2 of L. J. Leahy and W. L. Butsch, abstracted with permission of the authors.)

A white male infant, pregnancy and labor normal, was noted to be cyanotic, with rapid labored breathing shortly after birth. In an incubator with oxygen the temperature ranged from 99.2° to 101.4° F.: respirations were rapid (80 to 110 per minute). Examination revealed dullness and suppressed breath sounds over the right lower hemithorax. X-ray films were interpreted as showing atelectasis of the right upper and lower lobes, emphysema of the right middle lobe (Fig. 19–5, A, B). Bronchoscopy showed the right main bronchus nearly occluded in its lower portion by swollen mucous membrane and mucus. This was suctioned, and the bronchus was dilated. He was discharged, improved.

At 4 weeks, however, he was readmitted with increasing cyanosis and dyspnea. A diagnosis of pleural effusion, right, was made, and six successive thoracenteses were performed in the next 2 weeks. Each time clear, straw-colored fluid was withdrawn. X-ray film now showed a large fluid- and air-containing pocket in the right lower hemithorax (Fig. 19–5, C, D). Opera-

tion was performed at 7 weeks. The pleura over the right lower lung was thick and adherent. A thick-walled cyst was found containing straw-colored fluid and shaggy exudate. It lay contiguous with the lower esophagus for 4 cm. in the right costophrenic sinus, and sent a projection downward to the gastric cardia. The wall was thick, lined with typical gastric rugae, and contained layers of smooth muscle resembling that of the stomach. Postoperative course was uneventful.

**COMMENT.** In this case the correct diagnosis was not made immediately. The radiographic configuration of the cyst was at first not diagnostic, suggesting atelectasis and emphysema to those who saw it at the time. To us it resembles a greatly enlarged heart, and as such we might have been inclined to misinterpret it. After air had been introduced accidentally the proper interpretation became obvious.

## MEDIASTINAL TERATOMAS

The shadow of the enlarged thymus is the most common radiopaque mass visualized in the anterior mediastinum of the newborn. The enlarged thymus, however, appears to cause little, if any, trouble in the

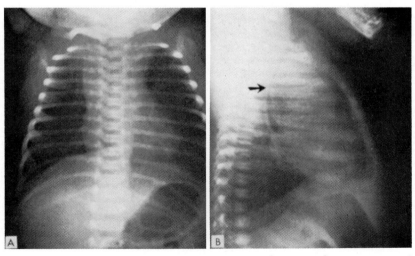

*Figure 19–7.* An 11-day-old male infant with severe respiratory distress and cyanosis since 2 days of age. *A,* Anteroposterior roentgenogram showing extreme hyperaeration of both lung fields and a wide superior mediastinum. *B,* Lateral roentgenogram showing extreme hyperaeration of the lungs and a mass filling the anterior mediastinum, producing posterior deviation and compression of the trachea (arrow). The tumor was excised and proved to be a benign teratoma lying behind a normal thymus gland and in front of the trachea. (Hope, J. W., and Koop, C. E.: Pediatr. Clin. N. Amer. 6:379, 1959.)

neonatal period. Thymoma has not been reported. When an anterior mediastinal mass is associated with respiratory distress in the newborn, the strong likelihood is that the lesion is a teratoma. All other anterior masses (lymphomas, lymphangiomas, substernal thyroids, and so on) occur with the utmost infrequency in this age period.

## FIBROSARCOMA OF THE LUNG

An unusual solid tumor of the lung in a newborn was reported to us in a personal communication from Sir Douglas Robb, of Auckland, New Zealand. As far as we can determine, this is the only fibrosarcoma of the lung thus far identified in a newborn.

CASE 19–2

(Case of Douglas Robb, from the Thoracic Surgical Unit, Green Lane Hospital, Auckland, N. Z. Personal communication to the author.)

"A male child, birth weight 8 lb., 5 oz. (3770 gm) was found to have its heart beat in the right chest and dullness over the left hemithorax. X-ray showed radiopacity of the left chest and heart displaced to the right. Barium swallow showed the cardia and stomach to lie below a normally placed left diaphragm, thus suggesting that the mass was of thoracic origin.

"On the second day of life a left thoracotomy displayed a yellowish spherical tumor occupying most of the lower lobe of the left lung, with fringes of lung tissue around. No adhesions, ...no pleural fluid,...the hilar structures were normal and not infiltrated and showed no enlarged glands. Left lower lobectomy was performed, recovery was uneventful and progress subsequently was good."

The specimen was examined by Dr. Stephen Williams, Pathologist. Sections showed the 6.5 by 6.0 cm tumor to be composed of poorly differentiated round and spindle cells arranged in sheets lying in various planes. Van Gieson's stain showed collagenous fibrils in some areas. Diagnosis was sarcoma, probably of fibroblastic origin.

COMMENT. The findings of dullness in one hemithorax with shift of the heart and mediastinum to the opposite side led to radiographic investigation. Identical signs might have been elicited from various solid tumors or fluid-filled cysts, or even from pleural effusion or chylothorax. The x-ray shadow indicated that a tumor was present,

and this was immediately removed. This assured the infant its maximum opportunity for complete cure.

## HAMARTOMA OF LUNG

Hamartoma is not a true neoplasm. It is a mass composed of the normal elements which make up an organ, combined in an abnormal manner. In the lung it is usually encapsulated and firm and ordinarily does not attain a great size. Under the microscope varying amounts of mesenchymal and epithelial elements are seen, often surrounding bits of cartilage. An abstract of one example in infancy follows.

CASE 19–3

(Case of Graham and Singleton, abstracted with permission of the authors.)

A white female infant born at term after normal pregnancy and labor, birth weight 7 pounds 4 ounces (3290 gm), seemed well during her 3-day nursery stay. At 6 weeks deep sternal retraction was seen. The time of onset of this symptom was not known.

Examination revealed shifting of the heart far to the right. There were no respiratory distress, no cyanosis, no murmurs, no abnormal heart sounds. A diagnosis of dextrocardia was made. On the following day the temperature rose to 103° F; cough appeared and later became severe and persistent. The infant began to vomit some feedings and to be mildly dyspneic. Breath sounds decreased on the left, and coarse and fine rales became audible on this side. X-ray study showed a homogeneous density filling the left hemithorax with mediastinal and cardiac shift to the right. The mass was anterior. With penicillin, oxygen and a transfusion she promptly became afebrile. Operation at 7½ weeks revealed a firm, rubbery left upper lobe and several large hilar nodes. Left upper lobectomy was done. The specimen was a firm mass with some aerated lung about the periphery. Under the microscope the septa were thick and cellular; the alveolar spaces were dilated and lined by tall cuboidal or columnar epithelium. Many spaces resembled bronchioles of an immature type. The diagnosis was hamartoma.

COMMENT. In this instance dyspnea appeared first, evidence of cardiac dislocation next, and pneumonitis supervened a bit later. X-ray examination revealed an intrathoracic mass. Despite its benign nature, immediate excision was imperative because its very size was producing pressure effects and infection, either of which might have caused early death.

## ACCESSORY AND SEQUESTERED LOBES

More than 200 cases of pulmonary sequestration have been reported in the literature; these were reviewed by Carter in 1969. They have rarely produced symptoms in newborn infants, and have usually been detected on chest films taken for other reasons. A sequestered lobe sometimes manifests itself in children or young adults by repeated infections in a fluid-filled cyst.

The malformation is slightly more common in males, and is distinctly more likely on the left side. Approximately two thirds of the cases involve the left lower lobe. Connections with the foregut may occur. Anomalous arteries from the aorta (above or below the diaphragm) usually enter the sequestered lobe, which does not receive pulmonary blood flow. Venous drainage is by the pulmonary veins or the azygos system. Complex congenital malformations coexist with extralobar sequestered lobes in 15 to 40 per cent of cases. Associated malformations are rare with intralobar sequestrations. Anomalous venous drainage, eventration of the diaphragm, and foregut duplications are among the more frequently associated conditions.

Usually, the sequestered lobe does not communicate with the tracheobronchial tree. This may occur, however, as in the infant, reported by Bozic, who also had atelectasis and hyaline membranes in all lobes except the sequestered one, which was perfused solely by the systemic circulation.

The most useful aid in diagnosis is a chest roentgenogram. It is helpful to have an angiographic study preoperatively to alert the surgeon as to the position of anomalous vessels.

The treatment is resection, because repeated infections are the rule.

Accessory lobes differ from sequestered ones in that they derive their blood supply from the pulmonary vascular system.

## CASE 19–4

A white female infant born after normal pregnancy and delivery seemed well at birth, but imperforate anus was discovered promptly. Me-

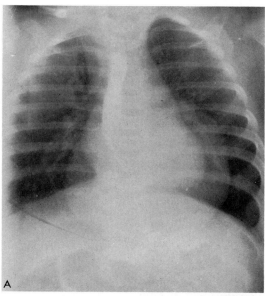

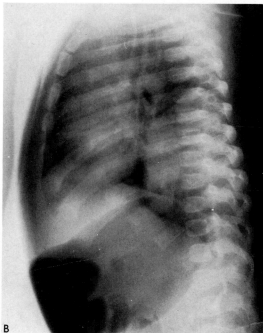

*Figure 19–8.* A, Anteroposterior view shows a homogeneous circular shadow surrounding the heart shadow. The heart appears normal, the lungs clear. B, In the lateral view the mass is seen to be disc-shaped, and to lie in the posterior mediastinum. This proved to be an accessory lobe.

conium was passed through a rectovaginal fistula easily until she was three months of age, when she was admitted to hospital for definitive repair. An x-ray film taken during this stay revealed a remarkable mass in the chest (Fig. 19–7). It lay behind the heart and did not impinge upon either trachea or esophagus. Operation (Dr. J. C. Handelsman) revealed it to be a spongy mass of unaerated lung tissue, deriving its blood via a branch of the pulmonary artery. This was removed with no difficulty. It was considered to be an accessory lobe.

## REFERENCES

Abell, M. R.: Mediastinal cysts. A.M.A. Arch. Path. *61*:360, 1956.

Adams, F. H.: Unusual case of bronchiogenic lung cyst simulating dextrocardia. J. Pediatr. *39*:483, 1951.

Bates, M.: Total unilateral pulmonary sequestration. Thorax *23*:311, 1968.

Boyd, G. L.: Solid intrathoracic masses in children. Pediatrics *19*:142, 1957.

Bozic, C.: Pulmonary hyaline membranes and vascular anomalies of the lung. Description of a case. Pediatrics *32*:1094, 1963.

Burnett, W. E., and Caswell, H. T.: Lobectomy for pulmonary cysts in 15-day-old infant with recovery. Surgery *23*:84, 1948.

Carter, R.: Pulmonary sequestration—collective review. Ann. Thorac. Surg. *7*:68, 1969.

de Paredes, C. G., Pierce, W. S., Johnson, D. G., et al.: Pulmonary sequestration in infants and children. A 20-year experience and review of the literature. J. Pediatr. Surg. *5*:136, 1970.

Ellis, F. H., Jr., Kirklin, J. W., Hodgson, et al.: Surgical implications of the mediastinal shadow in thoracic roentgenograms of infants and children. Surg. Gynecol. Obstet. *100*:532, 1955.

Eraklis, A. J., Griscom, N. T., and McGovern, J. B.: Bronchogenic cyst of the mediastinum. New Engl. J. Med. *281*:1150, 1969.

Ferguson, C. C., Young, L. N., Sutherland, J. B., and Macpherson, R. I.: Intrathoracic gastrogenic cyst—

Preoperative diagnosis by technetium pertechnetate scan. J. Pediatr. Surg. *8*:827, 1973.

Gerle, R. D., Jaretski, A., Ashley, C. A., et al.: Congenital bronchopulmonary foregut malformation. Pulmonary sequestration communicating with the gastrointestinal tract. New Engl. J. Med. *278*:1413, 1968.

Graham, G. G., and Singleton, J. W.: Diffuse hamartoma of the upper lobe in an infant: Report of successful surgical removal. A.M.A. J. Dis. Child. *89*:609, 1955.

Hope, J. W., and Koop, C. E.: Differential diagnosis of mediastinal masses. Pediatr. Clin. N. Amer. *6*:379, 1959.

Izzo, C., and Rickham, P. P.: Neonatal pulmonary hamartoma. J. Pediatr. Surg. *3*:77, 1968.

Kafka, V., and Beco, V.: Simultaneous intra- and extrapulmonary sequestration. Arch. Dis. Child. *35*:51, 1960.

Kraus, M.: Mediastinal mass. Path. Case No. 951 (No. 10,237). Case Rep. Child. Mem. Hosp. *15*:4061, 1957.

Kuipers, F., and Wieberdink, J.: An intrathoracic cyst of enterogenic origin in a young infant. J. Pediatr. *42*:603, 1953.

Opsahl, T., and Berman, E. J.: Bronchogenic mediastinal cysts in infants: Case report and review of the literature. Pediatrics *30*:372, 1962.

Pryce, D. M., Sellors, T. H., and Blair, L. G.: Intralobar sequestration of lungs associated with an abnormal pulmonary artery. Br. J. Surg. *35*:18, 1947.

Sabiston, D. C., Jr., and Scott, H. W., Jr.: Primary neoplasms and cysts of the mediastinum. Ann. Surg. *136*:777, 1952.

Smid, A. C., Ellis, F. H., Jr., Logan, G. B., and Olsen, A. M.: Partial respiratory obstruction in an infant due to a bronchogenic cyst. Proc. Staff Meet. Mayo Clin. *30*:282, 1955.

Spock, A., Schneider, S., and Baylin, G. J.: Mediastinal gastric cysts: A case report and review of the English literature. Am. Rev. Resp. Dis. *94*:97, 1966.

Starer, F.: The successful removal of an anterior mediastinal teratoma from an infant. Arch. Dis. Child. *27*:371, 1952.

Talalak, P.: Pulmonary sequestration. Arch. Dis. Child. *35*:57, 1960.

Veeneklaas, G. M. H.: Pathogenesis of intrathoracic gastrogenic cysts. Am. J. Dis. Child. *83*:500, 1952.

# 20   CHYLOTHORAX AND PLEURAL EFFUSION

**INCIDENCE.** Chylothorax is relatively rare in the neonatal period. We were able to find only eight cases reported to 1965, plus one of spontaneous pleural effusion without chyle. Subsequently, it is evident that the disorder is rare, but underreported, and appears to occur often enough to deserve mention as a cause of respiratory distress.

**ETIOLOGY.** In the adult, chylothorax almost invariably results from injury to the chest. One neonate reported had been born with the cord wrapped tightly about the neck, and a torn thoracic duct was discovered at autopsy. In the remainder no obvious difficulty was experienced during delivery. Minor trauma to the neck and chest cannot, however, be excluded even in apparently normal deliveries. The infant of Case III of McKendry et al., symptomatic from birth, was explored at 2½ months after three large aspirations had failed to relieve dyspnea. No tear in the thoracic duct was found, but serous fluid was observed to be weeping from the entire pleural surface. One supposes that in this case and perhaps in others blockage to lymphatic drainage from the lungs must exist. In one example of fatal issue neither a thoracic duct nor a cisterna chyli was discoverable at autopsy.

**DIAGNOSIS.** Dyspnea may be noted shortly after birth or at any time up to 2 weeks of age. In one case the first sign was observed as late as 7 weeks. About one half of the infants are symptomatic within 24 hours of birth. Tachypnea, dyspnea with retraction and cyanosis mark the onset. Dullness and diminution of breath sounds on one side with or without dislocation of the heart and mediastinum to the opposite side, depending upon the size of the effusion, are discovered. The effusion is usually on the right side. Bilateral effusion is rare.

X-ray films of the chest show opacification of one or both hemithoraces, the hazy homogeneous appearance suggesting fluid. Thoracentesis then reveals the presence of pleural fluid. *The fluid is chylous, i.e. milky and opalescent, only after fat-containing milk has been ingested.* In Stirlacci's case the first two taps produced clear yellow fluid, while subsequent specimens were chylous. Sakula recorded a similar sequence. Fluid is sterile, and contains about 4 per cent protein and some lymphocytes.

**PROGNOSIS.** One can never be sure how an infant will respond. Janet's infant recovered after one aspiration, Sakula's after two, Wessel's after 13. Three of the reported examples ceased pouring out pleural fluid after severe bouts of diarrhea.

The association, if any, is unclear. There were three deaths in the series, one at 20 days, another at 21 days. In this latter instance a leakage point was discovered in the posterior mediastinum. A third death occurred after 42 taps had been performed over a 2-month period. In this case no thoracic duct or cisterna chyli was found. The majority of infants have recovered after single or multiple thoracenteses. Usually there are no associated problems and no recurrences.

**TREATMENT.** Thoracenteses, repeated as often and as long as required, lead to eventual cure in most instances. If, after a reasonable period, continued tapping every 3 to 4 days does not seem to improve the infant, one is justified in considering exploration. A reparable tear in the thoracic duct might be found. We are not certain exactly what constitutes a reasonable period, but suggest that 2 months and 12 to 20 taps might be an adequate period of trial.

Continuous drainage via a chest tube can lead to protein depletion, inanition, lymphocyte depletion and impaired host defenses. If such treatment is needed to relieve symptoms, careful attention to nutrition is imperative.

Medium-chain-triglyceride formulas are useful in reducing chyle formation, hence the volume of chyle in the thorax.

**CASE 20–1**

A white male infant was born in the Johns Hopkins Hospital to a mother with pre-eclampsia, after labor had been induced by amniotomy 10 days before term. Labor had been short and uncomplicated. Birth weight was 7 pounds 15 ounces (3600 gm). The baby breathed and cried spontaneously and immediately, but was noted to be retracting deeply. Breath sounds were faint over the entire chest. His oropharynx, stomach and trachea were aspirated without improvement. Physical examination revealed dullness, almost flatness, to percussion everywhere. No breath sounds were heard over the right side and only faint ones over the left apex and base. There was deep retraction of the entire chest wall with each inspiration. The heart seemed normal in position; the sounds were good. The liver edge was 5 cm below the costal margin. X-ray film showed the right hemithorax to be completely opaque, the left almost completely so (Fig. 20–1). He was placed in an incubator with oxygen, 35 per cent, and high hu-

A

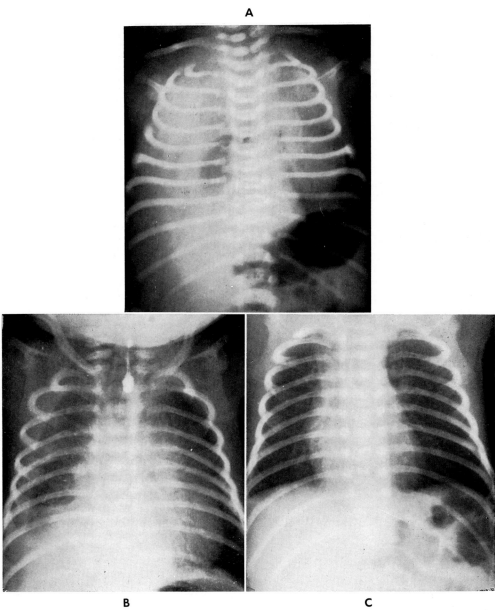

B                                                              C

*Figure 20–1.*    *A*, Anteroposterior view of chest made on the third day of life. Both lung fields are almost completely radiopaque, the right more than the left. The heart shadow is lost in the generally opacified chest. *B*, Two days later. The haziness had disappeared from the left side and cleared considerably on the right. What remains on this side is a broad pleural swath of increased density hugging the axillary wall. *C*, One week after *B*, on the twelfth day. All appears normal.

midity, given penicillin and streptomycin, and digitalized quickly with Cedilanid. He improved slightly over the next 2 days. X-ray film (third day) showed the left hemithorax to have cleared, but there was definite pleural effusion on the right, with shift of the heart to the left. Thoracentesis yielded 80 cc of clear straw-colored fluid, containing no bacteria, a few white blood cells and red blood cells. After this there remained but little respiratory distress. Steady improvement continued, and by the ninth day of life x-ray films were completely clear. Blood studies, urine examinations and tuberculin test were all negative. The infant has remained completely well.

**COMMENT.**   We have no notion as to the cause of this pleural effusion. We do know that it behaved very much as do the majority of cases of chylothorax, becoming apparent very early and disappearing rapidly. We must suppose that it belongs in the same category of disease, and that if taps had been performed later, after the beginning of milk feedings, the fluid would have been chylous.

## REFERENCES

Brodman, R. F., Zavelson, T. M., and Schiebler, G. L.: Treatment of congenital chylothorax. J. Pediatr. 85:516, 1974.

Chernick, V., and Reed, M. H.: Pneumothorax and chylothorax in the neonatal period. J. Pediatr. 76:624, 1970.

Gershanik, J. J., Jonsson, H. T., Riopel, D. A., et al.: Dietary management of neonatal chylothorax. Pediatrics 53:400, 1974.

Gwinn, J. L.: Radiological case of the mouth. Chylothorax in the newborn. Am. J. Dis. Child. 115:59, 1968.

Hashim, S. A., Rohott, H. B., Babayan, V. K., et al.: Treatment of chyluria and chylothorax with medium chain triglyceride. New Engl. J. Med. 270:756, 1964.

Janet, quoted by Sakula (vide infra).

McKendry, J. B., Lindsay, W. K., and Gerstein, M. C.: Congenital defects of the lymphatics in infancy. Pediatrics 19:21, 1957.

Perry, R. E., Hodgman, J., and Cass, A. B.: Pleural effusion in the neonatal period. J. Pediatr. 62:838, 1963.

Randolph, J. G., and Gross, R. E.: Congenital chylothorax. A.M.A. Arch. Surg. 74:405, 1957.

Sakula, J.: Chylothorax in the newborn. Arch. Dis. Child. 25:340, 1950.

Stewart, C. A., and Linner, H. P.: Chylothorax in the newborn infant. Am. J. Dis. Child. 31:654, 1926.

Stirlacci, J. R.: Spontaneous chylothorax in a newborn infant. J. Pediatr. 46:581, 1955.

Wessel, M. A.: Chylothorax in a two-week-old infant with spontaneous recovery. J. Pediatr. 25:201, 1944.

# PULMONARY HEMORRHAGE                    21

Among the many disorders afflicting the newborn in which pathogenesis is poorly understood, diagnosis difficult or impossible and therapy thoroughly unsatisfactory, pulmonary hemorrhage unquestionably deserves first rank.

**INCIDENCE.**   Landing discovered pulmonary hemorrhage, described as extravasated red blood cells in air spaces or septa, or both, in 68 per cent of lungs of 125 consecutive infants who died within the first week of life. Massive pulmonary hemorrhage was found in 17.8 per cent of autopsies (0.38 per cent of live births at The Johns Hopkins Hospital) by Esterly and Oppenheimer. In practice one sees only a few newborns who die with extensive pulmonary hemorrhage as the outstanding pathologic lesion. We encounter it perhaps three times a year.

**ETIOLOGY AND PATHOGENESIS.**   Pulmonary hemorrhage is more common in infants of low birth size than in those of average size, and is particularly common in infants of low birth weight for gestational age.

At times it is associated with evidence of bleeding elsewhere. In these cases it may be noted that puncture wounds made either for venipuncture or for subcutaneous or intramuscular injections continue to ooze for hours. No specific clotting defect is found in the blood of these infants, nor do they generally cease bleeding in response to transfusion of citrated or unmodified blood. Pulmonary hemorrhage may prove to be the cause of death in severe hemolytic anemia of the newborn or infants born of diabetic mothers. In none of these conditions do we understand the cause of bleeding into the lungs.

Rothman pointed out that pulmonary hemorrhage may follow labors during which uterine contractions are excessively vigorous. He believed that this may lead to increased blood volume in the fetus, producing capillary engorgement and rupture.

The finding of a low hematocrit on bloody fluid aspirated from the respiratory tract led Adamson et al. to suggest that the fluid was a filtrate from pulmonary capillaries, and indicative of their engorgement. Presumably asphyxia may lead to acute left ventricular failure in some infants.

Landing's elegant statistical analysis, referred to above, uncovers the fact that pulmonary hemorrhage is found more frequently in association with evidences of acute infection than with any other pulmonary lesion. It has long been contended that hemorrhage constitutes one of the early signs of pneumonia in the newborn. The literature contains many references to this so-called hemorrhagic pneumonia.

Aspiration of maternal blood can surely occur, as proved by the presence of maternal sickle cells in the alveoli but not in the vascular bed of an infant reported by Ceballos.

Evidence of increased intracranial pressure and anoxic brain injury was noted in association with pulmonary hemorrhage by McAdams.

We have encountered pulmonary hemorrhage, along with hemorrhage from other sites, in *E. coli* sepsis with extensive intravascular thrombosis, and once with intravascular thrombosis without any evidence of sepsis.

**DIAGNOSIS.** There is only one characteristic sign which distinguishes pulmonary hemorrhage from other disorders producing dyspnea in the newborn, and it is only present in half the proved cases. This is coughing up or regurgitating from the mouth or nose, or both, material containing blood. It may be brown and mixed with mucus or may resemble unmixed fresh blood. The infants usually have respiratory distress immediately after birth, but it may be delayed 3 days or more. They may or may not bleed excessively from venipuncture wounds. Physical examination reveals nothing diagnostic. Emphysema or atelectasis, or both, may be found, and medium to coarse rales are sometimes heard. Roentgenographic changes vary from massive consolidation to minimal streaking or patchy lesions.

**TREATMENT.** No therapeutic methods appear to be effective. We have utilized transfusions of citrated blood in several, direct transfusion in one, without altering the downhill course of the disorder. The prognosis is exceedingly grave.

## CASE HISTORIES

### CASE 21-1

A full-term white male infant, birth weight 6 pounds 2 ounces (2780 gm), was born with a loop of cord wrapped tightly about his neck. Cry was spontaneous, but dyspnea and cyanosis were noted after respirations had become established. Examination revealed multiple petechiae of the face, and tachypnea with retractions, but nothing else. Rapid irregular respirations continued, color remained dusky, and he frequently coughed up brownish mucoid material. Blood studies were not revealing. An electrocardiogram showed "T wave changes suggestive of myocardial ischemia," but was otherwise normal. X-ray film of the chest showed infiltration of both upper lobes and hyperaeration of both lower lobes (Fig. 21–1). At 46 hours of age apnea, cyanosis and flaccidity developed. The trachea was suctioned, some

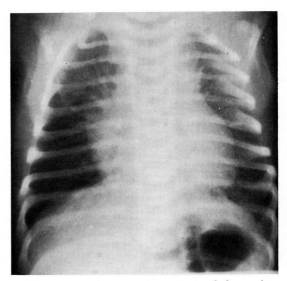

*Figure 21–1.* Anteroposterior view of chest taken on the second day of life. There is infiltration of both upper lung fields and hyperaeration of both lower fields. This combination of atelectasis and emphysema strongly suggests massive aspiration. In this infant autopsy revealed massive pulmonary hemorrhage.

reddish brown material was aspirated, oxygen under positive pressure was given, but he died 1 hour later.

Autopsy showed little more than massive hemorrhage throughout the lungs, into air spaces and septa.

**COMMENT.** This example was impossible to distinguish from a run-of-the-mill massive aspiration syndrome, with patchy atelectasis and emphysema as sequelae. The one suggestive difference was that brownish material was brought up from the lungs. Is it possible that the tightly wrapped cord about the neck induced increased blood flow through the pulmonary arteries and led to overfilling and rupture of capillaries?

CASE 21–2

A white male infant was born at the Women's Hospital of Maryland after a spontaneous delivery at the thirtieth week of gestation. Pregnancy and labor had been apparently normal in all respects. Amniotic fluid was clear, birth weight was 3 pounds 14 ounces (1760 gm), crying time less than 5 minutes. For a short time there was cyanosis of the face and head; respirations were 40 to 50 per minute. In the Isolette, with routine care for premature infants, all went well until the evening of the fourth day. At this time long periods of apnea began, during which the color became livid, then ashen. Examination showed nothing except a tendency to hold the head sharply retracted. Between spells color was fair while he was in oxygen, very dusky when taken out. Jaundice had been noted on the fourth day, became intense by the seventh day. On this day he suddenly vomited large amounts of bright red blood mixed with formula and after this became apneic, ashen and limp. After resuscitation, respirations recommenced, but were irregular and gasping, while the heart rate was slow. Endotracheal suction produced blood-stained material. Substernal retractions were noted after this procedure. A transfusion of 15 ml of type O Rh-negative blood was given, with brief improvement. Apneic spells recurred,

regurgitation of fresh blood continued, color deteriorated, and he died.

Autopsy showed massive pulmonary hemorrhage and moderate-sized subarachnoid hemorrhage.

**COMMENT.** This example seems to fall into an entirely different category from the first one cited. In that one the cord wrapped tightly around the neck; in this one prematurity and deep physiologic icterus were the possibly pathogenic abnormalities. In the first respiratory difficulty was apparent shortly after birth; in this it made its appearance on the fourth day. In the former the difficulty consisted of dyspnea with retraction, in the latter of apneic spells. Evidences of massive aspiration were clearcut in the first case, absent in the second. The only facts of which we can be certain are that the lung may be the site of massive bleeding in the neonatal period for a variety of reasons and that the disorder may manifest itself in a variety of ways.

## REFERENCES

Adamson, T. M., Boyd, R. D. H., Normand, I. C. S., et al.: Hemorrhagic pulmonary oedema in the newborn. Lancet *1*:494, 1969.

Ceballos, R.: Aspiration of maternal blood in the etiology of massive pulmonary hemorrhage in the newborn infant. J. Pediatrics 72:390, 1968.

Cole, V. A., et al.: Pathogenesis of hemorrhagic pulmonary edema and massive pulmonary hemorrhage in the newborn. Pediatrics *51*:175, 1973.

Esterly, J. R., and Oppenheimer, E. H.: Massive pulmonary hemorrhage in the newborn. I. Pathologic considerations. J. Pediatr. 69:3, 1966.

Landing, B. H.: Pulmonary lesions of newborn infants: A statistical study. Pediatrics 19:217, 1957.

McAdams, A. J.: Pulmonary hemorrhage in the newborn. Am. J. Dis. Child. *113*:255, 1967.

Rothman, P. E.: Intense uterine contractions, with special reference to massive pulmonary hemorrhage of the newborn. West. J. Surg. 65:308, 1957.

Rowe, S., and Avery, M. E.: Massive pulmonary hemorrhage in the newborn. II. Clinical considerations. J. Pediatr. 69:12, 1966.

# III

# Disorders of the Cardiovascular System

# GENERAL CONSIDERATIONS

*By Milton Markowitz*

In the 15 years since the first edition of this section was written, progressively more attention has been focused on the neonate with heart disease. It was apparent even then that pediatric cardiology and cardiovascular surgery would have to shift into the nursery eventually, because about one third of all infants born with heart defects died before one week of age. During the intervening years there has been a considerable educational effort directed at the early identification of infants with congenital heart disease. The development throughout the country of neonatal intensive care units and the means for speedy transportation to these units has fostered earlier diagnosis of cardiac, as well as other, problems of the newborn infant. No longer is any infant considered too ill for diagnostic study, especially with the development of newer noninvasive procedures. Improved methods for monitoring and correcting body temperature, hypoxia and acidosis have made diagnostic and surgical procedures much safer than in the past. Palliative, life-saving procedures are now available for a number of cardiac abnormalities. Moreover, by the use of hypothermia surgeons are now able to correct many malformations, even in the youngest age group. Clearly the time is rapidly approaching when the most complex defects will be amenable to total correction.

Although neonatal cardiology is dominated by congenital malformations, other cardiac conditions may affect the neonate. Primary myocarditis is no longer a postmortem oddity. The clinical features are recognizable, and preventive and therapeutic measures assume considerable importance. Disorders of cardiac rhythm are more common in older persons, but they present special problems in management when they occur in the newborn. This is particularly true of the paroxysmal arrhythmias. Early diagnosis and immediate treatment may make the difference between life and death.

In addition to a number of primary heart diseases, the cardiovascular system of the neonate is susceptible to disturbances peculiar to that period of life. Following birth there is a period of transitional circulation when the fetal pathways are still anatomically open and pathology elsewhere, especially in the lungs, can influence the hemodynamics of the circulatory system. Furthermore, the newborn myocardium may be unusually vulnerable to the effects of hypoxia, acidosis and other biochemical changes. These changes have been shown to depress myocardial function in newborn animals (Downing et al.) and may be the cause of heart failure secondary to neonatal asphyxia (Burnard and James).

## FETAL CIRCULATION

Knowledge of the fetal circulation has been derived mainly from cineangiographic studies in the human fetus by Lind and Wegelius. In recent years, Rudolph and co-workers have made many additional contributions. The general course of fetal blood through the heart and major blood vessels is depicted in Figure 22–1. Oxygenated blood from the placenta is carried by the umbilical veins to the inferior vena cava after passing through the ductus venosus or through the hepatic circulation. As the inferior vena caval blood enters the right atrium, the stream splits on the free margin (crista dividens) of the interatrial septum. The major portion of the stream passes through the foramen ovale directly into the left atrium where it mixes with a small amount of pulmonary venous blood before entering the left ventricle. From there, it is distributed to the myocardium, upper body and head. A smaller portion of the inferior vena caval blood enters the right atrium where it mixes with superior vena caval blood before going into the right ventricle. From there, because of the high pulmonary resistance, the blood largely

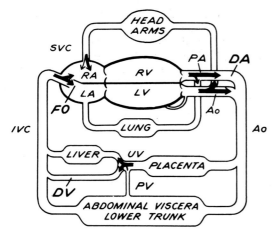

*Figure 22–1.* Diagrammatic representation of the fetal circulation. UV, umbilical vein; PV, portal vein; DV, ductus venosus; IVC, inferior vena cava; SVC, superior vena cava; FO, foramen ovale; RA, right atrium; LA, left atrium; RV, right ventricle; LV, left ventricle; PA, pulmonary artery; DA, ductus arteriosus; and Ao, aorta.

(Heymann, M. A., and Rudolph, A. M.: Effects of congenital heart disease on fetal and neonatal circulations. *In* Friedman, W. F., Lesch, M., and Sonnenblick, E. H. (Eds.): Neonatal Heart Disease. New York, Grune & Stratton, 1973.)

bypasses the lungs and goes into the descending aorta via the ductus arteriosus. Blood from the descending aorta supplies the abdominal fetal organs and lower half of the body.

The arrangement of the fetal circulation provides for differences in the oxygen concentration of the blood supplied to various fetal organs. Umbilical venous blood has an oxygen saturation of 80 per cent, which when mixed with the unsaturated blood from the lower half of the body yields a saturation of about 70 per cent in the inferior vena cava. As noted earlier, this well-saturated blood is diverted across the foramen ovale into the left side of the heart and out the ascending aorta. Thus, the coronary and cerebral circulations are provided with blood of the highest possible oxygen concentration. Right ventricular blood is a mixture of a small portion of the inferior vena caval stream and the unsaturated blood from the superior vena cava, resulting in an oxygen saturation of about 55 per cent. This less-well-oxygenated blood coming from the right ventricle supplies the lower half of the fetal body.

## NEONATAL CIRCULATION

Following occlusion of the umbilical vessels and removal of the low resistance placental vascular bed, there is a marked increase in systemic vascular resistance. At the same time, as the infant begins to breathe, there is pulmonary vasodilatation and a fall in pulmonary vascular resistance. Both of these events produce profound changes in the circulatory system. Right atrial pressure falls following elimination of the placental circulation, and left atrial pressure rises as pulmonary vascular return increases. As a result of the change in atrial pressures, there is functional closure of the foramen ovale. Anatomic closure may take several weeks (Christie). If within that time there is an increase in right atrial pressure, a right-to-left shunt may be re-established. At times vigorous crying or straining during the first few days of life may cause momentary right-to-left shunting through the foramen ovale.

With the fall in pulmonary vascular resistance and establishment of the pulmonary circulation, in full-term infants blood stops flowing through the ductus arteriosus 10 to 15 hours after birth (Rudolph and coworkers). Thereafter it remains anatomically open, and there may be ductal blood flow in either direction for several days under appropriate conditions (Adams and Lind; Rowe and James). The ductal shunt is one of the causes of heart murmurs recorded frequently during the first 12 hours of life (Braudo and Rowe). Complete obliteration of the ductus arteriosus may take several months. In one study the ductus was anatomically patent in 65 per cent at 2 weeks, in 44 per cent at 4 weeks, in 12 per cent at 8 weeks, in 3 per cent at 20 weeks, in 2 per cent at 32 weeks and in about 1 per cent at the age of 1 year (Christie). In a large group of infants, Mitchell showed that the ductus is rarely more than 2 mm in diameter after the first week of life. In patients with congenital heart disease the flow of blood through the ductus may be essential for life in certain types of cardiac anomalies. Nevertheless, Mitchell could not find evidence of a delay in the normal closure time of the ductus in infants with cardiac abnormalities dying within the first month of life.

In contrast to full-term infants, functional closure of the ductus is often delayed in premature infants (Danilowicz et al.). A recent survey showed an incidence of 15 per cent in infants under 1750 gm (Heymann and Rudolph). The ductus closes spontaneously in the majority of these infants. However, when the premature infant also has the respiratory distress syndrome, the patent ductus may cause congestive heart failure (see page 252).

In addition to changes in the patterns of blood flow from fetal to neonatal life, there are also changes in the pulmonary circulation. It was once thought that the high pulmonary vascular resistance during fetal life was due entirely to the tortuosity and muscle thickness of the small pulmonary vessels. Recent studies, however, suggest that the resistance in the small pulmonary arterioles is regulated chiefly by the $Po_2$. The pH and vasoactive substances such as catecholamines and bradykinin may also play a role. After birth, the increase in $Po_2$ to which the pulmonary vessels are exposed is the major cause for the dramatic reduction in pulmonary vascular resistance. Following the initial fall, there is a gradual decrease in resistance associated with the regression of the thickness of the medial smooth muscle in the pulmonary arterioles. In normal infants, the appearance of the vessels is similar to that in the adult within 3 to 5 weeks after birth (Heymann and Rudolph). Any disease state which causes a decrease in $Po_2$ may interfere with the pulmonary vascular maturation (Naeye and Letts).

The relation between the weight of the right and left ventricles during fetal and neonatal life has been studied by Emery and MacDonald. They demonstrated that left ventricular preponderance is present up to 30 weeks of fetal life. Thereafter the right ventricle is heavier than the left until 4 weeks after birth (Emery and Mithal). This may explain the normal right ventricular pattern seen in the electrocardiogram of the newborn infant. After the fourth week the left ventricle overtakes the right in weight and remains the heavier of the two chambers under normal conditions.

Recent hemodynamic studies have furnished important physiologic data in normal full-term infants. In a study by Moss et al. the pulmonary arterial pressures ranged from 32/10 to 68/38 mm of mercury and was equal or close to the systemic pressure up to 15 hours of age. Rudolph and his associates found a similar range of pulmonary pressures. The latter investigators recorded right atrial pressures from −3.0 to +4.5 mm of mercury, left atrial pressures from −2.0 to +7.0 mm and right ventricular pressures which varied from 33 to 80 mm. The systemic arterial pressures were 48 to 75 systolic and 28 to 40 diastolic.

## THE MANIFESTATIONS OF HEART DISEASE

A cardiac disorder is suspected when (1) a heart murmur is discovered, (2) cyanosis is present, (3) there are signs of heart failure or (4) there is an abnormal rate or rhythm. These are the cardinal signs of heart disease in the neonate. Much less commonly the initial suspicion is based on abnormalities in the peripheral pulses, cardiomegaly, or electrocardiographic changes. When several of these findings are present together, the diagnosis of a cardiac lesion is self-evident. Not uncommonly these manifestations appear as isolated signs, and it is necessary to distinguish them from physiologic variations and from certain noncardiac conditions. Each of these signs and some of their diagnostic implications are described below.

### HEART MURMURS

Murmurs are heard frequently during the neonatal period, particularly during the first day or two of life. Hallidie-Smith reported a frequency of 33 per cent on the first day and 70 per cent after 1 week. Braudo and Rowe heard murmurs in 60 per cent of babies examined an average of nine times during the first 48 hours of life.

Careful observations by Braudo and Rowe have shown that several types of murmurs can be distinguished. The most common is an ejection systolic murmur heard best over the pulmonary area and along the left sternal border. Less frequently there is a continuous murmur localized to the pulmonic region. The ejection systolic murmur is probably the result of flow across the pulmonic valve at a time when pulmonary blood flow is increasing markedly as the pulmonary vascular resistance is lowered. The continuous murmur may be due to flow through the ductus arteriosus, which may remain open for several days. Burnard heard murmurs more frequently in infants who suffered from birth asphyxia and attributed these murmurs to a larger ductal flow. Any disease state which decreases $PO_2$ or lowers blood pH increases pulmonary vascular resistance and increases the likelihood of a right-to-left shunt across the ductus arteriosus.

Heart murmurs which persist beyond the first day or two of life occur less frequently and should always direct attention to the possibility of a cardiac abnormality. In fact its detection may be the first confirmatory sign of heart disease in an infant with previously unexplained cyanosis or tachypnea. A heart murmur in the presence of these findings or associated with an inordinate tachycardia, cardiac enlargement or heart failure makes the diagnosis of congenital heart disease much more likely.

The intensity and location of the murmur will rarely suggest the precise nature of the anatomic defect. Wide diffusion over the precordium is not uncommon. The murmur associated with a stenotic lesion is more likely to be well localized. In defects with a left-to-right shunt the murmur may be variable and difficult to localize. With large shunts and increased pulmonary blood flow, pulmonary vascular resistance may remain high and the murmur may be soft and less characteristic (Rowe).

*Absence of a murmur does not exclude the diagnosis of heart disease.* Studies have shown that as many as 20 per cent of infants in whom death during the first month of life was due to proved abnormalities of the heart did not have heart murmurs (Ober and Moore).

The question of the prognostic significance of a heart murmur when it is an isolated finding is of considerable importance. Careful follow-up studies have shown that between 80 and 90 per cent of infants in whom a murmur had been discovered during the first week of life were entirely normal by the end of the first year (Richards and co-workers). In fact, in most infants the murmur had disappeared by the end of the first 3 months. As a general rule, the louder the murmur, the more likely its significance. Yet even a grade III to IV systolic murmur may disappear within the first few weeks or months of life. It is likely that these murmurs are due to a small ventricular septal defect which closed (Evans et al.; Li et al.).

The knowledge that heart murmurs in the absence of other cardiovascular findings may not denote heart disease should serve as a guide for the physician in his discussion with parents. The decision as to how fully one must discuss this finding will depend on the circumstances involved in each case. In some situations, particularly when adequate and close follow-up seems certain, it would appear wise to withhold the information entirely during this highly emotional period in the lives of parents. In the event that a frank discussion appears necessary, the parents can be assured of the high probability of a good outcome. Careful follow-up examinations are mandatory, however, since persistence of a loud murmur beyond the first 3 or 4 months of life almost always signifies the presence of some organic defect.

## CYANOSIS

Cyanosis of the newborn is an important clinical finding and its etiology should be sought after without delay. It may be due to pulmonary disease or airway obstruction, a congenital heart defect, central nervous disease, shock due to sepsis and a variety of less common conditions. Lees has written an excellent review of this subject.

Significant cyanosis must be distinguished from variations in skin color frequently seen in the newborn. Mottling of the skin due to vasomotor instability may come and go for weeks. Infants delivered with a cord around the neck or in a face presentation may have localized areas of bluish discoloration. Palms and soles may be blue from cold, but quickly pink up when warmed. During the first few days of life, infants may become dusky with vigorous and prolonged crying, possibly owing to momentary right-to-left shunting via the foramen ovale. Plethora associated with polycythemic states may be mistaken for cyanosis.

True cyanosis is usually central in origin; that is, arterial oxygen saturation is significantly reduced. Any one of five physiologic mechanisms may cause arterial unsaturation: right-to-left shunting, alveolar hypoventilation, diffusion impairment, ventilation-perfusion inequality and inadequate transport of oxygen by hemoglobin (Lees).

The common causes of arterial unsaturation from congenital heart disease are right-to-left shunting, obstruction to pulmonary blood flow and transposed vessels. When heart failure is also present, alveolar hypoventilation adds to the cyanosis. In infants with myocardial dysfunction without structural defects, cardiac failure may be the sole cause of cyanosis. Thus, there are many cardiac abnormalities which can cause cyanosis in the newborn and these will be discussed individually elsewhere in this section. Some general comments are included here on how to distinguish cardiac defects from the many other diseases associated with cyanosis.

Primary lung disease and airway obstruction are common causes of neonatal cyanosis. Tachypnea and intercostal retractions are more marked in such infants than in patients with cyanotic congenital heart disease. Infants with cyanosis due to pulmonary disease improve with oxygen, whereas those with cardiac venous-arterial shunts do not. However, this is not a point of distinction in patients with severe hyaline membrane disease who have very large ventilation-perfusion inequalities. A chest x-ray can help to exclude parenchymal disease and conditions causing mechanical interference; x-ray can also delineate cardiac size and depict the status of the pulmonary vascular bed. Blood gas and pH determinations may help distinguish varying hemodynamic states. For example, a carbon dioxide tension over 60 mm Hg should suggest a primary lung problem (Talner).

Newborns with central nervous system disease may be cyanotic from alveolar hypoventilation associated with intermittent periods of apnea. Additional signs of disturbed brain function are often present in the form of rigidity or flaccidity, and twitchings or frank seizures.

Cyanosis may accompany shock due to infections, adrenal hemorrhage or severe acidemia. Such infants are apathetic and hypotonic, and have very poor peripheral pulses. Severe hypoglycemic and hypocalcemic states may cause cyanosis, probably as a result of myocardial dysfunction. Anemia from hemolytic disease or hemorrhage can interfere with oxygen transport and thereby cause cyanosis. Congenital methemoglobinemia, a rare cause of cyanosis, is discussed on page 625.

## HEART FAILURE

Cardiac failure is a common manifestation of heart disease in infants less than 1 month of age. Since there is already a sudden and considerable increase in cardiac output at the time of birth, any significant increase in demand, such as can be created by a cardiac lesion, may result in heart failure soon after birth. The incidence and causes of heart failure among 1580 cases of congenital heart disease have been analyzed by Keith in an excellent review of this subject. Twenty per cent of the group who manifested failure did so during the first week of life. *Aortic atresia* was the leading cause, *transposition of the great vessels, coarctation of the aorta* and *patent ductus arteriosus* following in that order. Another 18 per cent failed between 1 week and 1 month of life. During this period *coarctation of the aorta* was the most common lesion, with *transposition of the great vessels* next in order.

Heart failure may result from postnatally acquired conditions. *Idiopathic paroxysmal tachycardia* is almost invariably associated with congestive failure when it occurs in the neonatal period. Indeed, more often than not the signs of failure call attention to the sick infant before the tachycardia is recognized. *Primary myocarditis* is still another cause. It occurs in its most malignant form in the newborn infant. Congestive failure may come on with great rapidity and result in sudden death before the condition is recognized. Extracardiac disease may also cause cardiac failure.

*Hypoglycemia* and *hypocalcemia* have been shown to produce congestive heart failure in the newborn. Infants severely *anemic* for any reason suffer from heart failure. An *arteriovenous fistula* is a rare cause. A case report of an infant with a cerebral arteriovenous aneurysm is cited elsewhere (p. 303).

Dyspnea is usually the first sign of failure. All too often it goes unrecognized at the outset. It may be the only manifestation of heart disease for some time before other signs become apparent. Initially there is an increase in respiratory rate. This ranges between 50 and 100 per minute, but extraordinarily rapid rates up to 150 may occur. As the failure progresses the tachypnea is associated with intercostal retraction. This is rarely as great as that seen with pulmonary disease. The paroxysmal form of dyspnea seen in cyanotic infants who are not in heart failure, but who suffer from anoxic spells, is uncommon in the first week, but may occur before the end of the first month.

Cyanosis often accompanies heart failure. Cyanosis from this cause is usually much less intense than the cyanosis due to *venous-arterial shunts.* Not infrequently, if a congenital defect with a left-to-right shunt is present, reversal of this shunt may occur with failure and thereby increase the cyanosis.

Persistent tachycardia in the range of 180 to 200 beats per minute is common. Gallop rhythm may be noted. The heart sounds may be poor, but this finding is often obscured in the restless tachypneic infant. Although some degree of cardiomegaly always accompanies failure, it is difficult to recognize the milder degrees of enlargement clinically or even on x-ray film. This problem is discussed more completely in the section on cardiomegaly (p. 225).

Enlargement of the liver is a cardinal manifestation of heart failure. This organ is easily palpable in young infants, and a change in its size is a valuable objective measurement of the degree of failure. It is often felt 1 or 2 cm below the costal margin in the normal newborn. As a consequence of either right- or left-sided failure, the liver edge becomes less sharp and extends down 3 cm or more. There is usually no tenderness over this organ. At times hepatic pulsations can be felt. Venous engorgement is not easily detectable and hence is of little aid. Peripheral edema is uncommon and is a poor prognostic sign when it does occur. Puffiness of the eyelids may be noted on occasion.

Pulmonary signs are variable. Although congestion normally diminishes resonance to percussion, this finding is not conspicuous in the newborn until the advanced stages of failure. On auscultation the breath sounds are often harsh over the upper lung fields and suppressed at the bases. There may be coarse and fine rales or rhonchi and wheezes.

In the absence of other evidence of heart disease it may be difficult to distinguish the signs of failure from *pulmonary disease* early in the course of an infant's illness. Cyanosis and some increase in respiratory rate and effort are common in both conditions. If rales are present, it may not be certain whether these are due to congestion or intrinsic lung disease. Likewise a readily palpable liver may be due to failure or to descent of this organ from overexpanded lungs. The differential diagnosis may be complicated by the fact that pulmonary edema is frequently the seat of bronchopneumonia and secondary heart failure may result from diffuse pulmonary disease. Close clinical observation of the infant's course will be repaid by the appearance of other signs of either pulmonary or cardiac disease which will make clear the distinction between these conditions.

### CARDIAC SIZE AND CONTOUR

An accurate clinical assessment of heart size in the newborn infant is far more difficult than in an older child. Percussion of cardiac borders in such a small chest is a trying task which at times is made inaccurate by increased resonance or dullness of adjacent or overlying lung. Even dextrocardia may be missed completely on the initial examination. Careful attention to the location of the apical impulse or the presence of an unusually forceful beat may be more helpful than percussion in the recognition of cardiomegaly. Even so, it is often not possible to tell whether the heart is enlarged or has been shifted from its normal position by extracardiac conditions. This displacement can result from atelectasis, emphysema, pneumothorax or diaphragmatic hernia, inter alia. These latter conditions as well as dextrocardia can be excluded by chest x-ray.

The chest roentgenogram is of value for determining heart size and pulmonary vascularity. Interpretation is often made difficult because of technical problems of accurate centering and because the high position of the diaphragm may give the heart a more horizontal appearance. Therefore it is not surprising that the cardiothoracic ratio of the normal neonate on routine examination may vary widely. In one study of 1000 healthy newborns this ratio varied from 44 to 74 per cent (Carter et al.). It is highly unlikely that this degree of variation would occur if special pains were taken to obtain adequate roentgenograms during quiet respirations after the first 24 hours of life. Although even under optimum conditions it may not be possible to judge slight degrees of enlargement, the experienced observer is able to detect true cardiomegaly with fair accuracy if the film is taken properly (Kurlander et al.). A cardiothoracic ratio of 0.60 is an accepted figure for the upper limit of normal.

Enlargement of the heart before birth is uncommon. Malformations associated with the obstruction of flow to the lungs will cause no unusual strain on the heart, since the lungs are bypassed during fetal life. Likewise shunt anomalies do not usually place a burden on the circulation, since there is normally considerable mixing of blood between the right and left sides of the heart. In general, cardiac enlargement occurs only when there is obstruction to flow on the left side of the heart. Therefore it is seen mainly with the group of anomalies associated with one or another form of *aortic atresia* (hypoplastic left-heart syndrome). Although the heart is normal in size at birth with most congenital defects, it may enlarge rapidly within a few days. This is true particularly in *transposition of the great vessels* and may also occur with *pulmonary atresia* and *severe pulmonary stenosis*. Whatever the nature of the defect,

if heart failure supervenes, there is always some degree of cardiac enlargement. Perhaps the only exception is seen in infants with *anomalous pulmonary venous return* of the subdiaphragmatic type, in which the heart is characteristically small in the presence of overt signs of congestive failure.

A careful analysis of the cardiac contour may be of help in making a diagnosis, particularly in cyanotic infants. An egg-shaped heart with a narrow base is fairly typical of *transposition of the great vessels*. A sharp concave angulation in the region of the pulmonary artery should suggest *truncus arteriosus* or *severe tetralogy of Fallot* (pseudotruncus). Unfortunately the base of the heart may be obscured by a thymic shadow, but this appears to occur less frequently when cyanotic heart disease is present.

Accurate assessment of pulmonary vascularity during the first 24 hours is difficult and, if possible, should be deferred until after the first day of life. Atelectasis or hyperaeration from various causes is common during the first day or two of life and may confuse the picture. Elevated diaphragms often accentuate lung markings and give the erroneous impression of increased blood flow or venous congestion. In general it is difficult to distinguish between pulmonary edema and increased vascularity from the linear markings alone. An assessment of the cross-sectional size of the blood vessels will serve as a more accurate guide. If the vessels seen "on end" are large, then increased pulmonary blood flow is present. If they also have a fuzzy or patchy appearance, then pulmonary congestion may be present as well.

## PERIPHERAL PULSES AND BLOOD PRESSURE

The pulse rate of a 1-day-old infant varies between 70 and 180, with an average of 125. The rate rises during the first week to 140, with a range of 100 to 190. Occasionally the pulse rate will reach 200 with crying. A persistent rate of 200 is abnormal and is seen with infections and heart failure. Sinus tachycardia should not be confused with paroxysmal tachycardia. In the latter the rate is usually between 220 and 300 and is constant. This is in contrast to the variations in rate noted with sinus tachycardia. A persistent heart rate below 70 is significant and is almost always due to congenital heart block. The clinical features of paroxysmal tachycardia and heart block are discussed in the chapter on arrhythmias (p. 283).

Careful palpation of the peripheral pulses should always be carried out. The radial and femoral pulses can be palpated in the normal newborn if sufficient time is taken for this examination. The femoral pulse is felt best about one fingerbreadth medial to the anterior superior spine of the pelvis. Weak or absent femoral pulses are diagnostic for coarctation of the aorta unless all the pulses are weak because of shock or severe heart failure. The radial pulses are often fainter than the femoral pulses when aortic atresia is present. They are particularly full with a large patent ductus arteriosus and truncus arteriosus.

Neonatal blood pressure can be measured best by the flush method of Goldring and Wohltmann. This technique consists in applying a 3 cm cuff around the forearm or calf, elevating the extremity, and blanching it with hand pressure or by a rubber bandage. Blanching is maintained while the cuff pressure is raised to 130 mm of mercury. The cuff is then deflated slowly and the extremity observed for flushing. The appearance of the first flush is recorded as the blood pressure. In a large study of normal newborns Forfar and Kibel found a mean arm pressure of 59.5 during the first 24 hours (S.D. [standard deviation] 12). The average leg pressure was 68 (S.D. 12). By 11 days of age the arm pressure rose to a mean of 88 (S.D. 13) and the leg pressure to 99 (S.D. 12). In this study there was considerable variation in the arm-leg pressure differential. The leg pressure was not infrequently equal to the arm pressure. In 10 per cent of the infants the leg pressure was actually lower, but this figure was rarely less than 75 per cent of the arm pressure. Since the results obtained using the flush technique can vary, some cardiologists prefer using a simple oscillometer (Rowe and Mehrizi).

The chief value of blood pressure determinations is in suspected coarctation of the aorta. In this condition the arm pressure may reach hypertensive levels even in the first week of life, but this is not an invariable finding. The majority of infants with this malformation have an arm-leg pressure differential of 20 mm of mercury or more, but at times there is no gradient between the pressures in the upper and lower extremities. Care must be taken in the interpretation of blood pressures recorded by the flush method. Variations occur with crying, when the cuff is deflated too rapidly, or when cyanosis is present. It is often necessary to do repeated determinations to avoid inaccuracies.

## ELECTROCARDIOGRAPHY

The electrocardiogram is a technically simple procedure in even the youngest infant. Bipolar and unipolar limb leads and precordial leads should always be recorded in every patient suspected of having heart disease. Care must be taken to use small electrodes for the extremities (3.5 by 2.0 cm) and for the chest (1.5 cm) and to select the proper electrode positions. The electrode paste must be removed between chest positions to avoid artefacts (Ziegler, 1948).

The electrocardiographic pattern of the normal neonate is fairly distinctive (Fig. 22–2). There is always a sinus tachycardia. The ventricular rate varies between 100 and 180, with an average of 130 per minute. The QRS axis in the frontal plane is toward the right, varying between 60 and 200 degrees. Right axis deviation may be absent during the first 48 hours in an occasional infant, and Walsh (1963A) has observed temporary left axis deviation in a small percentage of premature babies. The height of the P wave rarely exceeds 2.5 mv, and the P-R interval varies between 0.07 and 0.14 second, with an average of 0.11 second (Rothfield and co-workers).

The precordial leads show a normal right ventricular preponderance with R greater than S in $V_1$ and S greater than R in $V_5$. The range in amplitude for the R and S waves in the precordial leads is shown in Table 22–1. Although a Q wave may be seen as a normal variant if additional right precordial leads are taken ($V_4R$), it is rarely present in $V_1$ (Walsh, 1963B). The T waves

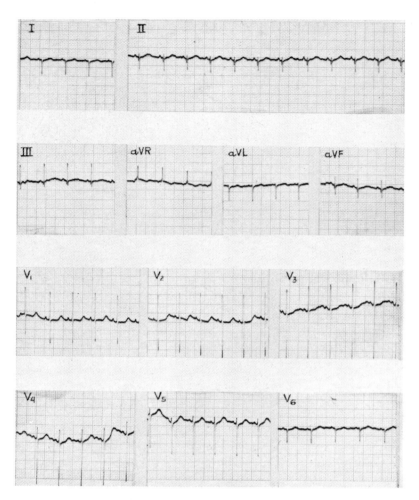

*Figure 22–2.* Electrocardiogram of a normal 2-day-old infant. The heart rate is 130. There is right axis deviation. The R wave in $aV_R$ is prominent. The electrical position is vertical. The T wave in lead $V_1$ is upright. There is a normal right ventricular pattern with R greater than S in $V_1$ and S greater than R in $V_5$.

are variable during the first 24 hours of life. They may be upright, diphasic or inverted in $V_1$. After 72 hours of age they are almost always inverted in $V_1$ and upright in $V_6$. On rare occasions the T wave may be upright in $V_1$ for the first week of life.

The electrocardiogram is indispensable for the diagnosis of arrhythmias. Atrial, nodal and ventricular premature beats and a wandering pacemaker are not uncommon and need cause no concern. Continuous electrocardiographic recordings have shown that virtually all newborn infants have mild sinus arrhythmia. The more serious disturbances, *heart block* and *paroxysmal tachycardia*, are discussed elsewhere (p. 283).

The absence of right axis deviation in the newborn is noteworthy, but is not necessarily diagnostic of heart disease. As has been noted already, a normal axis or even a mild left axis deviation may be seen during the first 3 days of life, especially in prematures. Persistence of a left axis deviation almost always signifies a cardiac abnormality. It occurs most commonly in *endocardial cushion defects* (ostium primum and atrioventricularis communis) and *tricuspid atresia*, but it may also occur in *pulmonary valve atresia* with an underdeveloped right ventricle.

Left ventricular preponderance should be suspected if there is (1) an absence of right axis deviation, (2) a horizontal electrical position of the heart, (3) deep S waves in $V_1$, (4) taller than normal R waves

**TABLE 22–1.** *Amplitude of R and S Waves in Precordial Leads from Right (V₁ and V₂) and Left (V₅ and V₆) Sides of Precordium, from Birth to 30 Days (Measurements in Millimeters)* *

| | Wave | V₁ | | | V₂ | | | V₅ | | | V₆ | | |
|---|---|---|---|---|---|---|---|---|---|---|---|---|---|
| | | Av. | Min. | Max. | Av. | Min. | Max. | Av. | Min. | Max. | Av. | Min. | Max. |
| 0–24 hours | R | 16.7 | 3.0 | 23 | 21 | 3.0 | 41 | 12 | 4.5 | 21 | 4.5 | 0 | 11 |
| | S | 10 | 0 | 28 | 22 | 1.0 | 42 | 12 | 1.5 | 30 | 4.5 | 0 | 3 |
| 1–7 days | R | 17 | 4 | 29 | 5 | 21 | 43 | 12 | 3.0 | 28 | 6.4 | 1.0 | 16 |
| | S | 11 | 0 | 25 | 21 | 1.0 | 36 | 7.6 | 1.5 | 16 | 3.2 | 0 | 13 |
| 8–30 days | R | 13.8 | 5 | 25 | 20 | 8 | 33 | 13.5 | 4.0 | 34 | 8.3 | 1.0 | 24 |
| | S | 7 | 0 | 17.5 | 17 | 3 | 28 | 5.9 | 2.0 | 14 | 2.6 | 0 | 10 |

*Adapted from Ziegler, R. F.: *Electrocardiographic Studies in Normal Infants and Children.* Springfield, Ill., Charles C Thomas, 1951.

in V₅ or V₆, (5) inverted T waves in V₅ or V₆ beyond the first 3 days, and (6) a delay in the intrinsicoid deflections over the left side of the chest of more than 0.04 second. It is unwise to make a diagnosis of left ventricular hypertrophy based primarily on the R/S ratio in V₁. Although this ratio is normally greater than 1, Keith et al. found a ratio of less than 1 in 18 per cent of normal newborns. Studies by this same group suggest that a deep S wave in V₁ signifies a left ventricular overload pattern and may occur in infants with the respiratory distress syndrome and low pulmonary vascular resistance.

A left ventricular pattern may be seen early in life in *tricuspid atresia, endocardial fibroelastosis* and *severe aortic stenosis.* It is occasionally seen in *truncus arteriosus, single ventricle, transposition of the great vessels* and *Ebstein's anomaly.*

It is often difficult to distinguish true right ventricular hypertrophy from the right ventricular preponderance normally present in the precordial electrocardiogram of the newborn. It should be suspected if there is (1) a qR pattern in V₁, (2) upright T waves in V₁ beyond the first week of life, (3) R waves in V₁ of a greater than average amplitude, (4) unusually deep S waves in V₅ and V₆, and (5) an intrinsicoid deflection of more than 0.03 second in V₁. Tall R waves in V₁ in association with upright T waves in the same lead have been described by Keith et al. in infants with the respiratory distress syndrome in

whom there is a high pulmonary vascular resistance.

The degree of right ventricular hypertrophy in the neonate will vary considerably with the kind and severity of the defect. It is marked in *aortic atresia* and *severe pulmonary stenosis* with a normal aortic root. A moderate degree of right hypertrophy is seen in the severe form of *tetralogy of Fallot* and total *anomalous pulmonary venous return* of the infradiaphragmatic type. It is less marked in *transposition of the great vessels.* It may be noted with a *single ventricle* or *truncus arteriosus.* Infants with a large *left-to-right shunt* with symptoms in the neonatal period often show right ventricular or combined ventricular hypertrophy. This is also true of infants with the *preductal type of coarctation of the aorta.*

## VECTORCARDIOGRAPHY

The QRS vector of the normal newborn is anterior, inferior and usually rightward. The direction of the inscription is clockwise in all three planes. The mean QRS forces are in keeping with the normal dominance of the right ventricle at this age. By the fourth day of life, a portion of the loop may be leftward and by the fourth week the QRS loop is well oriented to the left with a tendency toward a counterclockwise inscription in the horizontal plane. A lag in the normal evaluation of the vectorcardiogram suggests a right ventricular overload, whereas an acceleration suggests a left ventricular overload (Rowe and Mehrizi). Thus, serial vectorcardiograms may be helpful in overcoming the masking effect of the normal right ventricular preponderance in the neonatal period.

## ECHOCARDIOGRAPHY

Until recently, the use of ultrasound in diagnostic cardiology was limited to acquired heart disease, mainly in adults. However, recent studies have shown that echocardiography is a safe and accurate method of diagnosis of congenital heart disease in the newborn period. This noninvasive procedure is particularly attractive because of the risk of cardiac catheterization and angiocardiography in this age group. It is possible with echocardiography to identify the ventricular cavities, the ventricular septum and the presence of A-V valves, as well as the relationship of the mitral and semilunar valves (Chesler et al.). The echocardiographic criteria for normal newborn infants have been described (Meyer and Kaplan; Hagen and Deeley).

Several investigators have shown that the hypoplastic left heart syndrome can be diagnosed from the echogram with virtually 100 per cent accuracy (Meyer and Kaplan; Godman et al.). Infants with total anomalous pulmonary venous drainage have characteristic echocardiograms, and tricuspid atresia can also be readily diagnosed by ultrasound (Meyer and Kaplan). Preliminary studies suggest that dextrotransposition of the great vessels can be recognized by the altered spatial relationship of the great vessels (Gramiak et al.). Echocardiographic features of endocardial cushion defects and truncus arteriosus have also been described (Williams and Rudd; Chung et al.). Although additional experience is needed, it appears that ultrasound holds great promise for evaluating sick newborns in whom it is desirable to avoid catheterization if at all possible. It should prove to be especially valuable to exclude cardiac disease in patients who have cyanosis from noncardiac causes, as, for example, from the respiratory distress syndrome.

## CATHETERIZATION AND ANGIOCARDIOGRAPHY

It is often difficult to make an accurate anatomic diagnosis in the neonate with suspected heart disease from the history, clinical findings, x-ray and electrocardiogram. In asymptomatic infants, additional studies can be postponed until some future date when they can be done as an elective procedure. The most frequent example is the neonate with a heart murmur and no other clinical abnormalities. In sick neonates with suspected heart disease, a decision must be made regarding the need for cardiac catheterization and angiocardiography. Since these procedures are not without risk (Braunwald and Swan; Tooley and Stanger), the decision should be based on well-defined indications.

In their monograph Cardiac Catheterization and Angiography in Severe Neonatal Heart Disease, Gypes and Vincent list the following groups of neonates as candidates for emergency catheterization: (1) Infants who are cyanotic from the first hours of life and in whom cyanosis persists beyond the first day unaccompanied by significant labored breathing (it is dangerous to observe such infants until they do become symptomatic because clinical deterioration can proceed thereafter with alarming rapidity); (2) infants less than one week of age with signs of congestive heart failure and in whom there is no obvious non-cardiac explanation for heart failure; and (3) infants with respiratory distress in whom it is not possible to distinguish between pulmonary and cardiac disease from clinical and radiologic findings. In this latter group, it may now be possible to avoid catheterization on the basis of the echocardiographic findings (Godman et al.).

It cannot be emphasized too strongly that cardiac catheterization studies should be performed only in selected centers by personnel experienced in dealing with neonatal cardiac problems and in the general management of sick newborns. As Gersony and Hayes point out, "It should not be undertaken simply as an occasional addition to a cardiac surgical program for older children and adults."

# REFERENCES

Adams, F. H., and Lind, J.: Physiologic studies on the cardiovascular status of newborn infants. Pediatrics *19:*431, 1957.

Braudo, M., and Rowe, R.: Auscultation of the heart—early neonatal period. Am. J. Dis. Child. *101:*575, 1961.

Braunwald, E., and Swan, H. J. C.: Cooperative study of cardiac catheterization. Circulation 37 (Suppl. 3): 3–59, 1968.

Burnard, E. D.: A murmur from the ductus arteriosus in the newborn baby. Br. Med. J. *1:*806, 1958.

Burnard, E. D., and James, C. S.: Failure of the heart after undue asphyxia at birth. Pediatrics 28:545, 1961.

Carter, J., Cooper, G., Dammann, F., and Mitchell, F.: Roentgen evidence of normal heart and congenital abnormality in early infancy. J.A.M.A. *166:*337, 1958.

Chesler, E., et al.: Echocardiography in the diagnosis of congenital heart disease. Pediat. Clin. N. Amer. *18:*1163, 1971.

Christie, A.: Normal closing time of the foramen ovale and the ductus arteriosus: An anatomic and statistical study. Am. J. Dis. Child. *40:*323, 1930.

Chung, K. J., et al.: Echocardiography in truncus arteriosus. Circulation 48:281, 1973.

Danilowicz, O., et al.: Delayed closure of the ductus arteriosus in premature infants. Pediatrics 37:74, 1966.

Downing, S. E., et al.: Influences of arterial oxygen tension and pH on cardiac function in the newborn lamb. Amer. J. Physiol. *211:*1203, 1966.

Emery, J. L., and MacDonald, M. S.: The weight of the ventricles in the later weeks of intra-uterine life. Br. Heart J. 22:563, 1960.

Emery, J. L., and Mithal, A.: Weights of cardiac ventricles at and after birth. Br. Heart J. 23:313, 1961.

Evans, J. R., Rowe, R. D., and Keith, J. D.: Spontaneous closure of ventricular septal defects. Circulation 6:1044, 1960.

Forfar, J. O., and Kibel, M. A.: Blood pressure in the newborn estimated by the flush method. Arch. Dis. Child. *31:*126, 1956.

Gersony, W. M., and Hayes, C. J.: Perioperative management of the infant with congenital heart disease. *In* Friedman, W. F., Lersch, M. and Sonnenblick, E. H. (Eds.): Neonatal Heart Disease. New York, Grune & Stratton, 1973.

Godman, M. J., Tham, P., et al.: Echocardiography in the evaluation of the cyanotic newborn infant. Br. Heart J. 36:154, 1974.

Goldring, D., and Wohltmann, H. J.: "Flush" method for blood pressure determinations in newborn infants. J. Pediatr. *40:*285, 1952.

Gramiak, R., et al.: Echocardiographic diagnosis of transposition of the great vessels. Radiology *106:*175, 1973.

Gypes, M. T., and Vincent, W. R.: Cardiac Catheterization and Angiocardiography in Severe Neonatal Heart Disease. Springfield, Charles C Thomas, 1974.

Hagan, A. D., and Deeley, W. J.: Echocardiographic criteria for normal newborn infants. Am. J. Cardiol. *31:*137, 1973.

Hallidie-Smith, K. A.: Some auscultatory and phonocardiographic findings observed in early infancy. Br. M. J. *1:*754, 1960.

Heymann, M. A., and Rudolph, A. M.: Effects of congenital heart disease on fetal and neonatal circulations. *In* Friedman, W. F., Lesch, M., and Sonnenblick, E. H. (Eds.): Neonatal Heart Disease. New York, Grune & Stratton, 1973.

James, L. S.: Changes in the heart and lungs at birth. J. Pediatr. *51:*95, 1957.

Keith J. D.: Congestive heart failure: Review article. Pediatrics *18:*491, 1956.

Keith, J. D., Rose, V., Braudo, M., and Rowe, R. D.: The electrocardiogram in the respiratory distress syndrome and related cardiovascular dynamics. J. Pediatr. 59:167, 1961.

Kurlander, G. J., Petry, E. L., and Girod, D. A.: Plain film diagnosis of congenital heart disease in the newborn period. Am. J. Roentgenol. *103:*66, 1968.

Lees, M. H.: Cyanosis of the newborn infant. Recognition and clinical evaluation. J. Pediatr. 77:484, 1970.

Li, M. D., et al.: Spontaneous closure of ventricular septal defect. Can Med. Assoc. J. *100:*737, 1969.

Lind, J., and Wegelius, C.: Human fetal circulation, changes in the cardiovascular system at birth and disturbances in the postnatal closure of the foramen ovale and ductus arteriosus. Cold Spring Harbor Symposia Quant. Biol. *19:*109, 1957.

Meyer, R. A., and Kaplan, S.: Echocardiography in diagnosis of hypoplasia of left or right ventricle in neonatal congenital heart disease. Circulation 46:55, 1972.

Meyer, R. A., and Kaplan, S.: Noninvasive techniques in pediatric cardiovascular disease. *In* Friedman, W. F., Lesch, M., and Sonnenblick, E. H. (Eds.): Neonatal Heart Disease. New York, Grune & Stratton, 1973.

Mitchell, S. C.: The ductus arteriosus in the neonatal period. J. Pediatr. *51:*12, 1957.

Moss, A. J., Emmanonilides, G., and Duffie, E. J.: Closure of the ductus in the newborn infant. Pediatrics 32:25, 1963.

Naeye, R. L., and Letts, R. L.: The effects of prolonged neonatal hypoxemia on the pulmonary vascular bed and heart. Pediatrics 30:902, 1962.

Ober, W. B., and Moore, T. E.: Congenital cardiac malformations in the neonatal period; an autopsy study. New Engl. J. Med. *253:*271, 1955.

Richards, M. R., Merritt, K. K., Samuels, M. H., and Langmann, A. G.: Frequency and significance of cardiac murmurs in the first year of life. Pediatrics 15:169, 1955.

Rothfeld, E. L., Wachtel, F. W., Karlen, W. S., and Bernstein, A.: The evolution of the vectorcardiogram and electrocardiogram of the normal infant. Am. J. Cardiol. 5:439, 1960.

Rowe, J.: *In* T. K. Oliver Jr. (Ed.): Adaptation of extrauterine life. Report of the thirty-first Ross Conference on Pediatric Research. Columbus, Ohio, Ross Laboratories, 1959, p. 33.

Rowe, R. D., and James, L. S.: The normal pulmonary arterial pressure during the first year of life. J. Pediatr. 51:1, 1957.

Rowe, R. D., and Mehrizi, A.: The Neonate with Congenital Heart Disease. Philadelphia, W. B. Saunders Co., 1968.

Rudolph, A.M.: The changes in circulation after birth. Circulation *41*:343, 1970.

Rudolph, A. M., et al.: Studies on the circulation in the neonatal period. Pediatrics *27*:551, 1961.

Rudolph, A. M., et al.: Studies on the circulation of the previable human fetus. Pediatr. Res. *5*:452, 1971.

Talner, N. S.: Congestive heart failure in the infant. A functional approach. Pediatr. Clin. N. Amer. *18*:1011, 1971.

Tooley, W. H., and Stanger, P.: The blue baby—circulation or ventilation or both? (Editorial) New Engl. J. Med. *287*:983, 1972.

Walsh, S. Z.: Evolution of the electrocardiogram of

healthy premature infants during the first year of life. Acta Paediatr. Scand. (Suppl.) 145, 1963A.

Walsh, S. Z.: The electrocardiogram during the first week of life. Br. Heart J. *25*:784, 1953B.

Williams, R. G., and Rudd, M.: Echocardiographic features of endocardial cushion defects. Circulation *49*:418, 1974.

Ziegler, R. F.: A note on the importance of proper technique in the recording of the precordial electrocardiogram. Am. Heart J. *35*:769, 1948.

Ziegler, R. F.: Electrocardiographic Studies in Normal Infants and Children. Springfield, Charles C Thomas, 1951.

# 23 CONGENITAL HEART DISEASE
## By Milton Markowitz

**INCIDENCE.** Cardiac malformations occur in about eight of every 1000 births. Prospective studies of 56,109 births followed for an average of 3 years found an incidence of 8.1 per 1000 total births and 7.7 per 1000 live births (Mitchell and co-workers). Similar frequencies have been reported from other parts of the world (Carlgren; Landtman). Richards and co-workers reported about the same incidence 20 years ago, reflecting the lack of significant progress in our ability to prevent most cases of congenital heart disease. As noted above, cardiac malformations are more common in stillbirths than in live births. They are also more frequent in premature infants (McDonald).

The frequencies of different malformations are shown in Table 23-1. Ventricular septal defects are the most common by far, followed by atrial septal defects and patent ductus arteriosus. Next come valvular stenosis (pulmonary and aortic) and coarctation, followed by tetralogy of Fallot and transposition of the great vessels.

The order of frequency of cardiac anomalies recognized during the first month of life differs from that shown in Table 23-1. For example, transposition of the great vessels ranks high and aortic atresia (hypoplastic left heart syndrome), while an uncom-

mon anomaly overall, is the most common cause of death from heart disease during the first week of life (Table 23-2). On the other hand, the ostium secundum form of atrial septal defect is rarely recognized during the first month of life. Therefore, the findings in Table 23-2 reflect more accurately the cardiac anomalies physicians are most likely to encounter during the neonatal period.

**ETIOLOGY.** The cause of cardiac anomalies is not known in most cases. The rubella virus and the drug thalidomide are recognized cardiac teratogens. There is also suggestive evidence that dextroamphetamine may play a role (Nora et al.). It is likely there are other drugs, viruses and as yet unidentified teratogens in the environment which may act at a critical period early in embryonic development.

There is some evidence that heredity may be important. For example, Nora and Meyer found that 34 per cent of 417 patients with cardiac anomalies had one or more relatives with congenital heart disease, while in a matched control group 9 per cent of families had a positive family history. Twin studies also suggest that heredity may play a role (Nora et al.).

There are also known genetic syndromes which often have cardiac defects along

TABLE 23–1.   *Percentage Incidence of Different Malformations**

| | Calgren (1969) | Hay (1966) | Rose et al. (1964) | Michaelsson (1964) | Mitchell et al. (1971) | Mean |
|---|---|---|---|---|---|---|
| Ventricular septal defect | 43 | 34 | 31 | 22.5 | 29 | 31.9 |
| Atrial septal defect | 7.5 | 11.7 | 11 | 9.5 | 11.5 | 10.2 |
| Persistent ductus arteriosus | 8.5 | 7.7 | 7 | 12.5 | 7.5 | 8.6 |
| Pulmonary stenosis | 5 | 8 | 11 | 6 | 9.5 | 7.9 |
| Aortic stenosis | 7 | 4.2 | 8.5 | 6 | 3.5 | 5.8 |
| Coarctation | 7 | 5.3 | 3.5 | 6 | 6.5 | 5.7 |
| Fallot's tetralogy | 5 | 5.9 | 8 | 5 | 3.5 | 5.5 |
| Transposition | 6.5 | 5.6 | 2.5 | 3.5 | 2.5 | 4.1 |

*Modified from Campbell, M.: Incidence of cardiac malformations at birth and later. Br. Heart J. 35:189, 1973.

with other abnormalities. Congenital heart disease occurs in many single mutant syndromes, of which Ullrich-Noonan and Holt-Oram are examples. Cardiac defects are also common in children with chromosomal abnormalities. Half the patients with trisomy 21 (Down's syndrome) have congenital heart disease. However, single mutant gene syndromes and chromosomal abnormalities account for less than 6 per cent of cases with congenital heart disease. Thus, in most patients, there is no simple genetic explanation, nor are there recognizable chromosomal aberrations (Emerit et al.).

Other maternal factors may be important. Infants of diabetic mothers have an unusually high incidence of congenital heart disease (Mitchell et al.; Rowland et al.). However, it is not at all clear why diabetes is teratogenic. In an effort to reconcile genetic and environmental factors, Nora has proposed a multifactorial hypothesis, by which he means that there is a hereditary predisposition determined by many genes, plus an environmental trigger which acts on the predisposed individual.

**PREVENTION.**  The ability to prevent congenital heart disease is limited. Vaccination against rubella is effective and its widespread use could prevent the increased incidence of congenital heart disease which follows rubella epidemics.

Once a child with congenital heart dis-

TABLE 23–2.   *Percentage Incidence of Anatomic Types of Congenital Cardiac Defects in the Neonatal Period**

| Type of Malformation | Infants Surviving 1 Month of Life | Autopsied under 1 Month of Age |
|---|---|---|
| Transposition of great vessels | 16 | 10 |
| Aortic atresia or stenosis | 0 | 23 |
| Coarctation of the aorta | 11 | 13 |
| Ventricular septal defect | 20 | 7 |
| Tetralogy of Fallot | 16 | 5 |
| Pulmonary atresia or stenosis | 13 | 8 |
| Atrioventricularis communis | 4 | 5 |
| Anomalous pulmonary venous drainage | 0 | 4 |
| Mitral atresia or stenosis | 2 | 4 |
| Single ventricle | 4 | 3 |
| Truncus arteriosus | 2 | 3 |
| Tricuspid atresia | 2 | 2 |
| Atrial septal defect | 0 | 2 |
| Patent ductus arteriosus | 2 | 2 |
| Endocardial fibroelastosis | 0 | 2 |

*From Rowe, R. D., and Cleary, T. E.: Congenital cardiac malformations in the newborn period. Can. Med. Assoc. J. 83:299, 1960.

ease is born into a family, the parents often want to know the risk of a similar condition in future pregnancies and whether anything can be done to prevent it. Intelligent counseling depends on having a very complete family and genetic history and the knowledge of factors involved in determining risks.

Nora and co-workers have shown that the risk of recurrence depends on how common the defect is in the general population as compared to the number of affected family members. For example, if the family has one first-degree relative (sibling or parent) with a ventricular septal defect, then the recurrence risk is 4.4 per cent compared with a risk of 1.1 per cent for a less common anomaly such as Ebstein's anomaly. If there are two affected first-degree relatives, the recurrence risk increases. However, in most cases the risk of a recurrence is generally not sufficiently great to warrant the avoidance of future pregnancies.

**EMBRYOLOGY.** Much of the development of the heart occurs between the second and eighth weeks of embryonic life by a complex series of changes described briefly as follows. A vertical cardiac tube lying ventral to the gut tract is formed between the second and third weeks. The heart begins to take shape from this tube by constrictions and dilatations to form (cephalad to caudad) the bulbus cordis, primitive ventricle, primitive atrium and sinus venosus. During the fourth week the cardiac tube, which is now made up of the four regions noted above, twists and bends in a way which carries the primitive ventricle downward and forward and the atrium upward and backward. By the fifth week the base of the bulbus merges with the primitive ventricle, while its cephalic end enlarges to form the aortic sac or truncus arteriosus. During this same period the sinus venosus develops two horns into which drains much of the embryonic venous blood. Between the sixth and eighth weeks the sinus venosus becomes absorbed into the region of the right atrium.

While these external changes in the shape of the heart take place, internal partitioning begins between the fourth and fifth weeks through the formation of four septa. One septum divides the common atrioven-

tricular canal by the fusion of outgrowing endocardial cushions. Somewhat later the lateral margins of these cushions thin out to form the tricuspid and mitral valves. The atrial canal is divided by the septum primum, which grows down from the roof of the canal. This septum contains two openings: the lower opening, the foramen primum, progressively diminishes and disappears; the upper opening (future foramen ovale) is partially covered by a second atrial septum which grows out from the posterior wall. The common ventricular canal is divided by a muscular outgrowth from the ventricular wall. The muscular portion is joined at its ventral margin by a membranous extension from the bulbus cordis to complete the interventricular septum. The septum of the bulbus cordis develops from endocardial ridges and grows out in a spiral fashion to divide the aortic sac (truncus arteriosus) into the aortic and pulmonary trunks. Between the sixth and eighth weeks the aortic and pulmonary valves develop from further ridges of tissue along the walls of the bulbus cordis.

The vessels which lead to and from the heart develop during the same period. By the third week six pairs of aortic arches begin to take shape. The third, fourth and sixth arches enter into the development of the permanent vessels, but the others disappear. The third arch forms the internal carotid artery. The left fourth arch becomes part of the aortic sac of the bulbus cordis and forms the ascending portion of the aorta. The right fourth arch forms the innominate artery and the first portion of the right subclavian. The pulmonary arteries are formed from the sixth pair of arches. The right side of the sixth arch (right pulmonary artery) becomes disconnected from the aorta, while the left arch continues to connect the left pulmonary artery and the aorta (ductus arteriosus). It has been noted previously that the sinus venosus develops two horns into which drains the venous system of the embryo. The left horn loses its extracardiac connections and becomes the coronary sinus, which drains the heart itself. The right horn enlarges and forms the terminal portions of the inferior and superior venae cavae.

By the eighth embryonic week, the external shape of the heart, the internal structure and the vascular system are complete. Deviations may occur at any step along the way between the second and eighth week and may result in any one or combination of the following developmental errors: (1) aplasia or agenesis (complete failure of development); (2) hypoplasia (incomplete or defective development); (3) dysplasia (intrinsic abnormal development); (4) malposition; (5) dysraphia (failure of fusion of adjoining parts); (6) abnormal fusion; (7) inadequate resorption; (8) excessive resorption; (9) abnormal persistence of patency of vessels; and (10) abnormal (early) obliteration of vessels. The reader is referred to an excellent review by Van Mierop and Gessner for a more complete discussion of this subject.

## CARDIOVASCULAR DEFECTS: GENERAL CONSIDERATIONS

Virtually all cardiac malformations may at times cause signs and symptoms in the neonatal period. There is no completely satisfactory clinical classification for use as a basis for their presentation. In a treatise on the newborn it would seem appropriate to present cardiac anomalies in the order with which they are likely to cause difficulty in the first few weeks of life. Transposition of the great vessels heads the list, followed by the atresias (aortic, tricuspid and pulmonary) and coarctation of the aorta. Yet emphasis must also be placed on other malformations which, although much less likely to cause symptoms early in life, are nevertheless of great importance because surgical treatment may be imperative when the severe form of the defect is present. Pure pulmonic stenosis is perhaps the best example. In addition, it has been necessary to include briefer descriptions of still other anomalies which regularly enter in the differential diagnosis. The combined or bizarre lesions have been excluded.

In general, emphasis is placed on the clinical profile and the differential features. Case reports are utilized to demonstrate the more typical findings. A description of the course of the patient after the first month either is not included or is covered

briefly. Such descriptions are beyond the scope of this chapter and are available in several excellent texts on pediatric cardiology (Nadas and Fyler; Keith, Rowe and Vlad). The medical aspects of treatment are covered separately (p. 309). A differential diagnosis for the more common malformations and for some acquired lesions is presented in a separate chapter (p. 307).

## TRANSPOSITION OF THE GREAT ARTERIES

Transposition of the great arteries is one of the common and serious forms of congenital heart disease encountered in the neonatal period. In one series of infants with cardiac defects presenting during the first month of life, it was found in 10 per cent of autopsied cases and in 16 per cent surviving 1 month (Rowe and Cleary). Prompt recognition of this anomaly has assumed great importance since palliative and corrective surgery now make it possible to salvage many infants with transposition of the great arteries.

**PATHOLOGY.** The anatomy of the transposition complexes is most variable, and a number of classifications have been suggested (Lev et al.; Elliot et al.). It is beyond the scope of this text to review the entire subject, nor will a description of the incomplete forms, the Taussig-Bing syndrome, and the corrected transpositions be included. For the neonatologist it will suffice to consider the most common form (d-type), wherein the aorta arises from the right ventricle and lies anterior and to a variable degree to the right of the pulmonary artery, which comes off the left ventricle posteriorly. Communications between the greater and lesser circulations occur commonly and are of importance for the clinical picture and the prognosis. In careful morphologic studies of 60 cases Elliot and his associates found a ventricular septal defect in 22, patent ductus arteriosus in 34 and an interatrial communication in all. A significant number of patients have pulmonary stenosis as well. The heart is enlarged in all patients who live beyond the first few days. Right ventricular hypertrophy is found almost always, and in a smaller percentage left ventricular hypertrophy is present.

**HEMODYNAMICS.** Fetal development is not impaired by transposition of the great arteries. However, when the fetal shunts close after birth there are two separate circulations: the right ventricle pumps systemic venous return into the aorta and the left ventricle pumps venous return from the lungs into the pulmonary artery. Unless there is a communication between the circulations at the atrial, ventricular or ductal level, life cannot be sustained for very long. In the absence of a significant shunt, the arterial oxygen saturation is very low and cyanosis occurs early. Infants with a large ventricular defect have higher oxygen saturations and minimal cyanosis. In addition to a deficient oxygen supply to the tissues, transposition causes other handicaps. Unless pulmonary stenosis is also present, the lungs are overloaded and this eventually leads to pulmonary vascular disease. Cardiomegaly develops rapidly, and congestive heart failure occurs early.

**CLINICAL FEATURES.** The early appearance of cyanosis is the most characteristic feature of the transposition complex. It is usually noted at birth or within the first 24 hours of life. Thereafter the cyanosis deepens progressively until the infant is a dusky blue continuously. It is generalized except in the rare infant with a large patent ductus arteriosus with reversed flow causing less cyanosis over the lower half of the body.

Clubbing, though common in older infants with transposition, is never seen in the neonatal period.

The heart is normal in size at birth, but may enlarge rapidly over a period of a few days (Fig. 23–1). Thrills are uncommon. The auscultatory signs are not particularly distinctive. The second pulmonic sound may be normal, slightly accentuated or reduced in intensity. Heart murmurs are insignificant or absent unless there is an associated defect. A harsh systolic murmur along the left sternal border signifies the presence of a ventricular defect or pulmonic stenosis.

Signs of heart failure are frequently present. Seventeen per cent of a series of 108 cases were in failure during the first two weeks of life (Keith, Rowe and Vlad). Dyspnea, signs of pulmonary edema and enlargement of the liver are the classic findings.

The radiologic picture is often of diagnostic help. As has already been mentioned, the heart is normal in size at birth, but enlargement may occur within a few days. The base of the heart may be normal or narrow (Fig. 23–2). When enlargement is present, the characteristic oval or egg-shape contour may be noted. The pulmonary vasculature is increased except when pulmonary stenosis is also present.

The electrocardiogram is not distinctive. It may be entirely normal during the first few days of life. There may be evidence of

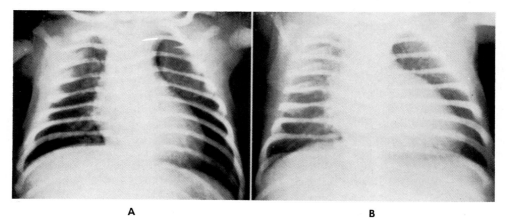

|      A      |      B      |

*Figure 23–1.* Transposition of the great vessels. *A,* Age 3 days. The heart is normal in size. Pulmonary vascularity is increased. *B,* Age 1 week. The heart is enlarged, and there is further increase in pulmonary vascularity.

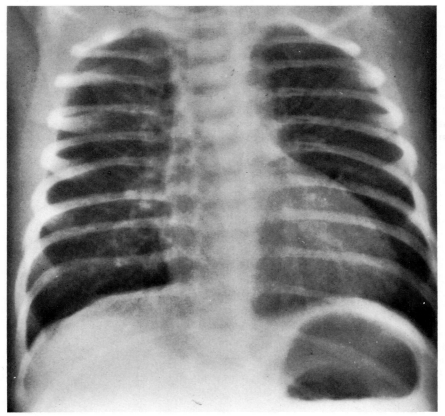

*Figure 23–2.* Transposition of great vessels in a 5 day old infant. Note narrow base and increased pulmonary flow. The heart is slightly enlarged.

mild right ventricular hypertrophy which becomes more prominent in infants with an intact ventricular septum or an associated pulmonic stenosis. Biventricular hypertrophy is more likely when there is a large communication between the right and left sides (Elliot et al.), but this combined pattern may take weeks or months to emerge.

**DIAGNOSIS.** Transposition of the great vessels should be suspected in every newborn infant with congenital heart disease when deep and unremitting cyanosis is the predominant feature. If, in addition to the cyanosis, the x-ray film shows a normal-sized heart initially, progressive enlargement, a narrow base and increased pulmonary vascularity, the diagnosis can be strongly suspected on these findings alone.

The differential diagnosis includes other cardiac defects which cause cyanosis in the neonatal period. *Tricuspid atresia* is a much less common malformation. The main points of difference are the decreased pulmonary vascularity and the left ventricular pattern of the electrocardiogram. Infants with *pulmonary atresia* with a normal aortic root or *severe pulmonary stenosis* may be markedly cyanotic and may have an enlarged heart and congestive failure. The diminished lung vascularity associated with these malformations is the distinguishing feature. The severe form of *tetralogy of Fallot* may cause cyanosis shortly after birth and may be impossible to distinguish from transposition with pulmonic stenosis. Finally the subdiaphragmatic form of *anomalous pulmonary venous drainage* will enter in the differential diagnosis. In this anomaly the heart is usually small and the lung fields show a characteristic passive engorgement.

The diagnosis of transposition can be

made with certainty by *angiocardiography*. This procedure should be carried out even in very young infants on an emergency basis if there is any suspicion of transposition and before the infant's condition begins to deteriorate.

**PROGNOSIS.** The outlook for infants with this anomaly is poor if untreated. Half of the infants die within a month and 90 per cent within the first year (Liebman et al.). The most malignant course is seen in infants with an intact ventricular septum. The presence of a ventricular septal defect may improve the prognosis somewhat, but even in this group life expectancy beyond 1 year is uncommon.

**TREATMENT.** Prompt treatment is needed for infants with transposition of the great vessels and an intact ventricular septum. The surgical creation of an atrial septal defect first introduced by Blalock and Hanlon in 1950 has been replaced by the balloon atrial septostomy technique of Rashkind and Miller. The latter procedure has made it possible to successfully palliate many critically ill infants. In some centers, it is performed at the time of catheterization in all infants who have transposition with or without a ventricular defect (Nadas and Fyler). It should be emphasized, however, that the balloon atrial septostomy, while a "medical" procedure, is not innocuous and should be done only by individuals experienced with this technique.

Not all infants are sufficiently improved by a Rashkind procedure, and in such cases the surgical creation of an atrial defect is indicated. Banding of the pulmonary artery is still another palliative procedure, and is required in infants with a large ventricular septal defect to minimize the chance of pulmonary vascular obstructive disease. There have been advances in techniques for corrective surgery. The Mustard operation, which redirects venous flow by the insertion of a pericardial baffle in the atrium, can now be done in infants less than 6 months of age (Barratt-Boyes et al.). Although there are still insufficient follow-up data on infants who have had a Mustard procedure early in life, Champsaur et al. have reported a 31 per cent mortality after 6 years of age in children who have had an atrial baffle operation after the first year of life. The ultimate corrective operation of switching the aorta and pulmonary artery has yet to be developed.

CASE 23–1

The patient was born after a full-term normal pregnancy, birth weight 7 pounds 10 ounces. Cyanosis was noted on the first day of life, and at 36 hours of age he was transferred to Hartford Hospital under the care of Dr. Leon Chameides.

Examination on admission revealed a dyspneic infant with marked intercostal retractions and severe generalized cyanosis. The lung fields were clear. The second heart sound was single and there were no murmurs. The peripheral pulses were all palpable and the remainder of the examination was negative. Chest x-ray showed a slightly enlarged heart with a narrow base and increased pulmonary vascularity. A clinical diagnosis of transposition of the great vessels was made, and cardiac catheterization was performed to verify the diagnosis and to perform a balloon septostomy.

The cineangiogram revealed the ascending aorta coming off the right ventricle. No ventricular defect could be demonstrated. Oxygen saturation in the aorta was 47 per cent. A balloon catheter was inserted into the left atrium, blown up with 3 cc of dye and forcefully pulled from the left atrium to the right atrium. This was repeated four times. At this point, the infant's color improved markedly and his respiratory distress diminished. The oxygen saturation in the aorta following the septostomy rose from 47 to 71 per cent. The infant was subsequently discharged home in good condition.

**COMMENT.** A clinical diagnosis of transposition of the great vessels was made on the basis of severe cyanosis on the first day of life, pulmonary plethora and a cardiac contour with a narrow base. Despite the infant's poor condition, he was able to tolerate the septostomy and was improved therefrom.

## THE HYPOPLASTIC LEFT-HEART SYNDROME (AORTIC ATRESIA)

The term "hypoplastic left-heart syndrome" was suggested by Lev to describe a group of malformations associated with some degree of underdevelopment of the left ventricle. These malformations include either singly or in combination aortic atresia, hypoplasia of the aortic arch, mitral valve atresia or stenosis and atresia of the transverse aortic arch.

The incidence of this syndrome among all congenital cardiac lesions is between 1 and 2 per cent (Keith, Rowe and Vlad). Yet it is the chief cause of death due to cardiac anomalies in the neonatal period. It was encountered in 23 per cent of an autopsied group of neonates reported by Rowe and Cleary. Although no adequate surgical procedures are available for this group of defects, it is important to differentiate them from operable lesions which may cause similar clinical findings.

**PATHOLOGY.** A number of pathologic lesions comprise this group. Among the 101 infants described by Noonan and Nadas there was hypoplasia of the aortic arch in 71, aortic valve atresia in 15, mitral atresia or stenosis in 9 and atresia of the transverse aortic arch in 6. The combination of aortic and mitral atresia is common. The right atrium and ventricle are always enlarged. An interatrial communication is usually present. The left ventricle is small and thick-walled. Not infrequently there is endocardial fibroelastosis of this chamber. The ductus arteriosus is usually widely patent.

**HEMODYNAMICS.** In the fetus, little or no blood is ejected by the left ventricle so that much of the blood is redirected to the right side of the heart. Hence, an enlarged right atrium and right ventricle are present at birth. After birth, there is no adequate systemic output because of the left-sided obstruction, and severe heart failure usually ensues within the first 24 hours of life.

**CLINICAL FEATURES.** The clinical findings of the entire group are sufficiently similar so that they can be described together. The infant may be in distress from birth or may appear normal for the first 12 to 24 hours of life. Rarely several days may go by before any difficulty is noted. An increase in respiratory rate is a common initial sign. As the dyspnea increases, the patient begins to appear very ill. There is always some tachycardia, often with a gallop rhythm. Heart murmurs are variable and may be absent. When present, they are heard best in the pulmonic area. Cyanosis

is usually present, but not infrequently the infant has a grayish, pale appearance. The peripheral pulses are weak. On occasion the radial pulses are less readily palpable than the femoral. Hepatic enlargement is striking, and peripheral edema may be noted. The blood pressure is low, with a narrow pulse pressure and with little difference between the arms and the legs. The clinical course is rapidly progressive, with death due to heart failure during the first week of life in the majority of cases.

Radiographic examination always reveals cardiac enlargement. This finding is usually present early. The hypoplastic left-heart syndrome is virtually the only malformation which causes cardiac enlargement at birth. The enlargement is both to the left and to the right. In one third of infants with aortic atresia reported by Watson and Rowe the cardiac contour was similar to that described with truncus arteriosus. The hilar shadows are increased, and congestion of the lung fields is the rule.

The electrocardiogram shows evidence of right ventricular hypertrophy in the majority of infants. The R waves over the right side are abnormally tall, and there is a delay in the intrinsicoid deflection over the same area. A qR pattern in $V_1$ is common, and tall peaked P waves are the rule.

**DIAGNOSIS.** The hypoplastic left-heart syndrome should be suspected in every infant who exhibits heart failure in the first week. It was the cause of failure in 44 per cent of the infants in this age group reported by Keith. It must be distinguished from other defects which may produce severe congestive failure early in life.

In *transposition of the great vessels* the heart is normal in size at birth, but enlargement and failure may occur within a few days. The intensity of the cyanosis is greater, the heart may have a characteristic egg shape, and the infant's course is not usually as rapidly progressive.

*Anomalous pulmonary venous return* of the infradiaphragmatic type is another cause of early heart failure. The heart is not usually enlarged in this condition. *Severe pulmonary stenosis* and *pulmonary valve atresia* may be distinguished by the diminished pulmonary vascularity.

Anomalies with a left-to-right shunt and

increase in pulmonary blood flow such as *patent ductus arteriosus* may also develop early heart failure. In patent ductus the pulses are full, the heart is rarely as enlarged as in the hypoplastic left-heart syndrome, and evidence of right ventricular hypertrophy is either absent or less striking.

It may be exceedingly difficult to distinguish *coarctation* from the hypoplastic left-heart syndrome. When severe congestive failure is present, all the pulses may be enfeebled and may give the erroneous impression of coarctation. The pulse differences may be more apparent after anticongestive treatment. The most distinctive finding is the pressure differential between the arms and the legs.

If the diagnosis is in doubt, special studies should be undertaken chiefly to distinguish this condition from cardiac lesions which can be palliated or corrected, and from non-cardiac conditions. When a hypoplastic left-heart syndrome is suspected, an echocardiogram should be obtained. This non-invasive procedure is well suited for these seriously ill infants and the diagnosis can be established without resorting to angiocardiography (Meyer and Kaplan; Godman et al.).

**PROGNOSIS.** Death from heart failure occurs in the majority during the first week of life. Among the 43 cases of aortic valve atresia reported by Watson and Rowe the average survival time was 4½ days. Infants with hypoplasia of the aortic arch may live somewhat longer.

**TREATMENT.** No adequate surgical procedure is available. Therapeutic measures such as oxygen and digitalis result in no or temporary improvement. Vigorous anticongestive treatment is indicated, however, while studies are carried out to prove the diagnosis.

CASE 23–2

A male infant was born after a full-term normal pregnancy. Birth weight was 8 pounds 2

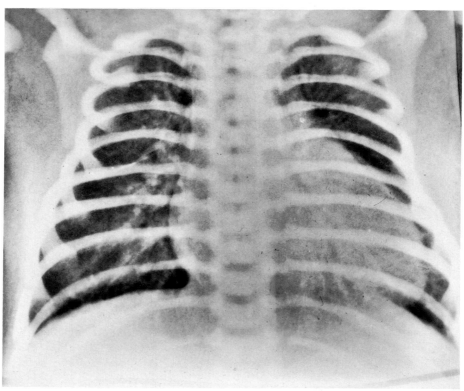

*Figure 23–3.*   Aortic atresia in a 2 day old infant. Note cardiac enlargement and congestive changes in the lungs.

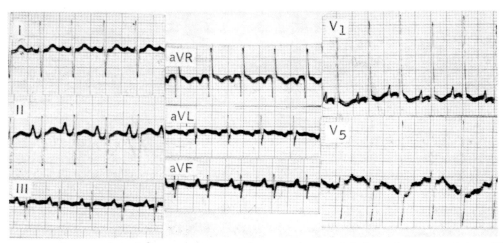

**Figure 23–4.** Electrocardiogram in aortic atresia and ventricular septal defect, taken at age 2 days. There is evidence of right ventricular hypertrophy with tall R waves in $V_1$. The P waves in lead II are tall and indicate right atrial enlargement.

ounces (3685 gm). His breathing time was 2 minutes and crying time 10 minutes. A soft heart murmur was noted at birth, but this disappeared after several hours. Later in the first day of life tachypnea, circumoral cyanosis and some enlargement of the liver were noted. He was digitalized. On the second day a grade II systolic murmur was heard over the precordium. He remained a dusky gray color in oxygen. Both the femoral and radial pulses were feeble. The arm and leg blood pressure was approximately 40. An x-ray film of the heart taken on the second day of life showed generalized enlargement with increased lung vascularity (Fig. 23–3). The electrocardiogram showed tall P waves and combined ventricular hypertrophy (Fig. 23–4).

During the first week of life the systolic murmur became loud and harsh. His response to anticongestive measures was never striking. The liver edge descended to the level of the umbilicus, and periorbital edema became apparent. He died on the 11th day.

Postmortem examination by Dr. T. Weinberg and staff revealed aortic atresia, agenesis of the mitral valve, a small left ventricular chamber, and interatrial and interventricular septal defects.

**COMMENT.** This infant demonstrated the early cardiac enlargement, right ventricular hypertrophy and intractable failure characteristic of aortic atresia. The cyanosis was never great; he had more of a dusky gray appearance. Loud heart murmurs are usually not present unless there are associated defects; septal defects were present in this case.

## TRICUSPID ATRESIA

Tricuspid atresia is a distinct clinical entity which can frequently be recognized early in life. It is seen in about 3 per cent of all patients with cardiac defects (Keith, Rowe and Vlad).

**PATHOLOGY.** Tricuspid atresia is a complex anomaly that consists of atresia of the tricuspid valve, hypoplasia of the right ventricle, and an interatrial communication. The opening in the atrial septum is the only means by which blood can leave the right atrium. The latter chamber is always enlarged. The left ventricle is enlarged and hypertrophied.

Tricuspid atresia is associated with transposition of the great vessels in 30 to 40 per cent of the cases (Tandon and Edwards). Hypoplasia of the pulmonary artery and atresia or stenosis of the pulmonary valve are present in a considerable number both with "simple" tricuspid atresia and when transposition is also present. An enlarged pulmonary artery occurs less frequently. A ventricular septal defect was found in 70 of 115 cases cited by Keith, Rowe and Vlad.

**HEMODYNAMICS.** Because of the atretic tricuspid valve and the underdeveloped right ventricle, the systemic venous return to the right atrium passes to the left atrium where the blood is mixed with the pulmonary venous return before entering the left ventricle. If a ventricular septal defect is present, blood will enter the right ventricle and the pulmonary artery. The degree of oxygen unsaturation depends on the size of the ventricular defect and the amount of pulmonary blood flow. Infants with pulmonary atresia or stenosis plus a small or absent ventricular septal defect will be severely cyanotic from birth. This is also true in tricuspid atresia combined with transposition of the great arteries and pulmonary atresia and stenosis.

CLINICAL FEATURES. Cyanosis is present at or shortly after birth in most infants with tricuspid atresia. The cyanosis varies in intensity. It is least severe in infants with an associated transposition of the great vessels and a large pulmonary blood flow. A loud, harsh systolic murmur heard best along the lower left sternal border is found at birth in about 50 per cent of the cases (Nadas). A systolic thrill is often palpable in the older infant, but is less common in the newborn. The second pulmonic sound is soft. Although severe congestive failure may occur in the older infant, it is much less common during the neonatal period unless the tricuspid atresia is accompanied by transposition of the great vessels. The liver is not enlarged in the absence of failure, but pulsations may be felt.

The heart is not usually enlarged in the neonatal period in simple tricuspid atresia. Enlargement may occur early when there is also pulmonary atresia or transposition of the great vessels with increased pulmonary blood flow. The typical contour for uncomplicated tricuspid atresia consists of a straight right border, a blunt high apex, and a concave left middle segment. Other variations in heart shape are not uncommon. This is particularly true for the neonatal period, when the radiologic examination is less helpful than in older infants with this defect. The pulmonary vascularity is reduced except when transposition of the great vessels is also present.

The electrocardiogram shows left axis deviation, left ventricular dominance or frank hypertrophy and tall P waves in almost all cases. Left axis deviation is often absent in patients with tricuspid atresia and transposition of the great vessels.

DIAGNOSIS. Tricuspid atresia should be suspected in all infants with cyanosis, diminished pulmonary vascularity and a left ventricular pattern in the electrocardiogram. *Pulmonary atresia* with an intact ventricular septum may cause identical clinical and laboratory findings. According to Keith, Rowe and Vlad, the main distinction is the vertical electrical position of the heart in pulmonary atresia in contrast to the horizontal position when tricuspid atresia is present. Occasionally *transposition of the great vessels, truncus arteriosus* and *single ventricle* may be associated with a left ventricular electrocardiographic pattern. The pulmonary vascularity is rarely reduced in these conditions. Other abnormalities involving the tricuspid valve, such as *Ebstein's disease* and *congenital tricuspid insufficiency,* are associated with marked enlargement of the heart, an uncommon finding in tricuspid atresia (Reisman et al.).

The diagnosis of uncomplicated tricuspid atresia can be suspected from the *echocardiogram* (Meyer and Kaplan). *Angiocardiography* will confirm the diagnosis. The dye will be seen to pass from the right atrium to the left atrium to the left ventricle, and a filling defect will be noted in the region of the right ventricle.

PROGNOSIS. This defect is a serious one and carries a poor prognosis. Of the 111 proved cases cited in one series, 17 infants died during the first month (Keith, Rowe and Vlad). Death results from heart failure or severe anoxia.

TREATMENT. Palliative surgery to relieve hypoxia is indicated early in severely cyanotic infants. Improvement can be obtained by creating a systemic pulmonary anastomosis (Waterston shunt) or by joining the superior vena cava to the pulmonary artery (Glenn procedure). Infants have been operated on successfully in the first week of life (Lambert et al.; Collins et al.). Fontan et al. have reported a method for a corrective procedure which involves joining the right atrium to the pulmonary artery by a homograft valve conduit from the right atrial appendage. Experience with this procedure is still very limited, but successful operations have been reported (Ross and Somerville).

## CASE 23–3

A white male infant was born 3 weeks postmaturely. The pregnancy was otherwise normal. Birth weight was 5 pounds 4 ounces (2385 gm). No abnormalities were noted at birth. Cyanosis was noted with crying on the second day of life. On the third day a grade II systolic murmur was heard along the sternal border. Mild cyanosis persisted during his stay in the nursery. His heart was not enlarged. The sounds were of normal quality. There was no evidence of heart failure. An x-ray film of the chest showed a normal-sized heart with clear peripheral lung fields (Fig. 23–5). The electrocardiogram showed left axis deviation and left ventricular hypertrophy (Fig. 23–6).

After his discharge from the nursery his cyanosis persisted, but he appeared to thrive. The cardiac findings remained unchanged. At 2 months of age spells of paroxysmal dyspnea began, and he was admitted to the Harriet Lane Home severely anoxic. An x-ray film of his chest showed minimal cardiac enlargement, a shallow pulmonary conus and clear lung fields. The electrocardiogram showed left axis deviation, a horizontal heart and left ventricular hypertrophy.

The diagnosis of tricuspid atresia was made. A right subclavian to pulmonary end-to-side anastomosis was done, and an interatrial septal defect was created (Dr. H. Bahnson). He showed great improvement and was comparatively well until 5 years of age.

Thereafter there was a progressive increase in cyanosis. Another anastomosis was carried out at 7 years of age, and he has again shown considerable improvement.

**COMMENT.** The appearance of cyanosis in the first few days of life is common in tricuspid atresia. The key to the diagnosis is the electrocardiogram, which demonstrates the left axis deviation, the horizontal heart and the left ventricular pattern typical of this malformation. Surgery was life-saving in this infant, who is still alive 12 years later.

## PULMONARY ATRESIA WITH A NORMAL AORTIC ROOT

Pulmonary atresia with a normal aortic root and an intact ventricular septum occurs in less than 1 per cent of all malfor-

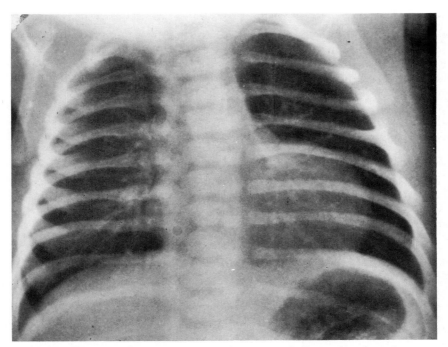

*Figure 23–5.* Tricuspid atresia. Film taken at 5 days of age. Note shallow right side and concavity in region of pulmonary artery. The lung fields are relatively avascular.

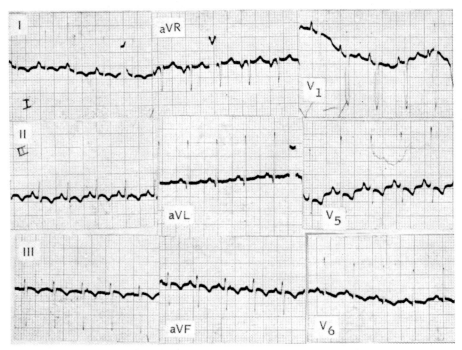

***Figure 23–6.***   Electrocardiogram in tricuspid atresia, taken at age 4 days. There is left axis deviation. The heart has a horizontal electrical position. The deep S waves in $V_4$ and inverted T waves in $V_5$ and $V_6$ indicate left ventricular hypertrophy.

mations (Keith, Rowe and Vlad), but because signs and symptoms are manifested early, it is a significant anomaly of the neonate. Early recognition is of great importance, since surgical intervention may be lifesaving.

**PATHOLOGY.** The obstruction is at the level of the pulmonary valve, which is represented by an imperforate membrane. The main pulmonary artery is patent, often smaller than normal and occasionally hypoplastic. The size of the right ventricle is variable. In about two thirds of the cases it is tiny and the tricuspid valve is proportionately small but not malformed. The remaining third have a normal or enlarged right ventricle and a malformed tricuspid valve (Davignon et al.). The right atrium is large, and an interatrial communication is always present. The left side of the heart is normal or slightly enlarged, and the ductus arteriosus is open.

**HEMODYNAMICS.** Since the pulmonary outflow is completely obstructed, blood can leave the right ventricle only by regurgitat-

ing back through the tricuspid valve into the right atrium and via an atrial defect into the left atrium. The pulmonary circulation depends almost entirely on a left to right shunt through patent ductus to the pulmonary artery. Arterial oxygen saturation varies with the amount of ductal flow, but clinical cyanosis is always present. Right ventricular pressure is elevated and right-sided failure frequently occurs in the first few days of life.

**CLINICAL FEATURES.** Cyanosis is a constant finding. It is often severe and appears on the first day or two of life. Heart murmurs may or may not be heard and are not usually distinctive. A single second sound is present. Dyspnea, hepatomegaly and other signs of congestive failure may occur early, but are often not as striking as the cyanosis.

On x-ray examination some degree of cardiac enlargement is almost always present. It is slight in patients with a hypoplastic right ventricle. Gross enlargement occurs in the group with a normally developed right ventricle. Right atrial enlargement may be obvious. The pulmonary vascular markings are diminished.

The electrocardiogram may be of aid in diagnosis. Tall, peaked P waves are the rule. The mean electrical axis of the QRS and the precordial leads will vary with the degree of development of the right ventricle. In infants with a small right chamber, the axis is farther to the left than normal for age. Indeed, frank left axis deviation was present in seven of 22 cases reviewed by Kiely et al. The R waves may be diminished over the right precordium, and the voltage over the left side of the chest may reflect a left ventricular preponderance. In infants with pulmonary atresia and a normally developed right ventricle, the axis is more likely to be normal, but there may be evidence of right ventricular overloading, indicated by a q wave in lead $V_1$ (Davignon et al.). Recent studies also suggest that echocardiography may be helpful in the evaluation of these patients (Godman et al.).

**DIAGNOSIS.** The diagnosis of pulmonary atresia with an underdeveloped right ventricle should be suspected in a neonate with significant cyanosis, decreased pulmonary markings and left ventricular dominance. Mainly it must be distinguished from *tricuspid atresia*. Usually the left ventricular pattern and left axis deviation are more prominent in tricuspid atresia and the heart has a horizontal electrical position in the unipolar limb leads (Keith, Rowe and Vlad). The less common variety of pulmonary atresia with a normal or hypertrophied right ventricle must be distinguished from isolated severe *pulmonary stenosis*. Benton et al. have suggested that patients with pulmonary stenosis have a "figure of 8" loop in the frontal vectorcardiogram which may aid in the diagnosis. *Tetralogy of Fallot* is rarely associated with severe cyanosis in the neonatal period, nor is there cardiac enlargement. *Transposition with pulmonary stenosis, single ventricle with pulmonary stenosis* and *pseudotruncus* will also enter into the differential diagnosis. The diagnosis may be proved by selective angiocardiography.

**PROGNOSIS.** Infants with pulmonary atresia die within the first days or weeks of life unless surgery is performed. However, recent advances in surgery have made it possible to improve long-term survival.

**TREATMENT.** Surgery should be performed as soon as the diagnosis has been established. Pulmonary valvulotomy will improve some infants who have an adequate right ventricular chamber. Unfortunately, the latter is present in a minority of infants with pulmonary atresia. In infants with a small right ventricle, Malm and his colleagues have carried out a combined pulmonary valvulotomy and a systemic-pulmonary artery shunt with successful results. More recently, this same group performed total correction with extensive infundibular resection of the right ventricular outflow tract, with 4.5 years survival in two of three infants.

CASE 23–4

(This case is abstracted with the kind permission of Dr. Lester Caplan of Baltimore.)

A white female infant was born after a full-term normal pregnancy. Birth weight was 6 pounds 13 ounces (3090 gm). Her condition at birth was normal. At 4 hours of age generalized cyanosis was noted. The cardiac examination was negative, and the lung fields were clear. At 12 hours a soft, precordial systolic murmur was noted, and there was a slight increase in the size of the liver. At 24 hours of age there was frank dyspnea and hepatomegaly. Cyanosis was prominent. The heart was not enlarged. The sounds were of good quality; the second pulmonic sound was single and was of average intensity. There was a short, soft, basal systolic murmur. The femoral pulses were normal. Digitalization was started.

An x-ray film of the chest was taken on the second day of life. The cardiothoracic ratio was not considered increased for this age, although the left lower cardiac border appeared a little full (Fig. 23–7). The electrocardiogram showed a left ventricular pattern with no axis deviation, absent R waves in aVR, and the R waves taller than the S waves in $V_5$ and $V_6$. The heart had a vertical electrical position (Fig. 23–8).

On the second day of life a louder systolic murmur was heard at the base. The signs of heart failure progressed, and the patient died on the third day of life.

Postmortem examination by Dr. T. Weinberg and staff revealed complete atresia of the pulmonic valve, a small, thick-walled right ventricle, an enlarged left ventricle and a patent ductus arteriosus.

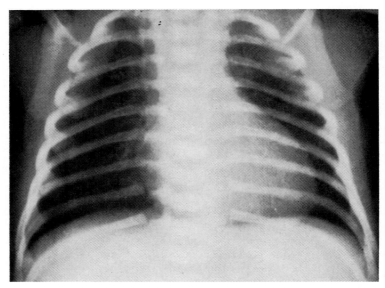

*Figure 23–7.* Pulmonary atresia. Film taken at age 2 days. The heart is slightly enlarged. Pulmonary vascularity is decreased.

**COMMENT.** The clinical features consisted of early cyanosis and heart failure, clear lung fields with little or no cardiac enlargement, and a left ventricular pattern in the electrocardiogram. The differential diagnosis was between tricuspid atresia (with or without transposition of the great vessels) and pulmonary atresia. The vertical electrical position of the heart is uncommon in tricuspid atresia and pointed toward a diagnosis of pulmonary atresia.

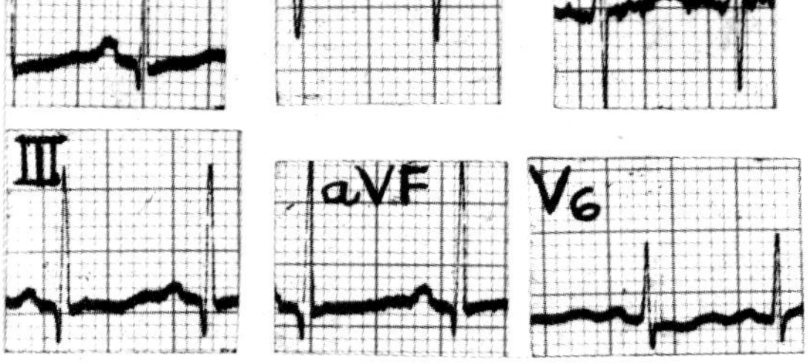

## COARCTATION OF THE AORTA

Coarctation of the aorta is an important cause of cardiac morbidity and mortality in the neonatal period. In Keith's excellent review of heart failure in infancy this malformation was the cause of failure in 10 per cent of the group less than 1 week of age and in 36 per cent between the ages of 1 week and 1 month.

This is a common anomaly. Nadas estimates that it occurs in 10 per cent of all congenital cardiac defects.

**HEMODYNAMICS.** Narrowing of the aorta causes obstruction to blood flow to the lower half of the body. There is a compensatory rise in systolic pressure in the upper extremities and a decreased systolic pressure in the legs. Other hemodynamic changes vary with the location of the insertion of the ductus and the presence of other defects. The pre-ductal or "infantile" coarctations are more likely to have associated anomalies and to cause difficulty in

*Figure 23–8.* Electrocardiogram in pulmonary atresia, taken at age 2 days, showing a left ventricular pattern with no axis deviation, absent R wave in a $V_R$, and R taller than S in lead $V_6$. The electrical position of the heart is vertical.

the neonatal period. When the aorta is narrow above the insertion of the ductus, the right ventricle acts as a systemic ventricle, pumping blood to the lower extremities through the ductus. Right ventricular pressure is high and right-sided failure is common. In the post-ductal or "adult" coarctations, there is left-to-right shunt from the aorta to the pulmonary artery. If a ventricular septal defect is also present, it may add to the already increased pulmonary blood flow, and left ventricular failure may occur early in infancy.

**PATHOLOGY.** Narrowing of the aorta may occur at any point distal to the innominate artery. In the infantile or preductal variety the aorta is coarcted above the entrance of the ductus arteriosus and may consist of a constricted point or a long, narrow segment. In the adult or postductal type the constriction is localized at or just below the entrance of the ductus.

Patency of the ductus is the most common associated anomaly. The ductus was open in 34 of 36 patients in the preductal group and in 13 of 54 in the postductal group among the cases reviewed by Keith, Rowe and Vlad. About one third of the patients have a ventricular septal defect. A variety of other anomalies may be found, and the more complex ones are seen in the preductal group. Endocardial fibroelastosis is also not uncommon.

The right ventricle is enlarged in almost all infants who die in the first weeks of life regardless of the type of coarctation. Left ventricular enlargement may also be present, but is far more common in older infants and children.

**CLINICAL FEATURES.** Symptoms appear during the neonatal period in a large number of patients with the preductal type. Although clinical disease this early is much less common in the postductal variety, it is not rare. This is particularly true if there is an associated large left-to-right shunt by means of the ductus arteriosus or a ventricular septal defect.

Signs and symptoms may be noted immediately after birth. This occurred in five of the 21 cases reported by Calodney and Carson. More frequently these infants appear normal at birth and show signs of cardiac insufficiency in the first days or weeks.

Wheezing and rapid breathing are common initial symptoms. These symptoms frequently go unnoticed in the nursery. Subsequently there is frank dyspnea, poor color and obvious failure to thrive. Cyanosis is prominent only if an additional malformation is present or if the heart failure is severe.

The heart is always enlarged, at times to a great degree. Heart murmurs are variable; they may be absent or insignificant. A loud systolic murmur and a thrill denote the presence of an additional defect. Pulmonary rales, hepatomegaly and edema are noted as the heart failure progresses.

The femoral pulses are weak or absent in all but the exceptional case, and this finding represents the most characteristic feature of this condition. The systolic blood pressure as determined by the "flush" technique is higher in the arms than in the legs. The pressure differential varies between 10 and 20 mm of mercury, and hypertensive levels may be recorded in the arms. Occasionally the arm and leg pressures are equal (Goldring et al.).

Radiologic examination reveals general cardiac enlargement. When the coarctation is preductal, cardiomegaly may be present at birth. Pulmonary congestion is common. There may be left or right axis deviation in the electrocardiogram, more often the latter. Right ventricle hypertrophy is common in preductal coarctation and probably begins in utero, since the increased work load is placed on the right ventricle (Ziegler and Lam).

**DIAGNOSIS.** Coarctation of the aorta should be considered in all infants with an enlarged heart or heart failure of unknown etiology. It should also be looked for in all cases of congenital heart disease. The chief clue to the diagnosis is recognition of diminished or absent femoral pulsations. The femoral pulses can always be palpated in the normal newborn if a careful examination is done. Elevation of the blood pressure in the arms above that found in the legs is a valuable confirmatory sign. The details of the "flush" technique for recording blood pressure as well as the normal blood pressure values are presented elsewhere (p. 227).

The differential diagnosis includes other

causes of heart failure in young infants in whom cyanosis is minimal or absent. *Aortic atresia, primary myocarditis, endocardial fibroelastosis, glycogen storage disease of the heart* and *anomalous left coronary artery* are in this group. The last two conditions rarely cause difficulty in the first month of life. The chief problem in diagnosis arises when the femoral pulses and the blood pressure are enfeebled by severe heart failure regardless of cause. The response to anticongestive treatment may bring out the femoral pulse and blood pressure differential when coarctation of the aorta is present.

The diagnosis can be established by *retrograde aortography.* The usefulness of this procedure even in the youngest infant was demonstrated by Keith and Forsyth. Cardiac catheterization and angiocardiography are not indicated unless other defects are suspected.

**PROGNOSIS.** Coarctation is a serious anomaly for the infant with symptoms early in life. Many of them do not survive the neonatal period. Of 14 patients reported by Goldring and co-workers, five died in 30 days or less. Numerous other reports bear out the poor prognosis, particularly for the preductal type. The great frequency of an associated left-to-right shunt is an additional reason for the high mortality rate. Although the postductal form may present symptoms early, death in the first month of life is uncommon.

**TREATMENT.** The surgical treatment of coarctation for older patients is well established. However, the indications for surgery in young infants are less clear. The "adult" or postductal variety may cause heart failure in 15 to 20 per cent of infants with coarctation (Nadas and Fyler). Such infants usually respond nicely to anticongestive treatment, and surgery can be postponed (Lang and Nadas; Freundlich et al.). Infants with preductal coarctation, who often have other defects, respond less well, and if after 72 hours of vigorous medical treatment there is little or no improvement, surgery is indicated. With recent improvements in technique, 70 to 80 per cent survive operation, while without surgery the mortality rate is extremely high (Sinka et al.; Litwin et al.; Meredith et al.).

CASE 23–5

An infant was born of a pregnancy which was complicated by severe hyperemesis. Labor was induced 2 weeks before term. Birth weight was 8 pounds (3625 gm). He breathed and cried

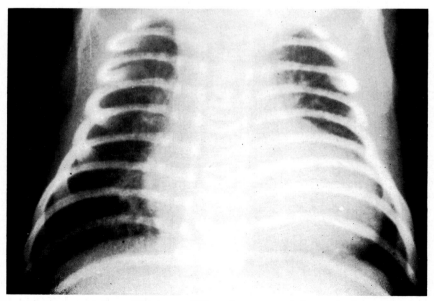

*Figure 23–9.* Infantile coarctation of the aorta. Film taken at age 3 days. The heart is enlarged to the left. There is considerable pulmonary congestion.

spontaneously. A facial nerve palsy was noted on the initial examination. On the third day of life there began an increase in respirations. Examination revealed an enlarged liver. No cardiac abnormalities were noted at this time. The following day he became cyanotic and the tachypnea increased. The heart was enlarged to the left. No murmurs were heard. The femoral pulses were not palpable. The blood pressure was 80 in the right arm and 50 in the right leg (flush method). An x-ray film of the chest showed cardiac enlargement and increased pulmonary vascularity (Fig. 23–9). The electrocardiogram revealed right ventricular hypertrophy. The infant did not respond to anticongestive measures and died on the fourth day of life.

The postmortem examination (Dr. Sadjadi) showed a greatly enlarged heart with dilatation and hypertrophy of the right ventricle. The aorta was coarcted proximal to the ductus arteriosus, which was widely patent. The foramen ovale was patent.

**COMMENT.** This infant presented with congestive failure as the initial sign of heart disease. The absent femoral pulses and the arm-leg pressure differential were the keys to the diagnosis of coarctation of the aorta. The presence of right ventricular hypertrophy noted on the electrocardiogram was confirmed at autopsy; this is a not uncommon finding in the infantile type of coarctation.

## TOTAL ANOMALOUS DRAINAGE OF PULMONARY VEINS

Total transposition of the pulmonary veins with drainage into the right atrium or one of its tributaries is not a common anomaly. It occurs in about 2 per cent of all autopsied patients with congenital heart disease (Darling et al.).

**PATHOLOGY.** Total anomalous pulmonary drainage may occur as an isolated anomaly or as part of a group of malformations. Of the 188 cases collected by Burroughs and Edwards, about one third had other major malformations, exclusive of an interatrial communication. The site of entry into the systemic venous system is variable. The most frequent sites are the left innominate vein, the right atrium and the right superior vena cava. Less commonly they enter the inferior vena cava, ductus venosus and portal or hepatic vein (infracardiac group). The latter sites are particularly germane to this discussion since neonatal difficulty is common in this group. Among 103 proved cases, anomalous venous drainage of this infracardiac type was noted in 12 per cent (Gott et al.; Keith, Rowe and Vlad). At autopsy the right side of the heart is dilated and hypertrophied, and an interatrial connection, either a patent foramen ovale or an atrial septal defect, is always present.

**HEMODYNAMICS.** When the pulmonary veins empty into the right atrium or its tributaries, the mixing of systemic and venous blood results in arterial unsaturation. The degree of unsaturation varies with the size of the interatrial communication and the amount of pulmonary blood flow. The less blood getting to the lungs, the more the unsaturation. Volume overloading of the right side of the heart leads to right ventricular hypertrophy and congestive heart failure. Of great importance is the degree of obstruction at the site where the transposed pulmonary veins enter. In all patients with infracardiac drainage and in some with supracardiac drainage, obstruction at the point of entry causes severe pulmonary venous congestion and early signs of heart failure.

**CLINICAL FEATURES.** The time of onset of the clinical manifestations varies with the size of the interatrial communication and the site of the anomalous connection. In the larger number the site of entry is in or near the right atrium, and a sizable atrial defect is present. These infants rarely have difficulty in the first days of life. If, on the other hand, the site of entry is some distance from the right atrium, the resistance to pulmonary venous return is strong. For this reason the infracardiac group are often in great difficulty from birth. Cyanosis is prominent. Dyspnea appears early, and gross signs of heart failure become apparent. The murmurs are variable and may even be absent. A quadruple rhythm is common, and the pulmonary second sound is accentuated.

The x-ray examination may be helpful. The heart is usually of normal size despite the gross evidence of heart failure. The lung fields are of particular interest. The interstitial tissue of the lungs is thickened and hazy, owing to edema secondary to pulmonary vascular congestion (Harris et al.).

The electrocardiogram will show right ventricular hypertrophy with an overload pattern.

**DIAGNOSIS.** Cyanosis and early heart failure in a newborn infant with a small heart should suggest anomalous drainage of the pulmonary veins below the diaphragm. The appearance of the lung fields may be of diagnostic help.

The intensity of the cyanosis is not unlike that seen in *transposition of the great vessels,* but the pulmonary plethora and a rapidly enlarging heart should distinguish this defect. *Pulmonary atresia* and severe *pulmonary stenosis* may also cause cyanosis and early heart failure. With these malformations the heart is often enlarged and

pulmonary vascularity is diminished. In *aortic atresia,* cyanosis is less distinct and the heart is grossly enlarged very early.

Dyspnea, cyanosis and the appearance of the lung fields may suggest *hyaline membrane disease,* aspiration or other pulmonary causes of the respiratory distress. In these conditions intercostal retraction, localizing pulmonary signs and the course of the patient will aid in the differential diagnosis.

The presence of this defect can be established by angiocardiography. In the case cited by Johnson and co-workers the contrast medium was seen to enter below the diaphragm in the region of the porta hepatis.

**PROGNOSIS.** Infants with pulmonary venous obstruction die within the first month of life unless surgical treatment is under-

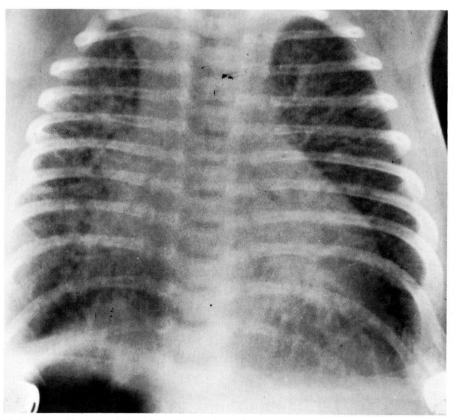

*Figure 23–10.* X-ray film of a 4 day old infant with total anomalous drainage of the pulmonary veins of the subdiaphragmatic type. Note the venous congestion of the lungs.

taken. Patients with other types of the anomaly are not usually symptomatic in the neonatal period.

TREATMENT. Cooley and Balas reported one of the first successful corrections in an infant with anomalous drainage into the inferior vena cava, by anastomosing the anomalous venous trunk to the left atrium. Other reports of successful surgical correction have been published recently (Jaffe et al.; de Leval et al.; Friedli et al.). The ability to save these infants emphasizes the need for early diagnostic investigation of these critically ill infants.

## CASE 23–6

(This case is abstracted with the kind permission of Dr. John Askin of Baltimore.)

A white male infant was born after a full-term pregnancy. The mother was Rh-negative, unsensitized. Birth weight was 6 pounds 14 ounces (3110 gm). No abnormalities were noted at birth. Slight cyanosis was noted during the first few hours of life. This was followed by the appearance of tachypnea and enlargement of the liver by the end of the first day. The heart was not enlarged, the sounds were of normal quality, and there were no murmurs. The infant was digitalized and placed in oxygen.

An x-ray film of the chest showed a normal-sized heart. The lung fields appeared congested with small areas of increased density (Fig. 23–10). The electrocardiogram revealed tall R waves over the right side of the precordium, indicative of right ventricular hypertrophy (Fig. 23–11).

There was slight improvement in congestive failure over the first few days of life, but fairly deep cyanosis persisted. At the end of one week dyspnea became prominent again, and the liver edge was palpated at the umbilicus. Pitting edema of the extremities developed. There was evidence of more severe right ventricular hypertrophy in subsequent electrocardiograms. A significant murmur was never heard in this patient. He died of heart failure at the end of the second week.

Postmortem examination by Dr. T. Weinberg and staff showed a slightly enlarged heart mainly due to an increase in size of the right atrium and ventricle. The pulmonary veins joined to form a common trunk which drained into the ductus venosus. The foramen ovale was patent.

COMMENT. This infant was seen in consultation with Dr. Catherine Neill, who suggested the correct diagnosis on the

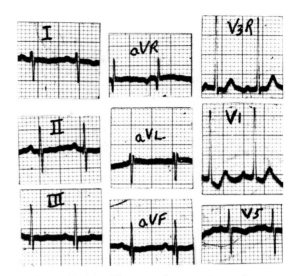

*Figure 23–11.* Electrocardiogram in total anomalous pulmonary return of the infradiaphragmatic type, taken at age 3 days. The tall R waves over the right side of the precordium denote right ventricular hypertrophy.

basis of cyanosis, early heart failure, a small heart and a right ventricular pattern.

## PATENT DUCTUS ARTERIOSUS

Patent ductus arteriosus is a common anomaly, second in frequency only to ventricular septal defect. In the past, it did not rank so high as a cardiac problem in the neonatal period because in most infants with a "classic" ductus, signs and symptoms are not recognized until later in life. In the previous edition, we noted that ductal closure was delayed in premature infants (Auld; Danilowicz et al.). Since that edition, a number of publications have appeared drawing attention to the high frequency of patent ductus in prematures generally and in ill prematures especially. Incidence figures vary among nurseries depending on diagnostic criteria, but reports indicate that from 10 to 25 per cent of infants under 2000 grams have clinical evidence of patent ductus arteriosus. The figure is much higher in infants with the respiratory distress syndrome (Zachman et al.; Kitterman et al.).

It is not clear why closure of the ductus is delayed in premature infants. It is well known that the ductus constricts with increased oxygen tension. It has been shown in animals that the less mature the fetus the greater the level of $Pa_{O_2}$ required to produce constriction (McMurphy et al.). There is suggestive evidence in animals that immature enzyme systems may be a factor in the decreased response to oxygen. It is also possible that the medial muscle layer of the ductus may be insufficiently developed in premature infants to effect adequate closure (Hornblad). Whatever the reasons for delay in closure in healthy prematures, pulmonary disease, or any other condition which diminishes oxygenation at the pulmonary level, increases the likelihood of a persistent patent ductus. The combination of respiratory distress syndrome and a significant shunt through the ductus has become a frequent and well-recognized clinical entity which often necessitates medical, and at times surgical, treatment.

**PATHOLOGY.** The ductus arteriosus comes off the left pulmonary artery and joins the aorta just below the origin of the left subclavian artery. In normal infants the ductus may remain anatomically patent for several weeks, but the opening is not larger than 2 mm after the first week of life (Mitchell). A wider patency which persists is considered abnormal. The open ductus varies widely in diameter and length. In a group of 23 infants described by Rudolph and associates, the ductus at the time of operation was between 4 and 10 mm in diameter, with an average of 7 mm. Infants who manifest symptoms from this malformation usually have cardiac enlargement involving both ventricles and the left atrium. Occasionally enlargement is localized to either the right or left ventricles. In full-term infants, other cardiac malformations are commonly associated with a patent ductus arteriosus, while in the premature, a patent ductus is a transient cardiovascular abnormality.

**HEMODYNAMICS.** The ductus is a vital fetal pathway. Closure of the ductus in utero may cause heart failure (Arcilla et al.). After birth, the ductus remains functionally open for 10 to 15 hours in healthy newborns, and such shunting which may occur during these early hours of life is of little physiologic significance. As has been noted, the ductus remains patent in prematures for longer periods of time and as the pulmonary vascular resistance falls, a gradient develops and blood flows from the aorta to the pulmonary artery. If the shunt is large, there is a volume overload in the pulmonary artery, left atrium and left ventricle. Left ventricular output falls and left atrial and pulmonary venous pressures rise. Pulmonary edema and congestive heart failure follow.

In infants with respiratory distress syndrome, pulmonary vascular resistance remains high during the active phase of the disease, and a significant ductal shunt does not begin until after the recovery phase. Many of these small infants develop signs of heart failure. Myocardial function may already have been compromised by the effects of hypoxia and acidosis associated with pulmonary disease, and the added burden of a left-to-right ductal shunt precipitates congestive heart failure.

**CLINICAL FEATURES.** A murmur heard best over the second left interspace is usually the first finding to arouse suspicion of a patent ductus arteriosus. Several different types of murmurs have been described: a high-pitched ejection systolic, a long crescendo systolic, a long systolic with "spillover" into diastole and a continuous murmur (Hallidie-Smith). The murmur may vary from day to day and even from hour to hour. The continuous murmur is common but transient, and it does not have the machinery quality heard in older infants and children.

In full-term infants a ductal murmur may be heard during the first 6 to 12 hours of life and is gone within a day in most babies. In premature infants, the appearance of a ductal murmur is delayed until pulmonary vascular resistance falls. In the respiratory distress syndrome, the resistance remains high until the onset of recovery so that auscultatory signs may not appear for some time. If the ductal shunt is large, the pulses are full, at times bounding, and the precordial impulse overactive. Signs of congestive failure may appear, and vary from merely an increase in respiratory rate to the full-blown picture of heart failure. Cardiac failure is more common in prematures with pulmonary disease and may appear between the first and fourth week of life. However, a large patent ductus in a full-term infant may cause heart failure and even death during the first few days of life (see Case 23–8).

In infants with large shunts, the heart is slightly to moderately enlarged on x-ray, and vascular markings are increased. Perihilar alveolar edema is an early sign of congestive heart failure but, in general, pulmonary signs of cardiac disease can be difficult to interpret when pulmonary disease coexists. There may be evidence of right ventricular hypertrophy, but more often than not the electrocardiogram is inconclusive.

**DIAGNOSIS.** The diagnosis of a patent ductus should be suspected in any premature infant with a systolic murmur over the pulmonic area, especially in those recovering from the respiratory distress syndrome. A bounding peripheral pulse is a valuable additional sign.

The differential diagnosis includes other defects with a left-to-right shunt. A ventricular septal defect may cause identical findings. The presence of a prominent systolic thrill favors the diagnosis of a ventricular defect but does not exclude a patent ductus. Ostium primum defect, atrioventricularis communis, single ventricle and truncus arteriosus must also be considered. A continuous murmur is not uncommon in truncus arteriosus. Premature infants with physiologic anemia may have a functional systolic murmur. Hypoproteinemia may also be present, causing mild edema which can be misinterpreted as congestive heart failure.

Further studies are usually necessary to establish the diagnosis but these can be postponed if the patient is not in failure or if congestive failure improves rapidly with medical treatment. Aortography is the procedure of choice since it is the least difficult to do. Recent studies suggest that serial echocardiography may also be useful in the assessment of infants with patent ductus arteriosus (Baylen et al.).

**PROGNOSIS.** In the premature infant with an open ductus, spontaneous closure occurs in virtually all patients, even in those who manifested heart failure. Girling and Hallidie-Smith found a mean closure time of 49 days, with a range of 11 to 112, in 33 premature infants with patent ductus.

**TREATMENT.** In view of the high incidence of spontaneous closure in premature infants, ligation of the ductus would appear to be unnecessary. However, there are reports of several series in which from 25 to 30 per cent required surgery (Edmunds et al.; Murphy et al.; Zachman et al.). Others feel strongly that surgery is rarely necessary and recommend a much more conservative approach (Krovetz and Rowe; Hallidie-Smith). There is general agreement that if heart failure cannot be controlled by medical management, then surgery is indicated regardless of age and weight of the infant. (See also Chapter 13.)

## CASE HISTORIES

### CASE 23–7

A white female infant was born after a pregnancy complicated by rubella in the first month. She was delivered at term. Birth weight was 7 pounds 5 ounces (3320 gm). No abnormalities were noted at birth. On the second day of life a precordial systolic murmur was discovered. There was no cyanosis, nor were any other cardiac abnormalities noted. From the very beginning the infant ate poorly and gained weight slowly. By the third week bilateral cataracts were first noted. The heart murmur appeared louder. An x-ray film of the chest showed generalized cardiac enlargement with some increase in pulmonary vascularity (Fig. 23–12). The electrocardiogram revealed tall R waves over the left side of the precordium which suggested some left ventricular hypertrophy.

At 1 month of life she was seen in cardiac consultation. She had barely regained her birth weight. There was some pallor, but no cyanosis. The respiratory rate was increased. Bilateral cataracts were present. The heart was enlarged to the left. The second pulmonic sound was loud. There was a grade 4 harsh precordial systolic murmur maximum at the third interspace on the left. Diastole was clear. The liver was enlarged. The peripheral pulses were all palpable and bounding. The arm and leg blood pressure was 95 mm by the flush technique.

The patient was digitalized with digoxin. She continued to eat poorly and was always in some degree of congestive failure. She was subsequently admitted to The Johns Hopkins Hospital, where a large patent ductus was divided at operation by Dr. H. Bahnson. Her postoperative course was excellent.

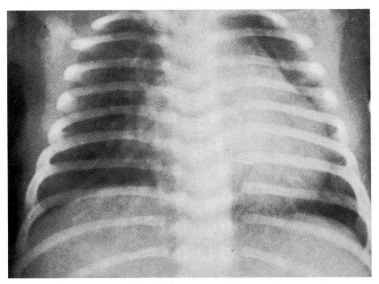

*Figure 23–12.*   Patent ductus arteriosus. Film taken at age 3 weeks. The heart is enlarged. Pulmonary vascularity is increased.

**COMMENT.** This infant had congenital heart disease and cataracts as sequelae of rubella in the first month of pregnancy. As a consequence of a large left-to-right shunt, she did poorly from birth, had cardiac enlargement by 3 weeks, and was in heart failure by the time we saw her at 1 month of age. This clinical course is not unusual in a patent ductus arteriosus with a large shunt.

CASE 23–8

A white female infant was born after a 44-week pregnancy. Labor was precipitous, and the amniotic fluid was meconium-stained. The breathing and crying times were delayed. She weighed 7 pounds (3175 gm). Directly after birth she was cyanotic and had increased, shallow respirations. Her lungs were clear. The heart sounds were normal, and there were no murmurs. Her color did not improve when she was in oxygen. At the end of 24 hours there was generalized spasticity, and her cyanosis persisted. Enlargement of the liver was noted, and there was an increase in the pulse rate.

An x-ray film of the chest showed generalized cardiac enlargement with some increase in pulmonary markings. The electrocardiogram showed abnormally deep S waves in lead $V_5$, suggestive of right ventricular hypertrophy.

The infant was digitalized with digoxin and appeared to respond over the next few hours with striking improvement in color. This response was not long sustained. The respirations again became labored, cyanosis returned, the heart rate became irregular, and death occurred at the end of the second day of life.

Postmortem examination by Dr. W. Lovitt and staff revealed an enlarged heart. The foramen ovale was open. The ductus arteriosus was 1.5 cm in length and 0.7 cm in diameter. There were no other cardiac abnormalities. The lungs were greatly congested. The cut surfaces were hemorrhagic, and the alveoli contained frothy material. Microscopic sections of the lung showed hemorrhagic congestion without other abnormalities. The brain showed venous congestion.

**COMMENT.** The clinical picture was a complicated one. The respiratory distress was thought to be due to aspiration complicated by heart failure, but the postmortem examination showed no evidence of pulmonary aspiration. The heart was enlarged, the ductus was widely patent, and there were congestive pulmonary changes. Although it cannot be stated with absolute certainty, the widely patent ductus may have played the primary role in this picture. Similar patients have been encountered by Keith, Rowe and Vlad. They suggest that the cause of death may be a malignant form of pulmonary hypertension with reverse flow through a large ductus.

## PULMONARY STENOSIS WITH NORMAL AORTIC ROOT

Pulmonary stenosis occurs as an isolated anomaly or as part of a complex of cardiac defects. The tetralogy of Fallot is a common example of the latter. The term is used here to describe patients with this anomaly in whom there is a normal aortic root and an intact ventricular septum, the so-called pure pulmonic stenosis. No distinction is made between the stenosis of the pulmonary valve and the much less common infundibular type, since these anatomic variants cannot usually be distinguished clinically in the neonate.

The incidence of isolated pulmonary stenosis is high. It was found in 10 per cent of Campbell's series of 1130 cases of congenital heart disease. Although many of these patients have murmurs from birth, only a small number with severe stenosis have symptoms during the neonatal period. This group is of considerable importance, however, since lifesaving surgery can be accomplished early in life.

**PATHOLOGY.** In the severe form of stenosis the cusps of the pulmonary valve are completely fused and project domelike into the pulmonary artery. This obstruction to the flow of blood results in hypertrophy of right atrium and right ventricle. Hypertrophy of the right ventricle can be so great as to markedly reduce the size of the right ventricular cavity to the point where it is functionally hypoplastic. The pulmonary artery may be dilated, but this is a less common finding in the neonate than in older infants. Patency of the foramen ovale is common. This opening may be large enough to allow a significant right-to-left shunt in some patients.

**HEMODYNAMICS.** Obstruction to pulmonary blood flow causes a marked increase in right ventricular pressure. If the pulmonary stenosis is severe, pressure overloading of the right side results in right ventricular hypertrophy and the early appearance of heart failure. There is also a right-to-left shunt through an atrial defect or the foramen ovale, causing a reduction in arterial oxygen saturation.

**CLINICAL FEATURES.** The majority of infants with severe pulmonary stenosis have murmurs from birth. But the charac-teristic, rough, diamond-shaped murmur at the pulmonic area is not present often in the neonatal period. It may be soft and heard early in systole at first and increase in intensity with age. It may not be localized to the pulmonic area. Occasionally the murmur is entirely absent (see Case 23–9). Diastolic murmurs are rare. A systolic thrill is almost always present in older patients, but may be absent in the neonate.

Cyanosis at birth is common when there is severe stenosis. It was present in 10 per cent of Campbell's series and in over 25 per cent of Keith, Rowe and Vlad's smaller group. The intensity of the cyanosis is variable. It may be prominent, but more often it is mild and intermittent, and increases with crying and feeding.

The rare infant with the most severe form of stenosis may be in great difficulty within a few days after birth. These infants are severely cyanotic, and signs of heart failure appear early. The heart is enlarged. On x-ray examination this enlargement is generalized. The contour is not distinctive. The poststenotic pulmonary bulge commonly seen in older infants cannot be identified. Pulmonary vascularity is reduced.

Electrocardiographic findings are variable in the neonatal period. At times there is clear evidence of right ventricular hypertrophy with a qR pattern and very tall R waves in $V_1$. A left ventricular pattern may be present early with emergence of right ventricular hypertrophy after the first month (Mustard et al., 1960). Tall P waves indicative of right atrial enlargement are a common finding.

**DIAGNOSIS.** It is extremely important to recognize the patient with severe pulmonary stenosis who manifests striking symptoms in the neonatal period and for whom corrective surgery should not be delayed. The diagnosis should be suspected in every infant with congenital heart disease in whom there is cyanosis and diminished pulmonary vascularity. It must be distinguished from other forms of congenital heart disease with diminished pulmonary vascularity. *Pulmonary atresia* with a normal aortic root may show an identical picture. The severe form of *tetralogy of Fallot* may mimic pure pulmonic stenosis, although the heart is usually smaller and has a more characteristic contour. It may not be

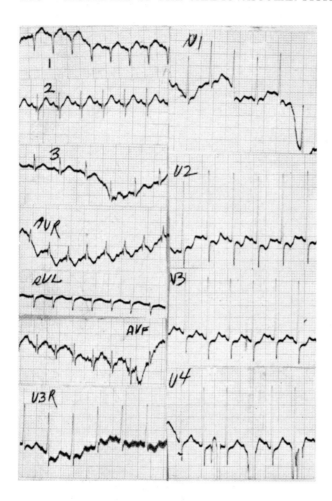

*Figure 23–13.* Electrocardiogram in severe pulmonic stenosis, taken at 4 days of age. There is right ventricular hypertrophy with tall R waves in $V_1$ and $V_2$.

possible to distinguish pure pulmonic stenosis from *transposition of the great vessels* and *single ventricle* when they are combined with pulmonic stenosis. Selective angiocardiography offers the best means for distinguishing these malformations and should be done without delay if pulmonic stenosis is suspected.

**PROGNOSIS.** This depends on the severity of the stenosis. Infants with symptoms in the first weeks of life always have severe stenosis and the worst prognosis. They usually die from congestive heart failure within the first year. Of the 10 deaths reported by Gibson and his co-workers, three were patients less than 1 month old and another four less than 1 year. In the milder and more frequent form of the disease the prognosis is much better.

**TREATMENT.** Direct-vision pulmonary valvulotomy is the procedure of choice. An operation is indicated if heart failure or severe cyanosis is present. Operation should be performed without delay when pulmonary stenosis is suspected. This can properly be considered an emergency procedure, since death can occur rapidly. Successful operations have been carried out in 5-day-old infants (Mustard et al., 1960). In general, earlier and more accurate diagnosis of congenital cardiac defects will result in an improvement in the present mortality rate among young infants with severe pulmonary stenosis.

CASE 23–9

A male infant was born after a full-term, normal pregnancy and an uneventful delivery.

Birth weight was 5 pounds 9 ounces (2535 gm). He breathed and cried spontaneously, and no abnormalities were noted at birth. Cyanosis with crying became apparent at 1 hour of age. This became progressively worse during the next day. No murmurs were heard, and the heart sounds were of normal quality. At 36 hours of age respirations became labored and there was enlargement of the liver. He was digitalized. There was no response to treatment, and he died at 3½ days of life.

An x-ray film of the chest was taken on the second day (Fig. 23–14). There were moderate generalized enlargement and very clear lung fields. An electrocardiogram was recorded on the second day. There was evidence of right ventricular hypertrophy with a qR pattern and tall R waves in lead $V_1$.

The postmortem examination (Dr. W. Lovitt and staff) revealed an enlarged heart. The right atrium was dilated. The right ventricle was enlarged, and the walls of this chamber were greatly hypertrophied. The pulmonary valves were severely stenosed, and there was a tiny patency in the center. The main pulmonary artery was large. The ductus arteriosus was patent, but not large. The foramen ovale was open. The left atrium and left ventricle were of normal size.

**COMMENT.** The clear lung fields and right ventricular hypertrophy suggested pulmonary stenosis, but the absence of a characteristic murmur made this diagnosis appear unlikely. This infant demonstrates early in life the enlargement, cyanosis and

heart failure which may result from severe pulmonary stenosis. Operative intervention would surely have been indicated if the correct diagnosis had been made.

## VENTRICULAR SEPTAL DEFECT

Ventricular septal defect is the most common cardiac malformation. Keith, Rowe and Vlad estimate that it occurs as an isolated malformation in about 20 per cent of children with congenital heart disease. In infants under 1 month of age, Rowe and Cleary found a similar incidence.

**PATHOLOGY.** Ventricular septal defect can occur as an isolated anomaly or as part of a more complex lesion. Examples of the latter group include truncus arteriosus, endocardial cushion defect and tetralogy of Fallot. These and other entities commonly associated with a ventricular defect are discussed separately.

The defect can occur anywhere in the ventricular septum, but most are found in the membranous portion. A smaller number lie in the muscular septum and are more likely to be multiple. The size of the opening is extremely variable. Some degree of overriding of the aorta is common in the membranous type. In young infants who die of this defect there is almost

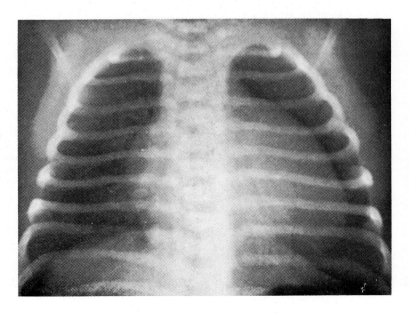

*Figure 23–14.* Severe pulmonic stenosis. Film taken at 2 days of age. The heart is grossly enlarged, and there is fullness along the upper left cardiac border. Pulmonary vascularity is reduced.

always dilatation and hypertrophy of the right ventricle.

**HEMODYNAMICS.** The size and direction of the shunt varies with the size of the defect and the pressure gradient between the ventricles. The latter is affected by the degree of pulmonary vascular resistance. In the first few hours of life when resistance is high, the shunt may be bidirectional, but a left-to-right shunt starts to develop fairly soon, increasing in volume over a period of several weeks. If the defect is large, and the pulmonary vascular resistance drops rapidly, pulmonary edema and left ventricular failure may develop in the first week of life (Rowe and Mehrizi).

**CLINICAL FEATURES.** The clinical findings will vary with the size of the defect, the volume of the left-to-right shunt and the amount of pulmonary vascular resistance. An overriding aorta (Eisenmenger complex) may play an additional role.

In infants with a small defect a soft heart murmur may be detected in the nursery, but it may not sound significant until two or three weeks of life. At that time the characteristic holosystolic harsh murmur along the lower left sternal border becomes apparent. A systolic thrill over the same area is common. The second pulmonic sound is normal and may be obscured by the loud murmur. The heart is not enlarged, and the electrocardiogram is normal. These infants are asymptomatic in the neonatal period.

Infants with large defects may appear ill as early as the third day of life. Twenty per cent of the Nadas series were sick practically from birth. Dyspnea and a tinge of cyanosis are common. A systolic murmur is present, but it is often softer and has more of an ejection quality than the classic murmur of ventricular septal defect. The second pulmonic sound is accentuated. Hepatomegaly and other signs of congestive heart failure may appear early. These infants feed poorly and are slow to gain weight. Some degree of cardiac enlargement and accentuated vascular markings are noted on x-ray examination. The electrocardiogram shows right or combined ventricular hypertrophy, more often the former in younger infants.

**DIAGNOSIS.** In infants with a small shunt the differential diagnosis centers about other causes of a precordial systolic murmur. It may not be possible to distinguish this anomaly from *patent ductus arteriosus* and *endocardial cushion defects* on the basis of the murmur or its location. The murmur of *pulmonic stenosis* with an intact septum has a late systolic accentuation, but in the young infant this may not be readily distinguished from the holosystolic murmur of a ventricular septal defect. Indeed it is not uncommon to have both malformations present. In the neonate with the mild form of *tetralogy of Fallot* a cardiac murmur may be the only finding. It generally is shorter and less harsh. There is no urgency to distinguish these defects in the asymptomatic infant, and studies can be done subsequently to clarify the diagnosis.

The infant with heart failure due to a ventricular septal defect must be distinguished from infants with other anomalies with increased pulmonary blood flow. *Patent ductus arteriosus* and endocardial cushion defects, particularly *atrioventricularis communis,* may cause a similar clinical picture. The finding of bounding pulses should suggest a patent ductus. The typical electrocardiographic tracing of the endocardial cushion defect is a valuable diagnostic aid. *Truncus arteriosus* with large pulmonary arteries and a *single ventricle* must also be considered in the differential diagnosis. As a rule, exclusion of the complex lesions associated with a ventricular septal defect cannot be accomplished without cardiac catheterization and cineangiography.

**PROGNOSIS.** There have been an increasing number of reports of the spontaneous closure of ventricular septal defects (Evans et al.; Nadas et al.). This probably occurs more frequently than is generally recognized and has been documented in patients who have been in heart failure in infancy (Wade and Wright). On the other hand, death during the first six months is not uncommon. Death may even occur in the first few days or weeks of life, especially in premature infants. The natural history of ventricular septal defects has been reviewed by Hoffman and Rudolph.

**TREATMENT.** Infants with isolated small defects do not require any specific treatment. However, close follow-up for the first few months of life is advisable, especially to reassure the parents that there is no need for concern and that the defect may close spontaneously in time.

The infant with a large defect should be observed closely for signs of heart failure so that anticongestive measures can be instituted without delay. If improvement does not occur or cannot be maintained, surgery should be considered. While surgical closure of the defect is the established treatment in older children, until recently the mortality was too high in young infants, and palliation by pulmonary banding was the treatment of choice. However, using deep hypothermia, Barratt-Boyes has successfully closed defects in 2 to 3 month old infants.

## TETRALOGY OF FALLOT

The tetralogy of Fallot is a common and well known cardiac malformation. It was found in 15 per cent of all defects among Abbott's cases. This incidence is disproportionately high for neonatal cardiac problems, since signs and symptoms are often delayed beyond the neonatal period.

**PATHOLOGY.** There is a tetrad of cardiac abnormalities: pulmonary stenosis, ventricular septal defect, an overriding aorta and right ventricular hypertrophy. The pulmonary stenosis is usually at the level of the infundibulum, but may occur anywhere along the pulmonary outflow tract. The degree of stenosis is variable. The septal defect is in the membranous portion and varies in size. The aorta straddles this defect and communicates with both ventricles. The right ventricle is invariably enlarged. Additional anomalies may be present. A right aortic arch occurs in 25 per cent. Rarely there is only one pulmonary artery.

**HEMODYNAMICS.** The right ventricular pressure is at systemic levels and there is a right-to-left shunt. The amount of cyanosis varies with the size of the ventricular defect and the degree of obstruction to pulmonary blood flow. If there is severe pulmonary valve stenosis or atresia, the pulmonary circulation depends on collateral flow from the aorta. The inability to

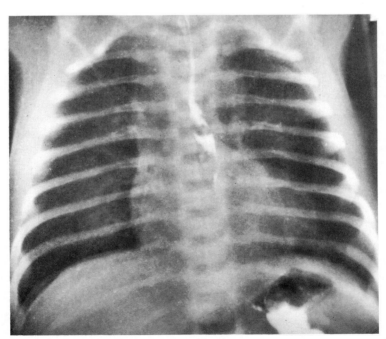

*Figure 23–15.* Severe tetralogy of Fallot in a 7 day old infant. Note concavity in region of pulmonary artery and avascularity of the lung fields.

deliver blood to the lungs on demand accounts for the "spells" these patients suffer. On the other hand, cardiac failure rarely occurs because the right ventricle is protected from a pressure overload by the ventricular septal defect.

**CLINICAL FEATURES.** Cyanosis is frequently absent in the newborn. According to Nadas, it is seen in about one third of the patients. The cyanosis is prominent only when obstruction to pulmonary outflow is severe. A systolic murmur is usually present, although it may not be apparent or sound significant during the nursery period. It may vary from a soft, early systolic murmur to a harsh, stenotic one. The more severe the pulmonic stenosis, the shorter and softer the murmur (Vogelpoel and Schrire). Usually the murmur is heard best along the mid left sternal border. Diastolic murmurs are uncommon. The second sound over the pulmonic area is soft.

Signs of congestive heart failure occur rarely in newborns with tetralogy. However, it may occur on the first day or two of life, if the pulmonary valve is atretic. Heart failure during the first weeks of life is also uncommon except in tetralogies that behave more like a large ventricular septal defect. These same infants may have large hearts. Otherwise the heart is not enlarged. The small heart with the tipped-up apex and concave pulmonary artery segment which is characteristic of this malformation may not be apparent during the neonatal period. Pulmonary vascularity may or may not be diminished.

The electrocardiogram may not be abnormal in the neonatal period. In the severe form of tetralogy, right ventricular hypertrophy may be recognizable by the persistence of an upright T wave in $V_1$. More often it takes weeks before the more classic findings of right ventricular hypertrophy emerge.

**DIAGNOSIS.** The well known classic features of the tetralogy of Fallot are not apparent during the first few days or weeks of life, and it is more difficult therefore to make a clinical diagnosis. Frequently cyanosis is not present. The heart murmur may sound soft and insignificant. When a loud murmur is present, it may not be distinguishable from the murmur caused by a

*ventricular septal defect* or other left-to-right shunt defects. The classic "coeur en sabot" contour is seen less frequently, and it is often difficult to assess the milder degrees of reduced pulmonary vascularity in the newborn. When cyanosis is present, tetralogy of Fallot must be distinguished from other malformations associated with diminished lung vascularity. In *severe pulmonary stenosis* and a normal aortic root, the heart is often clearly enlarged and right ventricular hypertrophy more prominent. *Tricuspid atresia* can be distinguished by the presence of left ventricular hypertrophy in the electrocardiogram. A *pseudotruncus arteriosus* with small pulmonary arteries, *pulmonary valve atresia, transposition of the great vessels* with pulmonary stenosis and *single ventricle* with pulmonary stenosis must be considered in the differential diagnosis and often cannot be excluded on clinical findings alone.

It should be clear from the foregoing that in order to establish a diagnosis of tetralogy of Fallot during the neonatal period further studies are often necessary. The mild case with a heart murmur only or with little or no cyanosis should not be subjected to these studies. The subsequent course will not infrequently make the diagnosis clear. More involved studies should be reserved for those infants with severe cyanosis in whom the diagnosis is in doubt.

*Angiocardiography* will reveal the dextroposed aorta and will define the degree of pulmonary stenosis. Such a study will help exclude transposition of the great vessels, truncus arteriosus and single ventricle.

**PROGNOSIS.** The mild form of tetralogy exhibits few or no symptoms during the first month of life. When there is severe stenosis, the usual course from birth is one of increasing cyanosis, feeding difficulties and failure to thrive. Death may occur during the first month of life, and survival beyond 1 year is uncommon unless successful operation has been performed. Death is due to anoxia, cerebral vascular accident, or some other complication such as brain abscess.

**TREATMENT.** Operation is indicated in the neonatal period when there is severe cyanosis as a result of pulmonary stenosis or pulmonary atresia. The surgical treatment of choice is the creation of an ascending aorta—right pulmonary artery shunt (Waterston shunt). Total or intracardiac repair has become a safe procedure for older children. However, excellent results are beginning to be reported for children under 1 year of age, one even as young as 4 weeks (Barratt-Boyes et al.).

## TRUNCUS ARTERIOSUS

A true truncus arteriosus is an uncommon anomaly, but it is one which often shows manifestation of heart disease during the first weeks of life. It was found in 11 patients among Nadas's 577 cases of congenital heart disease.

**PATHOLOGY.** In truncus arteriosus a single vessel arises from the heart. The size and origin of the pulmonary arteries arising from the single trunk vary greatly. They are rarely completely absent. There is always a ventricular septal defect, and not infrequently there is a single ventricle. The truncal valve is frequently deformed and incompetent.

**HEMODYNAMICS.** Each ventricle pumps blood through a common trunk. There is excessive blood flow to the lungs and, if the pulmonary vascular resistance falls rapidly, left ventricular heart failure can occur in the neonatal period. The degree of arterial oxygen unsaturation is variable and, when there is considerable mixing through a large ventricular defect, there may be only minimal cyanosis.

**CLINICAL FEATURES.** One commonly detects a heart murmur while the infant is still in the nursery. There is usually no or little cyanosis during this period unless the pulmonary arteries are hypoplastic. In fact there may not be definite cyanosis for several weeks or longer, except for an intermittent tinge of blue with crying. The murmur is loud and harsh and is not unlike that of a ventricular septal defect. A continuous murmur may be heard. A systolic thrill is not uncommon. The peripheral pulses are full. Mild tachypnea is often present from birth. These infants eat poorly and in general do not thrive. Signs of heart failure may occur in the first month of life.

X-ray examination of the heart shows lit-

tle or no increase in size during the first few days, although enlargement may subsequently occur during the first month. In some cases absence of the pulmonary trunk may cause a sharp angulation between the supracardiac shadow and the main body of the heart. Taussig pointed out that the width of the supracardiac shadow remains the same in the oblique views. Unfortunately the great vessel area of the heart is often obscured by thymus in the newborn, so that these features are less helpful in this age group. Increased pulmonary vascularity is common except when the pulmonary arteries are hypoplastic. The electrocardiogram is variable and may show left, right or a combined ventricular pattern.

**DIAGNOSIS.** It is usually not possible to make a clinical diagnosis of truncus arteriosus in the newborn with any degree of certainty. The majority of these infants are minimally cyanotic in the neonatal period. The systolic murmur is not unlike that heard in the *left-to-right shunt defects* and in a *single ventricle*. The presence of a continuous murmur is a most suggestive sign. It was found in more than half of Nadas's cases.

If truncus arteriosus is associated with large pulmonary arteries, heart failure may occur early. These patients resemble patients with a large pulmonary blood flow due to *ventricular septal defect* and *patent ductus arteriosus.*

When a truncus arteriosus is combined with underdeveloped or absent pulmonary arteries, cyanosis is present at birth. It is necessary to distinguish these infants from those with severe *tetralogy of Fallot, tricuspid atresia* and other anomalies with cyanosis and diminished pulmonary blood flow.

*Angiocardiography* will confirm the diagnosis. The common trunk is filled with dye and can be visualized as it comes off the base of the heart.

**PROGNOSIS.** Truncus arteriosus is a serious anomaly. Although death rarely occurs in the first month of life, survival beyond the first year is uncommon. Death results from severe anoxia or congestive heart failure.

**TREATMENT.** Successful surgery has been pioneered by the Mayo Clinic group, and the survival rate is improving steadily

(Mair et al.). Although the optimal age of operation is 4 years, corrective surgery can be carried out in 1 year old infants. The real problem is the very young infant who does not respond to anticongestive treatment. Pulmonary artery banding is recommended for these infants, although because of truncal valve incompetence, palliative banding may not be effective (Gelband et al.).

## SINGLE VENTRICLE

An absent or rudimentary ventricular septum results in a three-chambered heart with a single or functionally single ventricle. Signs of congenital heart disease may appear in the neonatal period when such a defect is present. It is not a common anomaly. It was found in about 2 per cent of both the Nadas and the Keith, Rowe and Vlad series of patients with congenital heart disease.

**PATHOLOGY.** In most cases with single ventricle the entire septum is absent and the tricuspid and mitral valves open into this common chamber. At times a rudimentary band or ridge may divide the inflow from the outflow area. Transposition of the great vessels is a common additional anomaly. Interatrial communications are also common, and at least one fourth of the patients have pulmonary stenosis.

**HEMODYNAMICS.** The common ventricle receives pulmonary and systemic venous blood. Unless pulmonary stenosis is present, there is excessive flow to the lungs, and heart failure may occur early. If severe pulmonary stenosis is present, cyanosis develops during the first few days of life.

**CLINICAL FEATURES.** Signs of congenital heart disease appear shortly after birth in most infants with a single ventricle. These signs vary in each patient. Cyanosis is variable in severity and may be absent entirely. It is more severe in infants with pulmonary stenosis. Loud precordial systolic mumurs are common. They have no characteristic localization. A systolic thrill is felt less frequently in the newborn than in older infants with this anomaly.

Cardiac enlargement is absent or not striking early in life. The cardiac contour is variable. If pulmonary stenosis is present, it may take on the characteristics of the tetralogy of Fallot. It may also resemble the contour seen in transposition of the great vessels, since this abnormality is commonly associated with a single ventricle. In either case the contour is less revealing in newborn than in older infants.

There is no characteristic electrocardiographic pattern. Either left or right axis deviation, or hypertrophy of the left or of the right ventricle may be present. In a large study of left axis deviation among patients with congenital heart disease Brink and Neill found left axis deviation in 20 out of 91 patients with single ventricle. These authors concluded that single ventricle was a common cause of left axis deviation among patients with cyanotic congenital heart disease. It is not clear, however, whether this finding is present in the neonatal period. A uniform pattern in all chest leads may occur. When it is present, and not due to a technical artefact, single ventricle should be suspected.

**DIAGNOSIS.** The variable clinical, x-ray and electrocardiographic picture makes the diagnosis of single ventricle most difficult. Infants with single ventricle and severe pulmonary stenosis have significant cyanosis early in life and may resemble those with *tricuspid atresia* and the severe form of *tetralogy of Fallot*. If, in addition to the cyanosis, there is some cardiac enlargement and early heart failure, *transposition of the great vessels, pulmonary atresia* and severe *pulmonary stenosis* will also have to be considered in the differential diagnosis. Infants with a single ventricle with questionable or no cyanosis and a significant systolic murmur may resemble those in the left-to-right shunt group, particularly those with *ventricular septal defect* and *patent ductus arteriosus*.

It is apparent from the foregoing that the clinical findings produced by a single ventricle may simulate the whole gamut of congenital cardiac defects. Further studies are almost always necessary. *Angiocardiography* will demonstrate a large single ventricle and delineate transposed great vessels when they are present. *Cardiac catheterization* will show a higher oxygen concentration in the ventricle than in the right atrium, and a ventricular pressure similar to the systemic pressure.

**PROGNOSIS.** As might be anticipated, the prognosis varies as much as the clinical picture. Nadas points out that infants with a single ventricle may die during the first week of life if there is a low pulmonary resistance and pulmonary overloading, or if there is extreme pulmonary stenosis. In the series reported by Van Praagh et al., 36 per cent of the infants died during the neonatal period. Patients with milder degrees of pulmonary stenosis have the best prognosis.

**TREATMENT.** Palliative treatment may be achieved by a Blalock-Taussig shunt when pulmonary stenosis is present. For patients with large pulmonary blood flow, Muller and Dammann recommended the creation of mild pulmonary stenosis. In older children it is now possible to create a prosthetic septum (Shigeru et al.; Edie et al.).

## ENDOCARDIAL CUSHION DEFECTS

The common forms of the atrial septal defect (ostium secundum) rarely cause signs or symptoms in the neonatal period, although heart failure in a 5 day old infant with ostium secundum has been reported (Ainger and Pate). On the other hand, defects in the lower portion of the septum (ostium primum) and a persistent common atrioventricular canal (atrioventricularis communis) frequently manifest cardiac signs early in life. Both malformations result from imperfect fusion of the endocardial cushions and are termed endocardial cushion defects.

**PATHOLOGY.** In the ostium primum syndrome the atrial defect is located just above the atrioventricular valves and is almost always associated with a cleft in the mitral valve. When there is a common atrioventricular canal, in addition to the above-mentioned anomalies, there is a defect in the ventricular septum and a cleft in the tricuspid valve. This results in a common opening between the atria and the ventricles. As a consequence of these malformations, all four chambers are often enlarged, and the pulmonary artery is dilated.

**HEMODYNAMICS.** Infants with a common atrioventricular canal (complete endocardial cushion defect), have bidirectional left-to-right shunts at the atrial and ventricular levels. Congestive heart failure occurs early. In partial endocardial cushion defect (ostium primum with or without a cleft in the mitral valve), there is a left-to-right shunt at the atrial level without significant hemodynamic consequences in the first few weeks of life. Over time, the presence of mitral regurgitation causes a left ventricular volume overload.

**CLINICAL FEATURES.** Infants with ostium primum defects do not usually appear ill at birth, nor do they often manifest difficulty during the first weeks of life. During this period the discovery of heart murmur is the only sign of a cardiac defect. The murmur is systolic in time, harsh, and widely distributed over the precordium. A short diastolic murmur may be heard. A thrill may be present. The second pulmonic sound is accentuated and widely split. The heart is usually not enlarged at this age. Pulmonary vascularity is increased.

Infants with atrioventricularis communis manifest symptoms much earlier. Tachypnea and intermittent cyanosis may be present from birth. There is a harsh systolic murmur over the precordium which is often loudest at the apex. A diastolic murmur is present occasionally. A thrill is not uncommon. The heart is overactive, and the second pulmonic sound is loud. There is generalized cardiac enlargement, and the left atrium may be large. The pulmonary segment is full. The vascular markings are prominent. Frank dyspnea and signs of congestive failure may appear early, and death during the first month of life is not rare.

One of the striking clinical features of atrioventricularis communis is its frequent association with Down's syndrome. Thirty per cent of the 55 patients described by Rogers and Edwards had this syndrome. Taussig found an equally high incidence.

The electrocardiogram in endocardial cushion defects is characteristic and is often of considerable diagnostic aid. The most striking feature is the left axis deviation, which is present at birth and is probably due to congenital conduction disturbance and not left ventricular hypertrophy (Toscano-Barbosa et al., Liebman and Nadas). Associated findings are an rsR′ pattern in the right chest leads, a prolonged P-R interval and tall P waves. The left ventricular or biventricular pattern seen in older infants and children is not usually present in the first weeks of life.

**DIAGNOSIS.** An endocardial cushion defect should be suspected in an infant with signs of a left-to-right shunt in whom the above-mentioned electrocardiographic findings are present. By this means it may be distinguished from a *ventricular septal defect* and *patent ductus arteriosus.* In infants with atrioventricularis communis, cyanosis, heart failure and pulmonary plethora may resemble the clinical picture of *transposition of the great vessels.* In the latter anomaly left axis deviation may be present occasionally. Angiocardiographic studies will distinguish these conditions.

**PROGNOSIS.** The prognosis with atrioventricularis communis is poor, in contrast to ostium primum defects. In the series of 47 patients collected by Rogers and Edwards death occurred in eight infants less than 1 month of age.

**TREATMENT.** Good surgical procedures have been developed for direct repair of ostium primum defects. Since the mortality rate is still high for young infants, operation is postponed whenever possible. There has also been considerable improvement in the surgical mortality for correcting atrioventricularis defects in children over 2 years of age (Rastelli et al.; Taguchi et al.; Wallace et al.). In very young infants partial constriction of the pulmonary artery to diminish pulmonary blood flow may result in some improvement. At best this procedure is palliative and the salvage rate low. However, since total correction in older children is now possible, vigorous efforts should be made to keep these infants compensated through infancy.

CASE 23–10

(This case is abstracted with the kind permission of Dr. Helen Taussig of Baltimore.)

A female Negro infant was born 3 weeks prematurely. The mother's pregnancy was complicated by hypertension. The infant was covered with meconium at birth. There was some

immediate respiratory distress and cyanosis which were attributed to aspiration. The initial examination showed clear signs of mongolism. The cardiac examination at this time was negative. Tachypnea and mild cyanosis persisted after the first day of life, and an intermittent precordial systolic murmur was heard. The heart was not enlarged clinically. The second pulmonic sound was exaggerated. The liver was not enlarged, and the femoral pulses were normal. An x-ray film of the chest showed some cardiac enlargement and an increase in lung markings. The electrocardiogram disclosed left axis deviation without evidence of ventricular hypertrophy (Fig. 23–16).

Because of persistent tachypnea the patient was digitalized. There was slow improvement, and she was discharged at 3 weeks of age. At 10 weeks of age she was readmitted with pneumonia and heart failure. In addition to pneumonitis, the x-ray film again showed cardiac enlarge-

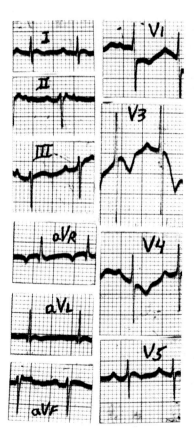

***Figure 23–16.*** Electrocardiogram in a case of atrioventricularis communis in a 6 day old with Down's syndrome. There is left axis deviation. At 10 weeks of age, in addition to the left axis deviation, there was evidence of combined ventricular hypertrophy.

ment with an increase in pulmonary markings. The electrocardiogram showed left axis deviation and evidence of combined ventricular hypertrophy. She recovered from her pneumonia and was followed up over a period of 8 months. She gained weight slowly. There was always some tachypnea present. The heart remained enlarged. The systolic murmur was grade I to II in intensity, was not particularly harsh, and was heard over the entire precordium. There were no thrills. Left axis deviation and combined ventricular hypertrophy were present.

**COMMENT.** The diagnosis was not completely established in this infant. She had Down's syndrome, and it is reasonable to suspect the presence of either an ostium primum defect or atrioventricularis communis. Either of these malformations, especially the latter, is commonly associated with Down's syndrome. There was good evidence of a left-to-right shunt with increased pulmonary blood flow. Heart failure may be present from the first few days as it was in this patient. Left axis deviation and combined ventricular hypertrophy are common findings with either the ostium primum defect or atrioventricularis communis.

## AORTIC STENOSIS

Congenital aortic stenosis has received increasing attention in recent years, mainly as a result of advances in the correction of this defect. The incidence of this anomaly among patients with congenital heart disease is between 2 and 3 per cent (Lambert et al., 1966). Although it is a far less common cause of cardiac morbidity in the neonatal period, infants with severe stenosis may manifest symptoms shortly after birth.

**PATHOLOGY.** Anatomically, there are two types of aortic stenosis: valvular and subvalvular. In the more common valvular type the thickened aortic cusps are fused to form a diaphragm with a small opening in the center. The subvalvular type consists of a fibrous ring below the aortic valves. If the stenosis is severe, hypertrophy of the left ventricle may occur early. Endocardial fibroelastosis of this chamber is frequently present. With the exception of coarctation of the aorta, other congenital anomalies are uncommon when the valvular type of stenosis is present.

**HEMODYNAMICS.** Obstruction to the flow of blood from the left ventricle causes a pressure load on that chamber, leading to hypertrophy. When the stenosis is very severe, coronary artery blood flow may be reduced.

**CLINICAL FEATURES.** Most patients with aortic stenosis have no symptoms in the neonatal period. A murmur is present at birth in about one fourth of cases (Downing). At this age the murmur does not have a characteristic location and is more commonly heard along the left sternal border. Later it shifts to the aortic area. The murmur is harsh, but its "stenotic" nature may not be apparent early in life. Although a thrill is common in the older patient, it is rarely present in the neonate. Similarly the second aortic sound is not noticeably diminished at this age. In the asymptomatic group the heart is not enlarged and the electrocardiogram may be normal.

A small group of infants with very severe aortic stenosis show symptoms in infancy which may date back to the first days of life. Intermittent cyanosis, dyspnea and signs of progressive heart failure are common in this group. The heart is enlarged. The electrocardiogram shows left ventricular or combined ventricular hypertrophy. In a patient described by Marquis and Logan electrocardiographic evidence of left ventricular hypertrophy was present at 3 days of age.

**DIAGNOSIS.** The usual criteria for a diagnosis in older patients are not present in the very young infant. The murmur is more often located along the left sternal border, there is no thrill, and the second heart sound over the aortic area is not strikingly diminished. The murmur may be similar to that heard with a *ventricular septal defect*, and it may also resemble that of *pulmonic stenosis* of the infundibular type, an *ostium primum defect* or a *patent ductus arteriosus*. In aortic stenosis, pulmonary vascularity is normal. It is diminished in pulmonary stenosis and increased when left-to-right shunt defects are present. Early left ventricular hypertrophy favors a diagnosis of aortic stenosis.

In some infants the heart murmur is absent or insignificant even though the aortic stenosis is of such severity that heart failure occurs in the first month of life. It is necessary to differentiate these infants from patients with *endocardial fibroelastosis* and *coarctation of the aorta.* The pattern of left ventricular hypertrophy occurs in both aortic stenosis and endocardial fibroelastosis and makes this differential diagnosis particularly difficult. The presence of good femoral pulses excludes coarctation of the aorta. It should be recalled that aortic stenosis is not uncommonly associated with the preductal type of coarctation and endocardial fibroelastosis.

When the diagnosis of aortic stenosis is a suspected cause of heart failure in the neonate, cardiac catheterization and angiocardiography should be performed without delay.

**PROGNOSIS.** When aortic stenosis causes symptoms in the neonatal period, the prognosis is poor. Of a total of 28 cases of congenital aortic stenosis described by Marquis and Logan, death occurred at 6 and 10 weeks of age in the two patients with early symptoms. The asymptomatic infants who have a heart murmur as their only manifestation of cardiac disease have a good prognosis. Their course is not described here.

**TREATMENT.** Rapid advances are being made in the surgical treatment of aortic stenosis. Various techniques are available. The procedure of choice for small infants is valvulotomy under direct vision, using a pump-oxygenator. Although this technique is still hazardous, the prognosis for young infants with heart failure is poor, and operation should be performed at the earliest age in this group. Collins et al. reported infants treated as young as 4 weeks of age.

CASE 23–11

An infant (a private patient of Dr. H. B. Taussig) was seen at the Harriet Lane Home at 1 month of life with an enlarged heart and rapid breathing. The patient was the result of a full-term pregnancy which was complicated by vaginal bleeding in the first trimester. Birth weight was 6½ pounds (2960 gm). A faint murmur was noted at birth, but she appeared well otherwise. On the ninth day of life the mother noted an episode of severe cyanosis following a period of hard crying. At 2 weeks of age the in-

fant was seen because of rapid breathing. A blowing systolic murmur of moderate intensity and enlargement of the liver were noted. An x-ray film of the chest revealed an enlarged heart. The patient was digitalized, and some improvement followed.

She was examined in Dr. Taussig's clinic at 1 month of age. There was tachypnea. Minimal cyanosis was noted after crying. The heart sounds were of poor quality. A grade II systolic murmur was heard along the lower left sternal border. It was transmitted to the neck and to the back. The peripheral pulses were strong. The liver was enlarged.

An x-ray film of the chest disclosed enlargement of the heart. The left atrium appeared enlarged in the esophagogram. The electrocardiogram showed low voltage in all leads. The T waves were inverted in leads I and II and in the left precordial leads.

The infant was seen in consultation with Dr. Taussig. The two diagnostic possibilities most seriously considered were endocardial fibroelastosis and anomalous left coronary artery. The patient was treated for congestive heart failure. Sudden death occurred at 2 months of age. Autopsy examination revealed aortic valvular stenosis and endocardial fibroelastosis of the right ventricle.

**COMMENT.** This patient demonstrated severe heart disease early in life as a result of aortic stenosis. As is often the case in the neonate, the clinical findings were atypical. The murmur was heard best along the left sternal border, there was no thrill, and the second aortic sound was normal. The electrocardiographic picture may have been modified by the presence of right ventricular endocardial fibroelastosis.

## MITRAL VALVE DEFECTS

Malformations of the mitral valve may be found in association with other cardiac abnormalities such as endocardial cushion defects (ostium primum and atrioventricularis communis), corrected transposition of the great vessels and the hypoplastic left-heart syndrome. This discussion is limited to isolated defects of the mitral valve, which occur much less commonly than combined anomalies. Starkey was able to find 11 "pure" cases of congenital mitral stenosis in the literature. More recently

Husson et al. reported 16 patients with isolated congenital mitral insufficiency.

**PATHOLOGY.** A variety of anatomic abnormalities of the mitral valve have been described. There may be simply a cleft in the anterior leaflet as an isolated defect. On the other hand, the leaflets may be normal, but the mitral ring may be widely dilated. Not infrequently the leaflets are thickened with little commissural formation and with short chordae tendineae. Accessory commissures may be present (Edwards and Burchell).

**CLINICAL FEATURES.** An isolated mitral valve defect which results in mitral regurgitation rarely causes any difficulty in the neonatal period. One of the patients described by Husson et al. had dyspnea and a significant heart murmur at 4 weeks of life. More often symptoms do not develop for months or years.

Infants with congenital mitral stenosis are much more likely to have difficulty in early infancy. A systolic murmur detected in the nursery may be the only finding initially. At times no murmur is present. A mid-diastolic or presystolic rumble is rarely heard early, but can be found eventually in the majority of patients. Within a few weeks or months after birth rapid respirations, sweating, minimal cyanosis and failure to thrive become apparent. Signs of congestive heart failure are present, and repeated bouts of respiratory infections are common.

The x-ray examination may reveal a large left atrium within days after birth. It was present by the fourth day in the case described below (Fig. 23–17). General cardiac enlargement and pulmonary congestion are other common findings.

The electrocardiogram shows some degree of right ventricular hypertrophy as well as right and left atrial hypertrophy.

**DIAGNOSIS.** Congenital mitral stenosis should be suspected in every infant in whom there is a large left atrium and evidence of pulmonary vascular obstruction. The diastolic murmur may be absent at first, and a regurgitant systolic murmur may be the only auscultatory finding. When the latter is present, it is necessary to exclude those malformations frequently associated with a mitral valve defect. The *atrioven-*

*tricular canal* anomalies often have distinctive clinical and electrocardiographic features. *Primary endocardial fibroelastosis* with or without mitral involvement can be distinguished by the presence of left ventricular hypertrophy. Although the mitral valve may be involved in the complex of defects which make up the *hypoplastic left-heart syndrome,* this poses no diagnostic problem, for these infants are in profound failure early and die within a week as a rule. Congenital mitral stenosis may be difficult to distinguish from *cor triatriatum* without more precise studies. The *cineangiogram* will show a large, poorly emptying left atrium with a narrowed mitral orifice.

**PROGNOSIS.** The prognosis will vary with the nature and severity of the mitral defect. As has already been mentioned, patients with congenital mitral insufficiency will only rarely have difficulty early. Infants with congenital mitral stenosis not infrequently die by six months of age (Ferencz et al.).

**TREATMENT.** Surgical treatment of mitral stenosis is indicated early in life if medical therapy does not bring the heart failure under control. Successful operations have been reported (Starkey).

CASE 23–12

A full-term male infant was born at Women's Hospital and weighed 8 pounds. The initial examination was negative. On the third day of life a grade III blowing holosystolic murmur was noted, and the infant was transferred to the Harriet Lane Home. A chest x-ray showed cardiomegaly, a large left atrium and definite venous congestion (Fig. 23–17). The electrocardiogram revealed broad flat P waves indicative of left atrial enlargement (Fig. 23–18). The patient was digitalized, and his clinical condition improved somewhat. By 4 months of age his respiratory distress became worse, however, and there was profuse sweating. At this time an apical diastolic murmur with presystolic accentuation was heard. A cine-angiocardiogram revealed a poorly emptying left atrium and a narrowed mitral orifice. An operation with digital fracturing of the mitral valve was carried out, but ventricular fibrillation developed and the infant died. Postmortem examination revealed stenosis of the mitral valve with shortening of the chordae tendineae. There was also fibroelastosis of the left atrium.

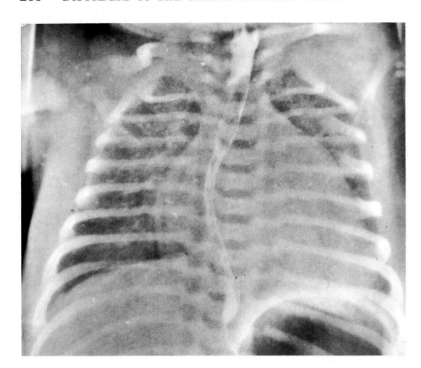

*Figure 23–17.* Mitral stenosis in a 4 day old infant. There is fullness of the middle left cardiac segment, the left atrium is enlarged, and there is heavy congestion of the lung fields.

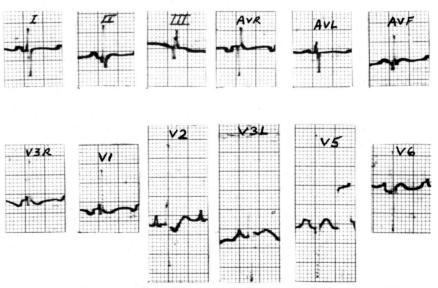

*Figure 23–18.* Four day old infant with congenital mitral stenosis. Note the flattening of the P waves in leads I and $V_5$ (P mitrale).

## ANOMALOUS ORIGIN OF THE CORONARY ARTERIES

Aberrant origin of either one or both coronary arteries from the pulmonary artery constitutes a group of rare cardiac anomalies. An anomalous right coronary artery is of little importance, since clinical disease does not usually result. In contrast, when both coronaries are aberrant, life cannot be sustained for long. Five cases have been described (Tedeschi and Halpern). Cyanosis and heart failure were present in all on the first day of life. The clinical picture was not characteristic, and the diagnosis was established only after death, which usually occurred within the first 2 weeks of life.

When the left coronary artery is anomalous in its origin, a more characteristic pattern of disease results and an antemortem diagnosis can be made. Although this anomaly does not usually manifest itself in the neonatal period, it can be a cause of death in the first week or two of life. With the increased interest in early screening for heart disease in the nursery, it is likely that infants with this abnormality will be detected earlier.

**PATHOLOGY.** The heart is grossly enlarged, owing to dilatation and hypertrophy of the left ventricle. The wall of this chamber may at times be extremely thin, even aneurysmal. The muscle appears pale. Microscopic examination shows extensive myocardial fibrosis of the left ventricle.

**HEMODYNAMICS.** As a result of the observations by Sabiston and his co-workers, it is believed that the physiologic disturbance is due to the flow of blood from the anomalous coronary in a retrograde manner toward the pulmonary artery; i.e., a coronary arteriovenous fistula. Rowe and Mehrizi suggest that this fistula may be operative in utero even though the clinical findings take several weeks to evolve. Insufficient coronary blood flow causes myocardial infarction and fibrosis leading to death in infancy.

**CLINICAL FINDINGS.** The infant appears normal at birth. Sudden death may occur in the first week (see Case 23–13), but this is exceedingly rare. Usually, severe symptoms are not noted until after the second month, but signs of difficulty may date back to the first few weeks. Irritability and slight difficulty in breathing, especially during feedings, are the earliest symptoms. Episodes of distress characterized by sweating, pallor and pain may occur. These paroxysms have been likened to attacks of angina pectoris. As the condition progresses, there develops an increasing and often an alarming degree of respiratory distress. The infant appears less well, his color becomes poor, and his weight gain diminishes.

On examination the baby appears dyspneic and anxious. Slight cyanosis about the mouth is common, but severe cyanosis is almost never present. There may be some precordial prominence indicative of cardiac enlargement. Rales and dullness are often present over the lower lung fields. There is always tachycardia. Murmurs are rarely heard. Enlargement of the heart is obvious except in the early stages of the illness. The liver is enlarged.

Roentgenograms show some degree of cardiac enlargement. This is usually not marked early, but in time the left ventricular enlargement becomes striking, and an aneurysmal dilatation may be present. Fluoroscopic examination confirms the enlargement of the left ventricle, and this is noted especially in the left anterior oblique view. The left cardiac border usually shows little pulsation. Hilar congestion is common.

The electrocardiogram may show a characteristic pattern within a few weeks of birth. The most significant finding is the presence of Q waves in leads I and aVL (Fig. 23–19). Inversion of the T waves in the standard limb and precordial leads is a common finding, but may be absent for several months.

**DIAGNOSIS.** It is difficult to make a clinical diagnosis early in the course of the disease. Mild or intermittent respiratory distress may suggest a *respiratory infection* rather than heart disease. Irritability and paroxysms of pain may not be unlike simple colic. The presence of heart disease often goes unrecognized until the signs of cardiac failure are full blown. At this point it is not difficult to make an antemortem diagnosis. Final proof can be obtained ei-

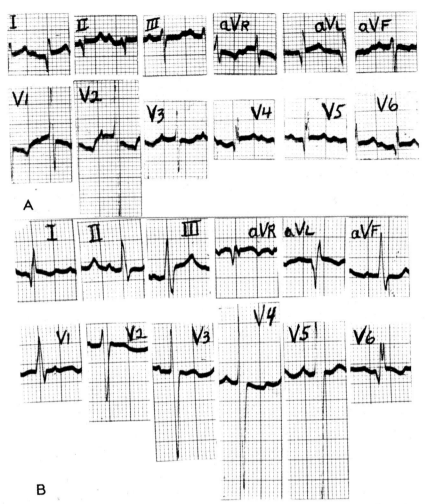

*Figure 23–19.*   A, Three week old infant with anomalous left coronary artery. Note deep Q waves in leads I and aVL. *B,* Same patient at 5 months. Note deeper Q waves in aVL and inversion of T waves in leads I and V₆.

ther by retrograde aortography or by the injection of contrast material into the pulmonary artery.

A dyspneic young infant with an enlarged heart without murmurs and with little or no cyanosis should always suggest the possibility of an anomalous left coronary artery. Left ventricular enlargement is characteristic. The absence of murmurs and cyanosis excludes other congenital lesions which may cause enlargement of the left ventricle. Palpable femoral pulsations rule out *coarctation of the aorta.* It is mainly necessary to differentiate this condition from *endocardial fibroelastosis.* The electrocardiogram usually makes this distinc-

tion possible. Whereas left ventricular strain is common to both, only an aberrant left coronary will show the QR pattern and inverted T waves in lead I (Lambert et al., 1955).

Myocardial infarction in the newborn infant with structurally normal coronary arteries has been reported (Arthur et al.). Although rare, this possibility must be considered when an infarct pattern is noted in the electrocardiogram. Talner and Campbell reported two newborn infants with evidence of anterolateral myocardial infarction at birth. One infant died and had a thrombus in the anterior descending left coronary artery.

**TREATMENT.** Some relief of heart failure may be obtained by oxygen and digitalis, but at best this is only temporary. Studies by Sabiston and co-workers have shown that in infants who develop a collateral circulation there may be a considerable "runoff" of arterial blood from the left coronary artery into the pulmonary artery by retrograde flow. Ligation of the left coronary artery would raise coronary artery pressure and improve the blood supply to the heart. Successful results have been reported, and this technique is the procedure of choice in patients with a demonstrable collateral circulation. For patients without a collateral circulation, Armer et al. have proposed a surgical method which utilizes the main pulmonary artery excised with the coronary ostium at its base and converted into a tube which is anastomosed to the aorta. Transplantation of the left coronary to the aorta would appear to be the ultimate procedure, but this has not yet been accomplished successfully.

**PROGNOSIS.** This anomaly has been described in adults, but these are not persons who had symptoms early in life. When difficulty develops early in infancy, the prognosis is poor. The majority of patients die by 6 months of life and almost all by 1 year. Advances in treatment may alter the outcome in the future. A greater degree of therapeutic success will depend not only on an improved surgical approach, but also on the ability to recognize this condition before extensive myocardial damage occurs. In this connection, *the presence of some difficulty in breathing in a young infant which is not otherwise explained should stimulate an investigation for possible underlying heart disease.*

CASE 23–13

(This case is abstracted with the kind permission of Dr. Ella Oppenheimer.)

An 8-day-old infant was admitted to the Harriet Lane Home with a sudden onset of rapid breathing. She was the result of a full-term normal pregnancy. No abnormalities were noted at birth, and her course in the nursery was uneventful. She remained well until the day of admission to the hospital, when blueness and rapid breathing were noted.

This infant was in extremis on admission. She was severely dyspneic. There was generalized cyanosis. The liver was enlarged. There were no other abnormal findings. She died shortly after admission.

A postmortem examination by Dr. Boyd revealed an enlarged heart. The left ventricle was dilated, flabby and pale. The left coronary artery arose from the base of the main pulmonary artery. The right coronary artery was normal. On cutting throuh the left ventricle there was evidence of an infarct (Fig. 23–20). Microscopic examination showed focal infarcts in the wall of the left ventricle with fresh muscle necrosis.

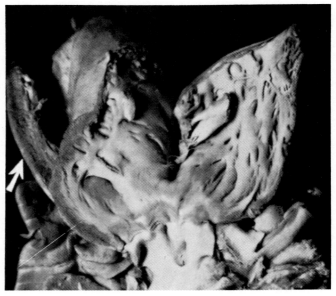

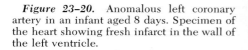

*Figure 23–20.* Anomalous left coronary artery in an infant aged 8 days. Specimen of the heart showing fresh infarct in the wall of the left ventricle.

# MALPOSITION OF THE HEART

## DEXTROCARDIA AND ISOLATED LEVOCARDIA

A right-sided heart (dextrocardia) is an uncommon anomaly. It is seen in about one in 10,000 adult patients (Lowe and McKeown). However, the incidence is surely higher in the neonatal population, since many infants with dextrocardia have associated cardiac defects of such severity as to preclude survival. The incidence of isolated levocardia (left-sided heart with malposition of the abdominal viscera or asplenia) occurs in about 1 per cent of patients with congenital heart disease (Campbell and Forgacs).

A variety of types of dextrocardia and isolated levocardia have been described, and the reader is referred to the elegant work of Van Praagh for a more complete exposition of this subject. In general, the classification of the different types depends on the location of the abdominal viscera, the position of the great vessels and the presence or absence of the spleen.

The most familiar form of dextrocardia is that associated with situs inversus and inverted but normally related great arteries. The diagnosis in these patients is often made by chance on physical examination or during the course of a routine chest film. The prognosis is excellent. However, the situation is often quite different for other types of dextrocardia as well as levocardia. The diagnostic approach to identifying each of the different anatomical types is beyond the scope of this text and the reader is again referred to Van Praagh. Suffice it to say that complete studies are indicated before any decision regarding surgical treatment can be made. The prognosis depends on the nature of the defects. Not infrequently, these are very complex, and death during the newborn period or in early infancy is not uncommon.

# EBSTEIN'S ANOMALY

This is a rare anomaly. Signs and symptoms may occur during the first 2 decades, but a number of patients with this anomaly have signs at birth. Since the diagnosis may be suspected in the neonatal period on the basis of electrocardiographic findings, a description of this anomaly is warranted.

**PATHOLOGY.**    The posterior and septal leaves of the tricuspid valve are displaced downward and are attached to the right ventricle. Thus this chamber is divided into a small lower portion and an upper portion which is partially combined with the right atrium to form one large chamber. A patent foramen ovale or an atrial septal defect is always present. The right ventricular wall is often thin, and the right atrium is dilated.

**HEMODYNAMICS.**    Blood is regurgitated from the right ventricle to the right atrium through the displaced tricuspid valve. Right atrial pressure is high, and heart failure may occur very early in life if there is massive regurgitation. Pulmonary blood flow is reduced and there is a right-to-left shunt through the foramen ovale. Arterial oxygen unsaturation results.

**CLINICAL FEATURES.**    The clinical picture is variable. Cyanosis may be present shortly after birth, but is rarely severe. A systolic murmur is common, but not particularly characteristic. A triple or quadruple rhythm occurs frequently and was present in two of the three infants reported by Yamanchi and Cayler. One of their patients had heart failure, and another had transient episodes of paroxysmal tachycardia.

Radiologic examination reveals generalized cardiac enlargement and decreased lung vascularity. The electrocardiogram may show either a left or right axis deviation, right atrial hypertrophy, incomplete or complete right bundle branch block and a left ventricular dominance. The small R waves over the right precordium, characteristic of this condition, may not become apparent until later in infancy.

**DIAGNOSIS.**    This rare malformation has to be distinguished from other causes of cyanosis and diminished pulmonary lung vascularity such as pulmonary stenosis or atresia, hypoplastic right ventricle and tricuspid atresia. Although there are other distinguishing features, the electrocardiogram provides the most help. The presence of complete right bundle branch block should always suggest Ebstein's anomaly. Unusual cardiac rhythms are heard in

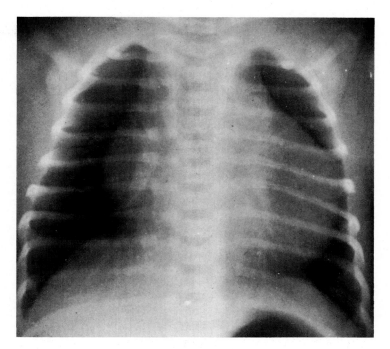

*Figure 23–21.* Ebstein's anomaly in a 2 day old infant. There is generalized cardiac enlargement, and the lung fields are avascular.

*anomalous pulmonary venous return,* but this malformation causes right ventricular hypertrophy.

*Cardiac catheterization* and *angiocardiography* are dangerous procedures when this anomaly is present, and deaths from cardiac arrhythmias have been reported. It may be necessary, however, to do limited right heart catheterization and selected venous angiograms to exclude severe pulmonary stenosis.

**PROGNOSIS.** Death during the neonatal period is rare. Keith, Rowe and Vlad report one patient who died at 3 days of age, and the patient reported below died at 4 days of life. The majority survive to the second or third decade of life.

**TREATMENT.** Anticongestive measures

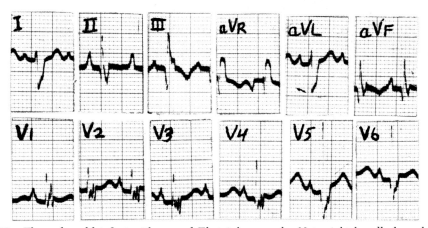

*Figure 23–22.* Three day old infant with proved Ebstein's anomaly. Note right bundle branch block, low R waves over the right precordium and tall R waves over the left precordium.

are indicated if heart failure is present. Infants with this anomaly often respond well to medical management. The three infants mentioned above thrived slowly for the first 2 months and thereafter gained normally (Yamanchi and Cayler). If heart failure is progressive, the creation of a shunt between the superior vena cava and pulmonary artery is the procedure of choice.

## CASE 23-14

A white female infant was born after a full-term normal pregnancy. Birth weight was 3.4 kg. Cyanosis was noted shortly after birth, and a systolic murmur was heard along the left sternal border. By 18 hours of age the heart was clinically enlarged, and there was hepatomegaly. The cyanosis was generalized and moderately severe. An x-ray film of the chest showed considerable cardiac enlargement and avascular lung fields (Fig. 23-21). The electrocardiogram showed right bundle branch block, a prolongation of the P-R interval, low R waves over the right precordium and a left ventricular pattern (Fig. 23-22). An angiocardiogram was done on the third day of life. This demonstrated a huge right atrium and a rudimentary right ventricle. On the fourth day of life a Glenn operation was attempted, but the infant expired before the procedure was completed. Autopsy examination showed Ebstein's anomaly of the tricuspid valve and left ventricular hypertrophy.

## REFERENCES

Ainger, L. E., and Pate, S. W.: Ostium secundum atrial septal defects and congestive heart failure in infancy. Am. J. Cardiol. *15*:380, 1965.

Armer, R. M., Shumacker, H. B., Lurie, P. R., and Fisch, C.: Origin of the left coronary artery from the pulmonary artery without collateral circulation. Pediatrics *32*:588, 1963.

Arcilla, R. A., et al.: Congestive heart failure from suspected ductal closure in utero. J. Pediat. *75*:75, 1969.

Arthur, A., Cottom, D., Evans, R., and Spencer, H.: Myocardial infarction in a newborn infant. J. Pediatr. *73*:110, 1968.

Auld, P. A. M.: Delayed closure of the ductus arteriosus. J. Pediatr. *69*:61, 1966.

Barratt-Boyes, B. G., et al.: Intracardiac surgery in neonates and infants. Circulation *43*:25, 1971.

Baylen, B. G., et al.: The critically ill infant with patent ductus and pulmonary disease—an echocardiographic assessment. J. Pediatr. *86*:423, 1975.

Benton, J. W., and others: Pulmonary atresia and stenosis with intact ventricular septum. Am. J. Dis. Child. *104*:161, 1962.

Blalock, A.: Surgical procedures employed and anatomical variations encountered in the treatment of congenital pulmonic stenosis. Surg. Gynec. Obstet. *87*:385, 1948.

Bopp, R. K., et al.: Surgical considerations for treatment of congenital tricuspid atresia and stenosis: With particular reference to vena cava-pulmonary artery anastomosis. J. Thorac. Cardiovasc. Surg. *43*:97, 1962.

Brink, A. J., and Neill, C. A.: The electrocardiogram in congenital heart disease, with special reference to left axis deviation. Circulation *12*:604, 1955.

Brock, R. C.: Pulmonary valvulotomy for the relief of congenital stenosis: Report of 3 cases. Br. Med. J. *1*:1121, 1948.

Burroughs, S., and Edwards, J. E.: Total anomalous venous connection. Am. Heart J. *59*:913, 1960.

Calodney, M. M., and Carson, J. J.: Coarctation of the aorta in early infancy. J. Pediatr. *37*:46, 1950.

Campbell, M.: Simple pulmonary stenosis. Pulmonary stenosis with closed ventricular septum. Br. Heart J. *16*:273, 1954.

Campbell, M.: Incidence of cardiac malformations at birth and later and neonatal mortality. Br. Heart J. *35*:189, 1973.

Campbell, M., and Forgacs, P.: Laevocardia with transposition of the abdominal viscera. Br. Heart J. *27*:69, 1965.

Carlgren, L. E.: The incidence of congenital heart disease in Gothenberg. Bull. Assoc. Euro. Pediatr. Cardio. *5*:2, 1969.

Champsaur, G. L., et al.: Repair of transposition of the great arteries in 123 pediatric patients. Circulation *37*:1032, 1973.

Collins, H. A., Harberg, F. J., Soltero, C. R., McNamara, D. G., and Cooley, D. A.: Cardiac surgery in the newborn. Surgery *45*:487, 1959.

Collins-Nakai, R., et. al.: Interrupted aortic arch in infancy. J. Pediatr. *88*:959, 1976.

Cooley, D. A., and Balas, P. E.: Total anomalous pulmonary venous drainage into inferior vena cava: Report of a successful correction. Surgery *51*:798, 1962.

Danilowicz, D., Rudolph, A. M., and Hoffman, J. I. E.: Delayed closure of the ductus arteriosus in premature infants. Pediatrics *37*:74, 1966.

Darling, R. C., Rothney, W. B., and Craig, J. M.: Total pulmonary venous drainage into the right side of the heart; report of 17 autopsied cases not associated with other major cardiovascular anomalies. Lab. Invest. *6*:44, 1957.

Davignon, A. L., Greenwald, W. E., DuShane, J. W., and Edwards, J. E.: Congenital pulmonary atresia with intact ventricular septum. Am. Heart J. *62*:591, 1961.

de Leval, M. R., et al.: Total anomalous venous drainage to superior vena cava associated with preductal coarctation of aorta. Br. Heart J. *35*:1098, 1973.

Downing, D.: Congenital aortic stenosis: Clinical aspects and surgical treatment. Circulation *14*:188, 1956.

Edie, R. N., et al.: Surgical repair of single ventricle. J. Thorac. Cardiovasc. Surg. *66*:350, 1973.

Edmunds, L. H., et al.: Surgical closure of the ductus arteriosus in premature infants. Circulation *48*:856, 1973.

Edwards, J. E., and Burchell, H. B.: Pathologic anatomy of mitral insufficiency. Proc. Staff Meet. Mayo Clin. *33*:497, 1958.

Edwards, J. H., Hamden, D. G., Cameron, A. H.,

Crosse, V. M., and Wolfe, O. H.: A new trisomic syndrome. Lancet 1:787, 1960.

Elliot, L. P., Anderson, R. C., Tuna, N., Adams, P., and Neufeld, H. N.: Complete transposition of the great vessels II. An electrocardiographic analysis. Circulation 27:1118, 1963.

Elliot, L. P., Neufeld, H. N., Anderson, R. C., Adams, P., and Edwards, J. E.: Complete transposition of the great vessels I. An anatomic study of sixty cases. Circulation 27:1105, 1963.

Emerit, I., de Grouchy, J., Vernant, P., and Corone, P.: Chromosomal Abnormalities and Congenital Heart Disease. Circulation 36:886, 1967.

Evans, J. R., Rowe, R. D., and Keith, J. D.: Spontaneous closure of ventricular septal defects. Circulation 22:1044, 1960.

Ferencz, C., Johnson, A. L., and Wiglesworth, F. W.: Congenital mitral stenosis. Circulation 9:161, 1954.

Fontan, F., et al.: Surgical repair of tricuspid atresia. Thorax 27:111, 1971.

Freundlich, E., Engle, M. E., and Goldberg, H. P.: Coarctation of the aorta in infancy. Analysis of a 10-year experience with medical management. Pediatrics 27:427, 1961.

Friedli, B., et al.: Infradiaphragmatic anomalous pulmonary venous return: Surgical correction in a newborn infant. J. Thorac. Cardiovasc. Surg. 62:301, 1971.

Gibson, S., White, H., Johnson, F., and Potts, W. J.: Congenital pulmonary stenosis with intact ventricular septum. A.M.A. J. Dis. Child. 87:26, 1954.

Girling, D. J., and Hallidie-Smith, K. A.: Persistent ductus arteriosus in ill and premature babies. Arch. Dis. Child. 46:177, 1971.

Godman, M. J.: Echocardiography in the evaluation of the cyanotic newborn infant. Br. Heart J. 36:154, 1973.

Goldring, D., Behrer, M. R., Thomas, W. A., McCoy, E., and O'Neal, R. M.: Clinical and pathological observations in infants with coarctation of the aorta and patent ductus arteriosus. J. Pediatr. 51:18, 1957.

Gott, V. L., Lester, R. G., Lillehei, C. W., and Varco, R. L.: Total anomalous pulmonary return. An analysis of thirty cases. Circulation 13:543, 1956.

Hallidie-Smith, K. A.: Murmur of persistent ductus arteriosus in premature infants. Arch. Dis. Child. 47:725, 1972.

Harris, G. B. C., Newhauser, E. B. D., and Gildion, A.: Total anomalous pulmonary venous return below the diaphragm. Am. J. Roentgenol. 84:436, 1960.

Hoffman, J. I. E., and Rudolph, A. M.: The natural history of ventricular septal defects in infancy. Am. J. Cardiol. 16:634, 1965.

Hornblad, P. Y.: Ductus arteriosus and the mechanism of closure. New Engl. J. Med. 282:566, 1970.

Husson, G. S., Blackman, M. S., Riemenschneider, P., and Berne, A. S.: Isolated congenital mitral insufficiency. J. Pediatr. 64:248, 1964.

Jaffe, H. S., et al.: Subdiaphragmatic total anomalous pulmonary venous drainage: Report of a successful surgical correction. Am. Heart J. 81:250, 1971.

Johnson, A. C., Wigelsworth, F. W., Dunbar, J. S., Siddoo, S., and Grajo, M.: Infradiaphragmatic total anomalous pulmonary drainage. Circulation 17:340, 1958.

Keith, J. D.: Congestive heart failure. Review Article. Pediatrics 18:491, 1956.

Keith, J. D., and Forsyth, C.: Aortography in infants. Circulation 2:907, 1950.

Keith, J. D., Rowe, R. D., and Vlad, P.: Heart Disease in Infancy and Childhood. New York, Macmillan Company, 1958.

Kiely, B., Morales, F., and Rosenblum, D.: Pulmonary atresia with intact ventricular septum. Pediatrics 32:841, 1963.

Kitterman, J. A., et al.: Patent ductus arteriosus in premature infants. N. Engl. J. Med. 287:473, 1972.

Kreidberg, M. B., Fisher, J. H., DeLuca, F. G., and Chernoff, H. L.: Pulmonary artery banding for persistent truncus arteriosus. J. Pediatr. 64:557, 1964.

Krovetz, L. J., and Rowe, R. D.: Patent ductus, prematurity and pulmonary disease. N. Engl. J. Med. 287:513, 1972.

Lambert, E. C., Canent, R. V., and Hohn, A. R.: Congenital Cardiac Anomalies in the Newborn. Pediatrics 37:343, 1966.

Lambert, E. C., MacManus, J. E., and Paine, J. R.: Indications for and results of cardiac surgery in infants. New York State J. Med. 55:2471, 1955.

Landtman, B.: Clinical and morphological studies in congenital heart disease: Review of 777 cases. Acta Pediatr. Scand. (Suppl.) 213:1, 1971.

Lang, H. T., and Nadas, A. S.: Coarctation of the aorta with congestive heart failure in infancy—medical treatment. Pediatrics 17:45, 1956.

Lev, M.: Pathologic anatomy and interrelationship of hypoplasia of the aortic tract complexes. Lab. Invest. 1:61, 1952.

Lev, M., Alcalde, V. M., and Baffes, T. G.: Pathologic anatomy of complete transposition of the arterial trunks. Pediatrics 28:293, 1961.

Lichtman, S. S.: Isolated congenital dextrocardia; report of two cases with unusual electrocardiographic findings; anatomic, clinical, roentgenographic and electrocardiographic studies of the cases reported in the literature. Arch. Int. Med. 48:683, 866, 1931.

Liebman, J., and Nadas, A. S.: The vector cardiogram in the differential diagnosis of atrial septal defect in children. Circulation 22:956, 1960.

Liebman, J., et al.: Natural history of transposition of the great arteries: Anatomy and birth and death characteristics. Circulation 40:237, 1969.

Lillehei, C. W., et al.: Direct vision intracardiac surgical correction of the tetralogy of Fallot, pentalogy of Fallot and pulmonary atresia defects. Report of first ten cases. Ann. Surg. 142:418, 1955.

Litwin, S. B., et al.: Surgical resection of coarctation of the aorta in infancy. J. Pediatr. Surg. 6:307, 1971.

Lowe, C. R., and McKeown, T.: An investigation of dextrocardia with and without transposition of abdominal viscera. Ann. Eugenics 18:267, 1954.

Mair, D. D., et al.: Selection of patients with truncus arteriosus for surgical correction. Circulation 46:144, 1974.

Malm, J. R., et al.: Results of surgical treatment of pulmonary atresia with intact ventricular septum. Adv. Cardiol. 11:18, 1974.

Manson, M. M., Logan, W. P. D., and Loy, R. M.: Rubella and other virus infections during pregnancy. Reports on Public Health and Medical Subjects, No. 101, London, 1960.

Marquis, R. M., and Logan, A.: Congenital aortic stenosis and its surgical treatment. Brit. Heart J. 17:373, 1955.

McDonald, A. D.: Congenital defects associated with prematurity. Arch. Dis. Child. 37:277, 1962.

McMurphy, D. M., et al.: Developmental changes in constriction of the ductus arteriosus. Pediatr. Res. 6:231, 1972.

Mehrizi, A., Hirsch, M. S., and Taussig, H. B.: Congenital heart disease in the neonatal period. J. Pediatr. 65:721, 1964.

Meredith, G., et al.: Management of coarctation of the aorta in the first six weeks of life. Thorax 25:413, 1970.

Meyer, R. A., and Kaplan, S.: Echocardiography in diagnosis of hypoplasia of the left or right ventricle in neonatal congenital heart disease. Circulation 46:55, 1972.

Miller, R. A., Baffles, T. G., and Wilkinson, A. A., Jr.: Transpositions of the great vessels: Diagnostic considerations and surgical therapy. Pediat. Clin. N. Amer. 5:1109, 1958.

Mitchell, S. C.: The ductus arteriosus in the neonatal period. J. Pediatr. 51:12, 1957.

Mitchell, S. C., Korones, S. B., and Berendes, V. W.: Congenital heart disease in 56,109 births. Circulation 43:323, 1971.

Mitchell, S., et al.: Etiologic correlates in a study of congenital heart defects in 56,109 births. Am. J. Cardiol. 28:653, 1971.

Montgomery, J. R., et al.: Congenital anomalies and herpesvirus infection. Am. J. Dis. Child. 126:364, 1973.

Muller, W. H., Jr., and Dammann, J. F., Jr.: The treatment of certain congenital malformations of the heart by the creation of pulmonic stenosis to reduce pulmonary hypertension and excessive pulmonary blood flow. Surg., Gynec. Obstet. 95:213, 1952.

Murphy, D. A., et al.: Management of premature infants with patent ductus arteriosus. J. Cardiovasc. Surg. 67:221, 1974.

Mustard, W. T., Keith, J. D., Trusler, G. A., Fowler, R., and Kidd, L.: The surgical management of transposition of the great vessels. J. Thorac. Cardiovasc. Surg. 48:953, 1964.

Mustard, W. T., Rowe, R. D., and Firor, W. B.: Pulmonic stenosis in the first year of life. Results of surgery. Surgery 47:678, 1960.

Mustard, W. T., Rowe, R. D., Keith, J. D., and Sirek, A.: Coarctation of the aorta, with special reference to the first year of life. Ann. Surg. 141:429, 1955.

Nadas, A. S., Scott, L. P., Hauck, A. J., and Rudolph, A. M.: Spontaneous functional closing of ventricular septal defects. New Engl. J. Med. 264:309, 1961.

Nadas, A. S., and Fyler, D. C.: Pediatric Cardiology. 3rd ed. Philadelphia, W. B. Saunders Company, 1972.

Noonan, J. A., and Nadas, A. S.: The hypoplastic left heart syndrome. Pediat. Clin. N. Amer. 5:1029, 1958.

Nora, J. J.: Multifactorial inheritance hypothesis for the etiology of congenital heart disease. Circulation 38:604, 1968.

Nora, J. J., Gilliland, J. C., Sommerville, R. J., and McNamara, D. G.: Congenital heart disease in twins. New Engl. J. Med. 277:568, 1967.

Nora, J. J., and Meyer, T. C.: Familial nature of congenital heart diseases. Pediatrics 37:329, 1966.

Nora, J. J., et al.: Risk to offspring of parents with congenital heart defects. J.A.M.A. 209:2052, 1969.

Nora, J. J., et al.: Empiric recurrence risks in common

and uncommon congenital heart lesions. Teratology 3:322, 1970.

Nora, J. J., et al.: Dextroamphetamine, a possible environmental trigger in cardiovascular malformations. Lancet 1:1290, 1971.

Oschner, J. L., Cooley, D. A., McNamara, D. G., and Kline, A.: Surgical treatment of cardiovascular anomalies in 300 infants younger than one year of age. J. Thorac. Cardiovasc. Surg. 43:182, 1962.

Potts, W. J., Smith, S., and Gibson, S.: Anastomosis of the aorta to a pulmonary artery. J.A.M.A. 132:627, 1946.

Rashkind, W. J., and Miller, W. W.: Creation of an atrial defect without thoracotomy. J.A.M.A. 196:991, 1966.

Rastelli, G. C., et al.: Surgical repair of the complete form of persistent common atrioventricular canal. J. Thorac. Cardiovasc. Surg. 55:299, 1968.

Reisman, M., Hipona, F. A., Bloor, C. M., and Talner, N. S.: Congenital tricuspid insufficiency: A cause of massive cardiomegaly and heart failure in the neonate. J. Pediatr. 66:869, 1965.

Richards, M. R., Merritt, K. K., Samuels, M. H., and Langmann, A. G.: Congenital malformations of the cardiovascular system in a series of 6053 infants. Pediatrics 15:12, 1955.

Rogers, H.: Recherches cliniques sur la communication congénitale des deux coeurs, par inocclusion du septum interventricularis. Bull. Acad. de Méd., Paris 8:1074, 1879.

Rogers, H. M., and Edwards, J. E.: Incomplete division of the atrioventricular canal with patent interatrial foramen primum (persistent common atrioventricular ostium). Report of five cases and review of the literature. Am. Heart J. 36:28, 1948.

Ross, D. N., and Somerville, J.: Surgical correction of tricuspid atresia. Lancet 1:845, 1973.

Rowe, R. D.: Maternal rubella and pulmonary stenoses. Pediatrics 32:180, 1963.

Rowe, R. D., and Cleary, T. E.: Congenital cardiac malformations in the newborn period. Can. Med. Assoc. J. 83:299, 1960.

Rowe, R. D., and Mehrizi, A.: The Neonate with Congenital Heart Disease. Philadelphia, W. B. Saunders Company, 1968.

Rowe, R. D., and Uchida, I. A.: Cardiac malformation in mongolism. A prospective study of 184 mongoloid children. Am. J. Med. 31:726, 1961.

Rowland, T. W., et al.: Congenital heart disease in infants of diabetic mothers. J. Pediatr. 83:815, 1973.

Rudolph, A. M., Mayer, F. E., Nadas, A. S., and Gross, R.: Patent ductus arteriosus. Pediatrics 22:892, 1958.

Rudolph, A. M., et al.: Formalin infiltration of the ductus arteriosus. A method for palliation of infants with selected congenital cardiac lesions. N. Engl. J. Med. 292:1263, 1975.

Sabiston, D. C., Neill, C. A., and Taussig, H. B.: The direction of blood flow in anomalous left coronary artery arising from the pulmonary artery. Circulation 22:591, 1960.

Shigeru, S., et al.: Successful total correction of common ventricle. Chest 61:192, 1972.

Sinka, S. N., et al.: Coarctation of the aorta in infancy. Circulation 40:385, 1969.

Starkey, G. W. B.: Surgical experiences in the treatment of congenital mitral stenosis and mitral insufficiency. J. Thorac. Cardiovasc. Surg. 38:336, 1959.

Taguchi, K., et al.: Surgical experience with persistent

common atrioventricular canal. J. Thorac. Cardiovasc. Surg. 55:501, 1968.

Talner, N. S., and Campbell, A. G. M.: Recognition and management of cardiologic problems in the newborn infant. In Friedman, W. F., et al. (Eds.): Neonatal Heart Disease. New York, Grune & Stratton, 1973.

Tandon, R., and Edwards, J. E.: Tricuspid atresia: A re-evaluation and classification. J. Thorac. Cardiovasc. Surg. 46:530, 1974.

Tanner-Cain, N., and Crump, E. P.: Situs inversus. Report of three cases and a review of the literature. J. Pediatr. 38:199, 1951.

Taussig, H. B.: Congenital Malformations of the Heart. New York, Commonwealth Fund, 1947.

Tedeschi, C. G., and Halpern, M. M.: Heterotopic origin of both coronary arteries from the pulmonary artery: Review of literature and report of a case not complicated by associated defects. Pediatrics 14:53, 1954.

Toscano-Barbosa, E., DuShane, J. W., Wade, G., and Wright, J. P.: Spontaneous closure of ventricular septal defects. Lancet 1:737, 1963.

Van Mierop, L. H. S., and Gessner, I. H.: Pathogenetic mechanisms in congenital cardiac malformation.

In Friedman, W. F., et al. (Eds.): Neonatal Heart Disease. New York, Grune & Stratton, 1973.

Van Praagh, R.: Malposition of the heart. In Moss, A. J., and Adams, F. H. (Eds.): Heart Disease in Infants, Children and Adolescents. Baltimore, Williams & Wilkins Co., 1968.

Van Praagh, R., Van Praagh, S., Vlad, P., and Keith, J. D.: Diagnosis of the anatomic types of single or common ventricle. Am. J. Cardiol. 15:345, 1965.

Vogelpoel, L., and Schrire, V.: Auscultatory and phonocardiographic assessment of Fallot's tetralogy. Circulation 22:73, 1960.

Wade, G., and Wright, J. P.: Spontaneous closure of ventricular septal defects. Lancet 1:737, 1963.

Wallace, R. B., et al.: Complete atrioventricular canal: Repair and results. Adv. Cardiol. 11:26, 1974.

Watson, D. G., and Rowe, R. D.: Aortic-valve atresia. J.A.M.A. 179:112, 1962.

Yamanchi, T., and Cayler, G. G.: Ebstein's anomaly in the neonate. Am. J. Dis. Child. 107:165, 1964.

Zachman, R. D., et al.: Incidence and treatment of the patent ductus arteriosus in the ill premature neonate. Am. Heart J. 87:697, 1974.

Ziegler, R. F., and Lam, C. R.: Indications for the surgical correction of coarctation of the aorta in infancy. Am. J. Cardiol. 12:60, 1963.

# MYOCARDITIS

## By Milton Markowitz

# 24

Myocarditis occurs in all age groups, but there is higher frequency in the first month than any other period of life. It is a well recognized entity with a clinical pattern sufficiently distinctive to make an antemortem diagnosis. Although often a fulminant disease, it is not invariably fatal, and early recognition and prompt treatment may alter the outcome.

INCIDENCE. For the 50 years following Fiedler's original description of primary myocarditis, only a few isolated cases had been reported in the first month of life. An exception was the report by Lind and Hultquist of five patients with myocarditis, four of whom were less than 3 weeks old. Since 1950 there has been a striking increase in the number of reported cases, particularly among newborn infants. Twenty-five newborns with myocarditis were reported within a 2-year period (Montgomery et al.; Javett et al.; Van Creveld and de Jager). Numerous other reports have since appeared (Kibrick and Benirschke; Sussman et al.; Robino et al.).

ETIOLOGY. Any infective agent can cause myocarditis, and examples of two uncommon etiologic agents, toxoplasma and staphylococcus, are described in case reports at the end of this chapter. However, viruses, chiefly group B Coxsackie, are the main cause of myocarditis in the newborn. The most conclusive evidence was presented first by Kibrick and Benirschke in a report of a 7-day-old infant with acute myocarditis and meningoencephalitis from whom a Coxsackie B virus was recovered. This same virus produced a similar myocardial lesion in suckling mice. By 1961 Kibrick was able to collect 54 cases in the neonatal period due to group B Coxsackie viruses. Of this group, 28 were infected during nursery outbreaks with the mother as the original source of the infection in many instances. Among the 26 sporadic cases there were a significant number in whom the infant's illness was associated with a febrile illness in the mother. There is some evidence that in a few patients the infection was acquired in utero, but the majority appear to have been acquired postnatally. However, asymptomatic infants in the nursery may also be a source of infection (Brightman et al.).

Neonatal myocarditis may be caused by viruses other than Coxsackie B. Herpes simplex virus has been isolated from the heart of a newborn infant dying of disseminated disease (Wright and Miller). Myocarditis may be caused by the rubella virus, although this agent has never been isolated from the heart. It has been suggested that rubella myocarditis occurs in utero and may progress after birth, leaving myocardial damage (Ainger, et al.; Harris and Nghiem).

**PATHOLOGY.** On gross examination the heart is enlarged and dilated. The cardiac muscle feels flabby and is often pale or nutmeg-like in color. Microscopic examination reveals a multicellular infiltration of the myocardium. Lymphocytes, large mononuclear cells, eosinophils and polymorphonuclear leukocytes are present in varying numbers with either patchy or diffuse distribution. Necrosis and fragmentation of muscle fibers may be present. Although rare in patients with primary myocarditis, involvement of the endocardium and pericardium may occur. When the Coxsackie virus is the etiologic agent, involvement of other organs, particularly the central nervous system, is common. Involvement of multiple organs is even more common with rubella and herpes viruses.

**CLINICAL FINDINGS.** The clinical course of young infants with myocarditis is variable. The initial symptoms may be mild and include lethargy, failure to feed, vomiting or diarrhea. Jaundice may be present, and evidence of a mild upper respiratory tract infection is sometimes noted. In the milder forms of the disease clinical manifestations may be limited to slight tachypnea, tachycardia and poor heart sounds. In the outbreak described by Javett and co-workers the course of the illness was occasionally biphasic with early signs of infection followed by temporary improvement. Frequently there are no premonitory

symptoms whatsoever. The infant becomes seriously ill very suddenly. Respirations increase, become labored, and are often accompanied by a grunt. The infant appears restless and anxious. The skin is pale, mottled and mildly cyanotic. The temperature may be slightly or greatly elevated or subnormal. The pulse rate is usually rapid, between 150 and 200, and weak. Occasionally bradycardia is present. The percussion note over the chest may be normal or hyperresonant. Dullness is uncommon. The breath sounds are usually harsh, and rales may be heard at the bases. Although there is always some degree of cardiac enlargement, it is often difficult to detect clinically. The heart sounds are mushy, particularly the first sound, and a gallop rhythm may be present. The liver is almost invariably enlarged. Edema is an uncommon finding, and venous engorgement is almost never detected. There may be signs referable to central nervous system involvement.

X-ray films of the chest show generalized cardiac enlargement as well as haziness of the lung fields. At times it is not possible to make the distinction between congestion and pneumonia. Electrocardiograms will often show abnormalities. Low-voltage QRS complexes and either low, isoelectric or inverted T waves are the most frequent findings. There may also be significant disturbances in conduction such as heart block, extrasystoles, and ventricular or atrial tachycardia. The electrocardiographic abnormalities are frequently transient. Although usually not helpful in the acute stage, viral studies should be carried out.

**DIAGNOSIS.** The diagnosis of myocarditis should be suspected in any neonate with a cardiac disorder in whom congenital heart disease has been excluded. The suspicion should be heightened if there is a known respiratory infection in the mother or proved viral illness in other nursery infants. The diagnosis can be confirmed by the recovery of virus from the nasopharynx and the stool or by the development of neutralizing antibodies.

The acute form of myocarditis is commonly mistaken for overwhelming *sepsis* or a severe *lower respiratory tract infection.* This is especially true for the latter, since cyanosis and respiratory distress may initially suggest pneumonia. Myocarditis should be suspected if there are an inordinate tachycardia, poor heart sounds with or without gallop rhythm, a degree of dyspnea out of proportion to the pulmonary findings, and cardiac enlargement on x-ray examination.

Myocarditis must also be differentiated from other cardiac conditions which may occur in the neonatal period: congenital heart disease with congestive failure precipitated by infection, the acute form of endocardial fibroelastosis, and paroxysmal tachycardia.

CONGENITAL HEART DISEASE. The absence of heart murmurs does not rule out this possibility. On occasion infants with a large left-to-right shunt have an insignificant murmur in the neonatal period. Coarctation of the aorta, a not uncommon cause of heart failure in the neonate, must always be excluded by careful evaluation of the arm-leg pulses and blood pressure.

ENDOCARDIAL FIBROELASTOSIS. In this condition there is usually left ventricular hypertrophy indicated in electrocardiographic tracings by high-voltage R waves in precordial leads taken over the left side of the heart. But the left ventricular pattern may not be as striking in the first few days or weeks of life. In myocarditis low-voltage complexes are characteristic and are the result of severe disturbances in myocardial function. Occasionally infants with endocardial fibroelastosis in severe failure may have low voltage temporarily.

PAROXYSMAL TACHYCARDIA. Congestive heart failure is frequently present, but in this condition the heart rate is usually much more rapid than in myocarditis. It must be borne in mind, however, that myocarditis may precipitate an attack of paroxysmal tachycardia (Lind and Hultquist).

Mild forms of myocarditis are particularly difficult to recognize. Signs of heart failure may not be prominent or may be absent entirely. The clinical manifestations may include pallor, slight increase in the respiratory rate, tachycardia and poor heart sounds. Such findings in an infant who has signs of infection and who appears to have a disproportionate degree of cardiac embarrassment should suggest the possibility of myocarditis. Although electrocardiographic studies may aid in the diagnosis, there is no specific pattern, nor does a normal tracing rule out the disorder.

TREATMENT. Young infants with myocarditis may become critically ill with such rapidity that treatment should be instituted as soon as the diagnosis is suspected. Minimal handling is essential, and laboratory studies should be deferred in the more severe cases. Oral feedings should be discontinued, and basal water and electrolyte requirement maintained by parenteral means during this critical period.

Oxygen therapy and digitalization should be started at once. The rapidly acting digitalis preparations should be used. For more complete details on digitalis dosage and anticongestive measures see the chapter on Treatment (p. 309). However, it should be emphasized here that patients with myocarditis may be unusually sensitive to digitalis and should be monitored carefully for toxicity.

Although the etiologic agent in myocarditis is frequently viral, bacterial infections of the lung are common, and antibiotics should be given. After the initial digitalization the patient should be maintained on digitalis until the heart has returned to normal size and the pulse is within normal limits.

PREVENTION. The fact that viral and bacterial agents may cause neonatal myocarditis emphasizes the need for preventive measures in carrying out nursery routine. The Coxsackie virus may cause minor or inapparent illnesses in adults and yet lead to serious, often fatal disease in newborn infants. Reports of outbreaks in nurseries suggest the infectious nature of this disorder. For these reasons stress must be placed on the absolute necessity for careful isolation of the mother and the newborn during the course of even mild respiratory infections.

PROGNOSIS. The prognosis in infants with fulminating disease is poor. Patients are on occasion "crib deaths" or arrive at the hospital moribund. Yet, even the severe form of the disease need not be invariably fatal. Four of the 10 patients reported by Javett and his associates and two of the three patients in another series recovered (Montgomery et al.). Suckling and Vogelpoel reported a 50 per cent mortality in 8 neonates. Among the 54 cases collected by Kibrick, 12 patients survived. Undoubtedly milder forms of the disease occur, and the recovery rate in this group is high. In a study of children 13 years after an attack of neonatal myocarditis, no clinical or laboratory abnormalities were found (Suckling and Vogelpoel). It is possible that, as the awareness of neonatal myocarditis as a clinical entity increases, earlier diagnosis and more vigorous supportive treatment will improve the over-all mortality rate.

## CASE HISTORIES

### CASE 24–1

A baby was delivered by cesarean section in the thirty-sixth week of a third pregnancy. There was severe preeclampsia with the first pregnancy followed by postpartum renal shutdown. The second pregnancy resulted in a spontaneous abortion during the first trimester. This third pregnancy was terminated because of severe periumbilical pain suggesting a ruptured uterus. No explanation for this symptom was found. The mother had low-grade fever on the second postoperative day, and this continued for one week. Her physical examination was negative except for nasal congestion and breast engorgement.

The infant weighed 7 pounds (3170 gm) at birth. He breathed and cried spontaneously, and his physical examination was negative. The infant was handled by his mother on her first and second postpartum days, but was isolated after the mother's fever had been discovered. He was well until the eighth day of life, when he suddenly refused his feeding and was found at that time to have a temperature of 101.4° F.

Physical examination revealed an acutely ill, listless infant with a pale grayish color and a weak cry. The respirations were 160 per minute, with little retraction. There was a tachycardia (200 per minute). The lung fields were clear. The heart was questionably enlarged. The sounds were of fair quality. There were no murmurs. The liver edge was 4 cm below the left costal margin. All the peripheral pulses were weak.

A diagnosis of heart failure probably secondary to primary myocarditis was made. He was placed in oxygen, was given large doses of antibiotics, and was digitalized intravenously with Cedilanid. There was no response to treatment, and he died 5 hours after the onset of illness. Before death he had two loose stools.

His white blood cell count was 13,600, with 60 per cent lymphocytes. The stool culture was negative. The postmortem blood and cerebrospinal fluid cultures were negative. The electrocardiogram disclosed low voltage in leads II, $V_5$ and $V_6$ with elevation of the S-T segments. The postmortem x-ray film revealed generalized cardiac enlargement.

An autopsy was performed by Dr. William Lovitt and staff. The single noteworthy finding was a patchy cellular infiltration throughout the myocardium. Viral studies were carried out at

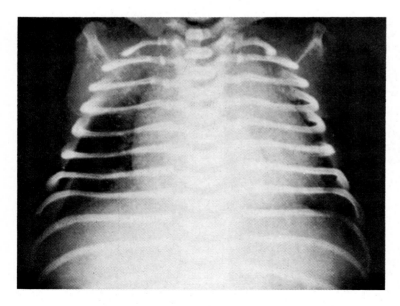

*Figure 24–1.* Generalized cardiac enlargement caused by toxoplasma myocarditis.

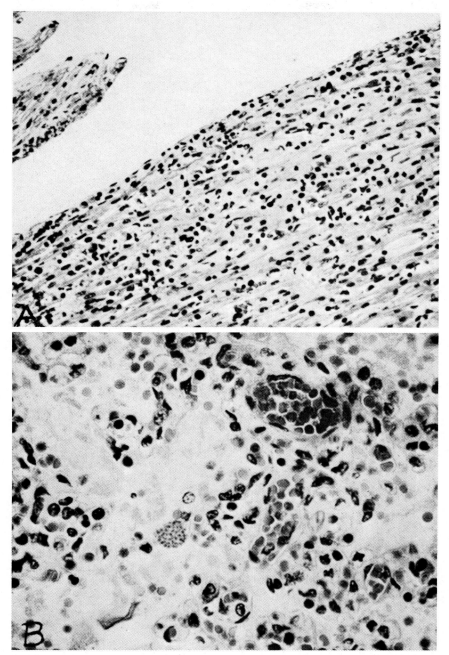

***Figure 24-2.*** *A*, Microscopic section of the heart showing diffuse cellular infiltration in the myocardium. *B*, Microscopic section of myocardium showing cellular infiltration and toxoplasma.

the University of Maryland virus laboratories through the kindness of Dr. Theodore Woodward and his staff. Cultures from the myocardium grew out Coxsackie virus, group B, type 2. Neutralizing antibodies for this virus were demonstrated in the mother's serum.

**COMMENT.** This is a typical story for the fulminant form of Coxsackie myocarditis. A nursery infant who is entirely well contracts his mother's mild or inapparent infection. Several days later there is sudden onset of heart failure. The type of onset, the absence of any evidence for a congenital cardiac defect and the diffuse electrocardiographic changes suggested the diagnosis of myocarditis. The Coxsackie virus isolated was group B, type 2. This is in contrast to the group B, type 4 Coxsackie, which has been the common offender reported in nursery outbreaks.

### CASE 24–2

(This case is abstracted with the kind permission of Drs. Harold Harrison and Abou Pollack of Baltimore.)

An infant was delivered after a 37-week pregnancy complicated by mild toxemia. The labor and delivery were uncomplicated, but meconium-stained fluid was noted. The birth weight was 6 pounds 6 ounces (2900 gm). A weak cry and cyanosis were noted at birth. The respirations were labored. There were many fine rales over the lung fields. The heart rate was 120 per minute, and the sounds were of fair quality. On clinical examination cardiac enlargement was not detected. The liver was enlarged to the level of the umbilicus. There was no edema.

Treatment with oxygen was started. Digitalization with lanatoside C was begun. Antimicrobial therapy was started. There was no response to treatment, and death occurred about 3 hours after birth. Blood and cerebrospinal fluid cultures were sterile. An x-ray film of the chest revealed a greatly enlarged heart (Fig. 24–1).

An autopsy was performed by Dr. Pollack. This revealed hydrothorax, hydropericardium, ascites and pneumonia. The heart was grossly enlarged. Microscopic sections showed a diffuse myocarditis characterized by interstitial infiltration of mononuclear lymphoid cells with a few polymononuclear leukocytes (Fig. 24–2, A). One muscle cell containing toxoplasma was found (Fig. 24–2, B). The alveoli showed foamy macrophages, some filled with toxoplasma. Similar lesions were found in the brain and the adrenals.

### CASE 24–3

An infant was delivered 3 weeks before term in an otherwise uneventful pregnancy. Delivery was complicated by a face presentation. The infant breathed and cried spontaneously. Birth weight was 4½ pounds (2025 gm). He appeared well until 12 hours of age, when a brief period of apnea occurred. He was then well until the fourth day of life, when a subnormal temperature (95° F.) was noted. He became lethargic and took feedings poorly, and mild jaundice developed. His physical examination was not remarkable. His blood cell count, cultures and chest x-ray were within normal limits. He was treated with antibiotics for possible infection. There was a gradual improvement until the twelfth day of life, when he again became lethargic and fed poorly. Examination revealed pallor and a relative bradycardia. The heart sounds were poor and at times barely audible. There was neither clinical nor x-ray evidence of cardiac enlargement. No murmurs were heard. The liver increased in size to 3 cm below the costal margin. An electrocardiogram revealed a bizarre pattern with major conduction disturbances consisting of an alternating atrioventricular

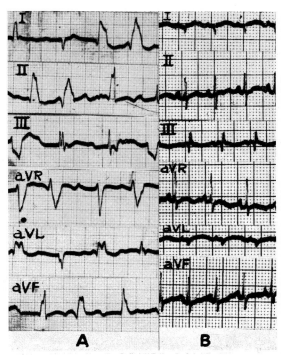

*Figure 24–3.* A, Standard and unipolar limb leads showing conduction disturbances with variable atrioventricular block, bundle branch block and multifocal ventricular complexes. B, Standard and unipolar limb leads showing return to normal rhythm 24 hours later.

block, bundle branch block and multifocal ventricular complexes (Fig. 24–3, *A*). He was treated with antimicrobial agents and oxygen. On the following day his over-all condition improved, the heart sounds were normal, and the electrocardiogram showed only some tachycardia (Fig. 24–3, *B*). He made an uneventful recovery.

**COMMENT.** The findings of jaundice, lethargy, loss of appetite and subnormal temperature in this premature infant suggested the presence of an infection. His course was biphasic, and the only signs of localization were related to the heart. These signs included a profound change in the quality of the heart sounds, evidence of early failure and a totally abnormal electrocardiogram. The biphasic nature of the illness was not unlike that reported by Javett and co-workers. The transient nature of the electrocardiographic findings is not unusual in myocarditis. Although the diagnosis was not proved, the findings strongly suggest the presence of myocarditis in this infant.

### REFERENCES

Ainger, L. E., et al.: Neonatal rubella myocarditis. Br. Heart J. 28:691, 1966.

Brightman, V. S., Scott, T. F., Westphal, M., and Boggs, T. R.: An outbreak of Coxsackie B-5 virus infection in a newborn nursery. J. Pediatr. 69:179, 1966.

Fiedler, A.: Ueber akute interstitielle Myocarditis. Zentralbl. inn. Med. 21:212, 1900.

Harris, L. C., and Nghiem, Q. X.: Cardiomyopathies. *In* Neonatal Heart Disease. New York, Grune and Stratton, 1973.

Javett, S. N., and others: Myocarditis in the newborn infant: Study of an outbreak associated with Coxsackie group B virus in a maternity home in Johannesburg. J. Pediatr. 48:1, 1956.

Kibrick, S.: Viral infections of the fetus and newborn. *In* M. Pollard (Ed.): Perspectives in Virology. Minneapolis, Burgess Publishing Co., 1961, Vol. II, pp. 140–157.

Kibrick, S., and Benirschke, K.: Acute aseptic myocarditis in the newborn child infected with Coxsackie virus, group B, type 3. New Engl. J. Med., 255:883, 1956.

Kibrick, S., and Benirschke, K.: Severe generalized disease occurring in the newborn period and due to infection with Coxsackie virus, group B. Pediatrics 22:857, 1958.

Lind, J., and Hultquist, G. T.: Isolated myocarditis in newborn and young infants. Am. Heart J. 38:123, 1949.

Montgomery, J., Gear, J., Prinslov, F. R., Kahn, M., and Kirsch, Z.: Myocarditis of newborn: Outbreak in a maternity home in Southern Rhodesia associated with Coxsackie group B virus infection. South African M. J. 29:608, 1955.

Robino, G., Perlman, A., Togo, Y., and Reback, J.: Fatal neonatal infection due to Coxsackie B₂ virus. J. Pediatr. 61:911, 1962.

Sussman, M. L., Strauss, L., and Hodes, H. L.: Fatal Coxsackie group B virus infection in the newborn. A.M.A. J. Dis. Child. 97:482, 1959.

Van Creveld, S., and de Jager, H.: Myocarditis in newborn caused by Coxsackie virus. Ann. Paediatr. 187:100, 1956.

Wright, H. T., and Miller, A.: Fatal infection in a newborn infant due to herpes simplex virus. J. Pediatr. 67:130, 1965.

# CARDIAC ARRHYTHMIAS

## 25

*By Milton Markowitz*

The heart rate in the normal newborn infant varies between 70 and 180 per minute with an average of 120 to 130 beats per minute. Sinus arrhythmia is not uncommon (Morgan and Guntheroth). Extrasystoles and bradycardia with nodal escape may occur, especially in prematures (Morgan et al.). Arrhythmias have been recorded in utero by fetal electrocardiography and may continue after birth (Hon and Huang). Most of these arrhythmias are not important and can be disregarded.

Significant disorders of rate and rhythm are encountered infrequently in the neonatal period. They are of two main types: the atrial tachycardias and heart block.

### ATRIAL TACHYCARDIAS

The term "atrial tachycardia" is used to include all forms of rapid heart action resulting from increase in the atrial rate. These include atrial flutter, nodal tachycardia and atrial tachycardia. The latter two are often grouped together under the heading of *supraventricular tachycardia*. A common pathogenesis was suggested by Prinzmetal for all the atrial tachycardias. These arrhythmias are described as one group with due note of any differences in incidence, diagnosis and treatment.

INCIDENCE. The frequency of the atrial tachycardias in the perinatal period is not known. In rare instances these arrhythmias have had their onset in utero. Eight newborn infants with flutter and three others with supraventricular tachycardia have been reported in whom a rapid and often irregular heart rate was noted before and continued after birth (Wilburne and Mock).

The postnatal occurrence of atrial tachycardias is not uncommon. A number of reports have been published since Hubbard's description of this arrhythmia in young infants. Of these, a considerable number have occurred within the first month of life. For example, Nadas et al. reported 41 patients in the pediatric age group, in 14 of whom the onset was within a few days or weeks after birth. Nadas had a striking preponderance of male infants in his series. Apley et al. described 13 infants with atrial tachycardia, and in nine the onset was noted between the sixth and thirty-fifth days of life. If these reports are representative of the incidence in individual hospitals, then atrial tachycardia may indeed occur more frequently in the neonatal period than is usually thought. In both the reports noted above supraventricular tachycardia was found far more frequently than atrial flutter. However, Moller et al. found 24 cases of congenital atrial flutter including three of his own. Twelve were recognized prior to birth, eight at birth and the remainder in the first week of life.

ETIOLOGY. A variety of etiologic factors may play a role in this group of arrhythmias, but in the majority no etiologic factor is found and the attacks must be considered idiopathic in nature. A small number have been described in association with congenital anomalies of the heart, but no particular anatomic defect predominates. It has been noted in infants with endocardial fibroelastosis and acute interstitial myocarditis. We have seen one infant with rhabdomyoma of the heart in whom paroxysmal tachycardia was the initial disturbance (Case 26–5). It is well known that persons with the Wolff-Parkinson-White syndrome (short P-R interval and abnormal QRS complexes) are subject to episodes of paroxysmal atrial tachycardia. We have seen one 4-day-old infant with paroxysmal tachycardia in whom the Wolff-Parkinson-White syndrome was readily apparent in the electrocardiogram after the tachycardia had been brought under control (Fig. 25–4). A 2-hour-old infant with this syndrome, but without paroxysmal tachycardia, has been reported (Walsh). An occasional patient may have repeated bouts of tachycardia and several months or years later show evidence of the Wolff-Parkinson-White syndrome.

CLINICAL FINDINGS. In contrast to that in older infants and children, the onset of symptoms in the neonate is fairly abrupt. It is usually marked by an increase in the respiratory rate and by the appearance of cyanosis in a previously well infant. From the very beginning there is either refusal to feed or an unwillingness to continue to do so for more than brief periods. Occasionally vomiting or low-grade fever may be present. The infant has an anxious expression and appears acutely ill. Cyanosis is at first mild and increases with the duration of the tachycardia, though the duskiness usually does not approach the severe cyanosis seen in certain kinds of congenital heart disease. At a later stage the color becomes ashen gray and the skin cold as a result of peripheral vasoconstriction.

The majority of the signs associated with atrial tachycardia are the result of heart failure. As has been noted, tachypnea is the presenting symptom. Respirations may range between 60 and 100 per minute and are accompanied by some substernal retraction. The lung fields often show fine or medium rales and some scattered areas of dullness as evidence of congestive changes. The pulmonary findings are variable, however, and usually cannot be differentiated from those of pulmonary infection, which is also not infrequently present.

Cardiomegaly occurs in the majority of infants. The increase in heart size can be detected clinically and may be proved by x-ray examination. This enlargement is always reversible unless organic cardiac disease is present. A soft systolic murmur may be heard over the precordium, although the rapidity of the heart may make it difficult to define. When present, the murmur is more often the result of cardiac dilatation than of an associated congenital defect.

Some enlargement of the liver is usually present, and indeed this organ may increase in size with great rapidity. Other signs of failure such as edema and fullness of the neck veins are rarely present in this age group, nor are they notable when they do occur. In rare cases, cardiac failure occurs in utero and the infant is born with massive edema (Silber and Durnin; van de Horst).

**DIAGNOSIS.** Recognition of the pronounced tachycardia is of course the key to the diagnosis, but this finding may be obscured by crying or respiratory sounds. The heart rate must be counted carefully by auscultation. The pulse should not be relied upon for this purpose. Although the normal rate of the young infant may approach 200 beats per minute with crying or other activity, the rate during an attack of tachycardia is always over 200 and usually ranges between 220 and 300 beats per minute. Persistence of this rapid rate during periods of quiet is of considerable diag-

nostic importance. In simple sinus tachycardia the heart rate may reach 200 in the neonate, but varies greatly with activity.

It is usually not possible to distinguish between supraventricular tachycardia and atrial flutter on clinical examination. When an extreme tachycardia is combined with periods of irregular rhythm, then atrial flutter with variable block is likely to be present. It is always necessary to perform electrocardiographic studies to determine the type of atrial tachycardia present.

**THE ELECTROCARDIOGRAM.** It is possible to distinguish between atrial and nodal tachycardia only if the relation of the P wave to the QRS complex can be identified. When this cannot be done, and it frequently cannot, then the tachycardia is designated as supraventricular. A heart tracing representative of this arrhythmia is shown in Figure 25–1. This record was made on a seven-day-old infant during an attack. The heart rate was approximately 300 per minute and perfectly regular. The P waves could not be identified. The QRS complex appeared normal. The T waves were inverted. Figure 25–1 also shows lead III in the same infant after termination of the paroxysm. The rate was 140 per minute. The P waves were well outlined, and the tracing is within normal limits.

The diagnosis of atrial flutter can be made by identifying the presence of small

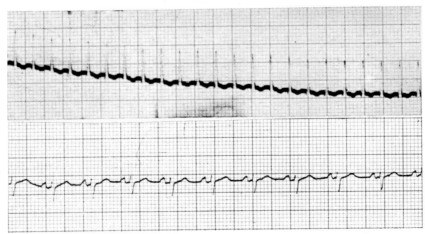

*Figure 25–1.* The upper tracing is lead III in a 7-day-old infant during a paroxysm of supraventricular tachycardia. The lower tracing (lead I) is in the same infant after the attack. This case history is not abstracted in the text.

F waves between the QRS complexes. The tracing has a characteristic "saw-toothed" appearance. Although the atrial rate is more rapid than in supraventricular tachycardia, the ventricles may beat at a slower pace. This is dependent on the degree of block. The electrocardiogram of an infant with flutter is shown in Figure 25–2. The atrial rate was 375 per minute, while the ventricular rate was between 110 and 180 as a result of a variable 3:1 and 2:1 block.

**TREATMENT.** An attack of paroxysmal supraventricular tachycardia in infants under one month of age is a medical emergency. Treatment should be started as soon as the diagnosis is made. Therapy is directed toward both the relief of heart failure and control of the tachycardia.

Oxygen is indicated and should be continued until termination of the paroxysm. If the restlessness is pronounced, morphine is of value. Because of vomiting and as-piration, it is important to discontinue oral feedings at the onset of the attack. Fluid requirements should be satisfied by intravenous administration of hypotonic fluids. Antibiotics are indicated in the presence of active infection, but only after naso-pharyngeal cultures have been taken.

Various methods have been used to terminate the tachycardia. None of them has been consistently successful. Reflex vagal stimulation by eyeball or carotid pressure is rarely effective in the young infants. Since these mechanical manipulations are not without danger, they should probably not be attempted in this age group.

Digitalis has proved to be of considerable value in infants and should be used initially in all cases. The more rapid-acting glycosides such as digoxin are preferred. In a certain number of patients digitalis may bring about improvement of heart failure and yet not terminate the paroxysm of tachycardia.

Countershock should be used in infants who fail to respond to digitalis in a reasonable period of time or who appear so ill that it does not seem judicious to await adequate digitalization. The use of external countershock is preferable to quinidine, metacholine or procainamide hydrochloride (Pryor and Blount).

**PROGNOSIS.** Paroxysmal tachycardia presents a serious threat to the life of a young infant. Death due to heart failure results unless the paroxysm is brought to an end. In the series of 13 infants with supraventricular tachycardia described by Apley and co-workers, three died in the midst of their initial attack.

It is not uncommon for the paroxysms to recur within 6 to 12 months after the original attack. Thereafter the prognosis is excellent in the idiopathic cases. On the other hand, in patients with the Wolff-Parkinson-White syndrome, attacks may recur for many years. A maintenance dose of digitalis should be given as a prophylactic measure for 6 to 12 months after the initial episode. Note that this regimen may not prevent recurrences in all cases and beta-adrenergic blocking agents may be useful in such patients (Rowe and Mehrizi).

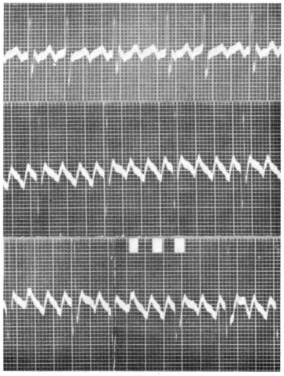

*Figure 25–2.* Standard limb leads during an attack of atrial flutter. (See text for details.)

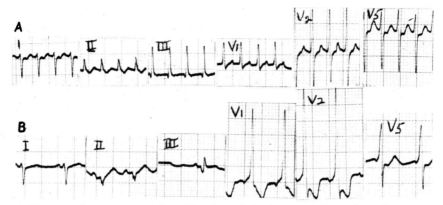

***Figure 25–3.*** Electrocardiogram in a 4-day-old infant. *A,* Supraventricular tachycardia. *B,* Tracing after the tachycardia stopped shows a typical Wolff-Parkinson-White pattern with a short P-R interval and a wide QRS. The delta waves can be seen just before the upstroke of the R waves in the precordial leads.

## CASE HISTORIES

### CASE 25–1

(This case is abstracted with the kind permission of Dr. Lester Caplan of Baltimore.)

An infant was the result of a 37-week pregnancy. At birth the amniotic fluid was stained with meconium. The infant weighed 7 pounds 13 ounces (3535 gm) and breathed and cried spontaneously. No abnormalities were noted on physical examination. The hospital course was unremarkable until the third hospital day, when one episode of vomiting occurred. The following day the infant appeared dusky and was noted to breathe rapidly. Examination revealed mild cyanosis, tachypnea (64 per minute) and a tachycardia. The heart rate was perfectly regular and too rapid to count accurately. The heart was not enlarged, and no murmurs were heard. The liver edge was 2 cm below the costal margin. There was no edema.

An electrocardiogram showed a regular heart rate of 300 beats per minute in all leads. The P and T waves were superimposed. There was a normal right axis deviation.

The infant was placed in oxygen and digitalized with 100 micrograms of lanatoside C intravenously, administered in two doses two hours apart. Six hours after the onset of treatment the heart rate was 124 per minute, the cyanosis had disappeared, and the liver edge could no longer be palpated. She was partially redigitalized with digitoxin and was then maintained on this preparation. There were no recurrences of tachycardia over the nine-month period of follow-up and there is no evidence of heart disease.

**COMMENT.** The fairly sudden onset of cyanosis and tachypnea associated with a heart rate of well over 200 is diagnostic of paroxysmal tachycardia. The electrocardiogram confirmed the clinical impression in this infant. The signs of early heart failure were already present at the time of diagnosis. The response to digitalis was rapid and complete.

## COMPLETE HEART BLOCK

Heart block may be discovered at birth or during the first days of life and is presumed to be congenital in origin. The acquired form of block is uncommon in this age group. It is occasionally seen in myocarditis and endocardial fibroelastosis. The description which follows is limited to congenital heart block.

**INCIDENCE.** Several hundred cases of congenital heart block have been reported. The discovery of this conduction disturbance at or shortly after birth, however, has been infrequent. In even rarer instances a diagnosis of heart block has been made before birth. Only 12 cases diagnosed antenatally have been reported exclusive of the case history appended (Moss and Litman).

**PATHOLOGY.** The pathology of congenital heart block has been reviewed by Lev. It may be associated with other cardiac abnormalities or occur as an isolated abnormality. In some cases there is no connection between the atria and the AV node, and in others the connection is intact but the branching portion of the AV bundle is absent. About 75 per cent of infants with congenital heart block have no other cardiac defects. In those who do, corrected transposition and atrial defect are the most common abnormalities (Nadas and Fyler).

**DIAGNOSIS.** The presence of antenatal heart block is suggested by the finding of a persistently slow fetal heart rate at any time during the last trimester of pregnancy. It can be distinguished from the bradycardia of fetal distress by the regularity and persistence of the slow rate, and by absence of a significant change in intensity of the heart sounds. An awareness of this entity and its recognition can avoid an erroneous diagnosis of fetal distress and unnecessary termination of pregnancy (Sanbey).

The finding of bradycardia during the first few days of life is diagnostic of congenital heart block. Although one may note a relative slowing of the heart during the first few hours of life in some infants with asphyxia pallida or severe intracranial lesions, the bradycardia is usually not of the degree seen in congenital heart block. In this latter group the heart rate is always less than 80 and often as low as 40 beats per minute. The infant may show no other abnormalities. This, however, depends on the kind and the severity of any associated cardiac anomalies. There may be cyanosis, cardiac enlargement and heart failure in infants with serious defects. On the other hand, bradycardia may be the only obvious sign of heart disease in the neonatal period, while other findings may become manifest during infancy and childhood. Frequently the bradycardia may be so mild as to escape detection at birth and remain to be diagnosed in later life.

The diagnosis can be readily established from the electrocardiogram. Congenital heart block is almost always of the complete type. The heart tracing will show the P waves appearing independently of the QRS complexes. The atrial rate is between one and two times as rapid as the ventricular rate. Otherwise the electrocardiogram is within the limits of normal, unless other cardiac abnormalities are present.

**PROGNOSIS.** The discovery of heart block in the very young infant is of prognostic importance. This finding may signify the presence of associated congenital heart disease, which may be so severe as to cause death within the first few days of life. Most infants with block have a rate between 40 and 80 beats per minute. In general a heart rate below 40 signifies a poor prognosis, even in the absence of other cardiac anomalies. With heart rates in the latter range, heart block per se does not place any additional strain on the heart. There is, however, the rare patient with congenital heart block who dies in the midst of a Stokes-Adams attack of syncope. These attacks are almost unheard of in infancy but may occur during childhood (Molthan, et al.). In almost all cases the heart block persists throughout life, but it may occasionally change in degree. In one patient the heart block disappeared entirely by the end of the first year. In a group of patients followed up by Campbell and Thorne for 25 years, cardiac function remained normal.

**TREATMENT.** No treatment is needed for the asymptomatic newborn with congenital heart block. Infants with very slow rates and reduced cardiac output have a poor prognosis. A pacemaker should be used without delay for these sick infants.

CASE 25–2

An infant was the result of a full-term pregnancy. Two months before term a fetal heart rate of 70 to 80 per minute had been noted by the obstetrician. During the last month, in addition to the bradycardia, there was thought to be a systolic murmur synchronous with the fetal heart. Labor was uneventful, and a 6 pound 5 ounce (2870 gm) female infant was delivered without difficulty. She breathed and cried immediately. There was no cyanosis. The heart was not enlarged, and there were no murmurs. The heart rate was 94 per minute shortly after birth and decreased to 80 within the first hour. The rhythm was perfectly regular. General examination was not remarkable.

An electrocardiogram taken during the first 24 hours showed complete heart block (Fig. 25–4). The ventricles were contracting at a rate of 90 per minute. The atria were beating independently at a rate of 140 per minute. The tracing was otherwise within normal limits. An x-ray film of the chest showed no abnormalities.

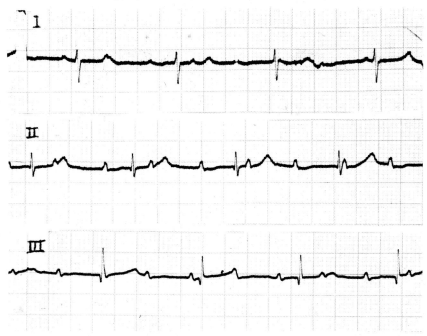

*Figure 25–4.* Age 4 days. Standard limb leads. Complete heart block is present. The ventricular rate is 90, the atrial rate 120.

At 2 weeks of age a systolic murmur was first heard along the left sternal border. This increased in intensity and by the sixth month of life had a loud, rough quality. The heart rate continued between 70 and 84 beats per minute. The child was followed up until 2 years of age. There was never any cyanosis, and her growth and development were normal. The heart was not enlarged, and the electrocardiogram continued to show complete atrioventricular dissociation. The murmur persisted. This was thought to be due to an interventricular septal defect.

**COMMENT.** This is an unusual example of congenital heart block which became evident 2 months before delivery. At birth, aside from the bradycardia, no abnormalities were noted. A murmur appeared subsequently, and a presumptive diagnosis of interventricular septal defect was made. The heart block and the murmur persisted for the 2 years of follow-up.

## REFERENCES

Apley, J., Conner, B. D., and Gibson, T. C.: Paroxysmal tachycardia in infancy. Arch. Dis. Child. *30*:517, 1955.

Campbell, M., and Thorne, M. G.: Congenital heart block. Br. Heart J. *18*:90, 1956.

Hon, E. H., and Huang, H. S.: The electronic evaluation of fetal heart rate. VII. Premature and missed beats. Obstet. Gynec. *20*:81, 1962.

Lev, M.: Pathogenesis of congenital heart block. *In* Neonatal Heart Disease. New York. Grune and Stratton, 1973.

Moller, J. H., et al.: Atrial flutter in infancy. J. Pediatr. *75*:643, 1969.

Molthan, M. E., et al.: Congenital heart block with fatal Adams-Stokes attacks in childhood. Pediatrics *30*:32, 1962.

Morgan, B. C., Bloom, R. S., and Guntheroth, W. G.: Cardiac arrhythmias in premature infants. Pediatrics *35*:658, 1965.

Morgan, B. C., and Guntheroth, W. G.: Cardiac arrhythmias in normal newborn infants. J. Pediatr. *67*:1199, 1965.

Moss, A. J., and Litman, N. N.: Congenital heart block. J. Pediatr. *48*:226, 1956.

Nadas, A. S., Daeschner, C. W., Roth, A., and Blumenthal, S. C.: Paroxysmal tachycardia in infants and children. Pediatrics 9:167, 1952.

Nadas, A. S., and Fyler, D. C.: Pediatric Cardiology. Philadelphia, W. B. Saunders Co., 1972.

Prinzmetal, M., Corday, E., Brill, I. C., Oblath, R. W., and Kruger, H. E.: The Auricular Arrhythmias. Springfield, Ill., Charles C Thomas, 1952.

Pryor, R., and Blount, G. G.: Refractory supraventricular tachycardia in infancy: External countershock termination. Am. J. Dis. Child. *107*:428, 1964.

Rowe, R. D., and Mehrizi: Disorders of heart rate and

rhythm. *In* The Neonate with Congenital Heart Disease. Philadelphia, W. B. Saunders Co., 1968.

Sanbey, A. O.: Congenital heart disease simulating foetal distress. Br. Med. J., 2:676, 1948.

Silber, D. L., and Durnin, R. W.: Intrauterine atrial tachycardia. Am. J. Dis. Child. *117*:722, 1969.

van der Horst, R. L.: Congenital atrial flutter and car-

diac failure presenting as hydrops foetalis at birth. S. A. Med. J. *44*:1037, 1970.

Walsh, S. Z.: Wolff-Parkinson-White syndrome in a healthy two-hour-old infant without paroxysmal tachycardia. J.A.M.A. *186*:14, 1963.

Wilburne, M., and Mock, E. G.: Paroxysmal tachycardia with onset in utero. J.A.M.A. *154*:1337, 1954.

# 26    MISCELLANEOUS CONDITIONS
## *Revised by Milton Markowitz*

## ENDOCARDIAL FIBROELASTOSIS

Endocardial fibroelastosis may occur as an isolated or primary condition or in association with a variety of congenital and acquired cardiac lesions. In the latter groups the clinical entity is that of the underlying cardiac disease and the fibroelastosis is a secondary finding on postmortem examination. The description which follows is limited mainly to infants with the primary or isolated form of endocardial fibroelastosis.

**ETIOLOGY.** The cause of primary endocardial fibroelastosis is not known. An old theory that it was the result of a fetal endocarditis secondary to maternal infection was discarded following studies by Gross. However, evidence has been presented suggesting that in utero Coxsackie B virus infection may play a role (Fruhling; Hastreiter et al.). This evidence is still inconclusive. The mumps virus has also been incriminated (Noren et al.; St. Geme et al.). However, infants with endocardial fibroelastosis lack antibodies to mumps, and mothers with proven mumps during pregnancy have not given birth to babies with this condition.

Anderson and Kelly presented fairly convincing evidence that the endocardial thickening seen in association with other congenital cardiac defects is due to abnormal currents of intracardiac blood under increased pressure. Nevertheless this hypothesis cannot account for its presence in the isolated form. The increasing number of reports of its occurrence in families and

multiple births points toward the possibility of genetic factors (Vestermark). Black-Schaffer and Turner challenged the concept originally advanced by Weinberg and Himelfarb that the primary defect is in the development of the endocardium. They believe that the basic lesion is a congenital defect in cardiac muscle and that the endocardial thickening is secondary to fibrin deposition. Some support for this hypothesis has been obtained from the demonstration of fibrin by electron microscopy within the thickened endocardial layers (Still and Boult).

**INCIDENCE.** The reports on incidence are confusing because of the inclusion of large numbers of cases with the secondary form of this disease. The study by Kelly and Anderson makes this distinction clear. In their series from the Babies Hospital there were 17 instances among 237 patients with congenital heart disease, an incidence of 7 per cent. Family occurrences were noted in three of the 17 cases. There are several additional reports which record the disease among multiple births and siblings (Case 26–2). The incidence in the general population is one case in every 5000 to 6000 births (Mitchell et al.). There does not appear to be any relation to birth weight, sex or race.

**PATHOLOGY.** Gross enlargement of the heart is a constant finding. The weight is increased, and there are hypertrophy and dilatation of one or more chambers. This is especially true of the left ventricle, which is the most frequent site of endocardial thickening. Involvement of the left atrium is fairly common, but less than half have an additional lesion of the right ventricle and right atrium. Fibroelastosis confined to the right side of the heart is rare. On gross examination the endocardium is diffusely thickened and smooth and has a porcelain-white appearance (Fig. 26–1). About half the cases show involvement of one or more valves, the mitral more commonly than the others. In contrast to the usual pattern of congenital abnormalities, there is a striking absence of other malformations.

Microscopic examination shows an increase in the fibrous and elastic tissue within the endocardium with some extension into the myocardium. When the valves are involved, the picture is similar to that of the endocardium. There is no evidence of inflammation in the heart. Pneumonia and signs of congestive failure are commonly associated autopsy findings.

**CLINICAL COURSE.** The majority of infants have their initial symptoms between the first and sixth months of life. A significant percentage show some difficulty from birth, and a case of heart failure in utero has been reported (Harris and Nghiem). In a series of 85 collected cases in which the age at onset was noted, 19 patients had difficulty within the first month, and in 13 of these cases signs or symptoms began at birth (Anderson and Kelly).

The clinical pattern of the disease falls into two fairly distinct types, acute and chronic. The mode of onset, symptomatology and course vary with each. In its most fulminant form the infant, previously well, may be discovered dead in his crib. The more typical acute case begins with the nonspecific symptoms of listlessness, failure to feed, vomiting or a mild cold. These are soon followed by onset of labored breathing. The physical findings are variable. Fever may be present, but is rarely high. The cardiac rate is variable. It may be slow if there is an associated heart block (see Fig. 26–2). In two reported cases heart block was present *in utero* (Anderson and Kelly). On the other hand, there may be an extreme tachycardia due to a paroxysmal atrial rhythm (Hung and Walsh). The heart sounds are often unusually forceful. Although the heart is always enlarged, clinical detection of enlargement may be difficult in the early stages. Signs of heart failure may not be prominent at the onset, but are almost always present at some time during the course of the disease.

The chronic form of the disease is the more common of the two types. The initial symptom is labored or wheezy breathing. *This may be present from birth.* Failure to gain weight and bouts of irritability are common. There may be intermittent cyanosis. The physical findings are those of a young infant in heart failure. Respirations are increased and grunting. There is flaring of the alae nasi and some intercostal retraction. Cyanosis is minimal or absent except as a terminal event. There may be abnormalities in the cardiac rhythm, as has already been noted. The heart is always enlarged. The heart sounds are of good quality and become muffled only when heart failure is advanced. A murmur is present in about a third of the patients, systolic in time and soft and nondescript in quality. The presence of a loud murmur should lead to suspicion of fibroelastic valvular involvement or an associated congenital defect. The liver is enlarged in the presence of heart failure. The blood pressure is either normal or low.

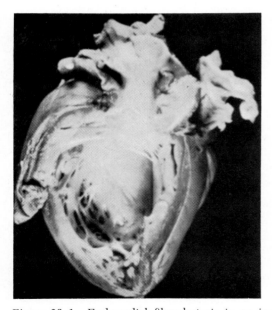

*Figure 26–1.* Endocardial fibroelastosis in an infant who died at age of 9 days. The endocardium of both ventricles is thickened and porcelain-white in appearance.

**LABORATORY FINDINGS.** Blood and urine examinations show no abnormality that can be related to the primary disease. The electrocardiogram is often of considerable diagnostic help in the chronic form of the disease. As might be anticipated from the pathology, evidence of left ventricular hypertrophy is common. Features which indicate hypertrophy are noted in the precordial leads over the left side of the chest ($V_5$ and $V_6$) and consist of abnormally tall R waves, prominent Q waves, prolonged intrinsicoid deflection and inverted T waves (Lambert and co-workers). Supraventricular or nodal tachycardia as well as partial and complete heart block has been recorded.

Roentgen examination of the heart reveals enlargement, especially of the left ventricle. In many of these infants left atrial prominence can be demonstrated on the esophagram. Angiocardiography may show little difference in left ventricular filling in systole and diastole. At times the increased thickness of the left ventricular wall can be appreciated.

**DIAGNOSIS.** Endocardial fibroelastosis should be suspected in the neonate if abnormalities of cardiac rhythm such as heart block or atrial tachycardia are present. In the most acute form it is difficult to make the diagnosis. These infants often resemble patients with sepsis or pneumonia. The presence of tachycardia, cardiomegaly and enlargement of the liver should lead to the suspicion of heart failure due to primary heart disease. Differentiation from primary myocarditis may be particularly difficult. The findings in both conditions are remarkably similar. One distinguishing feature is the strikingly low voltage noted on the electrocardiogram in severe myocarditis, but this may occur in endocardial fibroelastosis on occasion. The left ventricular pattern commonly found in endocardial fibroelastosis may be slight or absent in the acute case less than 1 week old (Case 26–1).

The chronic form of the disease may cause symptoms from birth, but the diagnosis is rarely suspected until the signs of heart failure are fairly well developed. At times the wheezing or labored respirations are wrongly interpreted as signs of asthma, an enlarged thymus or some other obstructive abnormality. The diagnosis should be suspected in any young infant with an enlarged heart, particularly when there is little or no cyanosis and no heart murmurs are heard. Absence of the latter signs should exclude most other forms of congenital heart disease. The presence of palpable femoral pulsations eliminates coarctation of the aorta. Infants with anomalous origin of the left coronary artery may have a similar clinical and roentgen picture. The electrocardiogram in this condition is often distinctive, however, and shows a pattern of coronary insufficiency with inverted T waves in leads I and II plus a prominent Q wave in lead I.

Glycogen storage disease of the heart is a rare cause of cardiac enlargement in infancy. Here the enlargement is usually globular, without specific chamber enlargement. The electrocardiographic pattern is more bizarre in glycogen storage disease, and a short P-R interval is often present. A specific diagnosis can be made by analysis of the glycogen content of skeletal muscle.

**TREATMENT.** This is directed toward the control of heart failure. Oxygen therapy is indicated. Oral feedings should be discontinued during the critical phase of the illness, and water and electrolyte requirements should be maintained by parenteral means. When oral feedings are begun, low solute formulas should be used as long as there is evidence of heart failure. Antimicrobial agents are indicated as a means of preventing secondary infection of the lungs. Digitalization should be started immediately. If the patient is extremely ill, one of the more rapid-acting digitalis preparations should be used. The prolonged use of digitalis has been recommended as an important aspect of therapy.

Diuretics should be reserved for infants who have clinical evidence of edema or who fail to respond to oxygen and digitalis. More complete details on the dosage of anticongestive drugs are presented elsewhere.

**PROGNOSIS.** A small number of patients fail to respond to all measures and die within 1 day to 2 weeks after onset of the illness. In a larger group the response to anticongestive treatment is good, even dramatic at times. Of 19 cases with symptoms before one month of life, 10 lived from 3 months to 3 years (Kelly and Anderson). In general, the earlier the onset, the worse the prognosis. Symptoms recur intermittently until death. The terminal illness is usually brief and is the result of heart failure often complicated by pneumonia. The prognosis in infants with the familial type of endocardial fibroelastosis is generally poor.

It is still not certain that endocardial fibroelastosis is an invariably fatal disease. Recently Linde and Adams described 17 patients in whom a presumptive diagnosis of primary endocardial fibroelastosis was made. Of these four have now had completely normal findings over a period of 3 to 10 years. Further observations will be necessary before the over-all prognosis in this condition is known. In the meantime early recognition and vigorous treatment hold forth the possibility of a favorable outcome in some patients.

## CASE HISTORIES

### CASE 26–1

A white female infant was born after a 36-week pregnancy. The mother was Rh-negative, unsensitized. Birth weight was 6 pounds 2 ounces (2780 gm). She was cyanotic at birth, but her color was recorded as normal by 12 hours. Thereafter she appeared well and was discharged from the nursery on the third day. After discharge she did poorly and failed to feed. She was readmitted to the hospital on the sixth day of life. She was jaundiced and febrile. The respiratory rate was 36, and rales were heard at both bases. The heart was not enlarged clinically, the sounds were of good quality, and there were no murmurs. The liver was not en-

larged. The femoral pulses were normal. There were several pustules in the groin.

The white blood cell count was 24,000, with an increase in polymorphonuclear cells. The blood culture was positive for hemolytic *Staphylococcus aureus*. The electrocardiogram showed a 2:1 heart block (Fig. 26–2). An x-ray film of the chest revealed a patch of pneumonitis at the right base. The heart was not enlarged.

She was treated vigorously for sepsis with antimicrobial agents and transfusions. She failed to respond and died on the third day of admission.

Postmortem examination by Dr. T. Weinberg and staff showed a patchy bronchopneumonia and diffuse endocardial fibroelastosis of both ventricles.

**COMMENT.** This case history demonstrates the difficulty in diagnosis of endocardial fibroelastosis during the neonatal period before the more classic signs of cardiac enlargement and left ventricular hypertrophy become apparent. The only cardiac disturbance noted clinically was heart block. Although there was obvious sepsis and pulmonary infection, the cardiac lesion probably played some role in the cause of death. We have seen other newborn infants die after a brief illness in whom endocardial fibroelastosis was the only postmortem finding.

### CASE 26–2

A six-week-old white female infant was admitted to the Sinai Hospital with grunting respirations of several hours' duration. She was born after a full-term normal pregnancy. There was a history of a 3 month-old male sibling who died

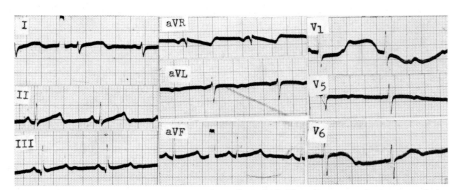

*Figure 26–2.* Electrocardiogram in an infant with endocardial fibroelastosis, taken at age 6 days, showing a 2:1 heart block.

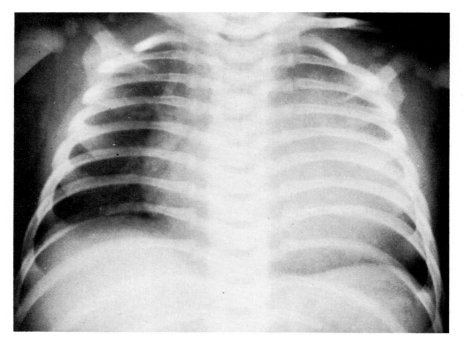

*Figure 26–3.*   Endocardial fibroelastosis in a 6-week-old infant. The heart is diffusely enlarged.

after a brief illness and in whom the diagnosis of endocardial fibroelastosis was made postmortem.

No abnormalities were noted at birth and except for being described as a poor feeder, her course was uneventful until just prior to hospital admission. Physical examination showed a dyspneic infant with circumoral cyanosis, tachy-

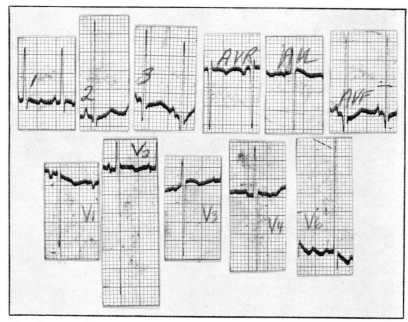

*Figure 26–4.*   The electrocardiogram in a 6-week-old infant with endocardial fibroelastosis. Note the deep S waves in $V_2$, tall R waves and inverted T waves in $V_6$.

cardia, good heart sounds, cardiomegaly and en-largement of the liver. An x-ray film of the chest revealed diffuse enlargement of the heart (Fig. 26–3). The electrocardiogram showed left ventricular hypertrophy (Fig. 26–4). She was treated vigorously with anticongestive drugs, showed a good response initially, but died suddenly on the fifth hospital day.

Postmortem examination revealed a greatly enlarged heart with diffuse endocardial thickening of the left ventricle (Fig. 26–5).

**COMMENT.** Endocardial fibroelastosis occurring in siblings has been reported on several occasions. In this family both in-

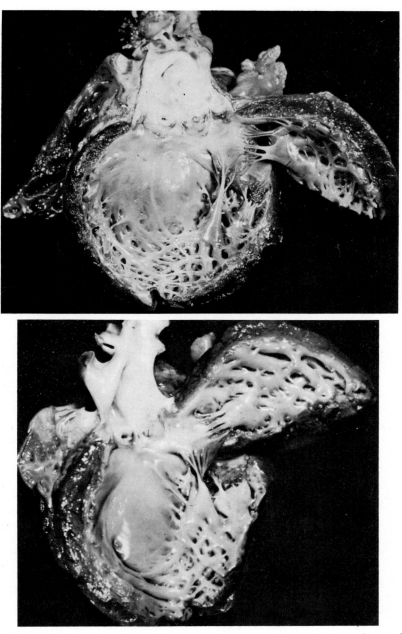

*Figure 26–5.* Endocardial fibroelastosis in siblings, ages 6 weeks and 3 months. In each case the endocardium of the left ventricle is thickened and porcelain-white in appearance.

fants appeared normal at birth and except for a somewhat slow weight gain, did well until the sudden onset of heart failure which resulted in their rapid demise. They represent the typical pattern of this disease seen in its most acute severe form. The prognosis among infants with a family history is said to be particularly poor.

## GLYCOGEN STORAGE DISEASE OF THE HEART

Glycogen storage disease of the heart is a rare condition which may manifest symptoms from birth. It is one of 11 types or subtypes of glycogenoses (type II) and it is the only type in which involvement of the heart is a major feature. It is transmitted through a single recessive autosomal gene. The defect is due to the congenital absence of alpha 4–6 glycosidase from intracellular lysosomes (Hers). This results in the accumulation of normal glycogen in lysosomal sacs, where it cannot be degraded by glycolytic enzymes.

PATHOLOGY. The heart is always enlarged, often to enormous proportions. The walls of both ventricles are thick, but the atria are normal. Microscopic examination shows infiltration of the muscle fibers with large vacuoles of glycogen. Varying amounts of glycogen deposition are also found in the skeletal muscles, liver, kidneys and central nervous system.

CLINICAL FEATURES. Symptoms were noted from birth in about one fourth of the 54 cases summarized by Ehlers et al. In the patient described at the end of this section, poor heart sounds, cardiomegaly and early signs of heart failure were noted within the first 12 hours of life (Rosenstein). More often the infant appears normal at birth, but goes on to have a history of poor feeding, lassitude and failure to gain weight. Hypotonia may be striking, and the tongue may appear thick. Cardiac enlargement is the rule. A systolic heart murmur may be noted, but it is often soft and variable. The liver is not usually enlarged.

The usual parameters for glycogen metabolism are normal, including glucose tolerance, response to epinephrine and glucagon. These infants do not suffer from hypoglycemia. Radiologic examination shows gross generalized cardiomegaly, although the heart need not be enlarged at birth. The electrocardiogram may show abnormalities at birth or after a period of some weeks. Unusually high voltage of the QRS complexes and the T waves is characteristic. There is evidence of left ventricular hypertrophy. However, a short P-R interval is the most distinctive electrocardiographic feature of glycogen storage disease. Caddell and Whittemore found that 86 per cent of their cases had a P-R interval of less than 0.09.

DIAGNOSIS. The diagnosis is rarely made in the neonatal period unless there is a family history of the disease. The early symptoms are ill-defined and, with the exception of intermittent episodes of dyspnea, do not suggest a cardiac abnormality. The patient is more likely to be several weeks or months old before the cardiac enlargement is detected. The diagnosis should be suspected in any infant with an enlarged heart, especially if the enlargement is great. Muscle weakness is an important additional clue. Macroglossia is often present and may be confused with cretinism or Down's syndrome.

This condition must be distinguished from other causes of cardiac enlargement in early infancy. The absence of cyanosis and significant murmurs will exclude many of the congenital defects. *Endocardial fibroelastosis* and *anomalous left coronary artery* are the two conditions which most frequently enter into the differential diagnosis. The left ventricular component in the x-ray film is more striking in both the above conditions, while the heart in glycogen storage disease is larger and more globular. All three entities may show a left ventricular pattern and striking T wave changes in the electrocardiogram. In the anomalous left coronary artery the electrocardiographic changes resemble more closely those seen with a posterior infarct. In endocardial fibroelastosis the T wave changes are restricted to the left side of the precordium, while they are often present in all leads in glycogen storage disease. A short P-R interval does not occur in endocardial fibroelastosis or with an anomalous coronary artery.

The diagnosis of glycogen storage disease can be confirmed by demonstrating increased glycogen in a biopsy of skeletal muscle. It can be more readily confirmed by examining blood lymphocytes for glycogen content (Nahill et al.).

**PROGNOSIS.** Death due to heart failure almost always occurs before the end of the first year. Among the 23 cases collected by Keith, Rowe and Vlad, two patients died during the first month of life.

**TREATMENT.** There is no satisfactory treatment for this condition. Anticongestive therapy and treatment of intercurrent infection should be instituted in an attempt to prolong life.

CASE 26–3

A 7¼-pound full-term white male infant was seen shortly after birth at Women's Hospital for a routine physical examination. The family history was remarkable in that two siblings died at 4 and 5 months of age in heart failure, and postmortem examinations revealed extensive deposition of glycogen in their myocardium. Examination at 1 hour of age revealed muffled heart sounds. A chest x-ray at 12 hours of age showed generalized cardiomegaly (Fig. 26–6). The electrocardiogram showed a P-R interval of 0.08 second, large biphasic QRS complexes and deeply inverted T waves in leads I, II and $V_2$ through $V_6$ (Fig. 26–7).

At 2 days of age the infant appeared hypotonic and the muscles had an abnormal firm quality. Respiratory distress, circumoral cyanosis, enlargement of the liver and pretibial pitting edema were noted. He was digitalized and treated with antibiotics. His response was poor; signs of increasing heart failure developed, and he died at 3 weeks of life.

Autopsy examination revealed an enlarged heart which weighed 110 gm. The atria were normal. The myocardium of both ventricles was thick, firm and pale. There were no valvular lesions. Microscopically, there was extensive glycogen deposition in the myocardium (Fig. 26–8), skeletal muscle, liver and kidneys.

**COMMENT.** This is an unusual example of glycogen storage disease of the heart in a third affected member of one family. Cardiac signs were present at birth, and hypotonia appeared early. The electrocardiogram showed the striking features of this condition.

## PERICARDITIS

Pericarditis in the newborn infant is a rare entity. A review of the literature by

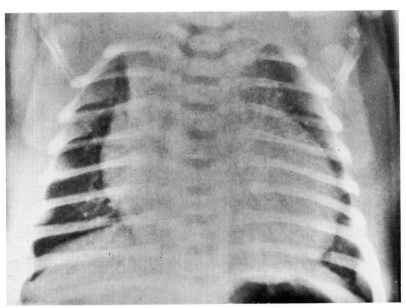

*Figure 26–6.* X-ray film of the chest of a 12-hour-old infant with glycogen storage disease of the heart. There is considerable cardiac enlargement.

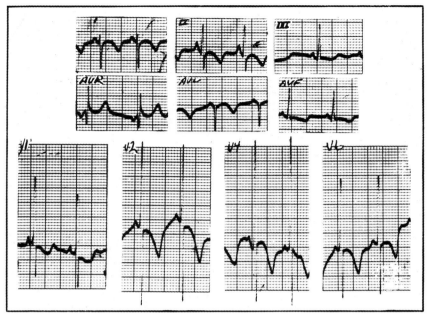

*Figure 26–7.* Electrocardiogram of a 1-day-old infant with glycogen storage disease of the heart. Note the short P-R interval, increased voltage and deeply inverted T waves in leads I, II, aV$_1$, and V$_2$–V$_6$.

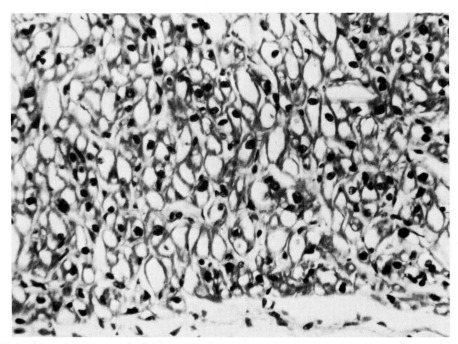

*Figure 26–8.* Microscopic section of the myocardium of an infant with glycogen storage disease of the heart. Note the vacuolization among the myofibers. These vacuoles were filled with glycogen when appropriately stained.

Valdés-Dapena and Miller revealed nine reported cases, to which they added two of their own. Pericarditis is usually caused by a bacterial infection which may be limited to the pericardium, but is more often part of a generalized infection. This may occur as an intrauterine infection or it may be acquired in the postnatal period. In our case pericarditis was due to a proved hemolytic staphylococcus infection which was almost certainly acquired from the mother after birth. Myocarditis and pneumonia were additional findings.

The *diagnosis* is rarely suspected before death. Although infection is suspected, it is more often thought to be sepsis or pneumonia. Signs of heart failure are common, but other signs of cardiac disease may or may not be present. In none of the cases was a pericardial friction rub heard. In one of the patients reported by Valdés-Dapena and Miller severe heart failure was present. The electrocardiogram showed inverted T waves in lead I without any specific changes suggesting pericarditis.

The *treatment* of pericarditis in the newborn is similar to that used in any infection in this age group. Broad-spectrum antimicrobial agents are indicated. If a pathogen is isolated from the blood stream or from the pericardium, a more specific antibiotic may be chosen. When heart failure is present, the usual anticongestive measures are used.

Case 26–4

An infant was the result of a full-term pregnancy. This was uneventful until 4 days before delivery, when the mother had a respiratory infection with fever. The delivery took place at another hospital and was uncomplicated. The birth weight was 7 pounds ¾ ounce (3220 gm). The infant appeared normal at birth. The day after delivery the mother's fever recurred, and a diagnosis of pneumonia was made. She nevertheless nursed the infant on several occasions. The infant was well until the fifth day of life, when a tachycardia was noted. Despite the unexplained tachycardia, the infant was discharged on the following day.

Several hours after discharge he had a temperature of 101° and refused feedings. That evening he was admitted to the Sinai Hospital. Examination revealed a vigorous infant with good color, but with definite respiratory distress. Respirations were 80 per minute. There were rales at both bases. No clinical enlargement of the heart was detected. The heart tones were of fair quality. There were no murmurs. Shortly after admission he became gravely ill. His color was ashen and mottled. Respirations became more rapid and grunting. The liver was palpable 4 cm below the costal margin. He was treated with antibiotics and oxygen. He worsened rapidly and died 2 hours after admission. An x-ray film of the chest showed infiltration in the right middle and lower lung fields and general cardiac

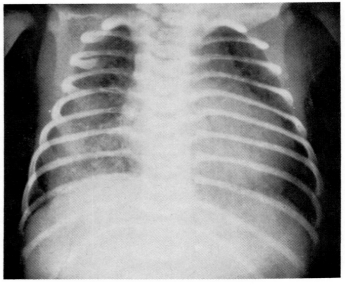

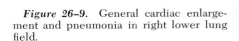

*Figure 26–9.* General cardiac enlargement and pneumonia in right lower lung field.

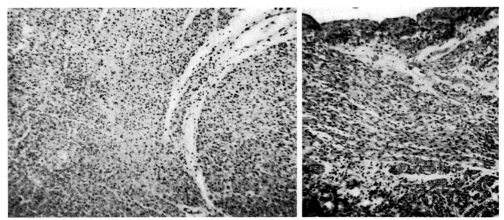

*Figure 26–10.* *A*, Section through the myocardium showing diffuse, polymorphonuclear infiltration. *B*, Microscopic section of the pericardium and myocardium. There is considerable cellular infiltrate.

enlargement (Fig. 26–9). Nose and throat cultures revealed *Staphylococcus aureus.* The blood and cerebrospinal fluid were sterile.

Postmortem examination by Dr. T. Weinberg and staff revealed gross and microscopic evidence of pneumonia of both lower lobes. The pericardial sac yielded 25 cc of yellow turbid fluid from which hemolytic staphylococci were cultured. The heart was enlarged and dilated. Microscopic examination showed a diffuse myocardial infiltration with polymorphonuclear cells predominating (Fig. 26–10, *A*). The inflammatory infiltrate extended into the pericardium (Fig. 26–10, *B*). Bacterial stains revealed grampositive cocci in the pericardium and myocardium.

COMMENT. This infant had a purulent pericarditis associated with myocarditis and pneumonia. The diagnosis of pneumonia was apparent, but cardiac disease was not suspected. The staphylococcus was proved as the pathogen. Since this infant was delivered in another hospital, it is not known whether this organism was isolated from the mother. Nevertheless the maternal illness was a likely source of infection.

## TUMORS OF THE HEART

Cardiac tumors are rare entities at best, but when they do occur, manifestations of heart disease are not infrequently present in the neonatal period. Several types of tumors have been described. Rhabdo-

myomas are the most common. They consist of numerous nodular areas which contain glycogen. They may occur in association with tuberous sclerosis. An intramural fibroma is less common, but has been reported in the neonatal period (Bigelow et al.). Myomas and sarcomas are exceedingly rare. The 23 cases reported in the literature under 1 year of age have been summarized by Rowe and Mehrizi.

The *clinical picture* is exceedingly variable. Arrhythmias are common with rhabdomyomas. In the patient cited at the end of this chapter paroxysmal atrial tachycardia was the presenting finding. Heart murmurs are usually not present. Heart failure is common. This often comes on with great suddenness. The heart may be normal or enlarged. Occasionally bizarre prominences distort the cardiac contour. The electrocardiographic findings are extremely variable. The tracing of a 7-week-old infant with rhabdomyomas is shown in Figure 26–11.

The *diagnosis* is rarely made during life. It should be suspected in any infant with tuberous sclerosis who shows evidence of cardiac disease, especially if a cardiac arrhythmia is present. The sudden onset of intractable heart failure in a previously well infant should suggest a cardiac tumor if the more common causes such as myocarditis and endocardial fibroelastosis can be excluded.

There is no satisfactory medical treat-

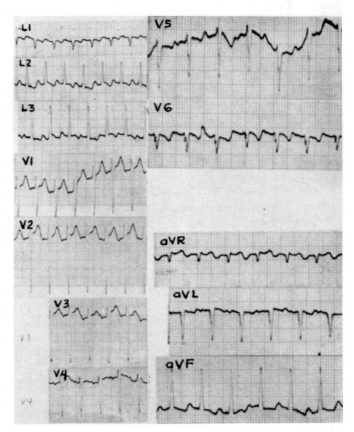

*Figure 26-11.* Age 7 weeks. Multiple rhabdomyomas of the heart. The electrocardiogram is abnormal. There is T wave inversion in the limb leads and over the left side of the precordium. The S waves are abnormally deep over the right and left sides of the precordium. The over-all pattern is bizarre.

ment for cardiac tumors. Successful surgical removal has been accomplished. Engle and Glenn reported the removal of rhabdomyosarcoma in a 4-month-old infant. He died on the eleventh postoperative day.

### CASE 26-5

(This case is abstracted with the kind permission of Dr. Jerome Fineman of Baltimore.).

An infant was admitted to the hospital at one month of age with heavy breathing of 1 day's duration. The patient was born 2 weeks prematurely. Birth weight was 5 pounds 5 ounces (2410 gm). He was normal at birth and appeared to be thriving until the sudden onset of his illness.

The infant was severely dyspneic and mildly cyanotic on admission. The respirations were 60, pulse 240, temperature normal. The heart was not enlarged. There were no murmurs. The liver was three to four fingerbreadths below the costal margin. The femoral pulses were normal. The electrocardiogram disclosed paroxysmal supraventricular tachycardia. The infant did not

respond to digitalis and died several hours after admission.

An autopsy was performed by Dr. Tobias Weinberg. The heart was of average size (weight 28 gm). On gross examination numerous nodules of varying size were seen within the walls of both ventricles and atria (Fig. 26-12). These masses protruded into the cavities of the chambers and were also noted beneath the pericardium. On cut section the nodules were yellowish gray in appearance. Microscopic section disclosed a loose cellular pattern with globular vacuolated areas which contained a small amount of glycogen.

**COMMENT.** This 1-month-old infant presented with the sudden onset of paroxysmal tachycardia and heart failure which did not respond to treatment. At autopsy multiple rhabdomyomas of the heart were found which undoubtedly were the cause of the arrhythmia. Sudden onset of heart failure in a previously well infant is not uncommon in infants with cardiac tumors.

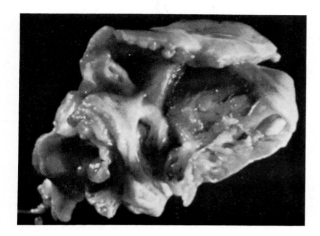

*Figure 26–12.* Age 1 month. Multiple rhabdo-myomas. Gross specimen of the opened heart shows numerous nodular masses within the walls of the ventricle and protruding into the chamber of the heart.

## ARTERIOVENOUS FISTULA AND HEART FAILURE

Arteriovenous fistula is a recognized, but rare, cause of heart failure in the newborn infant. An awareness of this entity is nevertheless important because survival depends on prompt recognition.

The site of the arteriovenous communication varies. Cerebral fistulas are the most common (Holden et al.; Hope and Izukawa). They have been found in the liver (Crocker et al.), internal mammary vessels (Glass et al.) and the skin (Cohen and Sinclair).

The pathophysiology of congestive failure in patients with arteriovenous fistulas has been studied by Elkin and Warren and others. The short-circuiting of blood decreases peripheral resistance, lowers diastolic pressure, increases cardiac output and causes cardiac enlargement.

Tachypnea is usually the first sign of difficulty, appearing between 1 and 4 days of age. This is followed by more overt signs of heart failure, and a rapid, downhill course is the rule. Cyanosis was present in all seven cases reported by Hope and Izukawa.

There may be gross evidence of a fistula such as the pulsating mass in the skin or over the cranium (Case 26–6). More often the site of the fistula cannot be seen or felt. However, a cranial bruit can be heard in virtually all cases of intracranial fistulae.

The neurologic findings are otherwise not remarkable.

The cardiac shadow is enlarged on x-ray, often to huge proportions. There may be electrocardiographic evidence of right atrial and ventricular hypertrophy. Cardiac catheterization studies by Hope and Izukawa showed a high superior vena caval oxygen saturation and a rapid return of the dye to the right heart, findings which should suggest the diagnosis of a cerebral A-V fistula.

The possibility of an arteriovenous fistula should be entertained in every neonate in congestive failure in whom primary heart disease has been excluded. Such infants should be examined scrupulously for a bruit over the lungs, the liver and particularly the cranium, since the head is the most common site. Prominent hemangiomas of the skin may suggest the presence of visceral hemangioma as well. If an intracranial fistula is suspected, the diagnosis may be confirmed by a cerebral arteriogram. Indeed, it would seem warranted to include a film of the skull in every infant who undergoes retrograde aortography for undiagnosed heart disease.

In general the response to digitalis and to other measures directed against heart failure is poor. The only treatment of value is surgical. Obviously this depends on the localization of the site of the fistula. If there is an intracranial lesion, ligation of one or both carotid arteries may be lifesaving.

Few infants have been salvaged because the diagnosis has not been made sufficiently early.

Case 26–6

An infant was born after a normal full-term pregnancy. Birth weight was 9 pounds (4077 gm). At the time of birth a large pulsating mass was noted over the right temporal region. A bruit and thrill were present over the mass. These findings disappeared after compression of the right carotid artery. At 36 hours of age the infant became cyanotic. The heart was enlarged on physical examination and in the chest x-ray (Fig. 26–13, A). Signs of congestive heart failure were present. An x-ray film of the skull demonstrated a defect in the right temporal region with a bulge in the same area (Fig. 26–13, B).

The patient was seen in consultation with Dr. David Clark and was thereafter transferred to the Harriet Lane Home. Rapid digitalization and venesection were carried out, and ligation of the right carotid artery was done. The infant died 1 hour after operation.

Autopsy examination was performed by Dr. Wagner of Lutheran Hospital. The common carotid artery was dilated. There was a gross abnormality in the floor of the right side of the middle cranial fossa. In this area there was a large cavity supplied by the middle meningeal artery which communicated with the lateral and right cavernous sinus. The heart was enlarged: weight 43 gm. The ventricular walls were hypertrophied. There were no other cardiac abnormalities.

# PERSISTENT PULMONARY HYPERTENSION OF THE NEWBORN

In recent years a number of reports have appeared describing full-term newborns who shortly after birth develop tachypnea, cyanosis, cardiomegaly and sometimes heart failure, and who therefore closely mimic infants with cyanotic congenital heart disease. Studies of these infants have revealed pulmonary hypertension and large right-to-left shunts through fetal channels, but otherwise anatomically normal hearts and without evidence of pulmonary parenchymal disease.

Various terms other than persistent pulmonary hypertension have been used to describe this clinical syndrome: persistent fetal circulation, persistence of fetal cardiopulmonary circulation, pulmonary vascular obstruction and progressive pulmonary hypertension. The incidence of this syndrome is not known, but it is probably more common than generally appreciated. Gersony has recently written a concise review of the subject.

**Etiology.** This syndrome has been described in infants with hypoglycemia not associated with maternal diabetes (Beard et al.). It also has been recognized in newborns with polycythemia and hyperviscosity (Gatti et al.; Gross et al.). In another series, Roberton and associates found a

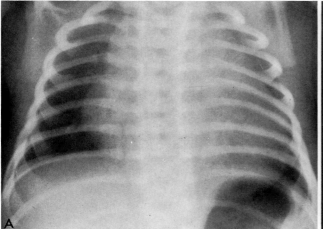 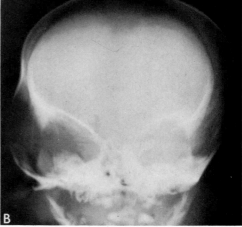

*Figure 26–13.*    Age 2 days. Cerebral arteriovenous aneurysm. *A,* X-ray film of chest demonstrates considerable cardiac enlargement. *B,* X-ray film of skull shows a bulge on the right side with defect of the outer margin.

high incidence of perinatal asphyxia, suggesting that intrauterine stress with hypoxia may be an important precipitating factor. It is likely there are a number of different factors which retard the normal changes in pulmonary vasculature either by pulmonary vasoconstriction or because of developmental abnormalities. The pathogenetic mechanisms are still not known, nor is it clear whether the disease in some of these infants who have a protracted clinical course bears any relationship to primary pulmonary vascular disease of older children (Burnell et al.; Levin et al.).

**PATHOPHYSIOLOGY.** In normal newborns, the pulmonary vascular resistance decreases rapidly after birth. Hemodynamic studies on infants with persistent pulmonary hypertension have consistently shown an abnormally high pulmonary vascular resistance along with arterial unsaturation at the ductal and/or atrial level indicative of right-to-left shunting. Cineangiographic and autopsy studies have revealed no evidence of other anatomical cardiac defects nor has there been evidence of pulmonary parenchymal disease. However, medial hypertrophy of the pulmonary arterioles has been a common finding (Siassi et al.; Levin et al.).

**CLINICAL FEATURES.** The clinical picture is fairly uniform and is that of a full-term infant who begins to breathe rapidly and have intermittent or persistent severe cyanosis shortly after birth. There are usually neither severe retractions nor grunting. Except for harsh bronchiolar breath sounds, the lung fields are clear to auscultation. A soft ejection systolic murmur is often present. Hepatomegaly is common, suggesting the presence of congestive heart failure. The peripheral circulation is usually normal.

Roentgenogram of the chest shows a mild to moderate degree of cardiac enlargement with normal pulmonary vasculature. The electrocardiogram may show a greater right ventricular preponderance than normal for the newborn, but the findings are often inconclusive. The blood gases reveal a decrease in arterial oxygen tension, often strikingly low, with only slight abnormalities of arterial pH and $PCO_2$.

The clinical course is variable. Infants who are going to survive usually improve rapidly within 3 to 6 days. Persistent cyanosis beyond that of the first week is a poor prognostic sign. However, the patient reported by Levin and his associates survived after a prolonged course. The prognosis in newborns with persistent pulmonary hypertension associated with hypoglycemia or polycythemia is generally good and the cardiopulmonary manifestations improve following treatment for the underlying condition.

**DIAGNOSIS.** The clinical manifestations of persistent pulmonary hypertension have to be distinguished from congenital heart disease and parenchymal lung disease. The occurrence in full-term infants, the degree of cyanosis without severe respiratory retractions, lack of improvement with adequate oxygenation and the absence of x-ray evidence of pulmonary disease should alert the physician to the diagnosis.

The distinction from cyanotic forms of congenital heart disease is often very difficult. Murmurs are rarely prominent in persistent pulmonary hypertension syndrome, but they may also be absent in congenital heart disease. Infants with cardiac defects of sufficient severity to cause tachypnea and cyanosis shortly after birth often develop frank congestive heart failure earlier. They are also more likely to have more distinctive electrocardiographic and x-ray findings than infants with persistent pulmonary hypertension. Nevertheless, it is often necessary to do cardiac catheterization and cineangiography to completely exclude a cardiac defect.

These studies can be avoided if there is evidence of hypoglycemia or polycythemia. Blood sugar and hematocrit determinations should be done in all infants with cardiopulmonary disease of uncertain etiology. It should be recognized, however, that hypoglycemia is not uncommon in infants with failure from congenital heart disease (Benzing et al.). Patients with either hypoglycemia or polycythemia can present with central nervous system manifestations. On the other hand, cyanosis may precede these manifestations. Cyanosis and signs of cardiac failure in a plethoric newborn should strongly suggest the persistent pulmonary hypertension syndrome associated with polycythemia and hyperviscosity.

**TREATMENT.** If the primary diagnosis is

hypoglycemia, glucose should be administered to maintain normoglycemic levels. In infants with polycythemia, a partial exchange transfusion, replacing whole blood with plasma, or a phlebotomy, is indicated.

The treatment of infants with persistent pulmonary hypertension in whom no underlying disease process can be identified is much less satisfactory. Oxygen therapy should be maintained and the concentration adjusted depending on the arterial oxygen tension. Since many of these infants are first suspected of having congenital heart disease, digitalis and diuretics are often administered, although there is no evidence that they influence the cause of the disease. There are a number of drugs which are known to influence pulmonary vascular tone, such as tolazoline, but the use of these agents is still experimental. Ventilatory assistance may be needed, but continuous distending airway pressure is contraindicated in this condition.

## THE HEART AND HEMOLYTIC DISEASE OF THE NEWBORN

Cardiac disturbances associated with hemolytic disease of the newborn are not uncommon. They are of two general types: (1) heart failure associated with severe anemia or from overloading the circulation during an exchange transfusion, and (2) arrhythmias or cardiac arrest while the exchange transfusion is in progress.

Profound anemia is a recognized cause of heart failure secondary to the associated anoxia. When it occurs in the neonatal period, it is almost always due to severe hemolytic disease. In addition to the extreme pallor, these infants exhibit peripheral edema, ascites, pulmonary congestion, poor heart tones and cardiac dilatation, often leading to death within minutes or hours after birth. Hogg studied the hearts of 40 infants who died of hemolytic disease and found an increase in heart weight, enlarged myocardial nuclei, varying degrees of endocardial fibroelastosis and occasional small infarcts. These findings were thought to be related to anemic anoxia.

Heart failure from circulatory overload is an uncommon but serious complication of the exchange transfusion. It may occur with mild hemolytic disease if excess blood is given. It is more likely to occur in infants who are markedly anemic at the start and probably at the brink of failure, which is then precipitated by the manipulations of the procedure or the quantity of blood injected if due caution is not observed. Congestive failure should be suspected if in the midst of the exchange transfusion the pulse quickens or slows markedly, respirations become grunting, the color worsens or frothing at the mouth appears. Any of these manifestations should be taken as a clear signal to stop the transfusion, measure the venous pressure, withdraw blood until the pressure falls below 10 cm and withhold the transfusion entirely or until the infant's condition improves.

Cardiac arrhythmias occur more commonly during exchange transfusion than is generally recognized and account for a significant proportion of deaths occurring during the exchange procedure. Examples of heart block, atrial, nodal and ventricular premature contractions, and ventricular fibrillation have been reported (Joos et al.; Taylor et al.). The occurrence of arrhythmias has not been correlated consistently with the severity of the hemolytic disease, the maturity of the infant, the temperature, age of the blood, acidosis, hypocalcemia, hyperkalemia or hypercitremia. Any of these, as well as unknown factors, may play a role. Arrhythmias have great clinical importance, since their appearance may herald the onset of cardiac arrest or precipitate congestive failure in infants who do not have severe hemolytic disease. In a large series of patients Van Praagh noted cardiac arrhythmias in 52 per cent of the patients who died.

It should be obvious from the foregoing comments that the management of infants with hemolytic disease must always include a careful assessment of the cardiac status prior to transfusion and an acute awareness that serious cardiac complications may occur during the course of the procedure or shortly after it has been completed. Before beginning the exchange, the venous pressure should be measured. In well-compensated infants it will range between 4 and 10 cm. If there is gross evidence of heart failure, sedimented cells should be given in aliquots of 5 to 10 ml after 10 to 20 ml of blood have been removed. In infants without clinical evidence of failure, if the venous pressure is above 10 cm with the infant in the quiet state, 10 ml more blood should be withdrawn than is given until the pressure is normal. During the course of every transfusion the infant should be observed clinically by the most senior physician in the team and by electrocardiographic monitoring. As has already been suggested, the transfusion should be stopped at once if *any one* of the following signs appears: 1) cyanosis, 2) grunting respirations, 3) significant change in pulse rate (tachycardia or bradycardia) and 4) any arrhythmia. Should cardiac arrest occur, closed-chest massage should be carried out, and, if this is unsuccessful, thoracotomy with direct massage should be performed. The complete recovery of two infants with cardiac arrest by open cardiac massage has been reported (Wallgren and Okmian).

## REFERENCES

Amatayahul, V., et al.: Association of hypoglycemia with cardiac enlargement and heart failure in newborn infants. Arch. Dis. Child. 45:717, 1970.

Anderson, D. H., and Kelly, J.: Endocardial fibroelastosis associated with congenital malformations of the heart. Pediatrics 18:513, 1956.

Beard, A., et al.: Neonatal hypoglycemia: discussion. J. Pediatr. 79:314, 1971.

Benzing, G., III, et al.: Simultaneous hypoglycemia and acute congestive heart failure. Circulation 40:209, 1969.

Bigelow, N. H., Klinger, S., and Wright, A. W.: Primary tumors of the heart in infancy and childhood. Cancer 7:549, 1954.

Black-Schaffer, B., and Turner, M. E.: Infantile hyperplastic cardiomegaly. Am. J. Path. 34:584, 1958.

Burnell, R. H., et al.: Progressive pulmonary hypertension in newborn infants. Am. J. Dis. Child. 123:167, 1972.

Cadell, J., and Whittemore, R.: Observations on generalized glycogenesis with emphasis on electrocardiographic changes. Pediatrics 29:743, 1962.

Cohen, M. I., and Sinclair, J. C.: Neonatal death from congestive heart failure associated with large cutaneous cavernous hemangiomas. Pediatrics 32:924, 1963.

Crocker, D. W., and Cleveland, R. S.: Infantile hemangioendothelioma of the liver; report of three cases. Pediatrics 19:596, 1957.

Di Sant'Agnese, P., Anderson, D. H., and Mason, H. H.: Glycogen storage disease of the heart. Pediatrics 6:607, 1950.

Ehlers, K. H., Hagstrom, J. W., Lukas, D. S., Redo, S. F., and Engle, M. A.: Glycogen-storage disease of

the myocardium with obstruction to left ventricular flow. Circulation 25:96, 1962.

Elkin, D. C., and Warren, J. V.: Arteriovenous fistulas: Their effect on the circulation. J.A.M.A. 134:1524, 1947.

Engle, M. A., and Glenn, F.: Primary malignant tumor of the heart in infancy. Case report and review of the subject. Pediatrics 15:562, 1955.

Fruhling, L., et al.: Chronic fibroelastic myoendocarditis of the newborn and the infant (fibroelastosis). Ann. Anat. Path. (Paris) 7:227, 1962.

Gatti, R. A.: Neonatal polycythemia with transient cyanosis and cardiorespiratory abnormalities. J. Pediatr. 69:1063, 1966.

Gersony, W. M.: Persistence of the fetal circulation: A commentary. J. Pediatr. 82:1103, 1973.

Gersony, W. M., et al.: "PFC" syndrome. Circulation 40(Suppl. 3):87, 1969.

Glass, I. H., Rowe, R. D., and Duckworth, J. W. A.: Congenital arteriovenous fistula between the left internal mammary artery and the ductus venosus. Pediatrics, 26:604, 1960.

Gross, G. P., et al.: Hyperviscosity in the neonate. J. Pediatr. 82:1004, 1973.

Gross, P.: Concept of fetal endocarditis. General review with report of illustrative case. Arch. Path. 31:163, 1941.

Hastreiter, A. R. and Miller, R. A.: Management of primary endomyocardial disease. Pediat. Clin. N. Amer. 11:401, 1964.

Hers, H. G.: Alpha glucosidase deficiency in generalized glycogen storage disease (Pompe's disease). Biochem. J. 86:11, 1963.

Hogg, G. R.: Cardiac lesions in hemolytic disease of the newborn. J. Pediatr. 60:352, 1962.

Holden, A. M., et al.: Congestive heart failure from intracranial arteriovenous fistula in infancy. Pediatrics 49:30, 1972.

Hope, R., and Izukawa, T.: Congestive cardiac failure and intracranial arteriovenous communications in infants and children. Aust. N. Z. J. Med. 3:598, 1973.

Hung, W., and Walsh, B. J.: Congenital auricular fibrillation in a newborn infant with endocardial fibroelastosis. J. Pediatr. 61:65, 1962.

Joos, H. A., Yu, P. N., and Miller, G.: Electrocardiographic changes during replacement transfusion. Am. J. Dis. Child. 88:471, 1954.

Kelly, J., and Anderson, D. H.: Congenital endocardial fibroelastosis. II. A clinical and pathologic investigation of those cases without associated cardiac malformations, including report of two familial instances. Pediatrics 12:539, 1956.

Lambert, E. C., Shumway, C. N., and Terplan, K.: Clinical diagnosis of endocardial fibrosis. Analysis of literature and report of four new cases. Pediatrics 11:255, 1953.

Lendrum, F. C.: The "pulmonary hyaline membrane" as a manifestation of heart failure in the newborn infant. J. Pediatr. 47:149, 1955.

Levin, D. L., et al.: Persistence of the fetal cardiopulmonary circulatory pathway. Pediatrics 56:58, 1975.

Linde, C. M., and Adams, F. H.: Prognosis in endocardial fibroelastosis. Am. J. Dis. Child. 105:329, 1963.

Mitchell, S. C., Forehlich, L. A., Banas, J. S., and Gilkerson, M. R.: An epidemiologic assessment of primary endocardial fibroelastosis. Am. J. Cardiol. *18*:859, 1966.

Nahill, M. R., et al.: Generalized glycogenosis type II (Pompe's disease). Arch. Dis. Child. *45*:122, 1970.

Noren, G. R., Adams, P., and Anderson, R. C.: Positive skin reactivity to mumps virus antigen in endocardial fibroelastosis. J. Pediatr. *62*:604, 1963.

Roberton, N. R., et al.: Severe respiratory distress syndrome mimicking cyanotic heart disease in term babies. Lancet *2*:1108, 1967.

Rosenstein, B. J.: Glycogen storage disease of the heart in a newborn infant. J. Pediatr. *65*:126, 1964.

Rowe, R. D., and James, L. S.: The normal pulmonary arterial pressure during the first year of life. J. Pediatr. *51*:1, 1957.

Rowe, R. D., and Mehrizi, A.: The Neonate with Congenital Heart Disease. Philadelphia, W. B. Saunders Company, 1968.

St. Geme, J. W., et al.: Experimental gestational mumps virus infection and endocardial fibroelastosis. Pediatrics *48*:821, 1971.

Siassi, B., et al.: Persistent pulmonary vascular obstruction in newborn infants. J. Pediatr. *78*:610, 1971.

Still, W. J. S., and Boult, E. H.: The electron microscopy of endocardial fibroelastosis. Arch. Dis. Child. *32*:298, 1957.

Taylor, W. C., Grisdale, L. C., and Stewart, A. G.: Unexplained death from exchange transfusion. J. Pediatr. *52*:694, 1958.

Usher, R.: The respiratory distress syndrome of prematurity. I. Changes in potassium in the serum and electrocardiogram and effects of therapy. Pediatrics *24*:562, 1959.

Valdés-Dapena, M., and Miller, W. H.: Pericarditis in the newborn. Pediatrics, *16*:673, 1955.

Van Praagh, R.: Causes of death in infants with hemolytic disease of the newborn. Pediatrics *28*:223, 1961.

Vestermark, S.: Primary endocardial fibroelastosis in siblings. Acta paediat. *51*:94, 1962.

Wallgren, G., and Okmian, L.: Successful resuscitation of two immature infants with cardiac arrest during exchange transfusion. Acta paediat. *50*:399, 1961.

Weinberg, T., and Himelfarb, A. J.: Endocardial fibroelastosis. Bull. Johns Hopkins Hosp. *72*:299, 1943.

# DIFFERENTIAL DIAGNOSIS OF NEONATAL CARDIAC PROBLEMS

# 27

*Revised by Milton Markowitz*

In the preceding chapters the distinctive features of a number of cardiac malformations have been described. There is, however, considerable overlapping of the clinical findings and it is often difficult to make a precise clinical diagnosis in the nursery. As a starting point, it is helpful to place neonates with suspected heart disease into three groups according to their major findings on physical examination, chest x-ray and electrocardiogram. In this way, the most likely diagnoses can be selected from the large and diverse number of lesions, and a judgment can be made regarding the need for cardiac catheterization and angiocardiography.

GROUP I: INFANTS WITH A HEART MURMUR AND NO OTHER EVIDENCE OF CARDIAC DISEASE. In a number of these infants the murmur will disappear during the first few weeks or months of life. If the murmur is due to a cardiac defect and there are no other findings, the diagnosis of the anatomical defect may be difficult. The intensity and location of the murmur are less diagnostic in the neonate than in older infants. All too often the systolic murmur is heard equally well over the entire precordium. This type of murmur is most likely caused by a left-to-right shunt. Among left-to-right shunt anomalies, *ventricular septal defect* is the most common, but it may be difficult if not impossible to distinguish from a *patent ductus arteriosus*. If the infant is a small premature and the murmur appears after the first week of life, a patent ductus is the likely diagnosis, especially if the peripheral pulses are full or are bounding. A systolic murmur is also heard in infants with an *endocardial cushion defect*. This anomaly should be strongly suspected if there is an unusual degree of left axis deviation on the electrocardiogram.

The majority of infants with *tetralogy of Fallot* do not have cyanosis in the neonatal period and therefore fall into this group. The heart murmur is often not as long or loud as that caused by a left-to-right shunt.

A reduction in lung vascularity and a typical cardiac contour may suggest a tetralogy, but unfortunately these findings are often less distinctive in the neonate. Less common anomalies such as *single ventricle* and *truncus arteriosus* may also have delayed cyanosis and should be included in the differential diagnosis. The presence of a continuous murmur after the first 24 hours of life should suggest the possibility of truncus arteriosus.

A definitive diagnosis cannot usually be made in neonates with group I defects without the help of cardiac catheterization or angiocardiography. These studies are not indicated in the newborn without symptoms or signs of heart disease other than a heart murmur. The clinical features often become more distinctive in later infancy, at which time properly selected diagnostic studies can be more readily accomplished.

**GROUP II: INFANTS IN WHOM CYANOSIS IS THE STRIKING CLINICAL FEATURE.** Cyanosis of the newborn may be due to pulmonary disease, a central nervous system disturbance, congenital heart disease or methemoglobenemia. Some of the distinguishing features among these various conditions have been discussed in a previous chapter so that this discussion will be limited to congenital heart disease.

The early appearance of cyanosis from congenital heart disease is due either to transposition of the great arteries or to anomalies causing severe reduction in pulmonary blood flow plus a right-to-left shunt. The latter include pulmonary atresia, tricuspid atresia, Ebstein's anomaly, severe isolated pulmonary stenosis and tetralogy of Fallot with pulmonary atresia or extreme pulmonary stenosis.

*Transposition of the great arteries* is the most frequent cause of cyanosis due to congenital heart disease in the newborn, and it is one of the most distinctive clinical entities. The cyanosis is usually severe. On x-ray examination the base of the heart is narrow, pulmonary vascularity is increased, and the heart becomes enlarged rapidly.

The difference in pulmonary vascularity on x-ray provides the main distinction between cyanosis due to transposition of the great arteries and the group of anomalies

characterized by diminished pulmonary blood flow.

In *pulmonary atresia* the heart is often enlarged shortly after birth, the pulmonary vascularity is clearly diminished, and there may be a transient left ventricular electrocardiographic pattern. Infants with *tricuspid atresia* have a normal-sized heart, diminished pulmonary vascularity, and left axis deviation and left ventricular hypertrophy. The severe form of *tetralogy of Fallot* is associated with reduced pulmonary vascularity and moderate right ventricular hypertrophy but little or no cardiac enlargement on x-ray film. Similar findings are present in a *single ventricle* with pulmonary stenosis. In isolated *severe pulmonary stenosis* the heart is enlarged early, pulmonary vascularity is reduced and there is right ventricular hypertrophy.

A careful evaluation of the physical findings, radiologic studies and the electrocardiogram will often suggest the correct diagnosis of the defects enumerated in group II. Infants in this group may deteriorate very rapidly and require further studies at centers experienced in the care of small infants with suspected heart disease. Infants with severe isolated pulmonic stenosis or pulmonary atresia are candidates for immediate operative correction. Palliative treatment can be accomplished for transposition of the great vessels, tricuspid atresia, severe tetralogy of Fallot and single ventricle with pulmonary stenosis.

**GROUP III: INFANTS WITH HEART FAILURE IN WHOM CYANOSIS AND MURMURS MAY OR MAY NOT BE PRESENT.** This group includes the hypoplastic left heart syndrome, coarctation of the aorta, total anomalous venous return of the infradiaphragmatic type and patent ductus arteriosus of prematurity. One condition that these lesions have in common is severe pulmonary venous congestion.

In the *hypoplastic left-heart syndrome* generalized enlargement of the heart is present at birth, heart failure occurs early and is profound, and right atrial and ventricular hypertrophy is present. *Coarctation of the aorta* should be suspected if femoral pulsations are absent or diminished or if there is a significant arm-leg blood pressure differential. In *total anom-*

alous pulmonary venous return of the infra-diaphragmatic group, there is early heart failure, a small heart and a very distinctive pattern of venous congestion of the lungs. Heart failure due to left-to-right shunts rarely occurs in the newborn period except for the *patent ductus arteriosus*, which is fairly common cause of failure in small prematures between the first and fourth week of life.

Heart failure may also be caused by myocarditis, endocardial fibroelastosis, glycogen storage disease, paroxysmal atrial tachycardia and arteriovenous fistula. In *primary myocarditis* the onset of the heart failure is fairly abrupt, the heart sounds are poor and there is low voltage in the electrocardiogram. In *endocardial fibroelastosis* there is usually some evidence of left ventricular hypertrophy. *Glycogen storage disease* of the heart rarely manifests overt cardiac signs in the nursery, but it should be considered nevertheless in any infant with a large heart and a bizarre electrocardiogram, especially if there is a family history. By simply counting the heart rate accurately, there should be no difficulty in excluding *paroxysmal atrial tachycardia* as a cause of failure. An *arteriovenous fistula* is a rare abnormality, but every neonate should be examined carefully for unusual bruits over the head, liver and lungs if there is unexplained cardiomegaly and congestive failure.

Infants with persistent pulmonary hypertension ("persistent fetal circulation syndrome") may have severe cyanosis and other findings resembling congenital heart disease. The simultaneous occurrence of hypoglycemia or polycythemia in an infant with suspicious cardiovascular findings should suggest this syndrome. However, in the absence of an underlying disease process, it is usually necessary to do further studies to exclude congenital heart disease.

If there is any question of the etiology of heart failure in the neonate or if the infant does not respond rapidly to medical treatment, definitive studies should be undertaken without delay to identify those conditions which may be amenable to surgical correction or palliation. These include patent ductus, coarctation, total anomalous pulmonary venous return and arteriovenous fistula.

# TREATMENT

*Revised by Milton Markowitz*

# 28

## MEDICAL MANAGEMENT

### CONGESTIVE HEART FAILURE

The signs and symptoms of heart failure have been described in a previous chapter. It was noted that 20 per cent of infants with congenital heart disease develop heart failure in the first week and in another 18 per cent it occurs between the first and fourth weeks of life (Keith). It is important to recognize failure in its early stages so that therapy can be begun as rapidly as possible.

**OXYGEN.** When heart failure is suspected, oxygen therapy is indicated if the arterial oxygen tension is low, even in the absence of clinical cyanosis. It should be administered in humidified atmosphere in concentrations of 35 to 40 per cent. Higher concentrations may be necessary for short periods of time. In premature infants it is important to monitor the level of arterial oxygen tension and adjust the oxygen concentration accordingly.

**DIGITALIS.** The cardiac glycosides are the chief therapeutic agents used to treat heart failure. Digoxin is the most widely used and the most satisfactory of the glycosides. It has the advantages of acting rapidly and of being available in oral and parenteral preparations. The recommended oral total digitalizing dose (TDD) for the full-term newborn is between 0.05 and 0.07 mg/kg. The parenteral dose is 75 per cent of the oral dose, or a TDD of 0.04 to 0.05 mg/kg. For parenteral administration, the intravenous method is preferred over the intramuscular, since the latter may cause muscle damage (Steiness et al.). Because the premature is less able to excrete or detoxify digitalis, the TDD for prematures should be reduced to 0.03 mg/kg (Levine and Blumenthal). In fact, studies by Levy and co-workers suggest that a similar dose is probably adequate for full-term infants and that the larger TDD usually employed is unnecessary, even though full-term infants appear to tolerate large doses. This subject has been reviewed recently by Soyka.

Since newborns tend to get very sick very rapidly, it is wise to plan for total digitalization over a period of 12 to 18 hours. Half the total digitalizing dose is given at once and one fourth at 6 to 8 hour intervals. The infant should be monitored with an EKG tracing before the final dose is given. The average daily maintenance dose of digoxin is 25 per cent of the total dose given in two divided doses daily.

It should be emphasized that the dosage schedules recommended above are only general guides and that digitalis tolerance varies with each infant and to some extent with the nature of the underlying disease. For example, infants with acute myocarditis are especially sensitive to digitalis. Care must be taken to avoid toxicity. Poor feeding rather than vomiting is an early sign of toxicity. The heart rate is the most valuable index and if the rate falls below 100 per minute, digitalis should be withheld. The EKG should be repeated at frequent intervals: premature beats and heart block are signs of toxicity. It is now possible to determine serum digitalis levels, and this should soon become a routine method to monitor patients on digitalis (Krasula et al.). A serum digoxin concentration in the range of 1 to 2 ng/ml is usually adequate.

**DIURETICS.** In general, diuretics are used when congestive heart failure does not respond rapidly to adequate doses of digitalis. The newer diuretic agents furose-mide and ethacrynic acid have replaced the mercurials. Both new drugs act by blocking the reabsorption of sodium to produce a natriuresis and diuresis. The advantages of these agents over the mercurials are their speed of action, independence from urinary pH and serum chloride concentration, and relative freedom from nephrotoxicity.

The dosages for furosemide and ethacrynic acid are 1 mg/kg/day intravenously and 2 to 3 mg/kg/day orally. The oral preparations are used for maintenance therapy usually on an every-other-day basis. Serum electrolytes should be monitored in patients receiving diuretics.

**ACID-BASE BALANCE.** In addition to serum electrolytes, the blood gases and pH should also be monitored in infants with heart failure. Hypoxia associated with poor cardiac output frequently causes lactic acidemia which should be corrected with sodium bicarbonate. Severe pulmonary edema may lead to respiratory failure, and the blood gases are a guide to the need for ventilatory support. If the $PCO_2$ is more than 60 mm Hg, nasoendotracheal intubation and ventilator therapy may be indicated.

**FEEDINGS.** Oral feedings should be withheld during the course of acute heart failure, since vomiting and aspiration are an ever-present danger in sick babies. During this acute phase the minimal fluid requirements should be satisfied by parenteral means. When the infant can tolerate oral feedings, and signs of cardiac insufficiency are still present, a low solute formula may be used.

**SEDATION.** Restlessness is less common in the newborn than in older infants with heart failure. Morphine is occasionally necessary. The dosage is 0.05 mg/kg.

**INFECTIONS.** Infections are common complications in patients with heart failure. Congested lungs are often the seat of bronchopneumonia. Great care should be taken to prevent infections, and strict isolation technique in the nursery or pediatric unit is mandatory. Since it is virtually impossible to tell when congested lungs are infected, therapeutic doses of appropriate antibiotics should be administered. Penicillin and kanamycin is the combination of choice unless cultures of the respiratory secretions indicate the need for other antimicrobial agents.

**ANEMIA.** Anemia may precipitate or aggravate congestive failure when there is an underlying cardiac lesion. Low hemoglobin may of itself cause anoxic heart failure if the anemia is severe or sudden. The classic example is seen in infants with the hydropic form of erythroblastosis who are in heart failure at birth. When the anemia is associated with primary heart disease, blood transfusion is used in conjunction with other measures. If, however, the anemia is the cause of failure, then blood transfusion may be the only treatment necessary. In either case several principles of treatment should be observed. 1) No attempt should be made to correct the anemia completely with a single transfusion. 2) A partial exchange transfusion should be given with sedimented blood, since blood with a high hemoglobin and a low plasma volume is an ideal substance for heart failure. 3) Close observation for the appearance of an elevation in pulse, pulmonary rales and an increase in liver size is necessary during the course of a transfusion. If heart failure from an underlying lesion is already present, it is wise to begin digitalization before the transfusion is begun. A safe dose of packed red blood cells is 5 ml per kilogram of body weight. A slightly larger amount may be used for subsequent transfusions if the presence or threat of failure has been overcome.

## SURGERY

Infants with congenital heart disease who are symptomatic in the first days or weeks after birth rarely survive until the first year of life without surgery. In fact, more than one fourth of infants born with anomalies of the heart and great vessels die before they reach one month of age, even with optimal medical management. Their survival depends on an early and accurate diagnosis, strict attention to hypoxia and acid-base balance, and palliative or definitive surgery.

Pediatricians and other primary care physicians have become aware of the importance of identifying these infants early and promptly transferring them under proper conditions to a center where an infant cardiac care program exists. Pediatric cardiologists are using the most sophisticated diagnostic techniques in the neonatal period, and an accurate diagnosis is usually possible even in the sickest infants.

Until a few years ago, surgery in the first weeks of life was limited almost entirely to palliative procedures. A few lesions could be corrected completely. Ligation of a patent ductus arteriosus and resection of aortic coarctation are two examples. However, most infants with potentially lethal defects could only be palliated: septostomy for transposition of the great vessels, pulmonary banding for large left-to-right shunts, and arterial shunts for lesions with severely reduced pulmonary blood flow. The development of palliative procedures certainly improved mortality and allowed correction at a later time. For example, in 1972 Edmunds and his associates reported on 61 infants operated within the first 6 weeks of life. Almost half (48 per cent) were alive 9 to 45 months after operation, respectable results for a group of patients who were not expected to survive early infancy without operation. Yet, there remained a sizable number of infants who could not be saved by palliation or in whom surgery could not even be attempted because of the complexity of the defects. Furthermore, there were many late complications of palliative operations.

Recent advances indicate that we are now entering an era of corrective surgery for even the youngest infants. The combination of deep hypothermia and limited cardiopulmonary bypass introduced by Hikasa and co-workers, and popularized by Barratt-Boyes and colleagues, provides the surgeon with a bloodless, motionless heart, permitting technical procedures not possible heretofore. Operating under these conditions, Castaneda and associates performed corrective surgery in 28 infants ranging from 1 to 90 days in age and from 2 to 5 kilograms in weight. There were only four hospital deaths among 26 infants with totally correctable lesions, such as ventricular septal defects (nine), transposition of the great arteries (six), tetralogy of Fallot (six), total anomalous pulmonary venous return (four), and aortic stenosis (one). Two of the 28 infants with non-correctable lesions (left ventricular tumor and truncus arteriosus) died.

These remarkable results indicate that the complete repair of the most complex cardiac defects will soon be possible for infants at any time after birth. We have reached the time when there is almost no limit to what surgery can accomplish if physicians will identify neonates who may have a cardiac defect and refer them without delay to a neonatal intensive unit where there are pediatric cardiologists and surgeons with experience and skill in the care of very small babies.

## REFERENCES

Barratt-Boyes, B. G., et al.: Intracardiac surgery in neonates and infants using deep hypothermia with surface cooling and limited cardiopulmonary bypass. Circulation 43:25, 1971.

Bernhard, W. F., et al.: Recent results of cardiovascular surgery in infants in the first year of life. Am. J. Surg. 123:451, 1972.

Casteneda, A. R., et al.: Open-heart surgery during the first three months of life. J. Thorac. Cardiovasc. Surg. 68:719, 1974.

Edmunds, L. H., et al.: Cardiac surgery in infants less than six weeks of age. Circulation 46:250, 1972.

Hallman, G. L., and Cooley, D. A.: Cardiovascular surgery in newborn infants: Results in 1050 patients less than one year old. Ann. Surg. 173:1007, 1971.

Hikasa, Y., et al.: Open-heart surgery in infants with an aid of hypothermia anesthesia. Arch. Jap. Clin. 36:495, 1967.

Krasula, R. W., et al.: Serum levels of digoxin in infants and children. J. Pediatr. 81:566, 1972.

Levine, O. R., and Blumenthal, S.: Digoxin dosage in premature infants. Pediatrics 29:18, 1962.

Levy, A. M., et al.: Effects of digoxin on systolic time intervals of neonates and infants. Circulation 46:816, 1972.

Mustard, W. T., et al.: Cardiovascular surgery in the first year of life. J. Thor. Cardiovasc. Surg. 59:761, 1970.

Soyka, L. F.: Digoxin: Placental transfer, effects on the fetus and therapeutic use in the newborn. Clinics in Perinatology 2:23, 1975.

Stark, J., et al.: Cardiac surgery in the first year of life: Experience with 1049 operations. Surgery 69:483, 1971.

Steiness, E., et al.: Plasma digoxin after parenteral administration. Clin. Pharmacol. Ther. 16:430, 1974.

# IV

# Disorders of the Gastrointestinal Tract

The newborn infant has accumulated by the time of birth a long experience in the acts of swallowing, gastric emptying and intestinal propulsion. From the fourth month of gestation, by which time the gastrointestinal tract is fully formed and its lumen patent, the fetus continually swallows amniotic fluid (estimated to be 20 ml/hour at term) and passes it through the stomach into the intestine. Extrauterine life presents the newborn with no new problems in this regard except defecation and the act of periodic glottic opening and closure for the purpose of breathing while eating. (See Neurogenic Stridor, p. 108.) The normal newborn sucks vigorously and swallows *almost* perfectly. The qualification is made because there is evidence that oily fluids leak into the tracheobronchial tree in many newborns during the act of normal deglutition. In 13 of 100 neonates DeCarlo et al. demonstrated distinct outlining of the lower respiratory tract after a mouthful of Lipiodol had been swallowed. In 11 this finding disappeared in 24 hours, but in two it persisted to 144 hours.

Frank and Gatewood have reported recurrent pneumonitis in three newborns owing to repeated aspiration of feedings. Cineradiography revealed incoordination in the act of swallowing at the level of the upper esophageal sphincter and overflow into the airway. All recovered after gavage feedings for no more than 2 weeks, after which swallowing was seen to be carried out perfectly.

Utian and Thomas reported two more serious cases of cricopharyngeal incoordination. Despite careful tube feeding their first infant died of aspiration pneumonia at the age of 5 months, having never regained the ability to swallow without spillage into the airway. Sections of the esophagus *postmortem* showed ganglia in the lower two thirds of its length but none in its proximal third. They suggest that this might have been a congenital aganglionosis analogous to Hirschsprung's disease.

Once in the esophagus, fluid is propelled into the stomach rapidly, and with few exceptions there is no reflux back to the esophagus.

The observations of Gryboski et al. suggest strongly that conditions favoring reflux are present in many newborns. Inferior esophageal sphincter mechanism pressures are low (−2 to +2 mm Hg) in the first 5 days, after which they quickly rise to +3 to +6 mm Hg.

The stomach empties intermittently, beginning within a few minutes and being complete between 2 and 4 hours. Meconium is passed within the first 24 hours. If it is not, obstruction should be suspected. For 2 or 3 days thereafter bowel movements consist of meconium, after which they become transitional for one day, then fecal.

Air enters the stomach of the newborn immediately after birth, and fills the small intestine in 2 to 12 hours and the large bowel within approximately 24 hours.

The newborn is able to digest all varieties of food as competently as is the older child. Within the past 30 years the age at which solid foods have been added to the diet has retreated from 6 months or later to 3 to 6 weeks. Some enthusiasts advocate feeding solids as early as the first week of life. Whether this is desirable is open to question, but there can be no doubt that the newborn is capable of ingesting, digesting and utilizing solid foods almost from the moment of birth. The pH of the gastric secretions is somewhat alkaline immediately after birth, almost surely because the stomach contains amniotic fluid. Within 2 to 3 hours it drops into the acid range, where it remains (Table 29–1).

Duodenal enzyme production of the newborn appears to proceed at a rate comparable to that of older infants except for amylase, which does not make its appearance for several weeks. Complete absence of or reduction in the quantity of duodenal enzymes beyond the first day is encountered in cystic fibrosis (mucoviscidosis) and

**TABLE 29–1.   *Acidity of Gastric Contents***

| | In Prematures | |
| Under 1 hr. | 6 hrs. | 24 hrs. |
|---|---|---|
| pH 7.7 | 2.6 | 3.7 |
| Range (3.0–8.0) | Range (1.4–7.1) | |

Incidence of achlorhydria: 6 hrs. = 25%; 24 hrs. = 69%.

| | In Term Babies (Vaginal) | | |
| Birth | 1 hr. | 4 hrs. | 24 hrs. |
|---|---|---|---|
| pH 5.8 | 3.5 | 3.5 | 2.8 |
| (4.0–7.5) | (2.0–5.0) | (1.5–5.5) | (1.3–4.0) |

Values in parentheses ±1 s.d.
Initial values in infants delivered by section are slightly more alkaline.
Data derived from Harries, J. T., and Fraser, A. J.: Biol. Neonat., *12*:186, 1968; and Avery, G. B., Randolph, J. G., and Weaver, T.: Pediatrics, 37:1005, 1966.

from the stools in complete intestinal obstruction.

## VOMITING

Regurgitation of the first few feedings offered may take place during the first day or two of life without arousing undue alarm. The newborn infant who vomits should, of course, be observed frequently and examined scrupulously for evidences of organic disease. In a fair number of cases no signs will be discovered to support such a diagnosis, and vomiting ceases on the third or fourth day. Ordinarily the withholding of milk constitutes adequate treatment, small quantities of water being substituted for milk for two to six feedings. Exactly why these infants vomit is not known. One of a variety of factors may be operative, including minimal intracranial injury, maternal medication and the swallowing of bloody or purulent amniotic fluid. If the last is suspected, lavage is indicated. The immaturity of the lower sphincter mechanism, noted above, may play an important part in this first-week vomiting.

Signs which suggest that vomiting may stem from organic disease are many and varied. Fever points toward parenteral or enteral infection. Failure to pass the first meconium stool within 24 hours suggests

intestinal obstruction. The converse is not true; i.e. *the passage of one or more meconium stools does not rule out complete intestinal obstruction.* This is especially true if the obstruction is high in the gastrointestinal tract. Abdominal distention points toward organic obstruction also. Again the converse is not true. *Complete obstruction, especially at the level of the duodenum or higher, may be present without distention.* Anorexia plus repeated vomiting may prevent completely the development of distention. The development of visible intestinal patterns upon the abdominal wall argues strongly in favor of organic obstruction, but is not absolutely pathognomonic.

Visible peristaltic waves moving from the left costal margin toward the midline indicate that the point of blockage is at or near the pylorus. When waves move from right to left, they arise in the bowel distal to the duodenum, and hence point to obstruction in the jejunum, ileum or colon. One small, palpable, firm mass, deep and just to the right of and either above or below the umbilicus, may represent a hypertrophic stenosed pylorus. Multiple firm masses scattered throughout a distended doughy abdomen characterize meconium ileus. A large palpable mass in one or the other flank suggests a malformed, hydronephrotic or infected kidney which might be the basis of vomiting. Spherical masses of cystic consistency may be cysts or duplications of the stomach or bowel. Rigidity of abdominal muscles is occasionally present in instances of peritonitis, but unfortunately this sign, useful in older patients, is often lacking in the newborn.

The nature of the material regurgitated furnishes useful clues to the location of obstruction. Pure mucus or a mixture of mucus and saliva alone denotes obstruction proximal to the stomach and suggests esophageal stenosis or atresia, rarely cardiospasm or esophageal diverticulum. Unaltered or coagulated milk, unstained with bile, points toward lax esophagus, hiatus hernia or obstruction at the pylorus or in the duodenum proximal to the ampulla of Vater. Bile-stained vomitus suggests narrowing or closure of the intestinal lumen distal to the ampulla. The presence of bile in vomitus is not absolutely diagnostic, but strongly suggests organic obstruction. Fecal vomitus indicates obstruction low in the intestinal tract.

When blood is mixed with the vomitus, it may be difficult to ascertain its source. It must never be forgotten that such blood may be maternal in origin, ingested with the amniotic fluid after placental hemorrhage, or ingested with the milk when the nipple is cracked and bleeding. Fortunately we are now able to differentiate fetal from maternal blood, since fetal red cells resist alkali denaturation.

Causes of vomiting in the newborn include, therefore, ill-defined ones which are self-limited in the first few days of life and a great variety of organic lesions causing obstruction at any point from the upper portion of the esophagus to the anus. These will be discussed in detail shortly. In addition, there are numerous others. Intracranial lesions, chiefly subdural hemorrhage and hydrocephalus, commonly produce vomiting. Infections of almost any system may be ushered in with vomiting, and in some of these, such as peritonitis, meningitis, pyelonephritis and hepatitis, vomiting may continue until the infection is controlled. Uninfected lesions of the genitourinary tract, mainly those which produce hydronephrosis, may in the newborn as well as in the older patient precipitate vomiting. Certain metabolic disorders, such as galactosemia and adrenal cortical hyperplasia, often cause vomiting. The list might be prolonged indefinitely to no particular advantage. Our only purpose in this paragraph is to point out that vomiting in the newborn may be a sign of disease in the gastrointestinal tract, but it may also, as in the older infant and the child, point to disease almost anywhere else in the body.

## CONSTIPATION

The first meconium stool is passed by 69 per cent of normal infants within 12 hours, by 94 per cent within 24 hours and by 99.8 per cent within 48 hours (Sherry and Kramer). Mangurten and Slade (1973) found no significant differences in their more recent study of preterm infants, and could discover "no relationship among birth weight, gestational age, Apgar score or age at first feeding and age at first stool." Failure to pass a stool within the first 24 hours must be regarded with suspicion. This may be the earliest sign of Hirschsprung disease (see p. 385).

After the first few days when pure meconium is passed, the newborn's stools consist of part meconium, part fecal matter for another day or two, after which they become entirely fecal. The number of stools passed by the normal infant is extremely variable, for some being as few as one every second or third day, for some as many as 10 per 24 hours. In general the stools of the breast-fed infant are more frequent and more liquid than those of the artificially fed infant. On the other hand, it is not too uncommon, nor is it abnormal, for a breast-fed infant to have stools at long intervals, every 24 or 48 hours or even longer. This does not represent constipation unless the stools then passed are hard and dry. At times this is the result of insufficient intake, but at other times even this is not the case. When intake is adequate and the nature of stool is not abnormal, infrequency of bowel movement may be completely ignored.

In some small newborns, especially prematures, constipation may become a real problem. Not only are stools passed at long intervals, but also, when passed, are small, hard and dry. Constipation in these tiny infants may produce anorexia, distention and vomiting, and should not be ignored. Rarely such constipation is so pronounced that true intestinal obstruction is produced. Laxative medication should be avoided, but a small saline enema when indicated is permissible and often effective. Reduction of fat content of the formula is at times helpful. The exact cause of the constipation is not known, but one suspects that weakness of intestinal and abdominal musculature may play an important role in its production. Infants of eclamptic mothers who may be hypermagnesemic are lethargic and flaccid, and may have a delay in passing meconium.

A most serious form of constipation in the newborn is that associated with cystic fibrosis, so-called meconium ileus. In this condition dry, inspissated or thick, gluey meconium may produce total obstruction at the time of birth or even *in utero*. This latter situation may lead to meconium peritonitis.

## DIARRHEA

Diarrhea is usually defined as the passage of numerous loose stools. This definition requires several qualifying statements. The breast-fed infant may pass as many as 10 or 12 loose movements in the course of 24 hours, yet eat well, gain well and behave perfectly normally. This is not a disease state and should not be termed diarrhea. Certain infants, on the other hand, may have but one or two loose movements in a day, yet look ill and become dehydrated and acidotic with great rapidity. A large quantity of fluid and electrolytes may become pooled within the intestinal lumen, where it represents a loss of body water and salts as complete as though it had been passed to the outside. Such a situation constitutes diarrhea and may be as hazardous as the passage of 15 or 20 loose stools in a day.

Diarrhea in the newborn is often due to enteral infection, although at times it may represent the intestinal response to parenteral infection. Rarely it is caused by disaccharidase deficiency, and even more rarely by deficiency of a monosaccharidase. These and other forms of diarrhea will be discussed in detail elsewhere. (See pages 784–786).

## HEMATEMESIS AND MELENA

The vomiting of blood or blood-stained gastric contents and the passage of bloody stools are not infrequent occurrences in the neonatal period. As mentioned earlier, the physician's first task is to determine whether this blood is maternal in origin or whether the infant himself is bleeding internally. As little as 3.0 ml. of blood ingested by the infant may produce one or more bloody stools which appear 7 to 17 hours after ingestion. By a simple test maternal blood may be distinguished from the infant's, a test based upon the low percentage of fetal hemoglobin (hemoglobin F) in the former and its high concentration in the latter.

The Apt test for the differentiation of fetal from adult hemoglobin is done as follows. Mix the specimen under study with an equal quantity of tap water. Either centrifuge the mixture or strain it through filter paper. If the supernate or the filtrate is pink, hemoglobin may be present. To 5 parts of this supernate or filtrate add 1 part of 0.25 per cent sodium hydroxide. The pink color should deepen and persist for more than 2 minutes if hemoglobin F is present. If it turns yellow within 2 minutes, it is hemoglobin A.

Fetal blood indicates one of a variety of lesions, and its source may be difficult, at times impossible, to determine. From retrospective pathologic evidence we know that bloody vomitus often stems from ulcerative esophagitis with or without lax esophagus, hiatal hernia or intrathoracic stomach. Peptic ulcer of the stomach or duodenum occurs in the newborn. Since it is not readily recognizable on physical examination or even radiographic contrast studies, diagnosis rests on exclusion of other causes of bleeding. These include deficiencies in the clotting mechanism and the group of generalized infections. Rarely the newborn bleeds from peptic ulcers in unusual locations, such as Meckel's diverticulum or gastrogenic cysts within the abdomen or thorax. Duplications of bowel often bleed. More uncommon is hemorrhage from the bowel due to intussusception which occurs, but with the utmost infrequency, in the neonatal period. Single or multiple polyps and hemangiomas of the bowel might conceivably do the same, but thus far they have not been reported at this early age. Multiple telangiectasia characteristically gives no symptoms until late in childhood. Pulmonary hemorrhage is often signaled by the issuance of blood from the mouth or nares, or both, and, unless the material is frothy, is difficult to distinguish from gastric bleeding.

An example in which ingestion of maternal blood caused definite symptoms follows.

CASE 29–1

A white female infant was born October 17, 1956, in the Hospital for the Women of Maryland after rapid spontaneous labor, about 37 weeks' gestational age. Birth weight was 3 pounds 15 ounces (1785 gm). When the membranes ruptured, 1¼ hours before delivery, thick, reddish-brown amniotic fluid gushed forth. The infant cried and breathed spontaneously. Shortly after delivery the abdomen was noted to be unusually full, and the infant passed a large, reddish-black, liquid stool. The abdomen remained full, but soft and doughy. No masses were felt, and no abnormal peristalsis was seen. Rectal examination was normal, but it induced passage of a large amount of reddened meconium. X-ray studies of the abdomen were normal. Stool and gastric contents contained blood whose hemoglobin was adult in type. Distention persisted, and appetite was poor for 4 days, after which all appeared normal. The infant was discharged on the eighth day.

COMMENT.    Melena developed in an infant whose mother's amniotic fluid was grossly bloody. She showed abdominal distention, poor appetite and tarry stools for four days, and thereafter was well. Blood in the stools proved to be maternal in origin.

## ANOREXIA

Some newborns eat poorly for a number of days for any one of a great variety of reasons. The reason in any particular case usually becomes obvious as one follows the course of the illness. An occasional newborn refuses to eat for an indefinite time, with no indication of underlying disease. This is not a matter of being unable to swallow, but seems rather to be due to a complete lack of the sensation of hunger. Severe brain defect such as hydranencephaly commonly causes this. So do less well defined brain disorders. In one child in our experience feeding had to be carried out by gavage for 3 months, after which appetite gradually became normal. This child developed slowly in the psychomotor field and has ended as an institutionalized mental defective. We are fairly certain that this is not the fate of all such severely anorexic newborns.

## REFERENCES

Avery, G. B., Randolph, J. G., and Weaver, T.: Gastric acidity in the first day of life. Pediatrics 37:1005, 1966.
DeCarlo, J., Jr., Tramer, A., and Startzman, H. H., Jr.: Iodized oil aspiration in the newborn. A.M.A. J. Dis. Child. 84:442, 1952.
Frank, M. M., and Gatewood, O. M. B.: Transient pharyngeal incoordination in the newborn. Am. J. Dis. Child. 111:178, 1966.
Gryboski, J. D.: Gastrointestinal Problems in The Infant. Philadelphia, W. B. Saunders Co., 1975.
Gryboski, J. D., Thayer, W. R., and Spiro, H. M.: Esophageal motility in infants and children. Pediatrics 31:382, 1963.
Harries, J. T., and Fraser, A. J.: The acidity of the gastric contents of premature babies during the first 14 days of life. Biol. Neonat. 12:186, 1968.
Illingworth, R. S.: Sucking and swallowing difficulties in infancy: Diagnostic problem of dysphagia. Arch. Dis. Childhood, 44:655, 1969.
Mangurten, H. H., and Slade, C. I.: First stool in the preterm, low birthweight infant. J. Pediatr. 82:1033, 1973.
Sherry, S. N., and Kramer, I.: The time of passage of the first stool and the first urine by the newborn infant. J. Pediatr. 46:158, 1955.
Sokal, M. M., Koenigsberger, M. R., Rose, J. S., Berdon, W. E., and Santulli, T. V.: Neonatal hypermagnesemia and the meconium plug syndrome. New Engl. J. Med. 286:823, 1972.
Utian, H. L., and Thomas, R. G.: Cricopharyngeal incoordination in infancy. Pediatrics 43:402, 1969.
Wolff, P.: The serial organization of sucking in the young infant. Pediatrics 42:943, 1968.

# 30    DISORDERS OF THE MOUTH, TONGUE AND NECK

Several minor disorders of the oral cavity may be disposed of briefly. Oral moniliasis will be discussed under Infections (p. 952).
*Tongue tie,* that universal condition of past generations, has been relegated to its proper place. The frenum binding the tongue to the floor of the mouth is recognized now to be short and not too elastic in

the normal newborn. The tongue need not be protruded far from the mouth in the course of the usual activities of the newborn infant, and shortness of the frenum does not hinder proper sucking and deglutition. The short frenum can be expected to lengthen over the course of the years. It need not be cut.

Infants may be born with one or more *erupted teeth,* commonly called *natal,* or one or more may erupt during the first month, hence *neonatal,* usually the lower incisors of the deciduous set. Reported incidence figures range from 1:5000 to 1:10,000 in most series. The abnormality is often transmitted as an autosomal dominant trait. Since only their crowns are calcified, while their roots are imperfectly formed, these teeth are almost always loose. They should be extracted.

*Cysts* large enough to be visible to the naked eye may be discovered in the mouths of 80 per cent of newborns. In decreasing frequency these *"Epstein's pearls"* or *"Bohn's nodules"* are present along the median palatal raphe, the maxillary alveolar ridge and the mandibular alveolar ridge. They may be ignored.

*Ranula* is a retention cyst of the sublingual salivary gland. It presents as a pea- to marble-sized mass on the anterior floor of the mouth filled with clear or yellow contents, pushing the tongue upward. Most will disappear in time; a few may have to be resected.

## CONGENITAL FUSIONS

In *ankyloglossia superior* the tongue is fused to the hard palate and the gums. Other anomalies are associated (See Chapter 95.)

A few infants have been born with partial or complete *fusion of the gums,* without other congenital anomalies. Snijman and Prinsloo's infant did well after a simple operative procedure.

## EPIGNATHUS

Epignathus is an extremely rare disorder. It defines any kind of growth arising from the upper jaw or palate and projecting from the mouth. The tumors may be polyps, hairy polyps, dermoids or teratomas. These are believed to arise from embryonal tissue rests, although some still consider them incomplete twins (sphenopagus or palatopagus).

Because of their location and size, some being as large as an orange or small grapefruit, they may cause respiratory difficulty and inability to take food. Most are benign (see Fig. 30–1).

*Treatment* must be directed first toward relief of dyspnea. An introduced airway may be adequate for short periods, but tracheostomy may be required if definitive attempts at cure are delayed. Feeding is best carried out by nasal catheter. Removal of the tumor is not difficult if the attachment is small, as in polyps, but may be practically impossible when the base is broad, as in some teratomas. Nevertheless surgical removal offers the only hope for cure.

## CONGENITAL EPULIS

This misnamed tumor arises from the upper or lower jaw, and its projection into the mouth may make closure difficult and sucking impossible. It is misnamed because in none of the reported cases has it arisen from the bone itself as in true epulis of older patients, but from the tissue overlying the bone. Langley and Davson found 23 cases in the literature, of which 15 arose from the maxilla, eight from the mandible. All but three were newborns, and all but three in whom the sex was known were females. They added three cases of their own.

The tumors were similar in appearance. They were covered with squamous epithelium, and packed with vascular connective tissue in which were encountered many large polyhedral or round cells with granular cytoplasm and a few elongated or spindle-shaped cells. In spite of the fact that myofibrils have never been seen in these cells, they have generally been assumed to represent myoblasts. The authors doubt that myoblastoma is their proper designation. In no instance has there been either local recurrence, invasion or metastasis.

Immediate surgical excision is indicated. The results are uniformly satisfactory.

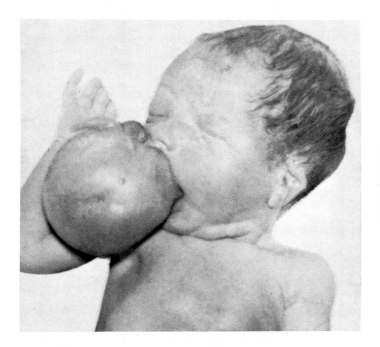

*Figure 30–1.* Infant with epignathus. The orange-sized mass attached to the maxilla protrudes grotesquely from the mouth. (Wynn, S. K., Waxman, S., Ritchie, G., and Askotsky, M.: A.M.A. *J. Dis. Child.*, 91:495, 1956. Reprinted with the permission of the authors.)

## NASOPHARYNGEAL TUMORS

Loeb and Smith estimate that at least fifty cases of nasopharyngeal tumors have been recorded in the world literature up to this time. Less than 10, discovered in the newborn period, have been successfully removed. Most of these have been simple hairy polyps or dermoids, a few more highly developed teratomas. Some have thin pedicles, but the rare teratoma may be broadly based far back on the palate or on the posterior pharyngeal wall, whence it may project out of the mouth or upward into the nasopharynx, or both. They arise from the midline or near it.

*Diagnosis* of dermoids not projecting externally may be made by careful examination of the pharynx. The tumor may be visible or palpable as a small sausage-shaped mass. Commonly freely movable, it may cause respiratory obstruction intermittently at those moments when it has got caught behind the soft palate, while its extrusion into the oropharynx may be accompanied by relief from dyspnea. In the example described by Dieter et al., only feeding difficulty was present from birth until the sixth day, at which time acute episodic respiratory distress began.

*Treatment* consists in immediate removal. Those dermoids with a thin pedicle may be removed easily with a snare. Those teratomas with a broad base, which are considerably less common, need to be shelled out surgically. The procedure is delicate and time-consuming, and tracheostomy prior to anesthesia is indicated.

## AGLOSSIA CONGENITA

An extremely rare congenital anomaly is absence, or almost complete absence, of the tongue. In Ardran and Kemp's example the floor of the mouth was covered with filiform mucosa resembling that of the tongue, and there were two lateral ridges and a small pyramidal mass in the midline of the posterior floor which contained some muscle. In addition there were micrognathia and syndactyly of the left hand.

The infant fed poorly at first but learned to feed after a time with the aid of gravity, suction by depression of the floor of the mouth and jaw and compression of the nipple by elevation of the floor of the mouth. Swallowing, visualized by cineradiography, was thereafter normal.

Taste is normal, and these children learn

to speak with only a few sounds imperfectly formed.

## CONGENITAL MACROGLOSSIA

Slight enlargement of the tongue may be noted at birth in some otherwise normal newborns, especially in those of short, stocky, muscular body build. For a few months the tongue may protrude slightly from a mouth not quite capacious enough to contain it. This is not true macroglossia.

INCIDENCE. True macroglossia is rare, indeed. We have never encountered one in our own practice and have seen remarkably few.

ETIOLOGY. Moderate enlargement is seen in Down's syndrome, in cretinism and in glycogen storage disease of the heart. In none of these is it sufficiently large to cause trouble in breathing or swallowing.

Huge thickening and overgrowth of the tongue to the point that it protrudes from a constantly open mouth, making feeding difficult and respiration noisy and partially obstructed, constitutes true macroglossia. Some of these are associated with macrosomia and omphalocele and a variety of other congenital defects, and these may suffer symptomatic neonatal hypoglycemia. They fit into the category of Beckwith's syndrome. The rest fall into two large pathologic groups, lymphangioma being the more common and muscular hypertrophy characterizing the remainder. In this latter variety the individual muscle fibers have been reported to be four or five times as thick as average ones.

DIAGNOSIS. Down's syndrome and cretinism will be ruled in or out in the usual fashion. The infant with glycogen disease will probably be limp and flaccid, and x-ray film will show cardiomegaly. Biopsy of skeletal muscle will reveal excess of glycogen in these babies. Macroglossia which is not symmetrical, but which is localized to one portion of the tongue, is almost surely lymphangiomatous, and is certainly that if it is associated with hygroma of the neck. Biopsy of the tongue should determine whether lymphangioma or muscle hypertrophy is the basic lesion.

TREATMENT. The lymphangiomatous form should be subjected to plastic surgery.

Recurrences are common and may necessitate further operations. Bronstein et al. preferred to wait out their case with muscular hypertrophy. Their patience was rewarded by a gradual shrinking in size of the tongue, which, along with growth of the mandible, made disproportion less and less obvious. Koop and Moschakis have seen three newborns among their eight cases of capillary lymphangioma of the tongue, all in association with nearby hygroma. They resected all, with tracheotomy when needed. They point out that these tongues are liable to a vesicular, hemorrhagic glossitis which they treat by electrodesiccation.

## BECKWITH'S SYNDROME

The presence of macroglossia in association with an omphalocele or other umbilical abnormalities and severe hypoglycemia was first described by Beckwith in 1963. This constellation of abnormalities, noted by a number of authors subsequently, is sufficiently characteristic to deserve the appellation of syndrome.

A repetition among sibships has been described in some instances, suggesting that it is an autosomal recessive trait. It has been noted both in white and black infants.

The infants may be born at term, or prematurely, and may be oversized for gestational age. Severe, symptomatic hypoglycemia may be present in the first days of life and persist for several months. The tongue is very large and persists that way, but becomes less apparent with postnatal growth of the face. There is a mid-facial recession and tendency toward exophthalmos. With increasing age, gigantism becomes apparent, and occasionally hemihypertrophy ensues.

A late complication is the tendency toward development of malignant neoplasms; adrenal carcinoma, Wilms's tumor and bilateral nephroblastomas have been reported.

PATHOLOGY. The brain is below expected weight; other organs are similar to predicted weight. Hyperplastic phenomena are noted in the kidneys and the islet cells and acini of the pancreas. The fetal zone of the adrenal cortex is prominent with cytomegaly and cortical cysts.

**TREATMENT.** Early recognition of the hypoglycemia and its correction with corticosteroids and glucose may improve the prognosis in this syndrome. The initial descriptions were of autopsied patients; the full clinical spectrum of the syndrome awaits further delineation (see page 523).

## PHARYNGEAL DIVERTICULUM AND PSEUDODIVERTICULUM

Congenital diverticula of the hypopharynx, running down into the mediastinum behind the esophagus and clinically simulating esophageal atresia with tracheoesophageal fistula, have been described. More recently pseudodiverticula, resulting from digital or instrumental trauma to the posterior pharyngeal wall during or after delivery, have also been reported.

In both conditions the anomalous tracts have been visualized after barium swallow.

Diverticula must be excised surgically. Pseudodiverticula may heal spontaneously, but they too may have to be repaired operatively.

## SIALADENITIS (INFLAMMATION OF THE SALIVARY GLANDS)

### SUPPURATIVE NEONATAL PAROTITIS

Suppurative parotitis strikes the newborn infant very rarely. Until 1970, 62 cases had been reported in the world literature, to which number Leake and Leake added 10. These had been encountered in the Boston Children's Hospital Medical Center in the preceding 25 years.

As a rule normal pregnancies and labors had preceded birth, and premature infants were involved a bit more often than expected. Swelling of one or both parotids, usually one, appears at any time from the first to the twenty-fifth day. Some babies have been quite well prior to the appearance of swelling, but the majority have suffered some illness; respiratory distress, dehydration, hyperbilirubinemia, pneumonitis or sepsis. It is widely believed that the dehydration, with cessation of flow from Stensen's duct, permits ascent of organisms from the mouth.

The offending organism is most often the *Staphylococcus aureus*, although *E. coli* and other coliforms have been responsible. Sepsis is not too uncommonly associated.

The parotid gland becomes swollen and the skin over it reddened, and there is usually low fever. Pressure over the gland forces purulent material from the orifice of Stensen's duct. Not infrequently, infection spreads to involve the other parotid or a submaxillary gland. Methicillin should be used until the organism is identified, and incision and drainage should be resorted to at the first sign of fluctuation.

Prognosis is good for uncomplicated cases.

### SUPPURATION OF THE SUBMAXILLARY GLANDS

Two examples of suppuration of a submaxillary gland were recently reported, not secondary to infection of the parotid gland. They seem to be the first on record. Swelling appeared beneath, in the region of the submaxillary gland, and pus could be expressed from the orifice of Wharton's duct beneath the tip of the tongue. In all other respects it behaves like suppurative parotitis.

## CONGENITAL BRANCHIOGENOUS ANOMALIES

Anomalous developments of the branchial arches may manifest themselves in a great variety of ways. The most obvious of these are 1) skin tags, 2) pits, 3), fistulas and 4) cysts. They are located for the most part in two sites, the preauricular region and anywhere along the anterior border of the sternocleidomastoid muscle, from mastoid to manubrium.

Skin tags should be removed for cosmetic reasons. Pits may be ignored. Fistulas may discharge mucoid or purulent material; they may penetrate deep in the neck to terminate near the pharynx and rarely may open into the pharynx. Cysts usually lie at the angle of the mandible but may be found low, just above the clavicle. Fistulas should be removed by careful, thorough dissection. Cysts should be extirpated early because they are prone to infection.

## MISCELLANEOUS LESIONS OF MOUTH AND NECK

*Micrognathus* is discussed under the First Arch Syndrome, as are *cleft palate* and *harelip*.

The *Klippel-Feil syndrome* is discussed under Disorders of Bones, Joints and Muscles (p. 907).

The neck is the site of diverse tumorous swellings, either present at birth or becoming manifest within the first few weeks of life.

*Sternomastoid tumor* can be seen and palpated within the body of the sternocleidomastoid muscle as a firm, smooth, generally ovoid mass. It does not usually appear until on or after the tenth day, grows for a few months, then recedes spontaneously within 4 to 8 months more. It may be accompanied or followed by *torticollis*, at times with cranial and facial asymmetry, oculomotor imbalance and high scoliosis. Its cause is not known and there is no general agreement as to correct treatment. Electromyography may be useful in arriving at a decision whether or not to excise the mass surgically.

*Goiter* may be visible and palpable at birth as a trilobed enlargement of the thyroid isthmus and its lateral lobes. The enlarged gland may be hypothyroid, euthyroid or hyperthyroid (see p. 504).

The neck is the favorite site for *cystic hygroma*, although identical cavernous lymphangiomata may arise in many other parts of the body. Its soft, bag-of-worms feel and its usual location external to the sternomastoid muscle on one side, between the mastoid and the acromial process, readily differentiates it from other cervical tumors (Fig. 30–2).

*Teratomas* are found not infrequently in the neck. Most often they are midline, as most teratomata tend to be, arising in or adjacent to the thyroid isthmus. Their very firm, cystic conformation may differentiate them from cystic hygroma,˙ but definitive diagnosis may be impossible prior to opera-

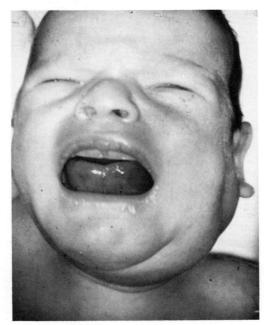

**Figure 30–2.**   Hygroma, neck and tongue.

tion. The percentage of malignancy is small (p. 107).

*Branchial cysts* (also called branchiogenic, lateral cervical or cervical thymic cysts), arise in the embryo from either the branchial groove, the thymic stalk or the pharyngeal pouch. They may be present at birth or may appear suddenly at any age. They lie beneath the sternomastoid muscle, but their anterior edge may bulge out from the muscle's anterior margin. They manifest a strong tendency to become infected and pus-filled. Sinniah et al. reported an extraordinary example in a baby, well at birth, who at 40 hours of age suddenly developed a large swelling on the left side of the neck along with respiratory distress and cyanosis. X-ray showed a large air-containing cyst which displaced the air passages and esophagus forward (Fig. 30–2). Excision resulted in cure.

We are apt to forget that the *thymus* is one of the organs which arises high in the embryo and must travel caudad before its two lateral buds join in the anterior mediastinum. Their descent may become arrested at any point in the journey. Most

**A**

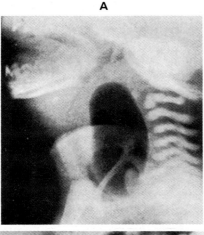

*Figure 30–3.* A, Lateral radiograph of the neck shows an air-containing cyst displacing the air passages and esophagus forward. B, Lateral view of the neck with patient quiet, demonstrating straight, unobstructed tracheal air column. C, Lateral view of neck with patient crying demonstrates mass lesion between the manubrium and the trachea displacing the lower cervical trachea backwards, and moderately narrowing this portion of the trachea. (From Thompson, R. E., and Love, W. G.: Persistent cervical thymoma apparent with crying. Am. J. Dis. Child. *124*:761, 1972.)

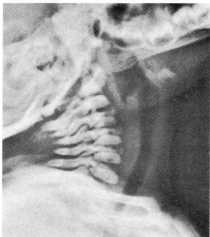

**B**

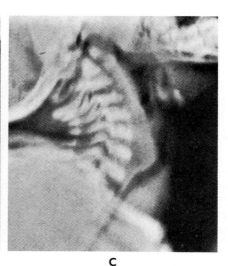

**C**

present as unilateral, soft, fleshy masses somewhere below the angle of the mandible along the anterior edge of the sternomastoid. Some descend much further and fuse at a point more caudad than is normal. Thompson and Love reported one such newborn in whom the mass made its appearance as an outpouching in the midline into the sternal notch, *but only when the infant cried* (Fig. 30–3).

*The spherical mass of thyroglossal duct cyst* lies in the midline deep in the neck and may extend backward to the base of the tongue, just above the larynx. It usually is cystic but may be solid and consist of thyroid tissue. Indeed it may represent all the thyroid tissue which the baby possesses. It is difficult to differentiate from teratoma. Very rarely the submental gland becomes enlarged, usually as a result of infection, and may present diagnostic difficulty: however, this gland lies anterior to the preferred site of thyroglossal duct cyst. Before surgical intervention one must make sure by radioiodine uptake studies that the baby has other functioning thyroid tissue.

## REFERENCES

Ardran, G. M., and Kemp, F. H.: Aglossia congenita. Arch. Dis. Child. *31*:400, 1956.

Baxter, C. F., Johnson, E. W., Lloyd, J. R., and Clatworthy, W., Jr.: Prognostic significance of electromyography in congenital torticollis. Pediatrics 28: 442, 1961.

Beckwith, J. B.: Extreme cytomegaly of the adrenal fetal cortex, omphalocele, hyperplasia of kidneys and pancreas, and Leydig-cell hyperplasia. Another syndrome? Presented to Western Society for Pediatric Research, November 11, 1963. Abstract read by title, American Pediatric Society, *41*:56, 1964.

Beckwith, J. B.: Macroglossia, omphalocele, adrenal cytomegaly, gigantism, and hyperplastic visceromegaly. Birth Defects: Original Article Series, V:188, 1969.

Bell, H. G., and Miller, R. G.: Congenital macroglossia: Report of two cases. Surgery *24*:125, 1948.

Bodenhoff, J., and Gorlin, R. J.: Natal and neonatal teeth. Pediatrics *32*:1087, 1963.

Brintnall, E. S., and Kridelbaugh, W. W.: Congenital diverticulum of posterior hypopharynx simulating atresia of esophagus. Ann. Surg. *131*:564, 1950.

Bronstein, J. P., Abelson, S. M., Jaffé, R. H., and von Bonin, G.: Macroglossia in children. Am. J. Dis. Child. *54*:1328, 1937.

Cataldo, E., and Berkman, M. D.: Cysts of the oral mucosa in newborns. Am. J. Dis. Child. *116*:44, 1968.

Cohen, M. M.: Congenital, genetic and endocrinologic influences on dental occlusion. Dent. Clin. N. Amer. *19*:499, 1975.

Combs, J. T., et al.: New syndrome of neonatal hypoglycemia. New Engl. J. Med. *275*:236, 1966.

David, R. B., and O'Connell, E. J.: Suppurative parotitis in children. Am. J. Dis. Child. *119*:332, 1970.

Dieter, R. A., Jr., Holinger, P. H., and Maurizi, D. G.: Angiofibromatous polyp of the pharynx. Am. J. Dis. Child. *119*:91, 1970.

Edson, B., and Holinger, P. H.: Traumatic pharyngeal pseudodiverticulum in the newborn infant. J. Pediatr. *82*:483, 1973.

Foster, J. H.: Congenital dermoid tumor of the nasopharynx. Ann. Otol. Rhin. Laryng. *53*:578, 1944.

Gellis, S., and Feingold, M.: Picture of the month. Am. J. Dis. Child. *115*:349, 1968.

Gifford, G. H., Jr., and MacCollum, D.: Facial teratoma in the newborn. Plas. Reconstr. Surg. *49*:616, 1972.

Girdany, B. R., Sieber, W. K., and Ozman, M. Z.: Traumatic pseudodiverticula of the pharynx in newborn infants. New Engl. J. Med. *280*:237, 1969.

Hajdu, S. I., Faruque, A. A., et al.: Teratoma of the neck in infants. Am. J. Dis. Child. *111*:412, 1970.

Hankey, G. T.: Congenital epulis (granular-cell myo-

blastoma or fibroblastoma) in a ten-weeks premature infant. Proc. Roy. Soc. Med. *48*:1015, 1955.

Irving, I.: Exomphalos with macroglossia: A study of 11 cases. J. Pediat. Surg. *2*:499, 1967.

Jacobs, P. H., Shafer, S. C., and Higdon, R. S.: Congenital branchiogenous anomalies. J.A.M.A. *169*:90, 1959.

Kesson, C. W.: Asphyxia neonatorum due to nasopharyngeal teratoma. Arch. Dis. Child. *29*:254, 1954.

Koop, C. E., and Moschakis, E. A.: Capillary lymphangioma of the tongue complicated by glossitis. Pediatrics *27*:800, 1961.

Ladd, W. E., and Gross, R. E.: Congenital branchiogenic anomalies. Report of 82 cases. Am. J. Surg. *39*:234, 1938.

Langley, F. A., and Davson, J.: Epulis in the newborn. Arch. Dis. Child. *25*:89, 1950.

Leake, D., and Leake, R.: Neonatal suppurative parotitis. Pediatrics *46*:203, 1970.

Loeb, W. J., and Smith, E. E.: Airway obstruction in a newborn by pedunculated pharyngeal dermoid. Pediatrics *40*:20, 1967.

Lofgren, R. H.: Respiratory distress from congenital lingual cysts. Am. J. Dis. Child. *106*:610, 1963.

Ochsner, A., and Ayers, W. B.: Case of epignathus. Surgery *30*:560, 1951.

Pannullo, J. N.: Congenital macroglossia, report of a case. Obst. Gynecol. 7:97, 1956.

Sinniah, D., and Somasundaran, K.: Lateral cervical cyst: A cause of respiratory distress in the newborn. Am. J. Dis. Child. *124*:582, 1972.

Smith, C. A.: Physiology of the Newborn Infant. 3rd ed. Springfield, Ill., Charles C Thomas, 1959.

Snijman, P. C., and Prinsloo, J. G.: Congenital fusion of the gums. Am. J. Dis. Child. *112*:593, 1966.

Thompson, R. E., and Love, W. G.: Persistent cervical thymoma, apparent with crying. Am. J. Dis Child. *124*:761, 1972.

Wells, D. H.: Suppuration of the submandibular salivary glands in the neonate. Am. J. Dis. Child. *129*:628, 1975.

Wynn, S. K., Waxman, S., Ritchie, G., and Askotzky, M.: Epignathus; survey. A.M.A. J. Dis. Child. *91*:495, 1956.

# DISORDERS OF THE ESOPHAGUS

# 31

The following classification of disorders of the esophagus which are encountered in the neonatal period is a modification of one suggested by Holinger, Johnston and Potts.

I. Congenital malformations of the esophagus
   A. Absence
   B. Atresia
      1. With tracheo-esophageal fistula
      2. Without tracheo-esophageal fistula

   C. Stenosis
      1. Fibrous stricture
      2. Web
      3. External pressure
   D. Duplication
   E. Hiatus hernia
      1. Short esophagus with intrathoracic stomach
      2. Sliding hiatus hernia
      3. Paraesophageal hernia

II. Abnormalities in neuromuscular control
  A. Cricopharyngeal incoordination
  B. Cardiospasm
  C. Achalasia
  D. Lax esophagus (cardiochalasia)
  E. Familial dysautonomia and other neurologic diseases
III. Compression or dislocation by neighboring structures
IV. Acquired lesions
  A. Erosion
  B. Peptic ulceration
  C. Rupture

## ABSENCE OF ESOPHAGUS

Several cases have been reported in which the entire esophagus, from hypopharynx to cardia, has been missing. Since this condition is incompatible with life and is at present uncorrectable, we shall not discuss it further.

## CONGENITAL ANOMALIES OF THE ESOPHAGUS

A classification of esophageal anomalies and their relative incidence is shown in Table 31–1. Note that esophageal atresia with distal tracheoesophageal fistula accounts for about 90 per cent of the total. Atresia without fistula and fistula without atresia account for most of the remainder. (These conditions are also discussed in Chapter 9, pages 110–115).

*TABLE 31–1. Anatomical Incidence and Survival Rate*

| Anomaly | Number of Patients | Number of Survivors |
|---|---|---|
| Esophageal atresia without TEF | 82 | 46 (56%) |
| Esophageal atresia with proximal TEF | 9 | 5 (56%) |
| Esophageal atresia with proximal and distal TGF | 7 | 5 (71%) |
| Esophageal atresia with distal TEF | 916 | 559 (61%) |
| TEF without atresia | 44 | 30 (68%) |

## ATRESIA OF ESOPHAGUS WITHOUT TRACHEO-ESOPHAGEAL FISTULA

Complete atresia of the esophagus rarely occurs as a solitary defect. The usual site of involvement is near the junction of the upper and middle thirds where the tubular structure suddenly narrows and becomes replaced by a fibrous cord. The length of the discontinuity or the fibrous cord varies from 1 to 5 or 6 cm. The lesion is caused by failure of this portion of the foregut to recanalize after it had become a solid structure in early embryonic life.

*Diagnosis* is based upon virtually the same criteria as those described for esophageal atresia with tracheo-esophageal fistula (p. 110). The cardinal signs are presence of inordinate quantities of mucus in the mouth and pharynx, prompt regurgitation of ingested or introduced fluids, and dyspnea either mild or severe. No air enters the gastrointestinal tract. Diagnosis may be confirmed by passing a catheter through the mouth or nose and meeting firm obstruction. One must be certain that the catheter is not coiling up within the pouch. Further confirmation is obtained by instillation of a few cubic centimeters of radiopaque material into the upper esophageal pouch.

Absence of air in the gastrointestinal tract rules out the presence of a fistulous communication between lower pouch and trachea. Since this is the most common of the compound defects, and since upper pouch fistulas are rare, absence of air in the abdomen should strongly suggest the diagnosis of simple atresia. This will be rendered considerably more likely if attempted ingestion of fluid does not induce paroxysmal coughing and dyspnea, since feeding when there is a direct connection between upper pouch and trachea almost always produces this response.

*Treatment* is surgical. We no longer feel as constrained to perform immediate definitive repair as we did 5 or 10 years ago. As soon as the diagnosis has been confirmed, two procedures must be initiated. The upper blind pouch must be kept emptied of nasopharyngeal secretions by continuous or oft-repeated suction, and gastrostomy must be performed both to reduce intragastric pressure, thus to forestall aspiration from below, and to supply fluid and protein-calorie requirements. Definitive repair, whether it be end-to-end anastomosis or interposition of a segment of bowel, may be delayed until the inevitable pneumonitis has been controlled, until the precise dimensions of the surgical problem have been delineated and until the tinier babies have gained some weight.

The results are about the same as those achieved in the repair of esophageal atresia with tracheo-esophageal fistula. Direct end-to-end anastomosis is the operation of choice. In many the distance between upper and lower pouch is too great for this procedure to be successful, and some less satisfactory and more complicated plastic repair will have to be undertaken. Several imaginative procedures have been tried in the attempt to avoid the interposition procedure. Shaffer and David had a serendipitous success when they sutured the ends of the pouches together. To their surprise, a fistula developed, which they were able to dilate by bougienage into a well-functioning channel.

## STENOSIS OF ESOPHAGUS

The lumen of the esophagus may be narrowed but not completely atretic. Narrowing results in the main from (a) congenital strictures, (b) webs, (c) external pressure and (d) acquired stenosis. The first two types are discussed together, since their etiology is roughly the same, as is their symptomatology.

**ETIOLOGY.** Both congenital strictures and webs in the neonate stem from imperfect evolution of the primitive foregut into the mature esophagus. In the complicated process of formation of the esophagus, usually at the point where the primitive

trachea and larynx bud off from the foregut, imperfect recanalization may take place. In some instances this failure was sharply limited to one point, and a weblike structure persists. In others the defect encompasses a length of 1 cm or more.

Stenoses are not limited to the junction of the middle and upper thirds of the esophagus. A number have been reported involving some or all of the lower third. A few are found at or just above the cardia. Some of these are acquired fibrotic narrowings that have resulted from reflux peptic esophagitis. Some fall into the not too well understood categories of cardiospasm and achalasia. This whole matter will be discussed in detail under those headings.

Vargas et al. described one 7-week-old infant who had vomited from birth and had aspiration pneumonia. Esophagram showed a stenotic area 3 cm above the diaphragm that never relaxed and would not permit passage of a filiform under direct guidance. Operation revealed 6 cm of intrathoracic stomach, a relaxed hiatus and a firm, doughnut-shaped ring of muscle at the esophagogastric junction. A myotomy and hernia repair led to complete cure.

**DIAGNOSIS.** The prime sign of esophageal stenosis is vomiting. The nature of esophageal vomiting is distinctive. It usually takes place during the feeding, after a few ounces or less of fluid has been ingested, or at the termination of a small meal. It may be repeated several times during the same meal, since it is unaccompanied by nausea and the hungry infant is willing and eager to attempt to eat again after his esophagus has been emptied. The returned material is completely unaltered in appearance except perhaps for an admixture of mucus from the oropharynx or, if ulceration has occurred, an admixture of fresh or old blood. The amount regurgitated is never great, although later, as dilatation progresses, it may exceed in volume the capacity of the normal esophagus.

The time of onset of vomiting is exceedingly variable and appears to depend almost entirely upon the degree of narrowing. Some infants with esophageal stenosis begin to vomit immediately after birth, after, that is, the institution of oral feeding. Some begin to vomit after a few weeks. A great many, perhaps the majority, do not begin to vomit until the attempt is made to add solids to the diet. Others can swallow both liquids and the thin purées commonly added first to the infant's diet, but cannot manage to swallow small lumps of food. In still others the onset of vomiting may be delayed for years until an unusually large object (for example, a large lump of meat, a coin or a marble), which would pass through the normal esophagus, becomes plugged in the stenotic stoma.

In many the vomiting is not at all constant, several meals entering the stomach with no difficulty, while one a day or fewer cannot be swallowed. In a few vomiting becomes intractable and swallowing of any type of food completely impossible. Some older children make pathetic efforts to help push the food into the stomach by introducing a hand deep into the pharynx.

The only other symptom may be pain. This may be complained of by older children or adults or may be evidenced in young infants by the facial expression and cry when the esophagus is overdistended, just before vomiting, or when the mucous membrane has become ulcerated. Vomiting commonly relieves the painful sensation.

Failure to gain is frequent, and actual loss of weight may be sustained in periods of intractable vomiting. As is to be expected, the smaller infants may rapidly become dehydrated and acidotic when obstruction is nearly complete.

The appearance of blood in the vomitus is due to the development of esophagitis with ulceration. This may be of the superficial erosive variety or the ulcers may be deep and linear.

The diagnosis is suggested by the nature of the vomiting. It must be verified by passage of a catheter and by fluoroscopic and x-ray studies. When attempting to pass a catheter, one must be exceedingly cautious, since it is not difficult to perforate a stenosed esophagus. The tube may be introduced through the nose or mouth and slowly inched forward until obstruction is met. It should then be withdrawn and the distance from naris or upper gum mea-

sured. Smaller and smaller bougies may then be introduced to see whether one will pass through with a minimum of pressure. It is safer when narrowing is extreme to make further attempts at passage under direct vision with the esophagoscope in place.

**RADIOGRAPHIC FINDINGS.** Fluoroscopy must be performed carefully lest minor grades of narrowing be missed. A thin barium mixture may be used, but, if this flows into the stomach rapidly, it should be followed by a thicker paste. The barium column may be seen to stop or hesitate, then to pass through the narrowed point in a thin stream or in narrow jets. Spot films will show, in the fibrous stenoses, symmetrical funneling to a narrow line followed by gradual widening of the opaque column. When a web is present, it may be visualized as a sharp shelf at the point of obstruction. The segment of esophagus proximal to the narrowed point soon becomes dilated.

**TREATMENT.** Rarely the original diagnostic catheterization may effect cure, as when a delicate web is torn by passage of the tube. This is the exception rather than the rule. In most cases bougienage must be repeated frequently and over a period of several years, the bougie being passed first through an esophagoscope. In those infants in whom even the finest bougie cannot be induced to traverse the stenosis, gastrostomy followed by retrograde bougienage may have to be resorted to. Segnitz, unable to penetrate the stenosis from either above or below, successfully performed a transthoracic repair of the stenotic area in a 1-month-old, 5-pound infant (Fig. 31–2).

## COMPRESSION OF ESOPHAGUS BY NEIGHBORING STRUCTURES

Other mediastinal masses, cystic or solid, may produce narrowing or dislocation of the esophagus. In this group are included, in addition to esophageal duplications, gastrogenic or enterogenic cysts, dermoids, anterior myelomeningoceles inter alia. More common, although still rare, causes of esophageal compression are anomalous blood vessels, such as right aortic arch, double

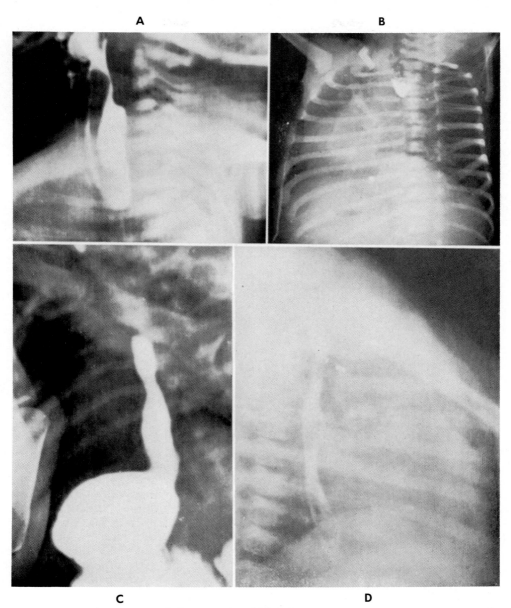

**A**

**B**

**C**

**D**

*Figure 31–1.* A, Esophagram recorded at 3 weeks of life, after increasing regurgitation since age of 2 weeks. Decided stenosis of esophagus is seen at about the junction of the upper and middle thirds. The esophagus proximal to the stenotic point is a little dilated. B, One week later, showing complete obstruction at the level of the stenosis. C, Preoperative regurgitation barium esophagram shows the lower limit of the stenotic area and a normal distal esophagus. At 5 weeks of age, attempted dilatations from above and from below after gastrostomy having failed, the stenosis was relieved by longitudinal incision followed by transverse closure. D, Postoperative barium esophagram at 6 weeks of age shows an adequate passageway. At the age of almost 1 year the patient was eating normally, and the esophagram was still normal. (Case of Dr. Richard H. Segnitz, Milwaukee, Wis. Reprinted with the kind permission of Dr. Segnitz, from Wisc. M. J. 55:447, 1956.)

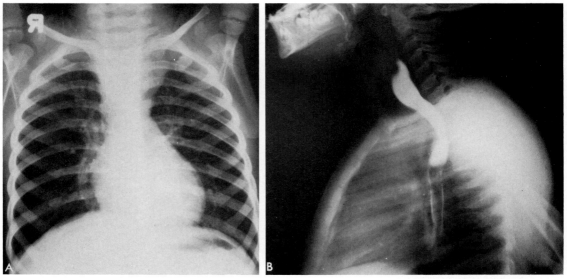

*Figure 31–2.* A, Anteroposterior view of chest shows a triangular shadow in the left upper lung field and deviation of the trachea to the right. B, Lateral view with barium in esophagus shows posterior displacement of the esophagus by a round mass. This proved at operation to be a cystic duplication of the esophagus.

This case is not abstracted in the text because the patient was not a newborn. She was a 2-year-old white infant who had had recurrent respiratory infections and respiratory distress since the age of 8 months. A soft mass could be seen in the left side of the neck when she strained or coughed. Cyanosis and dyspnea were marked. (Case of H. T. Langston, W. M. Tuttle and T. B. Patton. Prints reproduced with kind permission of Dr. Langston, from Arch. Surg. *61*:949, 1950.)

aortic arch, anomalous subclavian arteries and others. Since the symptomatology of all these is apt to be more closely related to the respiratory than to the gastrointestinal system, these are discussed in the section devoted to the former (p. 100 ff.).

## ACQUIRED STENOSIS

Newborn infants, like older ones, may suffer with strictures from ingestion of lye or other destructive chemicals but fortunately they seldom do. If they should, their management should be exactly the same as for other infants.

The most common form of acquired stenosis is that following *peptic ulceration of the lower esophagus* secondary to reflux of gastric contents. This entity is discussed in detail in the sections dealing with hiatus hernia and cardiochalasia (Chapter 31).

## ESOPHAGEAL DUPLICATIONS

Spherical or sausage-shaped cysts may be found in the mediastinum. Some have walls composed of mucosa, submucosa and muscular layers and are obviously duplications of some portion of the gastrointestinal tract. The histologic characteristics of a few of this latter group point to an esophageal origin. Most represent misplaced duplications of stomach or bowel.

The symptoms and signs are indistinguishable from those of other types of posterior mediastinal tumors. These are largely respiratory in nature, although dysphagia, vomiting and hematemesis may make up part of the clinical picture. Because of the preponderance of respiratory symptoms, this group has been described under Mediastinal Cysts and Tumors in Chapter 19.

## HIATUS HERNIA

It is customary to separate hiatus hernia into three categories: congenital short esophagus with intrathoracic stomach, sliding hernia, and rolling or paraesophageal hernia. This last seems to be almost entirely confined to age groups older than the newborn and will not be considered in detail in this chapter.

**INCIDENCE.** The difference in apparent incidence of partial thoracic stomach, whether this be due to congenital short esophagus or to sliding hernia, in England as opposed to the United States, is hard to understand. Here the disorder is considered rare. We ourselves encounter no more than one every few years, despite the fact that we have been making exhaustive efforts to discover examples. Yet Carré and his co-workers found 18 cases a year in Birmingham alone, and Thomson observed 48 cases from 1949 to 1955! Friedland et al., in California, confirmed a higher incidence after the introduction of the criteria of the British radiologists, suggesting that the diagnosis may have been missed in the United States.

**ETIOLOGY.** Congenital short esophagus was at one time believed to make up a large proportion of the hiatus hernia group. There followed a period when short esophagus was considered to have resulted almost always from fibrosing esophagitis. Botha, in 1958, after an exhaustive study of the anatomy of the normal newborn hiatus and a review of the pathology of partial intrathoracic stomach in young infants, reverted to the original position. He concludes that sliding hiatal hernia in adults is an acquired degenerative phenomenon, but in infants is due to congenital short esophagus or underdeveloped diaphragm. There is no way, he believes, to distinguish these latter two. We believe that the overall evidence suggests that intrathoracic stomach is based upon congenitally short esophagus rarely, upon fibrosis secondary to incompetent hiatus much more often.

Between the fourth and seventh weeks of gestation the esophagus elongates, and the stomach migrates rapidly in a caudal direction. Failure of complete elongation and migration leaves the esophagus short and the stomach completely or partially trapped above the diaphragm. Supradiaphragmatic stomach may be tubular and recognizable only by esophagoscope and in the x-ray film by the characteristic longitudinal rugal folds of its mucosa, separated from the esophagus above by a more or less well defined area of narrowing. More often the portion of intrathoracic stomach below the tubular esophagus and the hiatal constriction is tented and conical in shape.

The same picture may be produced by fibrosing esophagitis. Any of the conditions that permit reflux of acid peptic secretions of the stomach may result first in superficial erosions, and later in deep linear ulcerations which penetrate mucosa and muscular layers. The scarring that follows causes the esophagus to retract and shorten to a remarkable degree, and in this process the cardia is pulled upward through the hiatus.

The difference between congenital and acquired short esophagus would appear to be in the presence or absence of esophagitis. Unfortunately the hiatus is generally incompetent in the congenital form also, so that the supradiaphragmatic esophagus is subject to the same destructive influences. When this is true, the two conditions are virtually impossible to distinguish.

Botha completely re-examined the questions of the anatomy and physiology of the diaphragmatic hiatus in the neonatal period. He found that it differs in many important respects from the hiatus of adults. In the young infant the hiatus is small and fits the narrowed portion of esophagus snugly. It is generally composed of encircling fibers of two limbs of the right diaphragmatic crus that surround the esophagus and overlap to produce a constricted oblique tunnel. The muscle ring is firmly attached to the lower esophagus and cardia by a strong phrenoesophageal membrane.

The existence of a physiologically useful lower internal esophageal sphincter is now accepted by most observers. The muscular thickening is not localized as is the pyloric sphincter, but extends over a considerable but variable extent of the lower esophagus.

The combination of a small competent hiatus, reinforced by a lower esophageal sphincter, appears to Botha to be necessary in early life. The infant's supine position, his small stomach repeatedly filled with fluid and excess gas at short intervals, the abdomen subjected to sudden increases in intra-abdominal pressure produced by crying, straining at stool and hiccuping would lead to continual reflux were this not true.

Imperfect development of the hiatus therefore is a most important cause of cardiac incompetence.

**DIAGNOSIS.** It is possible to make the diagnosis of hiatus hernia within the neonatal period. Swyer observed 17 cases in infancy, and in seven of these the diagnosis was verified before the age of 1 month, in one as early as the fourth day of life.

The primary symptom is *vomiting.* The infants may begin to vomit from their first feedings, or the onset may be delayed weeks or months. Some babies regurgitate every meal; others do so intermittently. Only small quantities are brought back. Appetite remains strikingly good, so that refeedings are taken eagerly immediately after regurgitation. The formula is either unchanged or mixed with small quantities of mucus or blood. It is never coagulated, nor does it ever contain bile. Blood admixture may or may not appear early, but, if vomiting persists for weeks or months, it is almost sure to appear. Weight gain is slow or absent, and some babies lose weight and become dehydrated. The second symptom of importance, present in a large proportion of cases, is *anemia,* at times occult, in that bloodstained vomiting either has not occurred or has not been mentioned. *No anemia of undetermined origin has been investigated completely unless the lower esophagus and cardia have been well visualized by x-ray.* The third highly suggestive symptom is *persistent or recurrent lower respiratory infection,* again with or without overt vomiting. McNamara et al. stress this association in their recent report of 30 such patients who had gastroesophageal reflux, in 22 of whom supradiaphragmatic stomach was visualized. (They remind us that one normal radiographic study does not mean that a portion of the stomach does not ever slide above the diaphragm.) *Every persistent or recurrent pneumonitis deserves a careful cineradiographic study of the esophagus and cardia.*

Physical examination is unrewarding. The waves of hypertrophic pyloric stenosis have been seen and its tumor palpated in a fair number of these infants, but, when this is true, pyloric stenosis is a coexisting disorder, not an integral part of this clinical picture.

A stomach tube must be passed to rule out esophageal atresia or stenosis. In most cases the tube passes into the stomach readily. In some, especially if the first attempt to pass a catheter is not made until the infant is more than 1 month old, obstruction will be met at a point a few centimeters above the diaphragm. Most observers now believe that this low esophageal stenosis develops as a result of reflux and subsequent esophagitis. A few still believe it to be a concomitant congenital defect along with congenitally short esophagus and intrathoracic stomach. In still other cases the tube enters the stomach after a distinct hang at this same point, overcome by gentle pressure, after which it may be passed back and forth with great ease. Astley thinks that this represents cardiospasm which has resulted from esophagitis.

**ESOPHAGOSCOPY.** In the United States the esophagoscope has not been utilized freely in the differential diagnosis of these conditions in small infants. Some scattered observations have been made here, but many more have been reported from England. In Findlay and Kelly's series of nine cases endoscopy was performed in eight. In all these the esophagoscope traversed the widened upper esophagus, then detected the gradual funneling down of the stenotic area, which was easily distensible to permit its passage into another dilated pouch. This pouch of variable size, lying above the diaphragm, was lined with gastric mucosa and was certainly part of the stomach lying within the thorax. They decided that, in these instances at least, the stenotic point represented misplaced cardia and that its narrowing was due to variable cardiospasm.

Forshall was able to see gastric mucosa at times above and at times below the diaphragm when she did endoscopy on six of her cases of sliding hernia. As time passed these cardias ultimately became fixed at a point above the diaphragm. She argues from this observation that in most instances short esophagus with intrathoracic stomach is acquired rather than congenital, the shortening being due to esophagitis followed by fibrosis.

In paraesophageal hernia gastric mucosa

is not seen until the esophagoscope penetrates to a point below the level of the diaphragm.

By means of the esophagoscope esophageal complications are best recognized. These consist of esophagitis, with or without secondary fibrosis and stricture, and, rarely, peptic ulceration of the lower end.

**FLUOROSCOPY AND RADIOGRAPHIC EXAMINATION.** Definitive diagnosis of lower esophageal disorders can be made in vivo only by fluoroscopy and x-ray study. These examinations must be conducted with scrupulous care and a foreknowledge of the pitfalls. A simple barium meal with the infant supine often does not suffice. It has been suggested that at first a thin barium mixture be given (weight to volume ratio of 1:2). If this enters the stomach without hesitation, the stomach should be filled with it, and this should be followed by several swallows of a thicker paste (weight to volume ratio of 1:1). Multiple spot films or, better, a cineradiographic strip, should be taken in the erect, supine and Trendelenburg positions to determine whether reflux is present. Observations should then be made while gentle abdominal pressure is applied.

Stenotic areas in the esophagus will be visualized and the degree of narrowing and dilatation above ascertained. Unusual tightness or laxness at the physiologic cardia, a point 2 or 3 cm above the superior margin of the stomach, will be recognized. Unusual ballooning of the lower esophagus may be found, and spot films will show, by the rugal pattern, whether the dilated structure is lower esophagus or stomach. Irregularities in the mucosal pattern may indicate ulceration.

Cine-esophagography permits careful study of the films at leisure, and often demonstrates behavior of the barium column not appreciated at the moment of swallowing.

**PROGNOSIS.** The course of newborns with hiatus hernia is exceedingly variable. One can offer several generalizations about them as a group, but the fate of the individual within the group is unpredictable.

If untreated, as most of our infants were until comparatively recently, the majority would improve, even if the hernia continued to be demonstrable by x-ray in some for many years. A few would continue to vomit and in some of these esophagitis would develop. This would be signalized 1) by appearance of blood in the vomitus, 2) by persisting occult anemia, 3) occasionally by gross hematemesis or 4) by the symptoms of advancing esophageal stenosis. These in turn are recurrent, often intermittent vomiting, dysphagia, inability to

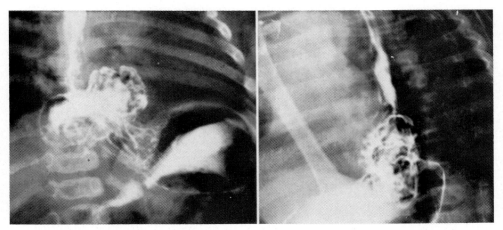

*Figure 31–3.* Views of esophagus and stomach taken at 1 week of age, in the Trendelenburg position. Both show the esophagus narrowing sharply as it enters the stomach, whose distinctive rugal pattern can be seen to lie well above the left diaphragm.

This infant began to vomit immediately after the institution of oral feeding. She was maintained in the semierect position for 7 weeks, by which time vomiting had ceased and weight gain commenced. At 1 year of age she seemed perfectly well.

swallow solids, complete esophageal obstruction by a bolus of food or recurrent pneumonitis from aspiration from the dilated proximal esophagus.

**TREATMENT.** All early cases, and this would obviously include all cases diagnosed in the neonatal period, should be treated at first medically and conservatively. The prime consideration should be the prevention of reflux, for if this can be accomplished, esophagitis and fibrosis will not follow. Reflux can best be obviated by maintaining the infant in the semi-upright position throughout the day and night. Held thus in a bosun's chair type of apparatus, or harnessed firmly to a tilted mattress, the infant soon becomes comfortable, eats well and sleeps peacefully. Vomiting usually ceases promptly upon change of position, but in some infants the feeding mixture will have to be thickened by the addition of cereal or banana powder in order to stop regurgitation completely. Antacids may be used freely to advantage.

In the minority in whom simple medical management fails to relieve reflux and regurgitation, operative intervention will have to be considered. This is especially true if admixture of blood with the vomitus indicates esophagitis or if this condition is seen to be present by esophagoscopy. The operator will attempt to mobilize the esophagus, fix the cardia at a point below the diaphragm and construct a competent snug hiatal ring.

The most difficult sequel of hiatal hernia to treat is the stricture that forms secondarily. This is not an important consideration in the neonatal period, since time is required for a tight stricture to develop. Nevertheless several authors have commented upon the rapidity with which stricture can form, and full-blown cases have been reported in infants as young as 4 and 6 weeks. An attempt may be made to handle these by postural therapy and repeated dilatations. The great hazard of perforation dictates the necessity of performing bougienage under direct esophagoscopic vision. Mercury-filled bougies may not be passed blindly until preliminary dilatation has been successfully accomplished. Dilatation in any event is not too successful an approach to the problem, and unless results are obtained quickly, and unless esophagoscopy demonstrates that the ulcerative

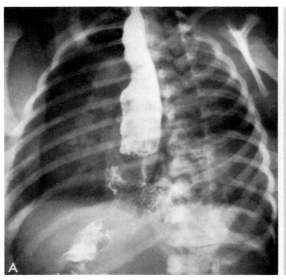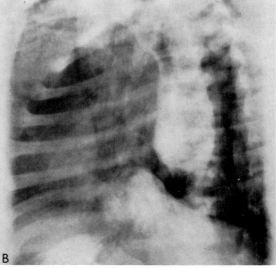

*Figure 31–4.* A, Supine film taken at 1 week of age after a barium meal. The greatly dilated esophagus narrows sharply several centimeters above the level of the diaphragm. *B*, Film taken in Trendelenburg position with abdominal pressure. The stenotic portion of the esophagus is about 1 cm long. Below it, but well above the diaphragm, lies a large pouch of the stomach.

This infant had multiple malformations, including cyanotic heart disease. She vomited intermittently from the second day of life until her death at eight weeks of age. Esophagoscopy showed a stricture of the lower esophagus.

process subsides completely, definitive operative intervention must be advised.

Roviralta believes that we subject too many children to operation. He selected 10 illustrative cases from his broad experience upon whom operation had not been performed for one or another reason. In four, described as total or subtotal, the greater part of the stomach lay above the diaphragm. All had vomited from birth, three with blood in the vomitus. Examined 9 to 20 years later, all were asymptomatic. In one the stomach had become completely intra-abdominal; in two some of the organ had re-entered the abdomen; in one no repeat radiogram was permitted. Six children with small and medium-sized hernias were similarly re-examined after many years, after nothing more than postural treatment. All were clinically well; in two no herniated stomach was seen; in two hernia was still present, but smaller; in two no repeat films were made.

Humphreys et al. have recently reviewed their own experience with hiatus hernia over the past 20 years. Of 34 cases, in infants and children, five were asymptomatic, discovered in the course of complete surveys because of the presence of other abnormalities. Eleven infants were treated medically, that is, 10 by posture alone, and one by posture plus several bougienages. All improved. Of seven of these who were studied some years later, the hernia could no longer be visualized in four. Eighteen were treated surgically and 15 of these did well. Three of four who had well developed stenoses at the time of operation did not do well, and required interposition operations later.

The authors conclude that postural treatment often suffices to relieve symptoms and that small hernias may become increasingly difficult to demonstrate; that hematemesis, melena, anemia and obstructive symptoms should make one think seriously of operative intervention; and that simple transthoracic repair of uncomplicated hiatus hernia is well tolerated by infants and children and can be expected to "give good results and negligible morbidity and mortality."

Lari and Lister (1972), in a more recent survey of 33 infants and children operated upon for hiatus hernia, stress a few points. One is that one may not delay operative intervention when medical management is clearly proving ineffective. The development of stricture renders operative cure less likely. The other is that gastrostomy and gastric fixation not only "improves the nutrition of a child before a major corrective procedure, but in a few cases may avoid more drastic operation."

## ACQUIRED LESIONS OF THE ESOPHAGUS

**ESOPHAGEAL EROSIONS.** The frequency of esophageal erosions at autopsy of infants was noted by Merriam and Benirschke, who found microscopic evidence of necrosis in 30 per cent of infants. It was most commonly associated with hyaline membrane disease, but was also noted in stillbirths. Instrumentation was not thought to be a factor in pathogenesis. More gross evidence of esophagitis in stressed infants had previously been described by Gruenwald. He found ulceration and hemorrhage in some instances, and felt that all these changes were manifestations of shock.

**PEPTIC ULCERATION, FIBROSIS AND SHORTENING OF THE ESOPHAGUS.** We have indicated in the foregoing section the extraordinary danger of peptic ulceration to the integrity of the lower esophagus when there is repeated gastro-esophageal reflux (p. 333).

**RUPTURE OF THE ESOPHAGUS.** Five newborns have by now been reported with rupture of the esophagus not produced by passage of a tube. In one instance rupture took place just proximal to a stenosing web, but in the other four, ruptures were spontaneous and unexplained.

In the example of Hohf et al., spitting up of bright red blood at 13 hours of age was the initial sign. This was followed by hydropneumothorax, treated by aspiration, then water-seal drainage. Diagnosis was indicated by passage of ingested milk through the drainage tube and verified by Lipiodol esophagram. The tear was repaired, and the patient recovered, but later had a stricture that required repeated dilatations.

# REFERENCES

Astley, R.: Oesophageal "spasm" in infancy. Proc. Roy. Soc. Med. *48*:1045, 1955.

Botha, G. S. M.: The gastro-esophageal region in infants: Observations on the anatomy, with special reference to the closing mechanism and partial thoracic stomach. Arch. Dis. Child. *33*:78, 1958.

Carré, I. J., Astley, R., and Smellie, J. M.: Minor degrees of partial thoracic stomach in childhood. Lancet *2*:1150, 1952.

Fleischner, F. G.: Hiatal hernia complex. J.A.M.A. *162*:183, 1956.

Forshall, I.: The cardio-esophageal syndrome. Arch. Dis. Child. *30*:46, 1955.

Friedland, G. W., Dodds, W. J., Sunshine, P., and Zboralske, F. F.: Apparent disparity in incidence of hiatal hernias in infants and children in Britain and the United States. Am. J. Roentgenol. Rad. Ther. Nucl. Med. *120*:305, 1974.

German, J. C., Mahour, G. H., and Woolley, M. M.: Esophageal atresia and associated anomalies. J. Pediat. Surg. *11*:299, 1976.

Gruenwald, P.: Asphyxia, trauma and shock at birth. Arch. Pediatr. *67*:103, 1950.

Gryboski, J. D., Thayer, W. R., Jr., and Spiro, H. M.: Esophageal motility in infants and children. Pediatrics *31*:382, 1963.

Hohf, R. P., Kimball, E. R., and Ballenger, J. J.: Rupture of the esophagus in the neonate. J.A.M.A. *181*:939, 1962.

Holder, J. M., and Ashcraft, K. W.: Esophageal atresia and tracheoesophageal fistula. (Collective Review.) Ann. Thorac. Surg. *9*:445, 1970.

Holinger, P. H., Johnston, K. C., and Potts, W. J.: Congenital anomalies of the esophagus. Acta Otolaryngol. Supp. 100, 100, 1951.

Humphreys, G. H., Wiedel, P. D., Baker, D. H., and Berdon, W. E.: Esophageal hiatus hernia in infancy and childhood. Pediatrics *36*:351, 1965.

Koop, C. E.: Recent advances in the surgery of oesophageal atresia. Progr. Pediat. Surg. *2*:41, 1971.

Langston, H. T., Tuttle, W. M., and Patton, T. B.: Esophageal duplications. A.M.A. Arch. Surg. *61*:949, 1950.

Lari, J., and Lister, J.: Some problems in surgical management of children with hiatus hernia. Arch. Dis. Child. *47*:201, 1972.

Mahour, G. H., Woolley, M. M., and Gwinn, J. L.: Elongation of the upper pouch and delayed anatomic reconstruction in esophageal atresia. J. Pediat. Surg. *9*:373, 1974.

Martin, L. W.: Management of esophageal anomalies. Pediatrics *36*:342, 1965.

Merriam, J. C., Jr., and Benirschke, K.: Esophageal erosions in the newborn. Lab. Invest. *8*:39, 1959.

Robb, D.: Congenital tracheoesophageal fistula without atresia but with large esophageal diverticulum. Austral. New Zeal. J. Surg. *22*:120, 1952–1953.

Rotch, T. M.: Three types of occlusion of the esophagus in early life. Am. J. Dis. Child. *6*:1, 1913.

Roviralta, E.: The natural evolution of hiatal hernias. Arch. Dis. Child. *39*:143, 1964.

Shafer, A. D., and David, T. E.: Suture fistula as a means of connecting upper and lower segments in esophageal atresia. J. Pediat. Surg. *9*:669, 1974.

Swyer, P. R.: Partial thoracic stomach and esophageal hiatus hernia in infancy and childhood. A.M.A. J. Dis. Child. *90*:421, 1955.

Vargas, L. L., Britton, R. C., and Goodman, E. N.: Report of a case of annular muscle hypertrophy at the esophagogastric junction. New Engl. J. Med. *255*:1224, 1956.

# 32

# DISORDERS OF NEUROMUSCULAR CONTROL OF THE ESOPHAGUS

Fleischner has summarized succinctly and persuasively the controversial problem of the physiology of the lower end of the esophagus. The anatomic cardia at the cardiac incisura probably has no sphincter function. This is reserved for that portion of the esophagus just at and extending from 1 to 2 cm above to 1 to 2 cm below the diaphragm. Although no true sphincter exists here in human beings, the muscular layers appear to be rather strong and exhibit a "sphincteric capacity," especially strong,

according to Botha, in very young infants. This "internal sphincter" is reinforced by the pinchcock action of the diaphragm itself, which acts as an "external sphincter" (Fig. 32–1). "In hiatal hernia, the dislocated 'internal sphincter,' deprived of its support by the diaphragmatic muscular ring, its 'external sphincter,' often becomes incompetent."

We have commented earlier (p. 339) upon the apparent physiologic immaturity of the lower sphincteric mechanism in the

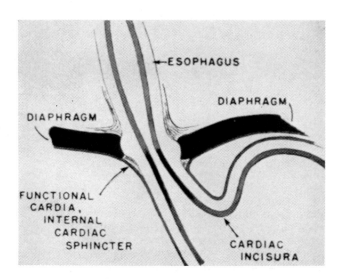

*Figure 32–1.* Diagram of a normal cardiac region. Esophagus is anchored to rim of esophageal hiatus of diaphragm by fibers of phreno-esophageal ligament. Incisura cardiaca (right lower arrow) indicates site of "anatomic cardia." Diaphragm forms external sphincter of "functional cardia" (lower left arrow). Internal cardiac sphincter is indicated by the diagrammatically exaggerated swelling of muscularis propria of esophagus. Variable zone of transition from esophageal to gastric mucosa is in black. (From Fleischner, F. G.: J.A.M.A. *162*:183, 1956.)

first 5 days of life which may permit reflux when intra-abdominal pressure is only slightly increased.

Other reasons have been advanced for cardio-esophageal incompetence based upon a rather imperfect understanding of the neuromuscular control of the so-called sphincter. Ingelfinger maintains that the sympathetic nerves have no effect whatsoever upon esophageal motility, whereas the vagus nerve, that is, the parasympathetics, maintains resting lower sphincteric pressure and regulates its response to swallowing. Why autonomic imbalance should occur in some infants, other than those in whom the nerve supply has been damaged, as in one of Astley's cases, is not known.

## CRICOPHARYNGEAL INCOORDINATION

We have already noted that not all newborn infants can swallow without at times aspirating some of the fluid into their tracheobronchial trees, and that in some infants this pharyngeal incoordination leads to recurrent pneumonitis. Matsaniotis et al. (1971) corroborated the original observations of DeCarlo and his collaborators by demonstrating such defective swallowing in 23 of 44 infants 6 days to 6 months old who were studied because of choking spells during feeding or persistent vomiting.

Blank and Silbiger (1972) found a variant of this condition in another newborn with a similar history. Her barium-swallow radiograms showed "a ringlike band at the entrance of the cervical esophagus suggesting a fixed mechanical obstruction. At esophagoscopy a transverse submucosal bar was seen which was indistinguishable from a normal cricopharyngeal muscle." They termed the condition *cricopharyngeal achalasia.*

## CARDIOSPASM

An impermanent constriction ring seen under the fluoroscope at the level of the lower esophageal sphincter may represent cardiospasm. In some infants this lies above a demonstrable hiatus hernia and the spasm is believed to result from the irritation of the refluxed gastric contents. In others no hernia can be seen. The following case exemplifies this latter situation.

CASE 32–1

A white male infant was born May 19, 1946, after a normal pregnancy, except for pneumonia in the third month, and a normal labor. Birth weight was 6 pounds 15 ounces (3150 gm), and he seemed completely normal at birth. In hospital he vomited many feedings, and impetigo developed. He was discharged on the seventh day, still regurgitating small quantities a few times a day. Stools were normal, three to four daily. At home regurgitation continued, but he gained 6 to 8 ounces weekly. On the twelfth day his mother noticed the escape of some grayish fluid from his nose and mouth immediately after a feeding, after which a severe "choking spell" occurred. He became very red and could not "catch his breath" for several minutes. After vomiting a small quantity of feeding he was relieved. These alarming spells recurred irregularly, once or twice a day, skipping an occasional day, until age 6 weeks, when we first saw him.

At age 6 weeks weight was 9 pounds (4080 gm). Physical examination was absolutely normal. During fluoroscopy (Dr. Whitmer B. Firor) barium mixture filled the esophagus to a point about 2 cm above the diaphragm. Here the column tapered to a point, beyond which thin tongues of fluid were shortly seen to fan out. After 10 minutes this trickling had filled the lower esophageal segment, whence it flowed freely into the stomach, but a sharp narrowing remained visible at the original point of obstruction. This disappeared in a few more minutes. Abdominal pressure in the supine and Trendelenburg positions then demonstrated no reflux into the lower esophagus (Fig. 32–2).

We were forced to assume that either cardiospasm or stenosis was responsible for the obstruction. A trial of atropine was decided upon, the drug being given in 1:1000 solution, one drop before each feeding, increasing by one drop a day up to the flushing point. Flushing ap-

peared at 6 drops, and this dose was maintained. Somewhat to our surprise, there was no further choking spell after atropine was begun, and regurgitation practically disappeared within 1 month. Fluoroscopy was repeated 20 days after the original examination, and the barium meal passed through to the stomach without hesitation. The child was followed up until the age of 8 years. During this time there had been no recurrence of vomiting.

**COMMENT.** This case must represent an instance of pure cardiospasm, responsive to atropine. Others in the literature have been cured, as was Astley's case, by a single bougienage, others by a short series of dilatations by stomach tube.

## ACHALASIA

Achalasia is an entirely different matter, although it too may present with repeated vomiting. At times vomiting is not a conspicuous feature, and the diagnosis is made because recurrent pneumonitis has called for a barium esophagram. Narrowing is seen at the hiatus, with moderate to advanced dilatation above the stenotic point.

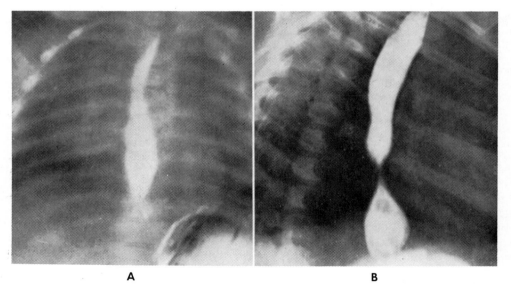

**A**        **B**

*Figure 32–2.* *A*, Barium swallow esophagram, made after the stomach had been filled with thin barium mixture. An additional mouthful is seen filling the upper part of the esophagus and coming to a stop at a constricted point a few centimeters above the cardia. Small tongues of the opaque mixture can be seen to fan out into the lower part of the esophagus. *B*, Ten minutes later. By now the lower esophageal segment had become filled, leaving the original constricted area still well defined. The rugal pattern of the lower segment is not characteristic of stomach.

Esophageal pressure and motility studies reveal that there is no increased tone of the lower sphincter area, but that tone within the body of the esophagus is reduced, and peristaltic waves are weak and ineffectual. The result is that stagnation of ingested food causes dilatation of the esophagus, at times to such a point that the term megaesophagus is justified.

Megaesophagus is a frequent complication of Chagas' disease, caused by infection with *Trypanosoma cruzi*. In this condition microscopic sections show loss of ganglion cells of the intrinsic neural plexus. Similar sparsity or absence of ganglion cells has been reported in idiopathic achalasia in some but not all affected adults, and not as yet in infants or children. Pathognomonic of achalasia in adults is a violent peristaltic response to tiny doses of acetylcholine. No similar studies have been reported in infants or children.

The following case exhibits what we believe are the characteristics of achalasia.

CASE 32–2

A black male infant was born October 14, 1949, after a normal pregnancy and delivery.

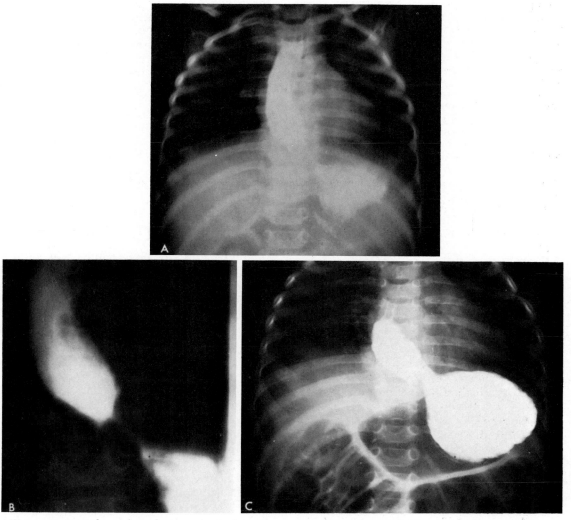

*Figure 32–3.* Films taken during a barium swallow examination. *A* and *B*, The constriction can be seen clearly and appears to be infradiaphragmatic. *C*, The lower segment looks as though it projects above the diaphragm. No rugal markings characteristic of stomach can be discerned in this segment.

Birth weight was 8½ pounds (3850 gm). At 2 weeks of age he began to vomit persistently, and this had continued ever since. Vomiting occurred immediately after feedings, and the material vomited was small quantities of unaltered food. He suffered two episodes of pneumonia in his first 6 months of life. At 6 months he weighed 9½ pounds (4300 gm), at 1 year 12 pounds (5450 gm). He had been studied and treated at a hospital in another city three times in all. He was admitted to the Harriet Lane Home August 15, 1951, aged 22 months.

His weight was 12 pounds (5450 gm). His condition was poor; there was much wasting, poor turgor and muscle tone, and he was irritable and uncooperative. "His only interest was in food," which he would take greedily and promptly vomit, forcefully and immediately after completion of the meal. The rest of the examination and all pertinent laboratory studies were normal. He was given continuous fluids intravenously for 3 days. On the fifth day a barium swallow revealed lower esophageal obstruction a few centimeters proximal to the cardia. No reflux from the stomach to lower esophagus could be demonstrated (Fig. 32–3).

Daily bougienage was instituted with bougies of gradually increasing size until by the twelfth day a no. 30 tube could be passed with ease. Improvement began almost at once, and vomiting diminished until it virtually ceased. Weight gain was rapid. Two months after admission he weighed 6.1 kg (13 pounds 7 ounces), and he was discharged. Two weeks later he weighed 15 pounds 14 ounces. He has remained well since.

**COMMENT.** Although this example was diagnosed as cardiospasm at a major pediatric center, one cannot be absolutely certain in retrospect that it does not represent either achalasia or congenital short esophagus, with acquired stenosis at the level of the hiatus. Esophagoscopy, motility studies and a trial of acetylcholine, which might have been diagnostic, were not performed. Careful studies for reflux and presence or absence of an intrathoracic portion of stomach were not performed after apparent cure of the stenosis.

The cure by repeated bougienage and the absence of longitudinal rugal markings in the lower esophageal segment suggest that achalasia may have indeed been the correct diagnosis.

**TREATMENT.** Cardiospasm may be mild and readily amenable to treatment, either by drugs or by a single dilatation. Achalasia is more commonly severe, is unresponsive to drugs and requires for its amelioration serial dilatations over a long period of time. Some of this latter group cannot be permanently benefited by bougienage, vomiting recurring after the completion of a long series of intubations. These infants have been subjected to a muscle-splitting operation at the cardia, the so-called Heller myotomy, similar to the Fredet-Ramstedt operation at the pylorus. Excellent results have been reported from the procedure.

## MEGAESOPHAGUS

A huge, dilated, tortuous esophagus may represent a terminal stage of congenital or acquired stenosis in the region of the lower sphincter, or of achalasia, whatever that may be. For other examples no explanation whatsoever is apparent. The case of Blank and Michael is illustrative. This infant, essentially healthy until 6 months of age, began to gag while eating, to wheeze and to cough, and respirations became noisy. Repeated studies revealed increasing dilatation of the entire esophagus with no evidence of obstruction below. The esophagus encompassed the trachea and obviously compressed it severely (Fig. 32–4). At autopsy hypertrophy of the muscularis mucosae and of the inner circular coat was seen, but not of the outer longitudinal muscle layer. Ganglion cells were normal in appearance and number. There was no inflammation or scarring. They could advance no adequate explanation for the megaesophagus, nor can we.

## CARDIOCHALASIA (LAX ESOPHAGUS)

In 1947 Neuhauser and Berenberg reported on 12 infants they had seen in the preceding 3 years in whom, they felt, there was relaxation of the hiatus portion of the esophagus with failure of the normal "sphincter" action of the cardia. They termed this condition cardio-esophageal relaxation or chalasia, and wondered whether it might be due to a temporary loss of proper autonomic control. British investigators have since described a great number of such cases. Forshall prefers the descriptive term "lax esophagus," since she believes

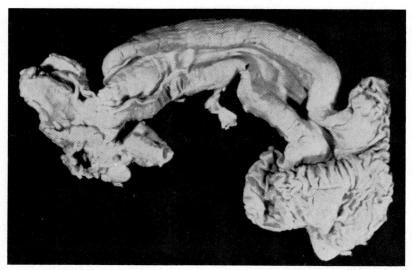

**Figure 32–4.** Megaesophagus, cause undetermined. (From Blank, E., and Michael, T. D.: Pediatrics 32:595, 1963.)

that the relaxation is not always limited to the hiatus region, but may involve the entire lower two thirds of the esophagus.

**DIAGNOSIS.** The only signs are regurgitation and vomiting. This begins usually in the first few days of life, almost invariably in the first week, invariably before the eighth week. It increases in frequency until it follows every feeding. In spite of this most of the infants appear well and hungry and gain weight fairly satisfactorily. Only a few fail to gain or actually lose weight. The vomiting is in general neither forceful nor projectile, but occasionally it is both. In some, projectile vomitus has been found to be caused by concomitant pyloric stenosis. Vomiting takes place often after the infant has been fed and returned to his crib in the prone or supine position. Mouthfuls may continue to be regurgitated from time to time throughout the interval between feedings. The vomitus contains no bile, but not infrequently blood appears in it.

Physical examination reveals no abnormalities.

A gastric tube meets no obstruction and slips into the stomach with the greatest ease.

**FLUOROSCOPY AND RADIOGRAPHIC EXAMINATION.** Definitive diagnosis depends upon x-ray examination. The barium meal passes through the esophagus with no hesitation. The lower portion of the esophagus appears dilated, thin-walled and flaccid. During inspiration the lower portion of the esophagus often fills with barium, whereas with expiration some is forced back into the stomach and some is forced upward into the mouth. Crying, struggling or light pressure upon the abdomen while the infant is supine produces reflux. This does not occur in the erect position. The dilated portion of the esophagus may be differentiated from supradiaphragmatic stomach by absence of the coarse rugae characteristic of the latter (Fig. 32–5). Esophagoscopy may be resorted to in order to verify this point.

**PROGNOSIS.** Response to therapy is usually dramatic. Forshall found recovery in 59 per cent of her cases to be rapid and satisfactory. Seven of her 58 patients died (one necrosis of the lower end of esophagus, one septicemia, one hematemesis, one inhalation of vomitus, one lung abscess, one gastroenteritis and one anesthesia death.) Four others had severe esophagitis with ulceration and stricture formation, and over the course of months the esophagus shortened, pulling a portion of the stomach into the chest. In these instances the shortened esophagus and intrathoracic stomach were unquestionably not congenital, but developed as a result of ulceration and fibrosis.

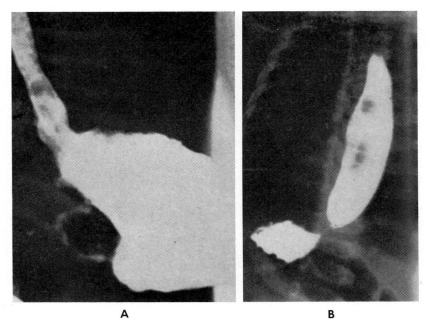

**A**                                                          **B**

*Figure 32–5.* *A*, At age 6 days. Moderate relaxation of cardia. Reflux filling produced by abdominal pressure. *B*, Age 3 months. Asymptomatic for 6 weeks. No cardio-esophageal relaxation or reflux filling. (From Berenberg, W., and Neuhauser, E. D. B.: Pediatrics 5:414, 1950.)

TREATMENT. Most infants respond promptly to simple change of position and the use of small, frequent thickened feedings. In mild cases we have found that it suffices to elevate the infant's head, by blocks under the crib legs or a pillow under the mattress, for an hour after each feeding. In some this is not enough, and more drastic steps must be taken in order to keep the baby constantly erect. Many types of "bosun's chairs" have been rigged up for this purpose. Infants may have to be kept in this apparatus for several months until a trial of the supine and prone positions proves them capable of retaining feeds while horizontal.

The sequelae of cardiochalasia are rare, but they may be identical to those caused by the reflux of gastric secretions in hiatus hernia.

Ulceration may result in severe anemia, for which transfusions are indicated. Shortening of the esophagus producing intrathoracic stomach requires surgical intervention with the object of mobilizing the esophagus, replacing the cardia below the diaphragm and tightening the hiatus.

## FAMILIAL DYSAUTONOMIA

Linde and Westover have called attention to the esophageal abnormalities one may expect in familial dysautonomia. Severe swallowing difficulties and recurrent pneumonitis, probably from aspiration, characterize many of these infants from birth. These observers noted, in addition to pharyngeal incoordination, weak peristaltic action which delayed esophageal emptying *in the supine position*. In the erect position gravity facilitated passage of food into the stomach. They found it necessary to feed each swallow to one of their infants in the supine position, so that milk could reach the hypopharynx, then to sit him up so that it could traverse the esophagus.

## REFERENCES

Astley, R.: Oesophageal "spasm" in infancy. Proc. Roy. Soc. Med. 48:1045, 1955.
Berenberg, W., and Neuhauser, E. B. D.: Cardioesophageal relaxation (chalasia) as a cause of vomiting in infants. Pediatrics 5:414, 1950.
Blank, E., and Michael, T. D.: Muscular hypertrophy

of the esophagus. Report of a case with involvement of the entire esophagus. Pediatrics 32:595, 1963.

Blank, R. H., and Silbiger, M.: Cricopharyngeal achalasia as a cause of respiratory distress in infancy. J. Pediatr. 81:95, 1972.

Botha, G. G. M.: The gastro-esophageal region in infants: Observations on the anatomy, with special reference to the closing mechanism and partial thoracic stomach. Arch. Dis. Child. 33:78, 1958.

Davies, W.: Cardio-chalasia in infancy. J. Pediatr. 41:467, 1952.

Fleischner, F. G.: Hiatal hernia complex. J.A.M.A. 162:183, 1956.

Forshall, I.: The cardio-oesophageal syndrome in childhood. Arch. Dis. Child. 30:46, 1955.

Gruenbaum, M.: Radiologic manifestations of familial dysautonomia. Am. J. Dis. Child. 128:176, 1974.

Ingelfinger, F. J.: The esophagus, March 1961 to February 1963. Gastroenterology 45:241, 1963.

Linde, L. M., and Westover, J. L.: Esophageal and gastric abnormalities in dysautonomia. Pediatrics 29:303, 1962.

Matsaniotis, M., Karpouzas, J., et al.: Aspiration due to difficulty in swallowing. Arch. Dis. Child. 46:788, 1971.

Messeloff, C. R., Shulman, H. I., and Buckstein, J.: Cardiospasm in infancy and childhood. Am. J. Dis. Child. 35:427, 1928.

Neuhauser, E. B. D., and Berenberg, W.: Cardioesophageal relaxation as a cause of vomiting in infants. Radiology 48:480, 1947.

Wyllie, W. G., and Field, C. E.: The aetiology of intermittent oesophageal regurgitation and haematemesis in infants. Arch. Dis. Child. 21:218, 1946.

# DISORDERS OF THE STOMACH    33

Those disorders of the stomach which have clinical importance in the neonatal period may be classified as follows:

I. Congenital anatomic defects
   A. Hypoplasia
   B. Diverticulum
   C. Duplication
   D. Atresia
II. Disorders of the pylorus
   A. Pylorospasm
   B. Hypertrophic stenosis of the pylorus
III. Peptic ulcer
IV. Gastric perforation

## HYPOPLASIA OF THE STOMACH (CONGENITAL MICROGASTRIA)

In two of our cases of esophageal atresia with tracheo-esophageal fistula (p. 110, Fig. 9–1) not only was the lower esophageal segment completely atretic but also the stomach itself was hypoplastic. The surgeon described them as "tiny and undeveloped." In these cases direct esophageal anastomosis was impossible because of the great length of atretic segment, and gastrostomy was performed as a preliminary to further plastic correction. The infants died after this procedure. It is prob-

able that the small size and poor functional capacity of the hypoplastic stomach contributed to the failure of the gastrostomy, hence to death.

In 1973 Blank and Chisolm reported a fascinating case of hypoplasia, without T-E fistula, which they termed congenital microgastria, in which the stomach was small and tubular, the duodenum maldeveloped and the cecum malpositioned and attached by bands to the abdominal wall and undersurface of the liver. Swallowed barium refluxed not only into the esophagus but also into biliary radicles in both lobes of the liver. At about 1 year of age, when she weighed 12¾ pounds (5.8 kg), the bands were cut and a gastrojejunostomy was performed. She improved slowly on frequent small pureed feedings, and at 27 years was the small but healthy mother of three normal daughters.

Dide had described a very similar case in 1894, and Caffey included one in the 1956 edition of his textbook. Two more examples were added to the literature in 1971. Malrotation and other congenital defects were present in most. The value of surgical intervention seems to depend more upon these associated anomalies than upon the gastric hypoplasia.

## GASTRIC DIVERTICULUM

Diverticula of the stomach are encountered not infrequently in patients 50 to 70 years of age, but may be discovered at any age. A few have been reported in the neonatal period.

Diverticula are commonly classified as either congenital, in which all the layers of the stomach wall are present and normal, or acquired, in which one or more layers are either missing or thinned and broken. The latter group may be subdivided into the pulsion type, caused by increased intragastric pressure, and the traction type, caused by the pull of adhesions to nearby inflammatory or neoplastic lesions. All three types have been seen in newborns.

No symptoms or signs stem from the diverticulum itself. The obstruction that causes rise in intragastric pressure, usually hypertrophic pyloric stenosis or duodenal narrowing, or the neighboring infected cyst or duplication which may produce traction diverticulum, is responsible for such symptoms as may be present. The diverticulum may rupture, however. In this event pneumoperitoneum and peritonitis follow and may be diagnosed in the usual manner.

## GASTRIC DUPLICATION

Any portion of the gastrointestinal tract may be duplicated in the course of its ontogenetic development. The most commonly accepted theory of pathogenesis is that advanced by Bremer. By about the sixth week of gestation much of the lumen of the gastrointestinal tract is occluded by rapid proliferation of the lining epithelial cells. These subsequently should all be reabsorbed and a single lumen re-established, but in a few fetuses a double lumen of variable size persists. Under these circumstances a portion of the tract may go on to develop as twinned structures. (More recent evidence, cited by Mellish and Koop, casts doubt upon Bremer's theory.) Duplications may be spherical or tubular, contiguous or distant, their lumens communicating or not with the nearby gastrointestinal tract.

The stomach is subject to duplication,

but is one of the less common sites. Some of the cysts produced by its duplication are left behind in the thorax (see Gastrogenic Cysts of the Mediastinum, p. 206) in the course of the stomach's normal caudad migration. A few arrive within the abdominal cavity. A few remain in both locations, the intrathoracic and abdominal cysts connected by a fistulous tract, which may penetrate the diaphragm or not.

*Symptoms* and *signs* may be minimal. The only finding may be a palpable cystic mass in the upper portion of the abdomen. Gastric duplications may produce intestinal obstruction, but they present in this way considerably less frequently than do duplications of the small bowel. Rarely, too, they may undergo peptic ulceration, and, if they communicate, hematemesis and melena may signal their presence.

*X-ray study* and *fluoroscopy* may show no abnormality in the absence of obstruction. Barium mixtures rarely fill the cavity of the duplication even when this communicates with the stomach. On occasion, however, one may be clearly seen in an upper gastrointestinal series study by a pressure defect involving stomach and bowel, as Figure 33–1 shows.

Differentiation from mesenteric cyst is difficult in uncomplicated cases, but obstruction renders the likelihood of the latter quite small, and hematemesis or melena points definitely toward duplication.

**TREATMENT.** Operative intervention and complete removal are indicated. Extensive resection of the stomach may be necessary if the duplication is tightly adherent. In spite of this, incomplete measures, such as marsupialization, cannot be countenanced.

## INTRINSIC OBSTRUCTION OF THE STOMACH (PYLORIC ATRESIA)

Up to 1971 the world literature contained 29 reports of congenital obstruction of the stomach due to atresia. In 19 of these cases a membrane completely occluded the prepyloric region, in three a fibrous cord joined the blind pyloric and duodenal ends, and in seven the blind ends were discontinuous. One infant of the first group

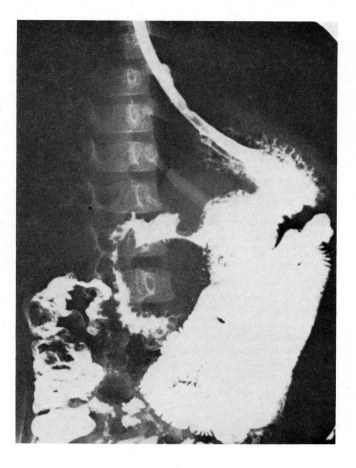

*Figure 33–1.* This 3-year-old boy had been well until 4 weeks before admission. Since then he had had bouts of vomiting and abdominal pain alternating with episodes of diarrhea. A vague, tender mass was palpable in the epigastrium. A gastric duplication half the size of the normal stomach was found attached to the greater curvature. (From Gwinn, J. L., and Barnes, G. R.: Am. J. Dis. Child. *113:*581, 1967.)

had a membranous partition proximal to the pylorus and a second in the duodenum a few centimeters distal to the pylorus. All of the cases presented with signs of high obstruction, but in this last one a visible and palpable cystic mass developed in the epigastrium on the second day of life. The sequestered portion of lower stomach and upper duodenum had become distended with accumulated secretions, and at operation resembled a tight cyst 5 cm in diameter occupying the pyloric portion of the stomach!

*Diagnosis* can be made only after exploration because of intractable vomiting from birth plus epigastric distention.

*Treatment* consists of excision of, or multiple radial incisions in, the membranous diaphragm. In some of these, gastroenterostomy may have to be performed because of obstructing edema. In the blind obstructions a shunt operation will surely have to

be performed. Gastroduodenostomy is preferable to gastrojejunostomy.

## PYLOROSPASM

Pylorospasm manifests itself by vomiting. Its onset is usually early, sooner than the usual onset of hypertrophic stenosis. It may begin after the first fluids have been offered or may be delayed until the end of the first week. It is usually intermittent, but may follow every feeding. It may be forceful, but is seldom projectile. Associated with vomiting is a definite diminution in capacity. A few infants seem unable to accept more than 1½ or 2 ounces at a time, a larger quantity causing discomfort and regurgitation. The pattern of a gastric bubble may appear in the left upper quadrant as one watches the abdomen during feeding, but this moves either not at all or sluggishly toward the midline. Most of us feel no pyloric tumor in this condition, but Craig, using an elaborate and time-consuming technique, was able to feel a contractile pyloric tumor in many infants who failed to gain and vomited repeatedly in the first two weeks of life. Constipation is not severe.

Fluoroscopic examination may demonstrate a short delay in peristaltic activity and beginning emptying of the stomach, but in some peristalsis is extremely active, and emptying may be completed unusually rapidly. No lengthening or narrowing of the pyloric canal can be demonstrated.

**TREATMENT.** Response to antispasmodics is generally excellent. Atropine has been our own drug of choice. One may begin with a dose of one drop of a 1:1000 solution of atropine sulfate 10 or 15 minutes before each feeding, increase by one drop each day until flushing appears, and revert to the previous day's dosage as the permanent one. Vomiting usually ceases within a few days, and capacity increases. After a week or two, seldom longer, the antispasmodic drug can ordinarily be discontinued without recurrence of symptoms. Antihistaminics have been used with success.

One should investigate carefully the possibility that pylorospasm may have been initiated or perpetuated by unfavorable environmental conditions. Relaxing the parents may effectively relax the infant's pylorus.

# HYPERTROPHIC STENOSIS OF THE PYLORUS

**INCIDENCE.** It is probable that the frequency of this disorder varies considerably from country to country and perhaps within different geographic sections of the same country. An incidence of 1 in 500 births would appear to represent an approximate over-all average.

Males are affected three to four times as often as females. Firstborns account for roughly half the cases, all other birth ranks for the remaining half. Blacks are decidedly less liable than whites. Premature infants have pyloric stenosis about as frequently as do full-term babies.

**ETIOLOGY.** Considerable doubt still exists about the cause of hypertrophic stenosis of the pylorus. Statistical evidence pointing to a genetic causation is suggestive, but far from convincing. It is, for example, difficult to ignore the implications of hereditary predisposition in the family reported by Burmeister and Hamilton. The father, almost surely, and four of his children suffered from hypertrophic pyloric stenosis. Evidence of its being an acquired disorder in our opinion counterbalances that in favor of heredity. Important are the lateness of onset of symptoms, absence of a palpable tumor prior to vomiting and steady increase in size of the tumor in proportion to the duration of vomiting, the preponderance of firstborns and the greater susceptibility of home-born over hospital-born (McKeown et al.). Also of significance in this respect is the fact that premature infants suffer the disorder at about the same postnatal age as do full-term babies. Pylorospasm seems to precede hypertrophy, and the success achieved by those who persevere in its treatment with antispasmodic agents suggests that the role of spasm is more than coincidental.

Rintoul and Kirkman, after studying 38 biopsy specimens and many controls, have observed that the myenteric plexus in the pylorus of the infant with hypertrophic stenosis contains no or sparse type I (Dogiel) cells. They were not certain whether this represented a congenital defect or whether it resulted from prolonged autonomic overstimulation, although they inclined toward the former hypothesis.

**DIAGNOSIS.** The cardinal signs of pyloric stenosis are vomiting, constipation, gastric peristaltic waves and pyloric tumor. Vomiting appears first and is followed within a shorter or longer time by the other signs.

Vomiting may begin at any time from birth to the eighth week of life or later. Most infants begin to vomit in the third, fourth and fifth weeks. We have seen a few who regurgitated their first few feedings while still in the newborn nursery, although days or weeks were to elapse before the diagnosis became certain. Onset beyond the sixth week is rare and becomes progressively rarer with the passage of time, but authentic cases have been reported in the second and third years of life. In premature infants the onset follows the same pattern postnatally, bearing no relation to true chronologic age.

At first vomiting follows feeding infrequently, but within days or weeks it increases in frequency until it follows virtually all. Early it may not be forceful, but it increases steadily in force until many vomits are projectile. Vomitus never contains bile. Rarely fresh or altered blood appears.

Stools begin to diminish in number when vomiting commences. Soon they become infrequent and dry, firm and scanty.

Gastric patterning becomes visible over the upper portion of the abdomen, and as the observer watches, preferably in strong light which strikes the infant obliquely from above, definite waves may be seen to march in slow, steady progression from the extreme left upper quadrant toward the midline. As one wave reaches the neighborhood of the umbilicus another forms slowly beneath the far left costal margin and makes its leisurely way toward the right. At times the gastric pattern may be accentuated and its movement initiated by feeding the infant an ounce or so of glucose solution or milk, then flicking the epigastrium sharply a few times with the fingernail.

In most instances of hypertrophic stenosis a definite tumor can be felt. Depending upon the degree of gastric dilatation, which in the fully developed case may be great indeed, the tumor will be felt either just at the umbilicus or well to its right, at its level, or above or below. It is best felt with the left hand pressing the right flank firmly upward while the right hand presses downward toward it. In this fashion the firm mass, the shape of an olive, may be caught and rolled between the two hands.

Throughout the course the appetite remains good.

**DIFFERENTIAL DIAGNOSIS.** Hypertrophic pyloric stenosis must be distinguished from congenital atresia or stenosis of the upper third of the duodenum, from cardiochalasia and from pylorospasm. *Atresia* or *stricture of the duodenum* distal to the ampulla of Vater permits bile to appear in the vomitus, a fact which effectively rules out pyloric stenosis. Complete atresia causes severe vomiting almost from the moment of birth. *Stenosis* proximal to the ampulla may be produced, but rarely, by annular pancreas (p. 375) or by external bands, usually in association with malrotation (p. 354) or by intrinsic incomplete stricture (p. 359). In these conditions the onset of vomiting may be delayed until the time when that of pyloric stenosis usually begins. In all there may be coexistent constipation, gastric patterning and left-to-right peristalsis. But in only one is a tumor to be felt. Further differentiation is afforded by roentgenography.

**FLUOROSCOPY AND RADIOGRAPHIC EXAMINATION.** Under the fluoroscope and in plain films the stomach will be seen to be dilated. A single large air bubble is visible in the left upper quadrant, extending beyond the midline to the right for a variable distance. If there were obstruction at some point in the duodenum, a double bubble would be visualized, the large gastric one and the smaller one to the right representing the dilated duodenal bulb. If, because of recent vomiting, there is little air in the stomach, an effervescent mixture may be administered in order to balloon the structures proximal to the suspected obstruction.

Hefke places great reliance upon the x-ray examination. In his own series the diagnosis made in 205 cases was confirmed by operation in 203 (99 per cent). His technique consists in emptying the stomach by gavage tube and instilling through the tube 2 to 3 ounces of a thin barium mixture. A film is taken in the right anterior oblique position after 5 to 10 minutes. If no barium has left the stomach by then, a similar film is taken 20 minutes later. He lays great stress on the pyloric opening time. If this exceeds 10 minutes, hypertrophic stenosis is likely; if it exceeds 30 minutes, it is almost certain. His second criterion is demonstration of a thin streak of barium, 1.5 to 2.5 cm in length, in the pyloric region, the so-called string sign. This is not often visualized in the anteroposterior exposure. It is present in the first film in two thirds of the cases, in the second in many of the remainder. As stated, if no barium has left the stomach by 30 minutes, the diagnosis is practically certain. He lays little stress upon the total emptying time, which may be delayed beyond the usual 2 to 4 hours in later cases, but may not be delayed in early ones. Other radiologists lay stress upon demonstrable bulging of the hypertrophied pylorus into the antrum.

TREATMENT. Most of us prefer to resort to surgery once the diagnosis has been established to our satisfaction. Some insist that diagnosis is never established until a tumor is consistently felt. Others are satisfied that the diagnosis is correct, even though in some infants no tumor becomes palpable, if there is persistent forceful vomiting, constipation, intense gastric peristalsis and x-ray evidence of delay in pyloric opening.

The operation of choice is the comparatively simple muscle-splitting procedure known as the Fredet-Ramstedt operation. Preoperative care consists in thorough rehydration with glucose and saline solution, with added potassium if necessary, until blood carbon dioxide, chloride, potassium and nonprotein nitrogen or blood urea nitrogen have returned to normal. Postoperatively, one withholds oral feeding for a short time, offers glucose solution after 8 or 12 hours, in 1/2-ounce quantities, increasing slowly and changing to a milk mixture 24 hours after operation. Continued vomiting

for a day or two is not unusual and need not cause alarm unless it persists into the third or fourth day.

How does one decide whether to treat hypertrophic pyloric stenosis medically or surgically? We would suppose that the circumstance of geographic location should be the most important factor. If one lives in or near a metropolis where a well trained surgeon and adequate preoperative and postoperative care are available, operative cure would seem to be simplest. The operation is easy, and the period of anesthesia short. Postoperative complications are rare. Within a few hours after operation the infant eats well and digests perfectly. He may be returned home in 7 to 10 days requiring no further special care.

Medical management, on the other hand, is possible but may consume 2 to 3 months. Antispasmodics are recommended, with frequent small feedings. Intravenous fluids may also be required. We believe that medical management is to be preferred only in outlying communities, in cases of unusual mildness, or in the rare instance in which hemophilia or some other disorder renders operation hazardous.

PROGNOSIS. Mortality in hypertrophic pyloric stenosis is now almost negligible, largely because of improved skills in surgery of the small infant with respect to preoperative fluid and electrolyte therapy, to anesthesia and to control of postoperative infection. Mortality rates as high as

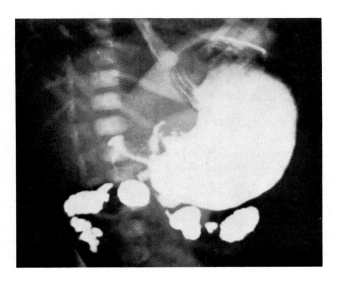

*Figure 33–2.* Oblique view of abdomen 30 minutes after ingestion of a barium meal. The stomach is still full, and only a little opaque material has escaped into the small bowel. A narrow line replaces the pyloric antrum and the first portion of the duodenum. This represents strikingly narrowed lumen and is a beautiful example of the "string sign" of hypertrophic pyloric stenosis.

21.5 per cent (Still) have decreased to less than 1 per cent in the most recent series reported.

## PEPTIC ULCER

Gastric or duodenal ulcers of the peptic type identical to those discovered in adults are encountered in the newborn. They are round or oval, sharply circumscribed, deeply punched out, with clean or rolled edges. Inflammatory reaction is absent or minimal. They may involve mucosa plus submucosa and muscular layers, and may even perforate serosa.

**INCIDENCE.** Ulcer is not common in infancy, but many more are found after death than have been suspected in vivo. In 1913, L. Emmett Holt, Sr., was able to find in the literature reports of 91 patients less than 1 year old. Of these, nine were neonates. By 1941 Bird, Limper and Mayer discovered reports of 243 cases in the total pediatric age group. Forty-two of these involved infants less than 14 days old. Lee and Wells encountered a peptic ulcer which had developed in the fetus in utero. Between 1949 and 1969, Seagram et al. found an average of five children per year admitted to the Hospital for Sick Children in Toronto with peptic ulcers. The lesion is rare in the first few years of life.

**ETIOLOGY.** Ulcer may develop in gastric mucosa wherever this might be found, in its normal location or in ectopic locations. In this latter category are included Meckel's diverticulum and gastrogenic cysts of either the thorax or abdomen, and intrathoracic portions of herniated stomach. It also may develop in nongastric mucosa that is bathed by gastric secretions, such as the proximal duodenum, the lower part of the esophagus of infants subject to reflux because of cardiochalasia or hiatus hernia, and near the stomata of surgical gastroenterostomies.

Why ulcer forms in the otherwise normal pyloric antrum or upper part of the duodenum is not known. In the newborn those conditions are not met that have been suggested as precursors and possible instigators of ulcer in the older child or the adult, except that gastric juice is highly acid after the first few hours of life. The opinion has become widespread that ulcer strikes more newborns who have suffered stormy deliveries and who have evidenced postnatal asphyxia than those delivered easily. No convincing proof of this contention has been gathered.

An occasional gastric ulcer results from erosion by the tip of an indwelling catheter.

**DIAGNOSIS.** In the neonatal period ulcer is recognized only by its disastrous complications, hemorrhage or perforation.

*Hemorrhage* is manifested by vomiting of fresh or altered blood, or by passage of fresh or altered blood by rectum. At times the loss of blood is considerable, causing rapid development of shock and a precipitous fall in the hematocrit level. At other times bleeding is more gradual and is recognized only by vomiting of dark brown-stained fluid or the passage of tarry stools. Most newborns who bleed into the stomach or duodenum lose blood by both routes; that is, by vomiting and by passage of blood by rectum.

Death may occur quickly from blood loss, or, if bleeding is not too massive and if replacement is prompt and adequate, recovery may take place. Hemorrhage may continue for 2 to 4 days, after which it commonly ceases, although at least one in our experience continued to bleed for seven days. Benzidine-positive stools may be passed for 3 or 4 days more, but this does not necessarily indicate continuation of bleeding.

*Perforation* may occur without prior bleeding or may follow hematemesis and melena. Most often, without premonitory signs of any kind, the newborn suddenly goes into profound shock. The abdomen rapidly distends and becomes full and tight. If shock is not too profound, the abdominal musculature becomes rigid, but this sign is often absent. Percussion reveals a tympanitic note throughout, tympany obscuring the normal area of liver dullness. In the case of Bird et al. the coincidence of bilateral inguinal hernia permitted the scrotum to be ballooned simultaneously by the air that escaped from the stomach. If death does not occur immediately, signs of peritonitis soon develop.

**FLUOROSCOPY AND RADIOGRAPHIC EXAMINATION.** Gastric and duodenal ulcers can be recognized by x-ray examination in the neonatal period only rarely. We have made many attempts to demonstrate them in newborns with hematemesis and melena and have rarely succeeded.

Perforation is readily demonstrable by x-ray film. Large amounts of free air can be visualized in the peritoneal cavity, and over the dome of the liver when films are taken in the erect posture.

**TREATMENT.** In the presence of hematemesis no food should be given by mouth until bleeding ceases. Fluids should be administered parenterally as needed. Blood lost should be replaced by transfusion repeated as often as necessary to keep the hematocrit level up to 35 to 40 per cent. Transfusions of 10 ml per kilogram may be given daily or as often as three times in 24 hours if absolutely necessary. If hemorrhage of great magnitude continues, there would appear to be no contraindication to use of a continuous drip of blood for 24 to 36 hours. We have never been forced to use this procedure for bleeding ulcer, but have utilized it for intractable bleeding of other kinds.

These infants should be watched assiduously for the first sign of perforation. If this occurs, with or without preliminary bleeding, immediate operation is imperative. Closure of the tear in the stomach or duodenum, if performed early, is simple and effective.

Scarring following ulceration, resulting in partial or complete obstruction of the first portion of the duodenum, has been encountered but once to our knowledge. In this case a bypass operation had to be performed 4 weeks after hematemesis had occurred on the first day of life (Floyd).

## GASTRIC PERFORATION

We cannot stress too strongly the importance of this disorder. Given a high enough index of suspicion, gastric perforation can be diagnosed promptly enough so that operative intervention will almost always be lifesaving.

**INCIDENCE.** By 1963 Reams et al. were able to find more than 100 cases in the literature, and by 1965 this number had risen to more than 150 (Shaw et al.). A great many have not been recorded. We ourselves encountered five cases in one year in Baltimore. It cannot therefore be considered rare.

**ETIOLOGY.** Many perforations are complications of peptic ulcer. Others have been attributed to birth trauma and a few to the ulceration caused by indwelling catheters. Some have been thought to follow rapid overdistention with gas in the course of positive pressure resuscitation, and some to the overdistention caused by obstructions distal to the stomach. Most of the remainder have been attributed to the rupture of weak points in the gastric wall where muscle was said to be congenitally deficient. This theory, first proposed by Herbut in 1943, gained wide acceptance. Shaw and his collaborators demonstrated in 1965 that all stomachs have potential points of weakness between the interlacing bundles of the muscularis externa, and that, after overdistention with air, rupture occurs at one or more of the weak points. The thin edge of the perforation will then show under the microscope only mucosa and submucosa, whereas the muscular layer will be found to have retracted 2 to 10 cm back from the mucosal edge. It appears then that this is not a congenital defect, but that the stomachs of all newborns are liable to rupture if intragastric pressure rises sufficiently. White believes that the supine position effectively seals air entrapped within the stomach, and that continued swallowing of more air may allow intragastric pressure to rise to dangerous heights. In the 3 years since newborns in the Johns Hopkins and Baltimore City Hospital nurseries have been maintained in the prone position not one case of gastric perforation has been encountered.

**DIAGNOSIS.** Low birth weight infants are more prone to gastric perforation than are term ones (58 of 90 in Reams' series, six of eight in Shaw's). Ordinarily, pregnancy, labor, and delivery have not been complicated, and the babies seem quite well at the outset. Symptoms appear usually on the third or fourth day, but may come as early as the second or as late as the eighth. Refusal of food, vomiting, respiratory distress and cyanosis may mark the onset, followed quickly by rapidly progressing abdominal distention.

Physical examination reveals moderate to extreme abdominal distention. The percussion note is usually tympanitic in the upper two thirds of the abdomen, obscuring normal liver dullness, but flat, and shifting with change of position, in the lower third. Often the distention is of such degree that respiration is embarrassed and cyanosis results. Pitting edema of the skin of the abdomen has been seen in several cases. There may be air filling the scrotal sac.

Flat films of the abdomen show excessive fluid and air within the peritoneal cavity. *One of the films must be taken in the erect position.* Much of the air can be recognized to be free; that is, not within the gastrointestinal lumen. A large air bubble will be seen above the dome of the liver, but below the diaphragm, with the infant in the erect position. When high obstruction coexists, the stomach may be seen to be dilated, or the characteristic double bubble of duodenal obstruction may be visualized.

TREATMENT. Operative intervention and closure of the rent must be performed immediately. Otherwise bacterial peritonitis will supervene and add a serious complication to an already sufficiently hazardous situation. When the most obvious tear has been repaired, others must be searched for meticulously, since they are not infrequently multiple. Then the operator must explore further for a basic defect, and, if this is found, he must correct it at the same time. Failure to follow through in this way led to the death of one baby whom we saw some years ago. One perforation was closed, but upon reoperation two days later two more were discovered, and the duodenal atresia which had been responsible for all three was then bypassed. Unfortunately it was then too late, and the patient did not recover.

Four of our last five patients survived. The prognosis in the series of Reams et al. was about 50 per cent survival if the patient was operated upon with 12 hours of onset, and 25 per cent if operated upon later.

## GASTRIC TERATOMA

Three instances of teratoma arising from the stomach have been reported in very young infants. None has been recognized in the neonatal period; indeed, all patients were 4 months old or slightly older. Since the tumors are undoubtedly congenital, it would appear to be only a matter of time before one is found within the first month.

Selman's example was discovered by palpation of the tumor. There were no other symptoms. The infant reported by Large et al. suffered severe hematemesis and melena, his hemoglobin level falling to 4.0 gm. A presumptive diagnosis of gastric duplication was entertained before operation. The baby of Handelsman et al. was brought to his pediatrician because of visibly increasing abdominal girth. He was constipated, anorexic and febrile, weak and poorly nourished. X-ray study showed calcified areas in an upper abdominal mass.

All these were benign and were removed along with a portion of the stomach wall to which they were broadly attached. All patients did well after removal of the tumor.

## REFERENCES

Benson, C. D., and Coury, J. J.: Congenital intrinsic obstruction of the stomach and duodenum in the newborn. A.M.A. Arch. Surg. *62*:856, 1951.

Bird, C. E., Limper, M. A., and Mayer, J. M.: Surgery in peptic ulceration of stomach and duodenum in infants and children. Ann. Surg. *114*:526, 1941.

Blank, E., and Chisolm, A. J.: Congenital microgastria: A case report with a 26-year follow-up. Pediatrics *51*:1037, 1973.

Bronsther, B., Nadeau, M. R., and Abrams, M. W.: Congenital pyloric atresia: A report of three cases and a review of the literature. Surgery *69*:130, 1971.

Burmeister, R. E., and Hamilton, H. B.: Infantile hypertrophic stenosis in 4 siblings. Am. J. Dis. Child. *108*:617, 1964.

Caffey, J.: Pediatric X-Ray Diagnosis. Chicago, Year Book Medical Publishers, 1956.

Corner, B. D.: Hypertrophic pyloric stenosis in infancy treated with methyl scopolamine nitrate. Arch. Dis. Child. *30*:377, 1955.

Craig, W. S.: Palpable contractile tumours in the newly born. Arch. Dis. Child. *30*:484, 1955.

Day, L. R.: Medical management of pyloric stenosis. J.A.M.A. *207*:948, 1969.

Dide, M.: Sur un estomac d'adulte a type foetal. Bull. Soc. Anat. Paris *66*:669, 1894.

Ducharme, J. C., and Bensoussan, A. L.: Pyloric atresia. J. Pediat. Surg. *10*:149, 1975.

Elgenmark, O.: Treatment of pyloric stenosis in infants with methyl-scopolamine nitrate. Acta Paediatr. 32:371, 1945.

Floyd, C. H.: Duodenal ulcer with intestinal obstruction in a newborn. J. Pediatr. 54:369, 1959.

Gross, R. E., Holcomb, G. W., Jr., and Farber, S.: Duplication of the stomach. J. Pediatr. 9:449, 1952.

Gruenwald, P.: Asphyxia, trauma and shock at birth. Arch. Pediatr. 67:103, 1950.

Gwinn, J. L., and Barnes, G. R.: Radiological case of the month. Am. J. Dis. Child. 113:581, 1967.

Handelsman, J. C., Rienhoff, W. F., III, and Ward, G. E.: Benign teratoma of stomach in an infant. A.M.A. J. Dis. Child. 90:196, 1955.

Hefke, H. W.: Reliability of roentgen examination in hypertrophic pyloric stenosis in infants. Radiology 53:789, 1949.

Henderson, J. L., Brown, J. J. M., and Taylor, W. C.: Clinical observations on pyloric stenosis in premature infants. Arch. Dis. Child. 27:173, 1952.

Holt, L. E.: Duodenal ulcers in infancy. Am. J. Dis. Child. 6:381, 1913.

Kellogg, H. G., Abelson, S. M., and Cornwell, F. A.: Perforation of the stomach in the newborn infant. J. Pediatr. 39:357, 1951.

Large et al., quoted by Handelsman et al.: Op. cit.

Lee, W. E., and Wells, J. R.: Perforation in utero of a gastric ulcer. Ann. Surg. 78:36, 1923.

Malmberg, N.: Hypertrophic pyloric stenosis — survey of 136 successful cases — with special reference to treatment with Scopyl. Acta Paediat. 38:472, 1949.

McCutcheon, G. T., and Josey, R. B.: Reduplication of the stomach. J. Pediatr. 39:216, 1951.

McKeown, T., MacMahon, B., and Record, R. G.: Evidence of postnatal environmental influence in the aetiology of infantile pyloric stenosis. Arch. Dis. Child. 27:386, 1952.

Meiselas, L. E., and Russakoff, A. H.: Bleeding peptic ulcer in infancy. Am. J. Dis. Child. 67:384, 1944.

Mellish, R. W. P., and Koop, C. E.: Clinical manifestations of duplications of the bowel. Pediatrics 27:397, 1961.

Ogur, G. L., and Kolarsick, A. J.: Gastric diverticula in infancy. J. Pediatr. 39:723, 1951.

Quinn, A. G.: Report of two ruptured gastric ulcers and one ruptured duodenal ulcer in 3 newborn infants. South. M.J. 1171, 1940.

Reams, G. B., Dunaway, J. B., and Walls, W. L.: Neonatal gastric perforation with survival. Pediatrics 31:97, 1963.

Rintoul, J. R., and Kirkman, N. F.: The myenteric plexus in infantile hypertrophic pyloric stenosis. Arch. Dis. Child. 36:474, 1961.

Rozenfeld, I. H., and McGrath, J. R.: Melena in the newborn infant. J. Pediatr. 40:180, 1952.

Rubell, E. B., Leix, F., and Clelland, R. A.: A case of perforated gastric ulcer in an eight-week-old infant. J. Pediatr. 40:337, 1952.

Saw, E. C., Arbegast, N. R., and Comer, T. P.: Pyloric atresia: A case report. Pediatrics 57:574, 1973.

Seagram, C. G. F., Stephens, C. A., and Cummings, W. A.: Peptic ulceration at The Hospital for Sick Children, Toronto, during the 20 year period 1949–1969. J. Pediatr. Surg. 8:407, 1973.

Selman, quoted by Handelsman and others: Op. cit.

Shaker, I. J., et al.: Aerophagia, a mechanism for spontaneous rupture of the stomach of the newborn. Am. Surg. 39:619, 1973.

Shaw, A., Blanc, W. A., Santulli, T. V., and Kaiser, G.: Spontaneous rupture of the stomach: A clinical and experimental study. Surgery 58:561, 1965.

Stern, M. A., Perkins, E. L., and Nessa, N. J.: Perforated gastric ulcer in a 2-day-old infant. Lancet 49:492, 1929.

Still, G. F.: Common Disorders and Diseases of Childhood. 4th ed. London, Oxford Medical Publications, 1924.

Svensgaard, E.: Medical treatment of congenital pyloric stenosis. Arch. Dis. Child. 10:443, 1935.

Touroff, A. S. W., and Sussman, R. M.: Congenital prepyloric membranous obstruction in a premature infant. Surgery 8:739, 1940.

White, J. Personal communication.

# 34

# INTESTINAL OBSTRUCTION

Complete or partial obstruction somewhere in the gastrointestinal tract from the first portion of the duodenum to the anus is not unusual in the neonatal period. Indeed, the bowel obstructs with surprising frequency even during the period of gestation. A variety of causes produce an identical clinical result. *Success or failure in salvage depends not nearly so much on discovering the exact pathogenetic mechanism or the precise localization of the ob-*

*struction as upon the promptness with which the symptomatic diagnosis is made and operative intervention instituted. On the other hand, a futile laparotomy is to be avoided if one can possibly do so.*

INCIDENCE. Santulli was able to collect from the records of the Babies Hospital of New York 134 cases of intestinal obstruction of all kinds, exclusive of imperforate anus, in the period of about 12 years from 1939 to 1952. Evans estimated that 3000 newborns in the United States suffer intestinal obstruction each year and guessed that the figure for the entire world would approximate 50,000 annually.

The majority of patients requiring emergency abdominal operation in the neonatal period are those with the various forms of intestinal obstruction (Holder and Leape).

Among the varieties of obstruction the intrinsic atresias are the most common. They are encountered approximately twice as frequently as stenoses. The favorite sites of atresia in order of frequency are the ileum, the duodenum, the jejunum and the colon. This last locus is involved rarely. Multiple atresias are fairly common. Errors in rotation and meconium ileus are the next most common causes. Aganglia, annular pancreas, intussusception, incarcerated hernias and a variety of other miscellaneous disorders are met, but rarely, in every large series.

**CLASSIFICATION.** The classification suggested by Santulli may be utilized, with minor modifications, for the sake of clarifying a complicated etiologic hodgepodge. Below is a free modification of his suggested schema.

*Causes of Intestinal Obstruction in the Newborn Infant*

I. Mechanical
   A. Congenital
      1. Intrinsic
         a. Atresia and stenosis
         b. Meconium ileus
         c. Hypertrophic stenosis of pylorus or duodenum (?)
         d. Cyst within lumen of bowel
         e. Imperforate anus
         f. Rupture of the bowel
      2. Extrinsic
         a. Malrotation with or without midgut volvulus
         b. Volvulus without malrotation
         c. Congenital peritoneal bands with or without malrotation
         d. Incarcerated hernias
         e. Annular pancreas
         f. Duplications of stomach or bowel
         g. Preduodenal portal vein and other anomalous vascular courses
   B. Acquired
      1. Intussusception
      2. Peritoneal adhesions
      3. Mesenteric thrombosis
      4. Meconium and mucus plugs

II. Functional
   A. Meconium and mucus plugs
   B. Due to defective innervation (Hirschsprung's disease)
   C. Necrotizing enterocolitis

**ETIOLOGY. INTRINSIC OBSTRUCTIONS.** Atresia and intrinsic stenosis may be attributed to failure of proper ontogenetic development. Between the fourth and tenth weeks of gestation the entire primitive gut, from proximal esophagus to distal colon, becomes solidified by ingrowth of epithelium which completely occludes the lumen. This cell cylinder rapidly disintegrates, producing vacuoles throughout its length, the vacuoles ultimately coalescing to reconstitute a continuous lumen. Failure of complete reabsorption leaves a residue of intraluminal tissue which, if sharply localized, ends as a weblike diaphragm or, if spread over some length of bowel, eventuates as a narrowed segment.

Another view, presented by Nixon, is that some intrinsic obstructions represent the end-results of some accident to the bowel in the latter part of gestation. Accidents include incarceration of the physiologic umbilical hernia, localized volvulus or intussusception, focal peritonitis and band formation. That such accidents occur in utero is well known; that they may account for single or multiple atresias, abnormalities of the mesentery and peritoneal bands seems likely from the evidence he presents. Dickinson has described and discussed an example of congenital ileal atresia with pseudocyst that illustrates neatly this presumed sequence of events. More recently Louw has produced atresias in animals after vascular insults to the intestine during development.

*Meconium ileus* is the second main cause of intrinsic obstruction. This earliest manifestation of the syndrome of cystic fibrosis, or mucoviscidosis, is caused by accumulation of abnormal meconium within the small intestinal lumen. Whether meconium is abnormally thick because of absence of pancreatic enzymes throughout fetal life or whether it is just one of many abnormally viscid secretions produced throughout the body in this disease state is still a moot question. Regardless of its pathogenesis, such diseased meconium acts as an impenetrable barrier to propulsion of air and fluids through the intestinal tract, and as a predisposing factor to perforation and meconium peritonitis. Oppenheimer and Esterly believe that intrauterine meconium obstruction produces interference with mesenteric blood supply, which in turn accounts for the large proportion of congenital anatomic defects found among these infants. These include intestinal atresia, volvulus, mesenteric defects and fibrous bands.

Meconium plugs may present as transient obstructions. Suppositories or a small saline enema may dislodge the white inspissated mucus and be followed by normal evacuation of meconium. Infants of mothers treated with magnesium sulfate are especially prone to have the "meconium-plug syndrome."

*Intraluminal cysts* are an infrequent cause of intrinsic obstruction in the newborn. They may be of two varieties, duplications of the bowel or retention cysts.

EXTRINSIC OBSTRUCTIONS. The chief cause of extrinsic obstruction lies in an error in rotation of the bowel. These are of three kinds: nonrotation, malrotation and reversed rotation.

Briefly summarized, the normal ontogenetic sequence is as follows. By about the fifth week of gestation the gastrointestinal tract is divided into a primitive foregut, which terminates just distal to the pylorus, the midgut, which ends a little distance beyond the ileocecal junction, and the hindgut. The midgut, which is to form the duodenum, jejunum, ileum and part of the ascending colon, is extruded into the umbilical cord, forced out by pressure of the rapidly enlarging liver. The mesentery fixes firmly the lower end of the foregut and upper end of the hindgut at points on the posterior abdominal wall that are near one another. This leaves the developing midgut suspended, as it were, by a narrow stalk, the duodenocolic isthmus. By about the tenth week the midgut begins to re-enter the abdominal cavity, completing its return in the short space of a week. The sequence of return is normally from proximal to distal, the most cephalad portion re-entering first, to the right of the superior mesenteric artery, and displacing the hindgut to the left, backward, then upward.

The cecum and adjacent colon are reduced last. The cecum migrates counterclockwise from its point of entry in the right lower quadrant to the left, upward, then across to the right upper quadrant. From the eleventh week onward the cecum gradually descends into the right lower quadrant and becomes fixed by fusion of its mesentery with the posterior parietal peritoneum. In its final position the midgut has rotated 270 degrees in a counterclockwise direction about the axis of the superior mesenteric artery from its original sagittal position within the umbilical cord, the duodenum being fixed behind and the transverse colon coursing over and in front of it (Fig. 34–1).

*Nonrotation* signifies that there has been no change in position of the bowel after its re-entry into the abdominal cavity. The duodenum descends sharply to the right of the superior mesenteric artery, the small bowel remains in the right side, the large bowel in the left. The cecum lies to the left of the midline. In *malrotation* there are irregular defects of rotation and fixation. In *reversed rotation* the distal midgut re-enters the abdominal cavity first and performs a 90-degree clockwise instead of the usual 270-degree counterclockwise rotation. In this condition the transverse colon passes behind the duodenum and superior mesenteric artery rather than in front of them.

Abnormal rotation of itself is not responsible for obstruction. This depends upon one of three coincidental factors. 1) The nonrotated midgut lies freely within the abdominal cavity, fixed only at the duodenum and proximal colon. The unattached cecum and small bowel are at liberty to swing in a wide arc in either direction, and, stimulated by the active peristalsis which follows the first ingestion of food, they often rotate in this fashion. The midgut may twist only a few degrees or may make as many as four complete turns. Obstruction depends not upon the amount of twisting, but upon the degree of kinking and vascular obstruction the twisting produces. Midgut volvulus usually obstructs the bowel at or near the duodenojejunal junction. 2) In malrotation misdirected efforts at fixation of dislocated segments of bowel

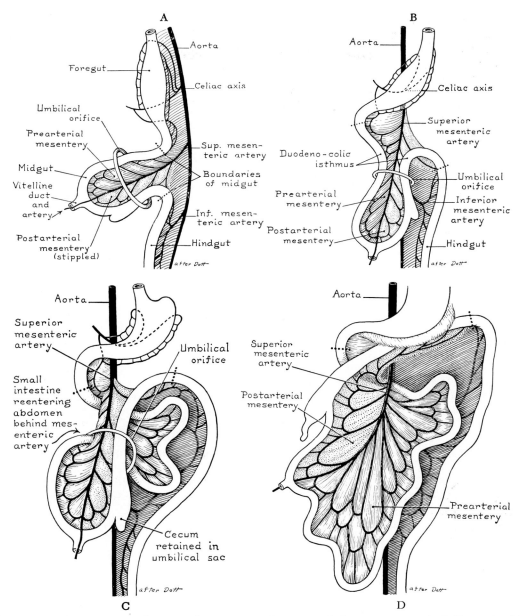

*Figure 34–1.* Diagrammatic drawings showing normal rotation of alimentary tract. *A,* Fifth week of intrauterine life (lateral view). The foregut, midgut and hindgut are shown with their individual blood supply supported by the common dorsal mesentery in the sagittal plane. The midgut loop has been extruded into the umbilical cord. *B,* Eighth week of intrauterine life (anteroposterior view). The first stage of rotation is being completed. Note the narrow duodenocolic isthmus from which the midgut loop depends and the right-sided position of the small intestine and left-sided position of the colon. Maintenance of this position within the abdomen after birth is spoken of as nonrotation. *C,* About the tenth week of intrauterine life, during the second stage of rotation (anteroposterior view). The bowel in the temporary umbilical hernia is in the process of reduction, the most proximal part of the prearterial segment entering the abdomen to the right of the superior mesenteric artery first, and the remainder of the bowel following in orderly sequence. The superior mesenteric artery is held forward close to the cecum and ascending colon, permitting the bowel to pass under it. As the coils of small intestine collect within the abdomen the hindgut is displaced to the left and upward. *D,* Eleventh week of intrauterine life at the end of the second stage of rotation. From its original sagittal position the midgut has rotated 270 degrees in a counterclockwise direction about the origin of the superior mesenteric artery. The essentials of the permanent disposition of the viscera have been attained. (From Gardner, C. E., Jr., and Hart, D.: Arch. Surg. 29:942, 1934.)

may lead to the formation of ectopic mesenteric bands. Obstruction, often partial, may be produced by these bands in loops of bowel over which they course. 3) In incomplete rotation the cecum may end up overlying a loop of small bowel. When the cecum is filled, the compressed intestine beneath it becomes obstructed.

Very rarely the bowel fails to differentiate into small and large intestine. Bennington and Huber have reported a very interesting example of undifferentiated intestinal tract, the infant dying after 13 days of severe uncontrollable diarrhea which began on the second day of life.

Congenital hernias may become incarcerated or strangulated in the neonatal period exactly as in later life. These hernias may be inguinal, diaphragmatic or internal. Rarely does an umbilical hernia become the site of obstruction.

Annular pancreas produces either no compression, or stenosis, or complete obstruction of the duodenum. It arises from a developmental anomaly. Normally the pancreas develops from three anlagen, a dorsal and two ventral pancreatic buds which form contiguous to the duodenum. The large dorsal anlage grows into the tail, body and superior portion of the head. Lecco believes that annular pancreas results when the left ventral bud becomes tightly attached to the duodenum, where, instead of rotating clockwise to meet the dorsal bud, it must stretch around the circumference of the bowel loop. Baldwin agrees, but suggests that the right bud also persists and completes the encirclement.

Duplications of the stomach or any part of the bowel may produce large cystic masses which, when filled, may compress adjacent loops to cause obstruction.

Intussusception is rare, but far from unknown in the first month of life. A few cases are initiated by an identifiable leader, such as an intraluminal mass or abnormal fixation of a segment of bowel, but, as in older infants, in most instances no initiating mechanism can be discovered.

NEUROGENIC OBSTRUCTIONS. As far back as 1901 Tittel pointed out the paucity or absence of ganglion cells of the myenteric plexus in some portions of the large bowel in several cases of megacolon. It was not until 1948 that this observation was confirmed by Zuelzer and Wilson, and Whitehouse and Kernohan. After this Swenson and his collaborators verified the etiologic role of aganglionosis or aganglia in Hirschsprung's disease by demonstrating 1) the failure of normal progression of peristaltic waves from splenic flexure to anus; 2) the absence of ganglion cells of the plexus of Auerbach in these same persons; and 3) the permanent cure of megacolon by excision of the aganglionic segment. Congenital aganglionosis, often familial in its distribution, is an important, if rare, cause of intestinal obstruction in the neonate. Since the colon does not become typically dilated and hypertrophied for several weeks or months after birth, diagnosis in the neonatal period is difficult. This is especially true in those bizarre instances in which aganglionosis involves not the usual site, the rectosigmoid colon, but more proximal segments of the colon or, even more rarely, portions of the small intestine.

DIAGNOSIS. Usually the correct diagnosis of intestinal obstruction can be made without too much difficulty. Vomiting, abdominal distention and constipation constitute as pathognomonic a triad in the newborn infant as they do in the older person. Nevertheless the intensity of these signs and their time of appearance vary according to the location and the completeness of the obstruction. Before discussing in detail the clinical pictures of particular lesions, some general comments might be in order. The problem with a vomiting, possibly distended, newborn is four-pronged. The pediatrician must 1) decide whether the illness is due to intestinal obstruction; 2) attempt to localize it; 3) try to arrive at an etiologic diagnosis; and 4) decide whether immediate operation is imperative. Although it is true that delay in advising operation is to be avoided, only slightly less desirable is the converse error of advising surgical exploration when sufficient factual evidence may be accumulated which contraindicates operation. *The most important single measure for the pediatrician is to insert a nasogastric tube to decompress the stomach and prevent vomiting and aspiration.*

The suspicion that intestinal obstruction

exists should arise in one's mind whenever vomiting, constipation or distention, or any combination of these signs, develops. *Vomiting* begins soon after delivery when an obstruction is high and complete, but may be delayed some days if it is low or incomplete. Vomitus contains bile if the obstruction is distal to the ampulla of Vater, none if it is proximal to it. Bile-stained vomitus is not an absolute sign of intestinal obstruction, but is highly suggestive. Not infrequently blood is mixed with vomitus, especially when the obstruction is high, but the presence of blood is not of itself a strong indication of obstruction. Occasional sporadic vomiting is less characteristic than vomiting after every feeding. If the infant regurgitates continually between feedings, the probability of obstruction is increased. Vomiting may be forceful or not. It is almost never projectile. Effortless regurgitation alone is not at all uncommon.

*Abdominal distention,* when present, is an exceedingly valuable sign. It may be noted at the time of delivery, but when considerable at that time, it more often indicates that perforation of the bowel had taken place before birth or that the fetus has ascites or a tumor. Ordinarily distention becomes apparent some hours after birth, reaching its maximum within 24 to 48 hours. The longer abdominal distention persists, the more likely it is that intestinal patterning will be seen through the abdominal wall. Such patterns, with visible peristaltic waves, are an almost certain indication of obstruction. In duodenal—or the rare gastric—obstruction, distention may be limited to the epigastrium, with or without a visible gastric pattern, or may be absent entirely. This absence of distention is caused by continuous emptying of the stomach by repeated vomiting and constant regurgitation.

*Constipation,* when present, is also a dependable sign. The normal newborn will pass a meconium stool within 12 hours, and almost never fails to do so by 24 hours. If he does not, obstruction must be suspected. On the other hand, the newborn with high obstruction almost invariably passes his normal complement of meconium stools. Even when obstruction is low

in the ileum, the bowels usually move several times within the first day of life.

Additional evidence can sometimes be gained by palpation of the abdomen. Distended, hypertrophied hollow viscera may sometimes be felt as vague, ill-defined tubular masses which can be rolled under the hand. Masses of hard or doughy consistency can often be felt scattered throughout the abdomen in meconium ileus, almost never in other forms of obstruction. A solid or cystic mass may upon occasion be the tumor responsible for obstruction.

The x-ray is the most useful ancillary diagnostic aid. Films should be taken in three positions: supine posteroanterior, erect posteroanterior and erect lateral. *No contrast medium should be used unless plain films have failed to substantiate the diagnosis. If doubt still exists, a barium enema series may be obtained, and only if the diagnosis is still uncertain should a contrast medium mixture be given by mouth.* Specific x-ray alterations will be described with each type of obstruction discussed later, but certain general deviations from the normal may be listed here. Normally, air enters and fills the stomach immediately after birth, the small bowel within 2 to 12 hours, and the colon within 18 to 24 hours. When obstruction exists, the air pattern may be seen to stop abruptly at one point, leaving the remainder of the bowel airless. The stomach and a loop or loops of intestine proximal to the point of obstruction may be dilated and, in the erect position, may show horizontal fluid levels. If the obstruction is low, a series of such dilated, air- and fluid-filled coils of intestine, each with its own fluid level, one above the other, makes a characteristic stepladder design. Obstruction at the pylorus produces one large bubble, the dilated stomach, whereas obstruction in the duodenum often produces a double-bubble picture, one bubble outlining the dilated stomach, the other the dilated loop of duodenum proximal to the obstruction.

When obstruction is incomplete (that is, in the stenoses or volvulus) dilated viscera may be seen above one point, and a trickle of gas may be visible below.

Barium enema may show the colon distal

to the locus of complete obstruction to be narrow and not readily distensible by the injected contrast mixture — so-called microcolon. Obviously the injected fluid does not progress cephalad beyond the obstructed segment.

Upper gastrointestinal series with contrast medium, performed only after the two foregoing studies have failed to supply a certain answer, may show moderate dilatation proximal to a locus of narrowing and a trickle of opaque liquid entering the bowel distal to the stenotic segment.

In meconium ileus a diffuse granular appearance may be noted, or minute bubbles of air may be apparent, mixed with the meconium which fills the small intestine.

## REFERENCES

Baldwin, cited by R. E. Gross and T. C. Chisholm.

Bennington, J. L., and Huber, S. L.: The embryologic significance of undifferentiated intestinal tract. J. Pediatr. *64*:735, 1964.

Clatworthy, H. W., Jr., Howard, W. H. R., and Lloyd, J.: The meconium plug syndrome. Surgery *39*:131, 1956.

Dickinson, S. J.: Origin of intestinal atresia of the newborn. J.A.M.A. *190*:119, 1964.

Emery, J. L.: The tryptic activity and presence of cornified squames in meconium as diagnostic aid in congenital intestinal obstruction. Arch. Dis. Child. *27*:67, 1952.

Evans, cited by D. C. Benson and I. J. Coury: Arch. Surg. *62*:856, 1951.

Gardner, C. E., Jr., and Hart, D.: Anomalies of intestinal rotation as a cause of intestinal obstruction. Arch. Surg. *29*:942, 1934.

Glover, D. M., and Barry, F. M.: Intestinal obstruction in the newborn. Ann. Surg. *130*:480, 1949.

Gross, R. E., and Chisholm, T. C.: Annular pancreas producing duodenal obstruction. Ann. Surg. *119*:759, 1944.

Gruenwald, P.: Asphyxia, trauma and shock at birth. Arch. Pediatr. *67*:103, 1950.

Holder, T. M., and Leape, L. L.: The acute surgical abdomen in the neonate. New Engl. J. Med. *278*:605, 1968.

Jones, T. W., and Schutt, R. P.: Alimentary tract obstruction in the newborn infant; a review and analysis of 132 cases. Pediatrics *20*:881, 1957.

Lecco, cited by R. E. Gross and T. C. Chisholm.

Louw, J. H.: Jejunoileal atresia and stenosis. J. Pediatr. Surg. *1*:8, 1966.

Nixon, H. H.: Intestinal obstruction in the newborn. Arch. Dis. Child. *30*:13, 1955.

Oppenheimer, E. H., and Esterly, J. R.: Observations in cystic fibrosis of the pancreas: II. Neonatal intestinal obstruction. Bull. Johns Hopkins Hosp. *111*:1, 1962.

Rack, F. J., and Crouch, W. L.: Functional intestinal obstruction in the premature infant. J. Pediatr. *40*:579, 1952.

Santulli, T. V.: Intestinal obstruction in the newborn infant. J. Pediatr. *44*:317, 1954.

Swenson, O., Neuhauser, E. B. D., and Pickett, L. K.: New concepts of the etiology, diagnosis and treatment of congenital megacolon (Hirschsprung's disease). Pediatrics *4*:201, 1949.

Tittel, K.: Ueber eine angeborene Missbildung des Dickdarmes. Wien. klin. Wchnschr. *14*:903, 1901.

Whitehouse, F. R., and Kernohan, J. W.: Myenteric plexus in congenital megacolon. Arch. Intern. Med. *82*:75, 1948.

Zuelzer, W. W., and Wilson, J. L.: Functional intestinal obstruction on congenital neurogenic basis in infancy. Am. J. Dis. Child. *75*:40, 1948.

# 35

# CONGENITAL INTRINSIC INTESTINAL OBSTRUCTION

## DUODENAL ATRESIA

Atresia signifies complete obstruction of a lumen, stenosis, narrowing and incomplete obstruction. Duodenal atresia is not a final pathological diagnosis. It may be caused by a number of defects, which in less aggravated form lead only to stenosis. The great majority of atresias are caused by intrinsic maldevelopment, and a substantial minority by annular pancreas. The other obstructive lesions are more apt to cause stenosis rather than atresia, and will therefore be discussed under that heading immediately below.

The diagnosis of duodenal atresia is not difficult. Vomiting begins within a few hours after birth, before ingestion of any fluids. It consists of pharyngeal, gastric and duodenal secretions containing at times mucus. Most atresias involve the second and third portions of the duodenum, so that vomitus almost always contains bile. Until feedings are begun vomiting takes the form of repeated regurgitations of small amounts. After a feeding the amount vomited may be large and moderately forceful, but this episode is followed by frequent, almost continual, regurgitations of small quantities. Distention, if present, is limited to the epigastrium, while the lower half of the abdomen remains flat. When epigastric distention is prominent, a pattern of the overfilled stomach can be clearly visualized. Rarely peristaltic waves move from left to right. As stated before, distention may be absent. The infant ordinarily passes one to three or more meconium stools in the first 24 to 36 hours. Thereafter bowel movements cease, although small quantities of thick mucus may continue to be passed from the rectum. No tumors are palpable within the abdomen.

The association of other, often severe congenital malformations with duodenal atresia is noteworthy. In a series of 157 neonates with duodenal obstruction, Young and Wilkinson reported other abnormalities in 70 per cent. In order of frequency they were Down's syndrome (21 per cent), annular pancreas, cardiovascular anomalies, malrotation, esophageal atresia, small bowel anomaly and anorectal lesions. Marked jaundice developed in about one third, and a few had biliary atresia. Many of the babies are born prematurely.

The familial occurrence of congenital duodenal atresia has been noted a small but significant number of times. Hyde, for instance, was involved with one family in which four siblings were born with the identical lesion. Mishalany et al. report a concurrence highly suggestive of an autosomal recessive type of inheritance. The parents of each of the affected babies in this remarkable family were first cousins, and all of the four parents descended from one great-grandfather and two great-grandmothers who were themselves sisters.

Radiographs of the abdomen show air in the upper half and complete airlessness elsewhere. No small or large bowel patterns are visible. Usually the air outlines two dilated hollow structures, the stomach and the upper duodenum, which are readily distinguished in the erect anteroposterior projection, and even more clearly outlined in the erect lateral position. At times this double bubble cannot be made out. Rarely there will be insufficient air in the stomach, because of continual regurgitation, to define clearly its outlines. Under these circumstances it is permissible to inject 10 to 20 cc of air through a gastric tube or to instill through the tube an effervescent mixture. This simple procedure may suffice to clarify an uncertain situation.

Neither barium enema nor upper gastrointestinal x-ray films should be needed to diagnose complete duodenal atresia, although a barium enema is useful before operation in order to ascertain the presence or absence of errors in rotation or to rule out the possibility of a second atresia lower in the bowel.

**TREATMENT.** Immediate operation, after restoration of fluids and achievement of good blood chemical values, is imperative. The operation of choice is side-to-side duodenojejunostomy. Gastroenterostomy relieves the obstruction, but digestive symptoms may persist for years because of the large blind duodenal loop.

**PROGNOSIS.** The chances of survival have increased considerably over the last few decades because of earlier diagnosis and operation, more adequate preoperative and postoperative hydration and blood chemical homeostasis, improved anesthesia, better operative techniques and better control of infection. Nevertheless the mortality rate remains high, varying from 30 to 65 per cent in the most recently published series. Many of the failures are unavoidable because of extreme prematurity or the concomitance of other serious congenital malformations.

## DUODENAL STENOSIS

Partial obstruction of the duodenum can be produced by intrinsic stenosis, annular pancreas, aberrant peritoneal bands either with or without malrotation, duodenal kinking (Chamberlain) or external pressure from a misplaced, malrotated, cecum. In a few cases an aberrant superior mesenteric

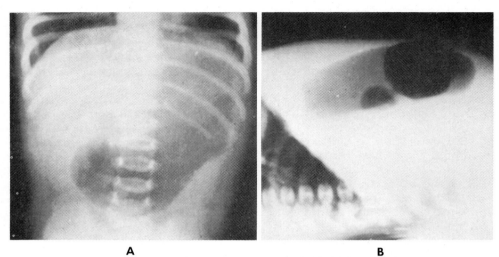

**A**                    **B**

*Figure 35–1.* *A*, Anteroposterior view in the supine position shows the distended stomach. If one looks carefully, one can see a second air bubble adjacent to the stomach above and to the right of the pyloric antrum. The rest of the bowel is completely airless. *B*, In the supine lateral position the large gastric bubble is seen, and within it two darker bubbles. These are surely the shadows made by the first and second portions of the dilated duodenum. There is a sharp fluid level.

These films are characteristic of duodenal atresia, as was the history. Vomiting began at 4 hours, followed by continuous regurgitation of dark brown fluid containing bile and blood. Meconium was passed several times and there was no distention.

artery has been the cause of the obstruction, and in even fewer a preduodenal portal vein. It is comparatively simple to localize the site of the narrowing, but differentiation between these various causes before operation is often impossible.

**DIAGNOSIS.** As one might expect, the symptoms of partial duodenal obstruction appear later and are more intermittent than are those of complete atresia. In the neonate vomiting may start at any time, but its onset is usually delayed until at least 4 days after birth. Onset at 10 days or at 1 month or at any time throughout childhood is not at all uncommon. Often only one or two feedings a day are lost, and there may be weeks or months during which no vomiting whatever occurs. Since most stenoses involve the third and fourth portions of the duodenum, the vomitus usually contains bile. Rarely it contains blood also, and blood may be passed *per rectum*. Stools may be normal in number and nature, or, during the periods when vomiting is prominent, constipation may be moderate to severe. Epigastric distention is also variable, as is visible gastric peristalsis.

Flat films of the abdomen, supine and erect, should be obtained immediately, but it is important to remember that in partial obstruction they may show nothing abnormal. If so, these should be followed by barium enema films. These may or may not show the cecum to lie in an abnormal position or to be excessively mobile. Only after these procedures have failed to provide diagnostic information is it proper to perform an upper gastrointestinal series with a thin barium mixture. With this the narrowed segment of bowel may be visualized, with or without dilatation of the loop proximal to it, and the contrast medium may be seen to trickle slowly into the intestine distal to the stenosis.

**TREATMENT.** Operation should be performed as soon as the diagnosis has been made. What is done will depend upon the situation encountered. Intrinsic stenoses should be bypassed by a duodenojejunostomy. Aberrant peritoneal bands should be divided. No attempt should be made to resect an annular pancreas, but it too should be bypassed. Malrotation should be corrected so far as is possible and the cecum fixed at or near its normal position.

CASE 35-1

A white female infant was born to a primiparous mother after a normal pregnancy and labor. Birth weight was 7 pounds 2 ounces (3230 gm). Crying and spontaneous breathing began promptly, and she seemed quite normal. Routine feedings began after 12 hours. On the third day she passed one loose brownish stool, and on the fourth day she was jaundiced and passed several stools of the same kind. That evening she began to vomit, and the temperature rose to 103.4°F. Examination (fourth day) showed an acutely ill, moderately jaundiced, dehydrated infant. The abdomen was scaphoid and soft, but bowel patterns were visible. When she was given fluids intravenously and subcutaneously, her temperature fell to normal by the next morning, but she continued to vomit greenish-yellow material and to pass brownish-green stools containing mucus. Examination (sixth day) showed now some abdominal distention, patterning with visible peristalsis and increased bowel sounds. A continuous intravenous infusion was given over the next few days, vomiting ceased, stools became normal, and hydration, and with it vigor, improved greatly. X-ray films taken on the eighth day showed distended loops of bowel lying mostly in the left side of the abdomen and little gas in the right half. Regurgitation diminished over the next 3 or 4 days, but never entirely stopped, while feedings were taken well and stools were few, but of normal color and consistency. Examination on the eleventh day showed her to be vigorous and hungry, with good skin turgor and good color. The epigastrium was full, and there was visible peristalsis in the upper part of the abdomen on both sides of the midline. X-ray gastrointestinal series using Lipiodol as the contrast medium on this day showed dilated stomach and duodenum with small quantities of the dye escaping into the distal bowel (Fig. 35-2). This obviously depicted a partial duodenal obstruction.

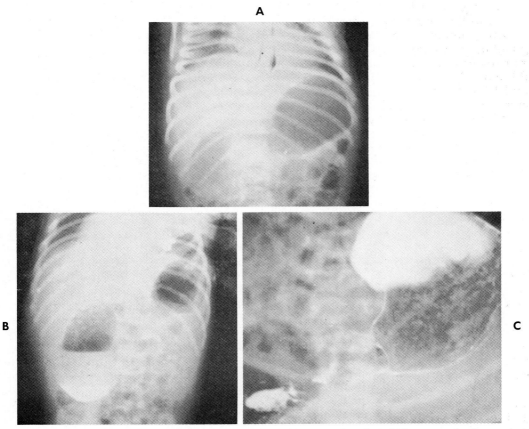

*Figure 35-2.* A, Anteroposterior film in the supine position shows a double-bubble pattern made up of stomach and hugely dilated duodenum. It shows, in addition, some air in the large and small bowels, indicating that obstruction cannot be complete. B, Anteroposterior film taken in the erect position after a barium swallow. A fluid level can now be seen in the dilated duodenum. C, After 1 hour a small mass of Lipiodol has passed out of the hugely dilated duodenum visible above it.

On that day operation was performed, intrinsic stenosis at the duodenojejunal junction was confirmed, and duodenojejunostomy was performed. The postoperative course was stormy because of persistent nausea. Wangensteen drainage and intravenous fluid therapy had to be continued for 8 days, after which glucose solution could be retained. This was slowly increased in quantity, changed to Alacta, and slow improvement set in. She continued to regurgitate upon occasion for 2 weeks after operation.

**COMMENT.** Onset of vomiting was delayed in this infant until the fourth day and followed 1 day of diarrhea. Dehydration with fever developed acutely and obscured the correct diagnosis. After this had been corrected the true nature of the disorder was manifested by repeated vomiting of bile-stained material while stools continued to be passed. Local signs were epigastric distention and visible patterning and peristaltic waves in this area. The whole added up to high intestinal partial obstruction. This impression was verified by a Lipiodol upper gastrointestinal x-ray series. In retrospect it seems clear that diagnosis could have been verified and operation should have been performed 4 or 5 days sooner. Much of the postoperative difficulty might have been avoided had this been done.

## JEJUNAL AND ILEAL ATRESIA

Congenital atresias involve the ileum most frequently, the duodenum next, the jejunum next and the colon least of all. Atresia occurs approximately twice as often as stenosis. Multiple points of atresia are not at all rare.

Etiology is discussed on page 353.

**DIAGNOSIS.** The clinical picture of jejuno-ileal atresia—the two are so similar that preoperative differentiation is impossible—varies in a few respects from that of duodenal atresia. Vomiting is likely to begin a bit later in life, usually at the end of the first day or during the second day, although abdominal distention has been noted in many immediately after birth. Distention becomes considerably more prominent, gradually increasing to involve the entire abdomen symmetrically. Vomitus in-

variably contains bile and may become fecal. Shrand argues with plausibility that the green staining of the amniotic fluid of his example of multiple jejunal atresia, and presumably of others, must have been due to vomiting in utero, not to meconium staining, for at operation the distal bowel was markedly narrowed and contained white meconium. After the lower bowel has emptied itself of its meconium no further stools are passed, but passage of five or six meconium stools is not unusual. The stools never become transitional or fecal. Percussion reveals tympany over the entire abdomen, including the flanks, but liver dullness, although elevated, is not obscured. With the stethoscope the sounds of hyperactive peristalsis are heard, although in a neglected late case they may be absent.

X-ray study shows many dilated loops of small bowel and no air in the large intestine. In the erect position one usually sees fluid levels in many of these dilated loops, at times in the characteristic stepladder pattern. Unless perforation has taken place no air can be discerned outside the intestinal loops, and no bubble will be seen above the liver. If a barium enema series is taken, microcolon is ordinarily seen, and the column of barium stops abruptly at the most distal locus of obstruction.

In differential diagnosis midgut volvulus, meconium ileus, aganglionosis and paralytic ileus must be considered seriously. It has become clear that jejuno-ileal atresia coexists with both volvulus and meconium ileus with surprising frequency. It is probable that prenatal volvulus leads to intestinal atresia by compromising mesenteric blood supply, and that prenatal obstruction by the thick, inspissated intestinal contents of cystic fibrosis may have the same effect. We shall review this problem after the symptomatology of these disorders has been described.

**TREATMENT AND PROGNOSIS.** Prognosis is still grave even when the diagnosis is made promptly and immediate operation is performed. In the most recent series the reported mortality rate of ileal atresia has been as high as 50 per cent or more, even in our best clinics. Part of this is due to the extreme prematurity of many of the pa-

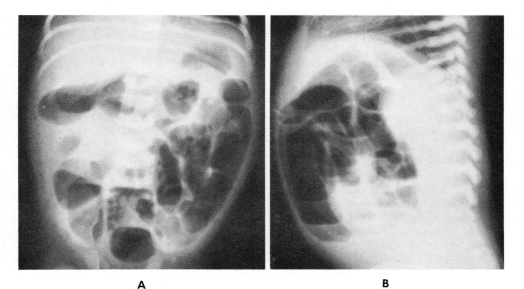

**A**                                    **B**

*Figure 35–3.* A, Supine anteroposterior flat film showing an irregular distribution of grossly dilated loops of bowel of varying sizes throughout the abdomen. The loop in the left lateral abdomen was misinterpreted as large bowel, but turned out at operation to be small bowel like all the others. B, Lateral erect film. In this position one can see the fluid levels in all the dilated loops of small bowel which produce the typical "stepladder" design of lower intestinal obstruction. Atresia was discovered in the ileum.

The history was equally typical, with vomiting and distention beginning at 17 hours, passage of a meconium plug but no further stools, and vomiting of bile-stained material.

tients, part to concomitant congenital defects. But a good deal of it is attributable to the fact that anastomoses made in the usual fashion often fail to function even though the stoma has been proved to be patent at the time of operation. Nixon believes that these poor results are due to paralysis of the hypertrophied segment proximal to the point of obstruction and suggests that results are much better when all the hypertrophied segment is resected and the anastomosis made with bowel of normal caliber proximal to it. Holder and Leape reemphasize the need to resect all the dilated bowel proximal to the obstruction and recommend that this be followed by end-to-end anastomosis.

## MECONIUM ILEUS

Meconium ileus is the form of intestinal obstruction in the newborn caused by abnormally thick tenacious meconium which is produced in cystic fibrosis. It is the earliest manifestation of this disorder, although most infants who prove later to be subject to cystic fibrosis, even in severe forms, have not manifested this particular sign. Its etiology has already been discussed (p. 353).

**INCIDENCE.** Meconium ileus is by no means common, but it ranks as the second or third most frequent cause of intestinal obstruction in the neonatal period. The atresia and stenosis group outrank it always and the malrotation group almost always in the large reported series. Shwachman et al. stated that 65 such patients were operated upon in the Children's Hospital of Boston from 1945 to 1955. They estimate that this disorder accounts for 15 per cent of all intestinal obstructions in the neonatal period. In Santulli's compilation of the cases seen at Babies Hospital of New York from 1939 to 1952, 20 of 134 congenital intestinal obstructions proved to be due to meconium ileus.

**DIAGNOSIS.** For the diagnosis of this condition an awareness of the physical status of previous children is of great importance. A history of congenital intestinal obstruction or cystic fibrosis in a sibling should immediately alert one to the possibility of meconium ileus. Fifteen of Shwachman and associates' 20 mothers had had one or more children before the birth of the one in question, and in five of these families a case of meconium ileus had been diagnosed. If one's suspicions are aroused, the diagnosis can conceivably be made before the signs of intestinal obstruction make their appearance.

If one has not been forewarned by the family history, the first suggestive sign is apt to be distention. This is noticed between 12 and 24 hours in most cases. Vomiting also occurs, but is not nearly so prominent as it is in the atresia group and does not make its appearance until the second day in most cases. Failure to pass meconium is absolute, but by the time this is noted the other signs have usually made their appearance.

On physical examination abdominal distention is the outstanding finding. Visible intestinal patterns are often discernible on the abdominal wall. On palpation these dilated loops can often be felt, but much more diagnostic is the presence of numerous hard masses throughout the abdomen. Some of these are sausage-shaped; most are hard or doughy balls, freely movable in any direction. Bowel sounds can generally be heard until late in the course. Digital examination of the rectum reveals a normal anus and sphincter and complete absence of meconium as far as the finger can penetrate.

X-ray examination is helpful. The dilated loops of small bowel confirm the presence of intestinal obstruction. In the erect position fluid levels are seldom seen in the uncomplicated cases. Tiny bubbles of gas may be seen mixed with the meconium in the distal small bowel in some cases and a diffuse granular appearance in others. The locus of obstruction can usually be made out to be in the distal small bowel.

Proteolytic enzymes are absent from the stools of all infants with complete obstruction. This renders this examination useless for differentiating this type from others. But newborn infants may show the characteristic elevation of sodium chloride in their sweat.

**COURSE AND PROGNOSIS.**  It is imperative that diagnosis be made and treatment instituted early, since complications supervene rapidly and frequently. These are per-

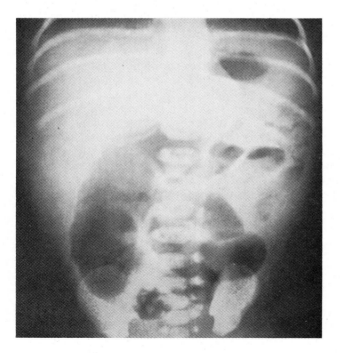

*Figure 35–4.*  Flat film of the abdomen taken in the supine position. The abdomen is distended, and the number of intestinal loops that are filled with air is small. A few of these are extraordinarily dilated. The point at which obstruction ends cannot be ascertained. At operation meconium ileus was found.

foration of the intestine with subsequent meconium and bacterial peritonitis, and volvulus. Indeed, both complications may have already occurred by the time of birth.

If relief of obstruction can be accomplished, these infants go on to development of the syndrome of cystic fibrosis in about the same fashion as do infants without meconium ileus. Shwachman et al. presented a long-range follow-up of 20 such children. As of 1956 11 had moderate to severe pulmonary disease, six mild, and three had no demonstrable pulmonary involvement.

**TREATMENT.** After the diagnosis has been established one is permitted to make some efforts to relieve the obstruction by medical means. This is especially true when the diagnosis has been made early and distention is not too great. Nonsurgical treatment until recently consisted of repeated enemas and gastric lavage, plus instillation of pancreatic enzyme by both routes. In 1969 Noblett suggested a new nonoperative method of treatment. She introduced Gastrografin per rectum under the fluoroscope until it penetrated the ileum. In her four babies the obstipation was relieved; and similar good results have since been obtained by others. But Gastrografin, because of its own high osmolality, causes an abrupt reduction in blood volume to such degree that it may be hazardous to life. If one uses it, fluid and electrolyte balance must be corrected first, and fluids instilled intravenously for a few hours during and after its use to keep serum osmolality below 290 mOsm per liter (Rowe et al.).

Gross pioneered the modern surgical treatment of these infants. Most surgeons now use the Bishop-Koop modification of his approach. "After resection of the dilated portion of the ileum an end-to-side Roux-en-Y anastomosis is performed, and the free end of the distal ileum brought out in the abdominal wall as an ileostomy." McPartlin et al., whom we just quoted, have achieved a 70 per cent short-term survival with this technique as opposed to 30 per cent before its adoption. One then irrigates the distal segment with acetylcysteine to clear it of its firm concretions. Anastomosis is carried out approximately two weeks later.

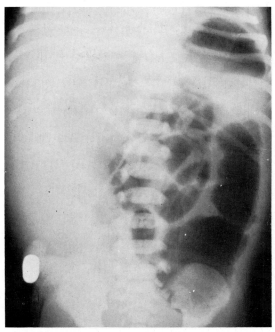

*Figure 35–5.* X-ray view of abdomen taken in the erect posture. The gas pattern is bizarre. Fewer loops can be seen than is usual, and these are almost confined to the left half of the abdomen; some are hugely dilated. No air is seen in the right half. There are no fluid levels, except in the stomach. The exact point of obstruction cannot be determined. At operation meconium ileus was found.

One of this infant's two siblings had died of intestinal obstruction in the neonatal period.

## CONGENITAL HYPERTROPHIC STENOSIS OF THE DUODENUM

Patton described an entity which had never been reported before and of which we have been able to find no further report. This is a hypertrophy of the muscularis of the first portion of the duodenum exactly analogous to the picture more commonly seen at the pylorus. The clinical history of his first case was indistinguishable from the usual story for hypertrophic pyloric stenosis. The second infant, after rallying from the shock of a difficult delivery, began to vomit at 2 weeks, and vomited more and more until 4 weeks, when he began to pass tarry stools, then tarry mucus only. Operation disclosed thickened duodenal muscularis. A muscle-splitting procedure was carried out, and the result was excellent, as it had been in his first case of the same nature.

## CYST WITHIN THE LUMEN OF THE BOWEL

Cysts of two varieties are encountered as obstructing elements within the bowel itself. Some are retention cysts derived from the secretory glands of the intestine, while others are duplications incorporated within the parent segment. We shall not discuss this disorder in detail because we have not encountered any cases causing obstruction in the neonatal period and because the symptom complex it produces is indistinguishable from all other partial obstructions.

## CONGENITAL DEFORMITIES OF THE ANUS AND RECTUM

The pediatrician need not be concerned too deeply with minute details of all the possible combinations and permutations that abnormal embryologic development may lead to in this area of the body. Essentially all that it is necessary to know is contained in the answers to three questions. Is there atresia with complete obstruction? Is there stenosis with partial obstruction? Is there a fistulous connection between lower bowel and urinary tract, genital tract or perineum? Later investigations should rule in or out concomitant upper genitourinary tract malformations, which are commonly associated.

**EMBRYOLOGY.** The proctodeum comprises the anus and a canal that extends cephalad a short distance to meet the blind end of the hindgut, which simultaneously moves caudad. At the seventh to eighth week of gestation these should make contact, separated only by the anal membrane. At the same time the lower urinary tract is developing alongside the lower intestinal tract, and the two anlagen are separated by the urorectal membrane. Malformations of the anus arise locally from maldevelopment within the proctodeum itself, while atresias, stenoses and fistulas arise from imperfect resolution of the anorectal membrane with or without concomitant failure of the urorectal membrane to separate completely the genitourinary and rectal anlagen.

**CLASSIFICATION.** Denis Browne classifies deformities of the anus into three groups, each containing several subgroups. Group I includes *stenosis of the anus,* in which the finger meets a fibrous ring just inside the junction of skin and mucosa, and the *microscopic anus,* which is exactly what its name implies. The *ectopic anus* (group II) is shifted well forward of its normal position to form a "shotgun perineum," with the edges of vagina and anus touching; the *vaginal ectopic anus,* in which the anus actually opens into the lower portion of the vagina (this should not be confused with imperforate anus plus rectovaginal fistula); and the *male ectopic anus,* which is a stenotic opening well forward of its normal position. Group III he calls the *covered anus,* with, in the female, no visible anal opening and feces passing freely through the vulva; and, in the male, a blue line running forward from the anal dimple, representing a sinus tract filled with meconium.

The classification of rectal and anal deformities most often utilized is that of Ladd and Gross. They divide them into four types.

Type   I — Stenosis at lower rectum or anus (incomplete rupture of anal membrane)

Type  II — Membranous form of imperforate anus (persistence of anal membrane)

Type III — Imperforate anus, and rectum ends as a blind pouch a variable distance from the perineum

Type IV — Anal canal and lower rectum form a distal pouch, separated from a blind rectal pouch by a variable distance

Fistulas are associated in a high percentage of cases (55 to 82 per cent of all reported series). Most of these involve the type III malformation, and, conversely, almost every type III deformity has an associated fistula. In the female these are almost always rectovaginal, rarely rectoperineal, never rectourinary. In the male, fistulas are almost always rectourinary, terminating in the bladder or urethra, and are only rarely rectoperineal. In Santulli's series of 62 cases the type III variety accounted for 53, type I for four, type II for three and type IV for only two examples.

**DIAGNOSIS.** Microscopic anus is obvious from the start resembling an imperforate anus with a tiny dot of meconium or stool visible at times in its center. Only a fine probe can be passed. A low stenosis usually does not cause symptoms within the neonatal period, difficulty in defecation and ribbon-like stools delaying their appearance ordinarily for several months. The reason may be that the stoma is large enough to permit passage of semiliquid and pasty stools characteristic of early life, but not of formed stools. When symptoms appear, digital rectal examination confirms the diagnosis.

So rare is the type II membranous diaphragm deformity that Potts has encountered only one in his entire career. The anus is normal in appearance; hence diagnosis usually awaits distention and vomiting, which begins at 24 to 48 hours of age. By then the bulging green or brown membrane may be visible at the anus, but, if not, it is readily palpable by the probing finger a few centimeters above the sphincter. If an x-ray picture is taken with the infant held upside down, a thermometer held in place within the anus as far as it will penetrate without forcing, the air in the lowermost loop of bowel will be seen to abut closely the thermometer bulb. This is true only provided one has waited at least 24 hours for air to have entered the entire large bowel and has held the infant inverted for at least 5 minutes so that its most distal loop has filled.

In the type III lesion one can see the anal dimple, but the anus is clearly imperforate. One expects to find a fistula, rectovaginal in the female, rectourinary in the male, rarely rectoperineal in either sex. One is almost never disappointed in this anticipation. X-ray studies with barium injected per vaginam or per urethram will confirm fistula, as will the appearance of meconium or flatus within the vagina of the female or the urine of the male.

The diagnosis of the type IV lesion, since the anus looks normal, awaits evidence of lower bowel obstruction, after which rectal examination may reveal the atresia. Thereafter plain x-ray films taken in the inverted position with the above-mentioned precautions should demonstrate the distance by which blind upper and lower pouches are separated.

**TREATMENT.** Briefly, all stenotic lesions are treated by repeated and long-continued dilatations; obstructive lesions with or without fistula must be treated surgically. In the case of membranous lesions surgery is simple, consisting merely in perforation of the diaphragm. Operative repair of the type III malformation in the female may be delayed months or years, since the rectovaginal fistula dilates adequately to permit passage of stools. The infant may require help in the form of mineral oil or Colace by mouth to keep the stools soft, and of periodic enemas whenever impaction threatens. The type III malformation in the male and the type IV malformation in either sex require immediate operation. The details of the various operative procedures depend upon the conformation of the defect. They will not be discussed here.

## RUPTURE OF THE BOWEL

The bowel, like the stomach, ruptures for a variety of reasons. Most common is rupture of a dilated loop proximal to an obstruction, either extrinsic or intrinsic. According to Thelander, the large bowel perforates twice as often as the small. In descending order of frequency stand colon, ileum, jejunum and duodenum, each of which outnumbers the stomach as the site of rupture.

Although most are explainable on the basis of obstruction, many demonstrate no such lesion. Trauma, diverticula and central nervous system damage have been blamed for spontaneous rupture without strong evidence to support these hypotheses. Obstructing mucus plugs have been seen in a few (see the following case). Sections taken from the edges of perforations most often show that these areas were weakened by absence or thinning of several layers of the intestinal wall without evidences of ulceration or infection. But a few perforations have always been noted to follow bacterial enteritis, and within the past decade a large number of such ruptures have been reported in association with a presumably new entity, necrotizing enterocolitis.

The clinical picture resembles that described for gastric perforation (p. 349). Briefly, it includes sudden development of distention, associated with refusal of food and with vomiting, and rapid supervention of shock. Blood may have been vomited or passed in the stool at the onset. Distention reaches a high degree, the abdominal wall becomes bluish and edematous, its veins dilated, and air often fills the scrotal sac. Flat films of the abdomen show an excess of air both within and without bowel loops and, in the erect position, an accumulation of air between the dome of the liver and the leaves of the diaphragm.

*Treatment* consists in immediate laparotomy, repair of the perforation and rapid search for additional ones, since multiple perforations are not uncommonly encountered, as well as search for a basic obstructive lesion. If one is found, it must be bypassed.

A few reported patients have recovered after operation. Our case, appended below, is another example of cure. Most patients die of peritonitis.

CASE 35–2

A 6 pound 8 ounce (2950 gm) boy was born to a known Rh-negative sensitized mother. Her first child was normal; her second had severe hemolytic anemia of the newborn, for which he received an exchange transfusion. He did well. This baby was slightly jaundiced at birth (bilirubin 6.7, indirect 4.3 mg per 100 ml), and his direct Coombs test result was 4+ positive. He was given an exchange transfusion at 4 hours. On the second day he was given another exchange transfusion because his blood bilirubin level remained high. On the fourth day he vomited several feedings and was anorexic, and that evening moderate distention was noted. After a saline enema a mucus plug was passed, but no stools. Flat films of the abdomen were taken (Fig. 35–6, *A*), but were read while wet, and their true significance was missed. The next morning the accumulation of air above the liver and the appearance of air within the peritoneal cavity, but outside bowel lumens, was recognized. He was transferred to the Harriet Lane

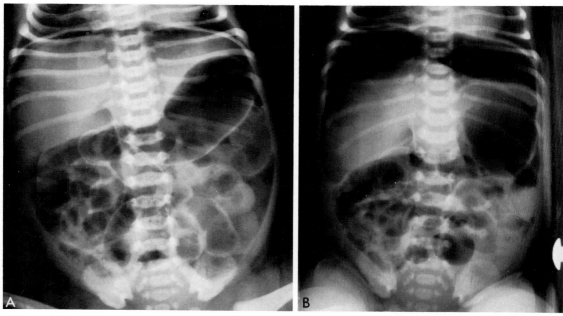

*Figure 35–6.* *A,* Anteroposterior view of abdomen taken in the erect position at 72 hours of age. There is air in the stomach and intestines, and one gets the distinct impression that some of the air is outside the lumen of the bowel. A layer of air is clearly visible above the liver and below the diaphragm. *B,* Ten hours later. By now there is a huge accumulation of air between the diaphragm and the liver.

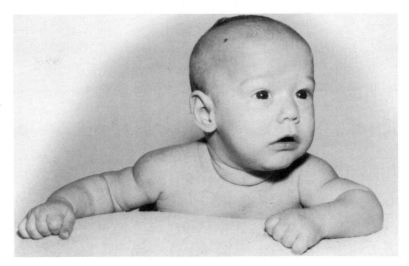

*Figure 35-7.* Photograph of the infant whose x-ray films are shown in Figure 35-6, taken at 4 months of age.

Home, where another film showed great increase in quantity of air leakage (Fig. 35-6, *B*).

Operation was immediately performed (Dr. D. C. Sabiston), and a ruptured spot in the ileum was discovered and repaired. He did well for 2 days; then vomiting and great distention recurred. At reoperation two more tears in the ileum were found and repaired. To our amazement he made a complete recovery after a stormy postoperative course. He was discharged at 4 weeks of age. The incision thereafter dehisced at one end, his liver and spleen remained large and his hemoglobin a bit low as a result of his hemolytic disease for the next 2 months, but by the age of 4 months he weighed 13 pounds (5900 gm) and seemed in all respects normal. Figure 35-7 is a picture of this miracle baby at this age.

**COMMENT.** This fortunate infant survived a serious episode of hemolytic anemia of the newborn due to Rh sensitization, followed by two successive catastrophic ruptures of the ileum. In the first of these, one puncture was discovered; in the second, two. The surgical disorder had no apparent connection with the medical one. It is not unlikely that the hard mucus plug, passed after an enema, was the obstructing element which caused dilatation and finally rupture of bowel loops proximal to it. The moral derived from this example is that perseverance in therapy is at times rewarded by unexpectedly excellent results.

# REFERENCES

Agerty, H. A., Ziserman, A. J., and Shollenberger, C. L.: Perforation of the ileum in a newborn. J. Pediatr. *22*:233, 1943.

Beck, W. C., and Chohany, G.: Duodenal atresia. J. Pediatr. *42*:432, 1953.

Boles, G. T., and Smith, B.: Preduodenal portal vein. Pediatrics *28*:805, 1961.

Boyden, E. A., Cope, J. A., and Bill, A. H., Jr.: Anatomy and embryology of congenital intrinsic obstruction of the duodenum. Am. J. Surg. *114*:190, 1967.

Browne, D.: Congenital deformities of the anus and rectum. Arch. Dis. Child. *30*:42, 1955.

Chamberlain, J. W.: Partial intestinal obstruction in the newborn due to kinking of the proximal small bowel. New Engl. J. Med. *275*:1241, 1966.

Di Sant'Agnese, P. A., Dische, Z., and Danilczenko, A.: Physicochemical differences of mucoproteins in duodenal fluid of patients with cystic fibrosis of the pancreas and controls. Pediatrics *19*:252, 1957.

el-Shafie, M., and Rickham, P. P.: Multiple intestinal atresias. J. Pediat. Surg. *5*:655, 1970.

Gross, R. E.: The Surgery of Infancy and Childhood. Its Principles and Techniques. Philadelphia, W. B. Saunders Company, 1953.

Gross, R. E.: An Atlas of Children's Surgery. Philadelphia, W. B. Saunders Co., 1970.

Holder, T. M., and Leape, L. L.: The acute surgical abdomen in the neonate. New Engl. J. Med. *278*:605, 1968.

Hyde, J. S.: Congenital duodenal atresia in four sibs. J. A. M. A. *191*:52, 1965.

Kalayoglu, M., Sieber, W., Rodnan, J. B., and Kiesewetter, W. B.: Meconium ileus: A critical review of treatment and eventual prognosis. J. Pediat. Surg. *6*:290, 1971.

Lee, C. M., Jr., and MacMillan, B. G.: Rupture of the bowel in the newborn infant. Surgery *28*:48, 1950.

McPartlin, J. F., Dickson, J. A. S., and Swain, V. A. J.: Meconium ileus: Immediate and long-term survival. Arch. Dis. Child. *47*:207, 1973.

Mishalany, H. G., Der Kaloustian, I. M., and Ghandour, M.: Familial congenital duodenal atresia. Pediatrics *47*:629, 1970.

Neuhauser, E. B. D.: Roentgen changes associated with pancreatic insufficiency in early life. Radiology *46*:319, 1946.

Nixon, H. H.: Intestinal obstruction in the newborn. Arch. Dis. Child. *30*:13, 1955.

Noblett, H. R.: Treatment of uncomplicated meconium ileus by Gastrografin enema: A preliminary report. J. Pediat. Surg. *4*:180, 1969.

Patton, E. F.: Congenital hypertrophic stenosis of the duodenum. J. Pediatr. *32*:301, 1948.

Potts, W. J.: The Surgeon and the Child. Philadelphia, W. B. Saunders Company, 1959.

Rowe, M. I., Furst, A. J., et al.: The neonatal response to Gastrografin enema. Pediatrics *48*:20, 1971.

Santulli, T. V.: The treatment of imperforate anus and associated fistulae. Surg., Gynec. Obstet. *95*:60l, 1952.

Scott, J. E. S.: Intestinal obstruction in the newborn associated with peritonitis. Arch. Dis. Child. *38*:120, 1963.

Shwachman, H., Pryles, C. V., and Gross, R. E.: Meconium ileus; a clinical study of 20 surviving patients. A.M.A. J. Dis. Child. *91*:223, 1956.

Strand, H.: Vomiting in utero with intestinal atresia. Pediatrics.

Thelander, H. E.: Perforation of the gastrointestinal tract of the newborn infant. Am. J. Dis. Child. *58*:371, 1939.

Touloukian, R. J., and Wright, H. F.: Intrauterine villus hypertrophy with jejunal atresia. J. Pediat. Surg. *8*:779, 1973.

Waggett, J., Bishop, H. C., and Koop, C. E.: Experience with Gastrografin enema in the treatment of meconium ileus. J. Pediat. Surg. *5*:649, 1970.

Waggett, J., Johnson, P. G., et al.: The nonoperative treatment of meconium ileus by Gastrografin enema. J. Pediatr. *77*:407, 1970.

White, H.: Meconium ileus: A new roentgen sign. Radiology *66*:567, 1956.

Young, W. F., Swain, V., and Pringle, E. M.: Long-term prognosis after major resection of the small bowel in early infancy. Arch. Dis. Child. *44*:465, 1969.

# 36

# CONGENITAL EXTRINSIC INTESTINAL OBSTRUCTION

This subgroup includes the various combinations and permutations of malrotation, as well as annular pancreas, incarcerated hernias and obstruction by masses outside the bowel. Malrotation may be present alone and may be asymptomatic for life, or it may become symptomatic because volvulus supervenes, owing to excessive mobility of bowel, or because aberrant bands compress a loop of intestine or because cecum overlies a loop and obstructs. Volvulus may occur in an apparently normal bowel or in a malrotated one. It is an extremely frequent complication of meconium ileus both prenatally and postnatally, as it is of duplication of the bowel. When volvulus is diagnosed, malrotation should be carefully ruled in or out, and when malrotation is discovered, the danger of volvulus and of other forms of obstruction must be kept in mind.

## MIDGUT VOLVULUS

This disastrous accident may take place in an infant whose small bowel has failed to re-enter the abdominal cavity in normal fashion and whose mesenteric attachments have not developed properly (see p. 355). The midgut lies free, attached to the posterior abdominal wall at only two points, the duodenum and the proximal colon, and is therefore liable to rotate on this narrow axis in either direction. When rotation occurs, it usually does so in a counterclockwise direction. It may twist only a few degrees or may make as many as three or four complete turns upon itself. Kinking of the entering bowel or of the emergent segment or of both may follow, but the point of obstruction is almost always at the duodeno-jejunal junction. The circulation to the twisted segment is often obstructed and leads to rapid development of gangrene.

**DIAGNOSIS.** Diagnosis rests upon sudden onset of vomiting and rapid development of distention. Vomiting ordinarily does not begin at birth, although an infant may rarely be born with volvulus, but is delayed until the third or fourth day in the early cases, and until a month or more in the late ones, or it may start at any time in between. Once begun, vomiting usually occurs after every feeding. The vomitus is bile-stained. The degree of distention depends in the first place upon the tightness of the volvulus and the consequent completeness or incompleteness of the obstruction, and in the second place upon the degree of vascular obstruction produced by the twisting. Obviously infants with complete obstruction and those whose mesenteric vessels have been occluded have the most severe form of abdominal distention. Since obstruction is often incomplete, all gradations of distention are seen.

Clinically, midgut volvulus can be suspected strongly when vomiting begins in an infant who had had no evidence of obstruction for 3 days or more and in whom the abdomen rapidly becomes greatly distended. Signs of shock will not be long delayed.

X-ray films of the abdomen are variable. One usually sees not quite complete obstruction in the third or fourth portion of the duodenum with moderate dilatation of the stomach and sparse, scattered accumulations of air in the small bowel. For the rest the abdomen appears full and homogeneously hazy. Barium introduced by enema may fail to penetrate beyond the transverse colon if the emergent loop is obstructed. If the radiopaque mixture reaches the cecum, it may demonstrate that this structure is displaced from its normal right lower quadrant location.

**TREATMENT.** Immediate operation is imperative. The danger is not so much that of high intestinal obstruction with its resultant blood chemical dislocations, although this is great, but the rapid development of gangrene of a large segment of bowel due to the vascular constriction caused by the twisted mesentery. The surgeon will have to decide how much, if any, of the involved intestine is no longer viable and will have to be resected. Extensive resection renders an already serious prognosis more grave.

## CASE HISTORIES

### CASE 36–1

A white male infant was born at the Sinai Hospital of Baltimore after an uneventful pregnancy, labor and delivery, at full term. He breathed and cried spontaneously and on the original examination at 2 hours of age was found to be healthy in all respects. Oral feeding was begun at 24 hours, and the first two bottles were taken well. Thereafter they were refused, and any attempt to force them caused vomiting. Later during the second day he began to regurgitate bile-stained fluid. He had passed meconium stools normally until 36 hours, after which there were no more. Examination at 48 hours showed him to be ill and anxious, the abdomen distended and tight. No bowel or stomach patters were seen. The note was tympanitic over the entire abdomen. An excess of bowel sounds was heard. X-ray film showed bizarre bowel patterns (Fig. 36–1). Operation was performed within a few hours (Dr. Howard Kern). On opening the peritoneum dilated loops of bowel promptly escaped through the wound and executed writhing movements for some moments. After this the bluish color of the bowel quickly returned to normal, and careful examination revealed no obstruction, no aberrant bands or vessels and no malposition. Postoperative course was uneventful, and the child remained well for the 12 years thereafter that we observed him.

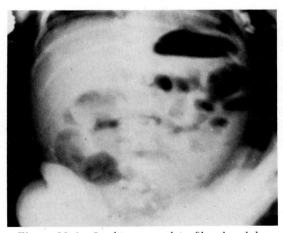

*Figure 36–1.* In this erect plain film the abdominal distention is obvious and the gas pattern bizarre. A gas bubble and fluid level can be seen in the left upper quadrant, defining moderately distended stomach. One greatly dilated loop of small bowel can be seen beneath it, and other smaller loops throughout the midabdomen and right lower quadrant. No large bowel can be visualized. This pattern strongly suggests midgut volvulus.

COMMENT. This was one of our earliest cases of neonatal obstruction. We would prefer now to have three x-ray views upon which to base a decision instead of the single one which we took then. The story was the typical one of midgut volvulus, vomiting and distention coming on soon after the first feedings were taken, the twisting no doubt initiated by the strong peristalsis induced by ingestion. It appears that at operation the twisted gut righted itself, and no evidence of malrotation could then be found. This probably represents a case of midgut volvulus without malrotation.

CASE 36–2

A white male infant was born at term weighing 8 pounds 11 ounces (3950 gm). Delivery had been effected by midforceps after transverse arrest, and he was flaccid and cyanotic at birth. After resuscitation he seemed fairly well. On the eighth day he began to regurgitate yellow-stained material. This continued throughout the next week, during which a flat film and gastroin-

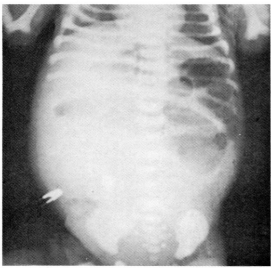

*Figure 36–2.* In this supine flat film the gas pattern is bizarre. Stomach cannot be defined with certainty, and the dilated bowel patterns of various sizes and shapes, confined to the upper part of the abdomen and mostly lying in the left upper quadrant, probably are all small intestinal loops. The remainder of the abdomen is homogeneously opaque and airless. This proved at operation to be midgut volvulus.

This case history is not summarized in the text. It was one of our earliest cases, and only this film was made.

testinal x-ray series were made and reported as normal. On the fifteenth day distention became prominent, vomiting increased, and he appeared ill. A barium enema x-ray film now showed evidences of malrotation (Fig. 36–3). Laparotomy revealed a 360-degree volvulus of the midgut, and aberrant bands and blood vessels producing obstruction to the third portion of the duodenum and acting as the pivot around which the bowel had rotated. The bands and vessels were severed, and the bowel was replaced into its normal position. Postoperative course was uneventful.

COMMENT. In this instance the partial obstruction was probably caused by aberrant bands and blood vessels. It became complete when volvulus supervened on the fifteenth day. This, then, is an example of malrotation without volvulus at first, with midgut volvulus later.

CASE 36–3

A white male infant, born after an uneventful pregnancy and labor, weighed 7 pounds 2 ounces (3239 gm) at birth. He behaved quite normally until 1 month of age, when he began to regurgitate feedings. At 5 weeks vomiting had become projectile, but was intermittent, lasting 1 day, remitting for 3 or 4 days. At 8 weeks moderate constipation appeared. Vomitus always contained bile. There was no evidence of abdominal pain. At this time he was admitted to the Sinai Hospital. Weight was 11 pounds 13 ounces (5360 gm), temperature 100.2° F. There had clearly been weight loss. The abdomen was full but not tight, and waves were seen to pass from the left costal margin to the umbilicus, but not beyond. Blood chemical determinations showed chloride 98, sodium 130, potassium 3.8 mg. per cent and carbon dioxide 23.3 mEq. per liter. X-ray films showed dilated stomach and first portion of the duodenum, partial obstruction at that point, and malrotation of the bowel (Fig. 36–4). Under the fluoroscope the misplaced cecum, lying in the left upper quadrant, was found to be freely movable. At operation a peritoneal band was found running from the cecum across the third portion of the duodenum, where it produced almost complete obstruction. This was divided, and no fixation was attempted. Postoperative course was smooth, and the infant has been perfectly well.

COMMENT. This example is typical in all respects of partial obstruction caused by an aberrant peritoneal band so often present with malrotation of the bowel. The

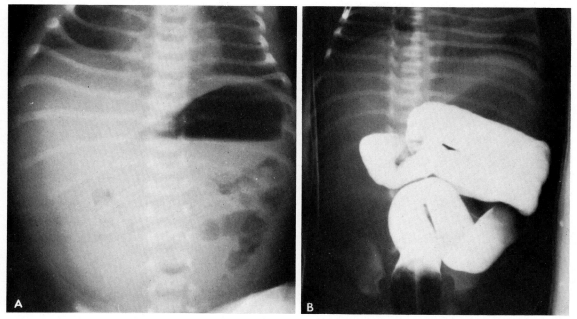

*Figure 36–3.* Films of abdomen taken on the fifteenth day of life. *A,* The erect anteroposterior flat film shows dilated stomach with fluid level, a small quantity of air in the small bowel in the left midabdomen, and a tiny bit to the right. The rest of the abdomen is airless, homogeneously opaque, and abdominal distention is obvious. *B,* Barium enema shows the large bowel lying almost entirely to the left and terminating in a cecum which lies in the upper part of the abdomen just to the right of the midline. *A* and *B* together make the diagnosis of midgut volvulus secondary to malrotation perfectly certain.

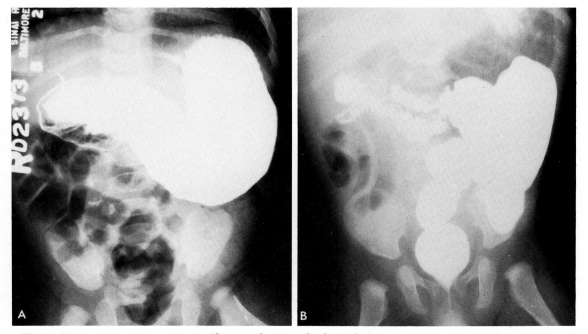

*Figure 36–4.* *A,* Barium meal x-ray film reveals a greatly distended stomach and first portion of duodenum, delayed emptying, and some dilatation of the air-filled intestinal loops in the mid- and right abdomen. Absence of gas in the left side is noteworthy. After 3 hours little barium has left the stomach and duodenum. *B,* Barium enema shows the large intestine to be of normal caliber, but lying almost entirely within the left side of the abdomen. What is probably cecum can be seen in the left upper quadrant. The bowel is obviously malrotated.

lateness of onset, intermittency and absence of severe constipation are characteristic. Finding the cecum in the upper part of the abdomen and hypermobile made the exact diagnosis almost certain. The other fairly strong possibility was that the filled cecum itself might have lain over the duodenum and produced the same clinical picture.

## INCARCERATED HERNIA

Herniated abdominal contents in the newborn may project into the thoracic cavity through the diaphragm, through the abdominal wall at the umbilicus or along the linea alba, through the inguinal ring or into internal defects of the mesentery. Diaphragmatic hernia has been discussed (p. 183). This variety seldom incarcerates. Umbilical hernia is also described (p. 394). We have never seen one of these become incarcerated, although a few have been reported beyond the neonatal period. Internal hernias can be diagnosed only at the time of operation for intestinal obstruction. They too are extremely rare in the neonatal period.

*Inguinal hernias,* generally of the indirect variety, are not at all an uncommon sight in the nursery or later in the neonate. Boys are affected much more often than girls. The right side is involved more frequently than the left, and bilateral hernias are found not uncommonly. The hernia may be complete or scrotal, abdominal contents descending into a wide-open funicular peritoneal process to fill the scrotum completely. Or it may be funicular, descending only to some point above the testis where the tunica vaginalis is sealed off. Other varieties, direct, femoral and encysted, are only rarely encountered.

*Diagnosis* may rest entirely upon detection of a mass in the inguinal region or within the scrotum. The mass generally appears intermittently, coming out after crying or straining and withdrawing during periods of sleep or inactivity. Later it may remain visible and palpable constantly. Many of these infants are extraordinarily irritable, crying as though in pain much of the day and night, for as long as 2 or 3 weeks before the hernia becomes apparent.

This circumstance undoubtedly has given rise to the lay belief that excessive crying causes hernia. It is probable that the reverse is true.

The superposition of vomiting, distention and, at times, the appearance of blood and mucus in the stools, upon anorexia, inordinate crying and the presence of an irreducible mass in the inguinal region, indicate that strangulation and complete intestinal obstruction have complicated simple incarceration.

*Differential diagnosis* from hydrocele is occasionally difficult. Hydrocele of the testis should not present much trouble, since in this disorder the enlargement clearly encompasses the testis, which can no longer be palpated, and the fluid-filled sac transilluminates brilliantly. In scrotal hernia the testis can be felt at the bottom of the mass, the whole is generally reducible, and light does not traverse it nearly so brightly. Hydrocele of the cord within the inguinal canal is often harder to differentiate, especially if a funicular hernia here is incarcerated and irreducible. Fortunately for one's conscience hydrocele and this form of herniation often coexist, so that exploratory operation can be advised without too much hesitation if one remains in doubt after careful examination and after attempted reduction has failed.

The mass in the inguinal canal proves on occasion to be a gonad. A few cases are on record in which the gonad discovered high in the inguinal canal turns out to be one of the sex opposite to that of the conformation of the external genitals. Thus a number of apparently female infants have been reported in whom the inguinal gonad was discovered to be testis. This situation is discussed in Chapter 56, on Sexual Differentiation.

**TREATMENT.** The accepted method of dealing with inguinal hernia is to advise operation. This must of course be done as an emergency if the mass cannot be reduced. If it can, one may wait a few days or weeks for a time suitable to the parents, but no longer. The danger of incarceration and strangulation hangs over one always, and the hazard of elective herniorrhaphy is so slim that procrastination is not to be condoned. Exceptions are at times made in the case of girls, in whom the prognosis for spontaneous closure appears to be appreciably greater than it is in boys.

Because hernia often appears later on the opposite side, more and more surgeons are exploring the other inguinal region after the first one has been repaired, and repairing that side too if the vaginal process is open. In 40 per cent it will be open, and one half of these would go on to develop hernia within months or years (Rowe, Copelson and Clatworthy, 1969).

White and his collaborators (1970) make a strong case in favor of performing inguinal herniography in children admitted for unilateral hernia in order to outline the opposite peritoneal sac. If this is also open, they believe, the potential hernia should be repaired with the overt one. We prefer to withhold opinion on this still unsettled question.

## ANNULAR PANCREAS

**INCIDENCE.** In 1954 Kiesewetter and Koop were able to discover 74 cases of annular pancreas in the literature and added six of their own. They commented that the condition had been described with regularity only in the preceding 10 years and suggested that it may be more common than this small total number suggests. By 1956 Frucht found the number to have increased to 100. It is discovered considerably more often in adults than in newborns, Rickham reporting a ratio of nearly nine older patients to one newborn. Males are affected much more frequently than females. Rarely, it may appear in siblings.

**DIAGNOSIS.** It must be remembered that annular pancreas 1) may not constrict the duodenum at all, 2) may constrict the duodenum sufficiently to produce duodenal stenosis, or 3) may completely block the duodenum. Thus it may cause no symptoms or it may simulate duodenal stenosis (p. 359) or duodenal atresia (p. 358). Indeed, it is not uncommonly associated with intrinsic duodenal atresia.

In the majority of instances ring pancreas encircles the second portion of the duodenum distal to the ampulla of Vater, but a few are situated proximal to the ampulla. In the former, vomitus is bile-stained; in the latter, not.

Jaundice is seen in a large proportion of neonates with this disorder. It is likely that jaundice is caused by compression of the common duct by the abnormally situated pancreas.

Concomitant congenital defects are frequently encountered, among which mongolism is prominent.

**TREATMENT.** Attempts to excise the constricting ring have been generally unsuccessful. This is due in part to the almost inevitable development of pancreatic fistula, in part to the fact that intrinsic stenosis or atresia often coexists. Gastroenterostomy is not recommended because the blind loop of proximal duodenum left behind must reflux into the stomach. The operation of choice is duodenojejunostomy.

CASE 36–4

A white male infant, born prematurely at home, birth weight 3 pounds (1360 gm), was admitted to the Harriet Lane Home Premature Nursery at 8 hours of age. He seemed vigorous,

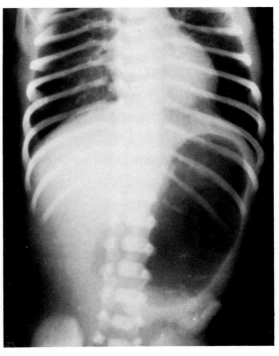

*Figure 36–5.* The supine plain anteroposterior film shows a hugely dilated stomach and a small bubble lying to its right which is the shadow of dilated first portion of the duodenum. No air is to be seen elsewhere in the abdomen. The diagnosis of complete duodenal obstruction can be made, but its cause, annular pancreas, had to be discovered at operation.

and his admission examination revealed no abnormalities. At 12 hours he began to drool bile-stained fluid. By 24 hours no meconium had been passed. At 36 hours glucose solution feedings had been vomited, and still no meconium had been passed. At this time fullness was noted in the left upper quadrant, but no peristaltic waves were seen. Plain x-ray films showed a hugely dilated stomach and the second bubble indicating duodenal obstruction (Fig. 36–5). At 45 hours laparotomy was done, and a completely encircling annular pancreas was found obstructing the second portion of the duodenum. Duodenojejunostomy was performed. Postoperative course was stormy because of wound infection and poorly functioning anastomosis, but ultimately satisfactory weight gain began. He was discharged at three months of age, weighing 5 pounds 4 ounces (2375 gm).

## DUPLICATIONS OF THE ALIMENTARY TRACT

Gross, Holcomb and Farber define duplications of the alimentary tract as "spherical or tubular structures which possess a well developed smooth muscle layer and are lined with mucous membrane, . . . are found at any level from tongue to anus and usually are intimately attached to some portion of the alimentary tube."

INCIDENCE. These authors have reported the largest series to be found in the literature. It comprised 67 cases seen at the Children's Hospital of Boston from 1928 through 1950. All but eight were under 2 years, and 25 per cent of the cases became manifest in the first month of life. In spite of the large concentration of cases at this hospital, duplications must be considered fairly rare.

PATHOLOGY. The wall of the cyst looks very much like wall of normal bowel. Only a few have gastric mucosa and secretions which resemble gastric juice. These have been described under Disorders of the Stomach (p. 344). The most common site of origin is the ileum and ileocecal valve region, the duodenum, jejunum, colon and rectum each supplying a small share of the total. Most are found within the abdomen, but a not inconsiderable portion remain entrapped within the thorax during ontogenetic descent. Double cysts are not rare, one being found within the abdomen, the other within the thorax.

Duplications may be tubes which branch from intestine to extend between mesenteric leaves, or double-barreled structures communicating at both ends. A few are cystic and lie free in the peritoneal cavity attached by only a mesenteric stalk. Most are spherical and contiguous to bowel, with which only the minority communicate. In perhaps one quarter to one third of cases defects of one or more vertebrae may be discovered by x-ray or at autopsy. These are indicative of notochordal maldevelopment.

ETIOLOGY has been discussed under Duplications of the Stomach (p. 344). But Favara, Franciosi and Akers (1971) have recently suggested that many, perhaps most, of the enteric duplications they found in the newborn had been caused by an intrauterine vascular accident. They were led to this conclusion by finding lesions highly indicative of vascular occlusions in most of their newborns with enterogenous duplications. These were intestinal atresias or stenoses, mesenteric defects and short, small bowel (p. 358). They do not think that this pathogenic mechanism is responsible for all duplications, pointing out that "theories of aberrant recanalization of the gut, persistence of enteric diverticula and notochordal maldevelopment remain important."

DIAGNOSIS. Enterogenous duplications upon occasion have been so large as to produce dystocia and prolonged second stage of labor. More often they manifest themselves by signs pointing toward intestinal obstruction, usually partial. Overt gastrointestinal hemorrhage is not uncommon, in the form of passage by rectum of blood mixed with stool, blood-stained mucus, tarry stools or fresh blood unmixed with bowel content. Occult hemorrhage may lead to severe anemia difficult to explain. Bouts of abdominal pain often distress the infant greatly. Duplications have initiated volvulus not infrequently and have less often served as leading points for intussusception.

Small cysts are generally neither visible nor palpable. Larger ones may be appreciated by fullness in one or another quadrant or by palpation of a vague abdominal mass or by local resistance to deep palpation. If obstruction coexists, its own signs will be superimposed upon those which pertain to the duplication itself.

Plain x-ray films of the abdomen reveal cysts if they communicate and are filled with air. If noncommunicating, or if communicating but not air-filled, their presence may be suspected by the discovery of distortions of bowel pattern caused by an interposed solid mass. Such distortions are visualized better in barium gastrointestinal series films. We append below one example in each of these two categories.

**TREATMENT.** Once the diagnosis is suspected, immediate operation is indicated. Complete excision of the duplication along with the segment of bowel to which it adheres is the operation of choice.

## CASE HISTORIES

### CASE 36–5

A 6 pound 8 ounce (2950 gm) white male infant was born uneventfully to a multiparous mother. His Apgar score at 1 minute was 10. On routine physical examination a mass was felt in the right lower quadrant. It was freely movable,

of cystic consistency. It was easily felt on rectal examination. Plain x-ray film showed a radiopaque shadow filling the right lower quadrant. (This film has been lost.) Intravenous pyelogram was normal. Operation was performed on the seventh day. A cyst containing clear fluid lay behind the cecum retroperitoneally, attached to the posterior abdominal wall by a short pedicle which seemed to arise from the root of the mesentery. Cyst and appendix were removed.

The surgeon was inclined to believe that this was a mesenteric cyst. Section showed it to be a cystic duplication of the intestine.

**COMMENT.** This duplication presented itself as a simple, palpable cystic mass without obstruction or bleeding. This variety is hard to differentiate preoperatively from mesenteric cyst, ectopic kidney or possibly ovarian cyst.

### CASE 36–6

A black female infant was born at home and brought immediately to the hospital, where the cord was cut and tied. She seemed well, but was admitted to the pediatric ward rather than the nursery because of the unsterile delivery. Admission examination revealed no abnormalities. By 24 hours no meconium had been passed, and there was slight abdominal distention. Rectal

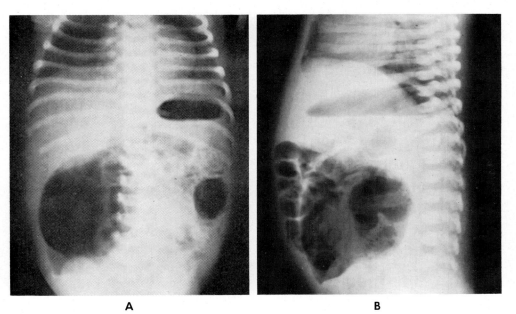

**A**  **B**

*Figure 36–6.* *A,* Anteroposterior view of abdomen in the erect position. A bizarre gas pattern is seen in which one can distinguish stomach, with fluid level, and a sparse scattering of gas throughout the small bowel. A large gas bubble filling the right side proved at operation to be a duplicated segment of colon. A smaller one on the left is probably a dilated loop of small bowel. *B,* Lateral view.

examination revealed a tight sphincter. A thermometer could be passed to its full length without difficulty. A 30-cc tap water enema was returned with a small amount of meconium and a large piece of tissue which appeared to be mucosal slough. The following morning the infant passed spontaneously a meconium stool. Now a vaguely defined mass could be felt filling the right lower quadrant. X-ray film showed some air in the stomach and a scattering of gas throughout mid-abdomen. The entire right half was occupied by one huge radiolucent bubble, and in the left there was a smaller such area resembling a dilated loop of small bowel (Fig. 36–6). During the evening of the second day distention increased, appetite diminished, and the baby vomited once. Operation was performed on the morning of the third day. A large duplicated segment of the colon was removed, along with several inches of colon to which it was tightly adherent, and a colocolostomy was performed. Postoperative course was essentially uneventful, and she was discharged well after 3 weeks.

**COMMENT.** This duplicated large bowel presented as a partial intestinal obstruc-tion. The vague mass became palpable on the second day, when by virtue of its connection with parent bowel, it filled with air and was readily visualized in the x-ray film. This fortunate circumstance makes diagnosis easy, but it is seldom present.

CASE 36–7

A white female infant was born after normal pregnancy and labor to a primiparous mother. Birth weight was 7 pounds 1 ounce (3200 gm). In the nursery she seemed entirely normal. At 2 weeks of age she passed a large tarry stool. After this she slept poorly and seemed to have frequent bouts of abdominal pain. After about 2 months these ceased. At 4 months they recurred, and she vomited a few times and slept poorly. She passed a small amount of bright blood by rectum on two occasions, and pain became incessant and colicky. There was no constipation or diarrhea, and vomiting was infrequent.

Physical examination on admission, age 5 months, showed her to be fairly nourished, weight 15 pounds 5 ounces (7050 gm), acutely ill, extremely pale, with continually recurring

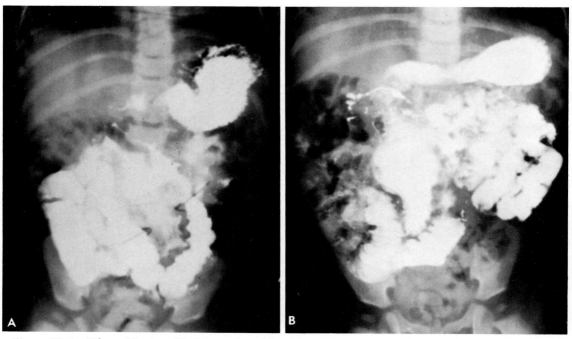

*Figure 36–7.* Films of barium-filled stomach and bowel show a persistent abnormality of pattern below the stomach. *A,* The pyloric cap is filled, but beyond this the duodenum appears to be almost empty. *B,* This same hiatus is apparent, and at this time the stomach seems to be flattened from below by some ill-defined mass. The duplicated segment of small bowel discovered at operation must have lain immediately caudad to the stomach, displacing it upward and normal small intestine downward.

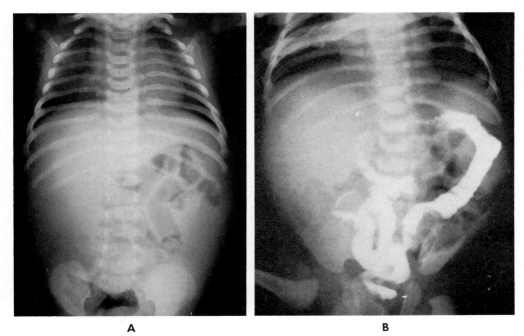

**A**     **B**

*Figure 36–8.* Films of another example of intestinal duplication not abstracted in the text. *A*, Flat anteroposterior supine film shows no air in the right side of the abdomen, and a bizarre, double-barreled pattern of small bowel in the left upper portion of the abdomen. *B*, After introduction of barium by enema the descending colon is seen to be narrowed and to be displaced to the left, while another portion of bowel is displaced to the right. Both loops seem to encircle a mass which contains neither barium nor gas. This mass proved at operation to be a duplication of the small intestine not connected with its parent bowel.

bouts of pain during which she cried out and drew her legs up over the abdomen. This was slightly distended, but not tight. No masses were felt, no points of tenderness, but there was some resistance to deep palpation in the left upper quadrant. Rectal examination was negative, and no blood or mucus appeared on the examining finger. Hemoglobin was 3.5 gm, red blood cell count 2.17 million, white blood cell count 16,000, with normal differential. She had several transfusions, and her general condition improved. Occult blood was discovered in the stool at all times. Flat films of the abdomen revealed nothing abnormal, but a barium gastrointestinal series showed a distinctly deranged pattern of bowel in the region of the duodenum (Fig. 36–7).

At operation a large duplicated segment of small intestine was discovered at about the junction of the jejunum and ileum, containing aberrant gastric mucosa, and communicating with the small bowel at its proximal end. This was resected along with a small segment of adjacent intestine to which it adhered, and an end-to-end anastomosis was performed. Postoperative course was uneventful.

**COMMENT.** This 5-month-old infant's earliest manifestation of trouble consisted in passage of a tarry stool at 2 weeks, followed by colicky pain. Throughout her long course she became severely anemic, although recognizable blood was passed on only three occasions. Clearly she was bleeding in occult fashion continuously. Diagnosis was suspected after seeing the films of the barium studies, but could be made with certainty only after exploratory laparotomy.

## REFERENCES

Abt, I. A.: Fetal peritonitis. M. Clin. N. Amer. *15*:611, 1931–32.

Astley, R.: Radiology of the Alimentary Tract in Infancy. Baltimore, Williams & Wilkins Company, 1956.

Bierman, C. W., Davis, J. K., and Biehusen, C.: Intestinal obstruction in a premature infant treated by resection and end-to-end anastomosis. J. Pediatr. *40*:474, 1952.

Favara, B. E., Franciosi, R. A., and Akers, D. R.: Enteric duplications, 37 cases: A vascular theory of pathogenesis. Am. J. Dis. Child. *122*:501, 1971.

Frucht, D. A.: Annular pancreas in infancy. Amer. J. Dis. Child. *92*:182, 1956.

Gross, R. E., Holcomb, G. W., and Farber, S.: Duplications of the alimentary tract. Pediatrics *9*:449, 1952.

Gryboski, J.: Gastrointestinal Problems in the Infant. Phila., W. B. Saunders Co., 1975.

Kiesewetter, W. B., and Koop, C. W.: Annular pancreas in infancy. Surgery *36*:146, 1954.

Montgomery, R. C., Poindexter, M. H., Hall, G., and Leigh, J. E.: Report of a case of annular pancreas of the newborn in two consecutive siblings. Pediatrics, *48*:148, 1971.

Patton, E. F.: Congenital hypertrophic stenosis of the duodenum. J. Pediatr. *32*:301, 1948.

Potts, W. J.: The Surgeon and the Child. Philadelphia, W. B. Saunders Company, 1959.

Prouty, M., and Waskow, W. L.: Duodenal compression by the mesenteric artery. J. Pediatr. *50*:734, 1957.

Rickham, P. P.: Annular pancreas in the newborn. Arch. Dis. Child. *29*:80, 1954.

Silverman, F. N., and Caffey, J.: Congenital obstructions of the alimentary tract in infants and children: Errors of rotation of the midgut. Radiology 53:780, 1949.

Small, W. T., and Berman, C. Z.: Annular pancreas producing obstruction in infancy. New Engl. J. Med. *251*:191, 1954.

# 37

# ACQUIRED INTESTINAL OBSTRUCTION

## INTUSSUSCEPTION

Intussusception is the invagination of one loop of bowel into a loop distal to it. The proximal segment, the intussusceptum, enters the distal portion, the intussuscipiens, as the tip of a glove finger may be inverted and pushed inside out up the length of the finger. The intussusceptum then travels down the bowel for a variable distance, at times reaching and even extruding from the anus. Intussusceptions usually originate in the ileum, though they may take off from the jejunum or the colon. Their danger lies only partially in the obstruction they produce. More important is intestinal gangrene from compression of the blood vessels that are carried along with the intussusceptum.

**INCIDENCE.** Although intussusception is a common cause of intestinal obstruction in infants, mostly male, 6 to 18 months old, it is exceedingly rare in the first month of life. Rachelson et al. (1955) were able to find reports of only 28 cases in newborns in the past 150 years. Our own experience has been limited to two cases.

**ETIOLOGY.** An obvious lead point is discovered in 6 to 8 per cent of all cases in most series; much less commonly in infants than in children and adults. These consist of Meckel's diverticula, polyps, intraluminal cysts, duplications and foci of lymphoid hyperplasia. A number of investigators have found an adenovirus in cultures from infants with intussusception much more often than from controls, and they postulate lymphoid hyperplasia as the trigger lead point. For the remainder no good reason has been advanced.

**DIAGNOSIS.** The cardinal symptoms of intussusception in infants are intermittent vomiting, accompanied by evidences of abdominal pain, a non-distended abdomen with a mass, usually in the right lower quadrant, and the passage of blood or blood-stained mucus per rectum. In the newborn, diagnosis is not so easy.

Talwalker, in 1962, reviewed painstakingly the case histories of 16 newborns with intussusception reported in the British literature and nine more unreported cases from English hospitals, and added one of his own. Vomiting and blood in the stools were almost always, but by no means always, present, while pain and palpable mass were almost always missing. Eight of 26 arose in the jejunum, an unusually high proportion of jejunals to ileocecals (see Tables 37–1 to 37–4).

X-ray study, in the newborn as in the older infant, reveals a characteristic picture. Flat films show the usual evidences of obstruction in the form of dilated loops of small intestine above and relative airlessness below the level of obstruction. Barium enema shows the column of opaque fluid to end in a meniscus, with a corkscrew pattern extending just proximal to the meniscus.

**PROGNOSIS.** Most of the reported patients died. This unfortunate result has often been due to the fact that the classic signs of intussusception have not all been present. The realization that this is the usual state of affairs in the newborn would without doubt lead to a greater awareness of the possibility, hence to more vigorous diagnostic efforts and probably to a higher percentage of cure. *The passage by a newborn of blood or blood-stained mucus, without discoverable cause in the anus or rectum, calls for proctoscopic inspection and a barium enema study.*

**TREATMENT.** Rarely a case may go on to spontaneous cure by sloughing of the entire intussusception and autoanastomosis. In the case of Rachelson et al. sloughing took place, and the gangrenous mass of inverted bowel was passed by rectum after nothing more than a few hours of anorexia! In this instance autoanastomosis did not follow, and anastomosis had to be accomplished later operatively.

The treatment of choice is operation after attempted reduction of the intussusception by hydrostatic pressure of a barium mixture

**TABLE 37–2. Intussusception — Symptoms (Continued)**

| Age at First Symptom | Number |
| --- | --- |
| Up to 48 hours | 15 |
| Up to 1 week | 5 |
| Up to 1 month | 4 |
| Total | 24 |
| Died soon after birth | 1 |
| Unusual presentation | 1 |

under the fluoroscope. Barium enema reduction alone is successful in a large number of cases occurring in older infants, but in infants less than 6 months old it is often unsuccessful. Zachary compiled some interesting figures apropos of this problem. The percentage of cure by barium enema was not high in the younger babies. Nevertheless the partial reduction obtained by hydrostatic pressure is useful in that it renders the subsequent operative procedure less traumatic, since much less "milking" of the bowel is required before reduction is accomplished. Talwalker's results with reduction in newborns were by no means bad. Unfortunately the authors of some of the largest recent reviews, such as Gierup et al., who report hydrostatic reduction successful in 81 per cent of 319 attempts — 85 per cent if done within 12 hours of onset — do not separate newborns from other infants and children.

Hayes and Gwinn have recalled to our attention the hazards of delay in arriving at the correct diagnosis, and remind us that *barium enema under fluoroscopy for diagnosis and possible reduction is not permissible as an office procedure.*

## PERITONEAL ADHESIONS

Obstruction may follow the development of adhesions between one hollow viscus

**TABLE 37–1. Intussusception — Symptoms**

| Symptom | Recorded | Not Present | No Mention |
| --- | --- | --- | --- |
| Vomiting | 20 | 2 | 1 |
| As first symptom | 14 | | |
| Bile staining | 9 | | |
| Blood in stools | 17 | 2 | 4 |
| As first symptom | 11 | | |
| Screaming | 5 | | |
| As first symptom | 4 | | |
| As only symptom | 1 | | |
| Mass felt per rectum | 2 | | |
| Mass felt abdominally | 4 | | |

Symptoms have not been recorded in three cases.

**TABLE 37–3. Intussusception — Treatment**

| | Total | Alive | Dead |
| --- | --- | --- | --- |
| Resection | 12 | 6 | 6 |
| Reduction | 10 | 7 | 3 |

*TABLE 37–4.   Intussusception – Types*°

| Type of Intussusception | Number | Method of Treatment | | | Causative Lesion |
|---|---|---|---|---|---|
| | | Reduction | Resection | None | |
| Ileocecal | 12 | 6 | 3 | 3 | 1 |
| Jejunal | 8 | 2 | 6 | – | 4 |
| Ileal | 3 | 2 | 1 | – | 1 |
| Colic | 1 | – | 1 | – | – |
| Site not mentioned | 2 | | | | |

°Tables 37–1 through 37–4 modified from Talwalker, Y. C.: Arch. Dis. Childhood. 37:203, 1962.

and another as a result of healed peritonitis of any kind. Inflammation may have resulted from bacterial infection, chemical irritation, such as bile peritonitis, or mechanical irritation, such as talc peritonitis. This variety of intestinal obstruction requires no further comment.

## MESENTERIC THROMBOSIS

Thrombosis of the mesenteric veins has been a well-recognized entity in adults since the forties. Pathologists have called our attention to mesenteric arterial thrombosis, most often involving the superior mesenteric artery, for almost as long. In the newborn we encounter both: the venous form almost always secondary to abdominal inflammatory disease, perhaps with dehydration, shock and increased blood viscosity playing a role; and the arterial form to emboli, either septic or non-septic, perhaps arising in the contracting ductus arteriosus. In the past decade this syndrome has surely been initiated by umbilical artery catheterization, a complication found not infrequently by both Kitterman and his associates and Neal and his. Fortunately only a few of these become symptomatic.

In 1953 Rothschild, Storch and Meyers reported a case of intestinal obstruction due to mesenteric artery occlusion in a newborn in which no lesion was found that could have initiated the process. The child was born by the breech at term. His condition was precarious during the first day, with flaccidity, cyanosis and subnormal temperature, gallop rhythm and enlarged heart. He improved for a few days, but on the fifth day began to vomit, and progressive jaundice and increasing distention de-

veloped. Barium meal series was interpreted as showing multiple obstructions, and laparotomy was performed. The peritoneal cavity contained much greenish fluid. Most of the small bowel was gangrenous with scattered areas of plastic exudate. No peristalsis was seen, and no arterial pulsation could be felt in the mesentery. The superior mesenteric artery was found after death to contain a tight thrombus formed before death.

The authors comment that the slow development of intestinal obstruction after a preliminary period of "looking sick" is characteristic of this condition. Blood in stools and bile-stained vomitus appear late, and distention is the final event.

It is difficult to pinpoint the exact cause of the superior mesenteric artery thrombosis. Possibly the breech delivery was responsible for "the precarious condition" after birth. The "progressive jaundice" suggested sepsis, but the authors do not report either antemortem or postmortem blood cultures.

Case 37–1

A white female infant was admitted to the Harriet Lane Home at 5 weeks of age. She had been born at home after an uneventful pregnancy and labor. Birth weight was 7 pounds 4 ounces (3290 gm). At 1 month, having been apparently well until then, she "got a cold," then began to refuse feedings and to vomit. Vomitus soon became yellow-green. Stools were normal, and there was no fever. Two days before admission, vomiting became almost incessant and changed to a coffee-ground appearance. This day she passed four loose reddish-brown stools. On the day of admission two tarry stools were passed. On examination she was acutely ill, dehydrated and acidotic, with a continuous weak cry. She regurgitated fecal vomitus continuously and during the examination passed two small currant-jelly stools. Breath sounds were suppressed at the right base, and here a few crackling rales were heard. The abdomen was distended and tense. No masses were felt. No x-ray studies were made, but after fluids had been administered intravenously for 6 hours she was operated upon. The peritoneum contained much brownish exudate which proved to be sterile on culture. The entire small bowel from the ligament of Treitz to the ileocecal valve was seen to be gangrenous, the mesenteric vessels thrombosed. An orange-sized cyst was discovered in the left side of the abdomen between the base of the mesentery and the descending colon. The cyst lay within the mesentery itself. It was excised. Microscopic examination showed its enterogenous structure. The infant did poorly and died on the third postoperative day.

**COMMENT.** The sequence of events in this case is difficult to understand. It must be assumed that in some way the presence of the duplication initiated mesenteric thrombosis, which in turn was responsible for intestinal gangrene. Possibly an antemortem vascular accident was responsible for both the duplication cyst and some defect in the mesentery and its vascular supply.

In a fascinating clinical-pathological conference, Oppenheimer and Avery discussed the case of a macrosomic infant with cyanosis from birth, who deteriorated suddenly on the twelfth day when she developed distention and evidences of intestinal obstruction. The final diagnoses were transposition of the great vessels, polycythemia and dehydration, and finally renal vein thrombosis and embolic thrombosis of the left iliac and small mesenteric arteries. The discussants pointed out that venous thrombosis in newborns is much more common in infants of diabetic than of non-diabetic mothers, and in infants with cyanotic heart disease. The mesentery artery thrombosis they attributed to emboli reaching visceral arteries instead of lungs because of the transposition.

## OBSTRUCTION DUE TO INSPISSATED FECES

Rack and Crouch reported the case of a premature in which obstruction developed

on the ninth day of life. Ultimately at operation the entire colon was found to be filled with a stony hard cast of inspissated stool. Constipation in prematures is not uncommon, and we are inclined to use saline enemas early when it does appear in them. It may be due simply to hypotonic abdominal and bowel musculature.

## PARALYTIC ILEUS DUE TO HEXAMETHONIUM BROMIDE

Hallum and Hatchuel described paralytic ileus in a premature infant whose mother had received hexamethonium bromide for toxemia.

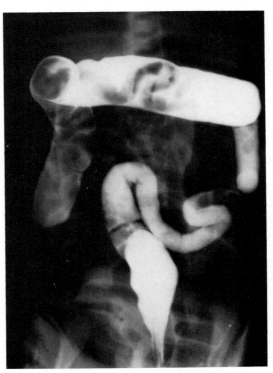

*Figure 37–1.* This case is not abstracted in the text. After a 6-cm long tenacious plug of firm mucus had been dislodged by saline enema on the second day of life, symptoms persisted. Shortly thereafter a barium enema was given which showed under the fluoroscope another obstructing plug at the splenic flexure. By the time the film was taken this plug had been dislodged by hydrostatic pressure and can be seen in the middle of the transverse colon. (We are indebted to Dr. Beryl J. Rosenstein for the summary and x-ray film of this case.)

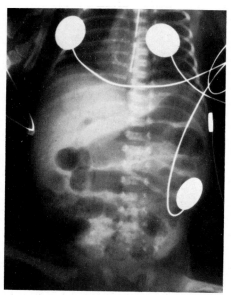

*Figure 37-2.* Abdominal distention and lethargy were noted in this 1200-gm infant 2 days after oral feedings were begun. Note thickness of the bowel wall and gas that has dissected into the biliary tract. Some gas is evident in the bowel wall (pneumatosis intestinalis).

## NECROTIZING ENTEROCOLITIS

Although undoubtedly enterocolitis has for many years been a sporadic problem among infants of low birth weight in particular, the larger number of prematurely born infants now surviving has increased the numbers of infants with this condition. In earlier editions of this book we spoke of enteritis with pseudomonas infection, which surely was one illustration of a larger spectrum of a disorder that has more recently been called necrotizing enterocolitis.

**ETIOLOGY.** Although the etiology remains uncertain, predisposing events include birth asphyxia, hypotension, respiratory distress, umbilical vessel catheterization, and patent ductus arteriosus: none of these conditions need be present. Early feeding of hyperosmolar formulas, particularly cow's milk, has been implicated, although the condition has been seen in infants fed only human milk.

**PATHOLOGY.** Affected areas of mucosal ulceration occur most often in the ileum or proximal colon. Perforation may occur, with gas (usually hydrogen) dissecting under the submucosa to give the radiographic picture of pneumatosis intestinalis (Fig. 37-2).

Thrombi of major vessels may or may not be present.

**DIAGNOSIS.** Infants under 1250 gm are most at risk. The disease usually presents soon after the initiation of oral feedings on the third to fifth day of life, but sometimes as late as the fourth week. Early signs are nonspecific, with temperature instability, lethargy, vomiting, apnea, and usually abdominal distention and ileus. Stools may be bloody but diarrhea is not usually present. Frequent radiographs facilitate diagnosis; pneumatosis intestinalis is present in about 80 per cent of reported cases.

**TREATMENT.** Oral feedings should be discontinued, and parenteral alimentation begun. Cultures of blood and stools are taken, and parenteral antibiotics are given as indicated. If perforation occurs, laparotomy, and sometimes bowel resection, is required. In some infants strictures occur at 2 to 3 weeks of age.

**PROGNOSIS.** With early recognition the disease is less than 20 per cent fatal. If medical management fails and resection is required, the mortality approaches 50 per cent.

## REFERENCES

Barlow, B., Santulli, T. V., et al.: An experimental study of acute neonatal enterocolitis. The importance of breast milk. J. Pediat. Surg. 9:587, 1974.

Book, L. S., Herbst, J. J., and Jung, A. L.: Carbohydrate malabsorption in necrotizing enterocolitis. Pediatrics 57:201–204, 1976.

Case Records of the Massachusetts General Hospital. Case 45–1973. N. Engl. J. Med. 289:1027, 1973.

Clark, E. J., Phillips, I. A., and Alexander, E. P.: Adenovirus infection in intussusception in children in Taiwan. J.A.M.A. 208:1671, 1969.

Clatworthy, H. W., Jr., Howard, W. H. R., and Lloyd, J.: The meconium plug syndrome. Surgery 39:131, 1956.

Danis, R. K.: Surgical Hazards with Hydrogen Peroxide. Presented at the Thirty-fifth Annual Meeting of the American Academy of Pediatrics, Surgical Section, Oct. 23, 1966.

Emery, J. L.: Abnormalities in meconium of the foetus and newborn. Arch. Dis. Child. 32:17, 1957.

Frantz, I. D., L'Heureux, P., Engel, R. R., and Hunt, C. E.: Necrotizing enterocolitis. J. Pediat. 86:259–263, 1975.

Gierup, J., Jorulf, H., and Livaditis, A.: Management of intussusception in infants and children: A survey based on 288 consecutive cases. Pediatrics 50:535, 1972.

Hallum, J. L., and Hatchuel, W. L. F.: Congenital paralytic ileus in a premature baby as a complication of hexamethonium bromide therapy for toxaemia of pregnancy. Arch. Dis. Child. *29*:354, 1954.

Hayes, D. M., and Gwinn, J. L.: The changing face of intussusception. J.A.M.A. *195*:817, 1966.

Hinden, E.: Meconium ileus with no pancreatic abnormality. Arch. Dis. Child. *25*:99, 1950.

Kitterman, J. A., Phibbs, R. H., and Tooley, W. H.: Pediatr. Clin. N. Amer. *17*:895, 1970.

Mayell, M. J.: Intussusception in infancy and childhood in Southern Africa. Arch. Dis. Child. *47*:20, 1972.

Neal, W. A., Reynolds, J. W., et al.: Umbilical artery catheterization: Demonstration of arterial thrombosis by aortography. Pediatrics *50*:6, 1972.

Necrotizing Enterocolitis in the Newborn Infant. Report of the Sixty-Eighth Ross Conference on Pediatric Research, Moore, T. D., ed. Columbus, Ohio, Ross Laboratories, 1975.

Oppenheimer, E. H., and Avery, M. E.: Clinical-pathological conference. J. Pediatr. *73*:143, 1968.

Prouty, M., Bruskewitz, H. W., and Schwei, G. P.: Intussusception in a newborn infant. J. Pediatr. *34*:487, 1949.

Rachelson, M. H., Jernigan, J. P., and Jackson, W. F.: Intussusception in the newborn infant with spontaneous expulsion of the intussusceptum. J. Pediatr. *47*:87, 1955.

Rack, F. J., and Crouch, W. L.: Functional intestinal obstruction in the premature newborn infant. J. Pediatr. *40*:579, 1952.

Rothschild, H. B., Storch, A., and Meyers, B.: Mesenteric occlusion in a newborn infant. J. Pediatr. *43*:569, 1953.

Rowe, M. I., Copelson, L. W., and Clatworthy, H. W., Jr.: The patent processus vaginalis and the inguinal hernia. J. Ped. Surg. *4*:102, 1969.

Schaffer, A. J., and Oppenheimer, E. H.: Pseudomonas (Pyocyaneus) infection of the gastrointestinal tract of infants and children. South. M.J. *41*:460, 1948.

Talwalker, V. C.: Intussusception in the newborn. Arch. Dis. Child. *37*:203, 1962.

Zachary, R. B.: Acute intussusception in childhood. Arch. Dis. Child. *30*:32, 1955.

Zachary, R. B.: Meconium and faecal plugs in the newborn. Arch. Dis. Child. *32*:22, 1957.

# INTESTINAL OBSTRUCTION DUE TO DEFECTIVE INNERVATION

# 38

## HIRSCHSPRUNG'S DISEASE (CONGENITAL MEGACOLON, CONGENITAL AGANGLIONOSIS)

The etiology of Hirschsprung's disease has been reviewed briefly on page 356. The pathologic criterion, as well as the cause of constipation by virtue of its effect upon orderly peristalsis, is absence of ganglion cells of the plexus of Auerbach in a segment of the large bowel. Passarge's data indicate that in some examples there is a strong familial incidence of aganglionosis, and that in other families other major defects, chiefly Down's syndrome, appear in excess, but that in most neither genic nor chromosomal factors are discoverable.

**INCIDENCE.** Congenital aganglionosis is one of the less common causes of neonatal intestinal obstruction, but is by no means an extreme rarity. Between 1950 and 1960 Kottmeier and Clatworthy found that 41 such patients had been admitted to one hospital, all proved by biopsy, of which 85

per cent had become symptomatic within the first week of life. Forty-five per cent were admitted to the hospital for the first time before the age of 3 months.

**DIAGNOSIS.** Vomiting, distention and constipation are the usual presenting signs. Diarrhea is prominent in about one fifth of all cases; it may be intermittent, alternating with periods of constipation, or constant, with no constipation whatever, or in the form of severe, often lethal enterocolitis.

Vomiting often begins on the first day but may be delayed until the third day or later. Distention may reach an advanced stage, accompanied by intestinal patterning. Meconium stools are usually passed for a variable number of days before constipation appears and becomes obdurate.

A characteristic story is that signs of obstruction develop and are relieved by enema. Thereafter the infant may be symptom-free for a period as short as a week or as long as 10 weeks, when vomiting, distention and constipation recur.

This cycle may be repeated a number of times until the clinical and roentgenologic picture becomes typically that of Hirschsprung's disease.

**CONFIRMATORY EVIDENCE.** Radiographic study early shows distended loops, throughout the abdomen, of both small and large bowel. In the erect posture numerous fluid levels may be seen. Often no point of obstruction can be distinguished. Barium enema fluid flows in freely and outlines a normal or slightly dilated rectosigmoid and colon. Only rarely in the first days or weeks of life does one see the characteristic narrowed rectosigmoid segment distal to a slightly dilated sigmoid segment, or the so-called pathognomonic "pigtail" sign. In Ehrenpreis' experience the typical caliber differential did not become apparent until 3 or 4 weeks of age in most, and until 8 or 9 months in some.

Highly suggestive in the first weeks, however, is the demonstration that barium remains in the lower bowel for 24 hours or more.

Kottmeier and Clatworthy correctly warn us not to accept the radiologic evidence of caliber differential as an absolute indication for operation. In their own experience several infants were operated upon mistakenly on that indication alone. In all of them resected bowel showed an abundance of ganglion cells.

The only certain method for the diagnosis of Hirschsprung's disease until recently has been the demonstration of absence of ganglion cells in a deep-muscle biopsy specimen of the rectum. But this technique too is subject to misinterpretation for a variety of reasons. Finding ganglion cells assures one that aganglionosis cannot be the correct diagnosis, but not seeing them may be a matter of too superficial a specimen, poor staining or some other error.

For this reason Tobon et al. have devised a comparatively simple manometric technique which graphically depicts the response of the internal sphincter to transient distention of the rectum by an inserted balloon. In the normal this sphincter relaxes after such distention; in Hirschsprung's disease it contracts. In so-called "functional constipation" resulting in

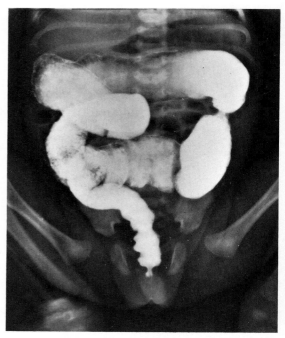

***Figure 38–1.*** Film to show rectosigmoid narrowing and dilatation of colon above. Anorexia and vomiting began in this infant at 1 day of age; he was in hospital 10 days and went home apparently well. He was at home for 5 days, during which he was anorexic and passed no stool whatever. No stool was found in the rectum, and the barium enema film taken on the thirtieth day of life is shown above. A Swenson procedure was done. He died on the fifty-fourth day of severe ileocolitis, a not uncommon complication of this disease.

"idiopathic megacolon" the sphincteric responses are absolutely normal. The authors believe that this test will supplant rectal biopsy as the definitive differentiating study between aganglionosis and the other poorly understood causes of severe constipation in infancy and childhood.

When aganglionosis involves proximal segments of the colon or the small intestine, the diagnosis is even more difficult. In these instances it will depend almost entirely upon the pathologic picture of biopsied or autopsied intestine. Total bowel aganglionosis can occur. Vomitus containing stool or barium from a barium enema makes the diagnosis probable. A fatal outcome is inevitable.

Stockdale and Miller reported two cases

in which recurrent diarrhea was the only symptom, while constipation, until then considered the pathognomonic sign, was absent and distention was minimal in one, moderate in the other. This observation probably demands that we biopsy the rectums of infants with severe recurrent diarrhea after all other causes have been ruled out.

**TREATMENT.** Definitive treatment of Hirschsprung's disease is operative. For a number of years after Swenson perfected the pull-through operation this was the only procedure used. Objections were then raised against it in view of persistent fecal incontinence, disturbances in bladder emptying and urinary incontinence in some of the survivors. The State operation, an end-to-end anastomosis of colon from above the aganglionic segment to the upper portion of the rectum, and the Duhamel operation, which bypasses the rectum, but leaves it in situ, were offered as substitutes. Many reports suggest superiority for the last. The Soave procedure involves excision of the rectal mucosa, with suturing of proximal normal bowel to the denuded rectum.

Most pediatric surgeons are loath to perform definitive repair until the infant has reached the age of 8 months or more, preferring to temporize by performing a colostomy.

An explosive form of enterocolitis may complicate the course of Hirschsprung's disease at any time, even after an apparently successful operation. It is often of such severity that fluid and electrolyte loss causes death within 24 hours. Its exact cause is unknown, but most agree with Swenson that the basic trouble is obstruction. In addition to rapid intravenous replacement therapy, rectal tubes and colonic irrigations must be used to empty the bowel. If these are unsuccessful, colostomy, perhaps even internal sphincterotomy, may be required to relieve obstruction and put an end to the diarrhea (Nixon).

# REFERENCES

Campbell, P. E., and Noblett, H. R.: Experience with rectal suction biopsy in the diagnosis of Hirschsprung's disease. J. Pediatr. Surg. 4:410, 1969.

Duhamel, B.: A new operation for the treatment of Hirschsprung's disease. Arch. Dis. Child. 35:38, 1960.

Ehrenpreis, T.: Hirschsprung's disease in the neonatal period. Arch. Dis. Child. 30:8, 1955.

Hiatt, R. B.: A further description of the pathologic physiology of congenital megacolon and the results of surgical treatment. Pediatrics 21:825, 1958.

Kostia, J.: Results of treatment in Hirschsprung's disease. Arch. Dis. Child. 37:167, 1962.

Kottmeier, R. K., and Clatworthy, H. W., Jr.: Aganglionic and functional megacolon in children: A diagnostic dilemma. Pediatrics 36:572, 1965.

Martin, L. W.: Surgical management of total colonic aganglionosis. Ann. Surg. 176:343, 1972.

McDonald, R. G., and Evans, W. A., Jr.: Hirschsprung's disease: Roentgen diagnosis. A.M.A. J. Dis. Child. 87:575, 1954.

Nixon, H. H.: Review article: Hirschsprung's disease. Arch. Dis. Child. 39:109, 1964.

Passarge, E.: The genetics of Hirschsprung's disease. New Engl. J. Med. 276:138, 1967.

Potts, W. J., Boggs, J. D., and White, H.: Intestinal obstruction in the newborn infant due to agenesis of the myenteric plexus (congenital megacolon). Pediatrics 10:253, 1952.

Rehbein, F., and von Zimmermann, H.: Results with abdominal resection in Hirschsprung's disease. Arch. Dis. Child. 35:29, 1960.

Santulli, T. V.: Intestinal obstruction in the newborn. Bull. New York Acad. Med. 33:175, 1957.

Soave, F.: Surgery of rectal anomalies with preservation of the relationship between the colonic muscular sleeve and the puborectalis muscle. J. Pediatr. Surg. 4:705, 1969.

Soper, R. T., and Figueroa, P.: Surgical treatment of Hirschsprung's disease: Comparison of modifications of the Duhamel and Soave operations. J. Pediatr. Surg. 6:761, 1971.

Stockdale, E. M., and Miller, C. A.: Persistent diarrhea as the predominant symptom of Hirschsprung's disease (congenital dilatation of the colon); Report of two cases. Pediatrics 19:91, 1957.

Swenson, O.: Congenital megacolon (Hirschsprung's disease); follow-up on eighty-two patients treated surgically. Pediatrics 8:542, 1951.

Tobon, F., Reid, N. C. R. W., Talbert, J. L., and Schuster, M. M.: Non-surgical test for the diagnosis of Hirschsprung's disease. New Engl. J. Med. 278:188, 1968.

Tobon F., and Shuster, M. M.: Megacolon: Special diagnostic and therapeutic features. Hopkins Med. J. 135:91, 1974.

# 39

# DISORDERS OF THE UMBILICUS

## GENERAL CONSIDERATIONS

The umbilical cord is a structure of the utmost importance to the fetus, serving as the sole channel bringing oxygen and nutriment to it and carrying from it carbon dioxide and waste products. Any accident that diminishes blood flow through this channel constitutes a grave hazard to the life or health of the fetus or newborn infant.

The prime danger in this regard is compression of the cord. This may take place when the cord, instead of floating freely within the amniotic fluid, becomes wrapped around the body, an extremity or the neck of the fetus. It may also follow when the cord is delivered before the baby; that is, in cases of prolapse of the cord. We must hastily point out the fact that looping about some portion of the fetus or being prolapsed does not necessarily mean that blood flow is impeded. In only a minority of these instances is looping so tight or is the prolapsed cord wedged so firmly between a fetal part and a bony prominence that true compression results. When it does, the obstetrician may note that the prolapsed portion, or the cord distal to a tight loop, is pulseless. The effects of such asphyxia upon the brain and respiratory system of the newborn infant have been discussed in other sections. One might add here that a tight loop about the neck jeopardizes the fetus no more than one about the wrist if blood flow is completely obstructed. If less tight, it is conceivable that a loop about the neck might obstruct venous return, while arterial flow is not diminished. Venous congestion, petechial hemorrhages and edema of the brain might be expected to follow, and this would have greater significance than similar congestive alterations in an extremity.

The second dangerous accident to the newborn is that the cord may tear during delivery. This hazard is discussed under Posthemorrhagic Anemia (p. 601). Other reasons for bleeding from the cord are treated in the same section.

The umbilical region is an extremely busy locale during embryonic life. Originally the widely open communication between the yolk sac and primitive gut, it ends up as a narrow aperture through which course the umbilical artery and vein, the vitelline duct and the urachus. In the interim the entire midgut has passed through it into a large physiologic umbilical hernia, has remained there some weeks and has ultimately returned to take up its proper position within the abdominal cavity.

After birth the umbilical arteries contract strongly, blood flow ceases and their lumens become narrow. Persistent pulsations, when they occur, are usually associated with hypoxia. Their intimal and medial layers undergo aseptic necrosis, the stump separates and granulation tissue develops and is quickly covered with epithelium.

It is our practice to ask the obstetricians to note the number of umbilical arteries on the page of information that accompanies each infant to the nursery, since the cord may dry quickly and make later identification uncertain. The condition occurs in about 1 per cent of single births and 7 per cent of twin births. Associated abnormalities occur in about one third of the infants and include all systems, but gastrointestinal obstructive lesions are among the most common. The question remains as to what the pediatrician does once a single artery is noted. A meticulous search for all possible congenital defects is indicated, with particular care to palpate the kidneys at a time when the infant is relaxed and the stomach not distended. At least one urinalysis is mandatory. Whether intravenous pyelography or cinecystourethrograms are indicated to search for associated urinary tract abnormalities is debatable, since one

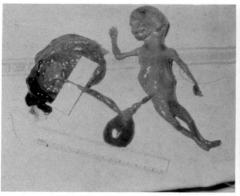
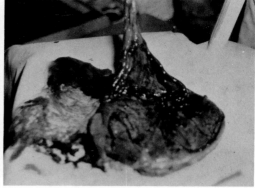

Fig. 39–1                         Fig. 39–2

*Figure 39–1.* Stillborn infant with umbilical cord and placenta attached. The cord is looped and is obstructed at the point of closure of the loop. The fetus is maldeveloped and macerated as a result.

*Figure 39–2.* Umbilical cord and placenta, showing the former's insertion into the latter after having divided into a number of fine branches. These branches in such a velamentous insertion are liable to be torn during delivery.

weighs the chances of discovering a significant treatable lesion against the hazards of irradiation to the gonads. Instances have been reported in which genitourinary anomalies have been discovered by pyelography on the sole indication of a single umbilical artery. Our preference is to examine carefully and follow the urine of such infants monthly, and defer roentgenographic studies until some other finding suggests urinary tract disease.

**CLASSIFICATION.** A large number of developmental errors may lead to imperfections in the umbilical region at the time of birth, and the umbilicus is liable to other postnatal disorders. These will be discussed in following order: 1) infection of the umbilicus, 2) septic umbilical arteritis, 3) granuloma of the umbilicus, 4) umbilical stomach, 5) omphalocele, 6) umbilical hernia, 7) congenital malformations of the vitelline (omphalomesenteric) duct, 8) congenital malformations of the urachus and 9) single umbilical artery.

## INFECTION OF THE UMBILICUS

We have become accustomed in this aseptic age to consider umbilical infection one of the archaic diseases which have virtually disappeared. Any practicing pediatrician can vouch for the fact that this is not true. Serous, purulent or sanguineous drainage from the umbilicus for a number

of days after the cord has separated is still a common complaint. Furthermore, clinically silent omphalitis and umbilical phlebitis and, more rarely, septic umbilical arteritis may be found after death to have served as portals of entry for sepsis of the newborn.

Tetanus neonatorum, having its origin in contamination of the cord stump, is still a great problem in primitive societies, but is encountered more and more rarely in medically sophisticated communities. This is discussed elsewhere (p. 802).

**DIAGNOSIS.** Omphalitis manifests itself by drainage from the umbilical stump or from its base at its point of attachment to the abdominal wall or from the navel after the cord has separated. Secretions may be thin and serous, sanguineous or frankly purulent. They must be differentiated carefully from the serous secretions of vitelline duct remnants or the urinous discharge of urachal remnants, and from the serous or serosanguineous discharge from umbilical papilloma. At times they are foul-smelling. Infection may remain restricted to the cord or may spread to involve the surrounding skin. Periumbilical redness and induration result, but true erysipelas, common a generation ago, is a rare sequel today.

**TREATMENT.** Simple omphalitis, without evidences of periumbilical spread, responds readily to local application of antibiotic compresses or ointments. Bacitracin and neomycin, or a combination of these, are the local antibiotics of choice. Oral or

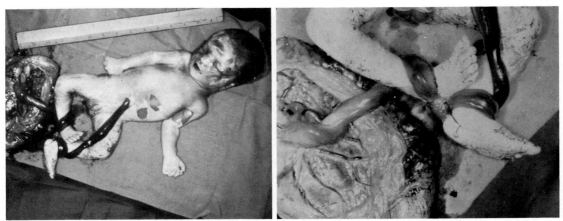

***Figure 39–3.*** All-over and close-up view of a lethal cord entanglement about the extremities of a stillborn fetus.

parenteral antibiotic medication is indicated if the discharge is frankly purulent or if any evidence of periumbilical spread appears. The hazards of generalized sepsis and metastatic infection of bone or lung, inter alia, must not be overlooked. Final choice of antibiotic will depend upon culture and sensitivity tests.

## SEPTIC UMBILICAL ARTERITIS

Forshall recalled to our attention this disorder, which was common at the turn of the century, but which is now comparatively rare. She pointed out that several clinical pictures may ensue from infection of the umbilical artery. Bacteria may invade, lie latent in or spread along the lumen, the inner necrosing coats or the mantle of loose connective tissue of the artery. Thereafter one of several courses may be followed. If both the iliac and abdominal ends are sealed, the infection remains localized and carries with it the implications of any septic focus. If the artery remains patent externally, the umbilicus drains purulent material. If the mantle zone becomes involved, spread from this region leads to peritonitis. Or infection may track along the course of the artery to point as an abscess in the scrotum or thigh. If the iliac end of the umbilical artery

remains patent, swarms of bacteria may be discharged into the blood stream to lead to rapidly fatal septicemia.

The etiology, pathogenesis and clinical course can best be illustrated by several case histories. Those that follow are taken from Forshall with the permission of the author.

### CASE HISTORIES

#### CASE 39–1

A white male infant whose early history is not known began to have purulent umbilical discharge at or before the age of 5 weeks. At 7 weeks he became fretful and anorexic and began to vomit. Within 36 hours of the onset he was very ill, pallid, with grunting respirations, in apparent shock. His abdomen was distended and tympanitic. A questionable mass and guarding were noted on the left side below the umbilicus. Peritonitis was suspected, laparotomy was done, and the abdomen was found to be full of seropurulent fluid. He died 48 hours later.

Autopsy showed a discharging but uninflamed umbilicus. The entire length of the left umbilical artery was swollen and full of blackish clot. There was a large, loculated periarterial abscess. *Staphylococcus pyogenes* was cultured from the arterial lumen, the abscess and the peritoneal exudate.

**COMMENT.** In this case the author believes that the mantle zone of the artery was infected in the immediate postnatal period. From here infection spread inward to invade the arterial lumen. By 5 weeks a large periarterial abscess had formed from which 1) pus was discharged through the umbilicus and 2) infection invaded the adjacent peritoneum. In this example the iliac end of the umbilical artery was closed.

CASE 39–2

A white male infant seemed well until the seventh day, when he began to bleed from the navel. On the ninth day he refused food and vomited, the vomitus containing blood. Admitted on the eleventh day, he was pale, collapsed and cold, obviously in shock. Petechiae were widespread, rales were heard throughout the lungs, and the abdomen was tightly distended. He died after eight hours in convulsion.

Autopsy showed no umbilical discharge, but the depths of the navel were purulent and hemorrhagic. *The umbilical arteries were patent throughout their length.* That part adjacent to the umbilicus was filled with black clot. Under the microscope the wall appeared normal, but masses of cocci were seen within the lumen. There was widespread periarteritis and early peritonitis. The lungs were solid with hemorrhagic pneumonitis. *Staphylococcus pyogenes* was found in the umbilicus and bronchial fluid.

**COMMENT.** Clearly the mantle zone was infected from birth, infection spreading to cause periarterial abscess and peritonitis. It also involved the lumen, and since the arteries were patent, masses of bacteria irrupted into the iliac artery and caused a virulent septicemia.

Another of Forshall's infants suffered a massive hemorrhage from the umbilicus at 21 days after having had a transient brownish discharge on the twelfth day. In this case iodized oil placed in the navel pooled in a cavity below and to its right. This proved to be an extraperitoneal pulsating mass, an aneurysm produced by weakening of the wall of the iliac artery by infection which had extended to it from the umbilical artery.

## GRANULOMA OF THE UMBILICUS

Serous or serosanguineous discharge from the umbilicus noted after the cord has separated suggests granuloma. If small, this can be seen only as a red button in the depths of the navel after it has been spread

open. Large ones project far out of the socket.

Granuloma must be differentiated from everted gastric or intestinal mucosa. The appearances may be remarkably similar. It has been pointed out that they have a different feel. When the tip of the finger is rubbed over a granuloma, the sensation is that of dry velvet, whereas mucous membrane feels velvety but moist, and a thin film of mucus comes away on the examining finger tip. More conclusive evidence is afforded by gentle probing. A granuloma is solid, but everted mucosa should permit the entrance of a fine probe at some point.

The *treatment* usually recommended is desiccation by silver nitrate. Performed with caution, this is satisfactory, but, since silver nitrate can burn normal skin, great care must be taken to touch only the granuloma with the point of the stick and to wash away the excess with moistened toothpick swabs after the application has been made.

## ABERRANT UMBILICAL STOMACH

In Cullen's monumental work on the normal and diseased umbilicus he comments that "several observers have reported mucosa at the umbilicus that more or less resembles gastric mucosa." He quotes Pillmans, who in 1882 observed "a 13 year old boy who exhibited a tumor the size of a walnut, bright red in color and covered with mucosa, present since birth. After he had eaten, the tumor would sometimes swell perceptibly, become redder, the mucosa thicker. A tenacious mucus was secreted, as much as 2 or 3 cc in 15 minutes. It was acid in reaction and digested fibrin at 39° C."

Wachter and Elman reported two cases of aberrant gastric mucosa at the umbilicus, present since birth, in white female infants 5 and 10 months old respectively. The first case presented an area of moist induration, 7 mm in diameter, surrounded by a partly cystic, partly solid mass about 5 by 5 cm. It drained clear fluid which was acid to blue litmus and congo red paper, and digested coagulated egg albumen. Removed in toto, the umbilical structure contained gastric mucosa. Their second case consisted simply of an indurated, reddened umbilicus which constantly drained an acid secretion. The authors point out that the diagnosis can be made at the bedside by a simple test proving that the discharge is acid.

It might be worth while to mention in passing that ectopic tissue of other varieties can be discovered in the umbilicus. For example, Harris and Wenzel have recently reported finding a small, spherical, firm red mass projecting from the surface of the cord 4 cm from the skin margin. This proved to be heterotopic pancreatic tissue plus intestinal mucosa.

### OMPHALOCELE (AMNIOCELE, EXOMPHALOS)

After the return of the midgut from the umbilical cord into the abdominal cavity by about the tenth week of gestation, the rectus muscles approach one another from above downward and close the larger circular defect originally present. At times this closure does not take place. Whether this is due to the circumstance that the abdominal cavity does not enlarge sufficiently to accept the returning bowel or whether for some reason the bowel does not re-enter, hence the muscular defect cannot close, is unknown.

Two types of exomphalos are now recognized, depending upon the time at which this failure of closure develops. If early, at about the third week of gestation, the defect is large and involves the midline from umbilicus cephalad, part or all of the way to the xiphoid process. This results in *omphalocele* or *amniocele* (Fig. 39–4). If later, at about the tenth week, the defect is smaller and is located at the umbilicus itself. This has been called *umbilical cord hernia* (Fig. 39–5). In both the protruding mass is covered by a thin transparent membrane composed of peritoneum and amnion. At times the membrane ruptures prior to and at other times during the delivery. In the latter case eviscerated intestine lies freely about the gaping hole in the abdominal wall (Fig. 39–7). This condition is called gastroschisis.

An important exception must be recorded to this statement as we originally wrote it. A *few hernias lie entirely within the base of the umbilical cord, are not obvious herniated masses covered by thin membrane, but are manifest only as swell-*

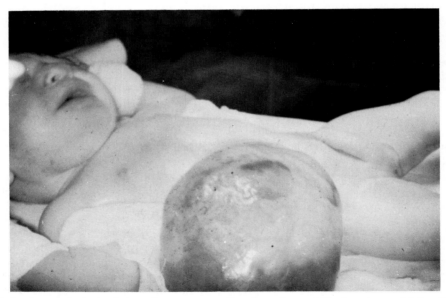

*Figure 39–4.* A grapefruit-sized mass is seen protruding from the umbilical region and lying limply on the abdomen. No specific structures can be identified without the mass in this photograph. It is covered by whitish, glistening membrane and is obviously an omphalocele.

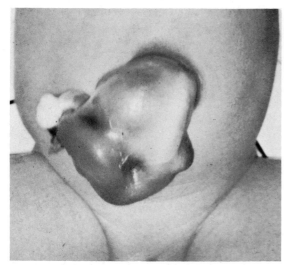

*Figure 39–5.* Showing a comparatively small mass protruding from the umbilical region. A loop of bowel can readily be recognized running around its lower margin. The mass is completely covered by shiny transparent membrane. This is clearly an "umbilical cord hernia."

*ings of the cord for a short distance from the skin margin.* Landor et al. have reported two cases in which such swellings were ignored and clamped, whereupon intestinal obstruction immediately ensued.

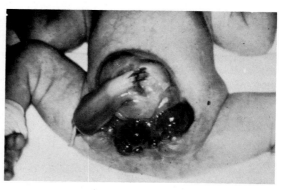

*Figure 39–6.* A combination of omphalocele and ectopia vesicae. The bright structure below the omphalocele is everted, exstrophic bladder.

One third to one half of all infants with exomphalos are born with other congenital defects. Many of these are local, examples being malrotation, Meckel's diverticulum and patent vitelline duct, but a good number involve the cardiovascular and other systems.

**DIAGNOSIS.** There is nothing that so closely resembles exomphalos that its diagnosis should be in doubt. The closest approximation to it would be patent omphalomesenteric duct with evagination of ileum. Here the protruding bowel is not

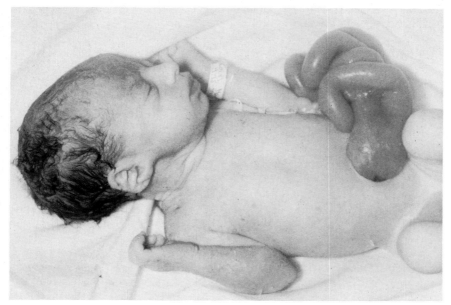

*Figure 39–7.* Omphalocele in which the containing amniotic-peritoneal membrane must have been torn away during delivery. Loops of bowel lie free upon the abdominal wall. (Case of Dr. Arnold Tramer of Baltimore, reprinted with his kind permission.)

covered by membrane. It consists only of one readily identifiable segment of small intestine, turned inside out, not of a mass of intestinal loops.

Small swellings of the umbilical cord near its attachment must be viewed with suspicion. They may be cysts of Wharton's jelly or hematomas or true hernias into the cord.

TREATMENT. Operative repair of small omphaloceles should be undertaken as soon as feasible. For larger lesions, usually over 6 cm in diameter, a plastic sheet is sewed around the edge of the defect. Steady pressure is applied over a matter of days to reduce the protrusion until surgical closure is possible. If surgery is contraindicated because of other lesions such as congenital heart disease, the sac may be painted with 1 to 4 per cent Mercurochrome to permit formation of a crust and protection from infection. Epithelialization will progress from the periphery inward, and will be complete in six to eight weeks. Surgery can then be deferred until the patient is several years of age.

PROGNOSIS. The prognosis is better for hernia into the cord than for omphalocele, although it is not bad when these latter are small. When they are large, and when they contain liver as well as intestine, the outlook is not good. In the latter situation an operative mortality rate of 60 per cent or more is to be expected. Even when these infants survive the primary closure, their general condition is precarious. The abdomen, protected by skin and a thin layer of subcutaneous tissue only, protrudes grotesquely, and their weight gain is slow. Many succumb to intercurrent infection or some other disorder before secondary closure can be attempted.

The outlook has improved with conservative and staged repairs to an overall survival of 70 per cent.

## GASTROSCHISIS

In this condition the abdominal contents are found floating in the amniotic liquid, presumably because of a defect in the abdominal wall lateral to the umbilicus. Occasionally they are edematous and matted; sometimes they are glistening as if only recently eviscerated.

TREATMENT. In about half the infants all the viscera can be returned to the abdomen. Intravenous alimentation may be required for some weeks before normal bowel function returns.

## UMBILICAL HERNIA

Umbilical hernia differs from omphalocele in that skin and subcutaneous tissue have covered the original defect, while separation of the rectus muscles has persisted.

DIAGNOSIS. Hernia is usually noted immediately after the cord has separated, although it may not attain its maximum size until the end of the first month or later. Umbilical hernias range in size from tiny ones as small as a marble to some as large as a grapefruit. The hernial aperture, located at or just above the umbilicus, may barely admit the tip of a finger or may measure 4 or 5 cm in diameter. The sac contains omentum alone or a loop of bowel from which a quantity of air can be squeezed back into the abdomen.

The diagnosis of umbilical hernias presents no difficulties. They should not be confused with ventral hernias, which appear in the midline at some point between the xiphoid and symphysis. These are protrusions, usually of omentum, through small defects in the linea alba, which seldom exceed the size of a pea.

TREATMENT. Small umbilical hernias may be left untreated, since their natural course is to close spontaneously within a few months to a year. We make an exception to this rule only in the case of infants who cry, cough or strain at stool excessively. When this is the case, or if hernias are of very large size, they should be taped firmly. We now prefer Scotch tape to adhesive, since it irritates the skin considerably less. Our own preference is for tight taping with three or four overlapping 2-inch strips extending from one lumbar region to the other over the inverted umbilicus to approximate the margins of the hernia.

Some umbilical hernias should be closed

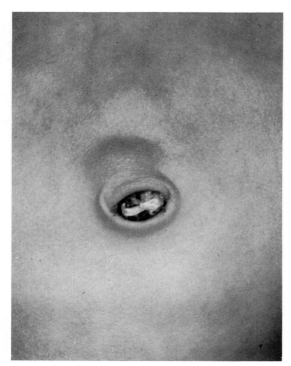

*Figure 39–8.* Two definite bulges are seen cephalad to the umbilicus, one above the other. Two distinct apertures could be felt in the midline. This represents a minor defect of the abdominal wall which was treated by taping.

surgically, but it is not easy to lay down arbitrary rules to designate exactly which ones. Large ones whose apertures measure 5 cm or more in diameter probably should be repaired early. Somewhat smaller ones

with apertures 2 to 5 cm across should be taped repeatedly and observed. If at the end of 6 to 8 months there has been no or little diminution in size, these too should be closed. Hernias smaller than 2 cm should never be operated upon unless they have not closed by the age of 4 years. There is room for wide difference of opinion in this matter.

## DEFECT OF ABDOMINAL WALL

Some herniations appear to be double or multiple, permitting omentum or bowel to protrude through more than one defect in the region of the umbilicus and above. These are not simple umbilical hernias, nor, since they are covered by skin, can they be termed omphaloceles. We call them, for want of a better name, defects of the abdominal wall. Figures 39–8 and 39–9 are of two infants with this defect. Treatment is surgical unless they are very small. In this event taping may be tried for a year or more and surgery resorted to only if there is no diminution in size.

## CAPUT MEDUSAE

Failure of fusion or obliteration of the abdominal portion of the umbilical vein early in fetal life demands enlargement of collateral umbilical vessels to carry oxygenated blood to the fetus. Prominent veins over

*Figure 39–9.* Large triangular herniation of and above the umbilicus. The bulge contained easily reducible bowel. A large aperture could be felt just above the umbilicus, and a second, smaller one several centimeters above it. Between them the rectus muscles were diastatic. This is a large defect of the abdominal wall demanding surgical closure.

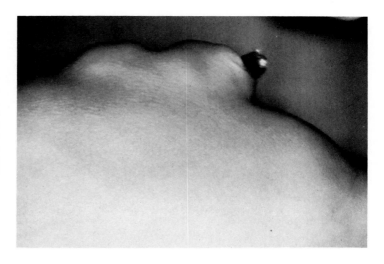

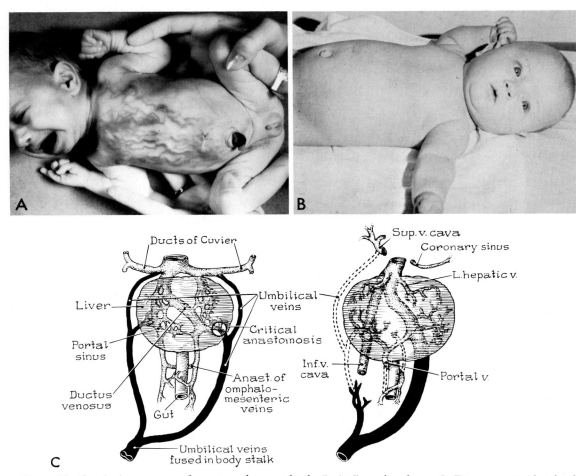

**Figure 39–10.**  *A,* Appearance of caput medusae at birth. *B,* At 5 weeks of age. *C,* Diagrammatic sketch of circulation through liver at time of birth.

the anterior abdominal wall, arranged spoke-like about the umbilicus, are striking at birth, and regress over the first weeks of life. White et al. published the only known instance of such an event in 1969. Their infant was only 2100 gm at term, but in all other respects was normal (Fig. 39–10).

## REFERENCES

Adams, F. H.: Omphalocele. J. Pediatr. 32:304, 1948.

Aitken, J.: Exomphalos: Analysis of a 10-year series of 32 cases. Arch. Dis. Child. 38:126, 1963.

Benirschke, K., and Bourne, G. L.: The incidence and diagnostic implication of congenital absence of one umbilical artery. Am. J. Obstet. Gynec. 79:251, 1960.

Benson, C. D., Penbirthy, G. C., and Hill, E. J.: Hernia into the umbilical cord and omphalocele (amniocele) in the newborn. Arch. Surg. 48:833, 1949.

Cullen, T. S.: Embryology, Anatomy and Diseases of the Umbilicus, Together with Diseases of the Urachus. Philadelphia, W. B. Saunders Company, 1916.

Cunningham, A. A.: Exomphalos. Arch. Dis. Child. 31:144, 1956.

Forshall, I.: Septic umbilical arteritis. Arch. Dis. Child. 32:25, 1957.

Grob, M.: Conservative treatment of exomphalos. Arch. Dis. Child. 38:148, 1963.

Gross, R. E.: The Surgery of Infancy and Childhood. Philadelphia, W. B. Saunders Company, 1953.

Gryboski, J.: Gastrointestinal Problems in the Infant. Philadelphia, W. B. Saunders Company, 1975.

Harris, L. E., and Wenzel, J. E.: Heterotopic pancreatic tissue and intestinal mucosa in the umbilical cord. New Engl. J. Med., 268:721, 1963.

Landor, J. H., Armstrong, J. H., Dickerson, O. B., and

Westerfeld, R. A.: Neonatal obstruction of bowel caused by accidental clamping of small omphalocele: Report of 2 cases. South. Med. J. 56:1236, 1963.

Lassaletta, L., Fonkalsrud, E. W., Tovar, J. A., Dudgeon, D., and Asch, M. J.: Management of umbilical hernias in infancy and childhood. J. Pediatr. Surg. 10:405, 1975.

Shuster, S. R.: A new method for the staged repair of large omphalocoeles. Surg. Gynecol. Obstet. 125:837, 1967.

Soave, F.: Conservative treatment of omphalocoele. Arch. Dis. Child. 38:130, 1963.

Wachter, H. E., and Elman, R.: Aberrant umbilical stomach: Report of two cases. A.M.A. J. Dis. Child. 87:204, 1954.

Wesselhoeft, C. W. Jr., and Randolph, J. G.: Treatment of omphalocoele based on individual characteristics of the defect. Pediatrics 44:101, 1969.

White, J. J., Brenner, H., and Avery, M. E.: Umbilical vein collateral circulation: The caput medusae in a newborn infant. Pediatrics 43:391, 1969.

# CONGENITAL MALFORMATIONS OF THE OMPHALOMESENTERIC (VITELLINE) DUCT

# 40

**EMBRYOLOGY.**   The yolk sac in the very small human embryo is a relatively large structure attached to its ventral surface, its cavity communicating directly with the primitive coelom. It soon shrinks and develops a long narrow stalk which becomes enclosed within the umbilical cord (Fig. 40–1). Its proximal end becomes connected with the primitive midgut, and for a time these two structures communicate freely. In the normal course of ontogeny the vitelline duct becomes obliterated and disappears.

Under adverse circumstances the duct or portions of it do not disappear. All the theoretical possibilities of imperfect obliteration are encountered in newborns. The entire duct may remain patent, leading to enteroumbilical fistula. A remnant of mucous membrane may persist at the umbilicus, producing a polyp. The proximal segment may fail to close entirely, leaving a Meckel's diverticulum behind. If the distal segment fails to obliterate, a draining sinus tract remains. When obliteration is complete at both ends, but imperfect somewhere in its midportion, an omphalomesenteric cyst forms. Finally, the duct may obliterate, but not be resolved, leaving behind a fibrous cord which courses from the umbilicus toward the ileum.

## PATENT OMPHALOMESENTERIC DUCT (ENTEROUMBILICAL FISTULA)

This condition manifests itself by drainage from the umbilical stump or from the umbilicus after the cord has separated. Dis-

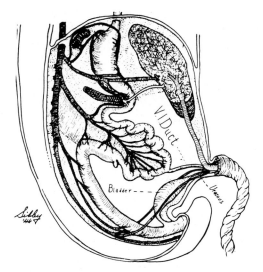

*Figure 40–1.*   Diagram showing the vitelline duct extending from the midgut to the umbilicus. At this stage the bladder is directly connected with the hindgut at the cloaca; on each side of the bladder the hypogastric arteries are visible. (From Sibley, W. L.: Arch. Surg. 49:156, 1944.)

charge may be noted as early as the first day or as late as the second week of life. Since the connection between the umbilicus and ileum is complete, gas and meconium, later fecal matter, will be seen to be extruded from the navel at irregular intervals. Careful inspection of the well cleaned area discloses a small orifice through which a fine probe can be passed with ease. There may be a bud or outpouching of the sinus tract, resembling a granuloma, in the center of which the orifice is situated. Injection of a few milliliters of radiopaque fluid permits visualization of the fistulous tract and confirms its communication with the small bowel. Simple fistulous connection between the ileum and umbilicus is not in itself too hazardous. It is true that constant contact with contaminated discharge often leads to omphalitis and periomphalitis, but with care this can be prevented. The great danger of this condition is that *evagination of small bowel* may take place, the attached segment of ileum literally turning itself inside out in the process of protruding through the umbilical orifice. The result is a T-shaped mass, whose external surface is intestinal mucosa, lying upon the abdominal wall.

Approximately 150 cases of enteroumbilical fistula had been reported by 1952, and 30 of these were complicated by prolapse of the ileum. The prognosis becomes approximately five times as grave when this complication occurs. Scaletter and Mazursky found that 20 of 113 (17 per cent) patients with simple fistula had died after operation, while 26 of 30 (87 per cent) died if evagination had already taken place. These figures indicate clearly that simple enteroumbilical fistula should be repaired surgically at once. Waiting until the infant grows larger in order to make the procedure easier cannot be condoned.

CASE 40–1

A male white infant was born after normal pregnancy and labor, weighing 9 pounds 10 ounces (4365 gm). He was treated repeatedly in the outpatient department for persistent bleeding of an "umbilical granuloma" by silver nitrate applications. At 10 days the cord had fallen away, but it had never healed. With straining, blood was discharged, estimated to amount to one teaspoonful. At times a white watery fluid

was seen to drain from it. From birth, appetite had been poor, vomiting frequent, and weight gain slow.

At four months of age he was hospitalized. Weight was now 13 pounds 5 ounces (6040 gm). At the umbilicus was a red exuberant mass resembling granulation tissue, measuring 1 by 1 cm. At its apex a dimple could be seen through which it was possible to pass a fine probe several inches (Fig. 40–2, *A*). The whole tract was resected on the ninth hospital day. Its distal end terminated in a Meckel's diverticulum arising from the ileum about 18 inches from the ileocecal valve (Fig. 40–2, *B*). Postoperative course was uneventful.

COMMENT. This, unfortunately, is an often-encountered story in cases of this sort. The supposed granuloma is treated by cauterizing agents. Failure to heal after months finally brings the realization that granuloma may not be the correct diagnosis. Those infants are fortunate who do not develop evagination and herniation of the ileum through the fistulous tract.

## UMBILICAL POLYP

In this disorder mucosal remnants of the omphalomesenteric duct persist at the umbilicus. The mucosa secretes mucus, but there is no discoverable orifice and no sinus tract.

After the cord has fallen away a bright red nodule is seen in the navel. This differs from granuloma in that it is moister. When the nodule is stroked, sticky mucus clings to the finger tip. The skin about the polyp is more likely to be excoriated than that about a granuloma. Biopsy should be performed if any doubt exists. The demonstration of mucous membrane characteristic of small intestine is pathognomonic.

*Treatment* of choice is cauterization, when one is absolutely certain that no sinus tract is present.

## OMPHALOMESENTERIC SINUS

In this variety of patency of the vitelline duct only the distal end remains lined with mucosa and in communication with the outside. The proximal segment may or may

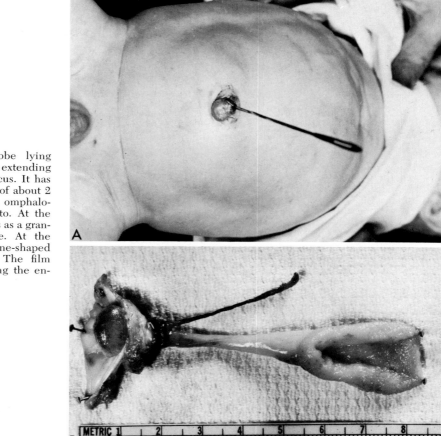

*Figure 40-2.* A, Probe lying within a fistulous tract extending inward from the umbilicus. It has been passed a distance of about 2 inches. B, The excised omphalomesenteric fistula in toto. At the umbilical end it presents as a granulomatous-looking bulge. At the ileal end it resembles a cone-shaped Meckel's diverticulum. The film showing barium outlining the entire tract has been lost.

not have persisted as an obliterated fibrous cord connecting the umbilicus with ileum.

The first sign is persistent discharge after the cord has separated. Discharged material is usually watery, but may be slightly bloody. At times there is bleeding of small amounts from the navel. Examination almost always discloses a red nodule projecting from the base of the umbilical well which at first glance resembles granuloma, but is actually pouting mucous membrane. One differential point between the two has already been mentioned; that is, that mucus clings to the examiner's finger tip in the latter case, but not in the former. Morgan noted another interesting phenomenon. As one watched, the polyp changed its shape intermittently. At times it would stand, become tense and protrude for a distance of 1 cm, while at others it would slowly draw inward and almost disappear from view. Careful inspection and exploration with a blunt probe disclose an orifice near the apex of the polyp. Injection of radiopaque material outlines the sinus tract.

*Treatment* consists in excision of the umbilicus and the sinus tract. The operator should explore the entire region between the umbilicus and small bowel for evidences of other anomalies along the course of the vitelline duct, and deal as indicated with any that might be found.

## OMPHALOMESENTERIC DUCT CYST (VITELLINE CYST)

When both the proximal and distal ends of the vitelline duct become obliterated, but a segment in the middle remains patent, an omphalomesenteric cyst forms from accumulation of its secretions. This variety of cyst must be distinguished from the many other kinds that are discussed elsewhere. Generally they present as visible and palpable masses buried shallowly within the abdomen just beneath the umbilicus. They are intimately tied to the navel. When grasped and moved from side to side or pressed inward, the umbilicus can be seen to pucker in conformity with their movement. They are spherical or ovoid, and their feel is distinctly cystic. Patency of the proximal end (i.e., Meckel's diverticulum) or of the distal end, as described in the previous paragraphs, or both, are not infrequently associated defects.

*Treatment* consists in surgical excision.

## MECKEL'S DIVERTICULUM

When the proximal, or intestinal, end of the omphalomesenteric duct fails to become obliterated completely, an outpouching of the ileum persists. The diverticulum may be as short as 2 cm or as long as 90 cm. It is usually tent-shaped, but it may be tubular. It may arise from any point of the small intestine as close as 3 cm proximal to the cecum or as far as 100 cm distant from it. The junction lies usually at some point in the ileum, rarely in the jejunum and exceptionally in the duodenum. It must arise from the antimesenteric side of the bowel, a fact that distinguishes Meckel's diverticulum from duplications. Its distal end usually lies free in the peritoneal cavity, but some are attached to the umbilicus by a fibrous cord, and a small minority remain patent to the umbilicus (omphalomesen-

teric fistula) (Fig. 40–3). Its structure simulates that of small bowel, with well defined mucosa, submucosa, muscularis and serosa. Unfortunately, it is the site, in about one fifth of the cases, of ectopic pancreatic or gastric tissue. Aberrant pancreatic tissue is usually present as a small mass in the wall, while gastric mucosa replaces or overlies the usual intestinal mucosa at some point or points. A pancreatic mass may act as a leader to produce intussusception. Gastric mucosa may cause peptic ulceration and bleeding; the latter is the sign which is almost always the presenting one if Meckel's diverticulum becomes symptomatic. The fibrous cord, if present, may produce intestinal obstruction. Rarely inflammation of the diverticulum may lead to peritonitis.

**INCIDENCE.** A Meckel's diverticulum can be discovered in 1.5 to 2 per cent of all persons. Only a small proportion of these ever become symptomatic, and when they do, this usually happens beyond the age of 4 months. Only exceptionally do they cause illness in the neonatal period. Males outnumber females by 3 to 5:1.

**DIAGNOSIS.** Hemorrhage from the bowel is the sign *par excellence* of Meckel's diverticulum. A few cases in older children and adults may produce the signs and symptoms of diverticulitis, but this condition has never been described in young infants. Hemorrhage is often sudden and catastrophic, causing a precipitous fall in the hematocrit level and a shocklike state within a few hours. The first few stools passed may be composed almost entirely of unchanged blood; later they become tarry. In other instances bleeding is constant and occult.

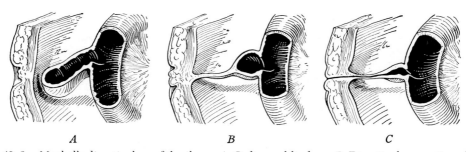

*Figure 40–3.*   Meckel's diverticulum of the ileum. *A*, Ordinary, blind sac. *B*, Diverticulum continued to umbilicus as a cord. *C*, Diverticulum, with fistulous opening at umbilicus (From Arey, L. B.: Developmental Anatomy. Revised 7th ed., 1974.)

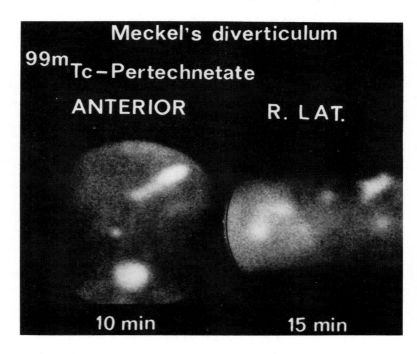

*Figure 40–4.* Anterior gamma camera view of abdomen of a 2-year-old infant. Note the small well-defined area of increased uptake located in right lower quadrant. The stomach and bladder are also visualized. On the lateral view, some radioactivity is evident on the diaper as well. (Courtesy of Dr. S. Treves, Children's Hospital Medical Center, Boston, Mass.)

Meckel's diverticulum must be differentiated from the other disorders that produce gross bleeding from the bowel. These are peptic ulcer, duplication and intestinal polyp for the most part. Intussusception, intestinal hemangioma and a few other even rarer entities may be responsible for an occasional case. Blood dyscrasias usually cause bleeding into the skin and from other sites simultaneously. Fissure in ano, proctitis and ulcerative colitis ordinarily do not lead to gross hemorrhage, blood loss being confined to the passage of bloody mucus or of stools containing a surface accumulation of blood. Polyps, too, are seldom responsible for massive hemorrhage, so that bleeding peptic ulcer and duplication are the only conditions left which are difficult to distinguish from bleeding Meckel's diverticulum. The most useful differential point is that hematemesis usually coexists with rectal bleeding in the case of peptic ulcer, whereas hematemesis is exceedingly rare in Meckel's diverticulum. The mass of duplication is sometimes palpable.

We no longer advocate barium studies, since they rarely demonstrate the lesion and may interfere with a technetium scan.

Scans after intravenous injection of $^{99m}$technetium pertechnetate are often, but not always, diagnostic of Meckel's diverticulum, since the technetium is concentrated in gastric mucosa.

**TREATMENT.** Blood replacement therapy is the prime indication in massive hemorrhage regardless of its cause. If bleeding ceases and the diagnosis has not been ascertained, it is permissible to keep the infant under observation and do nothing further. In the newborn a peptic ulcer, once healed, is not likely to cause further trouble. A second episode of bleeding at some future date suggests strongly some other diagnostic possibility, and Meckel's diverticulum takes first place in this list. Laparotomy is therefore indicated after a recurrent bout of hemorrhage. If a diverticulum is discovered, it must be excised. After its resection no further trouble is to be anticipated.

### REFERENCES

Brown, A. G., and Cain, F. G.: Evagination of ileum through patent omphalomesenteric duct. Am. J. Surg. 79:339, 1950.

Christie, A.: Meckel's diverticulum: A pathologic study of 63 cases. Am. J. Dis. Child. 42:544, 1931.

Clark, D. V.: Exstrophy of the ileum through a patent omphalomesenteric duct with strangulated umbilical hernia. J. Internat. Coll. Surg. 9:251, 1946.

Fox, P. F.: Uncommon umbilical anomalies in children. Surg., Gynecol. Obstet. 92:95, 1951.

Kittle, C. F., Jenkins, H. P., and Dragstedt, L. B.: Patent omphalo-mesenteric duct and its relation to the diverticulum of Meckel. Arch. Surg. 54:10, 1947.

Leonidas, J. C., and Germann, D. R.: 99m-Technetium pertechnetate imaging in diagnosis of Meckel's diverticulum. Arch. Dis. Child. 49:21, 1974.

Meguid, M. M., Wilkinson, R. H., Canty, T., Eraklis, A. J., and Treves, S.: Futility of barium sulfate in diagnosis of Meckel's diverticulum. Arch. Surg. 108:361, 1974.

Morgan, J. E.: Patent omphalomesenteric duct: Review of the literature and case report. Am. J. Surg. 58:267, 1942.

Scaletter, H. E., and Mazursky, M. M.: Congenital entero-umbilical fistula due to a patent vitelline duct. J. Pediatr. 40:310, 1952.

# 41      DISORDERS OF THE URACHUS

The urachus is that remnant of the allantois which extends from the bladder portion of the cloaca to the umbilicus. The urachus, like the omphalomesenteric duct, may remain completely patent throughout its length, or its proximal or distal end or its midportion may fail to obliterate.

**EMBRYOLOGY.** The allantois at first is an outpouching of the yolk sac from its caudal end and is in free communication with it (Fig. 41–1). Its internal end becomes attached to the primitive hindgut, and when the cloaca separates into the lower bowel and urinary system, this segment develops into a portion of the bladder. Its duct becomes incorporated into the umbilical cord, where it courses alongside the vitelline duct. The urachus normally persists as a musculotendinous structure situated between the transversalis fascia and peritoneum, but ordinarily its inner epithelial lining disappears.

Four types of anomalous development of the urachus have been described: 1) completely patent urachus, 2) patency of umbilical end (blind external type), 3) patency of vesical end (blind internal type), and 4) patency of midportion (urachal cyst).

**INCIDENCE.** All varieties are encountered rarely. By 1937 Herbst was able to find 140 cases in the literature. Three ex-amples were met in 200,000 admissions to the Children's Hospital of Boston.

## COMPLETELY PATENT URACHUS

The appearance of the umbilicus at birth is often normal. In some instances overgrowths of urachal remnants may present as protruding masses. In Nichols and Lowman's case, for example, there was a defect of the umbilicus with a protruding, elongated mass covered with overhanging skin, the center of which contained mucosa grossly resembling that of intestine. The mass was 6.5 cm long and 3.2 cm in diameter. Discharge from the normal or abnormal navel may appear at birth, within the first few days, or may be delayed several months. The fluid has all the characteristics of urine.

Diodrast or other radiopaque fluid injected into the orifice outlines the urachal tract and enters the bladder. Similarly, cystograms demonstrate the tract from below.

The only possible *diagnosis* with which patent urachus might be confused is patency of the vitelline duct. Careful observation of the nature of discharged material resolves doubt. Radiographic visualization supplies the final assurance.

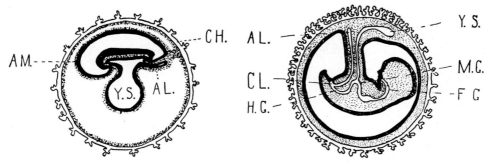

**Figure 41–1.** Diagrams illustrating formation of the allantois. The proximal portion of the allantois which extends from the cloaca to the umbilicus above the bladder is called the urachus. Abbreviations: *AL.*, allantois; *AM.*, amnion; *CH.*, chorion; *CL.*, cloaca; *FG.*, foregut; *H.G.*, hindgut; *M.G.*, midgut; *Y.S.*, yolk sac. (From Sibley, W. L.: Arch. Surg. *49*:156, 1944.)

*Treatment* consists in surgical excision of the umbilicus with the entire urachus and a small portion of the bladder. Results are usually good.

## BLIND EXTERNAL TYPE

When only the distal end of the urachus has failed to become obliterated, a draining sinus results. Drainage may become manifest immediately or, as is more usual, after the cord has separated, or only after several months. The discharge is watery, clear and yellow, and both looks and smells like urine. A nodule of aberrant mucous membrane may or may not be visible within the umbilicus, or projecting from it. At times a firm cord can be felt coursing beneath the skin and subcutaneous tissue in the direction of the symphysis pubis.

*Differential diagnosis* must be made between urachal sinus and omphalomesenteric sinus. The urinous discharge of the former is quite different from the serous, seromucous or serosanguineous secretion of the latter. Biopsy shows bladder-like mucosa in the former, intestinal mucosa in the latter. The sinus tract visualized by x-ray examination courses directly inward if it is vitelline duct, diagonally caudad and inward if it is urachus.

*Treatment* consists in surgical excision of the sinus tract.

## BLIND INTERNAL TYPE

Failure of obliteration of the proximal end of the urachus results in a diverticulum of the bladder near its fundus. This produces no symptoms and no disease, and hence has no clinical significance. It can be demonstrated only by cystogram. Nothing need be done about this condition.

## URACHAL CYST

Incomplete obliteration of the midportion of the urachus leads to the development of urachal cyst. At times this is a solitary defect, but not infrequently it is associated with persistent external or internal patency. Cysts may be present at birth, may grow slowly and become obvious at any time during infancy or childhood or may suddenly manifest themselves because of infection. Urachal cysts are highly susceptible to infection and, if not removed after the first episode, to repeated reinfection.

They present as spherical masses of variable size at some point between the umbilicus and the symphysis pubis. They feel and are superficial, since they lie extraperitoneally between the fascia of the transversalis muscle and the peritoneum. When they are infected, the surrounding skin and subcutaneous tissue are thickened, red and edematous, and often purulent material drains from the navel.

Plain x-ray film shows the round soft tissue mass within or just beneath the abdominal wall. If radiopaque material can be injected through an umbilical sinus, the entire cyst may be filled and visualized. Injection of Diodrast into the bladder may or may not fill the cyst from below.

Operation should be performed, preferably before the cyst becomes infected or, if this has already taken place, after infection has been controlled by compresses and antibiotics. The danger of surgical manipulation during active infection is that the peritoneum may be entered and general peritonitis ensue.

CASE 41–1

A white male infant was admitted to the Harriet Lane Home at 2 days of age because of an abdominal tumor and drainage from the umbilical cord. Pregnancy had been complicated by severe vomiting the first 5 months and bleeding at 3 and 6 months. Delivery was spontaneous 1 month before term, birth weight being 6 pounds (2720 gm). Physical examination revealed a small, slightly jaundiced infant whose abdominal wall was flaccid and deeply wrinkled. The flanks bulged loosely, the left more than the right. In the midline, extending from the umbilicus to symphysis, a mass could be felt, irregular, firm and cystic. The cord appeared clean, but at its base could be seen a 5-mm slit from which fluid resembling urine was oozing. Pressure upon the abdominal wall increased the quantity of discharge. The genitals were normal male in conformation except that the testes were undescended.

Urine was normal, hemoglobin 18.0 gm, nonprotein nitrogen 62, chloride 114, sodium 154, potassium 5 mg per 100 ml and carbon dioxide 20 mEq per liter.

X-ray studies included a urachogram taken after Lipiodol had been injected into the geni-tourinary tract through a catheter passed through the umbilical slit (Fig. 41–2, *A*), and a cystogram made in the usual fashion by injection from below (Fig. 41–2, *B*). Both showed identical pictures, including a patent urachus and a urachal cyst attached to an irregular shaped bladder.

Laparotomy revealed these conditions plus a hypoplastic right kidney, urethral stenosis, hypertrophy and dilatation of the left ureter, and hypoplasia of abdominal muscles.

The infant died on the twelfth day with severe uremia.

**COMMENT.** This case requires little comment. The multiple anomalies of the lower abdominal area included virtual absence of abdominal muscle and numerous malformations of the genitourinary tract. One of these was complete patency of the urachus from the bladder to the umbilicus plus a large midurachal cyst. Unfortunately the associated defects were lethal.

## REFERENCES

Herbst, cited by R. W. Nichols and R. M. Lowman: Patent urachus. Am. J. Roentgenol. 52:615, 1944.

MacMillan, R., Schullinger, J., and Santulli, T. V.: Pyourachus: An unusual surgical problem. J. Pediatr. Surg. 8:387, 1973.

Nichols, R. W., and Lowman, R. M.: Patent urachus. Am. J. Roentgenol. 52:615, 1944.

Sibley, W. L.: Cyst of the urachus. Am. J. Surg. 79:465, 1950.

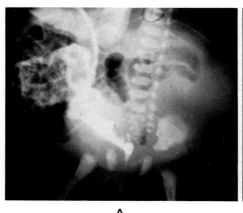
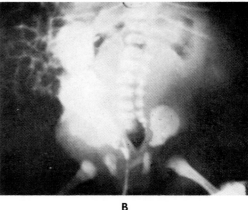

**A**                    **B**

*Figure 41–2.*   *A*, Urachogram showing a catheter traversing the patent urachus to a cyst adjacent to the bladder. The bladder is irregular in shape. *B*, Cystogram showing a catheter entering the bladder from the urethra, the contrast medium filling it and the urachal cyst above it.

# FETAL ASCITES, NEONATAL ASCITES AND PERITONITIS

# 42

## DYSTOCIA CAUSED BY FETAL ABDOMINAL ENLARGEMENT

Fetal abdominal enlargement may reach a size that calls for paracentesis or a destructive operation before delivery can be effected. Most are caused by accumulation of fluid within the peritoneal cavity, chiefly resulting from obstructive uropathy or meconium peritonitis. Rarely the fluid excess is contained within the uterus and vagina; that is, hydrometrocolpos which has developed antenatally. Some are due to organomegaly, enlargement of the liver caused by metastatic neuroblastoma leading this list. Polycystic kidneys have been found in a few. Rarer causes include congenital cirrhosis of the liver, portal vein obstruction, chylous ascites, Wilms' tumor and cysts of the liver.

## PERITONITIS

Two main categories of peritonitis are encountered in the neonatal period, chemical and bacterial. Together they comprise a considerable segment of the urgent surgical disorders of the first week of life. Rickham had to deal with 17 cases of peritonitis in the Newborn Surgical Service of the Alder Hey Hospital of Liverpool in the course of a 3½-year period in which 250 surgical cases were admitted (7 per cent). He suggests the following classification, somewhat modified.

*Peritonitis in the Neonatal Period*
I. Meconium peritonitis
  A. Group I (with intestinal obstruction)
    1. In lumen of gut (meconium ileus)
    2. In wall of gut
    3. Outside the gut (volvulus, hernia, bands, etc.)
  B. Group II (without intestinal obstruction)
    1. Defect in muscularis
    2. Vascular accident

II. Acute bacterial peritonitis
  A. Acute appendicitis
  B. Perforation of a hollow viscus
  C. Gangrenous bowel
  D. Trauma
  E. Septicemia
  F. Transmural infection from gastroenteritis
III. Bile peritonitis

## MECONIUM PERITONITIS

This is a "sterile, chemical and foreign body reaction resulting from leakage of bowel content into peritoneal cavity during late intrauterine or early neonatal period. Within 24 hours after birth the meconium may become contaminated . . . and the meconium peritonitis converted to a bacterial one" (White).

**INCIDENCE.** Although the disorder is not common, it is far from being an extraordinary rarity. Well over 100 cases had been reported up to 1950. Bendel and Michel discovered three cases in 108,000 live births in a 15-year period.

**ETIOLOGY.** As indicated in the classification, meconium may leak as a result of rupture of the intestine at some point proximal to obstruction, either intrinsic or extrinsic. In something less than half the reported cases no obstruction can be found to account for rupture. The tear may be obvious or may have healed over so perfectly that it cannot be distinguished at operation or autopsy. To explain bowel rupture without obstruction, various hypotheses have been advanced. The bowel wall may have been congenitally weak from localized defect or may have become weakened by a localized vascular accident or for some other reason. Trauma is not an important factor.

The most frequent predisposing lesions are atresia and meconium ileus. Stenosis does not lead to rupture. Cases have also been reported to follow intussusception, volvulus, incarcerated internal hernia, imperforate anus, and meconium plugs, among others.

The fetus begins to swallow amniotic fluid by about the third month of gestation. Within the next month meconium begins to form, reaching the ileocecal valve at 4 months, the rectum at 5 months. Theoretically, meconium peritonitis could occur at any time in the last 4 or 5 months of gestation.

**DIAGNOSIS.** If the bowel has ruptured before birth, abdominal distention at the time of delivery is the outstanding sign. The abdomen may be so huge that dystocia results, and the obstetrician has been forced in a number of cases to perform paracentesis before delivery can be effected. The infant is sick and cyanotic, and breathes rapidly and with grunting. The abdominal wall may be covered with dilated veins and may be bluish and edematous. Edema may extend to the flanks, scrotum or vulva. Anorexia, vomiting and constipation are prominent, although one or two meconium stools or masses of mucus tinged with blood may be passed.

The aforementioned description fits the great majority of infants born with meconium peritonitis. A minority are born in good or reasonably good condition, manifesting only a moderate degree of abdominal distention. A few of these will also show "hydroceles" at birth, "only to return at 4 weeks of age with hard scrotal . . . masses" (Berdon et al.). Radiograms of these show calcifications which may lead to the incorrect diagnosis of testicular teratoma. Only the additional finding of scattered abdominal calcifications indicates the proper explanation, that the scrotal fluid at birth was ascitic fluid which traversed the normally patent processus vaginalis and induced calcification. Calcified plaques here, as in the peritoneal cavity, can be expected to disappear within a few months.

If rupture occurs after delivery, the infant suddenly becomes obviously sick, and the signs enumerated above appear rapidly. In prenatal rupture with meconium peritonitis the physical examination reveals only fluid within the abdominal cavity, whereas if rupture takes place after birth, both fluid and air can be demonstrated within the peritoneum.

X-ray study in rupture occurring before delivery shows dilated loops of bowel in an almost completely opaque field; in postnatal rupture the picture is the characteristic one of pneumoperitoneum. In the first, scattered plaques of calcified material may be discerned throughout the abdomen.

**TREATMENT.** Unless the perforation has obviously healed spontaneously and no obstructive signs are present, immediate operation is indicated. If a tear is discovered, it must be repaired. Obstructive lesions must be searched for and bypassed where found.

**PROGNOSIS.** The outlook for recovery is poor. By 1956 (White) the number of survivors had reached 18. Many of the intrauterine ruptures cause stillbirth or a liveborn so sick that operative intervention is hopeless from the start. In others the matting together of intestinal loops and the great dilatation of segments of bowel prevent proper function even after good anastomosis has been effected. In still others superimposition of bacterial peritonitis diminishes the chance for survival.

CASE 42–1

A white male infant was born prematurely in a hospital in Havre de Grace, Maryland. Birth weight was 4 pounds 6 ounces (1940 gm). He did not breathe promptly and was placed in oxygen for several hours, after which he seemed reasonably well. He passed a meconium stool within 24 hours and took his first feedings well. On the fourth day his abdomen was moderately distended. Examination disclosed a hard golf-ball–sized mass in the left middle and lower quadrants which was thought to be ectopic kidney. X-ray film, however, showed it to be a calcified mass, and numerous others of smaller size were seen scattered throughout the peritoneal cavity (Fig. 42–1). The infant was transferred to the Harriet Lane Home and stayed 1 week, remaining afebrile, eating well, gaining weight and not vomiting. There was no distention, and no peristaltic waves were visible. Pyelograms, barium gastrointestinal x-ray series, sweat test, stool trypsin, and films of the long bones were all negative. The blood calcium was 11.6, phosphorus 6.6 and chloride 107 mg per 100 ml.

**COMMENT.** It seems clear that prenatal rupture of the bowel had taken place, setting up meconium peritonitis, and that the perforation had become sealed off. The chemical peritonitis subsided, leaving

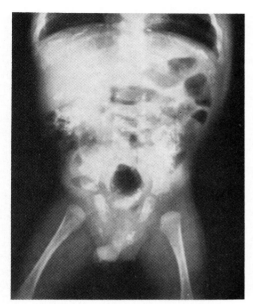

*Figure 42–1.* Flat film of the abdomen, made on the fourth day of life. One can see many areas of calcium deposition extending from the diaphragm to and including the inguinal canals. Clearly, some of these are situated outside intestinal lumen. There is no evidence of intestinal obstruction. The diagnosis is meconium peritonitis.

great calcium deposits behind. The example is out of the ordinary in that no illness to speak of followed and that a mass of calcified meconium was large enough to be readily palpable. More often one has to search the x-ray films carefully for small calcified deposits in order to make this diagnosis.

## BACTERIAL PERITONITIS

Invasion of the peritoneal cavity by bacteria may follow a long list of primary disorders. These include acute appendicitis, sepsis, omphalitis with spread inward via umbilical arteritis or periarteritis, and gastroenteritis. Peritonitis inevitably follows postnatal rupture of the stomach or intestine such as results from peptic ulceration, necrotizing enterocolitis, gangrene of the bowel due to volvulus, intussusception or mesenteric thrombosis, or occurs spontaneously, for no known reason.

Scott has reported six cases of peritonitis in infants 3 to 13 days of age, in whom the clinical histories consisted of vomiting but no diarrhea, distention, obvious intestinal obstruction without discoverable structural reason and, in five of the six, rupture and pneumoperitoneum. In all there was necrotizing inflammation of ileum, jejunum or colon. *E. coli* was grown from peritoneal swabs of four, and *E. coli* metastatic abscesses complicated one case. *Candida albicans* was seen in the intestinal sections of two. Two of the infants recovered, one after simple colostomy, and one after two resections of segments of gangrenous bowel and subsequent aspirations of osteomyelitis of the head of a femur. The author believes that overwhelming infection is the cause of this necrotizing enteritis but cannot decide whether bacteria—or fungi—invaded from the bowel lumen or from the blood stream (see also Necrotizing Enterocolitis, p. 384).

**DIAGNOSIS.** The signs of peritonitis are often overshadowed by those of the preceding disorder. Peritonitis adds little to the symptomatology of pneumoperitoneum or of gangrenous bowel subsequent to midgut volvulus. In the purer form, such as that which complicates gangrenous appendicitis or sepsis of the newborn, the onset is marked by anorexia, vomiting and progressive abdominal distention. On examination one may or may not be able to demonstrate free fluid within the peritoneal cavity by discovering dullness in the flanks, shifting with change of position. One does not expect to find in the newborn localized muscle spasm or general abdominal rigidity. Fever and leukocytosis are the rule in full-term infants, but not in those prematurely born.

X-ray examination can be helpful by demonstrating generalized distention of bowel loops with no obvious point of obstruction—unless obstruction is indeed the basis of the peritonitis—and a homogeneous opacity in the flanks and between bowel loops indicating free fluid.

**TREATMENT.** Any abdomen showing these signs will have to be laparotomized. If a primary disorder can be attacked surgically, this will be done. If not, drainage and vigorous antibiotic therapy will be the only recourse.

**PROGNOSIS.** In Rickham's series of 17,

seven infants died. This mortality rate of 40 per cent is probably better than that achieved in many other clinics.

## ACUTE APPENDICITIS

**INCIDENCE.** The appendix has been observed to be acutely inflamed at the time of birth at least twice and within the first few weeks of life approximately 10 more times. Neonatal appendicitis is therefore rare.

**ETIOLOGY.** No one knows the pathogenesis of appendiceal infection in the newborn.

**DIAGNOSIS.** The diagnosis was made easy for Reed. In his case, reported in 1913, an infant was born with an omphalocele through the transparent membrane of which cecum, small bowel and appendix could be seen. The appendix was visibly acutely inflamed! It was removed, the intestines were replaced, and cure was effected.

Jackson's case is obscured by the possibility that the infant had been given bichloride of mercury by mistake, so that we learn little about diagnosis from this history. In Hill and Mason's report an infant was born distended, all fluids offered were vomited, but meconium was passed freely. Distention became extreme, temperature rose to 102°, and he died on the third day. Autopsy showed a ruptured, inflamed appendix. Cultures from the peritoneal exudate after death were sterile. Other infants have been well for 3 to 4 days or longer, and have then begun to vomit and become distended, death occurring a few days after the onset. Polymorphonuclear leukocytosis has been found in several.

We encountered an example of Pseudomonas sepsis in a newborn in which death occurred after 5 days. At postmortem examination acute appendicitis was found among the multiple foci of infection.

**TREATMENT.** We have been unable to discover any report in which the inflamed appendix had been removed from a newborn, other than Reed's case. We have no doubt that soon this will be done, if it has not already been done, in view of our greater readiness to explore the abdomen in doubtful cases.

## BILE PERITONITIS

Davies and Elliott-Smith object to the term "bile peritonitis" to describe the disorder that arises from the escape of bile into the peritoneal cavity. They prefer "bile ascites," since, they say, no acute peritonitis results, but only an outpouring of fluid because of the higher osmotic pressure of bile.

**INCIDENCE.** This condition is an extreme rarity. We have been able to discover only five cases involving neonates.

**ETIOLOGY.** Adequate reasons for escape of bile were found in three cases. In one the common duct had ruptured just above a stenotic point in the common duct; in another, one of a group of tiny cysts at the junction of the cystic and common ducts had ruptured; and in the third the common duct had ruptured just proximal to the point where a gallstone lay. No cause was found in the other two infants.

**DIAGNOSIS.** The classic picture of bile peritonitis in the adult, sudden severe illness with abdominal distention, tenderness, fever and shock, was seen in only one of the foregoing cases. The others developed abdominal distention rapidly, the stools had been or became white, and mild jaundice appeared. Distention was accompanied in three of them by bilateral inguinal herniation, which was the reason why the infants were brought to the pediatrician. Free fluid was demonstrable in the peritoneal cavity by the usual physical signs. Why one infant became acutely ill at the onset while others were brought for consultation because of hernia alone is not understood.

Most of the infants were slightly jaundiced from birth, and stools had been noted to be without color. Hernias and abdominal distention made their appearance at 3 to 6 weeks of age. There was obvious discrepancy between the lack of color in the stools and the minor degrees of bilirubinemia and bilirubinuria found. Davies's comment about this point is that "the combination of white stools with only mild jaundice suggests that bilirubin is escaping elsewhere. Abdominal distention and shifting dullness suggest where it has gone."

**TREATMENT.** Three of the infants recovered quickly after laparotomy and drainage alone. Anastomosis of the common duct to the duodenum was successfully accomplished in the fourth. The fifth infant died without benefit of operation, although after death a stenotic common duct was found which could have been bypassed surgically. Clearly one should not rely upon drainage alone when bile peritonitis has been diagnosed, but careful exploration should be performed and any basic defect treated definitively.

## CHYLOUS ASCITES

**INCIDENCE.** Although accumulation of chyle within the peritoneal cavity is not too uncommon in adult life, it is a rarity in infancy. Nevertheless Kessel was able to find 31 cases reported up to 1952, when he added another to the collection. In many of these the onset was noted at birth or within the first few weeks of life. The disease is twice as common in males as in females.

**PATHOLOGY AND ETIOLOGY.** Pathologic alterations are limited to the abdomen in most cases. One case is on record in which chylous ascites was associated with chylothorax and lymphedema of one leg and the contralateral hand and forearm. Trauma, commonly a causative factor in adults, seems to play little etiologic part in the newborn. McKendry et al., who found great lymphatic channel dilatation and hypertrophy distally and little or none proximally, concluded that the factor responsible is failure of peripheral channels to communicate with the major ones. This congenital defect, if it indeed is this, appears to be irreversible in many, self-limited in others.

**DIAGNOSIS.** The abdomen has been noted to be swollen at birth in some cases, while in others swelling has begun a few days or weeks later. Kessel's infant was born "swollen all over," but by the age of 3 weeks all the edema had disappeared, while the abdomen remained full. In four examples scrotal swelling accompanied that of the abdomen, and in two of these tapping was accomplished via the scrotum. Lymphedema preceded the onset of abdominal distention by several weeks in one case.

Physical examination showed little more than abdominal fullness and the presence of fluid within the peritoneal cavity. Veins may become dilated over the surface of the abdomen. Appetite remains good, and vomiting does not occur unless a great excess of ascites causes tight distention.

Paracentesis results in a free flow of milky fluid with a high fat content and 3 to 5 gm of protein per 100 cc. The first few taps before the ingestion of milk may yield straw-colored fluid.

**COURSE.** The natural history of this disorder resembles closely that of chylothorax, to which it must be closely related. Some infants become well after one or two tappings. Scherer's infant was tapped 31 times in 2 months before outpouring of ascitic fluid finally ceased. An occasional baby has died of intercurrent infection with no apparent letup in ascites formation.

**TREATMENT.** Paracentesis may be required periodically to relieve distention. As much fluid should be withdrawn as comes out freely. Drainage should not be accomplished too rapidly. The interval between tappings depends entirely upon the speed with which the abdominal cavity refills. Little is gained by exploratory laparotomy. A low fat diet with medium chain triglycerides is often helpful in lessening the formation of chyle. Most patients undergo an eventual remission.

## REFERENCES

Abt, I. A.: Fetal peritonitis. Med. Clin. N. Amer. *15*:611, 1931.

Agerty, H. A., Ziserman, A. J., and Shollenberger, C. L.: Case of perforation of ileum in newborn infant with operation and recovery. J. Pediatr. *22*:233, 1943.

Bartlett, R. H., Eraklis, A. J., and Wilkinson, R. H.: Appendicitis in infants. Surg. Gynecol. Obstet. *130*:99, 1970.

Bendel, W. L., and Michel, M. L.: Meconium peritonitis: Review of the literature and report of a case with survival after surgery. Surgery *34*:321, 1953.

Berdon, W. E., Baker, D. H., Becker, J., and De Sanctis, P.: Scrotal masses in healed meconium peritonitis. New Engl. J. Med. *277*:585, 1967.

Byrne, J. J., and Bottomley, G. T.: Bile peritonitis in infancy. A.M.A. J. Dis. Child. *85*:694, 1953.

Ch'eng, Y. H., and K'ang, H. J.: Acute appendicitis in a newborn. Chinese M.J., *52*:876, 1937. Abstracted in Am. J. Dis. Child. *56*:895, 1938.

Connell, T. H., Jr., and Bogin, M.: Gangrene of the intestine occurring in utero: Report of a successful resection. A.M.A. J. Dis. Child. *87*:621, 1954.

Cowie, D. M.: The casuistry of chylous ascites and chylocele in sucklings and very young infants, with report of a case. Arch. Pediatr. *28*:595, 1911.

Davies, P. A., and Elliott-Smith, A.: Bile peritonitis in infancy. Arch. Dis. Child. *30*:174, 1955.

Fonkalsrud, E. W., Ellis, D. G., and Clatworthy, H. W., Jr.: Neonatal peritonitis. J. Pediatr. Surg. *1*:227, 1966.

France, N. E., and Back, E. H.: Neonatal ascites associated with urethral obstruction. Arch. Dis. Child. *29*:565, 1954.

Friedman, A. B., Abellara, R. M., Lidsky, I., and Lubert, M.: Perforation of the colon after exchange transfusion in the newborn. New Engl. J. Med. *282*:796, 1970.

Hill, W. B., and Mason, C. C.: Prenatal appendicitis with rupture and death. Am. J. Dis. Child. *29*:86, 1925.

Jackson, W. F.: A case of prenatal appendicitis. Am. J. Med. Sc. *127*:710, 1904.

Kessel, I.: Chylous ascites in infancy. Arch. Dis. Child. *27*:79, 1952.

Lee, C. M., Jr., and MacMillan, B. G.: Rupture of the bowel in the newborn infant; including case report of rupture in large intestine with recovery. Surgery *28*:48, 1950.

Marx, K., and Dale, W. A.: Neonatal ascites and obstructive uropathy. Pediatrics *27*:29, 1961.

McKendry, J. B. J., Lindsay, W. K., and Gerstein, M. C.: Congenital defects of the lymphatics in infancy. Pediatrics *19*:21, 1957.

Meyer, J. F.: Acute gangrenous appendicitis in a premature infant. J. Pediatr. *41*:343, 1952.

Nash, F. W., and Smith, J. F.: Fibrocystic disease of pancreas with meconium peritonitis at birth. Arch. Dis. Child. *27*:73, 1952.

Radman, M.: Dystocia due to fetal abdominal enlargement. Obstet. Gynecol. *19*:481, 1962.

Reed, E. M.: Infant disembowelled at birth—appendectomy successful. J.A.M.A. *41*:199, 1913.

Rickham, P. P.: Peritonitis in the neonatal period. Arch. Dis. Child. *30*:23, 1955.

Rosen, F. D., Smith, D., Earle, R., Janeway, C. A., and Gitlin, D.: The etiology of hypoproteinemia in a patient with congenital chylous ascites. Pediatrics *30*:696, 1962.

Scherer, C. A.: Ascites in infants. Internat. Clin. 2:3rd Series, 244, 1922.

Scott, J. E. S.: Intestinal obstruction in the newborn associated with peritonitis. Arch. Dis. Child. *38*:120, 1963.

Shnitka, T. K., and Sherbaniuk, R. W.: Congenital intussusception complicated by meconium peritonitis. Obstet. Gynecol. 7:293, 1956.

Sinclair, W., Jr., and Driver, M. M.: Meconium ileus, meconium peritonitis and volvulus of ileum with cystic fibrosis of pancreas. A.M.A. J. Dis. Child. *87*:337, 1954.

Stiennon, O. A.: Pneumatosis intestinalis in the newborn. A.M.A. J. Dis. Child. *81*:651, 1951.

Thelander, H. E.: Perforation of the gastrointestinal tract of the newborn infant. Am. J. Dis. Child. *58*:371, 1939.

Tow, A., Hurwitt, E. S., and Wolff, J. A.: Meconium peritonitis due to incarcerated mesenteric hernia. A.M.A. J. Dis. Child. *87*:621, 1954.

White, R. B.: Meconium peritonitis. A surgical emergency. J. Pediatr. *48*:793, 1956.

# V

# Disorders of the Genitourinary Tract

# 43

# GENERAL CONSIDERATIONS

*Revised by Warren Grupe*

**EMBRYOLOGY.** It is not possible to review the ontogeny of the urinary tract in detail in this place. Only a few facts will be recalled which have immediate bearing upon clinical disorders in the neonatal period.

MORPHOLOGIC DEVELOPMENT. The human kidney develops from the primitive nephrogenic ridge in three successive stages. The earliest stage, the pronephros, consists of a set of tubules in the 1.7-mm embryo. They join distally to form a duct which is the anlage of the mesonephric or wolffian duct. The pronephros degenerates, and more caudally differentiation of the mesonephros occurs. The importance of the two primitive kidneys is not clear, although it is thought that the mesonephros is capable of urine formation. It is the ureteric bud, arising from the caudal portion of the mesonephric duct and migrating cephalad, which makes contact with the metanephros, then through a series of dichotomous branchings induces the mass of metanephric cells to differentiate into the definitive kidney. The ureteral bud, in turn, forms the calyces, renal pelves and ureters. Defects in nephrogenesis have direct expression in congenital anomalies. For example, the absence of a kidney can reflect any one of several developmental arrests. Absence of the ureteric bud leads to an absence of both kidney and ureter. If the ureteric bud fails to make contact with the metanephros, a short blind ureter with a normal bladder insertion results. If the ureteric bud enters the mass of primitive tissue, but failure of induction or differentiation occurs, then one finds a nubbin of aplastic, non-functioning tissue at the end of an otherwise normal ureter. Failure of maturation of the primitive kidney may be associated with absence or anomalous development of gonads, sex ducts, adrenals and lung.

The development of the major and minor calyces is complete by about 10 weeks of gestation; the terminal collecting ducts appear in the subsequent weeks, and by 20 to 22 weeks nephrons are first seen with their collecting ducts near the medulla. Nephrogenesis starts at 7 to 8 weeks, and continues to about 35 weeks. Examination of the glomerular zones of the kidney provides one useful measure of the stage of gestation, at least to distinguish infants born before or after 35 weeks.

Electron microscopic studies by Vernier and colleagues show that glomerular capillaries form in situ in the endothelial cell mass. Foot processes arise by infolding of epithelial cell membranes, and are present in 30 per cent of the glomeruli in fetuses of 5 months of age.

The secretory and collecting tubules may not effect perfect juncture, and polycystic kidneys are the result. We cannot be sure that this is the proper explanation for this anomaly, but it seems probable. One or both kidneys may not complete normal ascent and may wind up in an ectopic location. If the ureteric buds fuse early in gestation, horseshoe kidney results, which is not only a single conjoint kidney, but also is generally one which sits lower than normal and in which the pelves face ventrally instead of medially. This is due to the fact that early fusion prevents proper ascent with its concomitant rotation. Not too rarely collecting systems, i.e., calyces, pelves and ureters, are duplicated; at times the entire kidney is a double structure, the ureters of which may join at some point in their course or may empty into the bladder or some abnormal site separately. Stenoses and strictures of the tubular structures are encountered with some frequency, most often at points of junction, but not always. Most of the difficulties these embryologic deviations produce are not associated with inability to function properly, although this statement is not true for polycystic or hypoplastic organs, but with their propensity for producing obstruction to outflow of urine. This in turn increases the possibility of infection and renders infection once acquired difficult to eradicate.

FUNCTIONAL DEVELOPMENT. Little is known about renal function in utero, since only recently has it been possible to keep catheters chronically implanted in fetal animal vessels and bladder to allow studies under physiological conditions. From studies made on abortuses, it is evident that by the third month of fetal life urine is formed; the urine is usually very dilute, with an osmolality of approximately 270 and a much lower urea and electrolyte concentration than is found in postnatal life.

The loop of Henle functions by the fourteenth gestational week, leading to a decrease in the volume and an increase in the quality of the urine produced; this change is accompanied by a continuing increase in glomerular filtration rate. In the early days after birth, urine of premature infants is rarely over 650 milliosmols, or approximately twice the osmolality of serum. When stressed, infants can concentrate more, but even full-term ones do not approach the ability of the adult in concentration. After birth also, urine osmolality will depend on feeding practices. With breast feeding, urine tends to concentrate somewhat on the second and third days of life, and then to achieve a steady range with an average specific gravity of 1.008. When the newborn is fed milk with a considerably higher content of phosphorus than is contained in breast milk, his relatively incompetent kidney cannot prevent its piling up in the blood, and tetany may result. Similarly, excesses of protein may lead to elevation of urea nitrogen in the serum.

The volume of urine produced by the normal fetus at term is not known, but it clearly is an essential source of amniotic liquid. Renal agenesis is regularly associated with oligohydramnios.

The average amount of urine in the bladder of a term infant at birth is said to be about 6 cc, with a wide range up to 44 cc. In the series of Sherry and Kramer, 17 per cent of infants voided first in the delivery room, and 92 per cent had voided by 24 hours. Almost all of them had voided by 48 hours.

The role of the kidneys in the regulation of acid-base balance of the fetus is not known, but it must be inconsequential since infants can be well developed and in normal acid-base balance at birth with agenesis of the kidneys. After birth, however, the kidney assumes the task of excretion of fixed acids. The pH of fetal urine is about 6; after birth the pH depends upon acid production by the fetus and the fluid intake. Acid-loading can increase the hydrogen-ion excretion; however, small premature infants are less able to excrete the hydrogen ions because of a reduced ability to excrete ammonium ions and phosphates. Infants fed human milk excrete about one tenth the amount of titratable acid as infants fed cow's milk, presumably because of the greater amount of phosphate in cow's milk. The renal threshold for bicarbonate has been shown by Edelman et al. to be lower in infants than in adults, consistent with the observation that plasma bicarbonate levels in neonatal life are lower than those in subsequent months.

In summary, no sudden renal morphologic events herald or accompany birth. Functional capability is increased with sudden demands of postnatal life upon the kidneys to become the organ of excretion and regulation of fixed acidity in the blood. The premature infant achieves the capability of the term infant some days after birth with respect to concentrating ability, but all infants require many months to reach levels of function comparable to that of the adult when comparisons are made per unit surface area.

Despite its limitations, the immature kidney does have the capability of altering function appropriately under stress. The homeostatic controls respond qualitatively but often require greater stimuli to initiate a response that is quantitatively more limited. A comparatively decreased glomerular filtration rate quantitatively hampers the neonate's ability to excrete excessive loads of a variety of substances including drugs. Glomerulotubular imbalance with glomerular preponderance defines tubular function at an even more reduced level, which is reflected in the infant's limited ability to conserve glucose, phosphates, bicarbonate and amino acids. Recent evidence would suggest that the extent of glomerulotubular imbalance may not be as great as previously described and that with optimum distribution of intrarenal blood flow, glomerulotubular balance may exist. Aptly suited for growth, the neonatal kidneys are functioning near their maximum capacity with little reserve for the stresses of disease, injudicious management or unrealistic expectations.

General remarks about the development of the genital tract will be discussed in Chapter 56.

## URINALYSIS

Examination of a fresh voided specimen of urine provides the most immediate information about the urinary tract and should be part of the physical examination of infants. The normal newborn urine is quite pale in color. Clouds of urates may be present in the first few voidings and may sometimes give the urine a pinkish tinge or stain the diaper a faint red. The benzidine test on the urine or diaper distinguishes between hemoglobin and urate stain. Specific gravity of the newborn's urine is ordinarily quite low. It may be factitiously elevated by high molecular weight solutes such as radiographic contrast material, sugars or protein. It may also be increased in children with cardiac failure, dehydration, respiratory distress and inappropriate ADH secretion. In the absence of exogenously administered solute, there is ordinarily a good correlation between urine osmolarity and specific gravity. Using small clinical refractometers, the specific gravity can be measured with as little as two drops of urine. The maximum concentrating ability of the premature is approximately 750 milliosmoles per liter (specific gravity 1.018). (See Table 43–1). Occasionally a full-term infant may reach as high as 1000 milliosmoles per liter (specific gravity 1.025). The inability of the newborn to concentrate the urine further is because growing infants normally excrete such a small solute load. Newborn infants attain the full capacity to concentrate urine by about 3 months of age. In the interim, their limited ability to concentrate influences their ability to tolerate either restricted intake or excessive insensible fluid losses. In older children the specific gravity increases markedly with water deprivation, while in young infants it may not. Therefore, urine volume may become a more useful parameter of hydration than specific gravity or urinary osmolality in the newborn.

## PROTEINURIA

Protein is normally found in small amounts in the urine of the newborn, varying between 30 and 75 mg in a 24 hour period, and a concentration not exceeding 10 mg per 100 ml. Proteinuria may be seen with asphyxia, cardiac failure, massive doses of penicillin, dehydration and in the presence of x-ray contrast media. Persistent proteinuria must be considered pathologic until proved otherwise and may be the first manifestation of renal disease. Massive proteinuria usually indicates glomerular injury. Persistent massive proteinuria in the newborn should alert one to consider congenital nephrotic syndrome. Renal biopsy may be necessary to establish the diagnosis. Tubular injury without glomerular disease usually results in a modest increase in protein excretion as well. Physiologic proteinuria of the newborn does not exist; it is probably an artefact related to the presence of urates. Doxiadis found a positive test for protein in less than 1 per cent of neonates after removal of urates from the urine.

Albumin is the most abundant of the plasma proteins in the urine, although other serum proteins can be easily identified. Tamm-Horsfall protein is a high molecular weight mucoprotein produced by the kidney; it may comprise as much as 25 to 40 per cent of normal urinary protein and seems to be a major constituent of urinary casts. Proteins do penetrate the normal glomerular basement membrane and have been shown by immunofluorescent technique to be reabsorbed in the proximal tubule. Administration of large amounts of plasma proteins or albumin to neonates can be associated with transient proteinuria, which may represent a saturation of the tubular reabsorptive mechanism.

A syndrome in young hypovolemic infants has been described in which transient renal obstruction seems to result from the precipitation of Tamm-Horsfall protein in the renal tubules; rarely acute renal failure may appear. This is detected on intravenous pyelograms by a prolonged nephrogram which may last for hours or days, as the radiopaque material is detained. Proteinuria has also been reported in children with cyanotic congenital heart disease in the absence of congestive heart failure. This proteinuria is thought to be related to increased venous pressure.

## HEMATURIA

Hematuria is not frequently seen in the newborn, with excretion rates usually less than 100,000 red cells per 12 hours. When hematuria is detected, its origin must be determined. Red blood cells can enter the urinary tract anywhere from the renal parenchyma to the urethra. The presence of red blood cell casts indicates glomerular disease. Other causes of hematuria include blood dyscrasias, infections, neoplasia, stones, trauma, congenital malformations, disseminated intravascular coagulation and anoxia. Hematuria can also be associated with nephrotoxic drugs. In the female, extraurinary sources such as the vagina must be excluded. Other causes in the newborn include renal vein thrombosis, renal arterial thrombosis, cortical and medullary necrosis, and obstructive uropathy.

In lower urinary tract bleeding with gross hematuria it is not uncommon that following centrifugation the reddish discoloration sediments to the bottom of the tube leaving a clear supernate. In glomerular disease, however, hemoglobinuria may also be present, producing a smoky or brownish color that does not sediment on centrifugation.

Radiologic examination, cystoscopy and renal arteriography may be necessary to establish the diagnosis in the newborn. If a urologic evaluation seems appropriate, it is generally more fruitful if the investigation is performed at that time when hematuria is present. It is rarely necessary to perform a renal biopsy to establish a diagnosis in the newborn.

## PYURIA

Pyuria, like hematuria, can appear from anywhere in the genitourinary tract. It can be present in glomerular disease, tubular disease, acidosis, interstitial nephritis, fever, dehydration and following instrumentation. White blood cell casts are always an indication of renal parenchymal disease.

Although commonly associated with urinary tract infections, pyuria can be associated with any type of inflammatory process within the genitourinary tract. In spontaneous voided specimens, pyuria occurs in only 2 per cent of normal newborn males and in 6 per cent of normal newborn females.

## CASTS

Casts are the only definitive evidence of upper urinary tract involvement. Cast formation can only take place in the lumen of the nephron. Red blood cell casts are most commonly seen in glomerular injury. White blood cell casts may be seen with infection, interstitial injury, tubular damage, or renal inflammation. Epithelial cell casts, which may be difficult to distinguish from white blood cell casts, are seen with tubular or interstitial injury. Broad casts, which develop in atrophied and dilated nephrons, are indicative of nephron death. Granular casts usually represent partially decomposed cellular casts. They can be seen in dehydration, interstitial injury or tubular injury. When cells are trapped within the substance of the casts, it indicates that these cells originated in the parenchyma of the kidney. Hyaline casts may occasionally be found normally or in states of dehydration; they are very common in massive proteinuria.

## RADIOGRAPHIC STUDIES

Evaluation of the anatomy of the neonatal urinary tract by intravenous urography can be difficult. Given the infant's relatively low glomerular filtration rate and poor ability to concentrate urine, visualization may be inadequate when standard intravenous contrast doses are used, and may not be entirely satisfactory even when the larger doses of radiopaque material which are the rule in pediatric radiologic settings are used. Since the radiopaque contrast agents commonly used have an osmolality approximately five times that of serum and a sodium concentration approximately one third of serum, excessive doses must be avoided, particularly in ill infants. However, 3 cc per kg of diatrizoate can be used safely unless the infant is markedly dehydrated. Contrast material is always injected intravenously; the intramuscular route is to be avoided. Urography can usually be successful in any infant with a urine creatinine concentration in excess of 15 times the plasma concentration with the anatomy shown to better advantage 5 to 7 days after delivery. The time sequence of the normal infant I.V.P. is elongated; the nephrogram persists longer than in the older child with pyelogram phase, beginning later and lasting longer as well.

The voiding cystourethrogram is important in outlining the bladder and urethra, and in determining the presence and degree of vesicoureteral reflux. A 15 per cent solution of diatrizoate, instilled at no more than 100 mm of water pressure by gravity drip infusion under fluoroscopic control in the unanesthetized child using a straight catheter (not a Foley), provides proper and safe filling and yields the most useful information.

Renal scans and renograms provide both anatomic and functional information about the kidneys. Their size, shape and location can be determined when conventional urography is contraindicated or unsuccessful. With the renogram, information about renal blood flow or parenchymal function and obstruction can also be determined. Ultrasonography is non-invasive, does not use radioactive materials and requires neither blood flow nor function. It is being increasingly used in localizing and measuring renal size, in identifying solid and cystic masses and as an aid in renal biopsy.

## CLINICAL EVALUATION OF RENAL FUNCTION

### GLOMERULAR FILTRATION RATE

It is particularly difficult, and often impossible, to accurately estimate glomerular filtration rate in the neonate by standard means owing to incomplete or inaccurate urine collections. Yet, creatinine clearance remains the most widely available assessment of glomerular filtration. When properly done, with accurately timed urine specimens, it can be quite reliable. The plasma creatinine concentration in healthy neonates is normally lower than in normal children. The creatinine clearance in the premature averages 25 to 30 ml/minute/1.73 m², and in the term neonate 35 to 40 ml/min/1.73 m²; this gradually rises to 65 to 75 ml/min/1.73 m² by 2 months of age. The serum creatinine in cord blood is usually in the range of 0.7 mg/100 ml, falling over the first few weeks of life to 0.3 to 0.4 mg/100 ml. In this light, a serum creatinine of 0.6–0.8 mg/100 ml, although below the upper limits of normal for a given laboratory, can reflect a glomerular filtration rate that is half normal for that infant. Diatrizoate may interfere with the laboratory determination of creatinine and give a falsely elevated result; therefore, adequate time for clearing diatrizoate from the plasma after intravenous urography should be allowed.

Although most standards for creatinine clearance have been devised on the basis of 24 hour collections, the production of creatinine is dependent on muscle mass and varies little throughout the day. Providing the time of voiding can be accurately determined and the collections complete, collection periods as short as 2 hours may be more practical in the nursery. A collection for creatinine clearance in which the infant's urinary excretion rate is less than 15 mg/kg/24 hours, should be considered incomplete and the result erroneous.

Clearances calculated according to a multi-compartmental analysis from the plasma disappearance of substances handled like inulin have been shown to have the accuracy of the creatinine clearance yet avoid the necessity of urine collections. Methods have been developed for $^{131}$I sodium iodothalamate and $^{51}$Cr–EDTA that appear quite accurate at very low doses of radiation.

### RENAL PLASMA FLOW

The measurement of renal plasma flow has little clinical diagnostic value in the nursery. It is ordinarily measured by the clearance of para-amino hippurate (PAH), which is virtually completely extracted by the kidney. The extraction in infants is less complete than in the older child, which causes underestimation of the true effective renal plasma flow. When corrected for body surface area, the renal plasma flow is still low at birth, but reaches mature levels by 6 months of age. It is felt that much of the improvement in glomerular filtration rate in the newborn is related to a decrease in renal vascular resistance and an increase in renal plasma flow.

## GLUCOSE

Normally, glucose is present in the urine in only trace amounts, below the detection levels of glucose oxidase-impregnated paper laboratory strips. Abnormal amounts of glucose in the urine are not interpretable without a simultaneous blood glucose. Glucose is both filtered and reabsorbed. The renal defect associated with glycosuria is a defect in tubular reabsorption, in which abnormal amounts of glucose appear in the urine at normal or only slightly elevated blood levels. This may occur as an isolated proximal tubular defect or in combination with aminoaciduria and phosphaturia. Renal glycosuria is not be to confused with diabetes mellitus. The tubular maximum for glucose (TmG) is lower in the newborn than in the adult. Determination of the TmG in the neonate is rarely necessary to establish the diagnosis. Glycosuria may also appear during intravenous infusions of glucose at normal rates because of the infant's relatively lower TmG.

## PHOSPHATE

An abnormal loss of phosphate in the urine may be the result of an intrinsic defect of the tubular reabsorption of phosphate or of increased parathormone activity. Hypophosphatemia is the rule in defects of phosphate reabsorption. If hyperparathyroidism is the result of hypocalcemia, elevation of the serum calcium by infusion will reduce parathormone secretion and thus increase the tubular reabsorption of phosphate.

## AMINO ACIDS

Amino acids are also reabsorbed by the proximal tubule. Characteristically, plasma amino acid levels are normal when there is a renal defect of amino acid reabsorption. They are elevated in the metabolic defects leading to overproduction, which results in a filtered level that exceeds the normal reabsorption capacity. Both the pattern and the amount of amino acids excreted varies with the age of the child. Infants normally have a higher excretion of amino acids, particularly threonine, serine, proline, glycine and alanine.

## HYDROGEN ION

The renal tubule excretes hydrogen ion in two phases. In the proximal tubule, hydrogen ion is produced by the dissociation of carbonic acid under the influence of carbonic anhydrase, and is excreted into the lumen to neutralize filtered bicarbonate. The system can handle a large quantity of bicarbonate against a low gradient. Defects in this system are manifested in a low threshold for bicarbonate. In the distal nephron, hydrogen ion is excreted in exchange for sodium or potassium. This system can handle a smaller quantity of hydrogen ion, but at a much greater gradient. Defects in this system are manifested in an inability to produce adequate amounts of titratable acid.

Proximal renal tubular acidosis can be either an isolated defect or combined with other proximal tubular defects such as aminoaciduria, glycosuria and phosphaturia. The isolated defect occurs predominantly in males and is characterized by a bicarbonate resistant, hyperchloremic acidosis. Should the blood bicarbonate fall below the renal threshold, an acid urine may be noted.

The normal newborn, in the first few days of life, may not be able to lower the urinary pH below 6.0. However, by the first week of life, urinary pH below 6.0 should be possible in face of a systemic acidosis. Also, the threshold for bicarbonate in the normal infant may be as low as 20 mEq/L, while the older child's threshold is usually 24 to 26 mEq/L. Occasionally a transient form of proximal tubular acidosis can be seen in severely ill infants that resolves as the infant's condition improves.

The diagnosis of proximal renal tubular acidosis is made by demonstrating both a

**TABLE 43–1.** *Evaluation of Renal Function in the Newborn*

| Function | Clinical Test | Premature | Full-term Neonate | Two Months | Adult | Age of Maturity |
|---|---|---|---|---|---|---|
| Glomerular filtration rate | Inulin clearance ml/min/1.73 M² | 40–60 | 30–50 | 70 | 120 | 12–18 months |
| | Creat. clearance ml/min/1.73 M² | 13–58 | 15–60 | 63–80 | 120–140 | 12–18 months |
| Renal plasma flow | PAH clearance ml/min/1.73 M² | 120–150 | 140–200 | 300 | 630 | 3–6 months |
| Proximal tubular reabsorption | Tm glucose mg/min/1.73 M² | | 60 | 170 | 300 | 12–24 months |
| Proximal tubule excretion | Tm PAH mg/min/1.73 M² | | 16 | 50 | 75 | 12–18 months |
| Distal tubule transport | Urine concentration (mOsm/kg) | 400–700 | 600–1100 | 700–1200 | 1400 | 3 months |
| | Maximum U/P Osm ratio | | 2.5:1 | 3.4:1 | 4:1 | 3 months |

low renal threshold for bicarbonate and the infant's capability to acidify the urine at bicarbonate levels below the threshold. Therapy consists of administering large amounts of either Shohl's solution or bicarbonate; amounts equivalent to 4 to 5 mEq/kg/day of bicarbonate may be necessary, given in divided doses throughout the 24 hours. The state is self-limiting and the infants do not develop rickets, renal stones or nephrocalcinosis. Growth can approach normal if vigorous treatment corrects the acidosis, although this level of control is difficult in the proximal form.

Distal renal tubular acidosis is usually an isolated defect occurring predominantly in females. Although it can be inherited as an autosomal dominant trait, it usually presents as an isolated circumstance in the absence of a family history. Most children are diagnosed after the neonatal period because of failure to thrive or polyuria, or during an episode of dehydration. These infants fail to produce an acid urine even in the face of profound systemic acidosis. Their ability to handle an administered ammonium chloride load is impaired. Therapy consists of Shohl's solution or bicarbonate equivalent to 1–2 mEq/kg/day. Most children require supplemental potassium as well. The defect is permanent and the infants may develop renal stones, nephrocalcinosis or rickets. Growth can be normal with sufficient control of the systemic acidosis, which is more easily attained in this form than in the proximal form.

Normal values for the clinically useful tests of several renal functions in the immature and mature newborn are listed in Table 43–1, compared with the normal adult and the age at which the function matures.

## REFERENCES

Arey, L. B.: Developmental Anatomy. 7th ed. (Rev.) Philadelphia, W. B. Saunders Company, 1974.

Brodehl, J., Franken, A., and Gellissen, K.: Maximum tubular reabsorption of glucose in infants and children. Acta Pediatr. *61*:413, 1972.

Brodehl, J., and Gellissen, K.: Endogenous renal transport of free amino acids in infancy and childhood. Pediatrics *42*:395, 1968.

Chantler, C., and Barratt, T. M.: Estimation of glomerular filtration rate from the plasma clearance of 51-chromium edetic acid. Arch. Dis. Child. *47*:613, 1972.

Cohen, M. L., Smith, F. G., Mindell, R. S., and Vernier, R. L.: A simple, reliable method of measuring glomerular filtration rate, using single, low dose sodium iothalamate I-131. Pediatrics *43*:407, 1969.

Dodge, W. F., Travis, L. B., and Daeschner, C. W.: Comparison of endogenous creatinine clearance with inulin clearance. Am. J. Dis. Child. *113*:683, 1967.

Edelmann, C. M.: Pediatric Nephrology: E. Mead Johnson Award Address 1972. Pediatrics *51*:854, 1973.

Edelmann, C. M., and Spitzer, A.: The maturing kidney. J. Pediatr. *75*:509, 1969.

Edelmann, C. M., Barnett, H. L., Stark, H., Boichis, H., and Rodriguez Soriano, J.: A standardized test of renal concentrating capacity in children. Am. J. Dis. Child. *114*:639, 1967.

Edelmann, C. M., Barnett, H. L., and Troupkou, V.: Renal concentrating mechanisms in newborn infants. Effect of dietary protein and water content, role of urea, and responsiveness to antidiuretic hormone. J. Clin. Invest. *39*:1062, 1960.

Edelmann, C. M., Boichis, H., Rodriguez-Soriano, J., and Stark, H.: The renal response of children to acute ammonium chloride acidosis. Peidatr. Res. *1*:452, 1967.

Edelmann, C. M., Rodriguez-Soriano, J., Boichis, H., Gruskin, A. B., and Acosta, M. I.: Renal bicarbonate reabsorption and hydrogen ion excretion in normal infants. J. Clin. Invest. *46*:1309, 1967.

Gatewood, O. M. B., Glasser, R. J., and Van Houtte, J. J.: Roentgen evaluation of renal size in pediatric age groups. Am. J. Dis. Child. *110*:162, 1965.

Greenberg, B. G., Winters, R. W., and Graham, J. B.: The normal range of serum inorganic phosphorus and its utility as a discriminant in the diagnosis of congenital hypophosphataemia. J. Clin. Endocrinol. *20*:364, 1960.

Greene, L. F., Feinzaig, W., and Dahlin, D. C.: Multicystic dysplasia of the kidney, with special reference to the contralateral kidney. J. Urol. *105*:482, 1971.

Hansen, J. D. L., and Smith, C. A.: Effects of withholding fluid in the immediate postnatal period. Pediatrics *12*:99, 1953.

Hurt, A. S., Jr.: Anomalies of the urinary tract in infants. Am. J. Dis. Child. *38*:1202, 1929.

Kathel, B. L.: Radioisotope renography as a renal function test in the newborn. Arch. Dis. Child. *46*:314, 1971.

Lyons, E. A., Murphy, A. V., and Arneil, G. C.: Sonar and its use in kidney disease in children. Arch. Dis. Child. *47*:777, 1972.

McCance, R. A., and Widdowson, E. M.: Normal renal function in the first 2 days of life. Arch. Dis. Child. *29*:488, 1954.

McCrory, W. W., Forman, C. W., McNamara, H., and Barnett, H. L.: Renal excretion of inorganic phosphate in newborn infants. J. Clin. Invest. *31*:357, 1952.

Moore, E. S., and Galvez, M. B.: Delayed micturition in the newborn period. J. Pediatr. *80*:867, 1972.

Parkkulainen, K. V., Hjelt, L., and Sirola, K.: Congenital multicystic dysplasia of the kidney: Report of 19 cases with discussion on the etiology, nomenclature, and classification of cystic dysplasia of the kidney. Acta. Chir. Scand. *244*:1, 1959.

Pratt, E. L., and Snyderman, S. E.: Renal water requirement of infants fed evaporated milk with and without added carbohydrate. Pediatrics *11*:65, 1953.

Rodriguez-Soriano, J., and Edelmann, C. M.: Renal tubular acidosis. Ann. Rev. Med. *20*:363, 1969.

Royer, P.: Explorations biologiques du metabolisme calcique chez l'enfant. Helv. Paediat. Acta *16*:320, 1961.

Sakai, T., Lenmann, E. P., and Holliday, M. A.: Single injection clearance in children. Pediatrics *44*:905, 1969.

Scriver, C. R.: Amino acid transport in the mammalian kidney. In Amino Acid Metabolism and Genetic Variation. Ed. Nyhan, W. L. pg. 327–340. McGraw Hill, New York, 1967.

Sherry, S. N., and Kramer, I.: The time of passage of the first stool and the first urine by the newborn infant. J. Pediatr. *46*:158, 1955.

Spence, H. M.: Congenital unilateral multicystic kidney: An entity to be distinguished from polycystic kidney disease and other cystic disorders. J. Urol. *74*:693, 1955.

Tausch, M.: Der Fetalharn. Arch. Gynaekol. *162*:27, 1936.

Thalassinos, N. C., Leese, B., Latham, S. C., and Joplin, G. F.: Urinary excretion of phosphate in children. Arch. Dis. Child. *45*:269, 1970.

Vernier, R. L., and Birch-Andersen, A.: Studies of the human fetal kidney. J. Pediatr. *60*:754, 1962.

Vernier, R. L., and Smith, F. G.: Fetal and neonatal kidney. In Assali, N.: Biology of Gestation. Vol. II. New York, Academic Press, 1968.

Woolf, L. I., and Nomen, A. P.: The urinary excretion of amino acids and sugars in early infancy. J. Pediatr. *50*:271, 1957.

# DISORDERS OF THE EXTERNAL GENITALS

# 44

*Revised by Warren Grupe*

## PHIMOSIS

The foreskin of the newborn is ordinarily of sufficient length to cover the glans penis completely. It extends beyond the tip and tapers down to a narrow point which, when spread apart, reveals an adequate orifice. At this age, and for 2 or 3 months more, the foreskin is fairly tight and rigid, and cannot be retracted without tearing. No attempt should be made to retract the foreskin at this time. Phimosis appears to be the normal condition in the neonatal period.

## SURGICAL CIRCUMCISION

The practice of circumcision has become almost universal in the United States. It is performed on the eighth day of life by orthodox Jews as a religious rite. On other infants it is usually done the day before discharge from the nursery; that is, on the third or fourth day of life. Some obstetricians have made early circumcision a fetish, reaching its reductio ad absurdum in one instance with which we are familiar in which the operation was performed when the hips had been delivered and pending expulsion of the upper half of the body!

The medical value of universal circumcision is still a moot question. No one will quarrel with its performance as a religious rite. The alleged advantages are prevention of permanent phimosis, the greater cleanliness afforded by elimination of the blind space in which smegma may collect and infection develop, a lower incidence of penile carcinoma later in life and virtual absence of carcinoma of the cervix in wives of circumcised men. But contraindications of some validity come to mind. The penile meatus, deprived of its protective cover, becomes liable to ulceration by ammoniacal urine, and ulceration not infrequently leads to meatal stenosis. A few instances of penile gangrene and more of near gangrene have followed the use of patented bell clamps. We ourselves have just been involved in a case of this nature as an expert witness for the defense. Of even greater moment is the suspicion that some cases of sepsis of the newborn originate at the site of surgical circumcision. The data purporting to show lowered incidence of subsequent carcinoma in both circumcised men and their wives are suspect, but fairly generally believed. Bolande, in a thoughtful review entitled Ritualistic Surgery—Circumcision and Tonsillectomy, concludes that arguments in favor of circumcision are not very convincing, but that "little serious objection can be raised . . . since its adverse effects seem minimal."

The pediatrician is seldom consulted as to the advisability of circumcision. When our advice has been sought, we have in latter years recommended that the operation not be done for other than ritual reasons. When it is not, we ourselves carefully attempt to retract the foreskin at subsequent monthly examinations, waiting to complete the retraction until it can be accomplished without trauma, and we then instruct the mother to perform the same procedure two or three times a week until the danger of adhesion is past.

## ULCERATIVE MEATITIS AND MEATAL STENOSIS

As far back as 1921 Brenneman taught that meatal ulceration occurred only in the circumcised baby. Mackenzie observed an incidence of such ulceration following circumcision in more than 20 per cent of 140 infants. Ulceration itself is of little consequence, although it does cause some discharge, bleeding, crusting and dysuria, since it clears promptly after the application of almost any bland ointment.

But it now seems incontrovertible that such ulceration leads to meatal stenosis of varying degree. Most of these cases cause no trouble, but some seem to be responsible for frequency, dysuria and perhaps enuresis, and a few, which have gone on to the stage of pinpoint meatus, may lead to obstructive symptoms and perhaps to an increased incidence of acute pyelonephritis.

## PREPUTIAL ADHESIONS

Surgical circumcisions are often incomplete and leave a fringe of foreskin behind. Mothers are ordinarily poorly instructed in the care of this region, with the result that preputial adhesions are permitted to form which become more and more fibrous and firm. One of the duties of the pediatrician at his monthly examinations is to tear these adhesions until glans and foreskin are thoroughly separated to anoint the raw areas with petroleum jelly and to instruct the mother in the performance of this procedure regularly until it is no longer necessary.

## MICROPHALLUS

The penis of the full-term newborn may appear to be very large or very small. Great care must be exercised in order to avoid error in judgment as to its actual size as contrasted with its apparent size. Commonly it projects 2 to 3 cm beyond the pubis. In some males it projects not at all, the glans alone being visible, flush with the pubic contour. These infants are usually very well nourished, and a penis of normal length and breadth can be palpated buried within the thick pad of subcutaneous fat. Rarely the phallus is indeed tiny, measuring less than 2 cm in total palpable length. These infants deserve careful consideration with respect to the other important indices of genital development. Special attention must be given to their chromosomal sex, to the presence or absence and position of gonads, to size and skin characteristics of the scrotum and to the structure of the urinary and genital excretory ducts. It is an easy matter to confuse an underdeveloped penis with an overgrown clitoris. If the testes are descended and if the urethra is completely penile and without hypospadias, small size of the penis need cause no alarm.

Guthrie, Smith and Graham have recently demonstrated that considerable penile growth can be induced in boys under three years of age by no more than four 3-weekly injections of Depo-Testosterone (25 mg each). After this observation shall have been verified it is probable that we should adopt this method in order to spare the child and his parents the problems of psychosexual adjustment that often follow persistent microphallus.

## MEGALOPENIS

When congenital adrenal cortical hyperplasia affects a male infant, penile overgrowth ordinarily does not commence until a year or more after birth. Rarely the penis has been noted to be larger than usual in the neonatal period. The observation that the penis is unusually large at birth calls for careful study of 17-ketosteroid excretion (see Chapter 54).

An extraordinary report appeared in the Case Reports of the Children's Memorial Hospital of Chicago (Andrews).

A 17-month-old white male infant was adopted at two weeks, at which time he was said to have been entirely normal except that his penis was much larger than usual. Unfortunately no measurements were recorded. It continued to grow until at the age of 17 months it was described as being the size of the penis of an adolescent boy. For 1 month he had suffered from colic and flatulence, and his urinary stream was noted to have become weak. The testes were normal in size and location; the prostate gland was enlarged. Intravenous pyelogram showed bilateral hydronephrosis and hydroureter and filling defects in the bladder. Operation revealed a mass in the bladder extending into the prostate and infiltrating the length of the penis. The tumor was thought to be ganglioneuroblastoma.

## TORSION OF THE PENIS

Congenital torsion of the penis is discovered extremely rarely as an isolated defect, somewhat more commonly when associated with other defects of the external genitalia. Hypospadias or epispadias is its usual concomitant. We have encountered one infant who had torsion of the penis, a slit-like balanitic hypospadias, hypoplasia of abdominal musculature, bladder neck obstruction, megacystis and megaureter. Stenosis of the meatus may coexist and may produce symptoms, but the torsion itself causes no difficulties.

The penis is twisted on its long axis, either clockwise or counterclockwise, so that

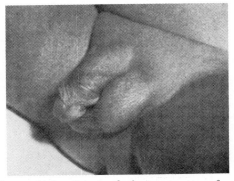

*Figure 44–1.* Counterclockwise torsion of penis with meatus at 2 o'clock. (Broussard, E. R.: J. Pediat. *46*:456, 1955.)

the frenum of the glans faces upward. In uncomplicated cases the meatus lies in the exact center of the tip of the glans, and urine is expelled forcefully and directly ahead (Fig. 44–1).

No treatment is indicated.

## HYPOSPADIAS

The penile urethra develops during the tenth to fourteenth weeks of gestation by progressive folding together of the edges of the urogenital groove from behind forward. The progression may stop short to leave the urethral orifice at some point between the scrotal raphé and the base of the glans penis. Figure 44–2 shows the loci where abnormal hypospadiac orifices are ordinarily situated.

Hypospadias is a very common condition, with an incidence of 1 in 700 newborn males. Although on theoretical grounds it implies a deficiency in fetal androgen synthesis or action, the large majority of affected infants have a normal potential for adult sexual function. The familial occurrence in 38 per cent of cases and the concordance rate of 50 per cent in twins found by Sorenson, together with the frequent occurrence in syndromes of multiple phenotypic abnormalities, suggest that many nonendocrine factors contribute to production of hypospadias. However, Aarskog, in 1970, reported that congenital adrenal hyperplasia, chromosomal abnormalities and maternal progestin ingestion accounted for 15 of 100 consecutive cases referred for evaluation. Other investigators have cited much lower yields. Application of specific radioimmunoassays of steroid metabolites, and recognition that the first 3 months of life is normally an active time for testosterone synthesis, may lead to a higher incidence of specific biochemical diagnoses in future series.

Hypospadias is subdivided into several types, depending upon the location of the meatus. The simplest form is the *balanitic* or *glandular*, in which the meatus is situated at the base of the glans penis. Usually this is asymptomatic and requires no treatment. Narrowing of the opening may upon occasion require dilatation or meatotomy. In the *penile* form the opening lies at some point between the glans and scrotum. Associated deformities usually found are absent ventral foreskin (hooded foreskin), ventral angulation of the shaft of the penis (chordee) and flattened glans. This type of deformity should be corrected surgically, but the first stage is not ordinarily performed until the age of 1 to 4 years. The remnant of foreskin should not be circumcised, since it may be useful in later plastic procedures. The *penoscrotal* and *perineal* forms demonstrate these deformities in greater degree. The penis may be underdeveloped, the scrotum bifid, the urinary meatus widely open and the testes undescended. In these forms the possibility of pseudohermaphroditism must be carefully explored. Staged operative reconstruction

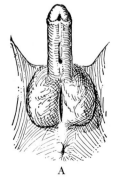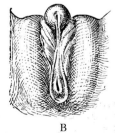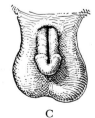

A                    B                    C

*Figure 44–2.*  Anomalies of the male genitalia. *A*, Hypospadias, showing in one drawing a composite of the common locations. *B*, Hypospadias, of a severe degree, in a false hermaphrodite. *C*, Epispadias. (Arey, L. B.: Developmental Anatomy. 7th ed., 1965.)

will be attempted some time after the first year of life.

In 1970 Hodgson described a new one-stage procedure for the correction of hypospadias in the distal third of the penile shaft. Others have gotten splendid results with this method.

## EPISPADIAS

When the urethra is displaced toward the dorsal aspect of the penis and opens at some point proximal to the glans, epispadias is present. The opening may consist of a small meatal orifice or of a long furrow which bisects the upper penile surface for some or all of its length. Epispadias is considerably less common than hypospadias and is generally but one small part of a massive defect which includes exstrophy of the bladder. Plastic repair of epispadias should be attempted at a later date, especially when incontinence of urine coexists.

## DIVERTICULUM OF THE MALE URETHRA

Congenital diverticula of the urethra are rare. Meiraz et al. recently described two examples. The diverticula arise at the penoscrotal junction and present at birth as swellings of variable size from which urine can be expressed. Diagnosis can be readily verified by injection of a radiopaque dye through the meatus. They endanger life because they produce obstruction which may eventuate in hydroureter and hydronephrosis, often with pyelonephritis. For this reason plastic repair must not be delayed.

## MEATAL ATRESIA

Failure to void during the first 24 hours of life should call first for careful examination of the penis. Obstruction to urinary outflow may be discovered in the form of absence of a meatal orifice. Fortunately the obstructing element in many instances consists of a membranous velum covering and sealing the opening. This can easily be

punctured with a fine hemostat and the meatus can be spread apart. Once opened, the orifice remains patent.

Other, more deeply seated, obstructions may be responsible for failure to void. Urethral atresia, with or without urachal patency, is a serious malformation which will have to be dealt with by the urologist. Vesical neck obstruction will be discussed later.

## UNDESCENDED TESTIS (CRYPTORCHIDISM)

It is customary to separate cryptorchid testes into 1) those whose descent has become halted at some point in their normal route from their original high paralumbar position to the bottom of the scrotum (arrested descent) and 2) those that arrive at an abnormal locus (maldescent). Descent may be arrested early, the testis remaining within the abdomen, or later, the gonad ceasing its progression at any point from the internal inguinal ring downward. In maldescent the testis may come to lie at some point in the upper part of the thigh or lower part of the abdominal wall or, more commonly, within the perineum.

**INCIDENCE.** Figures reported by various observers for nondescent range from 1 to 14 per cent (Robinson and Engle). Scorer examined 2700 newborn males and discovered 108 (4 per cent) examples of all stages of arrested descent.

In premature infants weighing 1000 gm or less, complete descent is not to be expected. As gestational age and birth weight increase, more and more testes will be found within the scrotum.

**PATHOGENESIS.** The testis arises early in gestation as an outgrowth of the urogenital ridge that bulges into the celomic cavity not far below the diaphragm. By the tenth week it has migrated caudad to lie at the boundary between the abdomen and the pelvis. There it remains until some time between the seventh and ninth months of gestation, when it passes through the internal inguinal ring and makes its way slowly down the processus vaginalis into the scrotum.

Failure to descend, according to Bongiovanni, may be due to primary testicular dysgenesis, ectopia, adhesion or shortness of spermatic vessels or premature tightening of inguinal rings. Disadvantages of high testes include delayed maturation of germinal elements, fibrosis of tubules, possible trauma, increased susceptibility to malignancy, although this is not great, and psychological trauma.

Descent is complete in most full-term newborns, but in a few not until after birth. Sixty of Scorer's 108 arrested ones finished descent by 1 month of age, another 29 some time between the second month and the end of the first year. The residue of 19 remained cryptorchid, three intra-abdominal, the rest within the canal.

**DIAGNOSIS.** The diagnosis can be made only by inability to see or palpate both testes in the scrotum. If both testes are undescended in a full-term newborn, one should give more than passing thought to the possibility of intersexuality. The size and conformation of the phallus and scrotum and the position and structure of the urethra and its meatus supply invaluable information as to this possibility. Yet Weldon et al. have seen five examples of cryptorchidism resulting from adrenal hyperplasia in whom there was *complete* masculinization of the external genitalia, with perfectly placed penile urethras (see Pseudohermaphroditism and Hermaphroditism, p. 512 et seq.).

**TREATMENT.** No treatment is indicated in the neonatal period for cryptorchidism per se. Suspicion of pseudohermaphroditism demands further studies, namely, 24-hour urinary ketosteroid and pregnanetriol excretion, serum electrolytes and buccal smears; and confirmation calls for appropriate therapy. Surgery is indicated if inguinal hernia, a not uncommon associated disorder, becomes obvious. During the course of operation for hernia the undescended testis will be brought down into the scrotum, if possible, and fixed in its normal position.

Lattimer et al. make the statement, in agreement with many if not all pediatric urologists, that "on the basis of histological, cellular kinetic and clinical studies, but most importantly the psychologic consider-ations, it appears best to initiate and complete the treatment both for true cryptorchid and for migratory testes between the fourth and fifth birthdays." The treatment for cryptorchidism is operative; that for migratory testes is by injections of gonadotropin.

## ANORCHIA

For the sake of completeness it should be pointed out that a few children who manifest "empty scrotum" suffer not from maldescent but from congenital absence of the testes. These babies will develop eunuchoidism and the often severe emotional problems of the sexually immature male. They can be identified by low plasma testosterone levels and by failure of this level to rise after chorionic gonadotropin stimulation. Treatment consists of testosterone therapy and intrascrotal placement of artificial testes.

## HYDROCELE

An accumulation of fluid about the testis constitutes a noncommunicating hydrocele or hydrocele of the testis. The processus vaginalis is sealed off tightly down to the testis itself, but a variable quantity of fluid occupies the space between the tunica vaginalis and tunica albuginea. If the amount is small, the testis appears to be moderately enlarged and may be relatively soft, but large collections may enlarge it tremendously and render it tense. The mass transilluminates brightly, but the dark round or oval shadow of the testis stands out sharply within it. The cord feels normal unless the processus is open for a distance proximal to the testis (infantile hydrocele), when this portion may be felt to be distended. The external inguinal ring is not dilated.

Communicating or congenital hydroceles, on the other hand, mean that the processus vaginalis is patent. It may be so for only a short distance below the inguinal ring, or patency may include the tunica vaginalis. In the former instance the cord appears thickened for some or all of its length below the ring, while in the latter instance apparent enlargement of the testis is added. It is difficult to determine the size of the inguinal ring in the presence of communicating hydroceles, but hernia often coexists and the conditions for herniation are by definition present. Campbell's schematic representation of the various types of hydrocele is informative (Fig. 44-3).

There should be no difficulty in differentiating scrotal hernia from noncommunicating hydrocele. Unless incarcerated, hernia varies in size, appears and disappears, often contains crepitant gas and does not transilluminate brightly. When it is incarcerated, one must rely upon nontranslucency and upon the fact that the testis lies free from the mass and below it, while the swelling can be followed as a firm tube

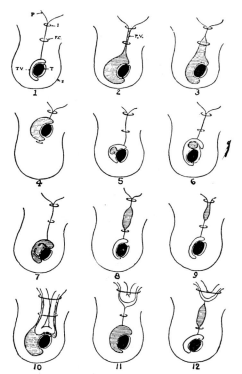

**Figure 44-3.** Schematic representation of types of hydrocele. *1*, Normal relationship. *2*, Congenital hydrocele. *3*, Infantile. *4*, Hydrocele of undescended testis. *5*, Hydrocele of testis. *6*, Hydrocele of epididymis. *7*, Bilocular. *8*, Hydrocele of cord. *9*, Hydrocele of hernial sac. *10*, With hernia (congenital type). *11*, Hydrocele of tunica vaginalis with hernia. *12*, Hydrocele of cord with hernia. (From Campbell, M. F.: Pediatric Urology.)

from the scrotum all the way into the inguinal canal. Communicating hydroceles which include the testis and the entire cord present a bit more difficulty, but their translucency and the relative absence of fluctuations in size—they may be slightly larger at night than in the morning—and visualization of the testicular shadow within the mass should make the distinction clear.

The finding of a small, firm, irreducible cystic mass within the inguinal canal just below the ring often gives rise to perplexity. For some reason fluid may become entrapped within the tunica vaginalis at this point to produce an acute hydrocele that is hard to distinguish from a small incarcerated hernia. If one can feel normally sized cord above it and an undilated inguinal ring, one can be sure that no hernia is present. If one cannot, and this seems to be the more common situation, differential diagnosis may be impossible without exploration.

The noncommunicating hydrocele seldom requires *treatment*. Huge ones which remain large and tense for many months are at times tapped. If fluid reaccumulates promptly, operative intervention may have to be considered. Communicating hydroceles are ordinarily watched closely and repaired only if herniation becomes apparent. The acute hydrocele of the cord may be repaired after exploration has ruled out the presence of strangulated hernia.

## TORSION OF THE SPERMATIC CORD

**INCIDENCE.** Peterson was able to find reports on 56 cases of torsion of testicle in the newborn period, up to 1961. Twenty-two of these were noted immediately after delivery, hence were torsions in utero. Testicular infarction is often spoken of as being of two types: those resulting from torsion, and idiopathic ones in whom no torsion is found at operation. Rhyne et al. argue convincingly that these also have resulted from torsion, but that spontaneous detorsion had taken place prior to operation.

**DIAGNOSIS.** In older children and in adults torsion commonly takes place within and distal to the reflection of the tunica vaginalis (intravaginal), whereas in the newborn the site is apt to be proximal to this point and extravaginal. This may account for the difference in symptomatology between these age groups, since the excruciating pain, often associated with nausea and vomiting, so characteristic of torsion in older patients is almost entirely lacking in newborns. In these the only findings are the objective ones of an enlarged, firm or stony hard mass in the scrotum, plus reddish or bluish discoloration and, at times, induration of the scrotal skin over the mass. This mass has been seen immediately after birth in many, or it has made its appearance at any time within the first few days of life. The right testis is involved much more often than the left, and bilateral involvement is not too uncommon. To our knowledge torsion of the testicular appendages (appendix testis and appendix epididymis) has not been reported in a newborn.

*Differential diagnosis* is comparatively simple. The only other disorders worthy of consideration are traumatic hematoma, strangulated hernia, hydrocele of the testis, orchitis and testicular neoplasm. The first two should present no difficulty in differential diagnosis. In hydrocele the mass is usually soft and fluctuant, though it may be tense; it transilluminates, and there is no discoloration of the overlying skin. Orchitis is an exceedingly rare localization of infection in sepsis of the newborn, and associated with it should be found some of the other manifestations of neonatal septicemia. Epididymitis is even rarer. Testicular tumors, usually dermoids, are rare in the neonatal period, and in them also discoloration and induration of the scrotum are not encountered.

**TREATMENT.** Treatment consists in immediate operation. It may be possible to save the organ by detorsion of the cord soon after twisting has occurred, but gangrene sets in so quickly and discovery is so often delayed by absence of pain in the newborn that this procedure is not often attempted. There would seem to be no good reason why the operator should not pause a few minutes to observe how well or poorly circulation returns to the testis after manual detorsion before taking the irreversible step of excision. Leape, however, was un-

able to save any one of seven examples he saw in the newborn period, one of which, incidentally, was bilateral. Orchiopexy should be performed on the uninvolved side after the affected testis has been removed.

CASE 44–1

A white male infant weighed 8 pounds 11 ounces (3950 gm) at birth, which was spontaneous and followed a completely normal pregnancy and labor. The initial physical examination was made at 12 hours of age. Everything was absolutely normal except for the scrotum and its contents. The right half of the scrotum was described as "dark reddish to blue, felt firm, contained a mass which seemed to be fixed to thickened scrotal skin and did not transilluminate." Temperature was 97° F. He was placid and obviously in no pain. On the third day of life a right orchidectomy was performed. The pathologic diagnosis was "hemorrhagic infarction of immature testis."

**COMMENT.** This example emphasizes the points already made. There was no pain or gastrointestinal upset. The testis was enlarged, but pathognomonic were the fixation to the scrotum, the discolored, thickened skin of that side of the scrotum and absence of translucency. These physical findings rule out neoplasm and hydrocele, while absence of fever, local tenderness and apparent illness effectually dispose of orchitis.

## LABIAL FUSION

True labial fusion is discussed fully under Pseudohermaphroditism (p. 513). It is a developmental defect and one at times dependent upon masculinization of the female external genitalia and excretory ducts by excessive androgen production in early embryonic life.

This should not be confused with another form of fusion not infrequently encountered in which the vaginal orifice is partially or completely obliterated by more or less tight adherence of the labia minora. This false fusion is effected by connective tissue adhesions, at first delicate, but later fibrous in consistency, which tie one labium to the other. Ordinarily this condition produces no symptoms, but in some patients it is the cause of frequency and dysuria.

The labia should be separated widely as part of the original neonatal examination and every few months thereafter. If this is done, adhesions can be torn painlessly while they are still delicate and friable. After months or years they may become so tough that the procedure will have to be carried out under anesthesia.

## HYPERTROPHY OF THE CLITORIS

See Pseudohermaphroditism and Hermaphroditism (Chap. 56).

## IMPERFORATE HYMEN

Absence of the one or two small openings normally present in the hymen leads to no trouble in the neonatal period unless the infant happens also to be one of those few who manufacture an excess of vaginal secretion shortly after birth. This combination may then produce hydrometrocolpos (Chap. 52).

## REFERENCES

Andrews, J.: Large penis. Clinical case no. 899. Case Rep. Child. Mem. Hosp. Chicago *14*:3824, 1956.

Bolande, R. P.: Ritualistic surgery—circumcision and tonsillectomy. New Engl. J. Med *280*:591, 1969.

Bongiovanni, A. M.: Diagnosis and treatment: The undescended testicle. Pediatrics *36*:786, 1965.

Brenneman, J.: The ulcerated meatus in the circumcised child. Am. J. Dis. Child. *21*:38, 1921.

Broussard, E. R.: Uncomplicated congenital torsion of the penis. J. Pediat. *46*:456, 1955.

Campbell, M. F.: Stenosis of the external urethral meatus. J. Urol. *50*:740, 1943.

Cecil, A. B.: Hypospadias and epispadias. Pediat. Clin. N. Amer. *2*:711, 1955.

Charnock, D. A., and Riddle, H. I.: Genital tract diseases in infants and children. Pediat. Clin. N. Amer. *2*:827, 1955.

Chiles, D. W., and Foster, R. S.: Torsion of the appendix testis in the newborn. Am. J. Dis. Child *118*:652, 1969.

Engel, R. M., and Scott, W. W.: Hypospadias: Experience with a new one-stage repair. Md. State Med. J. *20*:45, 1971.

Franzblau, A. H.: Torsion of the spermatic cord in the newborn. A.M.A. J. Dis. Child. *92*:179, 1956.

Gillenwater, J. M., and Burros, H. H.: Torsion of the spermatic cord in utero. J. A.M.A. *198*:1123, 1966.

Guthrie, R. D., Smith, D. W., and Graham, C. B.: Testosterone treatment for micropenis during early childhood. Pediatrics *83*:247, 1973.

Hodgson, N. B.: A one-stage hypospadias repair. J. Urol. *104*:281, 1970.

Klingerman, J. J., and Nourse, M. H.: Torsion of the spermatic cord. J.A.M.A. *200*:97, 1967.

Kolodny, H. D., Kim, S., et al.: Anorchia: A variety of empty scrotum. J.A.M.A. *216*:479, 1971.

Lattimer, J. K., Smith, A. M., et al.: The optimum time to operate for cryptorchidism. Pediatrics *53*:96, 1974.

Leape, L. L.: Torsion of the testis: Invitation to error. J.A.M.A. *200*:669, 1967.

Mackenzie, A. R.: Meatal ulceration following neonatal circumcision. Obstet. Gynecol. *28*:221, 1966.

Meiraz, D., Dolberg, L., et al.: Diverticulum of the urethra in two boys. Am. J. Dis. Child. *122*:271, 1971.

Peterson, C. G.: Testicular torsion and infarction in the newborn. J. Urol. *85*:65, 1961.

Rhyne, J. L., Mantz, F. A., Jr., and Patton, J. F.: Hemorrhagic infarction of testis in the newborn: Relationship to testicular torsion. A.M.A. J. Dis. Child. *89*:240, 1955.

Robinson, J. N., and Engle, E. T.: Cryptorchidism. Pediat. Clin. N. Amer. *2*:729, 1955.

Rubenstein, M. M., and Bason, W. M.: Complication of circumcision done with a plastic bell clamp. Am. J. Dis. Child. *116*:381, 1968.

Scorer, C. G.: A treatment of undescended testicle in infancy. Arch. Dis. Child. *32*:520, 1957.

Weldon, V. V., Blizzard, R. M., and Migeon, C. J.: Newborn girls misdiagnosed as bilaterally cryptorchid males. New Engl. J. Med. *274*:829, 1966.

# 45

# MAJOR CONGENITAL MALFORMATIONS OF THE GENITOURINARY TRACT

*Revised by Warren Grupe*

## EXSTROPHY OF THE BLADDER

This catastrophic malformation is fortunately rare. It has been estimated to appear once in 40,000 to 50,000 births. It occurs more often in boys than in girls. It is the result of a defect in ontogenetic development in which midline closure of the lower part of the abdomen fails to become complete. The resultant fissure involves not only abdominal wall, but also the bladder, urethra and penis or clitoris and labia. The bladder is no longer a closed sphere, but lies on the lower part of the abdomen as a bright red, everted corrugated sheet bulging outward. The trigone and ureteral orifices are exposed, and urine dribbles intermittently onto the mucous membrane surface. The penis is flattened and underdeveloped and deeply fissured on its dorsal surface; that is, it is involved in complete epispadias. The testes are usually undescended. In girls the clitoris is generally fissured and the labia are widely separated. The vagina is absent or is replaced by a rectovaginal cloaca. The symphysis pubis is often lacking, the pubic rami gaping widely apart. Inguinal hernias are often associated.

There is no difficulty in arriving at the correct diagnosis.

Therapy is surgical and consists of a primary orthopedic procedure calculated to approximate the rami, followed by plastic repair of such other defects as may be

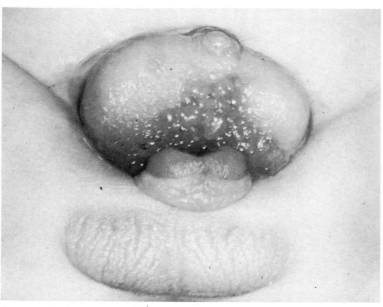

***Figure 45–1.*** Bulging everted bladder lying below the umbilicus. Beneath this a completely epispadiac penis is seen, while below this is a shallow, poorly developed scrotum devoid of testes.

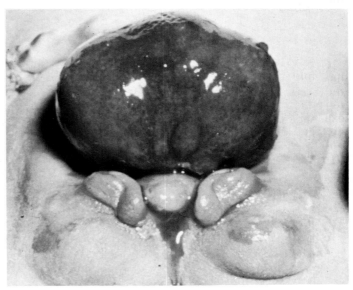

*Figure 45–2.* Bulging everted bladder lies on the lower part of the abdomen. Below it the three structures seen are a small, flattened phallus in the midline and widely separated labia to either side. Below and lateral to these are the bulges of indirect inguinal hernias. (Photograph of a case of Dr. Martin A. Robbins of Baltimore, reproduced with his kind permission.)

reparable. None of this is ordinarily undertaken until long past the neonatal period. Landau and Lattimer have advanced the age of first operative attack to as early as 3 to 6 months, at which time functional closure of the bladder is accomplished. They advise iliac osteotomies a week or two in advance of this procedure in order to effect closure of the wound more readily. In the interim the exposed bladder mucosa must be kept moist and protected from irritation and infection by thick pads moistened with normal saline solution.

The parents of these unfortunate infants require much support. The pediatrician and surgical confrère must devote as much time as is needed to bolster their morale. The may point out that although the situation is grave, it is not hopeless, and that newer approaches give promise that it may be possible to reconstruct the urinary outflow tract along more physiolo-

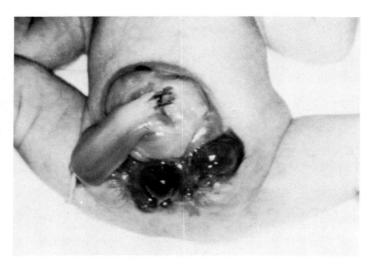

*Figure 45–3.* The umbilicus, with cord still attached, is herniated so as to form a large omphalocele. Beneath it lies the deep, dark red mucosa of everted bladder. The genitalia cannot be seen in this photograph. (This photograph is an enlargement of Figure 39–6.)

gic lines than has been accomplished in the past.

## ABSENT EXTERNAL GENITALS

Complete absence of external genitals has been reported on several occasions. We mention it only for the sake of completeness and append the photographs of one example (Fig. 45–4). Associated with this gross malformation were many internal ones, including complete absence of kidneys. The facies of this infant suggests the presence of that defect (see Fig. 45–5).

## CONGENITAL ABSENCE OF THE KIDNEYS (RENAL AGENESIS)

Congenital absence of one kidney causes no symptoms and is normally not discov-

ered in the neonatal period. We have recently encountered an example of Wilms' tumor in the only kidney a baby possessed.

Both kidneys may have failed to develop. This gross malformation is incompatible with life and therefore merits only the briefest of discussions. Certain clinical characteristics recognized by Potter are intriguing enough to warrant summarization.

**INCIDENCE.** The condition is more common than most of us realized. Amolsch was able to find 119 case reports in the literature up to 1937. Potter found 20 in 5000 consecutive autopsies on fetuses and newborns, an incidence of four per 1000 deaths, or 0.3 per 1000 births.

**DIAGNOSIS.** Almost all the subjects are male. Infants with bilateral agenesis fail to produce urine. The proportion in Potter's series was 17 males to three females. Associated with renal agenesis in a large percentage is gross malformation of the legs. In others hydrocephalus, meningocele,

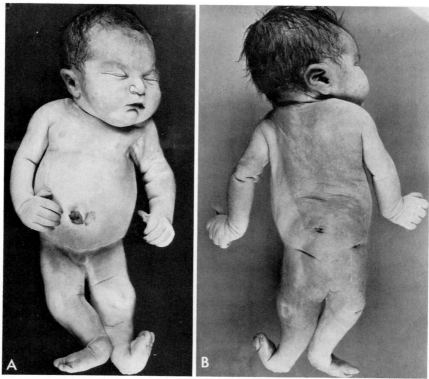

*Figure 45–4.*   Absence of external genitals, together with imperforate anus and facial characteristics suggestive of renal agenesis. (Case of J. D. Kirshbaum. Photographs reprinted with his kind permission from J. Pediatr. 37:102, 1950.)

multiple skeletal anomalies, arthrogryposis or imperforate anus exist, inter alia. Hypoplasia and immaturity of the lungs is a frequently associated finding. Oligohydramnios, often complete absence of amniotic fluid, is the rule, as is amnion nodosum.

While surveying her series Potter made the astute observation that these infants showed many characteristics which permitted diagnosis of renal agenesis in vivo. They were of low birth weight for gestational age. They looked prematurely senile. Their eyes were widely separated, and prominent epicanthal folds ran downward and then laterally below the eyes. The bridge of the nose was flattened, the chin receded, and the ears were large, floppy and low-set (Fig. 45–5). Potter's facies may be seen in association with other severe renal anomalies including aplasia, hypoplasia, dysplasia and multicystic dysplasia; these infants will have varying degrees of remaining renal function, produce urine and may survive the neonatal period. Pas-

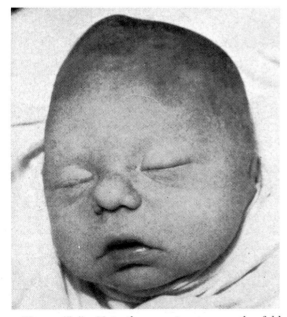

*Figure 45–5.* Note the prominent eyes, the fold sweeping in an arc from the inner canthus downward and outward, the depressed nasal bridge and retroussé nose and the low-set ears. In this case there was complete absence of the right kidney and hypoplasia of the left kidney. (Case of J. D. Kirshbaum. Photograph reprinted with the author's permission from *California Med. 71*:148, 1949.)

sarge and Sutherland have tabulated the pertinent data on three cases of their own—which, incidentally, showed no chromosomal aberrations—plus 20 of Potter's and 50 of Bain and Scott's (Table 45–1).

There have been two recent reports of association of bilateral and unilateral aplasia in the same families, and another in which one monoamniotic and monochorionic twin was born with no kidneys, while in his twin one was absent, the other ectopic and dysplastic. Neither twin had the facial features of Potter's syndrome, nor did they have hypoplastic lungs. There had been no oligohydramnios. The authors argue that the twins were protected from these complicating associated defects because the one functioning kidney among the four forestalled oligohydramnios. More and more students of this problem believe that the oligohydramnios is responsible, via excessive uterine pressure, for the pulmonary hypoplasia and for most of the other associated defects.

**PROGNOSIS.** One of Potter's 20 examples died before the onset of labor. Six died during labor. Those who were born alive died, usually cyanotic and dyspneic, at any time from 25 minutes to 11 hours after delivery. Often this form of death has been the result of pneumothorax, to the development of which the hypoplasia of the lungs predisposes. Dialysis is not generally instituted, since many die of their lung abnormality before uremia can intercede.

## CONGENITAL ABSENCE OF ABDOMINAL MUSCULATURE (THE TRIAD SYNDROME)

All or almost all the muscle mass that sheathes the abdomen may be missing at birth. At times only one side of the abdomen is involved; at others one or two of the definitive muscle groups are lacking.

**INCIDENCE.** About 200 cases have been reported to date. Total or subtotal generalized lack of muscle is encountered more often than localized forms, although the lower rectus group appears to be the one most severely affected, and the obliques attenuated, mostly in their medial portions (Rogers and Ostrow).

**TABLE 45–1.** *Renal Agenesis—Comparison of Data**

| | Infant 1 | Infant 2 | Infant 3 | Potter, 20 Cases | Bain and Scott, 50 Cases |
|---|---|---|---|---|---|
| Gestation, wk. | 34 | 32 | 37 | 36, median of 18 | 36 > 34 |
| Wt. gm. (lb., oz.) | 1910 (4, 3) | 1670 (3, 11) | 1920 (4, 4) | 700–3000 (1, 7–6, 6) Median:1645 | 1200–2350 (2, 6–5, 3) |
| Sex | Male | Male | Female | 17 males, 3 females | Not given |
| Presentation | Breech | Vertex | Breech | 6/18 breech | 30/49 breech |
| Absent amniotic fluid | + | + | + | 20 | Present in only one with iniencephaly |
| Unresuscitable | + | + | + | | |
| Survival time | 1 hr. | 2 hr. | 40 min. | 0–11 hr., 11 min. 1 hr., 38 min., median | 0–36 hr. 3 hr., 9 min., mean |
| Potter-face | + | + | + | 20 | 40 |
| Amnion nodosum | + | + | + | ? | 17/20 |
| Pulmonary hypoplasia | + (15.5 gm.) | ? (18.0 gm.) | + (10 gm.) | 20 3.2–20.0 gm. | 50 |
| Contracted joints, talipes, etc. | + | ? | + | 9/20 | 28/39 |
| Other severe skeletal abnormalities | − | − | − | 3 | − |
| Kidneys | Absent | Single nephron on one ureter | Cystic dysplastic | 0/20 | Absent 28/50; cystic dysplastic 17/50 |
| Ureters | Absent | 2 ureters | Present | 0/20 | Not stated |

*Passarge, E., and Sutherland, J. M.: *Am. J. Dis. Child.*, 109:80, 1965.

**ETIOLOGY AND PATHOGENESIS.** There is no hereditary predisposition. Males predominate in all series, with a ratio of 159 males to seven females at last count.

The musculature of the abdomen is derived from the original segmental myotomes by a process which involves splitting into epimere and hypomere, growth of the hypomere ventrad to surround the body cavity, fusion of segments and splitting into several layers. The whole process begins by about the fifth week and goes on until about the twelfth, when the anterior abdominal defect is finally closed by fusion of the rectus abdominis muscles. Failure to develop this musculature must follow some kind of damage to the embryo during the second month of gestation.

The disorder is often associated with other congenital defects, chief among which are those involving the testes (absence or nondescent), and the genitourinary tract, hence the term "Triad syndrome." These last are present so universally that most students of the problem were inclined until recently to believe that they were secondary to (i.e., caused by) the muscular deficiency. The modern consensus has swung away from this belief and holds that muscle hypoplasia and the urinary tract deformities arise independently from the same embryologic insult. Defects of this system include great distention of the bladder (megacystis), grossly dilated and tortuous ureters with massive reflux and hydronephrosis, often associated with dysplasia.

**DIAGNOSIS.** Many of the infants are moribund at birth. In one clinical-pathological conference at the Sinai Hospital of Baltimore Dr. Tobias Weinberg discussed three infants who had been born in 1953 and 1954. All three lived 1 hour or less. In addition to absent abdominal musculature, the first infant had anomalies of the feet, penis and scrotum, imperforate anus, polycystic kidneys, cystic urachus and a hugely distended bladder. The abdomen of the second looked and felt "completely flat, without tone, as though it were empty." Additional defects included arthrogryposis, cystic kidneys, hydronephrosis and hydroureter. The abdomen of the third infant was so greatly distended that he was thought to have ascites. Autopsy showed distention to be due to a huge bladder, bilateral megaloureter and hydronephrosis. Rogers and Ostrow stress that an association with patent urachus is not unusual and that the presence of an anatomic urethral obstruction "defines a lethal variant of this syndrome."

Infants less seriously affected are not so ill at birth. Their abdomens usually bulge, and the flanks sag limply. Characteristic is wrinkling and creasing of the skin of the abdomen, commonly spoken of as "prune-belly." The palpating hand meets no resistance, so that one can easily feel all the organs and the vertebral column. Usually many masses are palpable, large bladder, ureters and kidneys being readily felt.

**PROGNOSIS.** Most of the infants who survive the neonatal period are doomed to months or years of ill health caused by advancing chronic pyelonephritis, and early death in uremia. Rogers and Ostrow reported on the outcome of 20 cases, of whom 19 were male. Eight died between 5 hours and 3 months. Five of these demonstrated anatomic urethral obstruction and bilateral renal dysplasia. Twelve are still alive, aged 2 months to 25 years. Prognosis seems related to the degree of functioning renal tissue, the presence of obstruction and the success achieved in retaining adequate drainage of the urine and control of infection.

**TREATMENT.** Since there is so little muscle to work with, no reconstructive operations looking toward re-establishment of abdominal tone are possible. The best one can offer for this disability is the use of a tight binder. Surprisingly, the tone of the abdominal wall does seem to improve after the child has worn such a binder for several years. Antibiotic therapy should not be continuous for an indefinite period, but should be confined to short periods of intensive treatment when indicated.

McGovern and Marshall adopted an attitude which insists that "masterful inactivity" is entirely out of place in these infants. Many of them can be salvaged, they argue, if proper and immediate attention is paid to their genitourinary problems. By the time of birth the renal cortex may already have been thinned by excessive back pressure. This must be relieved at once, and these authors choose to effect relief by performing nephrostomies within the first few days of life. If the ureters are dilated and tortuous, they shorten, straighten and reimplant them at the same time or shortly thereafter. Later, if there still remains evidence of urinary reflux up one or both ureters, if the bladder remains large and its cystometric pressure increased, they operate again to revise the bladder neck.

Burke et al. added 19 examples to the 146 previously reported ones, including 18 boys and one girl. They found that of the 14 cases whose courses could be traced, nine were still alive. Of these nine, six had survived beyond 14 years, and five of these more than 20 years! Unlike McGovern and Marshall, they felt that those subjected to surgery had fared no better than those not operated upon, and that "close medical and urologic follow-up examination, with efforts to control or prevent bacteriuria and progressive renal failure, would seem to be most important in prolongation of life." Rogers' and Ostrow's conclusions are in agreement with these.

Patients with this anomaly have been successfully transplanted, using an ileal cutaneous conduit for urine drainage.

## FISTULOUS CONNECTIONS BETWEEN INTESTINAL AND URINARY TRACTS

Female infants born with imperforate anus often have fistulas connecting the lower bowel with the vagina (p. 366). This fortuitous and fortunate coincidence precludes the necessity in many instances for immediate operation, permitting its postponement until much later, when plastic procedures can be undertaken with an augmented probability of success.

The fistulas are less frequent in males with imperforate anus and, when they are present, they connect the rectum with bladder or urethra. They provide no relief for the immediate problem of intestinal obstruction. Indeed, they represent just one more congenital malformation which must be dealt with at once.

CASE 45–1

A white male infant was admitted on the second day of life. He had been born at home, uneventfully, after a normal pregnancy. The day after birth he began to cry and draw his legs up over his abdomen. A physician was called who discovered that the child had no anus and was passing flatus through his urethra. He had not vomited, nor had he passed fecal material from the urethral meatus. Examination showed a large, distended abdomen with loops of bowel

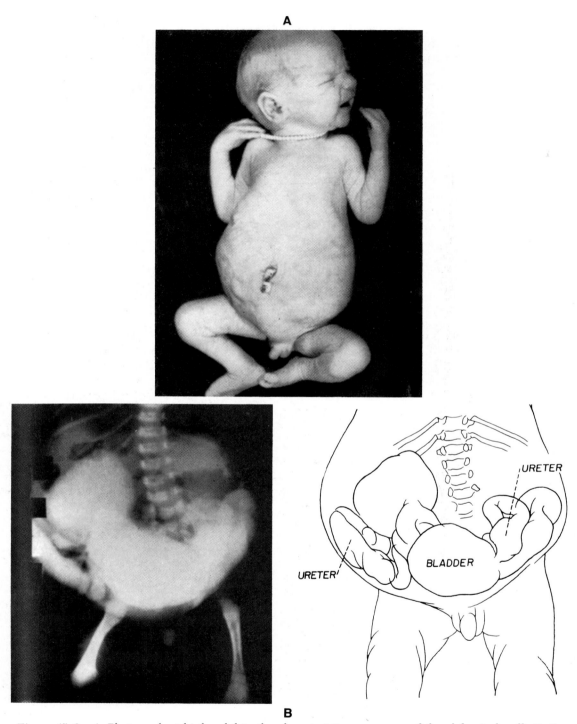

**Figure 45–6.** A, Photograph at birth exhibits the characteristic appearance of the abdominal wall. B, Cystogram performed via urethral catheter demonstrating bilateral urethral reflux, bilateral hydronephrosis, and hydroureter. (From McGovern, J. M., and Marshall, V. F.: Surg., Gynecol. Obstet. *108*:289, 1959.)

visible through its wall, with peristaltic waves traveling from right to left. The anus was replaced by a fold of redundant skin. The urine contained many pus cells and an occasional cast.

Plain film of the abdomen showed much gas and fecal material in the large bowel. In the upside down position a distance of 2 cm separated the opaque anal marker from the nearest gas-containing point in the rectum. Urethrogram showed a fistulous tract extending from the prostatic urethra to the rectum filled with opaque dye. Intravenous pyelograms showed no abnormality of the upper urinary tract.

An abdominal-perineal repair, double-barreled colostomy and division of the rectourethral fistula were performed. No long-term follow-up is available.

**COMMENT.** This is one example of fistula connecting the intestinal and urinary tracts in the male infant with imperforate anus.

### REFERENCES

Amolsch, A. L.: Bilateral metanephric agenesia: With a report of 4 cases. J. Urol. 38:360, 1937.

Bain, A. D., and Scott, J. S.: Renal agenesis and severe urinary tract dysplasia: Review of 50 cases with particular reference to associated anomalies. Brit. Med. J. 5176:841, 1960.

Burke, E. C., Shim, M. H., and Ketalis, P. P.: Prune-belly syndrome: Clinical findings and survival. Am. J. Dis. Child. 117:668, 1969.

Cain, D. R., Griggs, D., et al.: Familial renal agenesis and total dysplasia. Am. J. Dis. Child. 128:377, 1974.

Gellis, S. S., and Feingold, M.: Picture of the month: Congenital absence of abdominal musculature (prune belly). Am. J. Dis. Child. 109:571, 1965.

Kirshbaum, J. D.: Congenital absence of the external genitals (persistent primitive cloaca). J. Pediatr. 37:102, 1950.

Kirshbaum, J. D.: Facial characteristics of an infant without renal function. California Med. 71:148, 1949.

Kohn, G., and Borns, P. F.: The association of bilateral and unilateral renal aplasia in the same family. J. Pediatr. 83:95, 1973.

Landau, S. J., and Lattimer, J. K.: Functional closure of bladder exstrophy: A review of fifty cases. Pediatrics 31:433, 1963.

Mauer, S. M., Dobrin, R. S., and Vernier, R. L.: Unilateral and bilateral renal agenesis in monoamniotic twins. J. Pediatr. 84:236, 1974.

McGovern, J. M., and Marshall, V. F.: Congenital deficiency of the abdominal musculature and obstructive uropathy. Surg. Gynecol. Obstet. 108:289, 1959.

Passarge, E., and Sutherland, J. H.: Potter's syndrome: Chromosome analysis of three cases with Potter's syndrome or related syndromes. Am. J. Dis. Child. 109:80, 1965.

Potter, E. L.: Bilateral renal agenesis. J. Pediatr. 29:68, 1946.

Roberts, P.: Congenital absence of the abdominal muscles with associated abnormalities of the genitourinary tract. Arch. Dis. Child. 31:236, 1956.

Rogers, L. W., and Ostrow, P. T.: The prune belly syndrome: Report of 20 cases and description of a lethal variant. J. Pediatr. 83:786, 1973.

Texter, J. H., and Murphy, G. P.: The right-sided syndrome: Congenital absence of the right testis, kidney and rectus. Urologic diagnosis and treatment. Johns Hopkins Med. Bull. 122:224, 1968.

Ulson, A. C., Lattimer, J. K., and Melicow, M. M.: Types of exstrophy of urinary bladder and concomitant malformations. Report bases on 82 cases. Pediatrics 23:927, 1959.

# CONGENITAL MALFORMATIONS OF THE KIDNEY

# 46

*Revised by Warren Grupe*

### HYPOPLASTIC KIDNEYS, OLIGOMEGANEPHRONIA, DYSPLASIA, AND SEGMENTAL HYPOPLASIA

Hypoplasia of the kidneys has been defined as a congenitally decreased amount of normal renal tissue. Unilateral hypoplasia denotes a kidney which is less than 50 per cent of its expected weight, while bilateral hypoplasia is "severe" if the combined mass is less than half the weight expected, and "moderate" if it is one half to two thirds the average weight in proportion to total body weight and length (Rubenstein et al.). True hypoplasia is a rare occurrence in the human. The degree of dysfunction is determined by the total functioning mass of kidney. Tubular dysfunction is prominent in hypoplasia, with high volumes of dilute urine, acidosis and salt wasting. Lateral displacement of the nipples has been said to be an aid in diagnosis in the nursery.

The term "hypoplastic dysplasia" is used to describe kidneys which are small and manifest other evidences of embryonic maldevelopment.

Careful studies (Hodson et al.; Currarino; Gatewood et al.) have defined the normal in kidney size in all pediatric age groups as a ratio of kidney length to total body height and/or to vertebral body height, as determined by x-ray (Fig. 46–1). This should aid us in determining the pathogenesis of Schrumpfniere, or dwarfed kidneys. Kanasawa et al. are of the opinion that two quite different pathogenic processes lead to this same end result—one, chronic glomerulonephritis beginning very early in life, the other, chronic pyelonephritis affecting congenitally dysplastic kidneys. This matter will be discussed in greater detail in the pages devoted to chronic nephritis (Chap. 51).

## OLIGOMEGANEPHRONIA

An interesting subgroup of the renal dysplasias was described in 1962 by Royer and his collaborators. Because there were simultaneous hypoplasia and hypertrophy of the sparse nephrons present, they called the syndrome *oligoméganéphronie*. Characteristic is early renal failure which may then remain stable for many years. Early vomiting, later polyuria and polydipsia, failure to thrive, acidosis, proteinuria and renal loss of sodium and chloride are found almost invariably. Many develop rickets. Treatment is supportive and symptomatic.

Hypertrophy of the remaining nephrons is the usual reaction to loss of functioning renal parenchyma by whatever means. Thus, oligomeganephronia may be considered the expected response to insufficient nephron induction. Considered in this light, true hypoplasia could represent a dual developmental defect—first, an insufficient induction of nephrons by the advancing ureteric bud, and, second, an inability of the normal hypertrophy response.

## DYSPLASIA

Dysplasia on the other hand is more common and represents hypoplasia with disordered development of the metanephros. The majority of infants have associated abnormalities in the urinary tract, and it has been postulated on both experimental grounds and clinical observation that obstruction, while nephrons are imma-

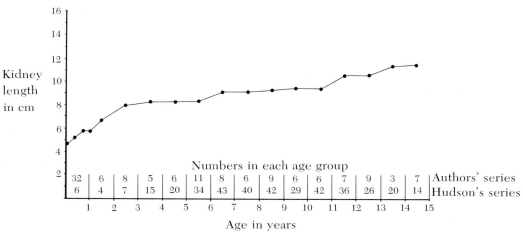

*Figure 46–1.* Length of kidney in presumed normals. (Modified from Baghdassarian et al.)

ture, is a major component in the abnormality, even though obstruction may no longer be demonstrable at birth. Dysplasia is a microscopic diagnosis characterized by primitive ducts, metaplastic cartilage, fetal glomeruli and tubules, and microcysts. Familial forms have been described. Dysplasia has also been associated with abnormal development in other organs, notably the central nervous system and lungs. It can be so severe as to mimic agenesis with oligohydramnios, Potter's facies, renal failure and death. Patients with dysplasia usually produce urine, while those with bilateral agenesis are anuric. Dysplasia has also been associated with imperforate anus and coarctation of the aorta.

Dysplasia may occur with macrocysts, and is not to be confused with the polycystic and microcystic diseases (see page 440 and page 472). Cysts may be unilateral or bilateral, diffuse or segmental, and there may or may not be association with other urinary tract abnormalities or obstruction. Separation of multicystic dysplasia, hypoplastic dysplasia and aplasia is not always possible, since the degree of overlap is so great in the clinical setting. Multicystic dysplastic and aplastic kidneys are nonfunctional while the degree of functional derangement in dysplasia is proportional to the amount of normally differentiated tissue. Multicystic dysplasia is the more severe and more common of these conditions (see page 440). When unilateral, the prognosis for complete recovery following nephrectomy is excellent. However, since obstructive abnormalities and non-cystic dysplasia can exist on the contralateral side, full investigation may be warranted.

## SEGMENTAL HYPOPLASIA

Segmental hypoplasia (Ask-Upmark kidney) is characterized by hypertension and localized areas of renal hypoplasia. It is the only one of the hypoplastic diseases accompanied by hypertension. The segment of hypoplasia is seen radiologically as a sharp cleft indenting the capsule during the nephrogram phase, and a "swallowtail" deformity of the adjacent calyceal system. Although it is considered by many to be a developmental abnormality, the role

of acquired injury, such as ischemia, or chronic pyelonephritis has not been excluded. The condition has been reported under the age of 2 years, but to our knowledge has not been reported in the newborn, which may be a function of its recognition rather than support for an acquired lesion. When unilateral and detected prior to the secondary development of more diffuse vascular disease, removal of the affected segment, or nephrectomy, is associated with disappearance of hypertension and complete recovery.

## DOUBLE COLLECTING SYSTEMS

Ureters may be doubled on one or both sides, either throughout their entire length or partially (Y-shaped ureters). Associated may be duplication of pelves and calyces, and renal mass may or may not be excessive.

A fair proportion of cases of recurrent pyuria in older infants and children is discovered to be caused by duplication of the urinary outflow tract. More often patients with this condition remain completely without symptoms or signs. Development of trouble depends upon whether obstruction of any degree exists. Such obstruction, if present, usually can be found to originate at the point of junction of the two ureters, at some abnormal point of emergence of one ectopic ureter or at the ureterocele, which complicates about 10 per cent of the cases. Ectopic emergence almost always involves the ureter that discharges the superior duplicated segment. Reflux up one ureter is common.

*Diagnosis* can never be made without complete urologic investigation. This may be undertaken because of the finding of an enlarged kidney, or of unexplained fever or pyuria.

*Treatment* will consist of the most conservative therapeutic measure appropriate to the situation discovered. Repeated dilatation of the stenotic juncture of the two ureters, occasionally attempted in older children, is not feasible in the newborn. Removal of the hydronephrotic or infected half of a kidney along with its ureter is indicated if the other half appears normal. If not, total nephrectomy must be performed.

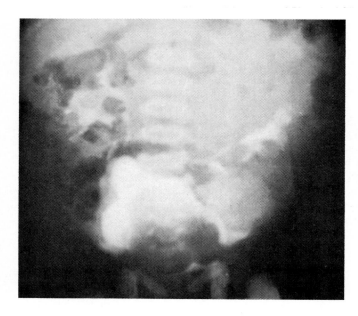

*Figure 46–2.* Intravenous pyelogram made on the fifth day of life. Two collecting systems can be seen on the right. The collecting system visible on the left is displaced far downward and appears to be flattened by an opaque mass above it.

CASE 46–1

A white female infant was born after an unremarkable pregnancy and delivery. The family history was interesting in that an aunt is said to have "three kidneys." Birth weight was 5 pounds 8 ounces (2500 gm), and the condition at birth was excellent. Abdominal distention was noted on the second day and was greater on the third day. At this time examination revealed a mass deep in the left upper quadrant which felt like an enlarged or displaced kidney. It was soft, rounded and smooth and extended almost to the iliac crest. Hemoglobin was 23.5 gm, white blood cell count 3560, with polymorphonuclears 53 per cent, stabs 11 per cent, lymphocytes 29 per cent, monocytes 5 per cent and eosinophils 2 per cent. Bleeding time was 3 minutes, clotting time 5 minutes. Flat x-ray film of the abdomen showed the stomach and bowel displaced anteriorly, the transverse colon inferiorly. An intravenous pyelogram showed displacement of the left calyceal system and pelvis downward and a double collecting system on the right (Fig. 46–2).

On the eighth day her temperature rose to 38.6° C, and she passed a tarry stool which was followed by others consisting almost entirely of fresh blood. Profound shock ensued and was controlled by oxygen, glucose, dextran and blood transfusions. On the following day laparotomy was performed. No bleeding site was found. The left kidney and ureter were found to be duplicated, the upper half of the left kidney hydronephrotic. This portion was resected. The right side was not explored.

The postoperative course was stormy. Bleeding from the bowel continued for 3 days, gross hematuria for 9 days. By the seventeenth day of life her hemoglobin had fallen to 11 gm, but she looked well and ate well.

She remained under our care for 5 years and is an apparently normal child. Repeat pyelograms showed the duplicated right kidney and the remaining half of the left kidney to be normal in all respects other than their peculiar conformation.

**COMMENT.** This newborn's illness presented with abdominal distention and an enlarged left kidney. Pyelogram revealed a mass displacing the left collecting system downward. The displacing mass proved to be the nonfunctioning hydronephrotic upper half of the duplicated kidney itself. The gastrointestinal bleeding is still unexplained, but may well have been due to peptic ulcer. The duplication of the right kidney has caused no trouble whatsoever.

## HORSESHOE KIDNEY

This condition is the result of fusion of the ureteric buds in embryonic life. It is often symptomatic because the ureters

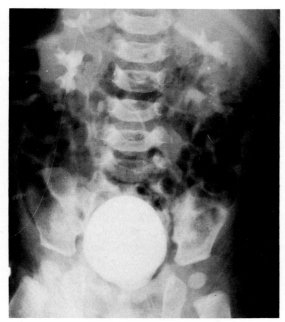

*Figure 46–3.* Film taken during the course of an intravenous pyelographic study. The left collecting system is definitely duplicated, and two ureters can be seen on that side. The same situation is almost surely present on the right. In spite of this the pelves are not enlarged, and all the calyces are delicate, sharply outlined and concave. There is clearly no obstruction to urinary outflow at any point.

This series of films was made in the course of a survey to determine the cause of vomiting. This was clearly an incidental finding that had no bearing on the chief complaint.

must cross the isthmus, at which point partial obstruction to urinary outflow may develop. Infection may follow.

**PATHOLOGY.** The fused mass lies closer to the midline and a bit lower than the site of the normal kidneys. Fusion has taken place at the lower pole in most cases, at the upper pole in less than 10 per cent. In the process the kidneys have not been able to complete their normal rotation, so that the pelves face anteriorly instead of toward the midline. The pelves are often extrarenal. The two collecting systems commonly develop normally, and ureters descend and enter the bladder in their proper positions.

**DIAGNOSIS.** At times the midline mass can be felt deep in the hypogastrium. More often suspicion is directed toward renal abnormality by the discovery of albuminuria

or pyuria, or by vomiting for which no obvious explanation can be found. Diagnosis is made by pyelography, either intravenous or retrograde. The characteristic malposition of pelves and visualization of a bridge producing one kidney mass rather than of two widely separated ones confirm the diagnosis.

**TREATMENT.** Nothing need be done unless infection of the urinary tract supervenes and cannot be controlled. When this complication exists, the urologist may attempt surgical correction. The single kidney should be divided and the two halves fixed in such positions as minimize urinary stagnation in any segment of the outflow tract. It may be necessary to resect a portion of the kidney mass which has been irretrievably damaged by chronic pyelonephritis.

## ECTOPIC KIDNEY

The ascent of the kidney from its low position in early fetal life to its permanent postnatal site has been described. At any point in this migration ascent may cease. The kidney may then lie within the pelvis or the lower part of the abdomen, and since rotation does not take place, the position of the renal pelvis and the course of the short ureter are abnormal.

*Diagnosis* depends upon palpation of a firm, fleshy, rounded mass in the lower part of the abdomen in a few instances or, in the majority, upon visualization of the malpositioned kidney by urography performed because of pyuria or abdominal symptoms. Symptoms are not caused by the ectopia itself, but by obstruction to urinary outflow or urinary infection which at times supervenes.

*Treatment* will be as conservative as possible. Removal of the kidney is necessary if pyelonephritis becomes chronic and incurable.

An even rarer defect in position is the *unilateral fused kidney,* or *crossed fused ectopia.* In this situation, as in horseshoe kidney, the ureteric buds fuse early in gestation, but one kidney ascends toward its normal position, carrying the other one across the midline and upward with it. This large mass can readily be felt deep in the lower part of the abdomen. Its particular hazard lies in the possibility that it may not be recognized at operation for what it is. Its removal would be a catastrophic error. We know of one instance in which the mass was irradiated intensively prior to operation for removal of a presumed Wilms' tumor.

## CYSTS OF THE KIDNEY

The kidney is the site of a large variety of cystic disorders. These can be classified, in ascending order of gravity, as solitary cysts, multiloculated cysts, multicystic kidneys and polycystic kidneys. Not included in this classification is the congenital microcystic defect which characterizes many of the examples of congenital nephrosis (see p. 471).

### SOLITARY CYSTS

Solitary serous cysts are found in 3 to 5 per cent of all autopsies. They are rarely observed by the clinician and become manifest only when they attain very large size. We have never seen an uncomplicated one in a newborn, but have found a large one associated with hydronephrosis due to vesical neck obstruction. In this case the diagnosis became clear only at the time of exploration, and the cyst was resected.

### MULTILOCULATED CYSTS

This term describes a kidney in which there are several or many disconnected solitary cysts. The parenchyma between them is intact, and there is left a considerable mass of functioning renal tissue.

*Diagnosis* is made by discovery of an enlarged kidney and demonstration of irregular distortion of the calyceal system on that side by pyelography. Exploration is required to clinch the diagnosis. Exploration will have to be done because of the difficulty in distinguishing these kidneys from those containing Wilms' tumors.

*Treatment* consists in resection of the large cysts.

### MULTICYSTIC KIDNEYS

This category differs from the preceding one in that cysts comprise all or almost all the mass of the kidney, there being practically no functioning renal parenchyma between them. The tissue between cysts is hypoplastic and dysplastic renal parenchyma. Calyces and pelves are deformed and the ureter is usually atretic or rudimentary, and does not communicate with the bladder. *Diagnosis* is suggested by palpating an enlarged kidney, in the left flank more often than the right, which feels irregularly nodular. The mass transilluminates brightly. The intravenous pyelogram shows no excretion of the dye on the side of the mass. One may see compensatory hypertrophy in the contralateral kidney. The lesion occurs usually in a male and is usually unilateral, although an incidence as high as 30 per cent of developmental anomalies in the contralateral kidney has been claimed. Diagnosis can be further substantiated by cystoscopy, during which procedure the homolateral ureteral orifice will not be seen, or if found, dye will not be able to be injected through it to the kidney. Such confirmation is ordinarily not necessary.

*Treatment* consists in removal of the affected kidney. When unilateral, complete recovery occurs.

### CASE 46–2

A white male infant was born after a normal pregnancy and short easy labor. He weighed 7 pounds 7 ounces (3380 gm), breathed and cried promptly and was scored 10 on the Apgar scale at 1 minute of age. Soon after birth he began to vomit thick, greenish mucus. Examination showed his abdomen to be moderately distended, but not tense. A large mass was felt deep in the left flank extending from the rib margin to the level of the umbilicus. It felt cystic above and hard and nodular at its lower pole. Urine was normal. Diagnoses of cystic kidney and Wilms' tumor were entertained. Flat film of the abdomen was of little help. An intravenous pyelogram showed a normal collecting system on the right except for displacement to the right and slight dilatation of the right ureter. No dye appeared within the left kidney at all. The bladder shadow seemed to be compressed from above on the left.

At operation a multilocular structure, 8 by 6 cm, replaced the left kidney. Cysts contained

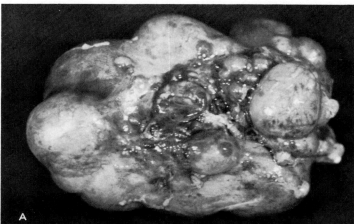

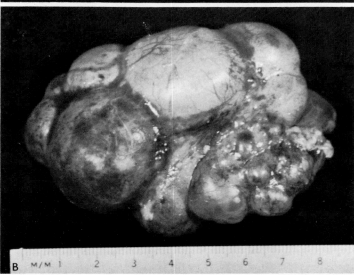

*Figure 46–4.* *A*, anterior view of multicystic kidney. *B*, medial view. The atretic ureter and blood vessels cannot be seen. (Case of Lipton, E. L., and Scordamaglia, L. J.: J. Pediat. *50*:730, 1957.)

clear fluid. Their walls were composed of fibrous tissue and contained a few glomeruli and tubules. Between cysts were focal areas of infantile glomeruli and tubules surrounded by an overgrowth of smooth muscle in which foci of myxomatous degeneration were noted.

The impression was hamartomatous malformation with cystic change.

This patient is now a tall, muscular, quite healthy young man.

**COMMENT.** This example is typical of all. A large irregular mass was easily palpable in one flank, and no dye was excreted after intravenous injection on that side. Wilms' tumor was excluded by its extreme rarity in the newborn period and by failure to excrete dye; renal vein thrombosis by

virtual absence of illness or of urinary changes and by the nodular feel; and hydronephrosis again by the irregular shape and by failure to visualize pooled dye in dilated calyces or pelvis. The vomiting, which is unusual, can no doubt be explained by the unusually large size of the tumor mass. Had trans-illumination been attempted, further evidence would have been obtained in favor of cyst or hydronephrosis and against Wilms' tumor or renal infarction.

## POLYCYSTIC KIDNEYS

This group of cystic lesions is entirely separable from those described above.

They are always bilateral, have no dysplastic elements morphologically and have a defined mode of inheritance. Polycystic disease should also be distinguished from other hereditary diseases that may be associated with cysts in the kidney. There is no therapy. Classification is still uncertain and morphogenesis is not clear. Often subdivided into neonatal, infantile, juvenile and adult types, it is probable that such subdivisions do not define distinct entities, though not all agree. However, on the basis of morphology, associated system involvement and mode of inheritance, at least two patterns emerge. It is often difficult to differentiate the two clinically in the nursery and thus impossible to provide intelligent genetic counseling.

### Infantile Polycystic Disease

This lesion can become clinically apparent at any age through childhood. In all cases, cysts are found in the liver as well as in the kidneys, although the degree of involvement of both organs may vary. Cysts may also be found in the pancreas and lungs, rarely in other organs. The length of survival seems to depend on the amount of functioning renal tissue. The more severely affected become evident soon after birth. The kidneys may be so large as to have interfered with delivery. Others may be stillborn, while others have Potter's facies and oligohydramnios. There may be associated abnormalities in the nervous, genitourinary, cardiovascular and pulmonary systems. Death during the neonatal period may be the result of uremia or of respiratory failure.

Other children may survive the neonatal period or not be detected until later in infancy. Hypertension is common in this group and may be associated with cardiac failure. Progressive renal failure inevitably develops. Portal hypertension, with a palpable liver and esophageal varices, may also develop. Some of these children live several years before uremia becomes evident.

In other children, generally older, hepatic involvement is the more prominent. In the past, these children have been grouped under "juvenile polycystic disease" or "congenital hepatic fibrosis." They may present with portal hypertension and esophageal varices, with the renal involvement almost incidental. Others will manifest hypertension or uremia, along with the evidence of hepatic dysfunction.

The lesion is inherited as an autosomal recessive. Morphologically, the renal cysts are uniformly distributed, fusiform and arranged radially. There is dilatation of the collecting ducts and distal nephrons with ectatic medullary ducts. There is relatively little fibrosis early. The kidneys are bilaterally enlarged by palpation, with a nodular, irregular feel. Urinalysis may show proteinuria, hematuria and decreased concentrating ability. The intravenous pyelogram shows delayed appearance of the contrast material, with a mottled, irregular nephrogram and distorted calyceal system. Retention of contrast material occurs in the cysts and occasionally pyelotubular back flow is seen on retrograde.

Both neonatal death and prolonged survival may be seen in one sibship, suggesting the different clinical courses to be reflections of the same genetic defect rather than separate entities. In other families, only a single pattern emerges, compatible with the different clinical progressions representing separate genetic abnormalities. Whether these subvarieties are truely distinct, or represent variations in the natural history of the same disease is still unclear.

### Adult Polycystic Disease

This is an extremely uncommon illness in the nursery, although it may appear in early childhood. It differs from the childhood types by an autosomal dominant pattern of inheritance and a relatively minimal hepatic involvement. The renal cysts are irregularly distributed, with both cortical and medullary cysts. Intravenous pyelography shows large, lobulated kidneys, with deformity of the pelvocalyceal system by the large cysts. Although progressive renal insufficiency eventually develops, this is unusual in childhood. Hypertension generally does not appear until renal insufficiency is advanced. Intravenous pyelography, which can detect cystic abnormalities in affected infants before the kidneys

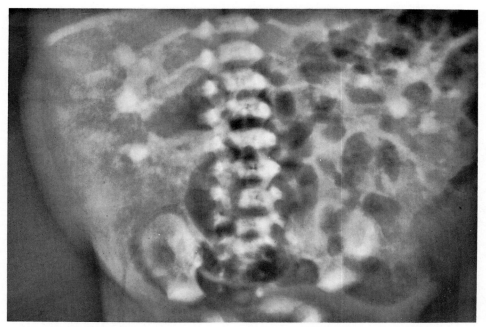

**Figure 46–5.** Intravenous pyelogram shows a bizarre distribution of calyces which are dilated and rounded. Separating some of the calyces are rounded radiolucent areas suggestive of cystic masses.

become palpable, should be performed on infants with a positive family history.

CASE 46–3

A white male infant was born after an uneventful labor, pregnancy and delivery. One of the two previous children had died at 11 months of age for reasons unknown. Birth weight was 7 pounds (3360 gm), and the condition at birth was excellent. On the second day of life large abdominal masses were palpated. He was sent home on the third day in spite of this finding. He was admitted to the Harriet Lane Home on the eighth day of life weighing 6 pounds 12 ounces (3230 gm). He was mildly icteric and acrocyanotic, his abdomen was distended, and a large mass was visibly and palpably filling each flank from costal margin to symphysis, the two almost meeting in the midline. They felt irregularly lobed, were freely movable and nontender. All else was normal.

Serum urea nitrogen level was 12 mg per 100 ml, bilirubin 10 (1.2 direct). Blood was normal, as were three urine specimens except for 2+ albumin in the first one. Intravenous pyelogram showed irregularity of calyces, with spreading of the major calyces (Fig. 46–5).

At age 2 months he was admitted in severe heart failure, and he died at 5 months of endocardial fibroelastosis. At autopsy polycystic kidneys were found.

## REFERENCES

Ahey, J. B.: Cystic lesions of the kidney in infants and children. J. Pediatr. *54*:429, 1959.

Baxter, T. J.: Polycystic kidney of infants and children: Morphology, distribution and relation of the cysts. *Nephron* 2:15, 1965.

Bernstein, J.: Heritable cystic disorders of the kidney: The mythology of polycystic disease. Ped. Clin. N. Amer. *18*:435, 1971.

Blyth, H., and Ockenden, B. G.: Polycystic disease of kidneys and liver presenting in childhood. J. Med. Genet. 8:257, 1971.

Branch, C. F.: Some observations on solitary cysts of the kidney. J. Urol. *21*:451, 1929.

Currarino, G.: Roentgenographic estimation of kidney size in normal individuals with emphasis on children. Am. J. Roentgenol. *93*:464, 1965.

Elkin, M., and Bernstein, J.: Cystic diseases of the kidney—Radiological and pathological considerations. Clin. Radiol. *20*:65, 1969.

Gatewood, O. M. B., Glasser, R. J., and Vanhoutte, J. J.: Roentgen evaluation of renal size in pediatric age groups. Am. J. Dis. Child. *110*:162, 1965.

Greenberg, L. W., and Nelsen, C. E.: Crossed fused

ectopia of the kidney Am. J. Dis. Child. *122*:175, 1971.

Hodson, C. J., et al.: Renal size in normal children. Arch. Dis. Child. *37*:616, 1962.

Kanasawa, M., Moller, J., Good, R. A., and Vernier, R. L.: Dwarfed kidneys in children. Am. J. Dis. Child. *109*:130, 1965.

Lieberman, E., Salinas-Madrigal, L., and Gwim, J. L.: Infantile polycystic disease of the kidneys and liver: Clinical, pathological and radiological correlations and comparison with congenital hepatic fibrosis. Medicine *50*:277, 1971.

Lipton, E. L., and Scordamaglia, L. J.: Congenital unilateral multicystic kidney associated with maternal rubella. J. Pediatr. *50*:730, 1957.

Orathanondh, V., and Potter, E. L.: Pathogenesis of polycystic kidneys. Arch. Path. *77*:459, 1964.

Peterman, M. G., and de la Pena, A.: Horseshoe kidney. Am. J. Dis. Child. *38*:799, 1929.

Royer, P., et al.: Pediatric nephrology. Philadelphia, W. B. Saunders Co., 1974.

Rubenstein, M., Meyer, R., and Bernstein, J.: Congenital abnormalities of the urinary system. J. Pediatr., *58*:356, 1961.

Sears. W. G.: Congenital cystic disease of kidneys, liver, and pancreas. Guy's Hosp. Rep. *76*:31, 1926.

Shapiro, I. J.: Congenital polycystic kidneys. J. Urol. *21*:308, 1929.

Van Acker, K. J., Vincke, H., et al.: Congenital oligonephronic renal hypoplasia with hypertrophy of nephrons (oligonephronia). Arch. Dis. Child. *46*:321, 1971.

Vlachos, J., and Tsakraklidis, V.: Glomerular cysts: An unusual variety of polycystic kidneys. Am. J. Dis. Child. *114*:379, 1967.

Vuthibhadgee, A., and Singleton, E. B.: Infantile polycystic disease of the kidney. Am. J. Dis Child. *125*:167, 1973.

# 47 HYDRONEPHROSIS

## *Revised by Warren Grupe*

Hydronephrosis denotes dilatation of the renal pelvis, usually associated with dilatation of the calyces emptying into that pelvis. Strictly speaking, any excess of fluid within the collecting system, calyces or pelvis, or both, must be considered hydronephrosis whether the total kidney volume is increased or not. In the majority of instances the one accompanies the other.

Hydronephrosis may be confined to the kidney by an abnormality of the ureteropelvic junction. This abnormality is obstructive, either intrinsic or extrinsic, in 80 per cent of infants, and functional in 10 to 15 per cent. In the remaining cases, no definitive abnormality of the ureteropelvic junction can be found. Hydronephrosis may also be accompanied by hydroureter, which can be either a primary ureteral abnormality, such as obstruction or infection, or an abnormality of the vesicoureteral junction leading to reflux. Congenital megaureter is always accompanied by reflux. Lesions of the bladder, such as megacystis, or of the urinary outlet, such as

urethral valves, can also result in hydronephrosis. Treatment depends on the clear definition of these possibilities. Each of these three situations deserves its own comments.

## OBSTRUCTION AT THE URETEROPELVIC JUNCTION

When hydronephrosis is limited to pelvis and calyces, one can be sure that an obstruction to the outflow of urine exists at the ureteropelvic junction. Such obstructions are by no means uncommon, and many are discovered in the neonatal period. Uson et al. reported upon 130, in infants and children up to 14 years of age, gathered from their own hospital. Thirty-nine were diagnosed before 2 years of age, and 16 of these earlier than 6 months. Males predominated by two to one, and both kidneys were involved in one fifth of the cases.

**PATHOLOGY.** Jewett divides all such

obstructive lesions into intramural, intraluminal and extramural groups, with intrinsic stenoses and aberrant renal arteries heading his list. Uson found 169 lesions in his cases, some examples manifesting more than one. There were 106 intrinsic stenoses, among which were found atresias, fibroses, muscle hypertrophies and mucosal valves. Among the extramural obstructions were 28 aberrant renal arteries and 21 fibrous bands or kinks. In two of his cases the anatomy of the region seemed perfect and the authors postulated, as had others before them, neuromuscular incoordination. Johnston in a similar study examined 36 hydronephrotic kidneys at surgery by measuring the intrapelvic pressure and the flow through the ureter. Mechanical obstruction was found in 29, functional obstruction in four and no cause was detected in three.

It is now quite clear that acute infections, even without underlying congenital obstructive defects, can and frequently do give rise to hydroureteronephrosis of considerable magnitude, and that one is justified in treating these with appropriate antibiotics and monitoring the outcome closely. Pais and Retik have noted reversible non-obstructive hydronephrosis in the neonate related to urinary tract infection, while Makker et al. have seen the same associated with generalized peritonitis.

The reason for the hydronephrotic changes with either obstruction or infection is not well understood. Although increased back pressure caused by the continued formation of urine seems logical, direct measurements of intrarenal hydrostatic pressures are not always elevated. Ischemic necrosis of papillae with subsequent re-epithelialization is commonplace. Some feel that the ischemia is predominantly arteriolar while others feel it is the result of venous congestion. In either state, the cause of ischemia is not clear, if not from increased intrapelvic pressure.

**DIAGNOSIS.** The diagnosis of congenital hydronephrosis in the neonatal period depends almost entirely upon discovery of a mass in the flank on one or both sides. Usually no symptoms are associated. Rarely gross hematuria is noted. Other infants may present with feeding problems, vomiting, failure to thrive, unexplained fevers or recurrent urinary tract infections. In any newborn with sepsis, the possibility of a congenital obstructive anomaly of the urinary tract must be excluded. Instances in which enlargement of the kidney or kidneys is extraordinarily advanced may manifest symmetrical abdominal enlargement or fullness in one or both flanks. The mass is situated deep in the flank, is easily caught and rolled between the anterior and posterior palpating hands, and is firm, round, regular and smooth. It is not tender. It moves with respiration. Large ones transilluminate brightly.

The discovery of such a mass on initial or discharge examination of a newborn calls for further study. The blood cell counts will not be found to deviate from the normal. Urine may be normal or may contain an excessive amount of protein, and white and red blood cells. Blood urea nitrogen may or may not be elevated. Intravenous pyelography may successfully outline the outflow tract and show dilatation of pelvis and calyces. It is important to continue to take films after intravenous injection of dye for four, eight or even 24 hours if necessary. Excretion of dye-containing urine may often be delayed, but is seldom lacking completely. Voiding cystogram may add important information, especially as concerns reflux. If doubt still remains, retrograde pyelograms will have to be made. These should clarify any remaining doubts.

**TREATMENT.** The approach taken is dictated by precise functional and anatomic definition of the lesion. The aim is to restore the continuity of the tract and establish the unobstructed flow of urine from the pelvis. Attempted dilatation by bougies introduced from below has no place in the therapy of ureteropelvic obstructions in the newborn. Occasional infants with a mild degree of obstruction, in whom there is no lower tract involvement, no infection and normal renal function, can be observed carefully, repeating the radiologic and functional evaluation at regular intervals. Some may resolve. In others, with more evidence of obstruction or renal parenchymal destruction, a surgical approach is preferred.

The surgical options include a primary repair of the ureteropelvic junction, pyelostomy or nephrectomy. Many different surgical procedures have been used with success; the approach in any given infant must be individualized, since no single operation or routine procedure is sufficient for the variety of defects that one encounters. A primary pyeloplasty will restore the tract to near normalcy and is the ultimate goal of a surgical program. In infants with a moderate degree of obstruction, no lesions of the lower tract, a normal amount of renal cortex demonstrated on urography, no compensatory hypertrophy on the contralateral side, normal renal function and no evidence of infection, a pyeloplasty should be considered as the initial approach. A high rate of success follows this procedure, with few complications. The result depends on the degree of intrinsic destruction. For example, the chance of success is generally better with extrinsic obstruction, such as an aberrant vessel or fibrous band, since the degree of obstruction is generally milder and the amount of intrinsic abnormality less. Some degree of intrinsic obstruction necessitating a pyeloplasty is always present even with a simple appearing extrinsic anomaly. With aberrant vessels, most operators will make every attempt to preserve the vessels while correcting the internal obstruction.

If the degree of obstruction is severe and the amount of renal damage marked, the chances of improvement with a primary repair of the ureteropelvic junction is small. Nevertheless, caution should be used in deciding the fate of that kidney. Marked hydronephrosis, with a markedly thinned cortex or contralateral compensatory hypertrophy or infection is probably best treated with nephrectomy. A temporary pyelostomy or nephrostomy is rarely necessary. It should be reserved for those situations in which the status of the kidney is in doubt, such as an acute infection with an otherwise moderate obstruction. Pyelostomy may also be helpful when there is a marked degree of hydronephrosis but with apparent good function and no contralateral compensatory hypertrophy; decompression may make a subsequent pyeloplasty technically easier. In any case, a kidney whose function is less than 20 per cent of the total renal function is probably sufficiently damaged to warrant nephrectomy.

If hydronephrosis is bilateral or if one or both kidneys appear reclaimable, the surgeon may choose to attempt plastic reconstruction of one or both kidney pelves. Uson and his co-workers were able to follow the courses of 51 of the infants and children upon whom they had performed pyeloplasties. Forty-three results were good and eight were poor, whereas 25 such children were lost to follow-up. During the same period 45 primary nephrectomies were performed. Bearn reported a newborn upon whom bilateral plastic repairs were performed in two separate operations 3 weeks apart, with excellent results.

## CASE HISTORIES

### CASE 47–1

A white male infant weighing 9 pounds (4225 gm) was born after long, slow labor by low forceps extraction, but breathed and cried promptly. Aside from a large caput the only abnormal finding was palpably enlarged kidneys, the left larger than the right. Re-examination on the third day again revealed the firm rounded mass in the left flank, undoubtedly a moderately enlarged kidney. Urine and routine blood examinations were normal.

Intravenous pyelogram (fifth day) revealed hydronephrosis of the right kidney, the kidney which seemed distinctly smaller by palpation, and an enlarged left kidney with normal calyces, pelvis and ureter (Fig. 47–1). During the procedure the infant voided, a beautiful urethrogram resulted, and the bladder neck could be seen to be normal. On that day urine contained 2+ albumin and occasional white and red blood cells. The blood urea nitrogen was 42 mg per 100 ml.

Cystoscopy and retrograde pyelography (sixth day) on the left side alone confirmed the fact that the left kidney, although enlarged, was normal.

The infant was discharged on the eighth day of life to be returned at the age of 3 months for further study and definitive therapy. This was not done.

**COMMENT.** This newborn with unilateral hydronephrosis was asymptomatic, his disorder having been discovered by physical examination. He manifested the not unusual finding of hypertrophy of the normal kidney producing enlargement greater than

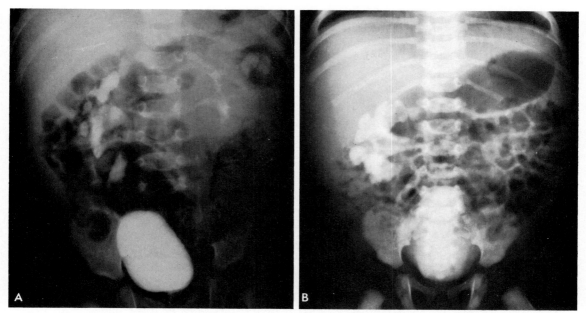

*Figure 47–1.*  A, Intravenous pyelogram made on the fifth day of life. The collecting system on the left appears to be perfectly normal. Calyces and pelvis of the right kidney are dilated, the calyces club-shaped. The right ureter cannot be seen. *B,* Later film shows that excretion from the right side is considerably slower than from the left. The enlargement and clubbing of calyces are more striking now, and the absence of right hydroureter strongly suggests obstruction at the ureteropelvic junction.

that produced by the disease on the opposite side. We have encountered this phenomenon on a number of occasions.

CASE 47–2

A white male infant was born by low forceps after a normal full-term pregnancy and uncomplicated labor. He cried and breathed spontaneously and seemed normal. Birth weight was 8 pounds 1 ounce (3650 gm). On the fourth day, examination prior to discharge revealed a mass deep in the left upper quadrant, plum-sized, round, firm and smooth. On the sixth day the mass had increased in size sufficiently to cause visible asymmetry of the abdomen.

A subcutaneous pyelogram made on the fifth day was unsatisfactory. An intravenous pyelogram the following day revealed a normal right kidney. The left kidney was enlarged, and dye was pooled irregularly within its outlines, but the calyceal system could not be defined.

The blood urea nitrogen was 25 mg, chloride 108 mg per 100 ml, and carbon dioxide-combining power 15.3 mEq per liter. Routine blood and urine examinations were normal.

Operation was performed on the seventh day through a transperitoneal approach. A greatly

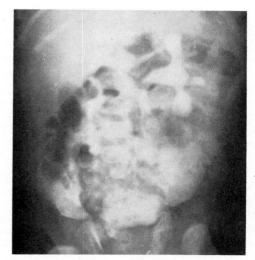

*Figure 47–2.*  Intravenous pyelogram made on the fourth day of life of an infant whose history is not abstracted in the text. The left kidney, palpably enlarged from birth, contains enlarged, pear-shaped calyces. The pelvis and upper portion of the ureter on that side are also dilated. No dye is visible on the right side. The reason for the nonfunctioning of the right kidney was not determined, since studies were delayed by a concomitant and severe congenital cardiac defect.

enlarged hydronephrotic left kidney was seen. Nephrectomy was performed. A tight, congenital intrinsic stricture of the ureteropelvic junction was found.

## URETERAL OBSTRUCTION

Obstructive lesions in the course of one or both ureters, leading to hydronephrosis plus hydroureter, but no megacystis, are exceedingly uncommon in the newborn period. One such case was described by Condit in 1956. It concerned a previously healthy 4-week-old infant who began to have unilateral convulsions which were difficult to control. Nonprotein nitrogen was found to be 137 mg per 100 ml of serum. After death the dilated ureters were seen to narrow sharply about 1 cm above their ureterovesical junction, and, at this point, thin semilunar valves were found within their lumens.

## BLADDER NECK OBSTRUCTION

One encounters obstructive lesions within the posterior urethra near the distal orifice of the bladder not infrequently in the neonatal period. Urethral obstructions are almost exclusively a male disease. They are present in larger numbers than diagnosed at or shortly after birth, since many are virtually asymptomatic until a later date. *It is imperative that the diagnosis of bladder neck obstruction be made and definitive therapy instituted at the earliest possible moment.* The infant's kidneys do not tolerate well the destructive effects of increased back pressure, especially when those of ascending pyelonephritis are superadded, as they frequently are.

**ETIOLOGY AND PATHOLOGY.** Since urine is formed and excreted from the fourth month of gestation onward, it is not surprising that trouble can be, and often is, manifest at the moment of birth when obstructive lesions have antedated delivery. Many examples of fetal and neonatal ascites have their origin in pre-existing bladder neck obstruction. In one extraordinary case (Rickham) the bladder had ruptured before birth, a circumstance which probably saved the patient's life, for the ureters and pelves, relieved of back pressure, were only moderately dilated. The bladder tear was closed, and the urethral valves subsequently repaired; the child seemed quite normal 5 years later!

Boys are affected considerably more frequently than girls. The pathologic lesions responsible for obstruction include a variety of congenital malformations. Valves of redundant mucosa arising from or near the verumontanum are by far the most common of these. Tsingoglu and Dickson found posterior urethral valves in 91 of 165 examples of lower urinary tract obstruction in infancy. Some valves are cusp-shaped, some filamentous, some resemble membranous diaphragms. The second-ranking congenital defect is ectopic ureterocele, the third, intrinsic stenosis or atresia of the orifice itself, producing symmetrical contracture or taking the form of a median bar of fibrous tissue running across the dorsal aspect of the posterior urethra. Hypertrophy of the vesical neck in which the thickening is muscular rather than fibrous has also been described but is rare as an isolated obstructive disease; most bladder outlet hypertrophy is secondary to urethral obstruction. The pediatrician need not concern himself unduly with the exact nature of the lesion.

**DIAGNOSIS.** Kretschmer and Pierson pointed out many years ago the ways in which posterior urethral or bladder neck obstructions become manifest. There are no physical findings that specifically indicate posterior urethral valves. Some cases have a completely silent course for many months or years only to be diagnosed, too late, after profound uremia had developed; some are admitted for failure to thrive. Some show symptoms of obstruction in the form of bouts of colicky pain preceding voiding, dribbling of urine, a small stream or obvious difficulty in starting the flow. In these a suprapubic tumor may be felt prior to voiding and may persist even after urination. Other infants develop ascending infection of the urinary tract, and the obstructive lesion may be discovered in the routine search for the cause of pyuria. Still other babies present themselves with gastrointestinal symptoms, chiefly anorexia and vomiting. Pylorotomies have been performed too often when the causative lesion has been in the genitourinary tract.

The newborn differs from the older infant in few respects in this regard. In most newborns the diagnosis is suggested by the finding of a tense cystic mass in the midline above the symphysis which may extend to or above the umbilicus. In 22 cases, Nesbit found the bladder palpable in all but one. In some children, either unilateral or bilateral flank masses representing hydronephrosis can also be palpated. Of the remainder, some vomit repeatedly. A fair number have bouts of abdominal pain which by careful observation may be seen to be associated with difficulty in voiding, and a few present with fever and pyuria. Demonstration of hesitancy in starting the flow of urine, poor stream, intermittency or dribbling is not easy, and hence is comparatively infrequent in the first month of life. Some nurseries, quite wisely, include among nurses' duties that of observing and recording in their reports the characteristics of the urinary streams of newborn infants.

Vesicoureteral Reflux. Reflux is a sign, not a diagnosis. It is common in the infant with outlet obstruction because the degree of obstruction is generally more severe. In children with milder degrees of obstruction diagnosis may not be made until later, and reflux is less common. Dysplasia is common in the immature kidney exposed to reflux; however, dysplasia can be seen with posterior urethral valves in the absence of demonstrable reflux.

Reflux can occur with primary abnormalities of the vesicoureteral junction, in the presence of duplicated collecting systems with ectopic ureteral insertions, or with ureteroceles. These inevitably require primary surgical repair of the ureterovesical insertion. Reflux secondary to infection, inflammation or infravesicular lesions, such as urethral valves, more often responds to correction of the primary problem, though occasionally surgical repair of the ureteral insertion is necessary.

Ascites with Obstructive Uropathy. France and Back pointed out that ascites in the neonatal period is associated with organic posterior urethral obstruction in a surprisingly high proportion of cases. Of 103 cases of neonatal ascites, there were 22 with dilatation of the urinary tract, and 18 of these infants were born with lesions obstructing urinary outflow at the bladder neck. In one of their own cases the ascites was fully developed at birth, the enlarged abdomen rendering delivery difficult. In others ascites appeared later. France and Back considered that transudation from thin-walled cysts on the kidney surface or from thinned-out areas in the dilated bladder or ureters was the source of the abdominal fluid. The diagnosis can be suspected by the discovery of a higher urea content in the ascitic fluid than in the blood plasma, and can be verified by a cystogram which shows leakage of contrast material from the bladder into the peritoneal cavity. Marx and Dale reported such a case in which tremendous ascites developed by the age of four weeks and subsided after indwelling catheter decompression of the bladder. Congenital valves were discovered and were resected at 8 months of age. Improvement followed.

By far the most reliable means of determining outlet obstruction is with the voiding cystourethrogram. Urethral valves can be clearly seen on voiding films, even when they are missed by cystoscopy; vesicoureteral reflux can also be determined best by this radiologic technique. It is important to obtain a voiding cystourethrogram prior to cystoscopy to determine which areas require special attention. Valves can be difficult to visualize by cystoscopy, and it becomes easy to confuse the secondary hypertrophy of the bladder neck as the primary lesion. Since surgical revision of the bladder neck is accompanied by a high incidence of sterility in the male, over-diagnosis and unnecessary surgery for want of a voiding cystourethrogram should be avoided.

The characteristic radiologic finding with urethral valves is dilatation of the posterior urethra just proximal to the valve, and poor filling of the urethra distally. The bladder neck is often prominent, giving the posterior urethra the appearance of a "spinning top." Reflux into one or both ureters is common, often accompanied by filling of the entire pelvocalyceal system, and can be associated with blunting and distortion of calyces. The bladder may show evidence of the obstructive process, with thickened walls and diverticulae, but at other times may show little change, presumably protected by the relief of vesicoureteral reflux at the expense of the kidneys.

Intravenous pyelograms in the neonatal period do not always adequately define the outflow tract. When they do, dilatation of the bladder will be seen with or without variable degrees of dilatation of ureters, pelves and calyces. Reflux up one or both ureters need not be seen early, but it almost always follows long-continued, increased intravesical tension as a result of loss of competence at the ureterovesical junction. This, together with the voiding urethrogram, defines the functional and anatomic condition of lower ureters, bladder and urethra with precision.

The passage of a rubber catheter may be difficult when the tip reaches the level of the stenosed bladder neck. *In many instances, however, the catheter passes into the bladder with the greatest of ease.* This is because mucosal flaps are situated so as to cause obstruction only from above downward; that is, they behave as check valves rather than stop valves.

Estimation of residual urine is not easy in the newborn, and offers little diagnostic help in the presence of diagnostic x-rays. The infant must be watched closely until he voids, promptly catheterized and the amount remaining in the bladder measured. In the normal there should be no more than 1 or 2 ml of residual urine.

The urine is not abnormal unless infection has supervened. Blood chemical determinations may fall within normal limits, but obstructions of sufficient magnitude rapidly lead to retention of nitrogenous end-products, with elevation of creatinine and blood urea nitrogen values.

The final diagnostic step is cystoscopy. The urologist skilled in the use of the infant's cystoscope will not only confirm the presence of posterior urethral obstruction by the appearance of the bladder, but also will determine its nature by direct inspection.

**TREATMENT.** Therapy is directed toward assuring quick and permanent relief from obstruction to urinary outflow. We stress the adjectives "quick" and "permanent" because halfway measures cannot be sanctioned. The kidneys of the newborn do not tolerate prolonged back pressure well, and when infection is added to pressure, their function may be irretrievably damaged in a short time.

Surgical removal of the urethral valves can be approached by one of several techniques. Most favor resection through the endoscope as the simplest and most effective method with the lowest morbidity. It is unusual that any surgical alteration of the bladder neck is necessary, and in the overwhelming majority the abnormal radiologic findings at the outlet resolve after simple excision of the valve. The same is true with the upper tracts, where reflux often disappears with no further surgery.

It may be technically impossible in rare circumstances to resect the valves through the cystoscope, and a more radical approach may be required, either by suprapubic cystotomy or by a perineal approach.

Repeated dilatation of the stenosis by bougienage from below may be, but often is not, adequate therapy. It cannot be expected to help when the basic defect consists of mucosal valves, nor does it relieve for more than a few hours or days many narrowings due to fibrous or muscular hyperplasia. Obstructions due to membranous diaphragms constitute the favorable exceptions.

## CASE HISTORIES

### CASE 47–3

A white male infant born at the Lutheran Hospital of Baltimore, at full term after a short labor, had dyspnea shortly after birth.

Examination at 4½ hours showed cyanosis and dyspnea with moderate subcostal retraction. This proved to be caused by pneumothorax, which cleared spontaneously within a few days and had no bearing upon the main problem. The abdomen was distended, particularly in the flanks, bowel patterns were seen, and a lemon-sized mass was palpable in the right upper quadrant below and distinct from the liver, deep in the flank. The bladder was felt as a symmetrical spherical mass extending to the umbilicus. The left kidney tip was barely felt.

Flat films of the abdomen revealed normal-sized, air-filled loops of bowel crowded downward by the mass.

*Catheterization was performed without meeting an obstruction,* and a large amount of normal urine was obtained.

Pyelography, by both intravenous and subcutaneous routes, was unsuccessful. Cystoscopy was then undertaken, and again no obstruction was met on introducing the cystoscope. The bladder wall appeared hypertrophied. The ureteral orifices were entered with ease, dye was introduced, and dilatation of calyces and pelves and tortuous dilated ureters were visualized (Fig. 47–3).

Blood urea nitrogen measured 15 mg per 100 ml.

Laparotomy was performed on the eighth day of life. A large cyst containing 75 ml of clear fluid was seen arising from the surface of the right kidney, as well as several smaller ones. These were resected. A suprapubic cystotomy was performed, and an indwelling catheter was fixed within the bladder.

Lethargy advanced to coma, and respirations became rapid and deep. The blood carbon dioxide-combining power fell to 10 to 15 mEq per liter; the sodium and chloride values dropped steadily. The infant died on the tenth day.

Autopsy revealed congenital urethral valves with two membranous cusps distal to the veru-

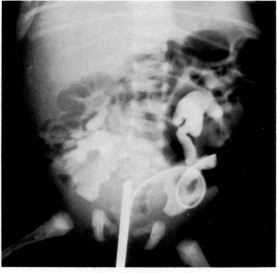

**Figure 47–3.** Retrograde urogram. The cystoscope can be seen in the bladder, and a catheter is in the left ureter. The right side has already been filled with dye. The bladder is enlarged, and both calyceal systems are greatly dilated and blunted. Both pelves are large. The right ureter cannot be visualized in this film, but the left ureter is dilated and tortuous.

montanum. Hypertrophy of the bladder, bilateral hydroureter and hydronephrosis were noted. A solitary cyst of the right kidney had been resected. The right testicle was undescended, and no left testicle could be found.

**COMMENT.** This infant was born with gross dilatation of the urinary tract due to congenital valves of the posterior urethra. He had additional congenital malformations of the genitourinary tract in the form of multiple cysts of the kidney and testicular maldevelopment. Noteworthy is the ease with which the catheter and cystoscope could be passed beyond this particular obstruction. The infant's chances for recovery would have been increased if voiding cystourethrogram had been made prior to operation and definitive repair of the bladder neck had been carried out promptly. The renal cyst could have been excised at some later date.

CASE 47–4

A white male infant was born after an uneventful pregnancy, labor and delivery. Birth weight was 7 pounds, 4 ounces (3490 gm), and he was rated 10 on the Apgar scale at 1 minute. Examined by his pediatrician at 8 hours, he was believed to be perfectly normal, but at 19 hours he vomited and thereafter seemed lethargic. At this time a cystic mass was palpable extending from symphysis to umbilicus. The rest of the physical examination was unrevealing.

Laboratory examinations were also within the limits of normal. No catheter could be passed per urethram, but it was possible to force a fine polyethylene tube into the bladder, to drain it and to inject Hypaque. The bladder was thick and trabeculated, and there was a small diverticulum on its anterior surface. A cineurogram was then performed. There was no ureteral reflux. On voiding, the posterior lip of the bladder neck was prominent, the posterior urethra was markedly dilated, and the dilated portion tapered down to a fine thread at the level of the external sphincter (Fig. 47–5). An intravenous pyelogram showed delayed excretion of dye, moderate hydronephrosis and hydroureter on the left and minimal hydroureter on the right.

Suprapubic cystostomy was performed (Dr. Hugh Jewett). No valves were seen, but the prostatic urethra was very narrow. Prostatotomy and dilatation of the urethra were performed, and the obstruction at the bulbomembranous junction was overcome so that a no. 12 French catheter could be passed into the bladder.

He bled freely into the urethra for 3 days, dur-

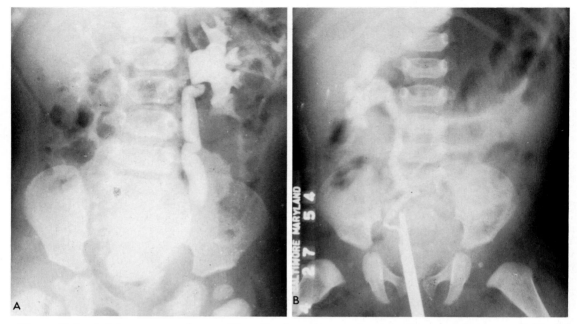

***Figure 47–4.***   A, Intravenous pyelogram. The collecting system on the right side cannot be seen well. The left ureter and pelvis are definitely dilated, but the calyces are concave and sharp. *B*, Retrograde pyelogram, right. On this side the reverse is true. The right ureter and pelvis are not at all or are questionably dilated, but the calyces are blunt and convex.

This was a 6-week-old infant whose symptoms of onset were diminution in number of voidings, episodes of stiffening and crying, and puffiness of the eyes. Bladder was not palpable but there were 30 ml of residual and a B.U.N. of 60. A median bar was found, and after resection the infant did well.

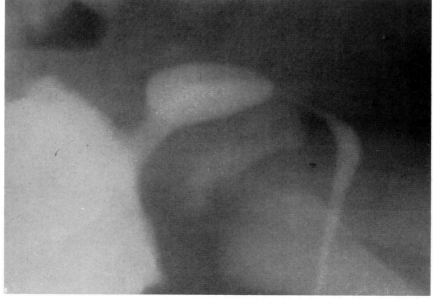

***Figure 47–5.***   One of the films of the cineurographic series shows the greatly dilated posterior urethra, which then tapers to a fine point at the level of the external sphincter. Its caliber remains threadlike for several centimeters and then reverts to normal.

ing which he was given 180 ml of blood. Thereafter a staphylococcal urinary infection supervened. This was controlled by Staphcillin, for which erythromycin was substituted later. When last seen at two months of age, he was voiding freely through the urethra, his serum urea nitrogen level was 12 mg per 100 ml, his urine was sterile, and he was eating and gaining well.

**COMMENT.** This case demonstrates the most common form of presentation of bladder neck obstruction in the neonatal period—the discovery of an enlarged bladder. It also illustrates how beautifully and precisely cineurography demonstrates the defect. Finally it appears to us to represent the ideal in treatment; that is, diagnosis within the first few days of life and definitive operative correction as soon as the diagnosis is confirmed.

## OTHER FORMS OF OBSTRUCTIVE UROPATHY

Obstruction to urinary outflow can be caused by a host of congenital abnormalities other than those discussed already as well as by the pressure of tumors contiguous to the ureters, bladder or even the urethra. There is not sufficient space available here to describe every variety that has been observed. Nor is there good reason to do this. The pediatrician will be on the qui vive for evidences of urinary obstruction; that is, palpable or visible enlargement of the bladder, ureters or kidneys, difficulty in passing urine, "colicky" abdominal pain just before voiding, unexplained vomiting and evidences of urinary infection as described in the paragraphs devoted to pyelonephritis (p. 786). The actual diagnosis of obstructive uropathy will then depend upon ancillary studies, including testing for residual urine, intravenous pyelography, cystoscopy, retrograde pyelography and cineurography. In the course of these studies not only the general diagnosis, but also the specific abnormality responsible for urinary obstruction, will come to light. Treatment will depend upon the outcome of these studies.

We append here only one further illustration from the multiplicity of varieties of this disorder one may encounter.

CASE 47–5

A white female infant was admitted to hospital at 7 days of age. The family history was unrevealing, pregnancy and labor had been uneventful, and her initial examination had been negative. She refused to nurse, had jaundice on the second day which disappeared after 2 days, and was discharged on the fifth day. At home she was lethargic and fed poorly. On the sixth day an attack of cyanosis necessitated admission to a hospital elsewhere. Here a loud systolic murmur was heard, and she was transferred to the Harriet Lane Home.

Examination on admission showed her to be well developed and nourished, hydrated, slightly dusky when out of oxygen, but with a good cry. The heart was not enlarged, but a loud systolic murmur could be heard, loudest in the third and fourth left interspaces. The liver was palpable one fingerbreadth below the right costal margin.

Hemoglobin was 15.2 gm, white blood cell count 22,650, with polymorphonuclears 56 per cent, lymphocytes 37 per cent, monocytes 7 per cent. Urine showed albumin 0, sugar 0, but the sediment contained 20 white blood cells per high-power field. Urine culture grew out a paracolon bacillus, later *Proteus vulgaris*. The blood nonprotein nitrogen measured 64 to 70 mg per 100 ml during the first week.

She responded well to penicillin given intramuscularly and tetracycline by mouth and began to eat well 3 days after admission. The cardiac study indicated that the lesion was probably an intraventricular septal defect. There was no evidence of heart failure.

An intravenous pyelogram revealed no excretion of dye on the right side. Excretion was good on the left, and on this side a tortuous ureter was visualized. On retrograde pyelography a large filling defect was seen in the bladder which was thought to represent a ureterocele of the right ureter. The left pelvis and calyces were dilated, possibly overfilled, the left ureter very tortuous (Fig. 47–6).

Suprapubic cystostomy with excision of the large ureterocele at the right ureterovesical junction was performed. Indwelling catheters were left in both ureters.

Over the course of the next month the urine became sterile, and function of the right kidney improved. Further pyelograms revealed more clearly the exact nature of the defect. The dilated right ureter crossed the midline and ended in an ectopic right kidney low in the left lumbar region.

After discharge, infection recurred and the function of the right kidney deteriorated progressively. When the infant was 5 months old,

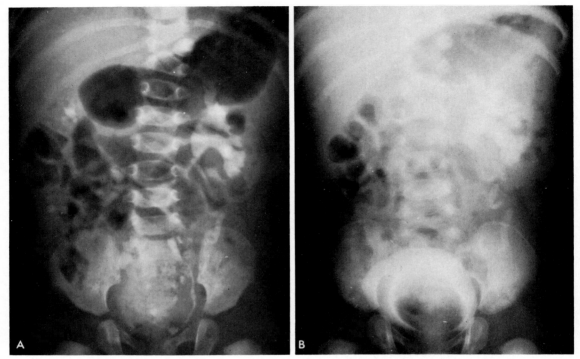

*Figure 47–6.* A, Intravenous pyelogram does not outline the right collecting system. On the left the calyces are dilated and somewhat blunted, and the pelvis is a bit dilated. The ureter, however, seems to be of normal caliber throughout its course. B, Retrograde cystogram and left pyelogram. A large filling defect is seen within the bladder. Again the left-sided hydronephrosis is visible.

the kidney was removed. Her subsequent course has been satisfactory in all respects.

**COMMENT.** The presenting symptoms in this infant were failure to eat well and cyanotic spells. There were no symptoms referable to urinary obstruction. Since she had a congenital heart defect in addition to pyelonephritis, it is difficult to be certain of the exact origin of her symptoms. Her pyelonephritis was improved, but not cured, by antibiotic medication and by removal of a large ureterocele. Ultimately the crossed ectopic, poorly functioning kidney had to be removed.

## CONGENITAL MEGALOURETER (MEGACYSTIS – MEGAURETER SYNDROME)

From time to time a case of pyuria is encountered in which the cause of persis-

tence of renal infection is great dilatation of the ureters without demonstrable obstruction. The bladder may also be dilated and hypotonic, while the ureteral orifices gape and permit free reflux of bladder urine. Usually associated are dilatation of pelves and blunting of calyces. This has been called the megacystis–megaureter syndrome. Chronic pyelonephritis invariably supervenes in this situation and is almost impossible to overcome.

**ETIOLOGY.** In some examples gross lesions of the spinal cord are responsible. Foremost are myelomeningocele or lipomyelomeningocele and dural or cord tears sustained during difficult breech extractions. The ureteral insertions in the bladder appear to be more laterally displaced, with a very short or absent intramural or submucosal tunnel.

A congenital imperfection of autonomic nerve control has been suspected in some, but no proof has ever been adduced for this hypothesis. Swenson suggested that megaloureter, like megacolon, with which it is occasionally associated, may be due to congenital defect of the pelvic parasympathetic system, associated with absence or underdevelopment of the intrinsic nerve supply of the ureters and bladder. He believes that he has demonstrated this defect in some cases. This observation has not been confirmed. Baker obtained electroureterograms of one case and found no alteration from the normal peristaltic pattern other than slightly lower voltage. He points out that the intrinsic nerve supply is not indispensable for orderly contraction, but that contraction waves seem to originate within muscle fibers independently.

In Swenson's series of 35 operated cases of megaloureter he found 17 aparasympathetic bladders (four of these had megacolon as well). Nine had absence of ureteral peristalsis, and four had cord bladders. Three had ureteroceles, while two were associated with agenesis of the musculature of the abdominal wall.

**DIAGNOSIS** is almost entirely dependent upon the discovery of urinary infection. Since infection may be delayed months or years, this condition does not often become manifest in the neonatal period. Final confirmation is made by intravenous urography and voiding cystourethrogram. Although very large, the bladder functions quite normally and empties completely. The apparent residual urine is the result of urine refluxed into the dilated upper tracts returning to the bladder post-void.

**TREATMENT.** If at all possible, urinary stagnation and reflux should be relieved. Several large series have shown a success rate in excess of 90 per cent when the insertion of the ureter into the bladder is revised. Since there is no abnormality of the bladder neck or the urethra in this condition, surgery in these areas is not needed, even if the bladder is very large.

The prognosis seems dependent on the amount of renal damage present initially. Often complicating urinary tract infections and pyelonephritis can be controlled by appropriate antibiotics, but infections tend to recur as soon as therapy is stopped. In some without surgical correction, infection can become chronic and intractable leading

to renal insufficiency. Following successful reimplantation of the ureter, progressive renal damage is unusual, even if subsequent infections occur.

Operations on the autonomic nervous system based upon the assumption that sympathetic-parasympathetic imbalance is the causative defect have been uniformly unsuccessful.

## REFERENCES

Askin, J. A., Reichelderfer, T., Salik, J., and Merritt, J.: Indications for excretory urography in children. Pediatrics 20:1033, 1957.

Baker, R.: Ureteral electromyography in congenital megaloureter. A.M.A. J. Dis. Child. 87:7, 1954.

Bearn, A. R.: Hydronephrosis in infancy. Arch. Dis. Child. 31:110, 1956.

Berman, L. B., Crotty, J. J., and Tina, L. U.: The pediatric implications of bladder neck obstructions. Pediatrics 28:816, 1961.

Condit, L.: Convulsions. Case Histories Child Mem. Hosp. Chicago 14:3803, 1956.

Flocks, R. H.: Lower urinary tract obstructions in infants and children. Pediat. Clin. N. Amer. 2:755, 1955.

France, N. E., and Back, E. H.: Neonatal ascites associated with urethral obstruction. Arch. Dis. Child. 29:565, 1954.

Jewett, H. J.: Upper urinary tract obstructions in infants and children. Pediat. Clin. N. Amer. 2:737, 1955.

Johnston, J. H.: The pathogenesis of hydronephrosis in children. Br. J. Urol. 41:724, 1969.

Kretschmer, H. L., and Pierson, L. E.: Congenital valves of the posterior urethra. Am. J. Dis. Child. 38:804, 1929.

Makker, S. P., Izant, R., Tucker, A., and Heymann, W.: Non-obstructive hydronephrosis associated with generalized peritonitis. N. Engl. J. Med. 287:535, 1972.

Marx, K., and Dale, W. A.: Neonatal ascites and obstructive uropathy: A case report with a four-year follow-up. Pediatrics 27:29, 1961.

Murnagham, G. F.: Experimental aspects of hydronephrosis. Br. J. Urol. 31:370, 1959.

Pais, V. M., and Retik, A. B.: Reversible hydronephrosis in the neonate with urinary sepsis. N. Engl. J. Med. 292:465, 1975.

Rickham, P. P.: Advanced lower urinary obstruction in childhood. Arch. Dis. Child. 37:122, 1962.

Swenson, O.: Congenital defects in the pelvic parasympathetic system. Arch. Dis. Child. 30:1, 1955.

Tsingoglu, S., and Dickson, J. A. S.: Lower urinary obstruction in infancy: A review of lesions and symptoms in 165 cases. Arch. Dis. Child. 47:215, 1972.

Uson, A. C., Cox, L. A., and Lattimer, J. K.: Hydronephrosis in infants and children. J.A.M.A. 205:323, 1968.

# 48

# RENAL VASCULAR THROMBOSIS
*Revised by Warren Grupe*

## RENAL VEIN THROMBOSIS

The renal vein may become thrombosed at any age, but the newborn is particularly prone to this disastrous accident.

**INCIDENCE.** In 1945 Abeshouse was able to find reports of 228 cases of this disorder in the literature. Ninety-eight of these had occurred in children, 90 in infants less than 2 months of age. This ratio has not changed with subsequent reports. The first diagnosis in vivo was made by Campbell in 1942. Currently, renal vein thrombosis is recognized during life with increasing frequency. It is not a common disorder, but it can no longer be considered a great rarity. Oppenheimer and Easterly, in reviewing 4000 consecutive neonatal postmortem examinations, found 14 infants with renal vein thrombosis of which five were infants of diabetic mothers.

**ETIOLOGY.** Thrombosis of the renal vein is usually divided into primary and secondary forms, the latter resulting from extension of the thrombus from the vena cava. The primary form, that in which thrombosis originates in renal veins themselves, is the one encountered in the newborn. The most important predisposing factors are dehydration and hypovolemia. Other factors include hypotension, low renal plasma flow, polycythemia, anoxia, septicemia and being born of a diabetic mother. In many cases no such predisposing disorder has been discovered, and congenital defect of the vein itself has been suspected, but not proved. Damage from a severely traumatic or breech delivery has also been seen. There is also clear evidence that the lesion can occur prenatally.

**DIAGNOSIS.** The characteristic sign of renal vein thrombosis is sudden enlargement of one kidney. This may occur during the course of severe diarrhea, or several days after a traumatic delivery, or in the midst of an illness suggesting sepsis of the newborn, or it may develop de novo. At times renal enlargement is unaccompanied by symptoms; at other times vomiting, abdominal distention, shock and fever may appear along with enlargement. These infants generally appear quite ill. Gross hematuria is frequently present, and may be the first sign; but hematuria may be microscopic and indeed may in many cases be absent entirely. The urine may contain an excess of protein and white blood cells, alone or in addition to red blood cells. Anuria or oliguria can be present.

The blood urea nitrogen level becomes elevated. Thrombocytopenia, when present, probably is the result, rather than the cause, of the thrombosis. Intravenous pyelography reveals complete absence of excretion of dye or only a slight opacification after a long delay on the involved side. If diagnosis is in doubt after this demonstration, further radiographic studies may add more precise information, as shown by Walters and Holder. Kidney photoscan with [197]Hg will show no function on the involved side. This, however, would be the case also with multicystic kidneys, with very advanced hydronephrosis and, at times, with huge Wilms' tumors. Transillumination may help distinguish solid from cystic masses, as may ultrasonography. But visualization of the renal vasculature by means of injection of radiopaque dye into a saphenous vein and cineradiography should supply the definitive answer (Fig. 48–1).

**TREATMENT.** The ideal treatment has until recently been considered to be immediate nephrectomy. Unfortunately operative intervention is at times contraindicated by concomitant disease such as active diarrhea with dehydration, or fever and severe jaundice with sepsis of the newborn. In two of our own cases operation was interdicted by the profound shock of concomitant adrenal hemorrhage in one and by the often associated thrombocyto-

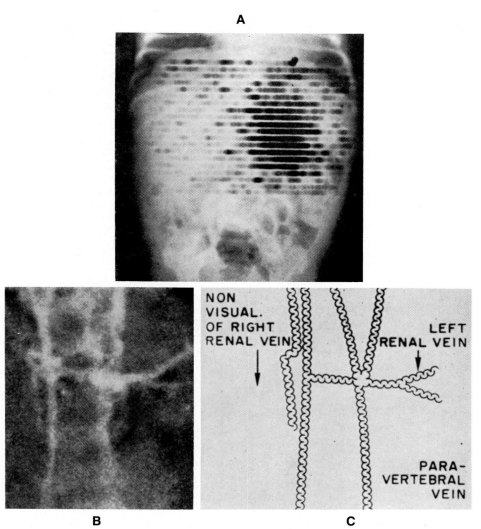

**Figure 48–1.** A, ¹⁹⁷Hg renal photoscan showed no function on the right with good function on the left. B, Venogram via the right saphenous vein using the cineradiographic technique showed filling of the paravertebral and left renal veins with no filling of the inferior vena cava or right renal vein. (From Walters, T. R., and Holder, T. M.: Am. J. Dis. Child. *111*:433, 1966.)

penia in the other. In such situations everything possible must be done to overcome the complicating disorder.

Recently Belman and his collaborators have recommended that unilateral renal vein thrombosis be treated medically. In the unilateral examples this means little more than good fluid and electrolyte balance control. Six of their seven infants so treated survived, and in only one of the survivors was the kidney found to be atrophic at one year of age. Ghai et al. recently reported thrombosis in one kidney of each

of a pair of conjoined twins. They did well after two exchange transfusions.

Bilateral thrombosis is much more serious. Two infants have been reported with recovery, one treated with renal vein and vena caval thrombectomies, the other by peritoneal dialysis, right nephrectomy, vena caval and left renal vein thrombectomies and heparin.

**PROGNOSIS.** Although the results are almost always excellent when nephrectomy is performed, the role for surgery must be questioned in view of the favorable results with conservative management. Many of these children are quite ill, toxic and febrile; supportive care to correct the primary disorders seems more valid than emergency surgery. Intrarenal thrombi with associated zones of hemorrhagic infarction are almost always present, making rapid correction of the large vessel thrombi of little consequence to the kidney. No clear case of unilateral thrombosis extending to bilateral involvement has been established. Our current recommendation is to support the patient with appropriate medical management with particular attention to hypovolemia. Anticoagulation has been used, but its effectiveness has not been established.

Of some concern have been reports of renal atrophy developing some months later, and the possibility of renal mediated hypertension, which may necessitate subsequent nephrectomy. Tubular dysfunctions, including proteinuria, amino aciduria, glycosuria, phosphaturia, metabolic acidosis with growth failure and rickets, have been reported as late sequelae of renal vein thrombosis.

## CASE HISTORIES

### CASE 48–1

(Case reported by Warren, Birdsong and Kelley.)

A white male infant was born by easy low forceps delivery after an uncomplicated pregnancy and labor. He remained well until the tenth day of life, when projectile vomiting began and he appeared distressed. Examination revealed a distended, tender abdomen. A mass, 9 by 4 cm in size, was felt in the left flank. Urine showed innumerable red blood cells and a 4+ albumin. Over the next few days albumin and red cells diminished, while white blood cells increased until their number was uncountable. In the blood the white cell count was 17,400, the blood urea nitrogen 52 mg per 100 ml. Intravenous pyelogram showed a normal right kidney and calyceal system, but no dye appeared on the left side.

Operation was performed on the eighteenth day. A large hemorrhagic kidney with its renal vein thrombosed was found and removed (Fig. 48–2). Postoperative course was uneventful.

**COMMENT.** This case is typical of the idiopathic variety of renal vein thrombosis. For no apparent reason and with no prece-dent illness one kidney suddenly enlarged, hematuria appeared, and blood urea nitrogen level rose. Vomiting, abdominal distention and probable abdominal pain were the accompanying signs and symptoms. Intravenous urogram showed loss of power to excrete dye by the involved kidney. Nephrectomy resulted in prompt cure.

### CASE 48–2.

(This case was reported by Avery, Oppenheimer and Gordon.)

A white male infant was delivered of a diabetic mother by cesarean section. He weighed 8 pounds 10 ounces (3930 gm) at birth. He required positive pressure resuscitation for 4 minutes, after which respirations become spontaneous, but were unduly rapid. At 34 hours jaundice was noted, the serum bilirubin measuring 15.8 mg, the hemoglobin 14.5 gm, but the direct Coombs test result was negative. On the third day a mass became palpable in the left flank, and the nonprotein nitrogen level was 88 mg per 100 ml. Urine showed 3+ albumin and three to five white blood cells per high-power field. On the fourth day he was still jaundiced, was lethargic and slightly cyanotic. There was no longer respiratory rapidity or difficulty. The mass had increased in size, extending from the costal margin to the iliac crest, deep in the left flank. Now the nonprotein nitrogen level was 92 mg, bilirubin 15.2 mg, of which 13 mg was indirect. Platelets numbered only 29,000 per cubic millimeter. Because of this last finding contemplated operation was postponed. Tachycardia and tachypnea with labored respirations developed, and puffiness appeared. Stools containing blood were passed. The liver edge descended two fingerbreadths below the costal margin. In spite of rapid digitalization he died.

Autopsy showed antemortem thrombosis of the left renal vein, extending into the inferior vena cava, and infarction of the left kidney.

**COMMENT.** In this example renal vein thrombosis complicated an undiagnosed illness characterized by initial apnea, subsequent dyspnea, cyanosis, jaundice and thrombocytopenia. There were proteinuria and pyuria, but no hematuria. The mother was diabetic. The thrombocytopenia may have resulted from the extensive intravascular clotting, as suggested by Avery et al.

### CASE 48–3

(Case history abstracted from Clatworthy, Dickens and McClave, with permission of the senior author.)

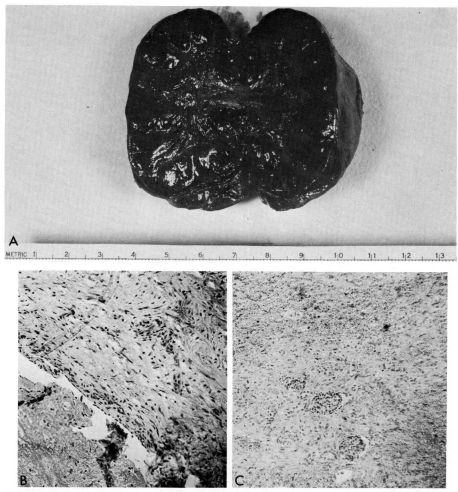

*Figure 48–2.* *A*, Photograph of gross specimens showing hemisected dark kidney which is infarcted throughout. *B*, Recent portion of thrombus in renal vein in lower left third of the field. Lines of Zahn, a few erythrocytes, and an occasional fibroblast are present. There is some retraction from the vein wall as the result of fixation. The opposite side of the thrombus (not shown) is adherent to the vein wall with early proliferation of fibroblast and endothelial cells. (Dark lines near middle and in the lower right corner in the portion of the thrombus shown and the lighter line across the vein line are artefacts.) *C*, Cortex of infarcted kidney, showing dilated capillaries containing fresh erythrocytes, which also are extensively extravasated into the tissue. There is dispersion and distortion of glomerular and tubular structures. Little evidence of necrosis is present.

A 7-day-old white male infant was admitted because of severe diarrhea which began on his third day of life. On the day of admission dehydration, cyanosis and shock had appeared. He was acutely ill. Respirations were rapid and deep. There was circumoral pallor and generalized cyanosis. The abdomen was soft, the liver edge down 1½ fingerbreadths, the spleen one, below the costal margin. Temperature was 98° F, pulse 150, respirations 40 per minute. The hemoglobin was 15.8 gm, and white blood cells numbered 11,000, with 56 per cent polymorphonuclears. Urine contained 200 mg of albumin per 100 ml, one to two white blood cells and four to five granular casts per high-power field. He was given plasma, then other fluids intravenously, as well as antibiotics. Temperature had risen to 101.4° F 12 hours after admission, but fell to normal by the third day, when the stools were also normal. On this day a rash appeared and medication was stopped, but a urine examination later in the day showed 40 to 50 white blood cells, 0 to three red cells, an occasional granular cast per high-power field and

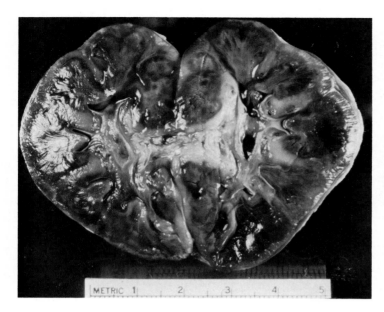

*Figure 48–3.* Sectioned left kidney to show swelling and deep dark discoloration due to hemorrhagic infarction. The intravenous pyelogram in this case showed a normal collecting system on the right, but no dye on the left side. (From Clatworthy, H. W., Jr., et al.: N. Engl. J. Med., *248*:628, 1953.)

120 mg of albumin per 100 ml. By the sixth day *E. coli* 0-111B was identified in the urine culture, and chloramphenicol was begun. Diarrhea recurred. On the eighth day a mass appeared in the left flank visibly and palpably extending down to the iliac crest. An intravenous pyelogram showed no dye on the left, a normal urogram on the right (Fig. 48–3). By the nineteenth day the mass was a bit smaller, but exploratory operation was performed. The perirenal fat was hemorrhagic and edematous, the left kidney swollen, tense and purple. The kidney was removed. The renal vein was thrombosed, the kidney infarcted.

**COMMENT.** Clatworthy points out that gross hematuria was not present in this case or indeed in most of the previously reported cases. His example clearly followed and was almost surely a result of diarrhea and dehydration. It was a particularly favorable one in that the onset was not explosive and never seemed to endanger the life of the infant. Many do not fit this pattern.

## RENAL ARTERY THROMBOSIS

Thrombosis of the renal artery is much less common than thrombosis of the renal vein. The clinical picture, however, is much the same in both conditions. Wood-

ward et al. alerted us to the fact that renal artery thrombosis, until now only a pathologic finding, can be diagnosed in vivo and treated successfully. Their two cases had failing hearts, then proteinuria, hematuria and hypertension. Azotemia was looked for and found in one. The kidneys were not enlarged. Pyelograms revealed no excretion of dye in the affected side. Operation was performed on one in the expectation of finding renal vein thrombosis, but the kidney was dark blue and not enlarged, and a thrombus was found in the main renal artery. In their other case the correct diagnosis was suspected, but the infant died before operation could be attempted. Removal of the kidney in their Case 1 resulted in cure.

The symptoms and signs of renal artery thrombosis are secondary to the renal infarction, and include an enlarged kidney, either anuria or oliguria, and hematuria. There may be evidence of thrombosis occurring in other organs including gangrenous areas of skin. Vomiting and abdominal tenderness may be seen; B.U.N. and creatinine may be either elevated or normal. There is usually variable function of the kidney by intravenous pyelography or renal scan. Renal artery thrombosis has also been associated with umbilical artery catheterization, particularly when hypertonic fluids have been administered. Early nephrectomy is probably not warranted since the extent of involvement is variable and the recovery cannot be predicted. Renal atrophy with or without hypertension can be a late sequela.

## PERIRENAL HEMATOMA

Perirenal hematoma may likewise simulate either renal vein or renal artery thrombosis. There may be a flank mass, a history of obstetrical trauma, anemia, hematuria, oliguria and a rising B.U.N. The importance of distinguishing this lesion is that a perirenal hematoma, unless evacuated, has the potential to organize and contract, leading to renal atrophy and hypertension of the sort seen experimentally after induced renal ischemia.

## WILMS' TUMOR

This discussion has been transferred from this section to that dealing with Malignancies (see pp. 1012–1014).

## REFERENCES

Abeshouse, B. S.: Thrombosis and thrombophlebitis of the renal veins. Urol. Cutan. Rev. *49*:661, 1945.

Avery, M. E., Oppenheimer, E. H., and Gordon, H. H.: Renal-vein thrombosis in newborn infants of diabetic mothers. N. Engl. J. Med. *256*:1134, 1957.

Belman, A. B., Susmano, D. F., Burden, J. J., and Kaplan, G. W.: Nonoperative treatment of unilateral thrombosis in the newborn. J.A.M.A. *211*:1165, 1970.

Campbell, M. F., and Matthews, W. F.: Renal thrombosis in infants: Report of two cases in male infants urologically examined and cured by nephrectomy at 13 and 33 days of age. J. Pediatr. *20*:604, 1942.

Clatworthy, H. W., Jr., Dickens, D. R., and McClave, C. R.: Renal thrombosis complicating epidemic diarrhea in the newborn: Nephrectomy with recovery. N. Engl. J. Med. *248*:628, 1953.

Fallon, M. L.: Renal venous thrombosis in the newborn. Arch. Dis. Child. *24*:125, 1949.

Fraley, E. E., Fish, A. J., and Najarian, J. S.: Bilateral renal vein thrombosis in infancy: Report of a survivor following surgical intervention. J. Pediatr. *78*:509, 1971.

Ghai, O. P., Singh, M., et al.: Acute renal failure following renal vein thrombosis in conjoined twins. Am. J. Dis. Child. *121*:57, 1971.

Gross, R. E.: Arterial embolism and thrombosis in infancy. Am. J. Dis. Child. *70*:61, 1945.

Oppenheimer, E. H. and Esterly, J. R.: Thrombosis in the newborn: Comparison between infants of diabetic and non-diabetic mothers. J. Pediatr. *67*:549, 1965.

Stark, H. and Geiger, R.: Renal tubular dysfunction following vascular accidents of the kidneys in the newborn. J. Pediatr. *83*:933, 1973.

Verhagen, A. D., Hamilton, J. P., and Genel, M.: Renal vein thrombosis in infants. Arch. Dis. Child. *42*:214, 1965.

Walters, T. R., and Holder, T. M.: Neonatal hyperbilirubinemia and renal vein thrombosis: Occurrence in a newborn infant of a diabetic mother. Am. J. Dis. Child. *111*:433, 1966.

Warren, H., Birdsong, M., and Kelley, R. A.: Renal vein thrombosis in infants. J.A.M.A. *152*:700, 1953.

Woodard, J. R., Patterson, J. H., and Brinsfield, D.: Renal artery thrombosis in newborn infants. Am. J. Dis. Child. *114*:191, 1967.

# HYPERTENSION
*By Warren Grupe*

# 49

Hypertension is very uncommon under 1 year of age and a rare occurence in the nursery, although its exact prevalence is unknown. Often its existence is first detected by the appearance of congestive heart failure. When discovered, a cause must be sought and established even if the blood pressure can be controlled by antihypertensive medication; essential hypertension in the neonate is so unusual as to be a virtual nonentity in this already uncommon clinical state.

The accurate determination of the blood pressure in the newborn can be difficult.

This probably has accounted as much for the absence of good surveys in normal infants as it has for the proliferation of techniques. The use of the Doppler ultrasound method has greatly enhanced the accuracy and simplicity of obtaining blood pressures in the small infant and appears, at the moment, to be the method of choice. A cuff approximating two-thirds of the length of the upper extremity should be used (in small infants, a 4 by 9 cm cuff works well), with the transducer placed over the brachial artery. In this fashion the blood pressure can be taken in the infant at rest. A cuff too small will overestimate the blood pressure, and a cuff too large will underestimate it. In general, the mean systolic blood pressure is slightly lower and the mean diastolic blood pressure is slightly higher with the Doppler technique than with the intra-aortic pressures, but the accuracy and reliability are excellent in the clinical situation. Normal pressures for neonates, obtained by umbilical artery catheter, are listed in Appendix V (p. 1063).

ETIOLOGY.    The most common cause of hypertension in the newborn is coarctation of the aorta (p. 246). For this reason, the blood pressure measurement should be obtained in both the upper and lower extremities; pressure normally should be higher in the leg than in the arm. Synchronism of brachial and femoral pulses is probably of more value in coarctation than attempting to judge the relative force of the femoral pulse. Renal vascular disease, usually renal artery stenosis, is the second most common cause. Cardiac failure without valvular disease has led in some reports to the initial diagnoses of myocarditis, endocardial fibroelastosis and cardiomyopathies, including glycogen storage disease, before renal artery stenosis has been detected. Raised intracranial pressure, from any cause, including tumor, subdural hematoma and meningitis, may cause an acute increase in blood pressure in the neonate. Pheochromocytoma and fibromuscular dysplasia have not been diagnosed in the newborn.

Hypertension has been reported in association with obstructive uropathy. Crossed renal ectopia with hypertension has been reported in a male infant with a left to right ectopia and one renal mass on the right.

This was associated with an imperforate anus and rectourethral fistula. Hypertension was corrected by removal of the ectopic kidney. There was hydronephrosis of the crossed left kidney, and arteriogram showed a small narrow renal artery. Another case was reported by Palmer et al. in a young patient with a solitary kidney and ureteropelvic obstruction. Peripheral and renal vein renin activity was normal. Removal of the obstruction resulted in a massive postoperative diuresis and cure of the hypertension. It was proposed that sodium and water retention, on the basis of renal insufficiency, suppressed the release of the expected increased amounts of renin.

Hypertension is not usual in patients with congenital anomalies of the urinary tract, however. Only infantile polycystic kidneys and segmental hypoplasia are commonly associated with elevated blood pressures. It is interesting that most patients with developmental anomalies such as hypoplasia or dysplasia seem quite resistant to the development of hypertension, even after the development of renal insufficiency. The reason for this is not evident.

Other causes of hypertension in the neonate include adrenal hyperplasia, fluid and electrolyte overload, neuroblastoma, Cushing's disease and primary hyperaldosteronism. These other causes are quite rare in the nursery. Systemic hypertension has also been reported following the ocular administration of 10 per cent phenylephrine in the neonate. Causes of hypertension reported in infancy are listed in Table 49–1.

## RENIN-ANGIOTENSIN SYSTEM

The renin-angiotensin system is undoubtedly involved in renovascular hypertension and has been implicated as a final common pathway in several other hypertensive states. Renin is released from the juxtaglomerular cells of the renal cortex in response to decreased renal plasma flow, decreased plasma volume or sodium depletion. An enzyme, renin acts on a liver produced glycoprotein substrate to release a decapeptide, angiotensin I. Another enzyme from lung converts angiotensin I to

**TABLE 49–1.  Causes of Hypertension in Infancy**

*Vascular*
  Coarctation of the thoracic aorta
  Coarctation of the abdominal aorta
  Anomalies of the renal pedicle, including arterial
    stenosis and hypoplasia
  Hypoplasia of the aorta
  Renal artery thrombosis

*Renal*
  Infantile polycystic kidneys
  Hypoplastic kidney
  Obstructive uropathy with hydronephrosis
  Crossed renal ectopia
  Acute and chronic renal insufficiency
  Renal tumors
  Medullary cystic diseases
  Multicystic kidney

*Other*
  Increased intracranial pressure
  Neural crest tumors
  Adrenogenital syndrome
  Cushing's disease
  Primary hyperaldosteronism
  Fluid and electrolyte overload
  Ocular phenylephrine

an octapeptide, angiotensin II, which both causes vasoconstriction and stimulates the adrenal cortex to produce aldosterone. Although the regulating mechanisms are not clearly defined, the advantage of this system in the maintenance of plasma volume, sodium regulation and intravascular pressure is obvious. The role of renin-angiotensin in the fetus and newborn is not clear. However, increased renal vascular resistance seems to be a major factor in the relatively decreased glomerular filtration rate and renal plasma flow in the neonate. Its role may also include maintaining functionally significant levels of aldosterone in a relatively refractory adrenal cortex.

Information about the renin-angiotensin system in the neonate is just becoming available. Based on morphology, it appears that the human fetus produces renin as early as the seventeenth week of gestation; sustained hypertension has been produced in the fetal lamb by renal artery constriction in utero, presumably related to the renin-angiotensin system. Using immunoassays, the level of plasma renin activity (PRA) 1 to 12 hours after birth is signifi-

cantly elevated compared to normal adult standards and is comparable to that found in adults following the combined stimulus of salt deprivation and upright position. Kotchen et al., using immunoassay, found that the mean PRA for the neonate is 8.8 ng/ml/hr $\pm$ 2.8 S.E.M. By 3 to 6 days, the PRA rises still higher to 11.6 ng/ml/hr. Three to 6 weeks later, activity falls slightly to 2.3 ng/ml/hr, but is still higher than in the average adult. Although some reports in prematures and term neonates do not find plasma renin levels to be different from those of older children, other groups measuring PRA in children between the ages of 2 months and 19 years have shown that PRA is higher in the younger children and gradually declines during the first 6 years to approximately adult levels. This decline with age does not seem to be related to an increase in sodium intake, since sodium excretion, corrected for body surface area, does not vary with age in normal children on normal diets.

Plasma renin substrate in the newborn is also significantly elevated over normal adult controls and seems to stay relatively stable between birth and 6 weeks of age. Plasma renin activity is dependent on both enzyme and substrate concentrations. However, it is probable that the increased PRA in the neonate is primarily a reflection of elevations of the enzymes rather than the level of substrate. The substrate concentration is only modestly elevated, while PRA is over 10 times that of the adult. Also, in 3- to 6-week-old infants, PRA is significantly lower than in the younger infant, while the elevated substrate concentration persists at roughly the same level.

Diagnostic and therapeutic decisions must allow for the higher normal levels of both PRA and substrate in the neonate. Like creatinine, the normal values for the laboratory are not always the normal values for the infant.

It is not clear if one can implicate the renin-angiotensin system in all hypertension of the newborn. For example, elevations of PRA are not universal in coarctation of the aorta, and the role of the kidney or renal plasma flow in this hypertensive state is controversial. The same is true for hypertension associated with either increased intracranial pressure or fluid and electrolyte overload.

**DIAGNOSIS.** The signs and symptoms of hypertension in the newborn are often non-specific until congestive heart failure develops. The infants can show irritability, anorexia, failure to thrive, vomiting, diarrhea, fever, respiratory distress, seizures, polyuria, hypokalemia, alkalosis and hypotonia. Since the initial findings are so protean, it becomes evident that accurate blood pressure determinations should be a part of the evaluation of the ill newborn, no matter what the initial impression.

Each of the causes listed in Table 49–1 must be considered and evaluated by appropriate radiologic and chemical techniques. The routine measurement in every infant of 17-hydroxysteroids, 17-ketosteroids, VMA, catecholamines and aldosterone secretion, without some other indication, most often increases the expense and postpones definitive therapy with little diagnostic return. Radiologic and electrocardiographic evaluations of heart size are important as is every effort to diagnose coarctation of the aorta. Urinalysis, tests of renal function and intravenous pyelography should also be done to determine the presence of renal parenchymal disease and congenital abnormalities of the urinary tract. Peripheral plasma renin activity is helpful if significantly elevated, but may be deceiving if normal. Since most reports of hypertension in the neonate in the absence of coarctation of the aorta are related to renovascular disease, a major effort to define this entity should be made.

The diagnosis of renal vascular hypertension is made best by arteriography, with which information about abnormal size, caliber and contours of the renal vessels becomes readily available. Accessory vessels become apparent as do areas of stenosis and/or post-stenotic diliatation. The nephrogram also provides the size and shape of the kidney and the homogeneity of its vascular supply. Renal vein samples for plasma renin activity should be taken at the same time as the arteriography.

When comparing the levels in both renal veins, a ratio of greater than 2 1/2 to 1 is highly suggestive of unilateral disease, and implies a good prognosis following

nephrectomy. Normal renal vein PRA does not clearly exclude unilateral disease, since blood from a small ischemic area may not be detected because of dilution of the blood from the remainder of the kidneys. However, selective sampling from branches of the renal vein is almost impossible in the infant. It is often difficult enough just to get a sampling catheter into the major renal vessels.

Reports of infants with renal vascular hypertension in whom rapid sequence pyelography has been used are insufficient to assess the value of this test. Reports in older children indicate that most, but by no means all, children with renal vascular hypertension will have some abnormality of either size or function, or in the appearance of contrast material in the affected kidney. Localized areas of poor or delayed visualization, as well as non-visualization, provide valuable information. It has been noted that delayed appearance of contrast material on one side, when coupled with increased density on the same side, is consistent with an abnormality of the renal pedicle. Since intravenous pyelography is difficult to assess in the newborn, it is unlikely that the rapid sequence pyelogram would negate the use of arteriography in an infant with hypertension. It would seem wise to proceed to aortography in a hypertensive newborn whether or not the pyelogram is suggestive of a renal lesion. Differential renal function studies are technically difficult in the child and practically impossible in the neonate. It would appear that tests such as the renogram, the urea washout pyelogram, and renal biopsy are of less value than the arteriogram in neonates with renal vascular hypertension. However, information on this is virtually non-existent.

Significant alteration of renal function indicates bilateral renal disease, either primary parenchymal involvement or secondary to hypertension. With any significant hypertension, secondary damage to cerebral, retinal and renal vessels can be expected. The renal lesion is a nephrosclerosis affecting primarily the afferent arteriole, but can progress to hyalinization of the glomeruli. The glomerular lesion is irreversible. Early control of hypertension seems to prevent progression of this secondary lesion, and in children the reversibility of the arteriolar damage appears more common than in the adult. Therefore, the clinical evaluation must be prompt and complete, but must also include consideration of bilateral or irreversible renal involvement.

**TREATMENT.** The major reason for pursuing the clinical evaluation to completion and to a precise diagnosis is to provide the opportunity for a surgical cure. When the result is unilateral artery stenosis, and if diagnosed early enough, nephrectomy is curative. Most feel that nephrectomy is better than attempts to reconstruct a renal artery, since most attempts to revascularize in the infant result in thrombosis of the repaired vessels. Bilateral stenotic disease is a more difficult problem. Some will attempt surgical repair on one side at a time with some reported success. There has been some success using autotransplantation in the treatment of bilateral disease. This has not been reported in an infant but has been performed successfully in an 8-year-old. Successful medical management may be a more prudent approach in bilateral disease, the surgical approach being reserved for those in whom control of the blood pressure cannot be maintained.

For those infants in whom surgery is not possible, pharmacologic agents become the mainstay of medical management. Treatment must be individualized, not only in terms of the type, amount or combinations of antihypertensive agents but also in terms of the goal of the specific therapy. For example, an infant with inoperable renal artery stenosis and renin-angiotensin-mediated hypertension should be considered in a different manner than one with chronic renal insufficiency whose major difficulty may be fluid and electrolyte excess.

Information about the long-term effects of antihypertensive drugs begun in infancy or about the effects of these agents on development in the immature is virtually nonexistent. The current controversy over whether reserpine is related to breast cancer is a typical example of the lack of information. Whether the drugs themselves have an influence on growth is not known.

Children with hypertension and normal renal function do not grow normally until the hypertension is brought under control. The mechanism whereby hypertension might alter growth is unknown. And the long-term effect of the treatment is also not certain.

When considering an approach to therapy one should keep in mind the pharmacologic effects and sites of action of the agents employed. Drugs that alter peripheral vascular resistance include thiazides, reserpine, hydralazine, methyldopa, guanethidine, diazoxide and nitroprusside. Drugs that interfere with the renin-angiotensin system include propranolol and methyldopa. Drugs that alter cardiac output include propranolol, hydralazine and reserpine. Drugs that decrease plasma volume include the thiazides, furosemide, ethacrynic acid and spironolactone.

Hypertensive emergencies should be treated with parenteral medication. The drugs available include reserpine, hydralazine, methyldopa, diazoxide and nitroprusside. Many infants will respond promptly to intramuscular reserpine and hydralazine, with the other medications being held in reserve; effect with these two agents should be seen within one hour of administration. Tachycardia from the hydralazine, and flushing, somnolence or irritability from the reserpine are the usual side effects.

In resistant patients, diazoxide, given rapidly intravenously, is the next step. To be effective, the drug must be administered by bolus within 30 seconds. The effect is almost immediate and may persist for hours after a single administration with no other antihypertensive drug. Few side effects have been reported. Transient tachycardia is usual. A report of non-fatal arrhythmia in an infant, related to diazoxide injected through a central venous line, is cause for concern. Thus, it is probably more prudent to use a peripheral vessel for diazoxide, even if a central catheter is available. Hyperglycemia and hyperuricemia have also been reported with diazoxide.

Parental nitroprusside has yet to fail to reduce blood pressure. Its effect is immediate (within seconds), the desired level of blood pressure can be virtually titrated by control of the intravenous rate, and hypotension from overdose can be reversed almost instantaneously by discontinuing the infusion. Its major drawback is also its main virtue; since changes in its effect are directly related to the rate of parenteral administration, it requires intense monitoring under constant observation by professional personnel familiar with its use. Experience with the drug is very limited in the neonate and side effects, other than hypotension, have not been well documented.

Dialysis or plasmaphoresis may be the most effective treatment for severe hypertension from fluid and electrolyte overload who does not respond to diuretics and restriction of intake.

In the medical management of persistent or chronic hypertension one should also keep in mind the etiology of the hypertension. Patients with fluid and electrolyte overload, either iatrogenic or related to renal insufficiency, should have their intake appropriately decreased and their output increased with diuretics. At the same time, consideration must be given to the potential of increasing the stimulus for renin release, by producing a low plasma volume; therefore, in an infant with renin-angiotensin mediated hypertension vigorous treatment with diuretics has at least the theoretical possibility of enhancing, rather than controlling, hypertension. It would seem more profitable in such a circumstance to consider those drugs known to suppress plasma renin activity, such as methyldopa or propranolol.

The starting oral doses for antihypertensive agents in common use are given in Table 49–2. These are a guideline; there is no routine dose, no routine order of increasing effectiveness, no fixed combination of agents. The best dose is one which attains the goal of a normal blood pressure with absent or clinically tolerable side effects and which is within the capability of the family to administer. The timing and frequency of medication are dependent on the diurnal variability of the infants' pressures and the duration of action of the medications. The aim should be to maintain as normal a blood pressure as possible throughout the day.

**TABLE 49–2.    Antihypertensive Medications in Neonates**

| Medication | Parenteral Dose | Oral Dose |
|---|---|---|
| Reserpine | 0.01–0.02 mg/kg I.M. | 0.02 mg/kg/day divided into 2 doses |
| Hydralazine | 0.15 mg/kg I.M. | 0.25 mg/kg/day divided into 3–6 doses |
| Methyldopa | 2–4 mg/kg I.M. or I.V. | 10 mg/kg/day divided into 3–4 equally spaced doses |
| Guanethidine | | 0.2 mg/kg/day single dose |
| Propranolol | | 1.5 mg/kg/day divided into 2–3 doses |
| Diazoxide | 3–5 mg/kg I.V. | |
| Nitroprusside | 0.004 $\mu$g/kg/min. I.V. | |

## REFERENCES

Belman, A. B., Kropp, K. A., and Simon, N. M.: Renal pressor hypertension secondary to unilateral hydronephrosis. N. Engl. J. Med. 278:1133, 1968.

Black, I. F. S., Kotrapu, N., and Massie, H. Application of Doppler ultrasound to blood pressure measurement in small infants. J. Pediatr. 81:932, 1972.

Bonomeo-Mcgrail, V., Bordiuk, J. M., and Keitel, H.: Systemic hypertension following ocular administration of 10% phenylephrine in the neonate. Pediatrics 51:1032, 1973.

Cook, G. T., Marshall, V. F., and Todd, J. E.: Malignant renovascular hypertension in a newborn. J. Urol. 96:863, 1966.

Coran, A. G., and Schuster, S. R.: Renovascular hypertension in childhood. Surgery 64:572, 1968.

Foster, J. H., Pittinger, W. A., Oates, J. A., et al.: Malignant hypertension secondary to renal artery stenosis in children. Ann. Surg. 164:700, 1966.

Goddard, C., Riondel, A. M., Veyrat, R., Megevand, A., and Muller, A. F.: Plasma renin activity and aldosterone secretion in congenital adrenal hyperplasia. Pediatrics 41:883, 1968.

Hernandez, A., Goldring, D., Hartmann, A. F., Crawford, C., and Reed, G. N.: Measurement of blood pressure in infants and children by the Doppler ultrasound technique. Pediatrics 48:788, 1971.

Hiner, L. B., Baluarte, H. J., Cote, M. L., et al.: Sodium balance and peripheral renin activity (PRA) in children. (Abstr.) Ped. Res. 9:375, 1975.

Imai, M., Igarashi, Y., and Sokabe, H.: Plasma renin activity in congenital virilizing adrenal hyperplasia. Pediatrics 41:879, 1968.

Kirkendall, W. M., Culbertson, J. W., and Eckstein, J. W.: Renal hemodynamics in patients with coarctation of the aorta. J. Lab. Clin. Med. 53:6, 1959.

Kotchen, T. A., Strickland, A. L., Rice, T. W., and Walters, D. R.: A study of the renin-angiotensin system in newborn infants. J. Pediatr. 80:938, 1972.

Ljungqvist, A., and Wallgren, G.: Unilateral renal artery stenosis and fatal arterial hypertension in a newborn infant. Acta Paediatr. Scand. 51:575, 1962.

Makker, S. P., and Lubahn, J. D.: Clinical features of renovascular hypertension in infancy: Report of a 9-month-old infant. Pediatrics 56:108, 1975.

Marie, J., Royer, P., Gabilan, J. C., and Vandevoorde, J.: Le traitement médical de l'hypertension artérielle permanente chez l'enfant. Ann. Pédiatr. (Paris) 4:251, 1965.

Mininberg, D. T., Roze, S., Yoon, H. J., and Pearl, M.: Hypertension associated with crossed renal ectopia in an infant. Pediatrics 48:454, 1971.

Palmer, J. M., Zweiman, F. G., and Assaykeen, T. A.: Renal hypertension secondary to hydronephrosis with normal plasma renin activity. N. Engl. J. Med. 283:1032, 1970.

Schmidt, D. M., and Rambo, O. N.: Segmental intimal hyperplasia of the abdominal aorta and renal arteries producing hypertension in an infant. Am. J. Clin. Pathol. 44:546, 1965.

Skinner, S. L., Lumbers, E. R., and Symonds, E. M.: Renin concentration in human fetal and maternal tissues. Am. J. Obstet. Gynecol. 101:529, 1968.

Snyder, C. H., Bast, R. B., and Platau, R. V.: Hypertension in infancy with anomalous renal artery. Pediatrics 15:88, 1955.

Stalker, P., Kotchen, T., Kotchen, J. M., and Holland, N. H.: Peripheral plasma renin activity (PRA) in normal children. (Abstr.) Ped. Res. 9:379, 1975.

Timmis, G. C., and Gordon, S.: A renal factor in hypertension due to coarctation. N. Engl. J. Med. 270:814, 1964.

Walker, C. H. M., West, P. J., Simons, S. L., and Whytock, A. R.: Indirect estimation of systolic and diastolic blood pressure in the newborn. Pediatrics 50:387, 1972.

Wernig, C., Schonbeck, M., Weidmann, P., et al.: Plasma renin activity in patients with coarctation of the aorta. Circulation 40:731, 1969.

# DIFFERENTIAL DIAGNOSIS OF ENLARGED KIDNEY

# 50

*Revised by Warren Grupé*

It is at times difficult to be sure whether a kidney is enlarged or not. During the initial physical examination on the first or second day of life one can often feel the lower poles of the kidneys. Indeed, it has been maintained that one should always be able to feel these, provided the examiner palpates deeply and assiduously, and that failure to feel one indicates that some abnormality is present. If we may be considered to belong to the category of the average examiner, we are constrained to admit that the average examination fails to discover a good many. In any event, palpability is not synonymous with enlargement.

A method of palpation proposed by Museles et al. takes only 30 seconds in the well relaxed infant. Palpating in both upper quadrants, the examiner supports the flank with one hand while palpating with the other. Moving the palpating hand medially, the first encounter is with the anterolateral aspect of the lower pole. The normal kidney is located above the level of the umbilicus. When the lower pole projects well below this level, the organ is either enlarged or dislocated downward. Since the long axis usually parallels the long axis of the body, medial displacement of the lower pole would suggest a horseshoe kidney. Palpation directly over the lumbar vertebrae, by moving the palpating hand medially, can detect the isthmus. Both lower quadrants are then examined for the presence of a pelvic kidney. Finally, the examiner places a hand in each flank, compressing medially and raising the hands slightly to allow the abdominal contents to pass between the fingers of the opposing hands. This helps in detecting a freely movable mass such as an intestinal duplication or a cyst.

On many occasions even the most experienced examiner will remain uncertain whether what he feels is abnormal. In the absence of symptoms or pathologic findings in the urine he may elect to wait and see what happens. If, on the other hand, the infant appears ill in any way, he will choose to make further studies in order to clarify the point. Determination of blood nonprotein nitrogen level and intravenous urography should suffice at the start.

An apparently enlarged kidney may be the result of one of a variety of pathologic processes. In the study by Museles et al., using the initial examination in 10,000 newborn infants, 71 infants had suspected renal anomalies by deep palpation, of which 55 (0.6 per cent of the total) were confirmed by x-ray. The most common abnormality encountered was horseshoe kidney, comprising 28 per cent of the anomalies found. Unilateral renal agenesis was the second most frequent finding, occurring in 26 per cent of the infants with anomalies. Other disorders included pelvic kidney (16 per cent), unilateral hypoplastic kidney (5 per cent), bilateral renal agenesis (3 per cent), polycystic kidneys (3 per cent), multicystic kidneys (3 per cent) and crossed renal ectopia (3 per cent). Other abnormalities to be considered include hydronephrosis, duplicated kidney, Wilms' or Wilms'-like tumors, renal vascular thrombosis, adrenal hemorrhage, adrenal tumors, meconium cyst, double collecting system, and duplication of the ileum. In the series by Museles et al. renal abnormalities accounted for 93 per cent of the anomalies found by deep palpation.

The general condition of the infant provides the first clue to differential diagnosis. Only renal vein thrombosis and adrenal hemorrhage would be likely to make the child ill. Wilms' tumor might if it were of long standing, and the congenital malformations might if they were already accompanied by urinary infection. This is not likely this early in life. The feel of the mass affords a second distinguishing point. A perfectly smooth, rounded mass is more likely to be hydronephrotic kidney than one of the others, but the infarcted and the downwardly displaced one may feel the same. Grossly irregular masses presenting one or more rounded knobs may contain embryoma or large cysts, the former feeling much harder than the latter. The surfaces of polycystic kidneys are apt to feel homogeneously and finely nodular, like the liver of Laennec's cirrhosis. Hugely enlarged kidneys have more chance of being hydronephrotic if smooth, the site of multiple cysts if nodular, than any of the others. Large cysts and the hydronephrotic kidney transilluminate brightly; the others do not.

Neuroblastoma seldom presents as unilateral kidney displacement alone in the newborn, although this may constitute part of the picture. The usual presenting sign is the huge, smooth liver of metastatic involvement; the primary tumor is not often felt.

Urine examination may be helpful. Albumin in excess is often found in polycystic kidney and renal vein thrombosis. Gross hematuria is pretty well restricted to renal vein thrombosis, although it may occur in some cases of hydronephrosis and of Wilms' tumor. The same may be said for microscopic hematuria, with the warning that its absence does not rule out these diagnoses. Pyuria and cylindruria are also found in infarcted kidneys and are present in the others only if infection has supervened.

The urea nitrogen level rises rapidly when the renal vein becomes thrombosed. It may be elevated early in hydronephrosis and in polycystic disease, but elevation commonly awaits a later date. Barring superimposed pyelonephritis, it should not be high in any of the other conditions under consideration.

Intravenous pyelography will demonstrate that the kidney enlarged because of infarction and the multicystic kidney are unable to excrete dye. We have recently seen a huge hydronephrotic kidney which excreted no dye; this must be rare. In all the other disorders the urogram, either intravenous or retrograde, and, if indicated, the cinecystogram should supply the definitive answer.

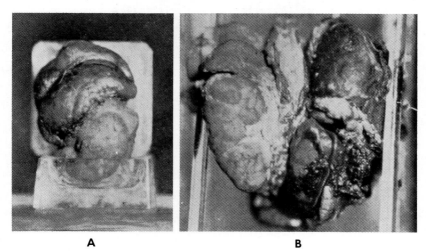

**A**        **B**

*Figure 50–1.* A, Hemorrhagic infarction of the right adrenal, which is in its normal position above the kidney. B, Posterior view. The left adrenal is intact; the right one is transformed into a hemorrhagic mass. The right kidney is pushed downward by hemorrhagic infiltration of perirenal tissues. Note the size of the right adrenal in comparison to the left adrenal and kidney. (Reprinted from Goldzieher, M. A., and Greenwald, H. M.: Am. J. Dis. Child. 36:324, 1928.)

Hydronephrotic or polycystic kidneys may be demonstrated by transillumination of the flank mass.

Kidney photoscan should help in distinguishing dislocated from enlarged kidneys, and multilocular cysts from multicystic or polycystic kidneys. Venogram, with dye injected from below, can rule renal vein thrombosis in or out with precision.

We have seen a case in which an erroneous diagnosis of polycystic kidneys was made when the correct one was bilateral adrenal hemorrhage. When the kidneys became palpable, toward the end of the first week of life, the history of neonatal distress was overlooked and the pyelograms were misinterpreted. Eight months later the appearance of calcification in both suprarenal regions led to revision of the original impression. Figure 50–1 indicates what great size hemorrhagic adrenals may attain.

The possibility of Wilms' tumor cannot be overlooked, but its rarity renders it an extremely unlikely cause of enlarged kidney in the first weeks of life. One must not, therefore intervene surgically until enough of these diagnostic methods have been employed to define the pathologic situation clearly. Headlong intervention is not called for. Even more important, x-irradiation and anticancer chemotherapeutic agents should be withheld unless pathologic evidence of malignancy is demonstrable.

# 51

# NEPHROPATHIES
*Revised by Warren Grupe*

## ACUTE PYELONEPHRITIS

This segment is to be found in the section devoted to Urinary Tract Infection (see page 786).

## CHRONIC NEPHRITIS AND NEPHROSIS

### GLOMERULONEPHRITIS

Glomerulonephritis in the neonate is an infrequent occurrence and is not as clearly understood as nephritis in the older child. The acute and the persistent glomerulonephritides common in childhood have not been established in the neonate by currently accepted techniques. Most reports of glomerular injury in the neonate are associated with the nephrotic syndrome (see page 471). In this circumstance minimal lesion glomerulonephropathy, focal segmental sclerosis, membranous glomerulonephropathy and diffuse mesangial sclerosis have been described. Other forms of renal injury that may also involve the glomerulus, include bacterial and non-bacterial pyelonephritis and hereditary nephritis.

One difficulty in evaluating glomerulonephritis in the neonate involves the characteristics of the immature renal glomeruli. In both humans and the experimental animal this includes a small diameter of the glomerular tuft with a narrow Bowman's space, splitting of the lamina densa, a nonfenestrated broad rim of the endothelial cytoplasm around the periphery of the glomerular tuft with a relatively narrow capillary lumen. Palisading of adjacent visceral epithelial cells over the capillary loop and broad extension of epithelial cytoplasm covering basement membrane is in contrast to the discreet foot processes noted in the older child or adult. In addition, glomerular senescence and hyalinization is common in the newborn, appearing to be a normal process of glomerular involution. Sclerotic glomeruli compromise approximately 10 per cent of the glomerular population in newborns dying of other diseases, although this has been reported in as high as 20 per cent of glomeruli. One may see the other hallmarks of nephron involution, including focal tubular atrophy and slight interstitial reaction. It is presumed that the mechanism of this normal glomerular involution is ischemia, but the hyalinized and sclerotic glomeruli can appear similar to those seen in chronic glomerulonephritis in the older child. Many of the clinical and pathologic descriptions of neonatal nephritis are difficult to evaluate in light of the current recognition of this normal involutional process. It is also quite possible that some examples of neonatal nephritis have been confused with renal cortical and medullary necrosis.

On occasion, acute and chronic pyelonephritis may also be associated with proliferative changes. This has raised questions about the relationship between infectious processes and neonatal glomerulonephritis.

Porter and Giles make out a strong argument in favor of the basic defect in their five cases being pyelonephritis rather than glomerulonephritis. In their Case I the pyelonephritis was acute and unmistakable. In their other four cases the alterations were older, death having occurred between 14 and 20 weeks of age, and were therefore more difficult to evaluate. In all five the urine culture was positive for *E. coli,* and in two the blood grew out the same organism. All met the pathologic criteria laid down by Weiss and Parker for the diagnosis of chronic pyelonephritis. They include 1) infiltration of interstitium with lymphocytes, plasma cells and eosinophils, 2) pericapsular fibrosis, with or without intracapsular crescent formation, and 3) colloid casts in dilated tubules lined by atrophic epithelium. They point out that their cases differ from chronic glomerulonephritis in that many glomeruli are unaffected, the glomerular tufts are often uninvolved where pericapsular fibrosis is evident, that involved glomeruli are apt to be found in wedge-shaped clusters and that interstitial inflammation is notable. Absence of much fibrosis they attribute to the relatively short course, and the presence of numerous crescents they discount with the statement that crescents seem to form more readily in infants that in adults and are found in many conditions other than glomerulonephritis.

These same authors wondered why all five of their patients were males when chronic pyelonephritis beyond the neonatal period is predominantly a disorder of females. They investigated the possibility of a congenital defect of the kidney being responsible for persistent infection and were gratified to find that in four of the five cases microdissection revealed the proximal tubules shorter than normal and almost devoid of convolutions. The fact that two of their patients were brothers strengthened their conviction that a congenital anomaly was at the bottom of the disorder.

Pyelonephritis that involves a hypoplastic or dysplastic kidney seems more likely to become chronic and progressive than the same infection that becomes lodged in a normal kidney.

Collins and others maintain, and the descriptions of the kidneys in their cases suggest, that chronic glomerulonephritis, whose pathogenesis is unclear, may be in some examples the correct pathologic diagnosis. Claireaux and Pearson disagree with Collins' conclusion, maintaining that the histologic alterations he described in the kidneys of his case, as in theirs, are compatible with chronic pyelonephritis.

Congenital syphilis can cause both an acute proliferative and chronic membranous glomerulonephropathy. The acute lesion is characterized by hematuria, proteinuria, cylinduria and moderate azotemia. The clinical diagnosis can be suspected when other stigmata of congenital syphilis are evident and positive serologic tests are noted. Renal biopsy discloses a proliferative glomerulonephritis with interstitial infiltrates of plasma cells and lymphocytes. The lesion usually responds completely to antibiotic therapy, with complete resolution of the glomerular lesion. Other infants with congenital syphilis may present with an infantile nephrotic syndrome including massive proteinuria, edema, hypoproteinemia and hypercholesterolemia. This also responds completely to antibiotic therapy (see page 829).

Nephritis has also been implicated in other congenital infections, including cytomegalic inclusion disease, Herpes virus, rubella virus and toxoplasmosis. These are usually mild both clinically and morphologically. The association of cytomegalovirus and toxoplasmosis with congenital nephrotic syndrome is not clear and is considered by some to be a coincidental or incidental finding.

Chronic glomerulonephritis has been described in newborns and in some cases has had a rapidly progressive course. Glomeruli are described as sclerotic and hyalinized, with severe epithelial proliferation and crescent formation. Tubular atrophy, casts, interstitial infiltrate, fibrosis and vascular sclerosis have also been described. The prevalence and incidence of this disorder in the nursery has not been established.

### INFANTILE NEPHROTIC SYNDROME

The infantile nephrotic syndrome is a heterologous group of diseases that may share in common only the fact that onset occurs in the first year of life. Although, with current knowledge, an exact classification is not entirely possible several distinct subgroups and several recurrent associations have been noted. It is clear that infantile microcystic disease (Finnish type) is not the only morphologic type and that the outcome of infantile nephrosis need not always be progressive loss of renal function leading inevitably to uremia and death. Because of the complexity of this group of diseases, renal biopsy is virtually mandatory for a diagnosis and to provide adequate guidance for therapy and prognosis. The presentation in these children differs little from that of the nephrotic syndrome in the older child. Massive proteinuria, often detected in the first specimen voided at birth, accompanied by hypoproteinemia, hypoalbuminemia and eventually anasarca are the hallmarks. Although hypercholesterolemia and hyperlipemia are also present, the serum lipids may not be as significantly elevated in the young infant as might be expected for the degree of hypoalbuminemia. The forms of infantile nephrotic syndrome have been subdivided on the basis of morphology, mode of inheritance, clinical course and response to appropriate therapy.

INFANTILE MICROCYSTIC DISEASE. This has been the most widely recognized form of infantile nephrotic syndrome, is probably still the most common lesion noted and has contributed most to the idea that infants with nephrotic syndrome will inevitably die of renal failure. It is a familial disease with an autosomal recessive mode of inheritance. It has been commonly reported in children of Finnish extraction but is by no means restricted to that lineage. Prematurity with a large edematous placenta is common, as is a high incidence of toxemia during the pregnancy. All die within the first year of life, though not usually of uremia; infections, diarrhea and severe electrolyte disorders are the rule. The characteristic lesion is microcystic dilatation of the proximal tubule, more so in the cortex than in the medulla; the dilated tubules have flattened epithelial cells and intact basement membranes. Microdissection studies have demonstrated the cystlike dilatations in the proximal tubule. Successful renal transplantation without recurrence of the original disease has been reported.

Confirming this diagnosis by biopsy is essential. Steroids and cytotoxic drugs are ineffective in the treatment of this lesion and, since infection is such a problem with these children, it is probably in the child's best interest that this form of therapy not be tried. Genetic counseling of the parents is very important, since there is one chance in four that subsequent children will be affected by the same lesion.

The disease has been diagnosed in both a 17-week and a 19-week fetus; in the 17-week fetus this was associated with a significant rise in α-fetoprotein in both amniotic fluid and maternal plasma.

MINIMAL LESION NEPHROTIC SYNDROME. This lesion is clinically and morphologically similar to the lipoid nephrosis more common in the older child. The nephrotic syndrome is not accompanied by persistent azotemia, hematuria, hypertension or evidence of systemic disease. The renal histology by light microscopy appears entirely normal; immunofluorescence microscopy shows no evidence of antibody deposition, and only fusion of the epithelial cell foot processes is seen by electron microscopy. Recovery from this disease, either spontaneously or following treatment with steroids, is not uncommon. Although some infants progress to chronic renal insufficiency, their course is longer than with the microcystic form of the disease. Clear definition by renal biopsy is important in planning treatment. No etiology is known and no hereditary pattern has been established.

FOCAL GLOMERULOSCLEROSIS. The nephrotic syndrome associated with this lesion is usually accompanied by microscopic hematuria. No etiology is known and there is no evidence of a pattern of inheritance. This is the third most common morphologic finding by biopsy of nephrotic infants. The lesion is usually steroid resistant and there is no clear evidence that steroids with cytotoxic agents alter the course or the prognosis of this lesion. A recurrence of this lesion has been seen in older children following renal transplantation.

DIFFUSE MESANGIAL SCLEROSIS. In most cases, the onset of this disease is beyond the neonatal period. The clinical course is that of a steroid resistant nephrotic syndrome with progressive loss of renal function. Renal insufficiency may not occur until the second year of life. Familial involvement may be present, although not clearly in all patients; the mode of inheritance has not been established. The renal pathologic features include diffuse mesangial sclerosis involving all glomeruli, with retraction of the glomerular tuft, which is surrounded by a crescent of epithelial cells. There is also interstitial inflammation and fibrosis. There are few reports of this lesion, and results with renal transplantation are not clear.

EXTRA-MEMBRANOUS GLOMERULONEPHRITIS (MEMBRANOUS GLOMERULONEPHROPATHY). This form has been described in a few infants, most often in association with congenital syphilis. A proliferative glomerulonephritis can also be seen in congenital syphilis (see page 829). In one patient immunofluorescent microscopy showed granular deposition of IgG, IgA, IgM, and β-1-C, suggesting that the renal lesion in congenital syphilis is immunologically mediated. Other reports have shown nodular deposition of IgG and fibrin without β-1-C. Light microscopy shows thickening of the glomerular basement membrane with minimal proliferation or infiltration. The tubules and interstitium are normal. The lesions respond well to penicillin, with complete recovery. Again morphological diagnosis becomes important in order to avoid the use of steroids or cytotoxic drugs.

Epimembranous glomerulonephropathy has also been seen in association with toxoplasmosis and cytomegalic inclusion disease. In others no cause can be identified.

INTERSTITIAL NEPHRITIS. One case, with onset at birth, has been described in which the primary renal abnormality was a chronic interstitial nephritis with widespread interstitial fibrosis. There were collections of lymphocytes in the interstitium but no plasma cells and no polymorphonuclear leukocytes, with no indication of an infectious etiology. The child had abnormal external genitalia and progressed to chronic renal failure and death at 9 months of age.

OTHER FORMS OF INFANTILE NEPHROTIC SYNDROME. Nephrotic syndrome has been reported in association with the nail patella syndrome, nephroblastoma and pseudohermaphrodism. Mercury intoxication, which may also be a cause, usually responds to withdrawal of the toxic agent. Although cytomegalovirus and toxoplasmosis have been described in association with the nephrotic syndrome, it is felt by many to be a coincidental finding rather than a cause.

With such morphologic heterogeneity, the differences in response to therapy, and the need for intelligent genetic counseling, clear diagnosis becomes important. Genetic counseling is clear only in the case of infantile microcystic disease, which has an autosomal recessive mode of inheritance. The nail patella syndrome and some cases

of diffuse mesangial sclerosis also appear to be familial. Some feel that even the minimal lesion form in the first year of life may be familial. Habib reports that four of seven children with minimal lesion disease and a family history of nephrosis had onset of their disease in the first year of life.

## RENAL CORTICAL AND MEDULLARY NECROSIS

It is appropriate to consider cortical and medullary necrosis together, since they are virtually indistinguishable clinically and often co-exist.

Bernstein and Meyer have recalled to our attention the pathologic finding of renal cortical or medullary necrosis in not a few newborns who succumbed within the first 2 or 3 days of life. Zuelzer had described this condition in newborns several decades earlier.

The disorder commonly follows serious illness at birth, including profound asphyxia from abnormalities of labor or delivery, severe anemia for any one of its usual causes or disseminated intravascular coagulation. To the usual signs of respiratory distress may be added later bouts of apnea, flaccidity and lethargy. Characteristic is complete anuria or, if urine is passed, it is scanty and contains protein and red blood cells. Edema does not appear but hypertension resistant to therapy can develop rapidly. The blood urea nitrogen and potassium levels rise, at times to great heights. Thrombocytopenia may be present as evidence of intravascular coagulation. Both conditions may have areas of focal necrosis in other organs. These infants commonly die before the fourth day of life. The prognosis seems to be related to the success with which the underlying cause can be treated as well as to the extent of renal damage. Vigorous supportive care, careful management of fluid and electrolyte balance and active handling of the renal failure, including peritoneal dialysis, have improved the outlook for these children. Bernstein and Meyer encountered two who survived the first month, one of whom developed and maintained persistent hypertension of high grade, the other of whom died. The kidneys of this patient showed extensive scarring which had resulted from the healing of widespread medullary necrosis.

These authors have no doubt that necrosis results from shock and diminution of glomerular blood flow. Should we not use plasma and blood more freely than we do in the treatment of the shocked asphyxiated newborn?

Reports of relatively longer survivals and recovery are increasing. Variable degrees of hypertension or persistent renal insufficiency may remain in these infants. Nephrocalcinosis may become apparent radiographically after several months; cortical necrosis produces symmetrical bilateral cortical calcifications, while healing medullary necrosis is recognized by deformed calyces and evidence of papillary necrosis.

## ACUTE RENAL FAILURE

Insufficient renal function, with or without decreased urine production, may occur in the newborn and be related to prenatal injury (such as eclampsia), dehydration, shock, sepsis, anoxia, intrinsic congenital renal abnormalities (such as hypoplasia and dysplasia), acquired renal disease, vascular accidents, cortical and medullary necrosis, acute tubular necrosis or nephrotoxic antibiotics. An exact diagnosis is not always possible yet vigorous and aggressive management has improved the chances of survival for these infants in recent years.

Delayed micturition may be manifested as anuria or oliguria (less than 15 ml/kg/day). The most common cause in infants is hypovolemia with inadequate perfusion of the kidneys. The other causes may be divided into those conditions in which insufficient urine is formed and those associated with obstructions to urine flow. These have been carefully reviewed by Moore and Galvez. Several authors feel that catheterization should be delayed in these infants for at least 48 to 72 hours, particularly in the absence of azotemia or elevated serum creatinine; others feel that urethral catheterization is the quickest way to determine if there has been urine formation. Although the exact risk to the infant of introducing infection with catheterization

has not been established, it must be considered in the decision since as high as 5 to 14 per cent of older hospitalized patients develop urinary tract infections following a single catheterization. The low incidence of serious problems in the series of Moore and Galvez when delayed micturition was the only sign indicates that a cautious and thoughtfully delayed approach may be very appropriate in this group of infants.

Hypoperfusion (prerenal azotemia) is usually recognized by a blood urea disproportionately high relative to the creatinine, a serum creatinine that is often normal, a low urinary sodium and a high urinary-to-plasma ratio for creatinine. Although intravenous or oral infusions of fluids and solutes can be successful, this should be attempted judiciously after positive evidence of hypovolemia is obtained. A therapeutic trial of 15 to 20 ml per kg of isotonic fluid given over a 4 to 6 hour period should be sufficient; a prompt increase in the hourly urine volume indicates the kidneys' capability to respond. Should there be little or no change in urine volume, yet a documented increase in the infant's weight, either Mannitol 0.5 mg per kg or Furosemide, 1 mg per kg may be given intravenously. Should no response be evident after these two measures, any further attempt to provoke urine by further fluid and electrolyte administration is to court disaster either by water intoxication or by overload of the cardiovascular system.

An abnormal urinary stream, a palpable bladder, a palpably enlarged kidney or evidence of a urinary tract infection with or without septicemia is certainly an indication of a structural abnormality requiring further investigation. A review of the symptoms and lesions of lower urinary tract obstruction in infants was reported by Tsingoglou and Dickson. In general, the most common symptoms were of a non-specific nature, with failure to thrive, vomiting and fever of unknown origin the most frequent. Acute retention or dribbling micturition were the most frequent signs related to the urinary tract. In this series, the peak incidence of urinary obstruction occurred in the first 2 weeks of life, with a rapid decline thereafter. The crude mortality was highest at 32.5 per cent in infants whose first symptoms were before 1 month of age and was 18 per cent in all cases with a follow-up of at least 1 year.

Radiologic and urologic investigation may be necessary before a diagnosis of obstructive uropathy (post-renal azotemia) can be made. Posterior urethral valves are the most common cause in males, while an ectopic ureterocele accounts for approximately 75 per cent in girls.

Treatment in the neonate is similar to that provided the older uremic child. Fluid and electrolyte balance must be carefully maintained, with careful monitoring of intake and output of both fluids and electrolytes. In the acute state, fluid intake should be equal to the insensible water losses plus the urinary output. Fluid balance can be most carefully monitored by changes in weight. Fluid intake should be adjusted to allow the infant to lose 0.5 to 1.0 per cent of body weight per day, if adequate calories cannot be provided. In the anuric or severely oliguric infant the administration of solute may not be necessary. In others, the administration of sodium, potassium and bicarbonate should be determined from changes in the serum levels and the urinary excretion. Urinary output can be estimated in the non-catheterized infant by weighing the diapers dry and re-weighing immediately following voiding. Peritoneal dialysis may be necessary for hyperkalemia when the plasma concentration exceeds 6 mEq per liter, signs of cardiovascular overload, hyponatremia, hypernatremia or severe metabolic acidosis. Ion exchange resin (Kayexalate) can be given by retention enema to remove potassium. Each gram of resin removes a milliequivalent of potassium; for each milliequivalent of potassium removed, a milliequivalent of sodium is gained. Hypertension should be treated by careful fluid and electrolyte balance and by appropriate medications. Efforts to maintain normal blood pressure should be made.

Peritoneal dialysis is sufficient to maintain an infant for several weeks. However, if renal insufficiency persists, hemodialysis, although technically difficult, should be considered. Finally, if the renal failure fails to revert, renal transplantation should be considered.

# REFERENCES

### Chronic Nephritis and Nephrosis

Allen, T. D.: Pathogenesis of urinary tract infections in children. N. Engl. J. Med. *273*:1421, 1472, 1965.

Beeson, P. B.: Experimental pyelonephritis: Influence of localized injury in different parts of the kidney on susceptibility to hematogenous infection. Trans. Assoc. Am. Physicians *70*:120, 1957.

Bernstein, J., and Meyer, R.: Congenital abnormalities of the urinary system. II. Renal cortical and medullary necrosis. J. Pediatr. *59*:657, 1961.

Boehm, J. J., and Haynes, J. L.: Bacteriology of "midstream catch" urines. Am. J. Dis. Child. *111*:366, 1966.

Claireaux, A. E., and Pearson, M. G.: Chronic nephritis in a newborn infant. Arch. Dis. Child. *30*:366, 1955.

Collins, R. D.: Chronic glomerulonephritis in a newborn child. A.M.A. J. Dis. Child. *87*:478, 1954.

De Luca, F. G., Fisher, J. H., and Swenson, O.: Review of recurrent urinary tract infections in infancy and early childhood. N. Engl. J. Med. *268*:75, 1963.

Grupe, W. E., Cuppage, F. E., and Heymann, W.: Congenital nephrotic syndrome and interstitial nephritis. Am. J. Dis. Child. *111*:482, 1966.

Hallman, N., and Jjelt, L.: Congenital nephrosis syndrome. J. Pediatr. *55*:152, 1959.

Hoffpauir, C. W., and Guidry, C. J.: Asymptomatic urinary tract infection in premature infants. Pediatrics *46*:128, 1970.

Hoyer, J. R., Michael, A. F., Jr., Good, R. A., and Vernier, R. L.: The nephrotic syndrome of infancy: Clinical morphologic and immunologic studies of four infants. Pediatrics *40*:233, 1967.

Kenny, J. F., Medearis, D. N., Jr., Drachman, R. H., Gibson, L. E., and Klein, S. W.: Outbreak of urinary tract infection due to Escherichia coli in male infants. Am. J. Dis. Child. *104*:461, 1962.

Kunstadter, R. H., and Rosenblum, L.: Neonatal glomerulonephritis and nephrotic syndrome in a 1,320 gm. prematurely born infant. A.M.A. J. Dis. Child. *88*:611, 1954.

Longio, L. A., and Martin, L. W.: Abdominal masses in the newborn infant. Pediatrics *21*:596, 1958.

Manley, G. L., and Collipp, P. J.: Renal failure in the newborn: treatment with peritoneal dialysis. Am. J. Dis. Child. *115*:107, 1968.

McCarthy, J. M., and Pryles, C. V.: Clean voided and catheter neonatal urine specimens: Bacteriology in male and female neonate. Am. J. Dis. Child. *106*:473, 1963.

Museles, M., Gaudry, C. L., and Bason, W. M.: Renal anomalies in the newborn found by deep palpation. Pediatrics *47*:97, 1971.

Norio, R.: Heredity in the congenital nephrotic syndrome. Ann. Paediat. Fenn. (Supp. 27) *12*, 1966.

Papaioannou, A. C., Asrow, G. G., and Schuckmell, N. H.: Nephrotic syndrome in early infancy as a manifestation of congenital syphilis. Pediatrics *27*:636, 1961.

Porter, K. A., and Giles, H. M.: A pathological study of five cases of pyelonephritis in the newborn. Arch. Dis. Child. *31*:303, 1956.

Pryles, C. V., Lüders, D., and Alkan, M. K.: A comparative study of bacterial cultures and colony counts in paired specimens of urine obtained by catheter versus voiding in infants with urinary tract infection. Pediatrics 27:17, 1961.

Reisman, L. E., and Pathak, A.: Bilateral renal cortical necrosis in the newborn: Associated with feto-maternal transfusion and hypermagnesemia. Am. J. Dis. Child. *111*:541, 1966.

Saccharow, L., and Pryles, C. V.: Further experience with the use of percutaneous suprapubic aspiration of the urinary bladder. Pediatrics 43:1018, 1969.

Sherwood, D. W., Smith, R. C., Lemmon, R. H., and Vrabel, I.: Abnormalities of the genito-urinary tract discovered by palpation of the abdomen of the newborn. Pediatrics 18:782, 1956.

Stansfeld, J. M.: Discussion on chronic pyelonephritis. Proc. Roy. Soc. Med. 47:628, 1954.

Sweet, A. M., and Wolinsky, E.: An outbreak of urinary tract and other infections due to E. coli. Pediatrics 33:865, 1964.

Weiss, S., and Parker, F., Jr.: Pyelonephritis: Its relation to vascular lesions and arterial hypertension. Medicine 18:221, 1939.

Wheeler, W. E.: Are there pathogenic E. coli? Pediatrics 33:863, 1964.

Worthen, H. G., Vernier, R. L., and Good, R. A.: The syndrome of infantile nephrosis. A.M.A. J. Dis. Child. 96:585, 1958.

***Infantile Nephrotic Syndrome***

Hallman, N., Norio, R., and Rapola, J.: Congenital nephrotic syndrome. Nephron *11*:101, 1973.

Hoyer, J. R., Mauer, S. M., Kjellstrand, C. M., Buselmeier, T. J., Simmons, R. L., Michael, A. F., Najarian, J. S., and Vernier, R. L.: Successful treatment of the congenital nephrotic syndrome by renal transplantation. Pediatr. Res. 7:293, 1973.

Hoyer, J. R., Michael, A. F., Good, R. A., and Vernier, R. L.: The nephrotic syndrome of infancy. Clinical, morphological and immunological studies of 4 infants. Pediatrics 42:33, 1967.

Kaplan, B. S., Bureau, M. A., and Drummond, K. N.: The nephrotic syndrome in the first year of life: Is a pathologic classification possible? J. Pediatr. 85:615, 1974.

***Acute Renal Failure***

Barratt, T. M.: Renal failure in the first year of life. Br. Med. Bull. 27:115, 1971.

Braunstein, G. D., Lewis, E. J., Galvanek, E. G., Hamilton, A., and Bell, W. R.: The nephrotic syndrome associated with secondary syphilis. An immune deposit disease. Am. J. Med. 48:643, 1970.

Chesney, R. W., Kaplan, B. S., Freedom, R. M., Haller, J. A., and Drummond, K. N.: Acute renal failure: An important complication of cardiac surgery in infants. J. Pediatr. 87:381, 1975.

Fine, R. N., Stiles, Q., DePalma, J. R., and Donnell, G. N.: Hemodialysis in infants under 1 year of age for acute poisoning. Am. J. Dis. Child. *116*:657, 1968.

Hill, L. L., Singer, D. B., Falletta, J., and Stasney, R.: The nephrotic syndrome in congenital syphilis: An immunopathy. Pediatrics 49:260, 1972.

Holliday, M. A., Potter, D. E., and Dobris, R. S.: Treatment of renal failure in children. Pediatr. Clin. North Am. 18:613, 1971.

Hoyer, J. R., Raig, L., Vernier, R. L., Simmons, R. L., Najarian, J. S., and Micael, A. F.: Recurrence of idiopathic nephrotic syndrome after renal transplantation. Lancet 2:343, 1972.

Kjessler, B., Johansson, S. G. D., Sherman, M., Gustavsson, K.-H., and Hultquist, G.: Antenatal diagnosis of congenital nephrosis. Lancet 2:553, 1975.

Manley, G. L., and Gollipp, J. J.: Renal failure in the newborn; treatment with peritoneal dialysis. Am. J. Dis. Child. *115*:107, 1968.

Meadow, S. R., Cameron, J. S., Ogg, C. S., and Saxton, H. M.: Children referred for acute dialysis. Arch. Dis. Child. 46:221, 1971.

Simila, S., Vesa, L., and Wasz-Hockert, O.: Hereditary onycho-osteodysplasia (nail-patella syndrome) with nephrosis-like renal disease in the newborn boy. Pediatrics 46:61, 1970.

# 52

# DISORDERS OF THE FEMALE INTERNAL GENITAL TRACT

*Revised by Warren Grupe*

## HYDROMETROCOLPOS

Hydrocolpos, or hydrometrocolpos, signifies an abnormal collection of fluid in the vagina and uterus due to a combination of excessive cervical and vaginal secretions and obstruction to the outflow of this material. It is more commonly encountered in the neonate than in any other period of life. It assumes great importance because misdiagnosis leads to totally unnecessary abdominal operative procedures. Diagnosis is simple and treatment often simpler.

**INCIDENCE.** Antell was able to find 21 cases in the literature up to 1952 and added one of his own. Radman et al. reported that among 25,000 admissions to the gynecological service of the Sinai Hospital of Baltimore there were two cases of hydrometrocolpos, both neonatal, one diagnosed at birth, the other at 9 weeks of age.

**PATHOGENESIS.** Excessive vaginal secretion is noted in many female newborns in the first few weeks of life. Its cause is believed to be transplacental transfer of estrogen from mother to fetus late in gestation. Commonly this secretion is discharged from the vagina; when bloody, it is spoken of as *pseudomenstruation*. If the vaginal introitus is obstructed, such secretions are dammed up and accumulate within the vagina and the uterus. Blockage may be effected by an imperforate hymen or by incomplete involution of the central portion of the vaginal plate. This latter leads to "imperforate vagina," a condition analogous to imperforate anus.

**DIAGNOSIS.** The presenting sign is often bulging at the vaginal orifice. When larger quantities of fluid accumulate, cystic tumors of considerable size may grow within the pelvis and abdomen. Signs of obstructed venous return may then appear, such as edema and bluish discoloration of the legs and lower part of the abdomen and visible dilatation of the veins and capillary network. Rarely the tumor may produce hydronephrosis or intestinal obstruction by pressure upon contiguous structures.

Diagnosis is made by visible and palpable bulging of the imperforate hymen, or of the perineum when the vagina is imperforate, associated with a lower abdominal cystic tumor.

Flat films of the abdomen show displacement of bowel by the mass. Pyelograms may show similar displacement of the bladder forward and of the ureters laterally.

**TREATMENT.** An imperforate hymen should simply be incised at the apex of the bulge. Nothing further is required. If the vagina is imperforate, other serious congenital anomalies, such as imperforate anus, often coexist, and an appropriate schedule of operative treatment will have to be drawn up for each case.

CASE 52–1

A white female infant, birth weight 6 pounds 12 ounces (3080 gm), was born after uneventful pregnancy and labor. She seemed perfectly well at birth. On the second day bulging of the

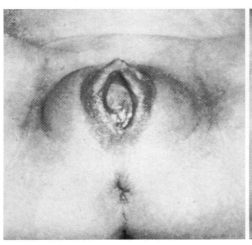
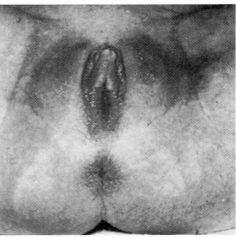

**A**    **B**

*Figure 52–1.* *A*, Appearance of external genitalia on admission. Note the bulge of the perineum, the widely spread labia and the bulging hymen between. *B*, After spontaneous rupture of the hymen. The labia majora are still prominent from edema, but the perineal and hymeneal bulging has disappeared, and the labia minora have assumed a more normal approximation.

vagina was noted when she cried or strained. The swelling was located behind and between the normal labia, was firm and was covered with pale translucent membrane. The consulting gynecologist felt that something more than simple imperforate hymen was involved, and advised that nothing be done at that time.

She was readmitted at 9 weeks of age. All had gone well until the day of admission, when the abdomen became progressively larger and no urine was passed. At this time the abdomen was distended and a globular tense mass was felt on the left side reaching from the pubis to the costal margin. A smaller, firm mass was palpated in the right lower quadrant of the abdomen. The veins over the abdomen were distended. A thin-walled cystic mass protruded from midvagina approximately 1.5 cm (Fig. 52–1, *A*).

After catheterization had evacuated 1200 cc of urine one could feel only one central mass with a small irregularity on its upper pole.

Flat film of the abdomen showed this spherical opacity which pushed the intestines upward. Intravenous pyelogram showed displacement of the ureters to either side (Fig. 52–2). The decision was made to explore the abdomen the following day, but suddenly the infant was found "floating in a yellowish fluid," and the tumor had disappeared. A hymenotomy was then performed, and she was discharged well three days later (Fig. 52–1, *B*).

**COMMENT.** A vaginal bulge was noted in this infant on the second day of life. Nothing was done, and the child remained well until the ninth week of life, when anuria and abdominal distention suddenly appeared. Still nothing was done, whereupon the baby took matters into her own hands and ruptured her imperforate hymen. The hymen was then incised, 9 weeks too late.

## OVARIAN CYST

**INCIDENCE.** Cysts of the ovary in the pediatric age group are not common. Costin and Kennedy discovered 200 cases reported to 1948 and added but 23 more from the wide experience of the Mayo Clinic. Reis and Koop found 25 ovarian tumors of all kinds in the records of the Children's Hospital of Philadelphia from 1947 to 1961. Ten of these were in babies less than 1 week old, and 10 more in those aged 1 week to 6 months. The great majority of these were cystic. Bower et al. were able to find 65 cases reported up to 1974. Their own example was the first in which ovarian cysts were bilateral.

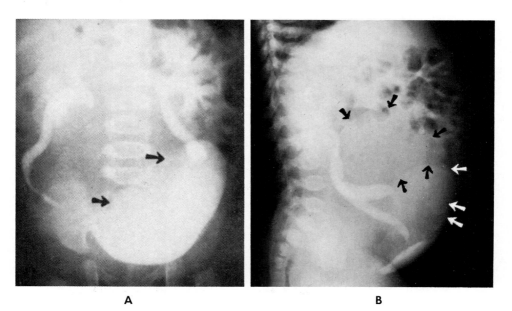

|   |   |
|---|---|
| **A** | **B** |

*Figure 52–2.*   A, Anteroposterior intravenous pyelogram showing bilateral hydroureter and hydronephrosis as well as dislocation of the bladder far to the left and of the right ureter far to the right. B, Lateral view with dye in the urinary collecting system shows the soft tissue mass, the hydrometrocolpos, dislocating the bladder downward and the ureters posteriorly.

**PATHOLOGY.** Most are cystic teratomas, some are follicular and a few are cystadenomas. Several students of the problem have stressed the important point that malignant ovarian tumors are exceedingly rare in the newborn period. Torsion of the pedicle occurs in 70 per cent of all ovarian cysts and produces the presenting signs and symptoms in many older children, but not often in the newborn. Cysts may rupture and lead to a picture simulating ascites, and peritonitis may follow rupture.

**DIAGNOSIS.** In at least two newborns the distended abdomen made delivery difficult. In the rest the diagnosis has been made by palpating a fluctuant mass in the lower part of the abdomen. One must attempt to distinguish this from other cystic masses. Catheterization should rule out distended bladder due to bladder neck or urethral obstruction. Careful examination of the vulva and perineum should dispose of the possibility of hydrocolpos (p. 476). Pyelography must be performed in order to exclude hydronephrosis of an ectopic kidney and hydroureter. Cyst of the urachus may or may not be suggested by the appearance of the umbilicus, and its more superficial position may be appreciated by careful palpation. Differentiation from this condition, as well as from mesenteric and pancreatic cyst, may have to await laparotomy.

If torsion complicates the picture, nausea and vomiting, fever, tenderness and guarding upon palpation of the lower abdomen may be added to the clinical picture.

**TREATMENT.** Immediate surgical removal is indicated. The dangers of malignancy, twisted pedicle and rupture render this decision mandatory.

## REFERENCES

Antell, L.: Hydrocolpos in infancy and childhood. Pediatrics *10*:306, 1952.

Bower, R., Dehner, L. P., and Ternberg, J. L.: Bilateral ovarian cysts in the newborn. Am. J. Dis. Child. *128*:731, 1974.

Castleman, B. (Ed.): Case Records of the Massachusetts General Hospital. Torsion with infarction of normal fallopian tube and ovary. N. Engl. J. Med. *284*:491, 1971.

Costin, M. E., Jr., and Kennedy, R. L. J.: Ovarian tumors in infants and children. Am. J. Dis. Child. *76*:127, 1948.

Davis, C. B., Jr., and Fell, E. H.: Double hydrometrocolpos and imperforate anus in the newborn infant. Am. J. Dis. Child. *80*:79, 1950.

Dooley, R. T.: Hydrometrocolpos: Report of a case in a newborn infant. Am. J. Dis. Child. *103*:692, 1962.

Ein, S. H., Darte, J. M., and Stephens, C. A.: Cystic and solid ovarian tumors in children. A 44-year review. J. Pediatr. Surg. *5*:143, 1970.

Graves, G. Y., McIlvoy, D. B., Jr., and Hudson, G. W.: Ovarian cyst in a premature infant. A.M.A. J. Dis. Child. *81*:256, 1951.

Kunstadter, R. H., Schultz, A., and Strauss, A. A.: Large ovarian cyst in a newborn infant. Am. J. Dis. Child. *80*:993, 1950.

Radman, H. M., Askin, J. A., and Kolodner, L. J.: Hydrometrocolpos and hematometrocolpos. Obstet. Gynecol. *27*:2, 1966.

Reis, R. L., and Koop, C. E.: Ovarian tumors in infants and children. J. Pediatr. *60*:96, 1962.

Smith, R. C.: Simple ovarian cyst in a newborn infant. Pediatrics *14*:232, 1954.

Tietz, K. G., and Davis, J. B.: Ruptured ovarian cyst in a newborn infant. J. Pediatr. *51*:564, 1957.

# VI

# Disorders of Mineral Metabolism and the Endocrine System

# 53

# DISORDERS OF MINERAL METABOLISM

*By John S. Parks*

## CALCIUM AND PHOSPHORUS METABOLISM

Greater than 90 per cent of the body's calcium is present in bone, where it forms a crystalline complex with phosphate and serves a structural function. Only 1 per cent of the total calcium is present in the extracellular fluid. Alterations in extracellular calcium concentration have profound effects on many cellular functions. Total serum calcium is normally maintained in the narrow range of 8.5 to 10.5 mg per 100 ml. Parathyroid hormone is the predominant factor in the regulation of calcium concentration. A fall in calcium concentration provokes release of PTH from the parathyroid gland. The hormone acts to elevate calcium concentration through several mechanisms. The most immediate effect is to increase renal tubular reabsorption of calcium and diminish reabsorption of phosphate. A second effect is to increase resorption of calcium and phosphate from bone by stimulating osteocyte and osteoclast activity. Parathyroid hormone indirectly increases calcium absorption from the intestine by increasing production of the active metabolite of vitamin D.

Vitamin $D_3$ is produced in the skin by the action of ultraviolet light on 7-dehydrocholesterol. Vitamin $D_2$ is provided artificially in many foods. Neither compound is active, as such, but must be converted to an active product by a series of two enzymatic hydroxylation steps. A liver enzyme converts vitamin D to the major circulating form, 1-hydroxy vitamin D. The kidney converts a small portion of this compound to the active form, 1,25-dihydroxy vitamin D. Parathyroid hormone increases the rate and extent of this reaction. The active form of vitamin D promotes intestinal absorption of calcium and plays a permissive role in the action of PTH on bone cells. Vitamin D resembles the steroid hormones in structure and molecular mecha-

nism of action, and, since it can be produced by the body, it is properly considered a hormone.

A third hormone, calcitonin, participates in the regulation of calcium metabolism. This small polypeptide is produced by the C-cells of the thyroid. Its actions on bone and kidney cells are, for the most part, antagonistic to those of PTH. Calcitonin concentrations are higher in the newborn period than at any other time in life. However, the known clinical states of calcitonin deficiency and calcitonin excess are not associated with abnormalities in serum calcium concentration.

### Calcium Homeostasis in the Fetus

During fetal development, the parathyroid glands arise from the embryonic third and fourth pharyngeal pouches. By mid-pregnancy, the human parathyroid glands have a histological appearance which strongly resembles that of adult glands, and they contain PTH as shown by their ability to induce bone resorption in a bioassay system. Fetal PTH levels are low throughout pregnancy but, at least in the sheep model system, they rise in response to a lowering of ionized calcium concentration (Smith, 1972). The placenta contributes to fetal calcium homeostasis and bone mineralization by actively transporting calcium into the fetal circulation (Twardock and Austin, 1972). Human umbilical cord total calcium, ionized calcium, and phosphorus levels are higher than maternal levels, and immunoreactive PTH is generally undetectable (Tsang et al., 1973). Calcium levels decrease progressively after birth, so that by 48 to 72 hours they are lower than those found in older infants and children. By 72 hours, a majority of full term infants have detectable PTH levels. The increase in PTH levels is followed by a rise in calcium levels (David and Anast, 1974). Renal phosphate clearance and cyclic AMP excretion, both markers of PTH action, increase over the same time span. The ability to release PTH in response to hypocalcemia is related to gestational as well as to postnatal age. Tsang et al. (1973) measured PTH levels in hyperbilirubinemic infants undergoing exchange transfusion. Ionized calcium levels dropped a mean of 1.5 mg per 100 ml during the procedure. Term infants greater than 52 hours of age showed a brisk rise in PTH, while younger infants and premature infants up to 3 or 4 days of age showed minimal PTH responses.

Fetal calcium homeostasis is influenced by maternal calcium levels, transport of calcium across the placenta, fetal parathyroid gland function and, in as yet undefined ways, by vitamin D metabolism. Abnormalities in maternal calcium homeostasis produce adjustments in fetal parathyroid function which may be entirely inappropriate for the newborn. The normal infant is born in a state of relative parathyroid insufficiency, and the premature is slower than the term infant in correcting this deficit.

## COMMON CAUSES OF HYPOCALCEMIA

EARLY NEONATAL HYPOCALCEMIA. Infants with an abnormal pregnancy, delivery or neonatal course are especially prone to develop hypocalcemia on the first or second day of life. Predisposing factors include prematurity, maternal diabetes, cesarean section, birth asphyxia, respiratory distress syndrome and bacterial sepsis. Tsang has reported on the influences of individual risk factors in a recent series of articles. Between 25 and 75 per cent of newborns in these high risk categories reach total calcium levels below 7.5 mg per 100 ml, and ionized calcium levels below 4.0 mg per 100 ml. Serum PTH levels are inappropriately low in the presence of hypocalcemia. Restoration of normocalcemia ultimately depends upon development of an appropriate PTH response. This process is moderately slow, requiring days to weeks. Infants of diabetic mothers are especially slow to respond, possibly because of relative maternal hypercalcemia and more prolonged suppression of fetal parathyroid activity (Tsang, 1972).

Most infants with early neonatal hypocal-

cemia show symptoms related to the conditions that put them at risk for the development of hypocalcemia. It is often difficult to decide whether a low serum calcium level or another factor is responsible for a given symptom. Chvostek and Trousseau signs and carpopedal spasm are of no help in recognizing neonatal hypocalcemia. A positive peroneal sign and ankle clonus may be more reliable indications. Tsang and Oh (1970) observed twitching of the extremities, a high pitched cry and hypotonicity more frequently in hypocalcemic than in normocalcemic premature infants. Seizures and apneic spells may occur and respond to calcium gluconate infusion. The only reliable means of detecting hypocalcemia is to obtain measurements of total and, if available, ionized calcium concentrations.

NEONATAL TETANY. Classic neonatal tetany, unlike early neonatal hypocalcemia, does not become manifest until some days or weeks after birth. Onset is usually delayed until the end of the first or the beginning of the second week of life. Most infants with this condition are otherwise quite normal, without a history of abnormal pregnancy or delivery. They generally leave the nursery, do well at home for a few days, and are brought back by their parents with an acute history of seizures, muscle twitching, feeding difficulty or labored breathing.

Tetany of the newborn virtually never affects breast-fed infants but follows one or more days of cow's milk feedings. Cow's milk contains 1220 mg of calcium and 900 mg of phosphorus per liter, as opposed to 340 and 150 mg, respectively, in human milk. Of significance, in addition to the greater load of both of these elements, is the differing ratio of calcium to phosphorus, being 2.25 to 1 in human milk versus 1.35 to 1 in cow's milk. In a prospective study, Oppé and Redstone found significantly higher phosphorus levels and lower calcium levels on the sixth day of life in infants fed cow's milk formulas. Infants who received adapted cow's milk formulas with a calcium to phosphorus ratio close to that of human milk had calcium and phosphorus levels identical to those of the breast-fed infants. An excess phosphate load tends to raise serum phosphorus levels and thus depress calcium levels.

Parathyroid hormone reverses this trend by diminishing renal tubular reabsorption of phosphorus and by its additional effects on serum calcium. It is reasonable to suppose that neonatal tetany reflects an abnormally delayed maturation of parathyroid function.

### RARE CAUSES OF HYPOCALCEMIA

MATERNAL HYPERPARATHYROIDISM. Prolonged intrauterine exposure to high calcium levels can produce prolonged suppression of the infant's parathyroid function. Bruce and Strong reported an infant whose mother had hyperparathyroidism and who was unable to maintain a normal serum calcium concentration throughout infancy. Maternal calcium and phosphorus levels should be determined whenever an infant has prolonged or refractory hypocalcemia, but the yield of positive results is generally small.

CONGENITAL ABSENCE OF THE PARATHYROID GLANDS. Taitz et al. reported an infant with congenital absence of the parathyroid glands and thymus who had severe neonatal hypocalcemia. As emphasized by DiGeorge, this condition represents faulty embryogenesis of third and fourth pharyngeal pouch structures. A right-sided aortic arch and absence of the isthmus of the thyroid are frequent associated anomalies. Defects in cellular immunity lead to severe infections and early death. The condition is not hereditary. Chest X-rays to look for a thymic shadow are part of the work-up for hypocalcemia. Absence of the parathyroid glands has also been reported in association with chromosomal abnormalities.

FAMILIAL CONGENITAL HYPOPARATHYROIDISM. Congenital hypoparathyroidism can also occur as an isolated finding. All familial cases have involved males, so that the condition seems to be transmitted as an X-linked recessive trait (Peden, 1960). Ordinarily, idiopathic hypoparathyroidism does not become apparent until well after infancy, when it can occur as an isolated finding or in association with multiple endocrine deficiencies and chronic mucocutaneous moniliasis. The autosomal dominant disorder, pseudohypoparathyroidism, is associated with multiple phenotypic abnormalities including short stature and a dramatic shortening of lateral metacarpal and metatarsal bones. This condition is due to renal insensitivity to PTH and it is generally not diagnosed in infancy.

MATERNAL OSTEOPOROSIS. Infants who are born to mothers with severe nutritional and environmental deficiency of vitamin D can be born with hypocalcemia and the bony changes of rickets. In contrast to all other forms of hypocalcemia, serum phosphorus tends to be low. Premature infants (Hillman and Haddad, 1975) and infants with malabsorption, biliary atresia and extensive bowel surgery can be considered to be at special risk for the early development of vitamin D deficiency rickets. Special attention to vitamin D supplementation is advisable in these groups.

HYPOCALCEMIA SECONDARY TO HYPOMAGNESEMIA. Davis et al. (1965) reported convulsions in an infant with hypocalcemia and hypomagnesemia. Serum calcium levels did not respond to calcium supplementation alone but rose when magnesium was given. Anast et al. (1972) have followed serum calcium, magnesium and PTH levels during treatment of an older child. Initially, both calcium and magnesium were low and PTH was undetectable. With magnesium supplementation, serum PTH rose to levels above the normal range within 2 days and this rise was followed by an increase in calcium levels. The conclusion in this patient and the patient of Suh et al. was that extreme hypomagnesemia produced a paralysis of parathyroid gland function. Factors predisposing to hypomagnesemia, and dosage schedules for magnesium concentration will be given in the section on magnesium metabolism.

LABORATORY DIAGNOSIS OF HYPOCALCEMIA. Direct measurement of serum calcium concentration is the most readily available means of documenting hypocalcemia. Values below 7.5 mg per 100 ml or 3.7 mEq/L are diagnostic. Total calcium levels may drop below 3.0 mg per 100 ml in severe cases. Roughly 50 per cent of the total calcium is ionized and is available to the cells. The proportion of ionized calcium is dependent to some extent upon serum protein concentration and upon pH, with a larger fraction being ionized at a lower pH. The McLean and Hastings nomogram for calculating ionized calcium is unreliable in infants (Brown et al., 1972). Sorrell and Rosen (1975) have reported striking discrepancies between ionized and total calcium in symptomatic children. Phosphorus levels are generally elevated in children and infants with hypocalcemia. Serum PTH levels by radioimmunoassay are low in virtually all categories of neonatal hypocalcemia except vitamin D deficiency. Hypoglycemia frequently accompanies early neonatal hypoglycemia.

**TREATMENT OF HYPOCALCEMIA.** Convulsions suspected to be due to hypocalcemia demand immediate treatment with an intravenous calcium preparation. A 10 per cent solution of calcium gluconate is commonly used for this purpose. It should be given slowly, at a rate of approximately one ml per minute, with continuous monitoring of cardiac rate. Injection should be stopped if the cardiac rate slows significantly, for there is a danger of cardiac arrest. In order to achieve cessation of convulsions or tremors, approximately 2 to 3 ml per kg may be required. It should be remembered that convulsions due to a variety of causes may cease with calcium administration and it is essential to document suspected hypoglycemia with a blood test.

Hypocalcemia with less dramatic symptoms should be treated in a less dramatic fashion. In newborns who are unable to take medications by mouth, intravenous supplementation with calcium gluconate may be employed in amounts providing 10 to 20 mg of elemental calcium per 100 ml. Extravasation of solutions containing calcium produces tissue necrosis and ectopic calcification (Lee and Gwinn, 1975). Uncontrolled infusion can result in cardiac arrest.

Oral calcium supplementation is the treatment of choice in most instances. The required dose is generally 50 to 100 mg of elemental calcium per kg per 24 hours in divided doses. Of the available calcium salts, calcium chloride is the best absorbed. It produces gastric irritation in concentrations above 2 per cent, and produces systemic acidosis when used in effective amounts, regardless of concentration. Calcium lactate, calcium gluconate and calcium gluconogalactogluconate (Neocalglucon) are generally used when more than 1 or 2 days of therapy are required. Attention should also be given to using adapted cow's milk formulas with phosphate contents approximating breast milk.

The required duration of calcium supplementation is highly variable, and each infant must be closely monitored for serum calcium levels during treatment and during attempts at withdrawal of treatment. Many of the rare causes of hypocalcemia are prolonged or even permanent. For long-term management of hypocalcemia, vitamin D or dihydrotachysterol is used in doses some 50 to 200 times the amount required to prevent rickets. Vitamin D can produce severe hypercalcemia and resultant renal damage and has no established place in the treatment of transient hypocalcemia. Human PTH is not available for the treatment of hypocalcemia, but may become available in the near future.

## RARE CAUSES OF HYPERCALCEMIA

**NEONATAL FAMILIAL HYPERPARATHYROIDISM.** Severe congenital hyperparathyroidism can occur as an autosomal recessive disease. The infants reported by Hillman et al. (1964) had hypotonia, failure to thrive, irritability and anemia. Serum calcium levels were above 20 mg per 100 ml. Removal of hyperplastic parathyroid glands was curative in the younger of the two infants. Parathyroid adenomas and ectopic production of PTH by nonparathyroid tumors are extremely rare in infancy.

**MATERNAL HYPOPARATHYROIDISM.** Just as the hyperparathyroid mother may produce hypoparathyroid babies with neonatal tetany, the hypoparathyroid mother may induce hyperparathyroidism in her fetuses in utero. Bronsky et al. (1968) added two cases of their own to the two previously reported. One showed marked demineralization of bones, especially the femora and humeri, with bowing and subperiosteal absorption (Fig. 53–1). In this, as in other cases, postnatal hypercalcemia has been mild or nonexistent. With virtually no therapy, the bony lesions disappeared by the age of 4 months.

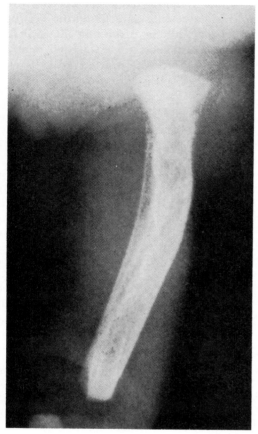

*Figure 53–1.* Note the bony demineralization, bowing and subperiosteal resorption, quite consistent with hyperparathyroidism. (From Bronsky, D., et al.: Pediatrics *42*:606, 1968.)

**HYPERCALCEMIA WITH SUBCUTANEOUS FAT NECROSIS.** Subcutaneous fat necrosis presents a distinctive appearance (p. 977), with discolored, lumpy and irregular areas distributed over the trunk and extremities. It generally does not become apparent until some days or weeks after a complicated delivery and difficult neonatal course. Hypercalcemia frequently accompanies this condition and may be severe, reaching levels above 20 mg per 100 ml. Baltrop's case was always a poor feeder, vomited intermittently and was one pound below birth weight at the age of 4 months. With restriction of calcium and vitamin D intake, his hypercalcemia and azotemia resolved. Other infants have not responded to these measures but have required prolonged treatment with prednisone.

**IDIOPATHIC HYPERCALCEMIA OF INFANCY.** The diagnosis of idiopathic hypercalcemia is generally considered after the neonatal period in infants with failure to thrive, developmental delay, muscular hypotonia with brisk reflexes, and an unusual "elfin" facies (Fig. 53–2). The forehead is high, the eyes wide-set, usually with squint and epicanthus, nose pinched and retroussé, with nares pointing forward, mouth wide and lips slack. The ears are large and low-set. Lenticular opacities due to calcium deposition may develop. The child may have a harsh systolic murmur due to supravalvular aortic stenosis.

Serum calcium is generally elevated in infancy, but tends to decline as the child grows older. Hyperphosphatemia and azotemia occur secondary to nephrocalcinosis and renal impairment. X-rays may show osteosclerosis of the skull and ends of the long bones.

Idiopathic hypercalcemia is usually divided into two forms, a mild one (Lightwood syndrome) and a severe one (Fanconi syndrome). The mild form tends to show recovery after measures are taken to reduce serum calcium, but the severe form produces irreversible mental retardation. The incidence of the mild form decreased dramatically in Great Britain after a reduction in the amount of vitamin D added to infant formulas. This latter observation provides the strongest evidence for the hypothesis that the condition may involve an unusual sensitivity to vitamin D. Other causes of intrauterine and early neonatal hypercalcemia may be responsible, as in the case of a patient who had the typical features of severe idiopathic hypercalcemia, but had elevated PTH levels and was found at surgery to have a parathyroid adenoma.

Treatment of idiopathic hypercalcemia involves reduction of calcium intake and total elimination of vitamin D from the diet, together with avoidance of sunlight. If hypercalcemia is severe, a 1 to 2 mg per 100 ml decline can usually be achieved with vigorous hydration. If additional reduction is required, saline loading and furosemide diuresis can be employed. Both measures should be used with great caution in infants with renal impairment. As in patients with subcutaneous fat necrosis,

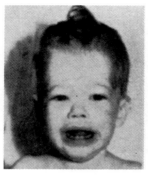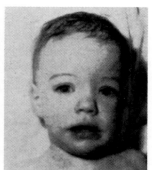

*Figure 53–2.* Photographs of two unrelated infants with idiopathic hypercalcemia, in order to show their striking facial similarity. The facies is described in the text. (From O'Brien, D., Peppers, T. D., and Silver, H. K.: J.A.M.A. *173*:1106, 1960. Reproduced with the kind permission of the senior author.)

prednisone treatment may be of value in the acute and long-term management of severe hypercalcemia.

## MAGNESIUM METABOLISM

Magnesium is the second most common intracellular cation and it is required for many enzymatic reactions, particularly those which also require ATP. About 50 per cent of total body magnesium is in bone, and most of the rest is intracellular. Normal serum magnesium levels lie between 1.5 and 2.8 mg per 100 ml (1.48 to 1.82 mEq/L). Roughly 35 per cent of total magnesium is bound to serum protein. Fetal magnesium levels are higher than maternal, due to active transport across the placenta. However, in experimental magnesium deficiency in rats, the fetus becomes relatively more deficient than the mother (Dancis et al., 1971). Following birth, there is a slight rise in magnesium levels in normal infants (David and Anast, 1974). Maintenance of normal magnesium levels requires normal absorption from the intestine and normal reabsorption by the renal tubule.

### HYPOMAGNESEMIA

Magnesium levels below 1.5 mg per 100 ml are seen in a variety of clinical settings (Tsang, 1972). Bowel resection and other situations requiring prolonged parenteral feeding can result in magnesium deficiency. Hypomagnesemia frequently accompanies severe malnutrition due either to malabsorption or to insufficient food intake. Hypomagnesemia has also been reported in association with isolated defects in intestinal absorption and in renal tubular reabsorption of magnesium. Hypomagnesemia and hypoparathyroidism frequently occur in the same infants, and magnesium administration is required in order to determine which is the primary and which is the secondary abnormality.

Hypomagnesemia is treated with magnesium salts, either parenterally or by mouth. The suggested intramuscular or intravenous dose of 50 per cent magnesium sulfate is 0.1 to 0.2 ml per kg, providing, respectively, 10 or 20 mg per kg of elemental magnesium. If given intravenously, the infusion should be slow and cautious, with electrocardiographic monitoring to detect acute disturbances, which may include prolongation of atrioventricular conduction time and sinoatrial or atrioventricular block. The magnesium dose may be repeated every 12 to 24 hours depending upon clinical response and monitoring of serum magnesium levels. Oral maintenance doses may be solutions of the chloride, sulfate or lactate salt calculated to provide at least 20 mg of magnesium per kg per day.

### HYPERMAGNESEMIA

Magnesium sulfate continues to be used in the management of eclampsia. Magnesium given to the mother readily crosses the placenta and causes elevation of fetal magnesium levels and depression of the newborn infant. Lipsitz and English (1967) studied 16 infants born to toxemic mothers who had received 16 to 60 gm of magnesium by continuous intravenous infusion for from 12 to 24 hours prior to delivery.

The mothers' blood levels of magnesium ranged from 3 to 14 mEq/L, and the babies' from 4 to 11.5 mEq/L. A majority of the babies were cyanotic, flaccid and unresponsive. Others had less severe signs, including delayed passage of meconium. Nine infants required tracheal intubation and respiratory support. The medication may or may not have played a part in the deaths of three of the 10 premature infants. There was no absolute correlation between cord blood levels and depth of depression, but symptoms disappeared within 24 to 48 hours pari passu with the steady fall in magnesium levels. Exchange transfusion has been advocated as a means of lowering magnesium more rapidly, and infusion of calcium salts has been used to antagonize some of the adverse effects of excess magnesium (Lipsitz, 1971).

More recently Outerbridge et al. (1973) reported the tragic case of a full-term newborn who was treated with an enema of 100 ml of a 50 percent magnesium sulfate solution for presumed hyaline membrane disease. 90 minutes later respiratory arrest occurred and his serum $Mg^{++}$ was 4.6 mEq per l. In spite of calcium and exchange transfusion the baby died at 46 hours of age.

There seems no room for doubt that magnesium enemas should no longer be used for the treatment of respiratory distress, and that it is dangerous for the obstetrician to continue the intravenous infusion of magnesium salts into toxemic mothers for more than 24 hours. Intramuscular injections and infusions for shorter periods may not be hazardous (Lipsitz, 1971).

## SODIUM METABOLISM

Both hypernatremia and hyponatremia may affect newborn infants. In both states convulsions and severe alterations in the sensorial state may be induced, either in the direction of obtunding the sensorium, ranging from unresponsiveness to coma, or of overstimulation, leading to irritability, irrational behavior and convulsions. Brain cells should become dehydrated as a result of hyperosmolality of the extracellular fluids in which they bathed, or swell from overhydration because of hypotonicity of these same fluids. Indeed Hogan et al. have shown that too rapid rehydration of rabbits with hypernatremia led to convulsions in 55 per cent of the cases, and in these an elevated water content of brain tissue was documented.

### HYPERNATREMIA

Serum sodium concentrations in excess of 160 mEq. per liter, usually associated with chloride levels greater than 110 mEq. per liter, are encountered in the newborn period as well as in later infancy and childhood. The most common causes of hypernatremia are:

1. *Severe diarrhea*, with loss of proportionally more water than sodium chloride in the intestinal discharges.

2. *Excessive intake of sodium salts.* This occurs fairly frequently when babies are treated for diarrhea with electrolyte solutions made up improperly or offered in excess. Taitz and Byers (1972) remind us that the use of heaping scoops, rather than level ones, of milk powder in the preparation of formula is often sufficient to produce dangerous hypernatremia. Insufficiently diluted liquid products can have the same effect (Abrams et al.). Serious epidemics of hypernatremia have been reported to follow the inadvertent substitution of salt for sugar in making up infant formulas in hospital milk rooms.

That the use of large quantities of sodium bicarbonate increases the risk of intracranial hemorrhage is strongly suggested by the study of Simmons et al. (1974). "Intakes of more than 5 mg per kg per 24 hours should be regarded as excessive."

3. *Nephrogenic diabetes insipidus.* In this condition excessive quantities of water are lost via polyuria.

Treatment consists in withholding sodium salts and *slow* rehydration for the hypernatremia, plus whatever other therapy seems indicated for the underlying condition.

### HYPONATREMIA

Serum levels of sodium below 135, usually but not always accompanied by levels of chloride below 95 mEq per liter, are discovered in a variety of conditions in the newborn infant. The presenting symptom of hyponatremia is, in the majority of cases, convulsions, but irritability, mental confusion and coma characterize some examples. Hyponatremia may be encountered under the following conditions:

1. *Severe burns.* Salt is lost in the profuse serous exudate from the denuded areas. It is our impression that this loss may be accentuated by treatment with silver nitrate, which exerts a specific leeching action upon the body store of sodium.

2. *Cerebrospinal fluid-to-ureter shunting* in the attempt to control advancing hydrocephalus.

3. *Acute adrenal insufficiency.* Sodium and chloride loss, along with hyperkalemia and elevation of blood nonprotein nitrogen, are characteristic of this syndrome (see pp. 494–497).

4. *Inappropriate antidiuretic hormone secretion.* This is uncommon in the newborn, but does occur in this age period. Feldman et al. described 3 infants in whom they attributed the problem to *asphyxia at birth.* Mor et al., with convincing documentation, ascribed the convulsions of their 6-week-old boy with severe pneumonia to inappropriate ADH secretion. The last example we saw was in an infant with a subdural hematoma. In this situation there is oliguria, high urine specific gravity, low sodium and chloride serum concentrations but normal potassium and non-protein nitrogen, and falling hematocrit and total serum solids.

5. *Water intoxication.* Not too long ago we discovered an example of this in a two-month-old infant. He had been fed a formula consisting of 13 ounces of evaporated milk, one-half gallon of water and some sugar. Since he always seemed hungry, he drank four or five eight-ounce bottles of water a day in addition. His calculated intake was 400 ml per kilogram per twenty-four hours!

We have also seen one newborn infant convulse for hours after birth until hyponatremia was discovered and rectified. His mother had received large quantities of 5 per cent dextrose without added salt for twenty-four hours or more prior to delivery.

6. *The congenital salt-losing syndromes.* Cheek and Perry reported in 1958 the first case of "transient salt-wasting" in a newborn. Since then similar cases, though perhaps not identical ones, have been reported under various names, such as pseudohypoadrenocorticism, possible infantile hypoaldosteronism, hypofunction of the adrenals in early life, saline diabetes because of congenital insensitivity of the renal tubule to aldosterone, and familial aldosterone deficiency.

These infants fail to thrive on the usual formulas. In addition to failure to gain, vomiting is often prominent, and evidences of shock supervene in some. Hyponatremia, hypochloremia and hyperkalemia invariably bring hyperadrenocorticism to mind, but normal 24-hour excretion of ketosteroids rules this out. Added salt, at first intravenously, later by mouth, in doses of 2 to 3 gm daily, causes improvement, and desoxycorticosterone (DCA, DOCA) in doses of 1 to 3 mg per day leads to more rapid weight gain and return of electrolyte concentrations to normal. After 1 to 2 years all supplemental salt and DOCA may be stopped. Quantities of supplements must be calibrated for each patient individually, and cessation of therapy must be determined by the trial-and-error method.

It seems clear that there is no defect in the renal tubules, but that there is some block in the pathway of aldosterone synthesis. David et al. found the block in their cases to lie in the hydrogenation of 18-hydroxycorticosterone, leading to an excessive urinary excretion of 18-hydroxytetrahydro compound A (18-OH-THA). Other defects have been described in other cases.

## IRON METABOLISM

The normal newborn should be born with an iron store of approximately 75 mg per kilogram of body weight (Widdowson and Spray). The serum iron concentration should fall within the range of 52 to 112 micrograms per 100 ml (Henry et al.). The subsequent fall of body hemoglobin content and its later rise, as well as the accompanying changes in body iron, are described later.

## CONGENITAL AND FAMILIAL IRON OVERLOAD

Increased body content of iron in the newborn has been reported to follow excessive hemolysis, multiple transfusions of blood and giant-cell hepatitis. Vitale, Opitz and Shahidi, to whom we are indebted for much of this brief summary, have described two siblings who were born with a marked body iron overload, along with multiple congenital anomalies, without evidences of excessive hemolysis. No measurements of iron were made on the first sibling, but his Kupffer cells were packed with iron-containing granules. He had in addition a peculiar facies, hypotonia, polycystic kidneys and megacephaly. He failed to thrive and died of pneumonia at 2½ months of age.

His brother had a similar facies, was hypotonic and failed to thrive. Serum iron concentration was found to be 270 micrograms per 100 ml. Liver, bone marrow and kidneys revealed heavy deposits of iron. Fed by gavage, he too died in respiratory failure at 6 months.

The authors concluded that this disorder is probably genetically determined but could advance no further explanation for its pathogenesis.

## COPPER DEFICIENCY

It can now almost surely be accepted as fact that copper deficiency exists and is not uncommon in severely malnourished infants. It is responsible for several signs: anemia, neutropenia, metaphysial flaring and periosteal reaction on x-ray, and low serum copper and serum ceruloplasmin levels. All of these are reversible by copper sulfate administered by mouth, but not by iron, folic acid or vitamin E.

Al Rashid and Spangler have reported one case in a newborn, and Seely et al. another in a 3 month old. Both were prematurely born, and in them the presenting sign was anemia, and there had been no precedent malnutrition or diarrhea.

## MENKES KINKY HAIR SYNDROME

In 1962 Menkes described a congenital constellation of defects, which included failure to gain, hypothermia, repeated infections, severe developmental and mental retardation and the characteristic sparse, brittle hair which gave the disorder its name. Under the microscope the hairs appear to be growing in a twisted fashion, the so-called pili torti. Ten years later Danks discovered that these babies suffered from a familial defect of copper absorption leading to hypocupremia and to lowered ceruloplasmin level. Copper salts by mouth has no effect but parenteral copper elevates these concentrations.

## MERCURY POISONING

Mercury poisoning due to the ingestion of mercury-contaminated foods, chiefly fish, has been recognized since 1940 or earlier. The congenital form was described more recently.

Snyder's (1971) example is typical. A large family ate a great deal of the meat of some hogs that had been fed seed grain impregnated with a methylmercury fungicide. Although three children became ill, their mother, who was pregnant, did not. After having eaten the contaminated meat during her third to sixth months of pregnancy, she delivered a full-term infant. Cyanosis and gross tremor appeared in the infant immediately after birth and lasted for several days. Both the baby's and mother's blood mercury levels were very high. He eventually developed myoclonus, abnormal encephalogram, hypotonicity and nystagmus.

Amin-Zaki et al. (1974) were able to describe a veritable epidemic from the identical cause, bread prepared from wheat treated with a methylmercury fungicide. At risk were 15 infant-mother pairs of whom six mothers and six infants became symptomatic. In the affected children motor and mental development were grossly impaired.

## REFERENCES

Abrams, C. A. L., Phillips, L. L., et al.: J.A.M.A. *232*: 1136, 1975.

Al-Rashid, R. A., and Spangler, J.: Neonatal copper deficiency. N. Engl. J. Med. *285*:841, 1971.

Amin-Zaki, L., Elhassani, S., et al.: Intrauterine methylmercury poisoning in Iraq. Pediatrics *54*: 1014, 1974.

Anast, C. S., Mohs, J. S., Kaplan, S. L., and Burns, T. W.: Evidence for parathyroid failure in magnesium deficiency. Science 177:606, 1972.

Baltrop, D.: Hypercalcemia associated with neonatal subcutaneous fat necrosis. Arch. Dis. Child. 38:516, 1963.

Bronsky, D., Kiamko, R., Moncada, R., and Rosenthal, I. M.: Intrauterine hyperparathyroidism secondary to maternal hypoparathyroidism. Pediatrics 42:606, 1968.

Brown, D. M., Boen, J., and Bernstein, A.: Serum ionized calcium in newborn infants. Pediatrics 49:841, 1972.

Bruce, J., and Strong, J. A.: Maternal hyperparathyroidism and parathyroid deficiency in child with account of effect of parathyroidectomy on renal function and of attempt to transplant part of tumor. Quart. J. Med. 24:307, 1955.

Dancis, J., Springer, D., and Cohlan, S. Q.: Fetal homeostasis in maternal malnutrition. II. Magnesium deprivation. Pediatr. Res. 5:131, 1971.

Danks, D. M., et al.: Menkes' kinky hair syndrome. Pediatrics 50:188, 1972.

David, L., and Anast, C.: Calcium metabolism in newborn infants. J. Clin. Invest. 54:287, 1974.

Davis, J. A., Harvey, D. R., and Yu, J. S.: Neonatal fits associated with hypomagnesemia. Arch. Dis. Child. 40:286, 1965.

DiGeorge, A. M.: Congenital absence of the thymus and its immunologic consequences, concurrence with congenital hypoparathyroidism. In Bergsma, D., and Good, R. A. (Eds.): Birth Defects Original Articles Series, No I, New York, The National Foundation, 1968, Vol IV.

Ghazali, S., Hallet, R. J., and Barratt, T. M.: Hypomagnesemia in uremic infants. J. Pediatr. 81:747, 1972.

Hillman, D. A., Scriver, C. S., Pedvis, S., and Shragovich, I.: Neonatal familial primary hyperparathyroidism. N. Engl. J. Med. 270:483, 1964.

Hillman, L. S., and Haddad, J. G.: Perinatal vitamin D. Metabolism II. Serial 25-hydroxyvitamin D concentrations in sera of term and premature infants. J. Pediatr. 86:928, 1975.

Lee, F. A., and Gwinn, J. L.: Roentgen patterns of extravasation of calcium gluconate in the tissues of the neonate. J. Pediatr. 86:598, 1975.

Lipsitz, P. J.: The clinical and biochemical effects of excess magnesium in the newborn. Pediatrics 47:501, 1971.

Lipsitz, P. J., and English, J. C.: Hypermagnesemia in the newborn infant. Pediatrics 40:856, 1967.

Menkes, J. H.: Kinky hair syndrome. Pediatrics 50:188, 1972.

Mor, J., Ben-Galim, E., and Abrahamov, A.: Inappropriate antidiuretic hormone secretion in an infant with severe pneumonia. Am. J. Dis. Child. 129:133, 1975.

Oppé, T. E., and Redstone, D.: Calcium and phosphorus levels in healthy newborn infants given various types of milk. Lancet 1:1045, 1968.

Outerbridge, E. W., Papageorgiu, A., and Stern, L.: Magnesium sulfate enema in a newborn. J.A.M.A. 224:1392, 1973.

Peden, V. H.: True idiopathic hypoparathyroidism as a sex linked recessive trait. Am. J. Hum. Genet. 12:323, 1960.

Permagent, E., Pietra, G. C., Kadotani, T., Sato, H., and Berlow, S.: A ring chromosome no. 16 in an infant with primary hypoparathyroidism. J. Pediatr. 76:745, 1970.

Seely, J. R., Humphrey, G. B., and Matter, B. J.: Copper deficiency in a premature infant fed an iron-fortified formula. N. Engl. J. Med. 286:109, 1972.

Simmons, M. A., Adcock, E. W., et al.: Hypernatremia and intracranial hemorrhage in neonates. Arch. Dis. Child. 47:257, 1972.

Smith, F. G., Jr., Alexander, D. P., Buckle, R. M., Britton, H. G., and Nixon, D. A.: Parathyroid hormone in foetal and adult sheep: The effect of hypocalcemia. J. Endocrinol. 53:339, 1972.

Snyder, R. D.: Congenital mercury poisoning. N. Engl. J. Med., 284:1014, 1971.

Sorell, M., and Rosen, J. F.: Ionized calcium: serum levels during symptomatic hypocalcemia. J. Pediatr. 87:67, 1975.

Suh, S. M., Tashjian, A. H., Matsuo, N., Parkinson, D. M., and Fraser, D.: Pathogenesis of hypocalcemia in primary hypomagnesemia: Normal end-organ responsiveness to parathyroid hormone, impaired parathyroid gland functions. J. Clin. Invest. 52:153, 1973.

Taitz, L. S., and Byers, H. D.: High calorie/osmolar feeding and hypertonic dehydration. Arch. Dis. Child. 47:257, 1972.

Taitz, L. S., Zarate-Salvador, C., and Schwartz, E.: Congenital absence of the parathyroid and thymus glands in an infant (III and IV pharyngeal pouch syndrome). Pediatrics 38:412, 1966.

Tsang, R. C.: Neonatal magnesium disturbances. Am. J. Dis. Child. 124:282, 1972.

Tsang, R. C., Chen, I., Friedman, M. S., et al.: Neonatal parathyroid function: Role of gestational age and postnatal age. J. Pediatr. 83:728, 1973.

Tsang, R. C., Chen, I., Hayes, W., Atkinson, W., Atherton, H., and Edward, N.: Neonatal hypocalcemia in infants with birth asphyxia. J. Pediatr. 84:429, 1974.

Tsang, R. C., and Oh, W.: Neonatal hypocalcemia in low birth weight infants. Pediatrics 45:773, 1970.

Twardock, A. R., and Austin, M. K.: Calcium transfer in perfused guinea pig placenta. Am. J. Physiol. 219:540, 1972.

# 54

## DISORDERS OF THE ADRENAL GLANDS

*By John S. Parks*

## GENERAL CONSIDERATIONS

The mammalian adrenal cortex is a dual endocrine organ, consisting of cortex and medulla within a common capsule. The two glands have distinct embryological origins and different functions. In the fifth week of fetal life, the primitive adrenal cortex is formed from cells of the coelomic mesoderm. A thin layer of more compact cells gradually surrounds the fetal cortex. This structure will eventually constitute the permanent, or definitive, adrenal cortex. During the seventh week, the cortex is invaded by ectodermal neural crest cells which aggregate to form a central cell mass, the adrenal medulla.

Adrenal cortical cells produce a variety of steroid hormones, and the medulla produces the catecholamines, norepinephrine and epinephrine. As a consequence of its special anatomic relationship to the adrenal cortex, the medulla is exposed to very high steroid levels in venous blood draining the cortex. Wurtman and Axelrod have shown that the enzymatic conversion of norepinephrine to epinephrine is enhanced by a high local concentration of cortisol. In all other respects, the adrenal cortex and medulla appear to function independently. Adrenal catecholamine deficiency in the neonatal period may contribute to hypoglycemia. The consequences of catecholamine excess are discussed in the section on neuroblastoma. This chapter will focus on development and function of the adrenal cortex.

Adrenal steroid production can be detected by the ninth week of gestation, and by the twelfth week the adrenal glands are fully as large as the kidneys. The primitive or fetal zone of the adrenal cortex accounts for most of its bulk. This zone involutes slowly during the third trimester and more rapidly after birth. Regulation of adrenal growth and function is inferred to be partly under the control of fetal pituitary ACTH, since anencephalic fetuses have hypoplastic adrenal glands. There is no intrinsic difference between male and female adrenal function in utero, and the adrenal does not contribute to normal genital differentiation. The fetal adrenal cortex is relatively deficient in $3\beta$-hydroxysteroid dehydrogenase, an enzyme required for the synthesis of C-21 glucocorticoids and mineralocorticoids. The primary role of the fetal adrenal appears to be production of inactive metabolites such as dehydroepiandrosterone sulfate, which the placenta can convert to estrogens. These estrogens may in turn help to maintain the pregnancy. Monitoring of maternal urinary estriol excretion has been used to provide insight into fetal and placental well-being in high risk pregnancies.

During the second half of pregnancy, the permanent adrenal cortex emerges as a distinct anatomic structure and begins to synthesize the glucocorticoids and mineralocorticoids that will be required for successful adaptation to extrauterine life (Fig. 54–1). Glucocorticoids, of which cortisol is the most important in man, play a major role in carbohydrate metabolism. They promote gluconeogenesis and synthesis of liver glycogen and act to elevate blood glucose levels. Levels of glucocorticoids in amniotic fluid show a marked increase between the thirty-sixth and fortieth weeks of pregnancy. Cortisol has enzyme-inducing capabilities that doubtless affect many organs and thus prepare the infant for postnatal life. This aspect of glucocorticoid action has been most completely delineated in the area of fetal lung maturation (Chapter 13). Prenatal increases in fetal cortisol production may also contribute to the initiation of labor.

Cortisol production is regulated by a hypothalamic-pituitary-adrenal homeostatic system. The hypothalamus produces a peptide corticotropin releasing factor which provokes release of ACTH from the pituitary. This system is activated by low circulating cortisol levels and by stressful stimuli. ACTH stimulates adrenal steroid production. High cortisol levels inhibit corticotropin releasing factor production or effect, or both, thus closing a negative feedback loop.

The glucocorticoid regulatory system is fully developed by birth. Although umbilical venous cortisol levels are lower than maternal levels, cortisone, corticosterone sulfate and 11-desoxycorticosterone sulfate levels are relatively high (Eberlein 1965; Baden et al., 1973). In the healthy newborn, cortisol levels remain relatively stable during the neonatal period, while levels of the other glucocorticoids decline. Perinatal stress, as exemplified by the respiratory distress syndrome, results in a rise in cortisol levels. Newborns also show an impressive cortisol response to administered ACTH (Gutai et al., 1972). Diurnal variation in plasma cortisol is not established during the neonatal period.

Mineralocorticoids differ from glucocorticoids in structure, activity, site of synthesis and regulation. Aldosterone is the most important natural mineralocorticoid in man. In contrast to cortisol, aldosterone lacks a 17-hydroxyl group and contains an aldehyde group at carbon 19. It acts to promote conservation of sodium and loss of potassium by renal tubules and sweat glands. Aldosterone deficiency results in hyponatremia and hyperkalemia. The hormone is produced by the zona glomerulosa, the outermost zone of the permanent adrenal cortex.

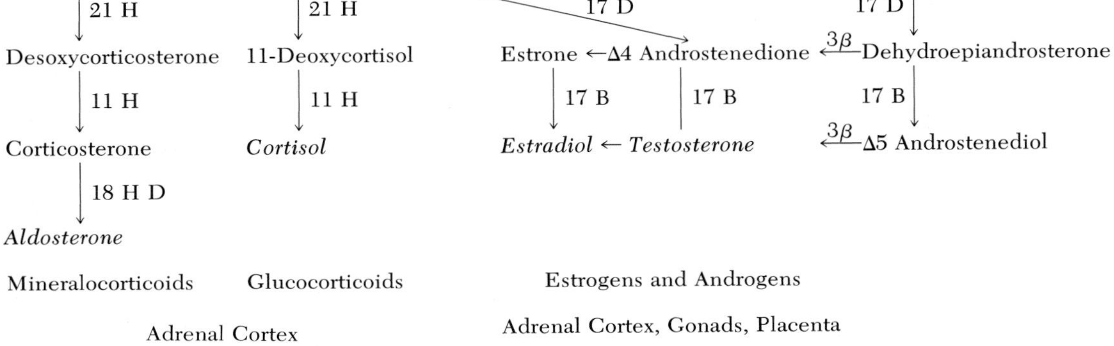

*Figure 54-1.* Steroid biosynthetic pathways.

ACTH contributes relatively little to the regulation of aldosterone synthesis. The main homeostatic mechanism involves release of renin from renal juxtaglomerular cells in response to diminished renal arteriolar pressure. Renin acts to increase angiotensin II which, in turn, increases aldosterone secretion and has a direct effect on vascular contractility. Increased pressure and volume acts to diminish renin production, thus closing the feedback loop. Low sodium intake and high potassium intake also enhance aldosterone secretion by a mechanism which is not dependent on the renin-angiotensin system.

The newborn is able to regulate aldosterone secretion in an appropriate manner. Kowarski et al. found that aldosterone levels in umbilical and newborn venous plasma were comparable to adult values. The levels rose to values above the adult range between 11 days and 1 year of age.

The fetus is not dependent upon endogenous glucocorticoid or mineralocorticoid production. Its needs can be met by transplacental passage of maternal hormones, and deficiencies, per se, are not evident at delivery. However, the catastrophic consequences of defective organogenesis or of enzymatic errors soon become apparent. Glucocorticoid deficiency can result in hypoglycemia within hours of birth, and mineralocorticoid deficiency manifests as salt loss and adrenal crisis within days or weeks.

### ADRENAL HEMORRHAGE

The large adrenal glands of the newborn infant are vulnerable to mechanical trauma during labor and delivery. Focal hemorrhage at the junction of the fetal zone and the permanent cortex is a common finding in infants dying of other causes (Boyd, 1967). Minor bleeding into the adrenal cortex may not produce symptoms but is often responsible for adrenal calcifications noted incidentally later in life. Massive adrenal hemorrhage is an uncommon but life-threatening event. Predisposing factors include high birth weight, prolonged or difficult labor, placental bleeding and perinatal anoxia. Adrenal hemorrhage may occur in premature infants without obvious trauma.

The adrenal may be the site of hemorrhage in infants with sepsis or with primary coagulopathies. In most published series, male infants outnumber females by three to one.

The affected infant shows signs of hypovolemic shock within the first few days of life. Pallor, apnea, hypothermia, listlessness and failure to suck are accompanied by a falling hematocrit and jaundice. A large flank mass may be palpated, more commonly on the right side. In 5 to 10 per cent of cases the hemorrhage is bilateral. The condition must be differentiated from renal vein thrombosis. In both conditions there may be azotemia, proteinuria and hematuria, but in adrenal hemorrhage the hematuria is of a lesser degree. Intravenous pyelograms reveal no function on the affected side when a renal vein or artery has been thrombosed. As shown in Figure 54–2, adrenal hemorrhage typically displaces the kidney downward and rotates it laterally, with flattening of the upper calyces.

Signs of adrenal insufficiency may be subtle and delayed. Hypoglycemia is a more common finding than is salt loss. Even with massive bilateral hemorrhage, functioning islands of zona glomerulosa cells are generally preserved. Destruction of greater than 90 per cent of the adrenal cortex is required to produce adrenal insufficiency.

Immediate management is directed at blood and volume replacement. Indications for steroid replacement include bilateral hemorrhage, failure to respond to volume expansion, hypoglycemia, polyuria, hyponatremia, hyperkalemia or an anticipated need from general anesthesia.

Within 1 to 3 weeks after the hemorrhage, a thin zone of calcification appears at the periphery of the gland. As blood and necrotic adrenal tissue are reabsorbed, the area of calcification shrinks and assumes the shape and size of the original gland. Such calcification may persist for life. Adrenal function generally improves with resolution of the hemorrhage. ACTH stimulation with measurement of plasma or urinary corticoid responses is indicated after the acute phase of the illness. Late adrenal insufficiency has been reported by Stevens, and one of Black and Williams' 8

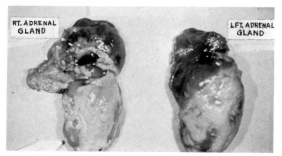

*Figure 54–2.* Kidneys and adrenal glands, with an enlarged hemorrhagic adrenal capping each kidney. The kidneys were also the sites of hemorrhagic necrosis, plus left-sided renal vein thrombosis.

This was an 11 pound 7 ounce boy born after excessive manipulation and traction and 22½ hours of labor. Asphyxia neonatorum was followed by facial twitchings, fever, and hematuria, and then convulsions. On the fourth day a large mass was palpable in the left flank.

cases developed renal vascular hypertension.

## Transient Adrenal Insufficiency

In 1946, Jaudon described a series of 14 infants with dehydration, salt loss and failure to gain weight. All responded to steroid replacement, and in each case it was eventually possible to discontinue treatment without a recurrence of symptoms. Others have reported additional infants with an apparent delay in maturation of adrenal cortical function. Bongiovanni described a premature infant with marked hyponatremia, hyperkalemia and no detectable serum cortisol or urinary corticoids. The infant did well on cortisol replacement and at age 6 months, following discontinuation of steroid treatment, he showed normal cortisol and aldosterone responses to ACTH. He has not developed adrenal calcifications. Kreines and De Vaux described a similar course in an infant born to a mother with Cushing's syndrome due to an adrenal adenoma.

The combination of hyponatremia, hyperkalemia and polyuria may occur in acutely ill infants under a variety of other circumstances which do not involve adrenal insufficiency. Infants recovering from hypovolemic shock and acute tubular necrosis

demonstrate these features, as do infants treated with furosemide without replacement of sodium. In doubtful cases, one may collect serum and urine specimens during a therapeutic trial of desoxycorticosterone acetate. This agent, given intramuscularly in a dosage of 0.5 mg per kg per day, provides a potent mineralocorticoid effect and does not inhibit pituitary ACTH or interfere with serum cortisol or urinary corticoid estimation. If steroid measurements do not support a diagnosis of adrenal insufficiency, and if serum sodium does not rise and serum potassium decline in response to desoxycorticosterone acetate, then the medication may safely be discontinued.

## Adrenal Hypoplasia

In the absence of pituitary gland function, the adrenal glands fail to develop normally. The adrenal glands of anencephalic infants weigh less than 0.5 gram at birth, as opposed to normal combined weights greater than 6 grams. Arrested development of the adrenals has been attributed to a lack of trophic stimulation by ACTH. Interestingly, the adrenal glands of anencephalic fetuses at mid-gestation are histologically normal, suggesting the involvement of non-pituitary factors in early adrenal morphogenesis.

Pituitary hypoplasia can also occur in infants without major central nervous system malformations. In these infants, severe hypoglycemia can result in death within the first 48 hours of life. Blizzard and Alberts described a male infant who had, in addition, microphallus and cryptorchidism. The association has been noted in several other cases and probably reflects a lack of trophic hormone stimulation of both adrenal and testis. Prompt glucocorticoid replacement is required.

Adrenal hypoplasia occurs as well in infants with anatomically and functionally intact pituitary glands. In 1965, Roselli and Barbosa gathered 23 cases of fatal congenital adrenal hypoplasia from the literature and added two of their own. Adrenal gland weight was abnormally low in all. There were several instances of multiple sibling involvement, suggesting an autosomal recessive mode of inheritance.

Early recognition, cortisol replacement and prolonged survival have permitted studies of the mechanisms that underlie familial adrenal hyperplasia. The disease is manifested in infancy or early childhood by hyperpigmentation as a consequence of elevated ACTH levels, and hypoglycemia as a consequence of glucocorticoid deficiency. In contrast to congenital adrenal hyperplasia, there is no excess of abnormal steroid metabolites. Mineralocorticoid production is generally unimpaired. Migeon et al. provided evidence that the disorder may result from an end organ unresponsiveness to ACTH. A possible defect might involve the adrenal membrane receptor for this polypeptide hormone. The family reported by Moshang et al. had features that suggested an inherited degenerative disease of the zona fasciculata and zona reticularis. Five of seven siblings were affected by the disease. Of these, two developed glucocorticoid deficiency some months after testing had shown normal adrenal function. Aldosterone excretion was normal in the basal state and rose after ACTH, indicating a normal response of the zona glomerulosa to the trophic hormone.

## Congenital Adrenal Hyperplasia

Adrenal steroid biosynthesis requires a sequence of enzymatic reactions which are illustrated in Figure 54–1. Genetically determined deficiency in the activity of any of the required enzymes results in a serious disease. This category of disease states has several features in common. Each condition is inherited in an autosomal recessive manner. Thus, multiple sibling involvement is common and recurrence risk in subsequent pregnancies is 25 per cent. There is no reliable or simple screening test for heterozygote carriers, and experience with prenatal detection has also been disappointing. The disorders begin before birth and persist throughout life. Each, with the exception of 18-hydroxysteroid dehydrogenase deficiency, involves hyperplasia of the adrenal cortex under the stimulus of elevated ACTH levels. Combined adrenal weights of 30 grams are not uncom-

mon. In each case, the disorder may be managed quite well with appropriate steroid replacement.

Clinical manifestations of adrenal hyperplasia depend upon the site and severity of the enzymatic block. With a block, precursors accumulate and are diverted into alternative metabolic pathways. Laboratory confirmation of a suspected defect involves measurement of these metabolites. The metabolites may have major physiologic effects, particularly on the differentiation of the external genitalia. For example, defects in 21-hydroxylase and 11-hydroxylase each lead to overproduction of androgens which produce virilization of female external genitalia. In other instances, the enzymatic defect impairs testicular testosterone synthesis and leads to undervirilization of the male fetus. Deficiency of 17α-hydroxylase has such an effect. The 3β-hydroxysteroid dehydrogenase defect demonstrates both features of congenital adrenal hyperplasia. Females tend to be virilized and males tend to be undervirilized at birth. The defects listed in Table 54–1 will be discussed individually.

## Deficiency of 21-Hydroxylase

Hydroxylation at the C-21 position is required for synthesis of mineralocorticoids and glucocorticoids. This enzymatic reaction is not involved in androgen or estrogen synthesis. The 21-hydroxylase deficiency is the most common form of congenital adrenal hyperplasia, accounting for 90 per cent of cases. In roughly 70 per cent the defect is partial or incomplete and permits synthesis of adequate amounts of aldosterone and cortisol to support life. In these children, the major clinical manifestations reflect androgen excess, but extreme stress may unmask partial adrenal insufficiency. Female infants demonstrate varying degrees of virilization, ranging from mild clitoral enlargement to severe clitoral enlargement with complete labial fusion and a phallic urethra. Males are formed normally at birth but show progressive virilization during infancy and early childhood with rapid linear growth, skeletal and somatic maturation, phallic enlargement and premature appearance of sexual

TABLE 54–1. *Enzymatic Defects in Adrenal Steroid Biosynthesis*

| Abbreviation | Enzyme | Virilization | Incomplete Masculinization | Salt Loss | Hypertension | Urinary 17-Ketosteroids | Predominant Abnormal Urinary Steroid |
|---|---|---|---|---|---|---|---|
| D M | 20,22 Desmolase | − | + | + | − | Low | Virtually absent Pregnenetriol |
| 3 β | 3β Hydroxysteroid dehydrogenase | + | + | + | − | Elevated | Tetrahydro DOC |
| 17 H | 17 Hydroxylase | − | + | − | + | Low | Pregnanetriol |
| 21 H | 21 Hydroxylase | + | − | ± | − | Elevated | Tetrahydro S |
| 11 H | 11 Hydroxylase | + | − | − | + | Elevated | Tetrahydro DOC |
| 18 HD | 18 Hydroxysteroid dehydrogenase | − | − | + | − | Normal | Tetrahydro corticosterone |

hair. The testes, however, remain infantile.

The remaining 30 per cent of affected children have a more severe defect of 21-hydroxylase and show signs of aldosterone deficiency early in life, with failure to thrive, hyponatremia, hyperkalemia, and, ultimately, vascular collapse. Here, too, there is a spectrum of severity with some untreated infants dying by 1 or 2 weeks of age and others failing to thrive for several months before diagnosis. Virilization of the female infant is a clinical clue which fosters early recognition and treatment. Male infants lack external markers of the disease and often die undiagnosed.

Congenital adrenal hyperplasia should be suspected in all infants with ambiguous genitalia, or a family history of this condition or of unexplained infant death, and in all infants with vomiting, sluggish feeding, dehydration or failure to thrive.

Diagnosis is established by demonstrating abnormal levels of the appropriate urine or plasma steroid metabolites and suppression by cortisol replacement. Urinary 17-ketosteroid excretion is greater than 2.5 mg per 24 hours and pregnanetriol excretion is greater than 0.5 mg per 24 hours after 3 to 5 days of age, when the normal newborn's level of these compounds have declined. Radioimmunoassay and gas liquid chromatography show elevations of 17α-hydroxyprogesterone and 11-ketopregnanetriol in serum and urine. It is vital that the steroid analyses be performed by laboratories that have defined normal ranges for infants. The usual assays are subject to interference in the low range and, while adequate for studies in adults, tend to give

a falsely high estimate of 17-ketosteroids and pregnanetriol in children. In the doubtful case, treatment may be initiated locally and the infant referred to a regional center for further studies. Routine steroid measurements do not differentiate between salt-losing and compensated forms of the disease. Elevated levels of plasma renin activity have been noted in the salt-losing form and may be a useful distinguishing characteristic. The usual practice is to monitor serum sodium and potassium levels closely during the first 2 weeks of life, waiting for salt loss to be expressed.

In the infant with severe salt loss, initial treatment requires volume expansion with isotonic saline in 5 or 10 per cent dextrose intravenously at a rate of 100 to 120 mg per kg per day with 25 per cent of this amount given in the first 2 hours. Plasma and vasopressor drugs may also be required. Simultaneously with the glucose-saline infusion, the mineralocorticoid desoxycorticosterone acetate (DOCA) should be given in a dosage of 0.5 mg per kg and repeated every 24 hours as indicated by state of hydration and by serum sodium and potassium levels.

Chronic medical treatment of congenital adrenal hyperplasia requires provision of sufficient cortisol to suppress adrenal androgen production and protect against stress. The required dosage is generally in the range of 15 to 25 mg per M² of hydrocortisone or cortisone acetate per day, given in three divided oral doses. Cortisone acetate may also be given intramuscularly every 3 days for long-term replacement. The dosage should be doubled during acute illnesses, and intramuscular cortisone acetate substituted in a dosage of 25 to 50 mg per $M^2$ per day during protracted vomiting or surgical stress. Inadequate dosage permits excessive production of androgens and excessively rapid growth and skeletal maturation. Overdosage produces slowing of growth and other features of Cushing syndrome.

Infants with proved or suspected salt loss should also receive mineralocorticoid replacement in the form of 9-fluorohydrocortisone (Florinef) orally in a dose of 0.025 to 0.1 mg per day. Suboptimal growth occurs with inadequate replacement, and excessive doses produce failure to thrive as well as hypertension.

Surgical correction of mild to moderate clitoral enlargement is generally not required. Clitoral size tends to remain stable or even decrease as the child grows. When indicated, surgery may be done at 4 to 12 months of age. Correction of labial fusion is probably best done around the age of 2 years. Some girls may require more complicated vaginoplasty at a later age. The prognosis for normal psychosexual development and reproductive function is excellent in boys and girls with 21-hydroxylase deficiency.

## DEFICIENCY OF 20,22-DESMOLASE

Conversion of cholesterol to pregnenolone is an essential step in the synthesis of mineralocorticoids, glucocorticoids, androgens and estrogens. Defects in this early set of reactions lead to severe salt and water loss and hypoglycemia. Male infants show incomplete virilization. Female infants have normal genitalia at birth, but will be incapable of producing estrogens at the time of puberty. No distinctive steroid precursors are present in serum or urine. The adrenal glands and gonads are enlarged and filled with cholesterol and other lipids, hence the name "lipoid adrenal hyperplasia." In the cases of Prader and Gurtner, and of Comacho et al., the defect was confirmed at autopsy. In other cases, perhaps with less severe defects, steroid treatment has permitted prolonged survival.

## DEFICIENCY OF 3β-HYDROXYSTEROID DEHYDROGENASE

Conversion of pregnenolone to progesterone requires oxidation at the 3 position and isomerization of a double bond from the Δ5 to the Δ4 position. Bongiovanni originally described several infants with defects in this crucial enzyme complex. The infants had severe salt and water loss and, despite adequate steroid replacement, did not survive infancy. Female infants were virilized and males had varying degrees of undervirilization. Urinary steroid metabolites were predominantly of the Δ4,3β-hydroxy configuration and included pregnenetriol and dehydroepiandrosterone. Subsequently several older children with partial defects of the enzyme have been described. Males have had hypospadias, and have developed gynecomastia at puberty. Schneider et al. report an elevated ratio of Δ5-androstenediol to testosterone, which provides evidence of persistent deficiency of testicular 3β-hydroxysteroid dehydrogenase activity and supports the hypothesis that the adrenal and testicular enzymes are under common genetic control. With increasing age, hepatic 3β-hydroxysteroid dehydrogenase activity increases under separate genetic control (Bongiovanni et al., 1971). This phenomenon explains the diminishing ratio of urinary pregnenetriol to pregnanetriol in older children with the defect. In infancy, 17-ketosteroids are markedly elevated, but pregnanetriol is elevated. This finding differentiates the defect from the more common deficiency of 21-hydroxylase. Glucocorticoid and mineralocorticoid replacement are required throughout life. Male fertility and female puberty have yet to be described in this syndrome.

## DEFICIENCY OF 11-HYDROXYLASE

Hydroxylation at the C-11 position is required for cortisol and aldosterone synthesis. As originally reported by Eberlein and Bongiovanni, deficiency of 11-hydroxylase results in virilization of the female infant together with a variable degree of hypertension. There is accumulation of the immediate precursors, 11-deoxycortisol (Compound S) and desoxycorticosterone (DOC) in the plasma and increased urinary excretion of their tetrahydro metabolites. Whereas compound S is biologically inert, DOC has mineralocorticoid effects and contributes to the hypertensive state. Neither compound is recognized by the hypothalamic-pituitary regulatory system. Hydrocortisone replacement suppresses ACTH production and thereby prevents further virilization and relieves hypertension. Monitoring of treatment requires management of urinary 17-ketosteroid or tetrahydro-S excretion.

## DEFICIENCY OF 17α-HYDROXYLASE

Hydroxylation at the C-17 position is required for cortisol, androgen and estrogen synthesis, but is not involved in the synthesis of mineralocorticoids. Biglieri described four adult females with lack of secondary sexual development, hyperkalemic alkalosis and hypertension who proved to have deficiency of this enzyme. They demonstrated excessive plasma levels of DOC and corticosterone and excessive excretion of their urinary metabolites. Aldosterone levels tended to be low, presumably due to inhibition of the renin-angiotensin system. Failure of pubertal development in females and defective virilization in males, as described by New, provide evidence that adrenal and gonadal 17α-hydroxylase activities are under common genetic control. Cortisol replacement inhibits ACTH production and relieves hypertension. Exogenous androgens or estrogens are required at the age of puberty.

## DEFICIENCY OF 18-HYDROXYSTEROID DEHYDROGENASE

The final steps in aldosterone synthesis involve hydroxylation and dehydrogenation at C-18. Deficiency at this level results in aldosterone deficiency and salt loss without any alteration in the synthesis of cortisol or the sex steroids. Ulick et al. described a patient with these features in 1964. Several authors have postulated that the transient salt wasting of infancy described by Jaudon might be due to delayed maturation of this enzyme. Appropriate therapy consists of a mineralocorticoid and supplemental sodium chloride. Glucocorticoid replacement is not required.

## ADRENAL OVERACTIVITY

Glucocorticoid excess results in hyperphagia, obesity and impairment of linear growth, together with hypertension, osteoporosis and polycythemia. The Cushing syndrome is exceedingly rare in infancy except as a result of administration of glucocorticoids or ACTH. The cases that have been reported show a preponderance of adrenal tumors, both adenomas and carcinomas. There may be overproduction of androgens as well as glucocorticoids. There is no suppression with administration of dexamethasone. Surgical treatment involves unilateral or bilateral adrenalectomy, with attendant glucocorticoid replacement to prevent acute adrenal insufficiency.

## REFERENCES

Baden, M., Bauer, C. R., Colle, E., Klein, G., Papageorgiou, A., and Stern, L.: Plasma corticoids in infants with the respiratory distress syndrome. Pediatrics 52:782, 1973.

Black, J., and Williams, D. I.: Natural history of adrenal haemorrhage in the newborn. Arch. Dis. Child. 48:183, 1973.

Blizzard, R. M., and Alberts, M.: Hypopituitarism, hypoadrenalism and hypogonadism in the newborn infant. J. Pediatr. 48:782, 1956.

Biglieri, E. G., Herron, M. A., and Brust, N.: 17-Hydroxylation deficiency syndrome. N. Engl. J. Med. 45:1946, 1966.

Bongiovanni, A. M.: Disorders of adrenal steroid biogenesis. *In* Stanbury, J. B., Wyngaarden, J. B., and Fredrickson, D. S. (Eds.): The Metabolic Basis of Inherited Disease. New York, McGraw-Hill Book Co., 1972, p. 857.

Bongiovanni, A. M.: Adrenogenital syndrome with deficiency of 3β-hydroxysteroid dehydrogenase. J. Clin. Invest. 41:2086, 1962.

Bongiovanni, A. M., Eberlein, W. R., and Moshang, T. M.: Urinary excretion of pregnanetriol and Δ5-pregnenetriol in two forms of congenital adrenal hyperplasia. J. Clin. Invest. 50:2751, 1971.

Boyd, J. F.: Disseminated fibrin thromboembolism among neonates dying within 48 hours of birth. Arch. Dis. Child. 42:401, 1967.

Camacho, A. M., Kowarski, A., Migeon, C. J., and Brough, A. J.: Congenital adrenal hyperplasia due to a deficiency of one of the enzymes involved in the biosynthesis of pregneneolone. J. Clin. Endocrinol. Metab. 28:153, 1968.

Eberlein, W. R.: Steroids and sterols in umbilical cord blood. J. Clin. Endocrinol. Metab. 25:1101, 1965.

Eberlein, W. R., and Bongiovanni, A. M.: Plasma and urinary corticosteroids in hypertensive form of congenital adrenal hyperplasia. J. Biol. Chem. 223:85, 1956.

Gutai, J., George, R., Koeff, S., and Bacon, G. E.: Adrenal response to stress and the effect of adrenocorticotropic hormone in newborn infants. J. Pediatr. 81:719, 1972.

Jaudon, J. C.: Addison's disease in an infant. J. Clin. Endocrinol. Metab. 6:558, 1946.

Kreines, K., and De Vaux, W. D.: Neonatal adrenal insufficiency associated with maternal Cushing's syndrome. Pediatrics 47:516, 1971.

Kowarski, A., Katz, H., and Migeon, C. J.: Plasma aldosterone concentration in normal subjects from infancy to adulthood. J. Clin. Endocrinol. Metab. 38:489, 1974.

Migeon, C. J., Kenny, F. M., and Kowarski, A.: The syndrome of congenital unresponsiveness to ACTH. Pediatr. Res. 2:501, 1968.

Moshang, T. M., Jr., Rosenfield, R. L., Bongiovanni, A. M., Parks, J. S., and Amrhein, J. A.: Familial glucocorticoid insufficiency. J. Pediatr. 82:821, 1973.

New, M. I., and Suvannakul, L.: Male pseudohermaphroditism due to 17α-hydroxylase deficiency. J. Clin. Invest. 49:1930, 1970.

Parks, G. A., New, M. I., Bermudez, J. A., Anast, C. S., and Bongiovanni, A. M.: A pubertal boy with the 3β-hydroxysteroid dehydrogenase defect. J. Clin. Invest. 33:269, 1971.

Prader, A., and Gurtner, H. P.: Das Syndrom des Pseudohermaphroditismus masculinus bei kongenitaler Nebennierenrinden-hyperplasie ohne Androgenüberproduktion (adrenaler Pseudohermaphroditismus masculinus). Helvet. Paediat. Acta 10:397, 1955.

Roselli, A., and Barbosa, L. T.: Congenital hypoplasia of the adrenal glands: Report of 2 cases in sisters, with necropsy. Pediatrics 35:70, 1965.

Schneider, G., Genel, M., Bongiovanni, A. M., Goldman, A. S., and Rosenfield, R. L.: Persistent testicular Δ5-isomerase-3β-hydroxysteroid dehydrogenase deficiency in the Δ5-3β-HSD form of congenital adrenal hyperplasia. J. Clin. Invest. 55:681, 1974.

Ulick, S., Gautier, E., Vetter, K. K., Markello, J. R., Yaffe, S., and Lowe, C. U.: An aldosterone biosynthetic defect in a salt-losing disorder. J. Clin. Endocrinol. Metab. 24:669, 1964.

Wilkins, L., Fleishman, W., and Howard, J. E.: Macrogenitosomia precox associated with hyperplasia of the androgenic tissue of the adrenal and death from corticoadrenal insufficiency. Endocrinology 25:385, 1940.

Wurtman, R. J., and Axelrod, J.: Adrenaline synthesis. Control by the pituitary gland and adrenal glucocorticoids. Science 150:1464, 1956.

# 55  DISORDERS OF THE THYROID GLAND

*By John S. Parks*

## GENERAL CONSIDERATIONS

Anatomic and functional development of the human fetal thyroid proceed rapidly during the first trimester. By 11 to 12 weeks of gestation, the normal thyroid gland has completed its caudal migration and the thyroglossal duct leading from the base of the tongue has been obliterated. Thyroid weight has increased to 0.05 per cent of total body weight, and this ratio will be maintained during further growth (Shepard, et al., 1964). Histologically, the gland's colloid-filled follicles resemble those of the adult thyroid. At this stage, the gland has developed the capacity to concentrate iodide from the circulation and synthesize the active thyroid hormones thyroxine (T4) and triiodothyronine (T3).

Using sensitive assays for T4, T3 and thyrotropic hormone (TSH), Fisher and others have provided detailed information about fetal thyroid function. Circulating T4 and TSH are detectable by 11 weeks but remain at low levels through 18 weeks. Between 18 and 22 weeks, there are abrupt increases in pituitary TSH content and serum TSH levels. This change may be due to the onset of thyrotropin releasing hormone (TRH) synthesis by the hypothalamus. Mean TSH levels remain high, at 8 to 10 $\mu$U per ml through term. In the fetus, as in the adult, less than 0.1 per cent of T4 and about 0.3 per cent of T3 circulate in the free form. The remainder is bound to thyroxine binding globulin (TBG) and other serum proteins. Fetal TBG levels increase during the second half of pregnancy under the influence of estrogens. However, the concentration of free as well as total T4 increases progressively and may exceed maternal concentrations as the fetus approaches term. Serum T3 arises from direct thyroidal secretion and from peripheral conversion of T4. The latter function appears to be diminished in utero. Fetal T3 levels are below 15 ng per ml prior to 25 weeks, and barely achieve detectable levels during the last trimester. There is minimal transfer of T4 or T3 across the placenta in either direction and TSH does not cross the placenta. At no time during pregnancy is there a correlation between maternal and fetal T4, T3 or TSH levels. The fetal hypothalamic-pituitary-thyroid system functions as an autonomous unit throughout gestation. Function is intensified during the last trimester, which is a critical period for brain growth and functional maturation.

Requirements for normal fetal thyroid function include an orderly sequence of thyroid organogenesis, a full complement of the enzymes necessary for thyroid hormone synthesis and an adequate supply of iodide. The fetus attempts to compensate for deficits in any of these areas by increasing TSH secretion and thus stimulating thyroid growth and activity. No help is available from the maternal circulation. Several factors which alter maternal thyroid function can, however, have adverse effects on the fetus. Either a deficiency or a great excess of maternal iodide ingestion can produce intrauterine goiter and hypothyroidism. Radioiodine in high doses can ablate the fetal as well as the maternal thyroid. Thiourea drugs used in the treatment of hyperthyroidism cross the placenta and interfere with fetal thyroid hormone synthesis. Finally, 7s immune gamma globulins are transported across the placenta. Maternal antibodies to thyroid tissues may inhibit and the long acting thy-

roid stimulator of thyrotoxicosis may inappropriately stimulate the gland.

The birth process evokes sudden changes in thyroid function. Serum levels of TSH rise to a peak of greater than 80 $\mu$U per ml in the first hour of extrauterine life. This brief surge of TSH, in turn, produces a more prolonged rise in T4 and T3 levels. Serum T4 peaks at approximately 15 $\mu$g per 100 ml and T3 reaches 400 ng per ml by 24 hours. Both values are considerably above the adult normal ranges of 4 to 13 $\mu$g per 100 ml for T4 and 50 to 200 ng per 100 ml for T3. Van Middlesworth's observations of elevated 24 hour thyroidal radioiodine uptake provide further evidence for physiologic hyperthyroidism in the neonate. Cold stress appears to be the most important stimulus to neonatal hypersecretion of TSH. Fisher and Oddie have observed blunted responses in infants who were kept warm after delivery. Premature infants also tend to have lesser degrees of physiologic hyperthyroidism. Levels of TSH decline to less than 20 $\mu$U per ml by 1 week, and T4 and T3 levels decline more gradually over the first month. At no time during infancy or childhood is the normal range for T4 below the normal adult range.

# CONGENITAL HYPOTHYROIDISM

## THYROID DYSGENESIS

**INCIDENCE AND ETIOLOGY.** The current incidence of cogenital hypothyroidism in the United States is between 1 in 5000 and 1 in 10,000 live births. The report of Dussault et al. of a neonatal screening program in the Province of Quebec identified seven hypothyroid infants among 47,000 who were tested. Disorganized embryogenesis leading to thyroid aplasia or hypoplasia is the most common cause of congenital hypothyroidism. In this group, there is no visible thyroid enlargement, and the diagnosis is considered because of clinical or laboratory findings of hypothyroidism. There is no single etiologic factor that accounts for thyroid dysgenesis. In contrast to inborn errors of thyroxine synthesis, there is seldom involvement of multiple siblings within a family. However, the risk is sufficiently high to justify early thyroid hormone testing in subsequent siblings. There may be a positive family history of chronic lymphocytic thyroiditis or hyperthyroidism, particularly on the maternal side. Blizzard reported a strikingly high incidence (29 per cent) of positive antithyroid antibodies in the mothers of hypothyroid infants. However, the great majority of mothers with antibodies give birth to infants with normal thyroid function. In some infants with thyroid dysgenesis there are other somatic abnormalities that indicate a more generalized disturbance of embryologic development. Prenatal infection has not been proven to be a major etiologic factor, but several reported infants have had both congenital toxoplasmosis and hypothyroidism (Andersen, 1960).

**DIAGNOSIS.** Hypothyroid infants are rarely born with all the full-blown characteristics of a cretin. Thyroid hormone is not required for fetal growth. Hypothyroid infants tend to be longer and heavier than average at birth. Lack of thyroid hormone is, however, reflected in slow skeletal maturation. Palpation of abnormally large anterior and posterior fontanels provides an early indication of delayed skeletal development. Subtle signs of hypothyroidism in the neonatal period include lethargy, a weak suck and poor feeding. Hypothermia and prolonged jaundice may raise suspicion of sepsis. Respiratory distress and cyanosis may also be noted. Contis et al. observed that the latter two findings, together with heart murmurs and low voltage P, R and T waves, led to a suspicion of congenital heart disease in one fourth of their series of hypothyroid infants. These findings were readily reversed by treatment.

Deviations from normal development become more apparent with age. Linear growth and weight gain are severely impaired. Feeding is listless, and the quantity of formula consumed is small. Constipation may be a very prominent complaint. Delay in motor and social development is particularly noticeable to experienced mothers. New parents may misinterpret these signs and report that theirs is an exceptionally good baby.

The complete picture of congenital hypothyroidism is unmistakable (Fig. 55–1)

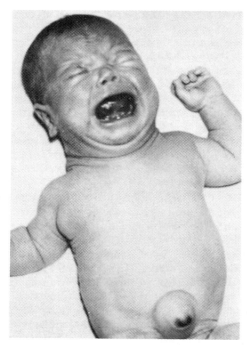

*Figure 55–1.* Athyrotic cretin at the age of four weeks. Only a few of his unusual characteristics can be distinguished from the picture. Noteworthy are the flattened bridge and uptilted tip of his shortened nose, widely separated eyes, puffiness about the eyes, large tongue and a large umbilical hernia.

and includes the following criteria. The facies is grotesque, owing to widely separated eyes with puffy lids, a short retrousse nose with flattened bridge, thickened tongue protruding from a mouth held constantly open and a low hairline over a corrugated forehead. The skin is remarkable for its pallor and coldness and is often mottled. Varying degrees of myxedema are found, chiefly involving the periorbital regions, the dorsa of the hands and the back of the neck. Excessive fat deposition may be apparent as a "buffalo hump" or as "fatty tumors" of the anterior neck. An umbilical hernia usually crowns a protuberant abdomen. The legs are short, the hands square and spade-shaped, the fingers stubby and broad. The pulse rate is slow, even in the presence of anemia. Behavior is as characteristic as appearance. Sluggish and unresponsive, the baby moves and cries little and hoarsely. The baby is slow to cry following an unpleasant stimulus, and the crying is not sustained.

Infants with complete thyroid agenesis may attain this extreme state of clinical hypothyroidism in as little as two months after birth. Others, with definite but ultimately inadequate remnants of thyroid tissue, may have a much milder and slower course.

**LABORATORY INVESTIGATIONS.** The most useful single test for investigation of suspected hypothyroidism is determination of total T4. Values below 6 $\mu$g per 100 ml by radioimmunoassay or competitive protein binding merit further investigation. In most cases, the total T4 value will accurately correlate with the available concentration of free thyroxine. The T3 resin uptake test provides a useful indirect measurement of TBG saturation. Normal T3 resin uptake values are entirely consistent with hypothyroidism, but greatly elevated values in the presence of low T4 values point to a deficiency of TBG. Measurement of T3 concentration is not required for the diagnosis of hypothyroidism. Measurement of TSH by radioimmunoassay is useful, particularly in the presence of equivocally low T4 values. After the first week of life, TSH values above 20 $\mu$U per ml provide firm evidence for primary hypothyroidism. The questions of the optimum screening test and the optimum time for screening remain to be resolved. Dussault's program in Quebec involves measurement of T4 in dried blood specimens obtained prior to discharge from the nursery. Klein and associates have measured TSH levels in cord blood specimens.

The anemia of congenital hypothyroidism may be macrocytic or normocytic and is associated with a low reticulocyte count which does not improve until thyroid replacement is begun. Hyperbilirubinemia, moderately elevated serum cholesterol and elevated blood urea nitrogen are common associated findings.

Additional tests are helpful in assessing the severity, duration and classification of hypothyroid states. X-ray films showing a lack of distal femoral and proximal tibial ossification centers suggest that the process began before birth. Some epiphyseal centers may be irregularly formed, fragmented or stippled. Uptake of radio-iodine at 24 hours is zero in athyreotics and generally less than 10 per cent in infants with thyroid hypoplasia. Iodine or technetium scans disclose a feeble uptake in the normal or at an ectopic location in a substantial number of infants who would otherwise be classified as having athyreosis.

**TREATMENT.** Synthetic L-thyroxine is the drug of choice for treatment of hypothyroidism. The cost is low and potency is more uniform than desiccated thyroid. Combinations of thyroxine and T3 produce unphysiologic and probably undesirable peaks of T3 shortly after ingestion. By contrast, a single daily oral dose of thyroxine produces steady, physiologic levels of both hormones. An appropriate starting dosage of L-thyroxine is 0.05 mg per day. The dose may be increased to 0.1 mg per day within days or weeks of starting therapy. This quantity is roughly equivalent to 60 mg of desiccated thyroid. A further advance to 0.15 mg per day may be made at 1½ to 2 years of age. The current recommended doses of thyroxine are much higher on a $\mu$g/kg or $\mu$g/M$^2$ basis than the 0.15 to 0.20 mg per day required to suppress TSH and maintain normal T4 levels in adults (Stock et al., 1974). Mestman et al. reported that suboptimal replacement in infants may permit normal linear growth without permitting normal mental development. Thyroxine doses lower than the 0.1 mg per day recommended by Bongiovanni (1963) may be used, so long as they are found, in the individual patient, to produce serum $T_4$ levels in the normal range for age and TSH levels below 8 $\mu$U per ml. Overdosage mimics many of the features of infantile hyperthyroidism including undue acceleration of bone age and premature craniosynostosis. Penfold and Simpson have noted the latter complication in children receiving as little as 0.2 mg of L-thyroxine per day.

**PROGNOSIS.** The initiation of thyroid hormone replacement brings rapid improvement in appearance, appetite, activity, skin color, myxedema and constipation. It is useful to warn the parents that their child will experience hair loss as a new crop of growing hairs displaces the resting hairs. With lifelong thyroid hormone replacement, the prospects for normal health and physical growth are excellent. However, optimism regarding mental development must be tempered by a knowledge of prior experience. Thyroid hormone deficiency during the proliferative phase of brain growth may result in permanent impairment of brain function. Human brain DNA content, and, therefore, cell number, undergoes a rapid increase in the third trimester and approaches an adult level by 5 years of age (Winick, 1968). Several recent studies of the outcome of hypothyroid infants emphasize the importance of early recognition and treatment (Collipp et al., 1965; Raiti and Newns, 1971; Klein et al., 1972). In these series, 74 to 82 per cent of children treated under 3 months and a minority of those treated after 3 months attained IQ's within the normal range. Even among those with normal intelligence, the frequencies of specific learning disabilities and of gross motor incoordination are increased in proportion to the delay in initiating adequate treatment.

## OTHER RARE CAUSES OF HYPOTHYROIDISM

Hypopituitary and hypothalamic disorders may cause hypothyroidism during fetal life. The thyroid gland does not seem to require TSH stimulation for normal embryologic development, and it continues to function at a low level in the absence of trophic stimulation. Deficiency of TSH usually occurs in association with a deficiency of growth hormone. Infants may present with neonatal hypoglycemia or with a slowing of linear growth. Serum T4 levels are not as low as in primary hypothyroidism, and the clinical findings are not as severe. Serum TSH is low in relation to T4 levels. Stimulation with synthetic TRH provokes a delayed and prolonged rise in TSH in those with hypothalamic defects and fails to elicit a TSH rise in those with true hypopituitarism. Treatment of hypothyroidism should be coordinated with a program of human growth hormone replacement.

Thyroidal resistance to pituitary TSH was postulated as a cause of hypothyroidism in a single patient described by Stanbury. Refetoff and associates have reported detailed studies on a family in which physiologic hypothyroidism reflected a variable tissue resistance to high circulating levels of free T4 and T3.

Familial thyroxine binding globulin deficiency is an X-linked trait which may be confused with hypothyroidism. Males who are homozygous for this trait have a nearly complete lack of TBG while hemizygous females have intermediate values. Serum total T4 levels are extremely low and T3 resin uptakes are high; however, free T4 and TSH levels are normal. Affected individuals are euthyroid and require no treatment.

## CONGENITAL GOITER

The normal thyroid gland cannot be seen nor can its outlines be palpated with assurance in the newborn. Visible and palpable thyroid enlargement is a clear and dramatic sign of abnormal intrauterine thyroid function. Goiter in the newborn can present formidable problems of management and differential diagnosis. Enlargement beyond the minimal degree is associated with evidence of tracheal compression. These signs include dyspnea with or without cyanosis, stridor and constant head retraction. Lateral x-rays of the neck and blood gas determinations are useful in deciding upon the need for and the techniques of airway management. Except in hyperthyroid infants, the use of L-thyroxine will bring about gradual reduction in size of the gland. Direct mechanical intervention may be required if the respiratory distress is severe. Alternatives include nasotracheal intubation, tracheostomy and partial thyroidectomy. In the latter case, either sectioning of the isthmus or partial resection of one or both lobes may be required. The infant shown in Figure 55–2 had an inborn error of thyroxine synthesis, but goiters of similar size may occur in several other conditions. Decisions regarding subsequent management require knowledge of the etiology of the goiter.

## INBORN ERRORS OF THYROID HORMONE SYNTHESIS

At least five distinct enzymatic steps are required for thyroid hormone synthesis and

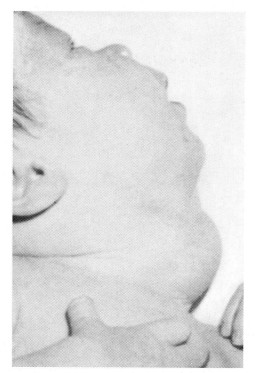

***Figure 55–2.*** Note the large mass bulging forward in the midline of the neck. No details of the cretinoid facies can be made out in this lateral view.

release. Genetically determined defects have been described for each of these steps. In each case, the disease has an autosomal recessive mode of inheritance. Although the term "familial goitrous cretinism" has been applied to this set of disorders, the term is misleading. Not all patients have visible goiters and not all are cretins in the sense of having severe congenital hypothyroidism. Development of goiter may precede or follow development of hypothyroidism. The subject is discussed in much greater detail in Stanbury's recent review.

The required steps in thyroid hormone synthesis are as follows: 1) selective trapping and concentration of iodide within the gland; 2) oxidation of iodide and covalent attachment to tyrosyl residues of thyroglobulin; 3) coupling of iodotyrosines to form T4 and T3; 4) cleavage of active thyroid hormones from thyroglobulin with secretion of hormones into the blood stream; and 5) recycling of intrathyroidal iodine by de-

halogenation of hormonally inactive iodotyrosines and iodothyronines.

Genetic deficiency in the iodide trapping mechanism produces a low T4 and a large thyroid gland which is incapable of taking up administered radioiodine. Salivary glands share the defect in iodide trapping and this fact has been used in diagnosis. The most common genetic defect in thyroxine synthesis involves oxidation and organification of iodide. When combined with sensorineural deafness, the disease is known as Pendred's syndrome. The gland rapidly concentrates administered radioiodine into a large pool of iodide which can be discharged by the administration of potassium perchlorate or thiocyanate. Defects in iodotyrosine coupling also produce a rapid uptake of iodine, but a definitive diagnosis can only be made by chemical studies of the excised gland. Patients with defects in thyroglobulin structure and breakdown of thyroglobulin may have a high level of protein bound iodine due to abnormal circulating iodoproteins. Infants with the dehalogenase defect also have high PBI levels due to circulating monoiodotyrosine and diiodotyrosine. In these two conditions, low T4 and elevated TSH levels indicate hypothyroidism.

Treatment of hypothyroidism due to inborn errors of thyroid hormone synthesis is identical to treatment of thyroid dysgenesis. Adequate thyroxine replacement will bring about nearly complete regression of goiter in young individuals. Prognosis for mental development depends both upon the severity of the defect and the duration of hypothyroidism prior to treatment.

### ENDEMIC GOITER

Congenital goiter has generally been common where goiter in older children and adults is also common. In many inland areas, the introduction of iodized salt has decreased the incidence of goiter in all age groups. However, iodine supplementation is not routine in West Germany, and Homoki and associates in Ulm recently reported on 45 goitrous newborns studied over a 16 month interval. Of these, one half had retarded bone age and elevated TSH, indicating congenital hypothyroidism. The authors advocated thyroid hormone replacement as a safe and effective means of reducing thyroid size and ensuring a euthyroid state.

## HYPERTHYROIDISM

The problems of the infant of a thyrotoxic mother start well before birth. The untreated mother is malnourished. Placenta and fetus share in this malnutrition and the outcome is likely to be either fetal death or premature delivery of an infant who is also small for gestational age. Proper management of the hyperthyroid mother requires either surgery or the use of marginally effective doses of antithyroid drugs. Radioiodine therapy is inappropriate because of the likelihood of ablation of the fetal thyroid. Iodides should never be used in treatment of the pregnant woman because they cross the placenta and produce fetal goiter. Concurrent use of thyroid hormone replacement and large doses of antithyroid drugs exposes the fetus to higher concentrations of these drugs without protecting against hypothyroidism.

The newborn infant may have definite thyroid enlargement. This may reflect intrauterine hypothyroidism due to transplacental passage of the methimazole, propylthiouracil or stable iodine used in treatment. If so, serum T4 levels will be normal or low and TSH levels will be high. If the T4 is very low, or if rapid shrinkage of the goiter is required for proper airway management, then treatment must be begun with full replacement doses of thyroxine. If neither of these criteria are

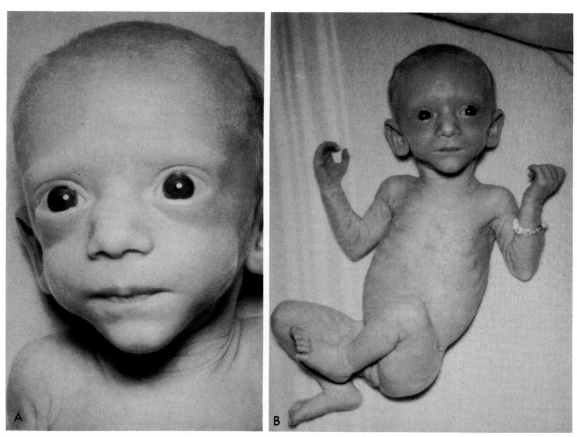

*Figure 55–3.* This transiently hyperthyroid infant of a hyperthyroid mother had a persistent stare and tachycardia, and failed to gain weight despite a ravenous appetite. Her thyroid gland was not palpable. (Photograph of a case of Drs. R. T. and J. Kirkland, reproduced with their kind permission.)

met, one can withhold treatment and follow the baby's progress.

Thyroid enlargement can also be a feature of neonatal hyperthyroidism. In this case, T4 will be high and TSH will be undetectable unless the infant is still under the influence of his mother's antithyroid medication. Serial measurements of T4 over a brief period will show a continuing rise in contrast to the normal infant's pattern of maximal T4 levels on the second day. In addition to goiter, clinical features of hyperthyroidism in the newborn period include an enormous appetite with failure to gain weight, diarrhea, hyperactivity, sweating, exophthalmos, tachycardia and cardiac failure (Fig. 55–3).

The etiology of neonatal hyperthyroidism has been thought to involve transplacental passage of LATS and other thyroid stimulating immune globulins. Despite several reported exceptions (Hollingsworth et al., 1972), most thyrotoxic infants have been born to thyrotoxic mothers and most have had a brief, self-limited course. Treatment is directed at reducing thyroid hormone synthesis and at minimizing the cardiovascular complications of the disease. Lugol's solution may be given in a dosage of 1 or 2 drops (6 to 12 mg of iodine) by gavage every 8 hours. If serial measurements of T4 show the iodine to be ineffective, or if the process fails to resolve within 4 to 6 weeks, propylthiouracil in a dosage of 5 to 10 mg per kg per day in three divided doses may be used. Digitalization and treatment with propranolol in a dosage of 2 mg per kg per day, as suggested by Smith and Howard, should be employed in infants with severe tachycardia and impending cardiac failure.

## REFERENCES

Andersen, H. J.: Studies in hypothyroidism in children. Acta Paediat. (Supplement) *125*:1, 1961.

Blizzard, R. M., Chandler, R. W., Landing, B. H., Pettit, M.D., and West, C. D.: Maternal autoimmunization as a probable cause of athyreotic cretinism. N. Engl. J. Med. *263*:327, 1960.

Bongiovanni, A. M.: The use and misuse of thyroid hormone in pediatric practice. Pediatrics *33*:585, 1964.

Collipp, P. J., Kaplan, S. A., Kogut, M.D., et al.: Mental retardation in congenital hypothyroidism: Im-

provement with thyroid replacement therapy. Am. J. Ment. Defic. *40*:432, 1965.

Contis, G., Nadas, A. S., and Crigler, J. F.: Cardiac manifestations of congenital hypothyroidism in infants. Pediatrics *38*:452, 1966.

Dussault, J. H., Coulombe, P., Laberge, C., Letarie, J., Guyda, H., and Khoury, K.: Preliminary report on a mass screening program for neonatal hypothyroidism. J. Pediatr. *86*:670, 1975.

Fisher, D. A.: Laboratory diagnosis of thyroid disease. J. Pediatr. *82*:1–9, 187–191, 1973.

Fisher, D. A., Hobel, D. J., Garza, R., and Pierce, C. A.: Thyroid function in the preterm fetus. Pediatrics *46*:208, 1970.

Fisher, D. A., Odell, W. D., and Hobel, C. J.: Thyroid function in the term fetus. Pediatrics *44*:256, 1969.

Hollingsworth, D. R., Mabry, C. C., and Eckard, J. M.: Hereditary aspects of Graves' disease in infancy and childhood. J. Pediatr. *81*:446, 1972.

Homoki, J., Birk, J., Loos, U., Rothenbuchner, G., Fazekas, A.T.A., and Teller, W. M.: Thyroid function in term newborn infants with congenital goiter. J. Pediatr. *86*:753, 1975.

Klein, A. M., Agustin, A. V., and Foley, T. P.: Successful laboratory screening for congenital hypothyroidism. Lancet *2*:77, 1974.

Klein, A. H., Meltzer, S., and Kenny, F. M.: Improved prognosis in congenital hypothyroidism treated before 3 months. J. Pediatr. *81*:912, 1972.

Mestman, J. H., Manning, P. R., and Hodgman, J.: Hyperthyroidism and pregnancy. Arch. Intern. Med. *134*:434, 1974.

Penfold, J. L., and Simpson, D. A.: Premature craniosynostosis—a complication of thyroid replacement therapy. J. Pediatr. *86*:360, 1975.

Raiti, S., and Newns, G. H.: Cretinism: Early diagnosis and its relation to mental prognosis. Arch. Dis. Child. *46*:692, 1971.

Refetoff, S., DeWind, L. T., and De Groot, L. J.: Familial syndrome combining deafmutism, stippled epiphyses, goiter, and abnormally high PBI: Possible target organ refractoriness to thyroid hormone. J. Clin. Endocrinol. Metab. *27*:279, 1967.

Shepard, T. H., Andersen, H. J., and Andersen, H.: The human fetal thyroid. I. Its weight in relation to body weight, crown-rump, estimated gestational age. Anat. Rec. *148*:123, 1964.

Smith, C. S., and Howard, N. J.: Propranolol in treatment of neonatal thyrotoxicosis. J. Pediatr. *83*:1046, 1973.

Stanbury, J. B., Rocmans, P., Buhler, U. K., and Ochi, Y.: Congenital hypothyroidism with impaired thyroid response to thyrotropin. N. Engl. J. Med. *279*:1132, 1968.

Stock, J. M., Surks, M. I., and Oppenheimer, J. H.: Replacement dosage of L-thyroxine in hypothyroidism; A re-evaluation. N. Engl. J. Med. *290*:529, 1974.

Van Middlesworth, L.: Radioactive iodine uptake of normal newborn infants. A.M.A. J. Dis. Child. *88*:439, 1954.

Wilroy, R. S., and Etteldorf, J. N.: Familial hyperthyroidism including two siblings with neonatal Graves' disease. J. Pediatr. *78*:625, 1971.

Winick, M.: Changes in nucleic acid and protein content of the human brain during growth. Pediatr. Res. *2*:353, 1968.

# 56 ABNORMALITIES OF SEXUAL DIFFERENTIATION

*By John S. Parks*

## GENERAL CONSIDERATIONS

Anatomic differentiation of the external genitalia is usually complete in the human infant by birth. This fortunate circumstance enables the obstetrician and proud parents to proclaim, "It's a girl" or, "It's a boy." Permanent gender assignment is made instantaneously. Occasionally, genital differentiation is incomplete or ambiguous. The physician's reactions to these medical emergencies will have an immense impact on the children and their families. It is important to have a sound understanding of normal sexual differentiation, to understand what can go wrong in development and to be able to initiate steps which will lead to appropriate gender assignment, diagnosis and management.

Two principles emerge in the consideration of embryologic sexual differentiation. The first is that sexual organs at all three levels—gonads, internal duct structures and external genitalia—develop from identical undifferentiated structures in the male and female fetus. The second principle is that the female form predominates unless opposed by active male determinants.

Male and female gonads develop from anlagen located on the urogenital ridge, next to the kidney and primitive adrenal. Primordial germ cells migrate into the gonads from the endoderm of the yolk sac. These cells later form either oögonia or spermatogonia. Prior to 6 weeks of gestational age, testis and ovary are indistinguishable. In the fetus with a 46 XY chromosome constitution, definite testicular differentiation occurs rapidly over the ensuing weeks. By 12 weeks, both testicular testosterone concentration (Reyes, Winter and Faiman) and the ability to enzymatically convert pregnenolone to testosterone (Siiteri and Wilson) are maximal. Proliferation and activity of fetal Leydig cells are stimulated by chorionic gonadotropin, which also reaches peak levels at this stage of pregnancy. Early development and function of the testis have important effects on genital development.

In contrast, ovarian differentiation occurs later and is not required for normal female genital development. In the fetus with a 46 XX chromosome complement, oöcytes appear at about the twelfth week. Primordial follicles, containing oöcytes surrounded by a layer of granulosa cells, are recognizable by the twentieth week. Reyes et al. were unable to detect the presence of either testosterone or estradiol in extracts of human ovary at any stage of fetal development. The biological effects of ovarian endocrine function prior to birth are unknown.

A schematic representation of fetal genital development is shown in Figure 56–1. At 7 weeks of gestation, the fetus has precursors of both male and female genital ducts. The mullerian ducts are anlagen of the fallopian tubes, uterus and proximal vagina. Wolffian ducts are anlagen for the epididymis, vas deferens, seminal vesicles and ejaculatory duct of the male. The brilliant experiments of Josso have shown that the fetal testis produces a locally active macromolecular hormone which induces regression of the mullerian ducts. This action cannot be mimicked by androgens. However, high local concentrations of testosterone, produced by the fetal testis, are required for further development of the wolffian ducts. Genital duct development is nearly complete by 12 weeks of gestation.

Male and female external genitalia are also identical during the second month of pregnancy. Three structures are easily recognizable, as shown in Figure 56–1. These structures are the genital tubercle, the genital folds and the genital swellings. Testosterone, and more specifically its active intracellular metabolite dihydrotestosterone, is required for male differentiation. Without testosterone, the genital tubercle re-

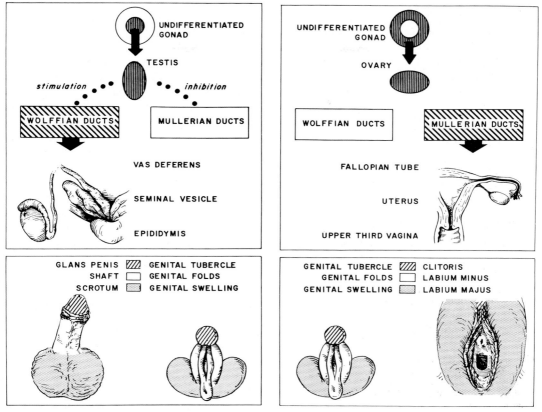

*Figure 56–1.* Outline of genital development. Note that gonadal development occurs from a common indifferent gonad, the internal genitalia develop from separate primordia present in both sexes, and the external genitalia develop in a continuous transformation of anlage common to both sexes. (From Federman, D. D.: N. Engl. J. Med. 277:351, 1967.)

mains small and forms the clitoris, the genital folds remain separate and form the labia minora, and the genital swellings form the labia majora. Virilization causes the genital tubercle to enlarge and form the penis. The genital folds fuse to form a phallic urethra, and the genital swellings fuse to form the scrotum. Fusion is complete by the twelfth week of gestation, but phallic enlargement continues to term.

Following birth, the pituitary gonadotropins LH and FSH rise to reach a peak at 1 to 3 months. In the male infant, there is an accompanying rise in testicular testosterone synthesis which has been shown by Forest et al. to produce plasma testosterone levels equivalent to those achieved in mid-puberty. This burst of activity is not accompanied by clinical signs of further virilization and is succeeded by a decline of tes-

tosterone to barely detectable levels by the end of the first year.

Most of the known errors of human sexual differentiation can be provisionally explained by genetic or biochemical alterations in the sequence of events outlined above. Federman and Grumbach have written excellent detailed reviews of this area. This discussion will follow the classification scheme shown in Table 56–1. The first category entails disorders of gonadal differentiation, usually in association with abnormal number or structure of the X or Y chromosomes. The second category involves virilization of the female fetus, and the third undervirilization of the male fetus. A fourth category involves anatomical defects which, in the majority of instances, do not have a definite chromosomal or hormonal etiology.

# DISORDERS OF GONADAL DIFFERENTIATION

## KLINEFELTER SYNDROME

Klinefelter syndrome is the most common sex chromosome anomaly, occurring once in 500 male births. The 47 XXY chromosome constitution arises through meiotic or mitotic nondisjunction, and is associated with advanced maternal age. Although the testes may be noticeably small during infancy, there are seldom any other genital abnormalities and the diagnosis is seldom made during childhood. Presenting features in older children and adolescents include mental retardation (in about 25 per cent), antisocial behavior, eunuchoid ha-

bitus and gynecomastia with variable virilization at puberty. Infertility is accompanied by the histological finding of hyalinization of the seminiferous tubules. Patients with the variant karyotypes 48,XXYY, 48,XXXY, and 49,XXXXY generally have severe mental retardation, and may be recognized earlier in childhood. De La Chapelle has reviewed 45 cases in which phenotypic males were found to have 46,XX karyotypes. Most had testicular morphology similar to that of 47,XXY males. However, Kasdan et al. have recently reported a family in which this karyotype was compatible with fertility.

## TURNER SYNDROME AND VARIANTS

Turner syndrome is defined as gonadal dysgenesis due to a missing or structurally defective X chromosome. The 45,X karyotype is associated with a high intrauterine mortality. Its frequency is 1 in 20 spontaneous abortuses, but only 1 in 2700 live newborn females. Infants with this condition often have distinctive physical features which have nothing to do with their gonadal abnormalities. The condition should be suspected and appropriate diagnostic tests should be done in female infants with webbing of the neck, edema of the extremities or coarctation of the aorta. Such an infant is shown in Figure 56–2. In this infant, as in the great majority with gonadal dysgenesis, the external genitalia and internal duct structures were unequivocally female. More subtle findings include low birth weight for gestational age, ptosis, hypertelorism, micrognathia, hypertension, cubitus valgus and dysplasia of finger and toe nails. In other children, somatic abnormalities are minimal and the condition is suspected because of short stature, failure of breast development and primary amenorrhea at the age of puberty.

Roughly 85 per cent of girls with gonadal dysgenesis have a 45,X karyotype, and the diagnosis can be made by finding a chromatin negative buccal smear. The remainder have either mosaicism, for example, 46,XX/45,X, or a structure abnormality of the X chromosome. Structural abnormalities include isochromosomes of either the short (XXpi) or long arm (XXqi), deletion of

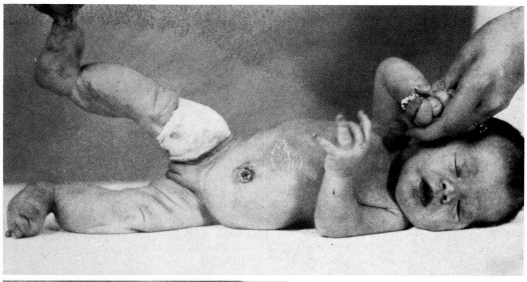

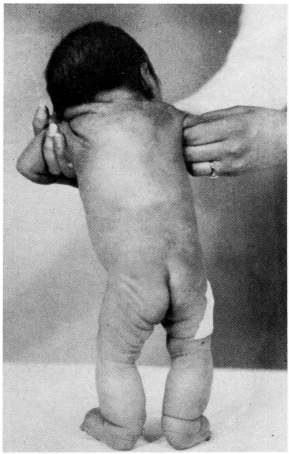

*Figure 56–2.* Edema of the feet extending to the midthigh, and of the hands. The neck is short, and the scalp hair extends to a low level. There are loose folds of skin over the neck.

In this infant an oral mucosal smear showed the chromatin-negative pattern. This is a typical instance of gonadal dysgenesis. (Reproduced from Pediatrics, *20*:743, 1957, with the kind permission of Dr. Melvin M. Grumbach, the author.)

the short (XXp⁻) or long arm (XXq⁻), and ring chromosomes. Mosaicism and structural abnormalities can be detected only by karyotyping.

Suspicion and confirmation of gonadal dysgenesis in a newborn infant confers an unusual responsibility upon the physician. There is seldom any doubt about gender assignment, for these infants are females. However, their ovaries have in most instances regressed to vestigial streaks by the time of birth. It is virtually certain that these girls will be short and infertile as adults. Chromosome findings are confusing to most parents and probably should not be mentioned during early discussions. The parents should be told that their child will be shorter than average and probably infertile, and will require hormone replacement at the age of puberty to foster a growth spurt, breast development and menstrual cycles.

Mosaicism involving the Y chromosome is less common than classical Turner syndrome, and produces a wider variety of phenotypes. Infants with 45,X/46,XY karyotypes commonly have ambiguous genitalia. Gender assignment should be in accordance with the expected potential for adult sexual function. Gonads generally consist of bilateral dysgenetic testes or a dysgenetic testis and a contralateral gonadal streak. Either or both gonads may have failed to produce mullerian inhibiting substance, and there may be a uterus and unilateral or bilateral fallopian tubes. Depending upon the extent and timing of intrauterine testosterone production, there may also be well-developed wolffian structures. Short stature and the somatic abnormalities of Turner syndrome are inconstant findings. Dysgenetic gonads are predisposed to neoplasia and should be removed at an early age. Hormone replacement at the age of puberty must be concordant with the sex of rearing.

## PURE GONADAL DYSGENESIS

Pure gonadal dysgenesis is a term applied to phenotypic females with bilateral streak gonads who lack the somatic stigmata of Turner syndrome. Karyotype may be either 46,XX or 46,XY. The 46,XX patients seldom show clitoral enlargement, may show some ovarian function at puberty and are not prone to gonadal neoplasms. This form of gonadal dysgenesis is transmitted as an autosomal recessive characteristic. Patients with 46,XY gonadal dysgenesis commonly have clitoromegaly at birth, virilize at puberty and are prone to develop gonadal neoplasms. Familial aggregations suggest X-linked recessive or male-limited autosomal dominant inheritance.

## TRUE HERMAPHRODITISM

True hermaphroditism requires the presence of both ovarian and testicular tissue in the same individual. The tissue may be present in the same or opposite gonads. In almost one half there is an ovotestis on one side and an ovary or testis on the other, in one fifth there are bilateral ovotestes, and in one third there is an ovary on one side and a testis on the other. The external genitalia are extremely variable, but roughly three fourths of patients have had phallic enlargement, generally with hypospadias, and have been raised as males. A uterus is usually present, and often is asymmetrical. Genital ducts develop in accordance with the function of the ipsilateral gonad. Chromosomal findings are varied and do not correlate with gonadal histology or external genital appearance. Benirschke et al. reported that of 108 patients, 61 were 46,XX, 23 were 46,XY and the remainder were mosaic. At puberty, some two thirds have breast development, two thirds menstruate, and a large proportion virilize. Male fertility has not been reported.

True hermaphroditism should be considered in any infant or child with ambiguous genitalia in whom an alternative explanation cannot be established from chromosomal, hormonal and radiologic contrast studies. Diagnosis requires laparotomy and biopsy of gonads. Management involves surgical removal of gonads, internal duct structures and features of the external genitalia which are incongruous with gender assignment.

## VIRILIZATION OF THE FEMALE FETUS

Virilization of the female fetus is the most common category of disorders producing ambiguity of the external genitalia. Its mechanisms and consequences are also the most easy to understand. Androgens may enter the maternal and fetal circulation following ingestion or as a result of a virilizing tumor. The female fetus may produce excessive androgens as a result of congenital adrenal hyperplasia. In these instances, the fetal ovaries and genital ducts are normal. Fusion of the genital folds and/or the genital swellings is a result of androgen exposure prior to the twelfth gestational week. Clitoral enlargement can occur with exposure at any time. Buccal smears are chromatin positive, and karyotypes are 46,XX. Medical management of congenital adrenal hyperplasia and surgical correction of anatomical abnormalities are followed by normal pubertal development and normal adult sexual and reproductive function.

## VIRILIZATION BY MATERNAL DRUGS

Virilization of the female fetus has been attributed to testosterone, the 19-nortestosterone progestins, progesterone, and even, paradoxically, diethylstilbestrol. In each case a fairly small proportion of exposed infants had clinically evident virilization. There was seldom evidence of virilization in the mother. It is not known which of these compounds act directly on the external genitalia and which act indirectly through altering androgen synthesis by the mother or fetus. It seems reasonable to speculate that differences in maternal, placental or fetal metabolism of the synthetic steroids may determine which infants are affected.

The incidence of this condition has diminished as the use of synthetic estrogens and progestins for management of threatened abortion has waned. However, the condition is still seen in offspring of women who unknowingly continue to take birth control pills following conception. Severity of virilization is quite variable, from mild clitoral enlargement to complete labial fusion with a phallic urethra. The infant will not show progressive virilization or accelerated growth and skeletal matura-

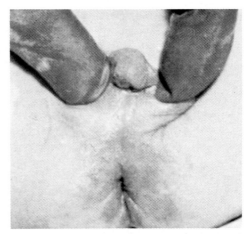

*Figure 56–3.* External genitals of an infant whose mother received large quantities of dehydroxyprogesterone in order to forestall abortion. One can see an enlarged clitoris, with no urethral meatus at its tip, a fused labioscrotum containing no gonads. The single urogenital orifice can be seen to open at the base of the phallus only when this is lifted away.

tion after birth. Even in the presence of a positive history of maternal hormone ingestion, it is mandatory to do a buccal smear and a 24 hour urine for 17-ketosteroids to exclude other possible diagnoses.

## VIRILIZATION BY MATERNAL OVERPRODUCTION OF ANDROGENS

Severe disorders of maternal androgen production generally preclude pregnancy. However, artificial induction of ovulation in a virilized woman, or development of a virilizing neoplasm during pregnancy, can set the stage for virilization of a female infant. In their review of 12 cases, Haymond and Weldon found only one case of adrenal tumor. The remaining 11 mothers had ovarian lesions. In most cases, the mother had clinical signs of virilization such as hirsutism, acne, clitoromegaly and deepening of the voice. In other cases, the fetus had a lower threshold for showing virilization than the mother. The clinical features of the offspring of virilized mothers are identical to those described above for girls whose mothers received sex hormones. Diagnosis requires demonstration of elevated urinary 17-ketosteroids or plasma testosterone in the mother, as well as exclusion of alternative diagnoses in the infant.

## Congenital Adrenal Hyperplasia

This category of diseases is discussed more fully in Chapter 54. Inherited enzymatic blocks in the synthesis of cortisol lead to overproduction of androgens and virilization of the female fetus. Defects in 21-hydroxylase, 3β-hydroxysteroid dehydrogenase and 11-hydroxylase can each produce this result. Buccal smear is chromatin positive, and urinary excretion of 17-ketosteroids remains above 2.5 mg per 24 hours. Treatment with cortisol suppresses adrenal androgen production and prevents further virilization and excessively rapid growth and skeletal maturation. In infants with salt-losing forms of congenital adrenal hyperplasia, cortisol and mineralocorticoid replacement are life saving.

## Undervirilization of the Male Fetus

Complete male genital differentiation requires the presence of testes, the ability of testes to produce testosterone and the ability of the genital anlagen to recognize and respond to testosterone. Defects can occur at each of these levels and result in genitalia that are either ambiguous or unambiguously female and discordant with a normal 46,XY male karyotype.

### Anorchia

In some male infants with cryptorchidism, testes cannot be found during careful surgical exploration. The presumption is that testicular function in utero was sufficient to initiate male genital differentiation but that the testes later underwent degeneration. The process may be analogous to the postulated mechanisms of thyroid dysgenesis. It has been referred to as the "vanishing testis" syndrome. Kirschner et al. have demonstrated, by selective venous catheterization and testosterone measurements, that some androgen production may persist despite the absence of morphologically distinct testicular tissue.

### Defects in the Synthesis of Testosterone

In several varieties of congenital adrenal hyperplasia the enzymatic defect is shared by adrenal and gonadal tissue. The result is undervirilization of the affected male due to impairment of fetal testosterone production. Specific defects include 3β-hydroxysteroid dehydrogenase and 17α-hydroxylase deficiencies discussed in Chapter 54. In these conditions, the enzyme deficiency impairs synthesis of cortisol as well as testosterone.

Defects may also occur in metabolic pathways unique to the synthesis of sex steroids. The 17,20-desmolase enzyme converts 17α-hydroxypregnenolone to dehydroepiandrosterone and 17α-hydroxyprogesterone to androstenedione. Deficiency, as in the family reported by Zachmann et al., leads to severe hypospadias, with or without cryptorchidism, and an elevated urinary excretion of 11-ketopregnanetriol and plasma level of 17α-hydroxypregnenolone. Occurrence in siblings and an "aunt" indicated X-linked recessive or male-limited autosomal dominant inheritance. Testosterone replacement will induce phallic growth and development of male secondary sex characteristics.

The next step in testosterone synthesis involves 17β-hydroxysteroid oxidoreductase, which converts dehydroepiandrosterone to Δ5-androstenediol and androstenedione to testosterone. Deficiency results in ambiguous genitalia and elevated levels of the two substrates for the enzyme. Puberty in the patients reported by Saez et al. was characterized by virilization and gynecomastia. The latter finding was attributed to elevated concentrations of the estrogen estrone.

# END ORGAN INSENSITIVITY TO TESTOSTERONE

### Deficiency of 5α-Reductase

The external genital anlagen of the fetus normally possess 5α-reductase activity and are able to convert testosterone to the active metabolite dihydrotestosterone. This transaction seems to be required for complete male genital development, and a defect at this level may explain an autosomal recessive condition known as "pseudovaginal perineoscrotal hypospadias." An interesting aspect of this condition, also known as the "penis at twelve" syndrome is marked virilization and phallic growth at puberty. In the adult, the ratio of circulating testosterone to dihydrotestosterone is increased.

### TESTICULAR FEMINIZATION

Recognition of testosterone or dihydrotestosterone by target tissues requires the participation of a cytoplasmic receptor protein which binds the steroid, enters the nucleus and interacts with nuclear chromatin to alter gene expression. Genetic disorders in the rat and mouse have been shown to involve receptor defects and closely parallel the human condition of testicular feminization.

In the complete form of the disorder, 46,XY infants have unambiguously female external genitalia. Unless there are inguinal hernias containing testes, recognition may be delayed until puberty, when these girls show normal breast development but lack sexual hair and fail to menstruate. The vagina ends blindly and the uterus and fallopian tubes are absent, reflecting the intrauterine production of and response to mullerian inhibiting substance. The disorder is familial, with multiple sibling involvement and occurrence in maternal aunts suggesting X-linked recessive or male-limited autosomal dominant inheritance. The gender assignment is unquestionably female. Gonads should be removed because of a high incidence of malignant degeneration. Estrogen replacement at puberty enhances breast development but does not induce menses, because there is no uterus.

Partial testicular feminization implies a partial defect in recognition of testosterone with an attendant partial inhibition of male genital differentiation. Wilson et al. have suggested that many familial cases of microphallus, hypospadias and gynecomastia with normal testosterone production at puberty fall in this category. They propose the term "familial, incomplete male pseudohermaphroditism, type I" to encompass conditions described separately by Reifenstein, Lubs, Gilbert-Dreyfus and Rosewater.

## ISOLATED ANATOMICAL ABNORMALITIES

### CRYPTORCHIDISM

For a discussion of cryptorchidism, see Chapter 44.

### PERSISTENCE OF MULLERIAN DUCTS

A fully developed uterus and fallopian tubes may be discovered incidental to surgery in phenotypic males with normal 46,XY karyotypes. The theoretical explanation of this finding is a failure of production or recognition of mullerian inhibiting substance. The condition may be transmitted as an autosomal recessive trait. Treatment consists of removal of organs that are discordant with the patient's gender.

## ANATOMICAL ABNORMALITIES IN ASSOCIATION WITH OTHER DEFECTS

Malformations of the external genitalia may be a part of a more complicated embryopathy. In females, genital abnormalities may be associated with imperforate anus, renal agenesis or congenital nephritis and other congenital malformations of the lower intestine and genitourinary tract. Drash and associates have reported an association between degenerative renal disease, Wilms' tumor and ambiguity of the external genitalia in males. Rimoin and Schimke's monograph has an excellent discussion of associations between genital abnormalities and largely non-endocrine syndromes. In many instances such infants have severe defects incompatible with life, but one still has the problem of assigning gender.

## EVALUATION OF INFANTS WITH AMBIGUOUS GENITALIA

It is extremely important that the evaluation of a newborn with ambiguous genitalia be carried out immediately after birth. A flow chart in Figure 56–4 indicates studies that can be carried out to provide a provisional diagnosis and a firm gender assign-

*Procedure*

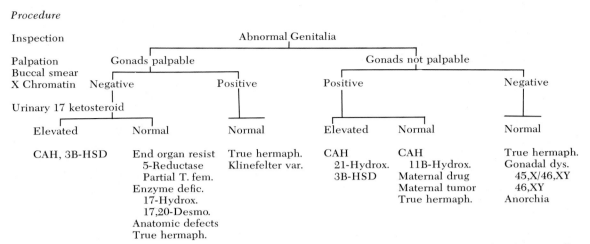

**Figure 56–4.** Investigation of the infant with ambiguous genitalia. Palpation of gonads is useful in that it usually is associated with an X chromatin negative buccal smear and a 46,XY karyotype. However, testicular non-descent can occur in virtually all of the enzymatic deficiency syndromes.

ment in the first 72 hours. The parents should be advised that their infant's genital development had not been completed by birth, that the baby is all girl or all boy and not a little bit of both, that tests will be done to determine the correct sex, and that announcement of the birth to friends and relatives should be delayed until the tests are returned.

Inspection of the external genitalia will reveal a phallic structure that is small for a male or large for a girl. There is likely to be chordee with hypospadias. The genital swellings may be fused or open. A urologic surgeon should be involved quite early in the examination of the infant. If the phallus shows little potential for penile function, a female gender assignment will be made regardless of further findings. However, the converse is not true. The degree of phallic enlargement should not preclude a female gender assignment. Palpation for gonads is extremely important, for these gonads are usually testes.

The buccal smear for determination of sex chromatin should be done on the first day of life. Although the number of positive chromatin bodies may be diminished in comparison to adult values, there should be no overlap of results between 46,XX females and 46,XY males. The chromatin positive infant should be considered to

have virilizing congenital adrenal hyperplasia until proved otherwise Lymphocyte karyotyping should be done on the same indications as the buccal smear, but analysis takes weeks rather than hours.

Determination of 17-ketosteroid and pregnanetriol excretion can be done in the first 72 hours. An alternative is to measure serum pregnanetriol by gas chromatography, as reported by Bongiovanni. Infants with congenital adrenal hyperplasia due to 21-hydroxylase or 3$\beta$-hydroxysteroid dehydrogenase will show an increase rather than a decrease in 17-ketosteroid excretion during the first week, with levels remaining above 2.5 mg per 24 hours.

History taking is extremely important. There should be a complete inquiry about all medications taken during pregnancy. Family history may reveal unexplained infant deaths among siblings of infants with salt-losing congenital adrenal hyperplasia. Infants with defects in testosterone synthesis or with partial testicular feminization commonly have hypogonadal maternal uncles, or maternal "aunts" with primary amenorrhea.

By 72 hours, a definite gender assignment will have been made in most cases. Chromatin positive infants will almost always be female. Those who do not have congenital adrenal hyperplasia, virilization due to maternal drugs or tumor, or associated birth defects will probably require laparotomy and gonadal biopsy in later infancy. Chromatin negative infants may have a male or female gender assignment depending on phallic structure. They will require karyotyping to exclude 45,X/46,XY mosaicism, further serum and urinary steroid measurement to define rare abnormalities of adrenal or gonadal steroid synthesis and contrast studies of the genitourinary tract to search for mullerian duct structures. Laparotomy and gonadal biopsy can safely be deferred to a later age.

The pioneering studies of Money and the Hampsons have shown that karyotype, gonads, internal ducts and hormones have very little to do with behavior and psychosexual inclinations. These features are chiefly influenced by gender assignment and home environment. If the parents are secure about their boy or girl, the gender role is firmly established in early infancy and can rarely be reversed. The physician's role is to be sure that the physical and hormonal state of the growing child is not seriously at odds with the gender assignment. In the girl with congenital adrenal hyperplasia, this involves glucocorticoid replacement, consideration of clitorectomy and vaginoplasty if needed in infancy, and continued follow-up after maturity. In the male with hypospadias and deficient testosterone production, it means surgical repair of hypospadias and evaluation of the need for testosterone replacement at the age of puberty. The genetic male with a female gender assignment needs protection from confusing information about chromosomes, and may require gonadectomy before puberty to prevent virilization.

## REFERENCES

Aarskog, D.: Clinical and cytogenetic studies in hypospadias. Acta Paediat. Scand. (Suppl.) *203*:1, 1970.

Benirschke, K., Naftolin, F., Gittes, R., Khudr, G., Yen, S. S. C., and Allen, F. H., Jr.: True hermaphroditism and chimerism. Am. J. Obstet. Gynecol. *113*:449. 1972.

Bongiovanni, A. M., Parks, J. S., Ranke, M., Kirkland, R., and Vaidya, V.: Gas-liquid chromatography in the diagnosis of congenital adrenal hyperplasia. J. Steroid Biochem. 5:467, 1974.

de la Chappelle, A.: Nature and origin of males with XX sex chromosomes. Am. J. Hum. Genet. *24*:71, 1972.

Drash, A., Sherman, F., Hartmann, W. H., and Blizzard, R. M.: A syndrome of pseudohermaphroditism, Wilm's tumor, hypertension, and degenerative renal disease. J. Pediatr. 76:585, 1970.

Federman, D. D.: Abnormal Sexual Development. Philadelphia, W. B. Saunders Company, 1967.

Forest, M. G., Sizonenko, P. C., Cathiard, A. M., and Bertrand, J.: Hypophyso-gonadal function in humans during the first year of life. I. Evidence for testicular activity in early infancy. J. Clin. Invest. 53:819, 1974.

Grumbach, M. M., and Van Wyk, J. J.: Disorders of sex differentiation. *In* Williams, R. H. (Ed.): Textbook of Endocrinology. Philadelphia, W. B. Saunders Company, 1974, p. 423.

Haymond, M. W., and Weldon, V. V.: Female pseudohermaphroditism secondary to a maternal virilizing tumor. J. Pediatr. 82:682, 1973.

Imperato-McGinley, J., Guerrero, L., Gautier, T., and Peterson, R. E.: An unusual form of male pseudohermaphroditism: A model of 5α-reductase deficiency in man. Science *186*:1214, 1974.

Josso, N.: Permeability of membranes to the mullerian-inhibiting substance synthesized by the human fetal testis in vitro: A clue to its biochemical nature. J. Clin. Endocrinol. Metab. *34*:265, 1972.

Kasdan, R., Nankin, H. R., Troen, P., Wald, N., Pan, S., and Yanaihara, T.: Paternal transmission of maleness in XX human beings. N. Engl. J. Med. *288*:539, 1973.

Kirschner, M. A., Jacobs, J. B., and Fraley, E. E.: Bilateral anorchia with persistent testosterone production. N. Engl. J. Med. *282*:240, 1970.

Money, J., Hampson, J. G., and Hampson, J. L.: Hermaphroditism: Recommendations concerning assignment of sex, change of sex and psychologic management. Bull. Johns Hopkins Hosp. *96*:253, 1955.

Reyes, F. I., Winter, J. S. D., and Faiman, C.: Studies on human sexual development. I. Fetal gonadal and adrenal sex steroids. J. Clin. Endocrinol. Metab. *37*:74, 1973.

Rimoin, D. L., and Schimke, R. N.: Genetic Disoders of the Endocrine Glands. Saint Louis, The C. V. Mosby Company, 1971.

Saez, J. M., Morera, A. M., dePeretti, E., and Bertrand, J.: Further in vivo studies in male pseudohermaphroditism with gynecomastia due to a testicular 17-ketosteroid reductase defect (compared to a case of testicular feminization). J. Clin. Endocrinol. Metab. *34*:598, 1972.

Siiteri, P. K., and Wilson, J. D.: Testosterone formation and metabolism during male sexual differentiation in the human embryo. J. Clin. Endocrinol. Metab. *38*:113, 1974.

Sorenson, H. R.: Hypospadias, with Special Reference to Aetiology. Copenhagen, Munksgaard, 1953.

Wilson, J. D., Harrod, M. J., Goldstein, J. L., Hemsell, D. L., and MacDonald, P. C.: Familial incomplete male pseudohermaphroditism, type I. Evidence for androgen resistance and variable clinical manifestations in a family with the Reifenstein syndrome. N. Engl. J. Med. *290*:1097, 1974.

Zachmann, M., Völlmin, J. A., Hamilton, W., et al.: Steroid 17,20-desmolase deficiency: a new cause of male pseudohermaphroditism. Clin. Endocrinol. *1*:369, 1972.

# 57

## DISORDERS OF CARBOHYDRATE METABOLISM

### *Revised by Marvin Cornblath*

This chapter is included in the section on disorders caused by endocrine dysfunction even though abnormalities in carbohydrate homeostasis may result from deficiencies in specific enzyme abnormalities (such as galactosemia, hereditary fructose intolerance and pre-term SGA), availability or utilization of multiple substrates (ketones, lactate, glycerol, alanine) as well as relative or absolute hyperinsulinism (transient diabetes mellitus, pituitary "aplasia," islet cell adenoma or hyperplasia). Single or multiple endocrine glands, such as the pancreas (through either insulin or glucagon), pituitary, thyroid, adrenal cortex and medulla, as well as the liver all play important roles in carbohydrate metabolism. One or several of these regulatory factors may operate to throw blood sugar homeostasis out of kilter. Sufficient clinical experience and laboratory data are now available to provide a useful clinical and pathological classification.

### GENERAL CONSIDERATIONS

It is necessary to understand the blood sugar pattern of the normal newborn before one can evaluate the deviations from normal. We shall not here go into details of the methodology involved, because this has been covered thoroughly by Cornblath and Schwartz and by others. It is sufficient to say that measurements of total reducing substances are not adequate; it is necessary to measure the true glucose levels in blood in order to understand properly the state of the carbohydrate metabolism.

The blood glucose level in umbilical cord blood is proportional to, but lower than it is in, maternal blood. The scatter at birth is great, depending upon a like scatter in the mother's blood, whether she has eaten recently or not, whether she has been receiving intravenous fluids or not, and so forth. This concentration drops initially to a mean level, in presumably normal full-term babies, of 55 to 60 mg per 100 ml at 2 to 4 hours. Cornblath and Reisner found a range of 30 to 120 mg in 95 per cent of these babies. From then on the mean curve rises until it reaches the 70- to 80-mg level from 72 hours onward. After this time a level in whole blood below 40 mg per 100 ml or exceeding 125 would be considered abnormal (Fig. 57–1).

All series include many blood glucose values in the 40's and 30's, a few in the 20's and an occasional one below 20 mg per 100 ml some time within the first 24 hours of life. Cornblath et al., in their 1961 study, found 14 per cent of their full-term infants born of normal mothers to have at least one true blood sugar level of less than 30 mg per 100 ml some time within the first 24 hours of life. More recently, Lubchenco and Bard found 11.4 per cent of a general nursery population with blood glucose levels less than 30 mg per 100 ml before 6 hours of age and prior to the first feed. None of these normal infants with blood sugar levels in the range considered hypoglycemic for older persons seemed the least bit discommoded by these low concentrations.

Agreement is general also with respect to the sugar concentration in the blood of low birth weight infants. Gittelman and Pincus found their mean level to be 39, with a range of 20 to 73 mg per 100 ml, whereas in an earlier study, utilizing exactly the same methods, they had reported a mean of 54.9 for full-term normals. Lubchenco and Bard found a greater incidence of blood sugars below 30 mg per 100 ml in preterm than in term infants, and Beard et al. reported an increased frequency with delayed feedings. Baens et al. carried on their study for a longer period and found that after the rise from 3 to 12 hours of age, the true blood sugar of their small infants fell to its lowest level on the third and fourth days, when the mean was as low as 39. They noted that a single hypoglycemic reading was not accompanied by signs or symptoms, but that repeated ones often were. Pildes and her co-workers found hypoglycemia (levels less than 20) in at least two successive readings in 5 to 6 per cent of all infants weighing less than 2500 gm at birth. All these infants fell below the fiftieth percentile for weight in relation to gestational age, and half of them fell below the tenth percentile. Of four sets of twins who were 25 per cent or more discordant in birth weight, and of whom the smaller weighed less than 2000 gm, hypoglycemia was found in the smaller twin. Thus, intrauterine growth retardation plays a great role in the production of neonatal hypoglycemia. It is likely that hypoglycemia can be forestalled in the infant of low birth weight, not always but often, by early feeding. If it has not been, it should be treated vigorously like all other neonatal hypoglycemias.

## THE HYPOGLYCEMIAS

Virtually everyone now accepts the definition of neonatal hypoglycemia as a whole blood sugar level of less than 30 mg per 100 ml (less than 35 mg in serum or plasma) in the first 72 hours of life, or of less than 40 mg (less than 45 mg in serum or plasma) after the third day, in full-term, full-size infants. In infants of low birth weight the lower figure of normal is set at 20 mg per 100 ml in whole blood or 25 in plasma or serum. One such reading is adequate for initiating therapy, but a second blood or cerebrospinal glucose analysis should be obtained. Two successive low readings must be obtained to establish a definitive diagnosis if the infant is asymptomatic.

**PATHOGENESIS.** There are many pathogenetic mechanisms involved in the production of hypoglycemia. The following list encompasses the majority.

1. Inadequate production or sparing of glucose
   A. Malnutrition
      1. Lack of glycogen or fat
      2. Lack of alternate substrates (i.e., ketones, glycerol, F.F.A.
      3. Lack of substrate or precursors, starvation, reduction in hepatic glucose output
   B. Block in gluconeogenesis
      1. Enzymatic immaturity or deficiency (i.e., fructose-diphosphatase)
      2. Excess insulin
      3. Homeostatic imbalance
2. Excessive utilization of glucose
   A. Hyperinsulinism
      1. Relative secondary to isolated or multiple endocrine deficiencies (e.g., hypothalamic deficiency or congenital hypopituitarism)
      2. Absolute or hyperinsulinemia
         a) Transient—IDM, erythroblastosis
         b) Persistent
            Islet cell adenoma, nesidioblastosis hyperplasia, Beckwith, "infant giant"

*Figure 57–1.* A total of 206 determinations of blood glucose levels were obtained in 179 full-sized infants (>2.5 kg) and a total of 442 determinations, in 104 low birth weight infants (<2.5 kg) throughout the neonatal period. (From Cornblath and Reisner, N. Engl. J. Med. 273:378, 1965.)

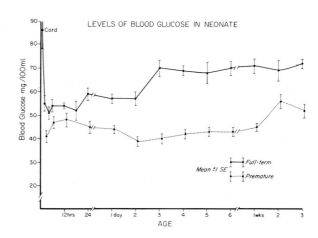

B. Hypermetabolism—small for gestational age
3. Functional, following
   A. Amino acid (i.e., leucine)
   B. Glucose
   C. Glucagon
4. Stress—requiring additional glucose
   A. Perinatal asphyxia—Term, appropriate or large for gestational age
   B. Anoxia, polycythemia
   C. Sepsis
   D. Hypothermia

We propose to discuss these various disorders in the sequence in which the attending physician would normally consider them.

First, the physician should perform blood glucose determinations on certain newborns routinely. They are mandatory for all infants of diabetic mothers and for all low birth weight babies who fall below the tenth percentile for gestational age. Such studies might well be done on all who fall below the fiftieth percentile, especially if an elevation of the hematocrit coexists. It is important that glucose values be done also on all infants with severe hemolytic disease of the newborn, before and often after exchange transfusion.

It would seem wise to perform regular observations of the glucose level on all undergrown preterm infants, perhaps all those weighing 1500 gm or less, through the first 4 days of life. We would recommend a few determinations on all hypothermic newborns, as well as on all macrosomic ones, especially if exomphalos is present (Beckwith-Wiedemann) or if associated with micropenis (Cornblath) or midline defects such as cleft lip or palate.

The attending physician will do this in order not to miss hypoglycemia, even if it is totally asymptomatic. There is no established schedule for the performance of these tests. Since hypoglycemia occurs as late as the third or even the fourth day in small, preterm or small for gestational age infants, clearly several tests should be made on them in the first 4 days. Infants of diabetic mothers, on the other hand, are usually only in jeopardy for the first 24 hours; therefore, determinations should be made at perhaps 2- to 4- hour intervals until it is evident that the initial drop is not to too low a level, or until the initial

fall has been followed by a substantial rise. In erythroblastosis fetalis frequent tests are particularly desirable after the beginning of exchange transfusions with ACD blood.

**CLASSIFICATION.** Recent data permit the differentiation of at least four clinical categories of neonatal hypoglycemia. As modified from Cornblath and Schwartz, these include the following categories:
   I. Early transitional
   II. Secondary
   III. Classical or transient symptomatic
   IV. Severe, recurrent or protracted

Category I occurs during the first 6 to 12 hours of life, is associated with perinatal distress, increased frequency of diabetes mellitus in the mother and moderately severe erythroblastosis, but with a normal frequency of toxemia and twins. There is no sex predilection. Delayed feedings may be important. Over 80 per cent of the infants are asymptomatic. The hypoglycemia is usually of short duration (<12 hours) and recurs infrequently. The hypoglycemia usually responds to relatively small quantities of glucose (<6 mg/kg/min).

Category II can be characterized as hypoglycemia associated with or secondary to a specific event, usually in a symptomatic infant. Thus, hypoglycemia has been reported with the following: 1) congenital and acquired defects in the central nervous system; 2) sepsis (Yeung); 3) congenital heart disease; 4) asphyxia, anoxia and preterminal; 5) hypothermia; 6) drugs to the mother; 7) abrupt cessation of hypertonic glucose; 8) endocrine deficiency (hypothyroidism and adrenal hemorrhage); 9) multiple congenital anomalies; and 10) hypocalcemia. These combinations are important because a low blood glucose should not eliminate the consideration of other pathology and some of the symptomatology and residual damage in the multiple entities enumerated may be secondary to hypoglycemia.

Category III, classical transient hypoglycemia, is associated with a high incidence of toxemia (hypertensive disease of pregnancy) in the mother and of twinning. The infants are usually small for gestational age; males predominate (2.5 ♂:1 ♀), and close to 80 per cent have clinical manifestations of hypoglycemia ranging from episodes of tremor, cyanosis, apnea and irritability to convulsions. Often associated with the hypoglycemia are 1) polycythemia (15 per cent), 2) hypocalcemia (12 per cent), 3) central nervous system pathology (10 to 15 per cent), and 4) cardiac enlargement with or without pulmonary edema (15 per cent). Treatment must be vigorous (8 to 10 mg glucose per kg per minute) and sustained for 48 to 72 hours or more, and as many as 10 per cent of the infants will have recurrent hypoglycemia later in infancy.

Category IV represents severe, recurrent or persistent hypoglycemia including specific syndromes associated with relative or absolute hyperinsulinism or specific enzymatic or metabolic abnormalities. A useful classification follows.

A. Hormone deficiencies
   1. Multiple—pituitary aplasia or hypoplasia
   2. Primary—pituitary, thyroid, adrenal cortex or medulla
B. Hormone excess—hyperinsulinism
   1. Exomphalos—macroglossia—gigantism syndrome of Beckwith-Wiedemann
   2. "Infant giants"
   3. Islet cell pathology including:
      a. Adenoma
      b. Nesidioblastosis
      c. Hyperplasia
      d. Leucine or other amino acid sensitivity
C. Hereditary defects in carbohydrate metabolism
   1. Glycogen storage disease, Type I
   2. Fructose intolerance
   3. Galactosemia
   4. Glycogen synthetase deficiency
   5. Fructose, 1-6 diphosphatase deficiency
D. Hereditary defects in amino acid metabolism
   1. Maple syrup urine disease
   2. Propionic acidemia
   3. Methylmalonic acidemia
   4. Tyrosinosis

Thus, hypoglycemia in the neonate may be of multiple etiology, pathogenesis, and significance.

## EARLY TRANSITIONAL HYPOGLYCEMIA (CATEGORY I)

Infants with this type of hypoglycemia include those with perinatal distress, delayed feeding, moderately severe erythro-

blastosis and those of mothers with gestational (IGDM) or with insulin dependent diabetes mellitus (IDM). It should be noted that hypoglycemia occurred before, during or following exchange transfusion in 18 per cent of infants with severe hemolytic disease (cord hemoglobin <10 gm/100 ml) (Raivio and Österlund, 1969). Only the IGDM and IDM will be discussed here.

INFANTS OF DIABETIC MOTHERS. Although as many as 50 per cent of infants of diabetic mothers (IDM) and 25 per cent of infants of gestational diabetic mothers (IGDM) have blood glucose levels of less than 30 mg per 100 ml during the first 2 to 6 hours of life, the majority of these infants show no untoward effects from their hypoglycemia. Many will recover spontaneously, others will respond dramatically to glucagon (300 $\mu$g or 0.3 mg per kg intramuscularly or intravenously, not to exceed 1.0 mg total), while a few have persistently low values which may be associated with clinical manifestations and require parenteral glucose to maintain normoglycemia (1 per cent to 10–20 per cent). Yet, there appears to be little if any correlation between low glucose levels and either mortality or morbidity. Many infants with low levels have been alert and lively when their blood sugar was at its lowest.

The multiple problems of the IGDM and IDM, including frequency of respiratory distress (p. 134), hyperbilirubinemia, polycythemia, hypocalcemia and perhaps hypomagnesemia as well as congenital malformations, make their hypoglycemia only one aspect of concern and management. Again, if the blood sugar remains low or coexists with symptoms, parenteral glucose support is indicated (see pp. 80 to 83).

## SECONDARY HYPOGLYCEMIA (CATEGORY II)

Hypoglycemia has been reported closely associated with or precipitated by a number of events, ranging from the abrupt cessation of hypertonic glucose infusion to infections and central nervous system abnormalities including congenital defects, birth injury, microcephaly, hemorrhage and kernicterus. Thus it is important that a hypoglycemic glucose level not eliminate the possibility of other pathology. Furthermore, some of the manifestations and damage in a number of neonatal pathological states may be due to associated hypoglycemia.

In three reported series (Koviosto et al., Fluge, and Gutberlet and Cornblath), of a total of 447 infants with hypoglycemic blood levels, 238 or 53.2 per cent were considered to have "secondary hypoglycemia."

## CLASSICAL TRANSIENT HYPOGLYCEMIA (CATEGORY III)

It was not until 1959 that the occurrence of hypoglycemia in groups of newborn infants other than infants of diabetic mothers was noted by Cornblath, Odell and Levin. They described eight infants born of mothers with toxemia who had tremors, cyanosis and occasionally convulsions in association with hypoglycemia. The time of recognition of symptoms was between 2½ hours and 7 days, with the peak between 24 and 48 hours. Since then, many clinics have described similar hypoglycemia in groups of infants, the majority of whom are of low birth weight for gestational age.

This syndrome is associated with an increased frequency of maternal toxemia and twinning, as well as central nervous system abnormalities (10 to 15 per cent), polycythemia (15 per cent), hypocalcemia (12 per cent) and cardiomegaly (15 per cent).

The symptoms of hypoglycemia include tremors, convulsions, bouts of apnea, apathy, refusal to feed, cyanosis, irritability and limpness, all of which are nonspecific and may exist for a variety of other reasons. Their nonspecific nature has led some to challenge their relationship to hypoglycemia. However, when two or more successive blood glucose values are low, and these symptoms disappear with the administration of parenteral glucose, it is hard to avoid the conclusion that they are related.

The frequency of hypoglycemia is 2 to 3 per thousand live births. Of infants less than 2500 gm birth weight, who have blood glucose levels determined daily, 5 to 6 per cent will show blood glucose levels of less than 20 mg per 100 ml on at least two occasions, according to Wybregt et al.

Once a blood glucose level of less than 30 mg per 100 ml is found in a full-term infant, or of less than 20 mg in one weighing less than 2500 gm, one repeats the determination if the baby is asymptomatic, and approximately 20 per cent are asymptomatic. If this is also low, or if the original low figure was accompanied by any of the above-mentioned symptoms, treatment is begun promptly. Symptomatic infants are given 0.5 to 1.0 gm per kg of 25 per cent glucose in water intravenously rapidly at the rate of 1.0 ml per minute, followed by a continuous infusion of glucose at the rate of 8 to 10 mg per kg per minute. Thus, for a daily fluid requirement of 65 to 85 ml per kg per day, use 20 per cent glucose water. After 12 to 24 hours add 40 mEq per liter of NaCl, and after 24 to 48 hours of intravenous therapy, add 1 to 2 mEq per kg per day of KCl. Oral feedings should be started as soon as the child's condition permits. Some infants remain hypoglycemic even after this amount of supplementary glucose. Glucagon is of no help to these babies, because their stores of glycogen appear to be exhausted. Diazoxide is not recommended because of its untoward side effects. Cortisone, on the other hand, may be very effective in raising the blood sugar level. If this is truly transient symptomatic hypoglycemia, both the added glucose and the cortisone will be able to be withdrawn after a few days.

Initial studies to be done when hypoglycemia is discovered and verified include a lumbar puncture to rule out intracranial bleeding, a hematocrit determination, a urinalysis for galactose or other reducing sugars and for acetone (with glycogen storage disease in mind) and a blood calcium. A roentgenogram of the chest for heart size is also indicated.

The blood sugar curve should be followed by determinations every 4 to 6 hours.

Further studies are indicated if the symptoms persist or recur. If the serum calcium is found to be below 7.0 mg per 100 ml, as it not infrequently is in these babies, calcium should be given as described for the hypocalcemias (p. 485).

All agree that symptomatic infants must be treated vigorously. Whether or not low blood sugar values are physiologic and without hazard in asymptomatic infants remains to be determined. Newborns may not respond to unusually low blood sugar levels with tremors or convulsions because of availability of other substrates such as ketones, lactate or glycerol to support cerebral function or because of some cerebral refractoriness comparable to their ability to withstand prolonged hypoxia. Indeed, the study of Anderson, Milner and Strich discovered "extensive degeneration of nerve cells in the central nervous system" in three infants who died with untreated hypoglycemia, whereas in three others whose hypoglycemia was corrected, but who died from other causes later, only slight abnormalities were found in the brain. For this reason it is advised that all hypoglycemic infants, symptomatic or not, be treated.

Follow-up of babies with transient hypoglycemia reveals that the great majority recover completely, although a few may have recurrences at some later date. In a prospective controlled 5 to 7 year follow-up of 39 hypoglycemic and 41 normoglycemic matched controls Pildes et al. found no differences in mean height or weight or EEG records. However, the hypoglycemic group had smaller head circumferences, a higher incidence of neurological abnormalities and a larger number of children with I.Q. scores below 86 than the control group. Asymptomatic infants had a better prognosis than did those with convulsions.

## SEVERE RECURRENT OR PERSISTENT HYPOGLYCEMIA (CATEGORY IV)

If hypoglycemia proves to be recalcitrant to the aforementioned management, or if it disappears only to recur promptly, one must begin a search for other causes, as outlined under Category IV earlier. Only a few of the syndromes in this category will be discussed here.

*Multiple Endocrine Deficiencies.* Associated with anterior pituitary "aplasia" or hypoplasia or perhaps a hypothalamic abnormality, at least 22 such patients have been reviewed by Sadeghi-Nejad and Senior, and Cornblath and Schwartz. The infants tend to have an increased birth weight (mean 3.81 kg for 14); males predominate 2:1; and in 20 per cent a sibling was affected to a varying degree. In addition to an 85 per cent frequency of severe symptomatic hypoglycemia in the first hours and days of life, jaundice, hypocalcemia, hepatomegaly and edema were relatively common. Another noteworthy abnormality in the males was a small phallus, or micropenis, reported in nine of 11 patients. A few infants had had midline deformities including clefts of the palate and lips. To date, the prognosis is guarded. A high index of suspicion must be maintained, and critical laboratory studies such as a blood sample for glucose, HGH, ACTH, cortisol, $T_4$, TSH and insulin must be done prior to initiating therapy. Therapy requires immediate parenteral glucose plus steroids. Further replacement therapy may be introduced as specific endocrine deficiencies are documented.

Recognizing its familial occurrence, Sadeghi-Nejad and Senior reported a patient who survived normally as a result of prompt therapy initiated on the basis of history of the death of a previous sibling. They suggest all future pregnancies be monitored with maternal plasma or urinary estriol values to anticipate affected fetuses.

### Hormone Excess–Hyperinsulinism

1. THE EXOMPHALOS-MACROGLOSSIA-GIGANTISM (EMG) SYNDROME OF BECKWITH-WIEDEMANN (page 521). Although not a constant finding, hypoglycemias of varying severity and duration have been reported in many of these infants during the first days of life. Much of the neonatal mortality and subsequent morbidity have been attributed to untreated hypoglycemia, but the evidence is far from conclusive. Carbohydrate tolerance tests and microscopic examination of the pancreas support the idea that hyperinsulinemia is responsible for the hypoglycemia.

This syndrome is characterized by omphalocele, muscular macroglossia, gigantism, visceromegaly and mild microcephaly, as well as diffuse cytomegaly of the adrenal fetal cortex and hyperplasia of the kidneys, pancreas and gonadal interstitial cells. Advanced bone age, abnormal insertion of the diaphragm, flame nevus of the face, earlobe fissures and hemihypertrophy also occur.

Over 50 patients have been reported and extensive reviews of the syndrome have been published.

2. "INFANT GIANTS" OR FOETOPATHIA DIABETICA. Infants with this syndrome, as reported originally by Hansson and Redin, have severe, intractable hypoglycemia that is refractory to all medical therapy and have required total pancreatectomy for metabolic control.

In the patients reported or known to us, birth weight usually exceeded 3800 grams, three quarters were female and the onset of clinical manifestations of hypoglycemia occurred shortly after birth and before 48 hours of age. Survivors are rare and tend to be retarded. Early recognition and total pancreatectomy offer the best prognosis.

3. ISLET CELL ADENOMA. Prior to 1959, only one neonate with questionable islet cell adenoma had been reported by Sherman in 1947. Since then, however, 13 infants with islet cell adenoma have been reported and others are known to us from CPC's or from difficult diagnostic consultations. Prior to 1967, three of five patients were diagnosed at autopsy; thereafter, only one of nine was so diagnosed and the age at surgery was significantly younger than before.

The sex ratio of males to females was 1.6 to 1, no infant was of low birth weight and mean birth weight was 3344 grams. In seven patients, diazoxide was ineffective in normalizing the blood glucose, as was every other type of medical therapy. The only diagnostic laboratory finding was a relatively high insulin to glucose ratio; that is, the plasma insulin values exceeded 10 microunits per ml when the blood glucose was less than 15 to 20 mg per 100 ml—thus a relative hyperinsulinism was apparent. Another diagnostic feature was that glucose infusion rates of 15 to 20 mg per kg per minute may be needed to attain normoglycemic glucose levels.

At operation, isolated tumors were found in 10 and two or more adenomata in three, thus the majority of infants had a partial to almost complete pancreatectomy. Six tumors were in the tail of the pancreas, three in the head, two in the body and two at the junction of the head and the body. The majority of infants had immediate hy-

perglycemia of quite significant magnitude following surgery, and this feature may be of diagnostic importance if the hyperinsulinism is due to discrete beta cell pathology.

Recently, diagnoses have been made earlier, and a number of infants are alive and well at follow-up. Others have moderate to severe neurological or mental defects, or both. Early diagnosis and therapy are critical and depend upon a high index of suspicion and reliable plasma insulin assays of blood obtained when the infant is hypoglycemic.

4. NESIDIOBLASTOSIS. Nesidioblastosis has recently been more frequently recognized as a cause of hypoglycemia, owing to the earlier and more aggressive surgical approach to hypoglycemia in infancy coupled with advances in understanding pancreatic histology by special staining (Yakovac et al.), electron-microscopy and specific immunofluorescent techniques (Orci and Zuppinger, in Cornblath and Schwartz, and Hirsh et al., 1976). Since 1971, the number of infants in whom this diagnosis has been verified by biopsy or pancreatectomy has increased (Yakovac et al., Harken et al., Grampa et al., Zuppinger, Hirsh et al., and Gabbay and Loo). The infants may present with the same broad spectrum of clinical manifestations as those associated with islet cell adenoma. The patients with severe hypoglycemia are equally refractory to all medical therapy including Diazoxide, growth hormone or steroids. There is a relatively high plasma insulin to glucose ratio here, as well. Recently, Hirsch et al. reported elevated plasma glucagon values in two patients, who responded normally to exogenous glucagon and had normal intravenous glucose tolerance tests. Since no laboratory tests are specific or diagnostic, early surgical intervention for biopsy or partial (75–85 per cent) pancreatectomy is indicated. If the hypoglycemia recurs, "total" pancreatectomy may be necessary (Harken et al.). At the time of surgery, special handling of the biopsy or surgical specimen is essential to prepare the tissue for electron-microscopy and immunofluorescent studies. Recently, in addition to the wide scattering of islet cells among ductular and acinar tissue

(Yakovac et al.), Orci and Zuppinger have demonstrated that the diffuse islet cells include beta cells containing insulin, alpha cells containing glucagon and D cells containing somatostatin. Thus, nesidioblastosis may provide important leads in understanding the interactions of these three hormones as well as the importance of organized surface contact between these cell types in regulating glucose homeostasis.

5. LEUCINE SENSITIVITY. This is not considered a specific cause of hypoglycemia and may be present with multiple types of beta cell abnormalities, either functional or structural. If present, a low leucine diet is diagnostic. Roth and Segal and Snyder and Robinson have reported patients in whom the details of successful dietary management can be found.

The hypoglycemia in some of these has responded to zinc glucagon, in some to diazoxide and in others to cortisone. In almost all, medication has been discontinued without further trouble after 2 to 7 months. Others have required pancreatectomy.

It is well known that hypoglycemia plays a role in the symptomatology of congenital galactosemia, hereditary fructose intolerance and the glycogen storage diseases. These disorders are discussed elsewhere. Hypoglycemia can also occur in certain hereditary defects in amino acid metabolism, including maple syrup urine disease, propionic acidemia, methylmalonic acidemia and tyrosinosis.

In 1963 Lewis et al. reported hypoglycemia caused by an inability to synthesize glycogen because of congenital and familial deficiency of the enzyme glycogen synthetase. Parr and others have since recorded another example. Their babies did not become symptomatic in the neonatal period, probably because they were receiving feedings throughout the night. Trouble appeared when night feedings were discontinued.

### THERAPEUTIC-DIAGNOSTIC TRIAL

In infants with severe, recurrent or intractable hypoglycemia, a diagnostic-therapeutic trial may lead to definitive specific medical therapy or surgical intervention at an early age. In addition to infusions of glucose, the following can be given in rapid sequence without discontinuing the prior therapeutic regimen:

| | |
|---|---|
| Hydrocortisone, P.O. or I.M. | 2–3 days |
| ACTH, I.M. | 2 days |
| Susphrine, I.M. | 2 days |
| Ephedrine, P.O. | 2 days |
| Human growth hormone, I.M. | 3–5 days |
| Diazoxide, 10 to 25 mg/kg/day P.O. | 3–5 days |

If there is no response, early pancreatectomy as recommended by Hamilton et al. is indicated. The spleen must not be removed.

## IDIOPATHIC SPONTANEOUS HYPOGLYCEMIA

If the disorder proves not to be transient and all the known causes of hypoglycemia have been eliminated by hormone, substrate and enzyme assays, one is justified in considering the diagnosis of idiopathic spontaneous hypoglycemia. This entity, first described by McQuarrie in 1954, has become even more rare since it became possible to measure the metabolic pathways necessary to maintain a normal blood glucose. After multiple endocrine deficiencies, relative or absolute hyperinsulinism and a variety of enzymatic defects have been sought in vain, a few infants, often siblings, will remain with no consistent or physiologic deviations from the normal to clarify the pathogenesis of the low sugar.

Treatment at first consists of steroids, then ACTH, followed by diazoxide and partial to complete pancreatectomy, depending upon severity, frequency of recurrence and clinical response.

## TRANSIENT DIABETES MELLITUS (TEMPORARY IDIOPATHIC NEONATAL HYPERGLYCEMIA)

Reversible diabetes mellitus is an almost unheard of phenomenon in any period of life except the neonatal. Gentz and Cornblath were able to find 50 reports of hyperglycemia in the first 6 weeks of life in the literature up to 1969. Of these, 11 appeared to be permanent diabetes, nine were uncertain and 30 were transient. Subsequently, additional patients have been reported by Milner and colleagues, including three siblings born over a 7 year interval.

This unusual syndrome also occurs in small for gestational age infants, who may present with marked dehydration and wasting, yet with a history of adequate food intake and no vomiting or diarrhea. Both sexes are affected equally, and a positive family history for diabetes is present in about one third of cases. Ketosis is mild and may appear after hydration. The diagnosis is based on glycosuria and hyperglycemia with blood sugars in excess of 250 mg per 100 ml. Where measured, acid-base derangements are not uncommon. Of 10 infants in whom electrolytes were measured, six had normal serum sodiums, one had hypernatremia and three were hyponatremic. Thus, the observations of Jung and Done of two infants with transient hyperglycemia secondary to hyperosmolarity and profound hypernatremia resulting from the ingestion of a concentrated formula are the exception and not the rule.

Although the exact etiology of this syndrome is unknown, several infants have had relative hypoinsulinemia; that is, inappropriately low plasma immunoreactive insulin values in view of the degree of the hyperglycemia. Thus, current data support the theory that a temporary delay in the maturation of beta cell function in the islet of Langerhans may be responsible.

In a few of the reported cases hyperglycemia was preceded by a period of symptomatic hypoglycemia.

The clinical course of a somewhat atypical infant with this disorder is exemplified by the case of Gentz and Cornblath.

This full-term white female had no F.H. of diabetes. Mother suffered an acute trauma on the day of delivery, resulting in a fractured mandible. Presentation was OA; delivery was accomplished by Kielland forceps rotation after caudal anesthesia. Apgar scores were 2 and 4. She was intubated and given sodium bicarbonate. Birth weight was 2780 gm and length was 49 cm.

At 5 hours generalized convulsions occurred. Blood sugar was less than 10 mg per 100 ml.

She was given intravenous glucose, 10 per cent, by continuous infusion, but convulsion recurred at 7 hours and blood sugar was still less than 10 mg per 100 ml. One gm of 50 per cent glucose was then administered quickly. Blood glucose rose to 25 mg per 100 ml but convulsion recurred. She was then given 15 mg hydrocortisone b.i.d., and the infusion of 10 to 15 per cent of glucose was continued. Convulsions continued through the fourth day in spite of dilantin, paraldehyde and pyridoxin.

At 5 days the blood sugar was more than 250 mg per 100 ml and hydrocortisone was discontinued. The fluid was changed to half-strength saline. Dehydration and lethargy followed, with marked glycosuria and moderate ketonuria. The blood sugar gradually rose to 2300 mg per 100 ml. At that time, plasma insulin values were 6 and 17 $\mu$U per ml (normal 2 to 20) and FFA values were 770 and 1250 $\mu$Eq per liter (normal 1000).

On day 6 she was given a total of 20 units of insulin, and blood sugar dropped to 170 and her dehydration, glucosuria and polyuria improved. Insulin was discontinued after 1 week, but was resumed when hyperglycemia recurred. Finally, at 40 days, insulin could be stopped for good. She was discharged at 4 months, and when seen at 7 months her growth and development were normal.

The authors comment that two of the previously reported cases of transient hyperglycemia of the newborn were found to be mentally defective at 4 and 8 years of age. They speculate that this result may have been attributable to overtreatment with insulin having resulted in hypoglycemic episodes.

These infants differ from true diabetics in the reversibility of their disease without recurrence in follow-ups of 3 to 25 years. For this reason some treat with insulin; some do not. We believe that insulin is indicated when hyperosmolality is great because of glucose levels that reach the level of 500 to 1000 mg per 100 ml, which they often do. This must represent a real hazard to the cells of the central nervous system, and possibly to the kidney. We say this because renal cortical necrosis and hyperglycemia have been found associated a number of times. These infants are usually insulin sensitive, and clinical improvement occurs with blood sugar values between 130 and 200 mg per 100 ml. Hypoglycemia must be avoided.

# REFERENCES

Anderson, J. M., Milner, R. D. G., and Strich, S. J.: Effects of neonatal hypoglycemia on the nervous system: A pathological study. J. Neur. Neurosurg. Psych. 30:295, 1967.

Arey, S. L.: Transient diabetes in infancy. Pediatrics 11:140, 1953.

Baens, G., Lundeen, E., and Cornblath, M.: Studies of carbohydrate metabolism in the newborn infant. VI. Levels of glucose in blood in premature infants. Pediatrics 31:580, 1963.

Beard, A. G., Panos, T. C., Marasigan, B. V., Eminians, J., Kennedy, H. F., and Lamb, J.: Perinatal stress and the premature neonate: II. Effect of fluid and calorie deprivation on blood glucose. J. Pediatr. 68:329, 1966.

Beard, A., Cornblath, M., Gentz, J., Kellum, M., Persson, B., Zetterstrom, R., and Haworth, J. C.: Neonatal hypoglycemia: A discussion. J. Pediatr. 79:314, 1971.

Benzing, F. III, Schubert, W., Hug, G., and Kaplan, S.: Simultaneous hypoglycemia and acute congestive heart failure. Circulation 40:209, 1969.

Case Reports of the Massachusetts General Hospital: Case 38–1962. N. Engl. J. Med. 266:1269, 1962.

Chance, G. W., and Bower, B. D.: Hypoglycaemia and temporary hyperglycaemia in infants of low birth weight for maturity. Arch. Dis. Child. 41:279, 1966.

Cochrane, W. A.: Idiopathic infantile hypoglycemia and leucine sensitivity. Metabolism 9:386, 1960.

Combs, J. T., Grunt, J. A., and Brandt, I. K.: New syndrome of neonatal hypoglycemia: Association with visceromegaly, macroglossia, microcephaly and abnormal umbilicus. N. Engl. J. Med. 275:236, 1966.

Cornblath, M., Joassin, G., Weisskopf, B., and Swiatek, K. R.: Hypoglycemia in the newborn. Pediat. Clin. N. Amer. 13:905, 1966.

Cornblath, M., Levin, E. Y., and Marquetti, E.: Studies of carbohydrate metabolism in the newborn. II. The effect of glucagon on the concentration of sugar in capillary blood of the newborn infant. Pediatrics 21:885, 1958.

Cornblath, M., Odell, G. B., and Levin, E. Y.: Symptomatic neonatal hypoglycemia associated with toxemia of pregnancy. J. Pediatr. 55:545, 1959.

Cornblath, M., and Reisner, S. H.: Blood glucose in the neonate and its clinical significance. N. Engl. J. Med. 273:378, 1965.

Cornblath, M., and Schwartz, R.: Disorders of Carbohydrate Metabolism in Infancy. 2nd ed., Philadelphia, W. B. Saunders Company, 1976.

Cornblath, M., Wybregt, S. H., Baens, G. S., and Klein, R. I.: Studies of carbohydrate metabolism in the newborn infant. VIII. Symptomatic neonatal hypoglycemia. Pediatrics 33:388, 1964.

Ehrlich, R. M., and Martin, J. M.: Diazoxide in the management of hypoglycemia in infancy and childhood. Am. J. Dis. Child. 117:411, 1969.

Farquhar, J. W.: The significance of hypoglycaemia in the newborn infant of the diabetic woman. Arch. Dis. Child. 31:203, 1956.

Filippi, G., and McKusick, V.: The Beckwith-Wiedemann syndrome. Medicine 49:279, 1970.

Fluge, G.: Clinical aspects of neonatal hypoglycaemia. Acta Paediatr. Scand. 63:826, 1974.

Garces, L. Y., Drash, A., and Kenny, F. M.: Islet cell tumor in the neonate. Pediatrics 41:789, 1968.

Geefhuysen, T.: Temporary idiopathic neonatal hypoglycemia. Pediatrics 38:1009, 1966.

Gentz, J. C. H., and Cornblath, M.: Transient diabetes of the newborn. Adv. Pediat., 16:345, 1969.

Gerrard, J.: Kernicterus. Brain 75:526, 1952.

Gittleman, I. F., and Pincus, J. B.: Blood sugar and citric acid levels in newborn infants. Pediatrics 9:38, 1952.

Graham, E. A., and Hartman, A. F.: Subtotal resection of the pancreas for hypoglycemia in an infant. Surg., Gynecol. Obstet. 59:474, 1934.

Grampa, G., Gargantini, L., Grigolato, P. G., and Ghiumello, G.: Hypoglycemia in infancy caused by beta cell nesidioblastosis. Am. J. Dis. Child. 128:226, 1974.

Grasso, S., Saporito, N., Messina, A., and Reitano, G.: Plasma insulin, glucose and free fatty acid (FFA) response to various stimuli in the premature infant. Diabetes 17(1):306, 1968.

Guest, G. M.: Infantile diabetes mellitus: Three cases in successive siblings, two with onset at three months of age and one at nine days of age. Am. J. Dis. Child. 75:461, 1948.

Gutberlet, R. L., and Cornblath, M.: Neonatal hypoglycemia revisited—1975. Pediatrics (in press) 1976.

Hamilton, J. P., Baker, L., Kaye, R., and Koop, C. E.: Subtotal pancreatectomy in the management of severe persistent idiopathic hypoglycemia. Pediatrics 39:49, 1967.

Hansson, S., and Redin, B.: Familial neonatal hypoglycemia: Syndrome resembling foetopathic diabetica. Acta Paediat., 52:145, 1963.

Harken, A. H., Filler, R. M., Av Ruskin, J. W. and Crigler, J. F., Jr.: The role of "total" pancreatectomy in the treatment of unremitting hypoglycemia of infancy. J. Pediat. Surg., 6:284, 1971.

Haworth, J. C., and Vidyasagar, D.: Hypoglycemia in the newborn. Clin. Obstet. Gynecol. 14:821, 1971.

Hazeltine, F. G.: Hypoglycemia and Rh erythroblastosis fetalis. Pediatrics 39:696, 1967.

Hirsch, H. J., Loo, S., Evans, N., Crigler, J. F., and Gabbay, K. H.: Investigation of nesidioblastosis using somatostatin. Soc. Ped. Res. 10:410, 1976.

Jung, A. L., and Done, A. K.: Extreme hyperosmolality and "transient diabetes." Am. J. Dis. Child. 118:859, 1969.

Keidan, S. E.: Transient diabetes in infancy. Arch. Dis. Child. 39:291, 1955.

Koivisto, M., Blanco-Sequeiros, M. and Krause, U.: Neonatal symptomatic and asymptomatic hypoglycaemia: A follow-up study of 151 children. Develop. Med. Child Neurol. 14:603, 1972.

Lewis, G. M., Spencer-Peet, J., and Stewart, K. M.: Infantile hypoglycemia due to inherited deficiency of glycogen synthetase in the liver. Arch. Dis. Childhood, 38:40, 1963.

Lubchenco, L. O., and Bard, H.: Incidence of hypoglycemia in newborn infants classified by birth weight and gestational age. Pediatrics 47:831, 1971.

Lucey, J. F., Randall, J. L., and Murray, J. J.: Is hypoglycemia an important complication of erythroblastosis fetalis? Am. J. Dis. Child., 114:88, 1967.

McQuarrie, I.: Idiopathic spontaneously occurring hypoglycemia in infants. A.M.A. J. Dis. Child. 87:399, 1954.

Norval, M. A., Kennedy, R. L. J., and Berkson, J.: Blood sugar in newborn infants. J. Pediat., 34:342, 1949.

Orci, L. and Zuppinger, K. A.: Nesidioblastosis. Chapter V Appendix. *In* Cornblath, M. and Schwartz, R.: Disorders of Carbohydrate Metabolism in Infancy. 2nd Ed. Philadelphia, W. B. Saunders Co., 1976.

Parr, J., Teree, T. M., and Larner, J.: Symptomatic hypoglycemia, visceral fatty metamorphosis and aglycogenosis in an infant lacking glycogen synthetase and phosphorylase. Pediatrics, 35:770, 1965.

Persson, B., Feychting, H., and Gentz, J.: Management of the infant of the diabetic mother. *In* Sutherland, H. W., and Stowers, J. M. (Eds.): Carbohydrate Metabolism in Pregnancy and the Newborn. Edinburgh, Churchill Livingston. 1975, pp. 232–248.

Pildes, R. S., Cornblath, M., Warren, I., Page-El, E., diMenza, S., Merritt, D. M., and Peeva, A.: A prospective controlled study of neonatal hypoglycemia. Pediatrics 54:5, 1974.

Pildes, R. S., Forbes, A. E., O'Connor, S. M., and Cornblath, M.: The incidence of neonatal hypoglycemia: A completed survey. J. Pediat., 70:76, 1967.

Pildes, R. S., Forbes, A. E., and Cornblath, M.: Studies of carbohydrate metabolism in the newborn infant. Pediatrics, 40:61, 1967.

Raivio, K. O., and Hallman, N.: Neonatal hypoglycemia. I. Occurrence of hypoglycemia in patients with various neonatal disorders. Acta Paediat. Scand. 57:517, 1968.

Raivio, K. O., and Osterlund, K.: Hypoglycemia and hyperinsulinemia associated with erythroblastosis fetalis. Pediatrics 43:217, 1969.

Reis, R. A., Da Costa, E. J., and Allweiss, M. D.: The management of the pregnant diabetic woman and her newborn infant. Am. J. Obst. & Gynec., 60:1023, 1950.

Roe, T. F., Kershnar, A. K., Weitzman, J. J., and Madrigal, L. S.: Beckwith's syndrome with extreme organ hyperplasia. Pediatrics 52:372, 1973.

Roth, H., and Segal, S.: The dietary management of leucine-sensitive hypoglycemia, with report of a case. Pediatrics, 34:831, 1964.

Sadeghi-Nejad, A., and Senior, B.: A familial syndrome of isolated aplasia of the anterior pituitary. J. Pediatr. 84:79, 1974.

Sadeghi-Nejad, A., Loridan, L., and Senior, B.: Studies of factors affecting gluconeogenesis and glycolysis in glycogenosis of the liver. J. Pediatr. 76:561, 1970.

Salinas, E. D., Jr., Mangurten, H. H., Roberts, S. S., Simon, W. H., and Cornblath, M.: Functioning islet cell adenoma in the newborn. Pediatrics, 41:646, 1968.

Sherman, H.: Islet cell tumor of pancreas in a newborn infant (nesidioblastoma). Am. J. Dis. Child., 74:58, 1947.

Smith, C. A.: The newborn patient (Clifford D. Sweet Lecture). Pediatrics, 16:254, 1955.

Snyder, R. D., and Robinson, A.: Leucine-induced hypoglycemia. Am. J. Dis. Child. 113:566, 1967.

Wybregt, S. H., Reisner, S. H., Patel, R. K., Nellhaus, G., and Cornblath, M.: The incidence of neonatal hypoglycemia in a nursery for premature infants. J. Pediatr. 64:796, 1964.

Yakovac, W. C., Baker, L., and Hummeler, K.: Beta cell nesidioblastosis in idiopathic hypoglycemia in infancy. J. Pediatr. 79:226, 1971.

Yeung, C. Y.: Hypoglycemia in neonatal sepsis. J. Pediatr. 77:812, 1970.

Zuppinger, K. A.: Hypoglycemia in childhood: Evaluation of diagnostic procedures. *In* Falkner, F., Kretchmer, N., and Rossi, E. (eds.): Monographs in Paediatrics. Basel, S. Karger, 1975.

# VII

## Inborn Errors of
## Metabolism

# 58

# GENERAL CONSIDERATIONS

## By Harvey Levy

One of the most exciting fields in medicine today is that of the inborn errors of metabolism, particularly within the newborn period. These disorders are becoming recognized more frequently as each month passes. Previously undiscovered disorders are being added to the list of known inborn errors of metabolism at an almost logarithmic rate. It is now apparent that inborn errors of metabolism represent not only a significant percentage of all known genetic disorders but also a growing percentage of detectable newborn diseases.

Two factors account for the increasing recognition of the significance in the neonatal period of inborn errors of metabolism. The first is that of greater availability and sophistication of methods for detecting and measuring biochemical substances in physiologic fluids. The second is that of an awareness, relatively recently acquired, that many inborn errors of metabolism are manifest as distinct and recognizable biochemical abnormalities in a newborn infant who is *entirely normal clinically*. Thus, timely treatment can prevent clinical manifestations from ever occurring in a number of these disorders.

Each inborn error of metabolism is genetic in origin. As in other genetic disorders, the basic abnormality is that of an abnormal or mutant gene. This gene, acting as a template, is responsible for the synthesis of an abnormal protein, which in inborn errors of metabolism is usually an abnormal enzyme. The abnormality in this enzyme is believed to be one of structure, so that it is deficient in its activity. The cause of this deficiency may be inadequate binding of substrate or, perhaps less commonly, insufficient amounts or inadequate binding of coenzyme. In such instances the result is usually demonstrable substrate accumulation in abnormally large amounts and reduced formation of product. Secondary effects such as accumulations of metabolites

of the substrate may also appear. An example of this is phenylketonuria (PKU), as illustrated in Figure 58–1, in which deficient activity of phenylalanine hydroxylase in the liver results in increased concentrations of phenylalanine and related metabolites in body fluids and tissues, and a concomitant decrease in the concentration of tyrosine, the product of phenylalanine hydroxylation. This deficiency of phenylalanine hydroxylase activity may be due either to an abnormality in the basic phenylalanine hydroxylase enzyme or, probably less commonly, to reduced amounts of tetrahydrobiopterin, a necessary cofactor for the enzyme. The basic problem in the latter case is also one of deficient enzyme activity, that of dihydropteridine reductase, which is responsible for the formation of tetrahydrobiopterin. The mechanism whereby clinical abnormalities occur in inborn errors of metabolism is presumed to be the accumulation of substrate and/or related metabolites, which in large concentrations may be toxic to certain body tissues. However, the precise mechanism whereby this toxicity occurs is not known

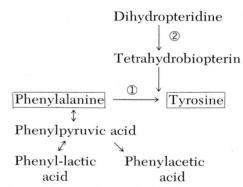

**Figure 58–1.** Pathway of phenylalanine metabolism illustrating the accumulation of phenylalanine and its metabolites and the reduced tyrosine formation. The two genetic deficiencies that have been found to cause this metabolic block are phenylalanine hydroxylase and dihydropteridine reductase.

and is under a great deal of study at the present time.

The excitement surrounding inborn errors of metabolism is based upon the recognition that for a number of them there is available management that may prevent irreversible clinical complications. Thus, mental retardation, liver disease and eye diseases that are now virtually not amenable to treatment may be prevented. Further, the potential for prevention of certain forms of heart and kidney disease, which also may be at least partly due to metabolic disorders, renders the entire field that much more exciting.

At the present time there are available two forms of specific treatment. The most important is that of a dietary change that results in a lowering of the concentrations of presumably toxic biochemicals in the body. The second involves the administration of a large amount of a specific vitamin that may be utilized as a cofactor by the enzyme in question. This latter therapy, which results in activation of the enzyme, is only possible when the enzymatic abnormality is such that the enzyme will respond to "flooding" by the cofactor. However, optimal effectiveness from either of these modes of therapy is often possible only when the metabolic disorder is discovered by routine newborn screening. An additional area that is therapeutic in a limited way is that of prenatal diagnosis. In this situation the presence of an inborn error of metabolism is suspected in the unborn fetus, perhaps on the basis of occurrence of the disorder in the family, and via amniocentesis and examination of the amniotic cells or fluid, the diagnosis is made. "Therapy" in this case is usually that of induced abortion which, while not treatment for the fetus, may be exceedingly important treatment for the family. An important exception to this has recently appeared in which intrauterine vitamin $B_{12}$ therapy was administered to a fetus affected with methylmalonic acidemia. If this form of therapy proves to be clinically efficacious, it may open an important new area for prenatal diagnosis. Other forms of therapy such as direct injection of enzymes and organ transplantation are being considered for certain disorders, although there is as yet no clear evidence that these methods can be effectively used. However, this is one of the most active and important fields under investigation and it can be anticipated that great advances may be made in the years ahead.

It is clear that routine newborn screening for a number of inborn errors of metabolism is an effective and desirable health measure. Already the vast majority of newborns within the United States and in many other countries are routinely screened for phenylketonuria. In addition, a growing number are being screened for galactosemia, maple syrup urine disease and several other inborn errors of metabolism. However, it is advisable to carefully select the type of error for which screening is desirable. For instance, certain inborn errors of metabolism may have strikingly prominent biochemical abnormalities and yet be clinically benign. Screening is unnecessary for such disorders, since no treatment need or should be given. In other disorders that produce clinical abnormalities the lack of preventive therapy militates against resources being devoted to their screening. Unfortunately, clear decisions regarding the nature and scope of routine newborn screening are currently made with difficulty, since there is to some extent a lack of information regarding the clinical consequences of many disorders and also a difference of opinion as to what may or may not constitute "therapy" in several given situations. These questions are under study at the present time and hopefully there will emerge over the next few years a clearer picture of proper newborn screening.

## SCREENING AND SPECIFIC DIAGNOSIS

As stated above, more and more newborns are being screened routinely for an ever increasing number of inborn errors of metabolism. At the present time, however, this screening does not include all newborn infants in the United States or any other country and certainly encompasses few of these disorders. In most areas of the United States a filter-paper blood specimen is obtained from the heel of newborn infants prior to nursery discharge. This specimen is usually sent to a central laboratory, where it is tested for evidence of phenylketonuria (PKU). In a few areas this specimen may also be subjected to a test for galactosemia, and in still fewer areas subjected to additional tests for disorders such as maple syrup urine disease (MSUD), homocystinuria, tyrosinemia and perhaps congenital hypothyroidism (cretinism). In the Canadian province of Quebec and in the state of Massachusetts a filter-paper urine specimen obtained from most newborn infants is also tested. This urine specimen is obtained by the mother when the infant is 2 to 4 weeks of age and sent to a central laboratory for tests that would detect those inborn errors of metabolism manifested in urine but not in blood. In Massachusetts, a filter-paper umbilical cord blood specimen is also obtained for the purposes of early diagnosis of galactosemia and detection of maternal phenylketonuria.

Whenever the possibility of an inborn error of metabolism is suspected in a newborn, either because of the family history of a particular disorder or because of clinical signs in the infant (to be discussed below), it is of utmost importance to contact the central screening facility or other experienced laboratory to determine whether or not tests that would detect metabolic disorders in the newborn are performed. If the test(s) desired is available at the laboratory, on either a routine or specific basis, it is then important to be certain that the proper blood or urine specimen from the infant is submitted. One must remember that if the infant is clinically ill and thus will not be discharged from the nursery at the usual age, the proper screening specimens should be obtained and sent to the laboratory no later than the fourth day of life. On a number of occasions when an infant has been clinically ill the blood specimen for screening purposes has not been obtained because of a general policy of obtaining this specimen only upon nursery discharge. In such instances the proper diagnosis has either not been made or has been delayed until irreversible damage or a terminal clinical state has supervened. In the case of PKU our worry is the opposite one — that we may have drawn the test specimen too early in life (see Chapter 60).

Many tests that might detect any one of a number of inborn errors of metabolism may not be available at a central screening laboratory. In such case it is important to determine whether these tests can be performed within the hospital laboratory or at another hospital or medical center within the area. Since certain of them are quite specialized, they may not be performed even within the area; in this case the physician should check with a medical center or screening laboratory to determine where they are available. Certain large laboratories are available for comprehensive screening for inborn errors of metabolism and will accept specimens from throughout the United States as well as from many other countries. In the first reference is listed a number of such regional facilities and the names and addresses of individuals who might be contacted in this regard.

The type of specimen that is most desirable depends upon the inborn error of metabolism suspected. For instance, phenylketonuria (PKU) is far more likely to be detected by examination of a blood specimen than a urine specimen. Conversely, argininosuccinic acidemia may be far more readily detected by testing urine than by an examination of blood. For other diseases, such as galactosemia, both blood and urine are desirable for a definite diagnosis. In general, however, whenever there is any reason to suspect an inborn error of metabolism both blood and urine should be submitted for examination. Often the filter-paper blood specimen sent for routine neonatal screening may be sufficient for a specific diagnosis, although in other instances it may be desirable to test a specimen of plasma, serum or liquid whole blood. Similarly, a urine specimen impregnated into filter paper may be sufficient for the detection of certain disorders, but often a liquid urine specimen is desirable. The determination of the type of specimen to be sent can only be accurately made after consultation with the laboratory at which the testing will be performed.

Certain clinical signs in the neonate should alert one to the possibility of the presence of an inborn error of metabolism. These signs, which are listed in Table 58–1, include prolonged and unexplained jaundice, lethargy, weight loss or failure of weight gain, vomiting, poor feeding and neurological signs such as convulsions or

**TABLE 58–1.** *Major Clinical Signs in the Neonatal Period That Suggest the Presence of an Inborn Error of Metabolism*

| Signs | Possible Disorder(s) |
|---|---|
| Jaundice<br>Hepatomegaly<br>Lethargy<br>Weight loss<br>Poor feeding | Galactosemia |
| Lethargy<br>Hypotonicity or spasticity<br>Vomiting<br>Poor feeding<br>Metabolic acidosis | Maple syrup urine disease<br>Methylmalonic acidemia<br>Isovaleric acidemia<br>Propionic acidemia<br>(Other) organic acidemias |
| Obstipation<br>Abdominal distention<br>Vomiting | Cystic fibrosis |
| Lethargy<br>Poor feeding<br>Hypotonicity<br>Hyperammonemia | Urea cycle disorder |
| Lethargy<br>Poor feeding<br>Hypotonicity<br>Poor respirations | Non-ketotic hyperglycinemia |

One important aspect of routine neonatal screening for inborn errors of metabolism should be added here. Screening is not diagnosis and should not be considered such. Screening is primarily for the purpose of eliminating all of those infants who clearly do not have a particular disorder, and for casting suspicion upon the few infants who might have the disorder. Consequently, screening tests are so constructed that out of the group of infants who yield "positive" tests and thus are suspected of having a disorder there may be only one or two infants who truly have the disorder. This construction is necessary for screening purposes so that "missing" an infant with a particular disorder will be avoided. Implicit within this design, however, is the realization that screening is only a process of sorting. Thus, any infant with a "positive" screening test should have additional testing by more specific means to determine whether or not the disorder is present. It is also important to realize that the vast majority of infants with "positive" screening tests do not have metabolic disorders. The families of these infants should be informed of this so that unnecessary diagnostic tests, treatment and anxiety may be avoided.

spasticity . At times a distinctive odor can be appreciated. Two general biochemical states can be associated with any one or a number of these signs and may be part of a number of different inborn errors of metabolism. These states are hyperammonemia and metabolic acidosis. Thus, among the first tests that should be obtained when one or more of these clinical signs appear are the determination of blood ammonia and of the state of acid-base balance. If the former is increased, there would be reason to suspect one of the urea cycle disorders. In the event of metabolic acidosis, maple syrup urine disease or one of the inborn errors of organic acid metabolism may be present. These disorders will be discussed in more detail later. Interestingly, a neonate with an organic acid metabolic disorder may have hyperammonemia as well as metabolic acidosis, although the hyperammonemia in this instance is usually less severe than that noted in association with the urea cycle disorders. Conversely, hyperammonemia is usually not present in the organic acid disorders.

## REFERENCES

American Academy of Pediatrics, Committee on Nutrition: Special diets for infants with inborn errors of amino acid metabolism. Pediatrics 57:783, 1976.

Ampola, M. G., Mahoney, M. J., et al.: Prenatal therapy of a patient with vitamin $B_{12}$-responsive methylmalonic acidemia. N. Engl. J. Med. 293:313, 1975.

Levy, H. L.: Genetic screening. *In* Harris, H., and Hirschhorn, K. (Eds.): Advances in Human Genetics. Vol. 4, New York, Plenum Press, 1973, pp. 1–104.

Milunsky, A., Littlefield, J. W., et al.: Prenatal genetic diagnosis. N. Engl. J. Med., 283:1370, 1441, 1498, 1970.

National Academy of Sciences, Committee for the Study of Inborn Errors of Metabolism: Genetic Screening. Washington, D.C. National Academy of Sciences, 1975.

Rosenberg, L. E.: Diagnosis and management of inherited aminoacidopathies in the newborn and the unborn. *In* Bickel, H. (Ed.): Congenital and Acquired Diseases of Amino Acid Metabolism. Clin. Endocrinol. Metabol. 3:145, 1974.

# 59

# INBORN ERRORS OF CARBOHYDRATE METABOLISM

*By Harvey Levy*

## GALACTOSEMIA

Galactosemia is one of the most dramatic of those inborn errors of metabolism that present clinical signs during the early days of life. Yet, the results of routine newborn screening for galactosemia indicate that this disorder may be almost as frequently "missed" in the newborn period as it is diagnosed. This is truly tragic, since the diagnosis of galactosemia may be at least strongly suspected on the basis of a urine test for reducing substances. Moreover, early diagnosis and prompt institution of a relatively simple therapy will likely lead to a normal life for an infant who is faced with the possibilities of neonatal death, cataracts, cirrhosis and mental retardation should the diagnosis not be made and therapy delayed for several months or perhaps not given at all. The salient clinical features of "classic" galactosemia in the neonate include jaundice, hepatomegaly, lethargy, poor feeding, failure to gain weight or actual loss of weight, and perhaps the vomiting of breast milk or formula. If prompt treatment is not given the neonate will generally become septic, usually with *E. coli,* and die by the age of 10 to 14 days. If death does not occur the untreated infant may spontaneously recover from all of the clinical signs but develop the chronic complications of cataracts, cirrhosis and mental retardation by 3 or 4 years of age. In untreated galactosemia, especially in the neonate, the urine is strongly positive for reducing substance (galactose) but negative on specific testing for glucose. Albuminuria and hyperaminoaciduria are also present. The specific diagnosis may be confirmed by careful blood examination, which will reveal a markedly increased galactose concentration and the absence of red blood cell galactose-1-phosphate uridyl transferase (transferase) activ-

ity. Treatment is the withdrawal of all foods containing lactose and galactose from the diet. When this treatment is instituted early in the neonatal period and continued throughout life, the prognosis for normal physical and mental development is excellent.

In recent years the field of galactose metabolism in man has become complicated by the recognition that increased blood galactose concentrations may be due to deficiencies of galactose metabolic enzymes other than transferase. These two entities, known as galactokinase deficiency and uridine diphosphate galactose 4-epimerase deficiency, will be discussed in following sections and the term "galactosemia" will be used to connote only the deficiency in transferase activity. Even within galactosemia itself, however, there are a number of variants, each representing a different genetic disorder. These variants, listed in Table 59–1, may or may not result in the clinical disease, depending upon the degree of residual transferase activity, and perhaps upon other factors as yet undetermined. Since galactose accumulates in both blood and urine both in "classic" galactosemia and the clinically significant transferase variants, the initial diagnostic means are identical as is the therapy.

**INCIDENCE.** Routine neonatal screening for galactosemia has indicated that the incidence varies from one case per 30,000 to less than one case per 100,000 screened infants. This variation depends to some extent upon the country in which the screening has been conducted, so that as in most other genetic disorders there would appear to be ethnic relation to the frequency. This difference in reported frequency may also be a result of differences in screening methods. It has become quite clear in the last few years that certain infants with galactosemia may be overlooked even in well

**TABLE 59–1.**    *Characteristics Regarding Variants of Galactose-1-Phosphate Uridyl Transferase*

| Variant | Erythrocyte Transferase Activity (% of Normal) | Starch-gel Electrophoretic Mobility (Related to Normal) | Other Biochemical Characteristics | Clinical Characteristics |
|---|---|---|---|---|
| "Classical" | 0° | — | — | Disease°° |
| Duarte | 50° | Faster | — | Benign |
| "Negro" | 0° | — | 10% activity in liver and intestine | Disease |
| Indiana | 0–45 | Slower | Unstable in heparinized blood and isotonic phosphate buffer | Disease |
| Rennes | 7 | Slower | — | Disease |
| Los Angeles | 140 | Faster | — | Benign |

°This represents the activity in individuals homozygous for the variant.
°°Jaundice, other neonatal signs with complications of cataracts, liver disease and mental retardation.

organized and well conducted screening programs.

**ETIOLOGY.**   There is abundant evidence that galactosemia in most if not all instances is transmitted as an autosomal recessive. The mutant gene is responsible for the formation of a transferase protein which is deficient in activity and in at least some instances abnormal in electrophoretic mobility. This would strongly indicate that the structure of the protein is abnormal, possibly in the substitution of a single amino acid residue, as is the case for sickle hemoglobin. Heterozygotes (carriers) usually have about 50 per cent of the normal red blood cell transferase activity, as expected, and often have abnormalities in the galactose tolerance curve; however, they are clinically normal.

**PATHOLOGY.**   Nothing specific is found in any organ upon biopsy or autopsy. Early in the disease the liver is enlarged and usually shows fatty metamorphosis of moderate to severe grade with no excess glycogen deposition. Later the alterations of portal cirrhosis are seen, including periportal fibrosis and bile-duct regeneration, which may progress to full-blown nodular cirrhosis of the Laennec type. The lenses may show the characteristic opacification of cataract formation.

**PATHOGENESIS.**   Galactose usually enters the body following the ingestion of lactose, the disaccharide of milk. When milk or a milk product is ingested the lactose is usually broken down by intestinal lactase to the monosaccharides glucose and galactose, which are then transported through the intestinal wall into the portal system and thus into the body. The galactose is normally metabolized to carbon dioxide via a specific metabolic pathway that consists of several enzymes (Fig. 59–1). In "classic" galactosemia, activity of the transferase enzyme is markedly deficient or virtually undetectable in erythrocytes, liver or cultured skin fibroblasts. As a result, galactose-1-phosphate accumulates in the cells of the body. This accumulated galactose-1-phosphate apparently inhibits the activity of galactokinase (product or feedback inhibition) so that galactose itself accumulates. Because galactose-1-phosphate does not leave the cell, it is only detectable in erythrocytes or within other cells of the body. Galactose, however, freely exchanges between intracellular and extracellular spaces, and therefore is detectable either within cells or within such extracellular areas as plasma or serum and urine. The free galactose within the ocular lens may be further metabolized to galactitol, which establishes an osmotic gradient through which fluid is then drawn into the lens. This results in swelling of the lens, denaturation and precipitation of lenticular protein and, eventually, cataract formation. It is believed that the damage to other organs, primarily brain, liver and kidney is a result of intracellular toxicity of galactose-1-phosphate. According to this theory galactose-1-phosphate accumulates in neu-

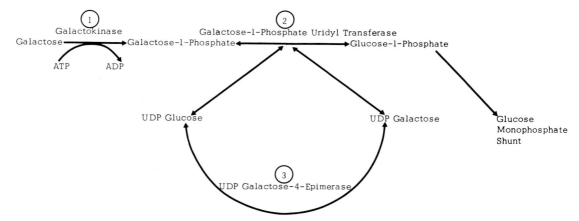

**Figure 59–1.**   Pathway of galactose metabolism. The known human disorders in this pathway are indicated by the numbered enzyme deficient in each disorder.

rons, hepatic cells and renal tubular cells, causing damage which eventually results respectively in mental retardation, cirrhosis and renal tubular malabsorption characterized by the Fanconi syndrome.

There are a number of secondary abnormalities which are probably related to the primary metabolic derangement but for which there is as yet no clear explanation. Most prominent among these is the marked hypoglycemia noted during the acute neonatal phase of galactosemia. It is conceivable that this is due to a disruption of gluconeogenesis, but the exact nature of the hypoglycemia has not yet been elucidated. Another prominent feature that has only recently been discovered is a mild but definite hyperaminoacidemia that affects virtually all of the measurable free amino acids in the blood.

**DIAGNOSIS.**   The clinical severity associated with galactosemia in the neonate varies markedly from no symptoms at all to very severe disease characterized by marked jaundice, hepatomegaly, weight loss and lethargy that if untreated will result in death. Recent studies have indicated that this clinical spectrum is associated with a spectrum of residual enzyme activity that varies from virtually undetectable in the very ill infant to as much as 10 per cent of residual activity in the infant who manifests no clinical disease in the neonatal period. Furthermore, the black infant may have the so-called "Negro variant," in which there is virtually undetectable activity in erythrocytes but perhaps some residual activity in liver, and in which there may be little or no symptoms in the neonatal period.

In the infant who is ill the greatest immediate danger appears to be that of sepsis, most often due to *E. coli.* As a result of routine newborn screening for galactosemia it has been recognized that a number of neonates with galactosemia have died with sepsis, the galactosemia being unrecognized until attention was called to it as a result of screening test abnormalities.

When the infant is affected clinically the usual history is that of jaundice beginning on the second or third day of life. This generally deepens and by the fifth or sixth day of life the infant is noted to have hepatomegaly, significant weight loss, lethargy and perhaps vomiting with a moderate degree of loose stools. Cataracts are usually not evident at this time. If milk is not withdrawn the signs worsen and sepsis may intervene, at which time death may be unavoidable. In some instances, however, sepsis may not develop and the signs of disease may spontaneously disappear despite the continuation of milk. In such patients the chronic abnormalities associated with galactosemia will develop later in infancy and childhood.

**LABORATORY INVESTIGATIONS.**   GALACTOSEMIA AND MELITURIA.   Within a few hours after the ingestion of milk, galactose can be demonstrated in blood and urine. The diagnosis can be readily made by testing a filter-paper blood specimen ("PKU" specimen) for galactose, using either a bacterial assay for galactose or a chemical method of galactose determination. These tests are most efficiently performed in a central laboratory as part of a routine newborn screening program for metabolic disorders and should be included in all such programs, as should screening for phenylketonuria, hypothyroidism and perhaps other disorders. The urine will also contain a large amount of galactose, and as a reducing substance will give a positive reaction to Benedict's solution. This is easily shown by testing the urine with a test tablet for reducing substance.

It is important to note in testing the urine that the commonly used dipstick methods utilize glucose oxidase and thus are specific for glycosuria. When such methods are used exclusively in the nursery, galactosemia will be entirely overlooked unless alternative testing methods are available. Whenever urinalysis is performed in the newborn the test for urinary sugar should always be for general reducing substances rather than the dipstick-type. If there is reducing substance in the urine a dipstick test for glucose should then be performed. In galactosemia this test will be negative or at most only slightly positive and thus consistent with the fact that most or all of the reducing substance is galactose. The identity of galactose in urine can be verified by paper chromatography and by specific methods of determination.

Two facts should be kept in mind when the urine is being examined in a case of suspected galactosemia. The first is that many normal babies (24 of 50 studied by Hayworth and McCredie) excrete detectable amounts of reducing substance in their urine in the first week of life, mostly from the third to fifth day. These include galactose, lactose and xylose. In a few the quantity is sufficient to produce a strong reaction with Benedict's solution. The other point is that the urine remains free of sugar in galactosemics unless milk is fed. This obvious fact can be overlooked when a sick infant is brought into the hospital and given only intravenous fluids. This has re-

sulted in delay in the verification of suspected galactosemia.

PROTEINURIA. Albumin appears in the urine within 48 hours after the ingestion of lactose or galactose and disappears about 5 days or so after their discontinuance. It may vary from a trace to a moderately large amount.

FORMED ELEMENTS IN THE URINE. Red blood cells, white blood cells and casts of various kinds may or may not be found.

HYPERAMINOACIDURIA. A marked increase in the excretion of virtually all free amino acids in the urine begins a few days after milk feeding has begun and reaches its maximum on about the tenth day. Although it is accompanied by a slight to moderate increase in the concentration of blood amino acids, the hyperaminoaciduria is clearly caused by renal tubular damage and a resulting reduced tubular reabsorption of amino acids rather than by "overflow" from the increased blood amino acid concentrations, since the latter is not of such degree that would produce the hyperaminoaciduria seen in galactosemia. The hyperaminoaciduria is not of a specific type and may be similar to that noted in small premature infants or those with renal tubular malabsorption due to the Fanconi syndrome or to vitamin D-responsive rickets. If milk feedings are stopped the hyperaminoaciduria will usually disappear in 5 to 7 days.

GALACTOSE TOLERANCE. After the oral ingestion of 1.25 or 1.50 grams of galactose per kilogram of body weight the galactose concentration increases to an inordinately high level and remains markedly elevated for as long as 5 hours. Figure 59–2 shows the galactose tolerance curve of the patient whose history follows. At the end of 3 hours the blood galactose concentration was 153 mg per 100 ml, at which point the blood measurements in this 2-week-old infant were discontinued.

Galactose tolerance tests should probably not be performed in infants with proven galactosemia or who are even suspected of having galactosemia. For clinical diagnosis and therapy galactosemia can be very adequately studied on the basis of response to milk feedings. A loading dose of galactose produces marked accumula-

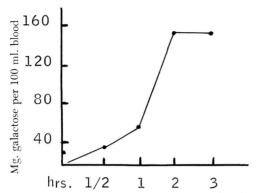

***Figure 59–2.*** Galactose tolerance curve of infant with galactosemia.

tions of galactose and galactose-1-phosphate, as well as marked hypoglycemia, in such infants and could result in irreversible organ damage. Furthermore, enzyme assays of the readily available erythrocytes and cultured skin fibroblasts will almost always determine the specific type and degree of galactosemia, making a galactose loading test unnecessary. As the infant gets older additional information can be rather simply obtained by once again feeding milk and measuring the concentrations of galactose in blood and urine following this feeding.

GALACTOSE-GLUCOSE RELATIONS. An inverse relation exists between the levels of galactose and glucose in the blood. During the course of a galactose tolerance test glucose concentration falls while that of galactose rises, and vice versa. At the height of galactose concentration appreciable hypoglycemia may be present, with glucose levels as low as 20 mg per 100 ml or less and symptoms appearing. As noted previously, the precise cause of hypoglycemia has not yet been ascertained.

LIVER FUNCTION. One of the first signs of galactosemia is neonatal jaundice. By the fifth day of life this jaundice is usually of moderate degree, with total serum bilirubin concentrations of approximately 14 to 18 mg per 100 ml. If the galactosemia remains untreated serum bilirubin will usually increase in concentration, and by 7 to 9 days of life the concentration may be as high as 20 mg per 100 ml or higher. It was formerly believed that the bilirubin

was generally of the direct-reacting (conjugated) type, suggesting that the hyperbilirubinemia is on the basis of liver damage, perhaps obstructive in type. Recent evidence, however, indicates that the hyperbilirubinemia of the neonate may be predominantly indirect-reacting (unconjugated) in many instances. This could still be explained by liver damage in that the bilirubin conjugating mechanism could be inhibited by galactose-1-phosphate or other toxic metabolites that may accumulate in galactosemia. Other indicators of liver function, such as the levels of SGOT and serum alkaline phosphatase, may be elevated but this is usually of a mild degree and may not occur until the second week of life. Within a few days after the discontinuance of milk the serum bilirubin concentration will begin to recede as will the other indicators of liver malfunction.

RENAL FUNCTION. There is no gross evidence of reduction of kidney function. The blood urea nitrogen concentration, the specific gravity of urine, and the excretion of sodium, potassium and chloride remain within normal limits. In the younger infants Komrower et al. demonstrated a moderate degree of renal acidosis, which disappeared with advancing age.

BLOOD ELEMENTS. There is usually little or no alteration in the indices of hematologic function. In particular, evidence of hemolysis is almost always absent. Hemoglobin usually remains normal, as does the reticulocyte count. If neonatal sepsis intervenes, however, any of the hematologic signs of this complication may be present. These signs include anemia, evidence of hemolysis, alterations in the white blood cell count and thrombocytopenia.

TREATMENT. Treatment consists of the complete discontinuance of milk and milk products from the diet at the moment the diagnosis is established. This means that breast feeding or feeding of any milk-containing formula or whole milk must cease and a non-milk formula be substituted. Several non-milk formulas are available, two of the most popular being Nutramigen* and CHO-free.** If there is signifi-

---

*Mead, Johnson Laboratories, Evansville, IN 47721.
**Syntex Laboratories, Palo Alto, CA 94304.

cant hypoglycemia and if the infant is feeding poorly or is dehydrated it may be wise to institute nonspecific intravenous fluid therapy for replacement and maintenance. At least two blood cultures should be obtained, and antibiotic therapy effective against *E. coli* and other gram-negative organisms should be begun *before* the results of the blood cultures are available. The latter is of particular importance, since sepsis is so commonly associated with galactosemia.

The galactosemic individual will probably have to remain on a diet that restricts the intake of lactose and galactose for the remainder of his life. This means that milk and milk products are to be avoided. In contrast to many other inborn errors of metabolism, foods high in protein, such as meat and fish, may be readily ingested. Thus the diet in galactosemia can be relatively easily administered and tolerated without problems or complications.

**PROGNOSIS.** Unless the diagnosis is made during the first week or two of life the infant may die with sepsis. Even should the infant survive, the outlook with respect to life will be poor unless galactose is withdrawn before hepatic cirrhosis reaches the irreversible stage. It is impossible to state with exactness just how soon this is, since cases vary widely in severity. Hepatomegaly and cataracts may regress and disappear after having been present for surprisingly long periods. Each day that the infant is subjected to the toxicity of galactose and its metabolites must be considered to diminish his chances of making a perfect recovery.

The prognosis with respect to mental development is not yet known with certainty; however, there would appear to be little doubt that the frank mental deficiency noted in untreated or late-treated galactosemia is to a great extent if not entirely a result of the disease. This mental deficiency is largely or completely preventable by early and correct treatment. The diagnosis can and should be made early in the neonatal period; a delay of a week or two may mean the difference between mental normality and mental retardation. The rapidly growing brain of the newborn cannot be insulted for many days with impunity.

CASE 59–1

A white male infant was born at the Women's Hospital of Maryland October 6, 1953, with a birth weight of 8 pounds 4 ounces (3740 gm) after a normal pregnancy and uncomplicated delivery at term. He breathed and cried spontaneously. His mother elected not to breast-feed, and he was offered an evaporated milk, Dextrimaltose formula. No difficulties were encountered, and he was discharged on the fifth day.

The father and the mother are both in good health. The father had one child by a previous marriage who is living and well. This was the mother's first pregnancy. The parents are unrelated.

From the moment the child arrived home on the fifth day, vomiting and semisolid stools were noted, The following day jaundice appeared. He was always hungry and ate well, but most of the feedings were vomited. By the twelfth day there had been a weight loss of 1½ pounds, and he was admitted to the Sinai Hospital for study.

Physical examination on the twelfth day revealed that he was vigorous but irritable. There was mild jaundice of the skin and sclera but no fever or other evidence of infection. The abdomen was full but not tight, the liver edge being palpable three finger-breadths below the right costal margin. It was very firm. The spleen was not palpable. The rest of the examination was negative.

He was observed in the hospital on a routine milk diet for 1 week. During this week vomiting, loose stools and failure to gain persisted. The liver remained large and firm, and the spleen enlarged to one finger-breadth below the costal margin. Jaundice was never deep and all but disappeared within 5 days.

Eye consultation (Dr. Arnall Patz) at 2½ weeks of age revealed "a central refractile zone about the nucleus of each lens which forms a fine circle about the lens . . . this is typical early lenticular opacity of galactosemia."

On October 31, when the infant was 26 days old, milk was withdrawn from the diet and Nutramigen substituted. There was an immediate and striking change. Feedings were retained, weight gain began and the liver shrank rapidly. The urine was free of galactose within 48 hours.

Serologic test for syphilis was negative. X-ray films of long bones and the chest were negative. Blood culture was sterile. Hemoglobin was 13.0 gm, white blood cells 22,000, with normal differential. Fasting blood sugar was 132, blood urea nitrogen 84, bilirubin 3.2, direct 2.5, indirect 0.7, all expressed in mg per 100 ml. Urine contained reducing substance 3+, fermentation test was negative, osazone test positive for galactose. Galactose tolerance test revealed the following levels: fasting 14, $1/2$ hour 25, 1 hour 67, 2 hours 148, 3 hours 153 mg per 100 ml. (Fig. 59–2). Coombs tests were negative. Both mother and child belonged in blood group O, Rh negative.

He was readmitted for study at 16 months of age, at which time his liver was found to be palpable one finger-breadth below the costal margin. Otherwise there were no physical abnormalities, the eyes showed no residual opacity whatsoever, and psychometry revealed normal mental development. The galactose tolerance was unaltered. Growth and development have been absolutely normal until the present. His mother gave birth to a second child who was not fed milk until a determination of the enzyme transferase, kindly performed for us by Dr. Isselbacher of the National Institutes of Health, showed that he had adequate amounts of that enzyme in his red blood cells. He was then offered a routine evaporated milk diet, upon which he is thriving.

**COMMENT.** This infant was sent into hospital at the age of 12 days with the tentative diagnosis of galactosemia. This suspicion was fostered by 1) vomiting and mild diarrhea beginning several days after milk feeding was begun, 2) late appearance of mild jaundice, 3) rapid enlargement of the liver without concomitant or proportionate splenomegaly and 4) absence of any evidence of infection or hemolysis. Diagnosis was confirmed, and withdrawal of galactose-containing foods was followed by rapid improvement, with recession of hepatomegaly and dissolution of the early cataracts.

In spite of the excellent result we are dissatisfied with our handling of the case in one particular. We believe that 13 days is a needlessly long time to have elapsed between admission of the infant and withdrawal of galactose. One week should have been more than sufficient to make the diagnosis with assurance. In this child the extra week of galactose feeding apparently made no difference; in a more severe case it might have.

We are pleased, on the other hand, with our handling of the second child in the family. He was never offered milk until we were certain, after enzyme studies, that he could metabolize it properly. Had he been galactosemic, this would have represented the ideal in the prophylactic treatment of galactosemia.

## GALACTOKINASE AND UDPGal-4-EPIMERASE DEFICIENCIES

Galactose may be increased in blood and urine as a result of deficient activity of galactokinase or USPGal-4-epimerase (Fig. 59–1). Galactokinase deficiency has been identified in the newborn as well as in older children and adults. In contrast to galactosemia, galactose-1-phosphate does not accumulate in galactokinase deficiency. In the untreated state cataracts will develop during early childhood. Unlike galactosemia, however, there are no neonatal symptoms, and other complications such as liver disease and mental retardation do not occur. The diagnosis may be suspected upon finding large amounts of galactose in the blood or urine and confirmed by the finding of markedly reduced or absent galactokinase activity in erythrocytes. The treatment is identical to that for galactosemia in that milk and other foods containing lactose must be excluded from the diet. Neonatal screening that utilizes an assay for galactose should detect galactokinase deficiency as well as galactosemia. It is important to identify and begin treatment of this disorder in the neonatal period in order to prevent the formation of cataracts.

UDPGal-4-epimerase (epimerase) deficiency has been described in only one infant. While ingesting milk this infant accumulated a moderate amount of galactose in blood (8–10 mg/100 ml) and an even larger amount of galactose-1-phosphate in erythrocytes. The infant remained well, without cataracts or other signs of galactosemia, suggesting that this may be a benign disorder. The diagnosis is confirmed by the finding of reduced epimerase activity in erythrocytes.

## GLYCOGEN STORAGE DISEASES

As Cori pointed out as early as 1952, a number of different metabolic lesions may lead to the same effect, abnormal accumulation of glycogen in various tissues. At that time Cori delineated four distinct types, and since then at least two others have been recognized. Some of the forms infrequently manifest in the neonatal period, while others never become symptomatic until later in life. For this reason only three of the subtypes merit discussion within this volume.

## Von Gierke's Disease (Hepatorenal Glycogenosis, Cori's Type I)

Von Gierke's disease is a disorder of carbohydrate metabolism in which glycogen accumulates strikingly in the liver and kidneys, and to a lesser degree in other organs.

**INCIDENCE.** Although von Gierke's disease is rare, it is the most common of the subtypes. It manifests itself in the neonatal period so infrequently, however, that we ourselves have never encountered a case in an infant that young, and have discovered only one symptomatic neonatal case in the literature (vide infra).

**PATHOGENESIS.** Von Gierke's disease is transmitted genetically as an autosomal recessive. The basic defect lies in congenital absence or deficiency of the enzyme glucose-6-phosphatase. This enzyme is not found in the blood cells, and therefore the deficiency can only be demonstrated in liver or intestine.

**DIAGNOSIS.** Symptoms commonly do not appear until several months after birth, when abdominal enlargement, loss of appetite and vomiting occur. In some instances the onset is marked by "sinking spells" that resemble and later prove to be hypoglycemic episodes.

The example reported by Calvin is of special interest to the neonatologist.

An enlarged, smooth liver was found at original examination soon after birth. There was a little vomiting during the first week, but nothing at all abnormal during the second and third weeks. At 3½ weeks, vomiting recurred, and listlessness developed. Examination showed nothing but lethargy and a liver enlarged to three finger-breadths below the costal margin. The infant took no food for the first 12 hours and began to have generalized convulsions at this time. The blood sugar level was found to be 10 mg per 100 ml, the urine acetone 4+. Intravenous glucose solution controlled convulsions and diminished lethargy. An epinephrine test revealed a flat curve. The infant did fairly well on a high protein, low carbohydrate food (pro-tein milk) but at six weeks, anorexia, vomiting, apathy and convulsions reappeared. The blood sugar level fell to 12 mg and could not be raised. An exploratory laparotomy was performed in the hope that a pancreatic islet cell tumor might be found and removed. Death followed. Autopsy showed glycogen storage disease of the liver and kidneys.

Von Gierke's disease is suspected because of hepatomegaly with or without sinking spells or convulsions. Withdrawal of food for a few hours leads to hypoglycemia and acetonuria. The blood lactate and pyruvate levels are high. The diagnosis is confirmed if an epinephrine injection fails to elevate the blood sugar level or elevates it only slightly. Coincidental laboratory findings include elevated serum levels of lactate, ketone bodies, total lipids, cholesterol and free fatty acids almost invariably. Liver biopsy supplies further assurance if most of the liver cells are vacuolated and the vacuoles can be shown to contain glycogen. Finally, the absence or paucity of glucose-6-phosphatase may be demonstrated in enzyme assay of liver tissues.

**PROGNOSIS.** Many infants fail to gain and grow adequately, dying of hypoglycemia and acidosis within the first years of life. A few, who are less severely afflicted, survive but their growth remains stunted and they become anemic and prone to repeated infections. If they live beyond 4 years, their prognosis progressively improves (Van Creveld and Huijing).

**TREATMENT.** Although therapy is not very successful, it is not without value. Afflicted infants may be supported slightly better on high protein, low carbohydrate diets. Feedings should be given every 3 or 4 hours, day and night for many months. The carbohydrate should be glucose or its polymers. Hypoglycemic episodes must be treated vigorously with parenteral fluids containing much glucose. The use of cortisone or its derivatives over a long period has not been of striking benefit.

## Generalized Glycogenosis (Pompe's Disease, Cori's Type II)

This type of glycogen storage disease is almost always determined by its effects upon the heart (massive cardiomegaly, early heart failure). It has therefore been discussed fully with the disorders of the cardiovascular system (p. 296).

Pompe's disease should be considered in the differential diagnosis of every cardiomegaly. Additional suggestive clinical evidence for this diagnosis includes weakness, hypotonia and hyporeflexia or areflexia of skeletal muscles and enlargement of the tongue. Failure to grow and gain weight precede the onset of cardiac failure. The muscular weakness, due to interference of function by massive glycogen deposition, has on occasion been of such degree as to suggest myasthenia gravis. The diagnosis must be considered in every case of macroglossia. Diagnosis can be inferred by bizarre electrocardiographic changes in the greatly enlarged heart (Caddell and Whittemore), and confirmed by muscle biopsy or by the discovery of a low level of alpha-glucosidase activity in leukocytes (Huijing et al.).

## CORI'S DISEASE ("DEBRANCHER" ENZYME DEFICIENCY OR CORI'S TYPE III)

To our knowledge this variety has never been diagnosed in the first month of life, but Hug et al. have reported a case in which tremendous hepatomegaly was found incidental to an acute febrile illness in a 7-month-old infant. It is likely that this sign could have been discovered months earlier.

In this type there is no cardiomegaly (because glycogen does not accumulate in smooth muscle) and no muscular weakness or hypotonia (because glycogen accumulation in striated muscle, though excessive, is not nearly so abundant as it is in Pompe's disease). Fasting hypoglycemia and hyperlipemia may be present. Hepatomegaly and failure to grow and gain normally are often the only clues.

The pathogenetic defect is deficiency of amylo-1,6-glucosidase, the "debrancher" enzyme. Diagnosis is suggested by a positive double glucagon test; that is, a failure of blood sugar to rise after glucagon has been administered after a 12-hour fast, but a normal rise when it is administered shortly after a meal. In this test if outer branches are available, glucagon can in-

duce phosphorylase to degrade them, but after these have been used up, the inner branches are not susceptible to cleavage in the absence of the "debrancher" enzyme. Diagnosis can be ascertained by a demonstration that amylo-1,6-glucosidase activity is markedly reduced in the patient's tissues.

## ESSENTIAL BENIGN FRUCTOSURIA

Fructose may be excreted in the urine in nephrosis and in some forms of liver disease. Fructosuria also appears in some persons who are deficient in the enzyme fructokinase, which catalyzes the transformation of fructose into fructose-1-phosphate. This disorder is transmitted as an autosomal recessive. Diagnosis is made by finding melituria in the presence of normal blood glucose levels and glucose tolerance curves, by identifying the sugar as fructose and by demonstrating prolonged and high curves of blood fructose concentration after its ingestion or intravenous administration. The disorder is asymptomatic. No treatment is required.

## HEREDITARY FRUCTOSE INTOLERANCE

This disorder is quite rare and virtually never is manifested in the neonatal period. The clinical symptoms of vomiting, hypoglycemia and hepatomegaly present when fruit or sucrose, each of which contains fructose, is ingested. The disorder is transmitted in an autosomal recessive manner and is due to a deficiency in liver aldolase B. Following the ingestion of fructose in such patients both fructose and fructose-1-phosphate accumulate in the body. In addition to the clinical findings, laboratory findings include a reduction in serum phosphate concentration and a picture of the urinary Fanconi syndrome with proteinuria, glycosuria and generalized hyperaminoaciduria. The diagnosis is based upon the characteristic clinical and laboratory findings following the ingestion of food containing fructose. Diagnosis may be confirmed by a fructose tolerance test in which the ingestion of a loading dose of fructose induces not only an abnormally high and prolonged blood fructose tolerance curve, but also, and more significantly, a reduction in serum phosphate and perhaps blood glucose concentrations. It should be noted that a fructose tolerance test in an affected infant should only be done in the hospital under carefully controlled conditions with intravenous fluid administered, since marked hypoglycemia can occur during this test. Treatment of this disorder is complete elimination of fruits, sugar and other fructose-containing foods from the diet.

## REFERENCES

Caddell, J. L., and Whittemore, R.: Observations on generalized glycogenosis, with emphasis on electrocardiographic changes. Pediatrics 29:743, 1962.

Calvin, J.: Glycogen storage disease. Am. J. Dis. Child. (Abstr.) 86:63, 1953.

Cori, G. T., and Cori, C. F.: Glucose-6-phosphatase of the liver in glycogen storage disease. J. Biol. Chem. 199:661, 1952.

Dancis, J., Hutzler, J., et al.: Absence of acid maltase in glycogenesis type 2 (Pompe's disease) in tissue culture. Am. J. Dis. Child. 117:108, 1969.

Donnell, G. N., and Lann, S. H.: Galactosemia: Report of four cases. Pediatrics 7:502, 1951.

Donnell, G. N., Collado, M., and Koch, R.: Growth and development of children with galactosemia. J. Pediatr. 58:836, 1961.

Gitzelmann, R.: Deficiency of uridine diphosphate galactose-4-epimerase in blood cells of an apparently healthy infant. Helv. Pediat. Acta 27:125, 1972.

Hammersen, G., Houghton, S., and Levy, H. L.: Rennes-like variant of galactosemia: Clinical and biochemical studies. J. Pediatr. 87:50, 1975.

Haworth, J. C., and McCredie, D.: Chromatographic separation of reducing substances in the urines of newborn babies. Arch Dis. Child. 31:189, 1956.

Howell, R. R., Ashton, D. M., and Wyngaarden, J. B.: Glucose-6-phosphatase deficiency. Glycogen storage disease. Pediatrics 29:553, 1962.

Hug, G., Krill, C. E., et al.: Cori's disease (amylo-1,6-glucosidase deficiency): Report of a case in a Negro child. N. Engl. J. Med. 268:113, 1963.

Huijing, F., van Creveld, S., and Loosekoot, G.: Diagnosis of generalized glycogen storage disease (Pompe's disease). J. Pediatr. 63:984, 1963.

Kalckar, H. M., Anderson, E. P., and Isselbacher, K. J.: Galactosemia, a congenital defect in a nucleotide transferase. Biochim. Biophys. Acta 20:262, 1956.

Kelly, S.: Septicemia in galactosemia. J.A.M.A. 216:330, 1971.

Koch, R., Acosta, P., et al.: Nutrition in the treatment of galactosemia. J. Am. Diet. Assoc. 43:216, 1963.

Komrower, G. M., Schwarz, V., et al.: A clinical and biochemical study of galactosemia: A possible explanation of the nature of the biochemical lesion. Arch. Dis. Child. 31:254, 1956.

Laron, Z.: Essential benign fructosemia. Arch. Dis. Child. 36:273, 1961.

Levy, H. L., Pueschel, S. M., and Hubbell, J. P., Jr.: Unconjugated hyperbilirubinemia. N. Engl. J. Med. 292:923, 1975.

Levy, H. L., and Shih, V. E.: Screening for galactosemia. N. Engl. J. Med. 287:723, 1972.

Nadler, H. L., Inouye, T., and Hsia, D. Y.-Y.: Classical galactosemia: A study of fifty-five cases. In Hsia, D. Y.-Y. (Ed.): Galactosemia. Springfield, Ill. Charles C Thomas, 1969, pp. 127–139.

Sadeghi-Nejad, A., Presente, E., et al.: Studies in type I glycogenosis of the liver. The genesis and disposition of lactate. J. Pediatr. 85:49, 1974.

Segal, S., Blair, A., and Roth, H.: The metabolism of galactose by patients with congenital galactosemia. Am. J. Med., 38:63, 1965.

Shih, V. E., Levy, H. L., et al.: Galactosemia screening of newborns in Massachusetts. N. Engl. J. Med. 284:753, 1971.

Smetana, H. F., and Olen, E.: Hereditary galactose disease. Am. J. Clin. Path. 38:3, 1962.

Thalhammer, O., Gitzelmann, R., and Pantlitschko, M.: Hypergalactosemia and galactosuria due to galactokinase deficiency in a newborn. Pediatrics 42:441, 1968.

Van Creveld, S., and Huijing, F.: Glycogenosis. Memorias del XII Congreso Internacional de Pediatria, Vol. II, 554, 1962.

Willems, C., Heusden, A., et al.: Hypertyrosinémie avec hyperméthioninémie néonatales dan un cas d'intolérance au fructose. Helv. Paediat. Acta 26:467, 1971.

# INBORN ERRORS OF AMINO ACID METABOLISM

# 60

*By Harvey Levy*

Routine newborn screening and other testing programs are still uncovering new disorders and variants of known disorders within this category. Most of the detectable free amino acids in the body are involved in one or another of these disorders, either directly or indirectly. It is neither necessary nor desirable to discuss them all in a general text such as this. A number are very rare and therefore are not likely to be encountered by any one individual. Others, however, are more likely to be seen either as a result of routine newborn screening for metabolic disorders or because of their presentation with clinical abnormalities in the newborn period. It is important to note that for many of these disorders therapy is available that may prevent irreversible clinical damage, but for optimal effectiveness it must be instituted during the early days or weeks of life. It is also important to realize that the diagnosis of many of these disorders may be difficult and must be confirmed by experienced laboratory personnel before therapy can be begun. A laboratory such as this is probably available in only one or two places within each state or region and should be contacted whenever a question concerning one of these disorders arises.

## PHENYLKETONURIA

Phenylketonuria, often called PKU, is an inborn error of metabolism involving the amino acid phenylalanine. If treatment is not begun in the neonatal period or at least fairly early during infancy brain damage with mental retardation almost invariably results. The early institution of dietary therapy, well before symptoms have appeared, will prevent the mental retardation that would otherwise result. Thus, it is of utmost importance that this disorder be diagnosed in all affected neonates by the routine screening of blood specimens.

**INCIDENCE.** Based on the results of routine newborn screening for PKU within the United States and in many other countries, the general frequency is about one in 15,000 individuals. However, among different countries and even among different states within the United States this frequency seems to vary between one per 6000 and less than one per 25,000. These differences presumably relate to genetic variations among different ethnic groups. Thus, the highest frequencies are reported in Ireland and among Americans of Irish descent, while it is rarely found among Blacks and Jews. Approximately 1 to 2 per cent of individuals currently institu-

tionalized for mental retardation are found to have PKU.

**ETIOLOGY AND PATHOGENESIS.** PKU is inherited in an autosomal recessive manner. It is estimated that 1 to 2 per cent of the population are carriers of the gene. In the affected state the genetic abnormality results in an almost total lack of phenylalanine hydroxylase activity, which in turn results in an inability to convert phenylalanine to tyrosine (see Fig. 58–1), permitting a marked accumulation of phenylalanine in the blood, other body fluids and tissues. The urine may contain excessive amounts of phenylalanine and its metabolites, which include phenylpyruvic acid, phenyllactic acid, phenylacetic acid, phenylacetylglutamine and o-hydroxyphenylacetic acid. However, in the neonatal period there may be little or no urinary excretion of at least the first three of these phenylalanine metabolites, owing to the fact that their formation is dependent upon activity of phenylalanine transaminase, an activity that may be low until the infant is several months of age.

It appears that the brain damage noted in untreated PKU is either a direct or an indirect result of the accumulation of phenylalanine or its metabolites, or of both. Thus, when these concentrations have been controlled by use of a special diet, mental retardation and other manifestations of brain damage do not appear. Although the precise mechanism of this brain toxicity is not known, the most generally accepted theory is that the phenylalanine exerts toxicity directly on the neurons. Another theory is that of direct toxicity not of phenylalanine but of its metabolites; still another theory suggests that the toxicity is secondary to a general reduction in intracellular amino acid concentration produced by an inhibition of cellular uptake of amino acids exerted by increased phenylalanine. Regardless of which of these theories is correct, reduction in the accumulation of phenylalanine and its metabolites by the low-phenylalanine diet currently in use would seem to be the proper available form of therapy.

**DIAGNOSIS.** Routine newborn screening for PKU is a necessity because clinical signs of this disorder do not appear until brain damage is already irreversible to some degree. There is no greater incidence of complications during the prenatal, perinatal and neonatal periods among phenylketonurics than one would find in the general newborn population. Affected infants usually appear entirely normal. Clinical symptoms that may be associated with PKU, including irritability, eczema and signs of brain damage, usually are not seen until the infant is several months of age, when the brain damage may already be to some extent irreversible. The so-called "musty" odor of the urine is rarely detected until late in infancy or even in childhood in the untreated patient.

Diagnosis in the neonatal period must always be made by the demonstration of an increased phenylalanine concentration in blood. If it is already known that PKU is present in the family, particularly in a sibling, the suspicion of PKU must be especially high, since the disorder is inherited. For instance, if a sibling is known to have PKU each parent is presumably a carrier for the gene and thus the chances of any other child having PKU are one in four. Even when there is no family history of PKU a blood test should be performed on the newborn infant. In most states there is a general statewide program for testing all newborn infants for PKU. Usually a filter paper specimen of blood is obtained from a heel puncture and sent to a central state laboratory. There, the specimen is usually examined by the Guthrie Bacterial Inhibition Assay or by a fluorometric assay for phenylalanine. In most infants with PKU the blood phenylalanine concentration, which is normally 2 mg per 100 ml or less, will be at least 8 mg per 100 mg or greater by the third day of life. However, an occasional PKU infant will have only a slight degree of phenylalanine increase. In order not to overlook this occasional infant it is important that another blood specimen be obtained on all newborn infants whose blood phenylalanine concentration is at least 4 mg per 100 ml or greater.

It is important to remember that the urine of a newborn infant with PKU rarely has a detectable increase in phenylalanine and its metabolites. Thus, the urine ferric chloride test that responds to phenylpyruvic acid, which may be effective in detecting PKU in older infants and children, is almost always ineffective in detecting PKU in the newborn period. Consequently no currently available urine test should be relied upon for the detection of PKU in the newborn infant.

In the course of newborn screening for PKU a repeat blood specimen must be requested from a number of infants who have no metabolic disorder, including PKU. This is an unfortunate but seemingly inevitable aspect of such screening. A number of entirely normal newborns will have blood phenylalanine concentrations that may be as great as 4 or even 6 mg per 100 ml in the first specimen of blood. Since infants with PKU may also have a mild elevation of this degree during the first days of life, all such infants must be retested. In this repeat blood specimen the infant with PKU who is on a normal diet should have a blood phenylalanine concentration well above 6 mg per 100 ml and often will have a concentration that is in excess of 20 mg per 100 ml, whereas the normal infant will have an entirely normal blood phenylalanine concentration.

Recently there has been a good deal of discussion concerning the optimal age for obtaining this blood specimen. The general practice is to obtain the specimen at the time of discharge from the nursery. Since this is usually on the third day of life and since the concentration of blood phenylalanine is usually elevated in the infant with PKU by that age, there is generally no problem in detecting PKU by this method. However, many infants are currently being discharged from newborn nurseries on the second day of life and on occasion even sooner. Since elevation of the blood phenylalanine concentration in an infant with PKU depends to some extent upon the length of time he has been ingesting protein, there is concern that infants with PKU whose blood has been obtained on the first and second day of life may not manifest the biochemical abnormality. The extent to which this concern is valid is not yet known, and a recent study from California would suggest that many infants with PKU may even have an elevated blood phenylalanine concentration by the first day of life. It is probably best to obtain a second blood specimen from all infants whose blood was initially obtained on the first or second day of life even if the phenylalanine concentraion in this first blood specimen is normal.

The detection of an increased blood phenylalanine concentration in a newborn infant, while usually indicative of PKU, may be associated with other metabolic disorders. For instance, phenylalanine may be increased as part of the generalized increase in the blood amino acid concentration in an infant who is ill with galactosemia. In at least one infant this increase in phenylalanine was the first indication of the presence of galactosemia. Newborn infants who are quite ill and dehydrated from other metabolic disorders, such as maple syrup urine disease, may also have an increase in the blood phenylalanine concentration. As in galactosemia this is usually associated with a general increase in the concentration of all detectable blood amino acids. Whenever an infant is found to have increased blood phenylalanine by the Guthrie test, other tests, such as paper chromatography or quantitative amino acid analysis, should be performed to determine whether the blood phenylalanine increase is a specific finding indicative of PKU or whether other amino acids are increased as well, which should lead to the suspicion of another metabolic disorder. Since the treatment of PKU can be difficult and may be exceedingly hazardous to an infant who does not have PKU, the diagnosis of this disorder should never be made and the treatment should never begin unless one is absolutely certain that he is dealing with phenylketonuria.

**TREATMENT.** Once developmental retardation and other signs of brain damage have become manifest treatment may be of little or no benefit. Ground lost during the early period of rapid cerebral development can never be completely regained. Ideal treatment consists, as it does in galactosemia, in preventing any brain damage.

When the diagnosis of phenylketonuria has been clearly confirmed by several different diagnostic criteria, the infant should be given a low-phenylalanine diet. This treatment regimen, particularly in its early stages, must be planned and monitored carefully under the guidance of physicians, dietitians, nutritionists and others who are experienced and knowledgeable in the treatment of PKU. Initially the regular infant formula is discontinued and a synthetic diet low in phenylalanine is substituted. It is important to remember, however, that this synthetic diet must not be given alone but must be supplemented with a certain amount of milk in order to supply the infant with his minimum phenylalanine requirements. If this is not done the body will quickly be depleted of phenylalanine, reflected in an undetectable blood phenylalanine concentration, and severe complications such as brain damage and even death can result. The amount of milk necessary as a dietary supplement varies from one infant to another and must be added to the diet on the basis of the blood phenylalanine concentration. In general this concentration should be maintained within a range of 4 to 8 mg/100 ml. Later in infancy the foods added to the diet should be low in protein, generally fruits and vegetables.

In most treatment centers a low phenylalanine diet is continued until the child is about 4 or 5 years of age, at which time, it is believed by many, the brain is no longer susceptible to damage resulting from untreated PKU. Consequently, high protein foods such as meat, fish and milk are gradually introduced until the child is on an essentially normal diet. Studies have indicated that, though the accumulation of phenylalanine and related metabolites then becomes as great as in a child with PKU who had never been treated, there is no evidence of brain damage occurring as a result of discontinuing the diet.

It seems that for optimal effectiveness the infant should be started on the low phenylalanine diet by the age of 3 weeks. It is strongly recommended that treatment be carried out and monitored in a center where similar cases are being managed. The busy pediatrician simply cannot supervise such patients adequately.

## HYPERPHENYLALANINEMIAS

Aside from phenylketonuria there are other inborn errors of metabolism which are associated with reduced activity of liver phenylalanine hydroxylase and which result in mild to moderate degrees of increased blood phenylalanine concentration in the untreated state. These were formerly considered under the rubric of phenylketonuria but are clearly distinct entities.

### "Atypical Phenylketonuria"

An infant whose blood phenylalanine concentrations in the untreated condition are consistently greater than 12 mg per 100 ml but less than 20 mg per 100 ml is usually considered to have this entity. The initial newborn screening test often reveals a lower phenylalanine concentration than in the true phenylketonuric. The frequency of this condition is lower than that of phenylketonuria and may be in the order of approximately 1:30,000. In the United States "atypical PKU" seems to be more common among those of Italian descent than among other ethnic groups. It is not known to what extent clinical complications may occur in this disorder, although it is believed that if left untreated lowered intellectual performance or a mild degree of mental retardation may result. In most centers a low-phenylalanine diet is administered to such infants just as in phenylketonuria. However, since these infants have a greater tolerance for phenylalanine than the infant with PKU, it is important to remember that the diet in these infants must be monitored with particular care.

### Persistent Mild Hyperphenylalaninemia

As is "atypical phenylketonuria," this entity is usually genetically distinct from phenylketonuria. The infant with persistent mild hyperphenylalaninemia (PMH) in the untreated state has a blood phenylalanine concentration consistently greater than the normal 2 mg per 100 ml but no greater than 12 mg per 100 ml. The frequency of this condition seems to be similar to that of "atypical phenylketonuria," about 1:30,000. It appears to have some ethnic distribution, having a much higher frequency among Ashkenazi Jews in Israel and in the United States than does phenylketonuria. The importance of this

entity is that it seems to be clinically benign and thus probably should not be treated. Consequently, it must be differentiated from "atypical phenylketonuria" and true phenylketonuria.

### Maternal Phenylketonuria

During the last few years it has been discovered that women with phenylketonuria who receive no dietary therapy during pregnancy may bear non-phenylketonuric offspring who are mentally retarded and perhaps microcephalic. The reason for this is not clear but it is presumed that the increased phenylalanine and metabolites that may cause brain damage to any affected individual may also cross the placenta in such a mother and cause prenatal brain damage to the fetus. This entity is of potentially great importance, since as a result of newborn screening programs there will be in the decades ahead a number of women who have PKU but who are mentally normal and thus who will want to bear children. Will all such women have offspring who are mentally retarded?

It now appears that those women who have true phenylketonuria with blood phenylalanine concentrations of 20 mg per 100 ml or greater and perhaps some women with "atypical phenylketonuria" may be in such danger. Women who have persistent mild hyperphenylalaninemia and perhaps women with "atypical phenylketonuria" whose blood phenylalanine concentrations are not greater than 14 mg per 100 ml seemingly may bear normal children. Furthermore, there are now a number of reported instances of apparently normal offspring resulting from pregnancies in which the mother with phenylketonuria received a low phenylalanine diet during pregnancy, with control of the blood phenylalanine concentrations at levels of less than 12 mg per 100 ml. Additional information must be accumulated before proper decisions can be made concerning the finding of increased blood phenylalanine in pregnant women. At the present time, however, one should keep in mind that all mothers who have borne one or more mentally retarded children should themselves be tested for phenylketonuria. If phenylketonuria is found, the mother and her family should be so advised in order that family planning decisions or decisions regarding a low phenylalanine diet during future pregnancies can be made.

## MAPLE SYRUP URINE DISEASE (BRANCHED-CHAIN KETOACIDURIA)

This is an inborn error of metabolism involving the so-called branched-chain amino acids (leucine, isoleucine and valine). It is inherited in an autosomal recessive manner. The basic enzymatic defect appears to be in the mechanism concerning activity of the three branched-chain α-ketoacid decarboxylases. As a result the untreated infant develops an accumulation not only of the three branched-chain amino acids but also of their corresponding ketoacids. The latter presumably cause a severe metabolic acidosis which, if untreated, can result in neonatal death. The frequency of maple syrup urine disease is not known but seems to be less than one per 100,000.

There are at least three different disorders within the "maple syrup urine disease" category. The first and most dramatic is that termed *maple syrup urine disease* itself. In this entity the infant usually has a normal prenatal and perinatal history. On about the third day of life, he may be noted to be lethargic. By the fourth or fifth day of life, vomiting, increased lethargy, poor feeding and perhaps neurologic signs such as opisthotonos appear. Metabolic acidosis is clearly evident by this time. If treatment is not begun, the course of the infant is progressively downhill. The neurologic signs increase, with the appearance of convulsions and marked hypotonia. Death ensues by the age of 2 weeks in almost all such infants. The second entity, known as *intermediate maple syrup urine disease,* is usually totally asymptomatic within the neonatal period. Such infants appear to be normal until they are several months old, at which time developmental lag is noted. Subsequently frank mental retardation becomes obvious and episodes of metabolic acidosis, often mild and associated with acute febrile illnesses, develop. The third entity, known as *intermittent maple syrup urine disease,* is also asymptomatic during the neonatal period, and usually remains asymptomatic even later in infancy and early childhood except when there is an acute febrile episode or trauma, such as that due to surgery or an accident. During these episodes severe metabolic acidosis with all of the acute signs of maple syrup urine disease may occur. Several such affected individuals have died during these acute episodes.

**DIAGNOSIS.** As in virtually all other inborn errors of metabolism, the most effective means of diagnosing maple syrup urine disease is by routine newborn screening. In several states, the blood specimen that is obtained for PKU screening is also tested for increased blood leucine concentrations in order to detect maple syrup urine disease. In an infant with the severe form of maple syrup urine disease, this may be the only effective means of instituting therapy before irreversible brain damage or death has occurred. For infants with other forms of maple syrup urine disease, this may be the only means by which the disease is suspected before other irreversible changes have occurred.

If there is a suspicion of maple syrup urine disease on the basis of either clinical signs or a family history, blood and urine specimens should be obtained and sent to a laboratory where the proper testing can be performed. During acute episodes in any form of maple syrup urine disease, the branched-chain amino acid concentrations in blood, particularly leucine, will be far greater than the normal 2 mg per 100 ml, perhaps as high as 40 mg per 100 ml, or even greater than 50 mg per 100 ml. The urine may have an odor reminiscent of maple syrup. The branched-chain ketoacid concentration in the urine will be exceedingly high and may be detected by a screening test using the dinitrophenylhydrazine reagent. When this reagent is added to a normal urine there will be no change but when it is added to a urine containing a large concentration of ketoacids, the dinitrophenylhydrazones will be formed, resulting in a cloudy precipitate. Amino acid analysis of the urine will often reveal increased branched-chain amino acids.

In the intermediate form of maple syrup urine disease, the only finding may be that of increased blood leucine concentration except during acute episodes, when all of the other findings appear. In the intermittent form of this disorder, blood amino acids as well as urine amino acids and ketoacids may be perfectly normal in concentration except during acute episodes. Thus, this latter type of maple syrup urine disease may be particularly difficult to diagnose and often can be suspected only on clinical grounds. In the neonatal period, the blood leucine concentration should be increased in the severe and intermediate forms of maple syrup urine disease at any time after the first or second day of life but may be entirely normal in the intermittent form of maple syrup urine disease.

**TREATMENT.** In general, the treatment of any form of maple syrup urine disease is dietary. The diet must be reduced in branched-chain amino acid content, especially that of leucine, and is exceedingly difficult to prepare and administer. The dietary therapy should only be attempted at a medical center staffed by physicians and others who have the time and knowledge to deal properly with this difficult disorder. The basic diet consists of a mixture composed of the necessary free amino acids and excluding the branched-chain amino acids, proper minerals, a carbohydrate and a fat such as corn oil. This basic diet must be prepared in a way that will be reasonably palatable and must be supplemented with a small amount of milk or other food containing the branched-chain amino aids as well as low-protein foods such as fruits and vegetables.

It has recently been discovered that an occasional infant with the intermediate form of maple syrup urine disease responds to supplemental amounts of vitamin $B_1$ (thiamine). The cofactor metabolite of thiamine is normally necessary for the proper activity of the branched-chain decarboxylases. In individuals with maple syrup urine disease who are thiamine responsive, it is probable that in some way the increased thiamine activates the enzyme to some degree. Unfortunately, more individuals with maple syrup disease of any form seem to be unresponsive to thiamine.

# SULFUR AMINO ACID ABNORMALITIES

There are several different disorders within this group. All are due to a specific metabolic block within the methionine metabolic pathway. Their clinical importance seems to range from none whatsoever to severe clinical disease. Each is seemingly inherited in an autosomal recessive manner. All may be detectable in a newborn screening program for metabolic disorders if the proper methods are used, and are currently so screened for in a number of states within the United States and in several other countries.

## Hypermethioninemia

Increased blood concentrations of methionine may be induced in a perfectly normal neonate by the feeding of a high protein diet. This is a transient state that will disappear within 2 or 3 days after the high protein diet is discontinued. If the increased protein ingestion is continued hypermethioninemia will also spontaneously disappear by the time the infant is about 3 months old. No clinical abnormality is known to result from hypermethioninemia.

Increased blood concentrations of methionine are also related to neonatal liver disease of the "hepatitis" type. It is presumed that the hypermethioninemia as well as the tyrosinemia that is seen in association with this type of liver disease are secondary to hepatocellular damage. These amino acid abnormalities are important only in that they may serve as indicators of the presence of liver disease and perhaps also as measures of the severity of damage.

A recent inborn error of metabolism known as methionine adenosyltransferase deficiency has been described in which there is a specific hypermethioninemia. The two infants reported with this disorder have been entirely normal without any therapy aimed at reducing the accumulation of methionine in the blood. Thus this may very well be a benign condition.

## Cystathionine Synthase Deficiency

This disorder, usually referred to as "homocystinuria," is due to a deficiency in activity of the enzyme cystathionine synthase and results in the accumulation of methionine in blood and homocystine in blood and urine. It is transmitted as an autosomal recessive and has a frequency of probably one per 50,000 to one per 100,000 of the population. It does not usually appear in the neonatal period. Later in infancy, however, the propensity for thromboembolic phenomena present in this disease may result in cerebral thrombosis with signs of stroke. Thus, infants with acute cerebral thromboses should always be tested for the presence of this disorder. If untreated the disorder leads to brain damage with mental retardation, dislocation of the ocular lenses, various severe skeletal abnormalities with osteoporosis and thromboembolic phenomena later in life. However, the clinical manifestations are highly variable, and some individuals may escape the severe manifestations of brain damage and even the severe skeletal abnormalities.

Diagnosis is based upon the presence of homocystine in the urine and an elevated blood methionine. It is particularly difficult to diagnose in the neonate, as such small infants may not have the hypermethioninemia associated with this disorder. Conversely, other infants with cystathionine synthase deficiency may have hypermethioninemia but lack the homocystinuria. Consequently, for effective diagnosis the blood should be tested for methionine concentration, and homocystine should be sought in the urine.

Treatment may be difficult and should be administered only at centers staffed by experienced people. A number of affected individuals (perhaps as many as 50 per cent) seem to be biochemically responsive to supplemental amounts of vitamin $B_6$ (pyridoxine). In such individuals large amounts of pyridoxine, perhaps in association with a modified low-methionine diet, may be all that is necessary to control the biochemical manifestations. Individuals who are resistant to pyridoxine should be treated with a low-methionine diet.

### Cystathioninuria

This inborn error is caused by a deficiency of the enzyme cystathionase and is associated with an accumulation of cystathionine in blood and urine. There are two forms; one is responsive to supplemental amounts of pyridoxine and the other is resistant to this vitamin. Diagnosis is made on the basis of a persistent increase of cystathionine in urine as well as on the demonstration of detectable amounts of cystathionine in blood. Present evidence would indicate that this is a benign disorder with no clinical consequence in either the early infantile or later periods of life.

### TYROSINEMIA

Tyrosinemia, an increase in the concentration of the amino acid tyrosine, may be present either transiently or persistently in the newborn.

### Transient Neonatal Tyrosinemia (TNT)

This entity is said to occur in as many as 5 to 10 per cent of all newborns. It is caused by delayed maturation of the enzyme parahydroxyphenylpyruvic acid oxidase, an enzyme responsible for the conversion of parahydroxyphenylpyruvic acid to homogentisic acid. When activity of this enzyme is reduced, parahydroxyphenylpyruvic acid and tyrosine, its immediate precursor, accumulate. In addition, there is a secondary accumulation of other metabolites of tyrosine, including parahydroxyphenyllactic acid and parahydroxyphenylacetic acid. A markedly increased concentration of tyrosine is noted in the blood, sometimes in excess of 20 mg per 100 ml (normal blood tyrosine concentration is less than 4 mg/100 ml). Tyrosine and the metabolites noted above are present in greatly excess quantities in the urine.

There are several interesting characteristics of this common disorder. First, transient neonatal tyrosinemia is considerably more frequent among premature than among fullterm infants. This is presumably related to a greater tendency for immaturity of many or most enzyme systems among prematures. Second, this entity is clearly related to a high protein intake. Since most protein contains a fairly large quantity of tyrosine, an increased protein intake would presumably result in a greater body load of tyrosine, possibly in excess of that which can be metabolized by the residual enzyme activity. Third, the deficient enzyme is dependent to a degree upon the presence of vitamin C (ascorbic acid), and it has been found that supplemental quantities of ascorbic acid may result in its activation and thus may reverse the abnormal tyrosine and tyrosine metabolite accumulations.

Transient neonatal tyrosinemia usually appears after the first week of life when the protein intake has been increased beyond that of the first days of life. In susceptible infants the tyrosinemia usually reaches its peak during the second or third month of life, especially when the protein intake has been rather markedly increased at that time. There is presently some debate as to whether any clinical consequences occur as the result of transient neonatal tyrosinemia. Although some authors have reported a slightly reduced intellectual performance among children who had transient neonatal tyrosinemia, others report no such reduction at all. At the present time it is probably advisable to limit the protein intake of all infants to less to 6 gm per kg of body weight and to maintain a daily ascorbic acid intake of 25 to 50 mg so as to lessen the chances for significant neonatal tyrosinemia to occur.

This entity can occasionally confuse the results of newborn screening for phenylketonuria. A marked elevation of tyrosine in transient neonatal tyrosinemia may secondarily result in an increase in the blood concentration of phenylalanine, the immediate precursor of tyrosine (see Fig. 58–1). When this occurs the finding of an increased phenylalanine concentration in a newborn blood specimen may be mistakenly thought to be due to phenylketonuria. However, if a blood amino acid analysis is performed the differentiation between phenylketonuria and transient neontal tyrosinemia is unmistakable, the former being associated with a normal or low tyrosine concentration and the latter with a markedly increased tyrosine concentration. Thus, this analysis should be performed on all infants whose initial newborn screening test suggests phenylketonuria.

## Hereditary Tyrosinemia

This is a little understood metabolic disorder, which is probably genetically determined and inherited in an autosomal recessive manner, though this is not clear. Equally unclear is the precise enzymatic defect which seemingly lies at the level of liver parahydroxyphenylpyruvic acid oxidase. However, some infants with manifestations of this disorder have also had deficient activities of liver tyrosine transaminase. The major biochemical manifestations are those of increased tyrosine and methionine in blood and increased tyrosine and tyrosine metabolites in urine.

Affected infants are usually clinically normal until the end of the first month or two of life, when jaundice and hepatomegaly are noted. At this time liver function tests are abnormal and there may be a urinary pattern of the Fanconi syndrome with glycosuria, generalized hyperaminoaciduria and proteinuria. Within the next few weeks the signs of hepatic and renal disease progress and radiographic changes of rickets are noted. If untreated, death due to liver disease occurs later, during the first year or perhaps during the second year of life. Unlike transient neonatal tyrosinemia hereditary tyrosinemia does not respond to ascorbic acid. A diet that is low in phenylalanine and tyrosine may control the biochemical abnormalities and result in reversal of the renal abnormalities and rickets but, except in a few isolated cases, has not been effective in reversing the progression of liver disease.

There is much debate on whether hereditary tyrosinemia is a primary inborn error of metabolism that produces the clinical complications noted above or whether the biochemical abnormalities are secondary to a peculiar and perhaps specific type of liver disease. It is certainly true that severe hepatocellular disease can result in an accumulation of tyrosine and tyrosine metabolites, which disappear when the liver disease improves. It is also true that infants with inborn errors of metabolism that do not primarily involve tyrosine but that do affect the liver, such as hereditary fructose intolerance (see Chapter 59), may also have the biochemical findings of tyrosinemia. It is equally true that there are many instances of severe infantile liver disease that are not associated with tyrosinemia or, if so, are not also associated with renal abnormalities and rickets.

### Tyrosinosis

This may be a second inborn error of tyrosine metabolism. Only a few cases have been reported. There is some evidence that it is a single entity associated with a deficiency of cytosol tyrosine transaminase and that the accumulations of tyrosine in blood and urine and of tyrosine metabolites in urine are secondary to this deficiency. Despite the latter accumulations, which are identical to those noted in hereditary tyrosinemia, there are no abnormalities of liver, kidney or bone. However, all of the reported patients have been mentally retarded. Clinically the mental retardation appears to be very much like that noted in phenylketonuria, with developmental delay becoming obvious during the first year of life and frank intellectual retardation becoming manifest during the second and third years. In addition, most affected children have had a peculiar keratosis of the palms and soles and a keratitis of the cornea. Treatment has not yet been successfully given, though presumably the disorder would respond biochemically to a diet low in phenylalanine and tyrosine. If an analogy to phenylketonuria can be made it would seem that the diet would have to be instituted during the early weeks of life for optimal effectiveness. As in hereditary tyrosinemia, ascorbic acid is not effective in the treatment of tyrosinosis.

## UREA CYCLE DISORDERS

This group of inborn errors of metabolism will be specifically discussed in this chapter because dramatic and severe clinical symptoms may appear during the neonatal period. Each disorder is associated with a specific enzymatic deficiency within the Krebs-Hensleit urea cycle, a cycle whereby the human converts ammonia to urea, the latter to be excreted in urine as a waste product. This is an extremely important cycle within the body, since a block within this cycle will result in an increased level of ammonia and consequently the clinical symptoms of hyperammonemia or ammonia intoxication. Thus, all of the disorders within the urea cycle may have similar clinical symptoms. These include lethargy, poor weight gain or weight loss, vomiting, hypotonia or even neonatal collapse and unresponsiveness if the blood ammonia concentration becomes markedly increased during the first day or two of life. Symptoms of lethargy, poor weight gain, vomiting and developmental delay may not appear until later in infancy in the milder forms of any of these disorders.

Treatment consists of a low protein diet to reduce the elevated blood ammonia concentration. If the symptoms are severe, especially in the neonatal period, death will rapidly occur unless rather dramatic treatment is given. In certain reported instances this form of therapy has consisted of exchange transfusion or peritoneal dialysis, or both.

### Ornithine Transcarbamylase (OTC) Deficiency

Unlike most inborn errors of metabolism this is X-linked. Thus affected male infants, who are hemizygotes, have virtually no activity of this liver enzyme and become severely hyperammonemic during the first days of life. Characteristically these infants are born as normal individuals but by the second or third day of life develop symptoms of marked lethargy and hypotonia. Amino acid analysis of blood reveals reduced citrulline and arginine but, strangely, no increase in ornithine. There is also a large amount of orotic acid in urine. Despite dramatic treatment in a few cases no male infant with this disorder has lived longer than 2 months. Females with this disorder are heterozygotes and thus have approximately 50 per cent of normal enzyme activity in the liver. They usually do not manifest signs of hyperammonemia during early infancy, but later in life, especially during times when the protein intake has been increased, they may become hyperammonemic with vomiting, lethargy and ataxia. Treatment of these individuals is reduction of protein intake.

## Citrullinemia

This is probably inherited in an autosomal recessive manner and is associated with a deficiency of the enzyme argininosuccinic acid synthetase. The major observable biochemical abnormality is that of an increase in the blood and urine concentration of citrulline. Only a few cases have been described. The disorder may present in infancy, and signs of hyperammonemia may be present or clinical signs may appear later in life.

## Carbamyl Synthetase Deficiency

This seemingly autosomal recessive disorder is caused by a deficiency of the first enzyme within the urea cycle. Severe signs of hyperammonemia may develop early in infancy and be clinically indistinguishable from ornithine transcarbamylase deficiency; however, in contrast to the latter, there is no orotic acid in the urine. Treatment of the few reported cases has had limited effectiveness.

## Argininosuccinic Acidemia

This is perhaps the most frequent urea cycle disorder. It is autosomal recessive and is associated with a deficiency of argininosuccinase, an enzyme that can be measured in red blood cells as well as in cultured skin fibroblasts. Marked elevations of argininosuccinic acid are noted in urine, and increased concentrations of this amino acid may be detected in the blood. There are several forms of this disorder. The first presents in the neonatal period with severe hyperammonemia, and huge accumulations of argininosuccinic acid; collapse with unresponsiveness has invariably resulted in death despite therapeutic attempts. The second presentation is that of the infant who is clinically normal during the first month or two of life but by the third or fourth month develops signs of developmental lag, hepatomegaly and often peculiarly sparse and coarse hair. Signs of brain damage and liver disease progress, often

with the onset of convulsions later in infancy. If treatment is not given until after clinical manifestations have appeared, these infants will probably die by the end of the first year or during the second year of life. The third presenting picture is that of the infant who has argininosuccinic acidemia but no clinical abnormalities. These infants have been discovered as a result of routine newborn screening for metabolic disorders. Whether or not they represent a clinically benign form of argininosuccinic acidemia has not yet been determined.

## Argininemia

This is associated with a deficiency of arginase, an enzyme that can also be measured in red blood cells. Only a very few cases have been reported. The major clinical symptoms have been a progressive neurologic degeneration, usually appearing in late infancy or early childhood and marked by developmental delay, ataxia and spasticity. A mild hyperammonemia has also been noted in most cases.

# HYPERGLYCINEMIA

This is not a disorder per se but a biochemical abnormality noted in a number of disorders that may produce clinical signs in the neonatal period. When associated with ketosis and metabolic acidosis, the hyperglycinemia is termed "ketotic" and may be secondary to any one of a group of inborn errors of organic acid metabolism. Hyperglycinemia may also be present as an isolated but striking finding in the absence of ketosis and acidosis and, when so, is called non-ketotic hyperglycinemia.

### THE KETOTIC HYPERGLYCINEMIAS

Signs of metabolic acidosis usually develop during the first or second week of life. The infant may vomit, feed poorly, be lethargic and fail to gain weight. Studies of blood will reveal, in addition to the metabolic acidosis, a glycine concentration that will be two to six times normal. Urinary glycine will be markedly increased but there will be no other amino acid abnormality. Tests for urinary ketones, such as that using the Acetest* tablet or the Keto-stix*, will be positive. The basic disorder present, however, is one involving a defect in the metabolism of an organic acid. These disorders will be discussed in Chapter 61.

## NON-KETOTIC HYPERGLYCINEMIA

Several clinical syndromes have been described in association with hyperglycinemia in the absence of ketosis and acidosis. These are sufficiently distinct as to suggest that this form of hyperglycinemia, like the ketotic hyperglycinemias, may also be a secondary finding. However no specific disorder involving compounds other than glycine has yet been discovered in an individual with non-ketotic hyperglycinemia.

ACUTE NEONATAL TYPE. The clinical picture in this disorder is one of the most striking in neonatal medicine. The infant, who is usually born after a normal pregnancy, appears to be normal for the first 24 to 36 hours of life. At this time he begins to appear lethargic, and by the end of the second day is so inactive and hypotonic as to be characterized as having "acute neonatal collapse." A respirator is often necessary. Biochemical studies fail to reveal acidosis or hyperammonemia. In fact, the routine biochemical findings are surprisingly normal for such a serious clinical state. Amino acid studies reveal a markedly increased blood glycine concentration, sometimes as great as 10 times normal, and a huge urinary excretion of glycine. The CSF contains an even greater increase in glycine than is present in blood, resulting in a relatively low plasma to CSF glycine. Studies of short-chain fatty acids and other organic acids have revealed normal findings. Measurements of glycine oxidase in the liver of a few patients have revealed reduced activity, though it is not yet clear whether this is a primary or secondary finding.

Specific and effective therapy for this disorder has not yet been devised. Despite efforts that have included exchange transfusion and peritoneal dialysis, almost all of these infants have died within a few weeks of birth. The one infant in our experience who has survived has severe brain damage and is in an almost vegetative state. Recently, it has been suggested that early and massive treatment with sodium benzoate may reduce the glycine accumulations and may also improve the clinical status, though this has not yet been given adequate trial.

INFANTILE TYPE. These infants appear to be normal until 1 to 2 months of age, when poor head control and other signs of developmental lag become evident. Myoclonic seizures often develop shortly thereafter. As in the acute neonatal type, biochemical studies reveal a specific increase in blood and urinary glycine as well as a reduced plasma to CSF glycine ratio. The glycine accumulations, however, usually are less marked than those noted in the acute neonatal type, with blood glycine often being no greater than two to four times normal. A diet specifically low in glycine content may be effective in controlling this disorder, though adequate trials have not yet been conducted. Since a few affected infants have had a bizarre comatose response to the administration of L-valine, it is possible that valine is in some way related to this disorder. However, no specific valine metabolic defect has yet been described in such individuals.

OTHER FORMS. An unusual type of spinal motor neuron disease causing weakness of the legs and beginning in childhood or adolescence has been described in several patients with non-ketotic hyperglycinemia. There might also be a benign form, though this has not been clearly ascertained.

---

*Ames Company, Elkhart, IN 46514

## REFERENCES

Avery, M. E., Clow, C. L., et al.: Transient tryosinemia of the newborn: Dietary and clinical aspects. Pediatrics 39:378, 1967.

Bank, W. J., and Morrow, G. III: A familial spinal cord disorder with hyperglycinemia. Arch. Neurol. 27:136, 1972.

Berman, J. L., and Ford, R.: Intelligence quotients and intelligence loss in patients with phenylketonuria and some variant states. J. Pediatr. 77:764, 1970.

Bickel, H., Gerrard, J., and Hickmans, E. M.: The influence of phenylalanine intake on the chemistry and behavior of a phenylketonuric child. Acta Paediat. *43*:64, 1954.

Campbell, A. G. M., Rosenberg, L. E., et al.: Ornithine transcarbamylase deficiency. A cause of lethal neonatal hyperammonemia in males. N. Engl. J. Med., *288*:1, 1973.

Carson, N. A. J., and Raine, D. N. (Eds.): Inherited Disorders of Sulphur Metabolism. S.S.I.E.M. Symposium No. 8. Edinburgh, Churchill Livingstone, 1971.

Carton, D., DeSchrijver, F., et al.: Argininosuccinic aciduria. Neonatal variant with rapid fatal course. Acta Paediat. Scand. *58*:528, 1969.

Dobson, J., Koch, R., et al.: Cognitive development and dietary therapy in phenylketonuric children. N. Engl. J. Med. *278*:1142, 1968.

Dunn, H. G., Perry, T. L., and Dolman, C. L.: Homocystinuria. Neurology *16*:407, 1966.

Gaull, G. E., and Tallan, H. H.: Methionine adenosyltransferase deficiency: New enzymatic defect associated with hypermethioninemia. Science *186*:59, 1974.

Gelehrter, T. D., and Snodgrass, P. J.: Lethal neonatal deficiency of carbamyl phosphate synthetase. N. Engl. J. Med. *290*:430, 1974.

Gentz, J., Jagenburg, R., and Zetterström, R.: Tyrosinemia. An inborn error of tyrosine metabolism with cirrhosis of the liver and multiple renal tubular defects (deToni-Debré-Fanconi syndrome). J. Pediatr. *66*:670, 1965.

Gentz, J., Lindblad, B., et al.: Dietary treatment in tyrosinemia (tyrosinosis). Am. J. Dis. Child. *113*:31, 1967.

Goldsmith, L. A., Kang, E., et al.: Tyrosinemia with plantar and palmar keratosis and keratitis. J. Pediatr. *83*:798, 1973.

Grant, D. B., Alexander, F. W., and Seakins, J. W. T.: Abnormal tyrosine metabolism in hereditary fructose intolerance. Acta Paediat. Scand. *59*:432, 1970.

Guthrie, R., and Susi, A.: A simple phenylalanine method for detecting phenylketonuria in large populations of newborn infants. Pediatrics *32*:338, 1963.

Hartlage, P. L., Coryell, M. E., et al.: Argininosuccinic aciduria: Perinatal diagnosis and early dietary management. J. Pediatr. *85*:86, 1974.

Holtzman, N. A., Meek, A. G., and Mellits, E. D.: Neonatal screening for phenylketonuria. I. Effectiveness. J.A.M.A. *229*:667, 1974.

Holtzman, N. A., Mellits, E. D., and Kallman, C. H.: Neonatal screening for phenylketonuria: II. Age dependence of initial phenylalanine in infants with PKU. Pediatrics *53*:353, 1974.

Holtzman, N. A., Meek, A. G., et al.: Neonatal screening for phenylketonuria: III. Altered sex ratio; extent and possible causes. J. Pediatr. *85*:175, 1974.

Holtzman, N. A., Meek, A. G., and Mellits, E. D.: Neonatal screening for phenylketonuria: IV. Factors influencing the occurence of false positives. Am. J. Pub. Health *64*:775, 1974.

Kang, E. S., Sollee, N. D., and Gerald, P. S.: Results of treatment and termination of the diet in phenylketonuria (PKU). Pediatrics *46*:881, 1970.

Kaufman, S., Holtzman, N. A., et al.: Phenylketonuria due to a deficiency of dihydropteridine reductase. N. Engl. J. Med. *293*:785, 1975.

Kennaway, N. G., and Buist, N. R. M.: Metabolic studies in a patient with hepatic cytosol tryosine aminotransferase deficiency. Pediat. Res. *5*:287, 1971.

Levy, H. L., Mudd, S. H., et al.: Cystathioninuria and homocystinuria. Clin. Chim. Acta *58*:51, 1975.

Levy, H. L., Nishimura, R. N., et al.: Hyperglycinemia: In vivo comparison of non-ketotic and ketotic (propionic acidemic) forms. II. Valine response in non-ketotic hyperglycinemia. Pediat. Res. *6*:395, 1972.

Levy, H. L., Shih, V. E., et al.: Hypermethioninemia with other hyperaminoacidemias. Am. J. Dis. Child. *117*:96, 1969.

Levy, H. L., Shih, V. E., et al.: Persistent mild hyperphenylalaninemia in the untreated state: A prospective study. N. Engl. J. Med. *285*:424, 1971.

Levy, H. L., and Shih, V. E.: Maternal phenylketonuria and hyperphenylalaninemia. A prospective study. Pediat. Res. *8*:391, 1974.

MacCready, R. A., and Levy, H. L.: The problem of maternal phenylketonuria. Am. J. Obstet. Gynecol. *113*:121, 1972.

Martin, H. P., Fischer, H. L., et al.: The development of children with transient neonatal tryosinemia. J. Pediatr. *84*:212, 1974.

Menkes, J. H., and Avery, M. E.: The metabolism of phenylalanine and tyrosine in the premature infant. Bull. Johns Hopkins Hosp. *113*:301, 1963.

Menkes, J. H., Hurst, P. L., and Craig, J. M.: A new syndrome: Progressive familial infantile cerebral dysfunction associated with an unusual urinary substance. Pediatrics *14*:462, 1954.

Menkes, J. H., Welche, D. W., et al.: Relationship of elevated blood tyrosine to the ultimate intellectual performance of premature infants. Pediatrics *49*:218, 1972.

Nyhan, W. L. (Ed.): Heritable Disorders of Amino Acid Metabolism. New York, John Wiley & Sons, 1974.

Scriver, C. R., Mackenzie, S., et al.: Thiamine-responsive maple-syrup-urine disease. Lancet *1*:310, 1971.

Scriver, C. R., and Rosenberg, L. E.: Amino Acid Metabolism and Its Disorders. Philadelphia, W. B. Saunders Co., 1973.

Shih, V. E.: Early dietary management in an infant with argininosuccinase deficiency: Preliminary report. J. Pediatr. *80*:645, 1972.

Short, E. M., Conn, H. O., et al.: Evidence for X-linked dominant inheritance of ornithine transcarbamylase deficiency. N. Engl. J. Med. *288*:7, 1973.

Snyderman, S. E., Sansaricq, C., et al.: The therapy of hyperammonemia due to ornithine transcarbamylase deficiency in a male neonate. Pediatrics *56*:65, 1975.

Szeinberg, A., Cohen, B. E., et al.: Persistent mild hyperphenylalaninemia in various ethnic groups in Israel. Am. J. Dis. Child. *118*:559, 1969.

Trijbels, J. M. F., Monnens, L. A. H., et al.: A patient with nonketotic hyperglycinemia: Biochemical findings and therapeutic approaches. Pediat. Res. *8*:598, 1974.

Van Der Zee, S. P. M., Trijbels, J. M. F., et al.: Citrullinaemia with rapidly fatal neonatal course. Arch. Dis. Child. *46*:847, 1971.

# 61 INBORN ERRORS OF ORGANIC ACIDS

*By Harvey Levy*

It is generally false to distinguish disorders of organic acids from those of amino acids. The organic acids involved are intermediary metabolites within amino acid metabolic pathways. There are two important reasons, however, for making such a distinction. First, in the organic acid disorders metabolic acidosis, often striking and frequently presenting in the neonatal period, is a prominent finding, whereas metabolic acidosis is not usually one of the complications of a primary aminoacidopathy. Second, in organic acid disorders it is an organic acid rather than an amino acid that is most prominently abnormal. Thus, if tests are conducted for amino acids only, as is often the case, the organic acid disorders may be overlooked.

The most frequently detected organic acid disorders are due to defects in the metabolic pathways of the branched-chain amino acids. These disorders are often associated with hyperglycinemia (see Chapter 60), although this is not a constant finding in all patients.

## ISOVALERIC ACIDEMIA

This disorder has been termed the "sweaty foot syndrome," owing to the offensive odor noted on the body and in the blood and urine of affected individuals. It is caused by a specific defect in the metabolism of leucine. As a result of this defect, isovaleric acid, a short-chain fatty acid, accumulates in the body and may be detectable in the blood, urine and CSF. The free isovaleric acid is presumably responsible for the unique odor reminiscent of dried sweat or rancid cheese.

This disorder usually presents with metabolic acidosis in the neonatal or early infantile period. It is characterized by vomiting, lethargy and weight loss. The "sweaty foot" odor is often detectable at this time, although it can be difficult to distinguish unless it is sought. If untreated or if treated only with supportive measures the acute symptoms may disappear and the infant remain clinically normal until infection, unusually high protein intake or some other intercurrent event precipitates another acute episode of metabolic acidosis. Recurrent metabolic acidosis is the hallmark of isovaleric acidemia, as it is with the other organic acid disorders. Death may occur during any one of these acute episodes. Mental retardation seems to result frequently unless specific therapy is given.

The diagnosis is made on the basis of the demonstration of increased isovaleric acid in serum or plasma and of isovalerylglycine in urine. The latter may be more striking than the former, though a testing laboratory should be able to identify either compound.

Aside from supportive therapy with fluids and other measures during acute episodes, isovaleric acidemia may be controlled with a diet that is specifically low in leucine. In one individual treated from the neonatal period the frequent episodes of metabolic acidosis and the mental retardation were seemingly prevented.

## PROPIONIC ACIDEMIA

This disorder, like isovaleric acidemia, is marked by recurrent episodes of metabolic acidosis, usually beginning in the neonatal period. It is due to a defect in the isoleucine metabolic pathway and is characterized by increased concentrations of propionic acid and related metabolites in blood and urine. No unusual odor is associated with this disorder and it is most readily diagnosed upon the demonstration by short-chain fatty acid analysis of markedly increased propionic acid in serum or plasma. There is also a decided tendency for hyperglycinemia and ketone-positive urine to be associated with this disorder, making this perhaps the most likely of the organic acid disorders to be associated with "ketotic hyperglycinemia."

Death and mental retardation are common sequelae. Treatment with a diet low in the content of branched-chain amino acids, methionine and threonine has been given with success in a few cases. Some patients may at least partially respond to supplemental biotin, since the enzyme propionyl-CoA carboxylase, which is deficient in propionic acidemia, utilizes biotin as a cofactor.

## METHYLMALONIC ACIDEMIA

This organic acidopathy seems to present in one of two ways. The first and most striking presentation is that of severe metabolic acidosis beginning on the second or third day of life. This has generally ended in neonatal death despite supportive therapy. The second presentation is that of metabolic acidosis beginning at the age of 5 to 8 weeks in an infant who was previously healthy. This usually coincides with an increase in the amount of protein ingested. This second and somewhat delayed presentation may also end in death unless vigorous supportive therapy is given.

Methylmalonic acidemia may be due either to a defect in methylmalonyl-CoA mutase (or, rarely, methylmalonyl-CoA racemase), which is responsible for the conversion of methylmalonyl-CoA to succinyl-CoA within the metabolic pathway of valine, or to lack of normal synthesis of deoxyadenosyl-$B_{12}$, the $B_{12}$ coenzyme for the mutase. The diagnosis is made by the demonstration of increased methylmalonic acid in urine. The blood ammonia level may also be elevated during acute episodes of metabolic acidosis, presumably as a secondary phenomenon.

Treatment depends to a great extent on whether or not there is a biochemical response to supplemental amounts of vitamin $B_{12}$. All patients with methylmalonic acidemia should be given such a trial. If there is a response (which would suggest the presence of either a $B_{12}$ metabolic block or a mutase abnormality at the site of coenzyme binding), the patient could be treated with supplemental vitamin $B_{12}$ alone. Otherwise, a diet low in valine should be given.

Other organic acid disorders that may be important in the neonatal period include $\beta$-methylcrotonyl-CoA carboxylase deficiency, $\alpha$-methylacetoacetyl-CoA thiolase deficiency, pyruvic acidemia, succinyl-CoA: 3 ketoacid CoA transferase deficiency and possibly pyroglutamic acidemia and glutaric aciduria. Each is characterized by recurrent metabolic acidosis and by the urinary excretion of the affected organic acid.

## REFERENCES

Brandt, I. K., Hsia, Y. E., et al.: Propionicacidemia (ketotic hyperglycinemia): Dietary treatment resulting in normal growth and development. Pediatrics 53:391, 1974.

Hsia, Y. E., Scully, K. J., and Rosenberg, L. E.: Defective propionate carboxylation in ketotic hyperglycinaemia. Lancet 1:757, 1969.

Kang, E. S., Snodgrass, P. J., and Gerald, P. S.: Methylmalonyl coenzyme A racemase defect: Another cause of methylmalonic acidemia. Pediatr. Res. 6:875, 1972.

Levy, H. L., Erickson, A. M., et al.: Isovaleric acidemia: Results of family study and dietary treatment. Pediatrics 52:83, 1973.

Stern, J., and Toothil, C. (Eds.): Organic Acidurias. Edinburgh, Churchill-Livingstone, 1972.

Stokke, O., Eldjarn, L., et al.: Methylmalonic acidemia. A new inborn error of metabolism which may cause fatal acidosis in the neonatal period. Scand. J. Lab. Clin. Med. 20:313, 1967.

Tanaka, K.: Disorders of organic acid metabolism. *In* Gaull, G. E. (Ed.): Biology of Brain Dysfunction. Vol. 3. New York, Plenum Pub. Co., 1975, pp. 145–214.

# 62

# INBORN ERRORS OF LIPID METABOLISM

*By Harvey Levy*

With the increasing interest in precursors of atherosclerosis, especially those leading to coronary artery disease and to strokes, lipid abnormalities are gaining wider attention. Most of this attention is being focused on the possible role of increased blood cholesterol and triglyceride concentrations in the production of atherosclerosis. In terms of therapy, there is now widespread acceptance of the concept that control of these factors, perhaps beginning in early infancy, may be the most effective way to prevent clinical complications.

Routine newborn screening for increased lipid concentrations in blood, especially that of cholesterol and triglycerides, has been strongly considered and even instituted on a limited trial basis. Whether or not such screening can truly identify those affected is a matter of dispute. Recent evidence might suggest that this is not possible with currently available methods, at least when umbilical cord blood is used. In this rapidly advancing field, however, it is likely that future developments will render testing for lipid disorders a worthwhile addition to current routine newborn screening.

## FAMILIAL HYPERLIPOPROTEINEMIA

There are now at least five seemingly distinct disorders in this group, classified as types I through V. Each type is characterized by a particular lipoprotein accumulation. Although clinical signs are rarely present in the neonatal period, an awareness of these disorders is important even in early infancy, since in some instances it may be desirable to begin therapy at that time to prevent later clinical complications.

Type II hyperbetalipoproteinemia is by far the best known and most common of these disorders. In the homozygous state it is characterized by a markedly elevated concentration of plasma cholesterol and a moderately increased plasma triglyceride concentration. Xanthomas (yellowish fatty nodules) are usually present on the eyelids or over the elbows, extensor tendons of the hands and the Achilles tendon. These xanthomas have been noted at birth. Ischemic heart disease and other complications of severe atherosclerosis develop in childhood or adolescent years.

Even though homozygous type II hyperbetalipoproteinemia is relatively rare, the heterozygotic state may have a frequency as high as 1 per cent of the population. These individuals will also have increased plasma cholesterol and triglyceride concentrations, though the degree of increase will be less than that noted in homozygotes. The most striking finding among heterozygotes is a tendency to develop severe atherosclerosis with ischemic heart disease and other complications beginning in the middle adult years.

## LIPIDOSES

This category includes those inborn errors of metabolism that are characterized by an abnormal accumulation of lipids within certain cells of the body. This is to be distinguished from the inborn errors of lipid metabolism discussed previously in which the lipid accumulations are in the lipoprotein form and circulate freely through the body. The lipidoses are often included within the broader category of lysosomal disorders (which also includes the glycogen storage diseases and the mucopolysaccharidoses), since the defective enzymes are those that are located in the lysosomes of the cell. This is in contrast to other inborn errors of metabolism in which the enzyme in question is located in the mitochondria or cytosol of the cell.

In the lipidoses, lipid material fills the neurons, and structurally related glycolipids, polysaccharides or glycoproteins accumulate in other tissues. There is often severe and progressive damage to brain and other organs, usually resulting in death. There is as yet no effective therapy for any of the disorders, although enzyme replacement is being actively pursued on an experimental basis. Programs of heterozygote detection and prenatal diagnosis are being conducted for at least one of these disorders (Tay-Sachs disease).

Clinical signs in most of the lipidoses often appear in infancy but usually later than the neonatal period. Consequently they will not be considered in detail here. However, some discussion is in order for the few that are particularly well-known or that do present as neonatal disease.

TAY-SACHS DISEASE. This is the most common and best known of the lipidoses. It is transmitted in an autosomal recessive manner and is most common among Ashkenazi Jews, though it occurs infrequently in other ethnic groups. $GM_2$ ganglioside accumulates in neurons, causing severe and progressive mental and motor deterioration, usually beginning at age 4 to 6 months. Death is inevitable and usually occurs between 2 and 5 years of age. There is no known treatment. Fortunately antenatal diagnosis is now possible (see pages 30–33).

GM$_1$ GANGLIOSIDOSIS (TYPE 1). Although this disorder is very rare, it is considered here because it is one of the few lipidoses that may present with clinical signs in the neonatal period. $GM_1$ ganglioside accumulates in neurons. Throughout the reticuloendothelial system and other visceral organs such as the kidney there are foam cells. Shortly after birth the infant is noted to be lethargic, to suck and feed poorly, and to gain weight slowly. Developmental delay is obvious within the first weeks of life. The symptoms are progressive, with death occurring at 1½ to 2 years of age.

OTHER LIPIDOSES. Gaucher's disease of the infantile, or type 2, form usually presents at about 3 to 4 months of age with hepatosplenomegaly and failure to thrive. On occasion (about 10 per cent of all cases) the affected infant will be abnormal at birth, with lethargy and poor feeding as well as hepatosplenomegaly. Cerebrosides accumulate in many tissues of the body. The disease is progressive, with death at 1 to 3 years of age.

In the infantile, or type A, form of Niemann-Pick disease the infant may be noted to have prominent eyes and hepatomegaly within the first days of life. This disease is progressive, with the development of marked hepatosplenomegaly and severe neurologic manifestations. Death occurs at 1 to 4 years of age. Sphingomyelin is the lipid that accumulates in the affected tissues.

Wolman's disease is characterized by vomiting, failure to thrive and hepatosplenomegaly in the first week or two of life. An additional and striking finding is that of calcification of the adrenal glands. It is characterized by the storage of neutral lipids such as cholesterol in the affected organs. The disease is progressive, with death at 2 to 14 months of age.

## REFERENCES

*Familial Hyperlipoproteinemia*
Fredrickson, D. S., and Levy, R. I.: Familial hyperlipoproteinemia. *In* Stanbury, J. B., Wyngaarden, J. B., and Fredrickson, D. S. (Eds.): The Metabolic Basis of Inherited Disease. 3rd ed., New York, McGraw-Hill Book Co., 1972, pp. 545–614.
Ose, L.: L.D.L. and total cholesterol in cord-blood screening for familial hypercholesterolaemia. Lancet 2:615, 1975.

*Lipidoses*
Kolodny, E. H.: Heterozygote detection in the lipidoses. *In* The Prevention of Genetic Disease and Mental Retardation. (A. Milunsky, Ed.). Philadelphia, W. B. Saunders Co., 1975, pp. 182–203.

# 63

# MISCELLANEOUS INBORN ERRORS OF METABOLISM

*Revised by Harvey Levy*

## CONGENITAL HYPOPHOSPHATASIA

Alkaline phosphatase concentrations in blood and tissues are diminished in the presence of hypothyroidism and of scurvy. Rathbun, in 1948, described an infant in whom this enzyme was virtually absent from birth. He termed the resulting disorder congenital hypophosphatasia.

**INCIDENCE.** The condition is very rare. Approximately 10 cases had been reported up to 1960, and a few more have been described since then. Most of the infants became symptomatic from 6 months to 2 years of age. In only two that we are familiar with was the disease full-blown within the neonatal period, while one or two others began to show nonspecific symptoms within the first month. In at least two the bony alterations were visible in x-rays of the mother's abdomen made at the thirteenth week of gestation.

**ETIOLOGY.** The basic defect lies in inability of osteoblasts to produce alkaline phosphatase. Two siblings have been involved at least twice among the few recorded cases. McCance and Fairwether made the diagnosis in one fetus by prenatal x-ray films taken because an older sibling had died of hypophosphatasia. The alkaline phosphatase level is diminished and hypercalcemia often develops. An excess of ethanolamine phosphate is found in the urine of homozygotes, and an intermediate amount in that of heterozygotes. It is clearly a hereditary disorder whose exact mode of inheritance has not been ascertained.

**PATHOLOGY.** The deficiency of alkaline phosphatase results in failure of deposition of calcium salts in growing bones. At the epiphysial ends of the long bones and the costochondral junctions of the ribs the picture which results resembles closely that of florid rickets. Osteoid is abundant, but remains uncalcified. A similar lack of calcification involves the membranous bones of the skull. The kidneys in some of the autopsied cases have revealed changes which were not considered to have been causative. Sobel et al. found the phosphatase activity of the costochondral junction to be less than one fifteenth that of similar tissue from a child with active rickets, one seventh that of normal infants.

**DIAGNOSIS.** The earliest symptoms make their appearance at birth rarely, or some weeks or months after birth. One would suppose that the degree of deficiency of the enzyme dictates the time of onset. Failure to gain weight and vomiting are the first signs of trouble. Drowsiness and dehydration follow, as do enlargements at the wrists and ankles and beading of the ribs suggestive of active rickets. Hypotonia is generally marked. In several infants the fontanel has become full and tense, although the cerebrospinal fluid was found to be normal. Shedding of erupted teeth has been the first sign noted in some older children. Serum alkaline phosphatase concentrations are markedly reduced. Urine amino acid analysis may reveal the presence of phosphoethanolamine.

Rathbun's case merits brief summarization both because of its historical interest as the original description and because it is one of the two of which we are aware which became full-blown in the neonate.

A white male infant was born at term, weighing 9 pounds 11 ounces (4394 gm), after an uneventful pregnancy and labor. He was breast fed, took the breast fairly well, but lost steadily. By 3 weeks, his weight had fallen to 7 pounds 5 ounces (3316 gm). At this time it was noted that he became blue on crying, and for the 11 days preceding he had seemed to be in pain, especially when handled. For 3 days short crying spells were followed by coarse, jerking movements lasting 3 to 5 minutes. Examinations at 3 weeks showed poor nutrition and acute distress. The head was soft, "like a balloon full of water." The costochondral junctions were enlarged, producing a definite rachitic rosary. The lower ends of the radius and ulna were prominent, the tibiae and fibulae bowed.

Serum calcium determinations ranged from 10.9 to 13.6 mg per 100 ml, phosphorus from 4.4 to 6.9 mg except terminally, when this figure rose to 10.5 mg. The nonprotein nitrogen concentrations were similarly normal. All determinations of serum alkaline phosphatase were either 0 or exceedingly low, the highest one reaching 0.7 Lowrey-Bessey unit (normal for the age being 5 to 15 units). X-ray films of the bones showed flaring at the ends of the ribs, much demineralization of all the skeleton, including the skull, and irregularities at the ends of the long bones, all highly suggestive of active rickets.

Therapeutic trials of percomorph oil in large doses, thyroxin and testosterone failed to raise the alkaline phosphatase level or to improve calcification. The infant died after a series of convulsions. Autopsy showed the bone changes described above. In the grossly normal kidneys the collecting tubules were distended with casts, and in some areas their epithelium was eroded and focal inflammatory reaction surrounded these damaged tubules.

**TREATMENT.** No medications tried have improved the disorder.

**PROGNOSIS.** The most severely affected infants become ill early and die quickly. The others survive a number of years only to become dwarfed and grotesquely deformed. They resemble children with vitamin D-resistant rickets. Premature shedding of teeth is characteristic.

## PSEUDOHYPOPHOSPHATASIA

Scriver and Cameron described a fascinating variant of this disease. Their baby presented all the signs of congenital hypophosphatasia except lowered alkaline phosphatase in the blood. The bones on x-ray looked rachitic, there was premature loss of deciduous teeth, and hypercalcemia and phosphoethanolaminuria were present. The other remarkable aspect of this case was that at 9 months spontaneous healing of the bones began, possibly but by no means certainly in response to steroid therapy, and by 20 months they seemed almost normal and remained so thereafter. Calcium fell to normal, but the phosphoethanolamine output continued to be excessive.

## NEPHROGENIC DIABETES INSIPIDUS

This term has been used to describe a familial condition in which there is excessive loss of water from the kidneys due to congenital inability of the renal tubules to reabsorb water. However, no other metabolites are lost in excess. The blood chemical alterations are secondary results of the water loss.

**ETIOLOGY.** In the few families reported only boys have been involved. The defect is therefore sex-linked, transmitted through the female to the male. It probably entails absence or deficiency of one or more enzymes concerned with water reabsorption by the tubules.

**DIAGNOSIS.** Waring, Kajdi and Tappan pointed out the following clinical characteristics. The disorder becomes manifest shortly after birth. There is erratic and unexplained fever, constipation is persistent, vomiting is prominent, and there are polydipsia and polyuria which are unaffected by Pitressin. Dehydration appears rapidly when fluid intake is curtailed. The blood chemical determinations show high levels of sodium, chloride and nonprotein nitrogen. In crises of dehydration the carbon dioxide-combining power falls to low levels. Urine is voluminous when intake is adequate, and its specific gravity seldom exceeds 1.010. It contains no excess of protein, carbohydrate or cellular sediment.

The above-mentioned authors found an increased skin resistance in several of their affected infants.

**TREATMENT.** No curative therapy is available. The infants must have access to unlimited quantities of water. Flax and Gersch's 2-week-old boy had fever whenever his intake fell below 2000 ml per day. At 18 months this same child normally consumed 3½ quarts of water in addition to his milk and other dietary fluids. During episodes of fever the fluid requirement is even greater. Parenteral fluids must contain a minimum of sodium chloride.

Within the past few years some amelioration has been effected. Treatment with drugs of the benzothiadiazine series induces some diminution of urinary output and some increase in its specific gravity. Brown and his co-workers were able to achieve even better results with ethacrynic acid, even in the presence of fairly liberal sodium intakes.

## MYASTHENIA GRAVIS

Myasthenia gravis can exist in two forms in the neonatal period. Approximately 12 per cent of infants of myasthenic mothers show a transient form and constitute most of the cases. Rarely, a permanent form is manifest initially in the neonatal period. This dichotomy is exactly analogous to the one which obtains in neonatal thrombocytopenic purpura.

**INCIDENCE.** About 80 cases of the transient neonatal form affecting infants of myasthenic mothers had been reported by 1970. The condition is very rare. Of the several hundred cases of the juvenile form, a small minority manifested signs as early as the first week of life. This form of the disease is thought to be a recessive genetic defect.

**ETIOLOGY.** The physiologic defect leading to increased muscle fatigability is not known. Whatever the defect is due to, acetylcholine deficiency, cholinesterase excess or the presence of some curare-like antagonist to acetylcholine at the motor end-plate, it is counteracted temporarily by Prostigmin and neostigmine. Efforts to identify neuromuscular blocking activity in the serum of myasthenic patients have not been successful. In an extensive review of neonatal myasthenia gravis published in 1970, Namba et al. concluded that "it seems probable that the disease is due to a maternal environmental influence which still remains to be identified."

**DIAGNOSIS.** Both forms, when they involve the newborn, make their appearance at birth or on the second or third day of life. Symmetrical muscle weakness is the outstanding feature, involving the entire body and face. The infants are limp, motionless or nearly so, their muscles almost completely without tone. The face is flat and expressionless, the cry is weak, sucking feeble and swallowing difficult. In contrast to older patients, ptosis and extraocular weaknesses are not commonly seen. The Moro response is poor; the deep reflexes are diminished or absent.

Differential diagnosis at this stage may be difficult unless the mother is myasthenic. If she is, the assumption that the infant also is myasthenic is natural and probably correct. If the mother is normal, intracranial injury, amyotonia congenita (Oppenheim's disease) and nuclear agenesis (Moebius's syndrome) will have to be ruled out. The depressed sensorium of the infant with flaccid weakness due to birth injury is absent in the myasthenic. The latter is clearly conscious, but weak. Amyotonia congenita poses a more difficult problem. Here the generalized weakness and areflexia coupled with unimpaired sensorium simulate myasthenia perfectly. The muscles of respiration are apt to be affected more commonly and more profoundly in the amyotonic, but they may also be in the myasthenic. Diminution or absence of creatine in the urine is diagnostic of Oppenheim's disease. The bilateral facial nerve palsy, often associated with extraocular palsies, of Moebius's syndrome might be suggestive of myasthenia, but the absence of generalized weakness and the presence of other congenital deformities should make this distinction clear.

*All these confusing syndromes can be differentiated from myasthenia gravis by alleviation of the weakness by administration of an anticholinesterase.* Neostigmine methylsulfate in doses of 0.05 to 0.5 mg intramuscularly or subcutaneously produces improvement in 10 to 15 minutes that lasts several hours. Edrophonium chloride, 0.5 to 1.0 mg intramuscularly or subcutaneously, relieves weakness within minutes, but the effect is of brief duration (i.e., several minutes).

**COURSE AND PROGNOSIS.** The outlook for the newborn with the neonatal form is good, provided one makes the diagnosis promptly and treats properly. Cases last as short a time as a few hours or as long as 7 weeks. Once muscle strength has returned, it never again is lost. Infants with the juvenile form can be expected to suffer from the disease for life. Their affliction is not quite so severe as is that of adults, crises are infrequent, and periods of remission may be frequent and long. Death in respiratory failure can take place in either form.

**TREATMENT.** Constant treatment with drugs is not indicated unless difficulty with sucking or breathing ensues. Neostigmine is usually effective intramuscularly or subcutaneously, in initial doses of 0.1 mg when given as neostigmine methylsulfate. The drug should be given 10 to 20 minutes before a feeding if the infant is weak. As the infant improves, the medication can be given by nasogastric tube. The need for medication may persist for 1 to 115 days, with a mean of 28 days, according to Namba et al.

Periodic attempts to withdraw the drug should be made. In the neonatal form withdrawal without return of symptoms will be successfully accomplished some time between 1 and 8 weeks of age. In the juvenile form treatment will almost always be required for life, except during periods of remission. The advisability of thymectomy in these children will not have to be considered until much later in life.

## CYSTIC FIBROSIS

Cystic fibrosis, also known as cystic fibrosis of the pancreas and mucoviscidosis, is an inherited disorder that affects many different organs of the body, most notably the lungs and the pancreas. It is probably an inborn error of metabolism, though the precise metabolic system(s) involved has yet to be defined.

**INCIDENCE.** The disease is inherited in an autosomal recessive manner. In the United States it is far more common among whites than among Blacks, having an incidence of approximately 1 per 1600 in whites to 1 per 3000 in Blacks. In general, it has a similar frequency among most white populations in Europe. It is very rare in Oriental peoples.

**PATHOPHYSIOLOGY.** The most prominent biochemical abnormality found is that of increased concentrations of $Na^+$ and $Cl^-$ in sweat. The viscosity of mucus secreted by many exocrine glands is markedly increased. This leads to inspissated mucus in many organs, including the trachea and bronchial tree, the pancreas, the intestinal tract, the bile ductules and ducts

of the liver, and the testis. The viscid mucus in the tracheobronchial system leads to chronic pulmonary infection. In other organs the outflow tracts become chronically obstructed and the secretions collect within the organ, causing tissue damage. In the pancreas this results in a reduction in the flow of digestive enzymes to the intestine. In the liver biliary cirrhosis may eventually occur.

The basic defect in cystic fibrosis has not yet been proved. Recent studies have focused on the ability of serum or the media of cultured skin fibroblasts from patients with cystic fibrosis to inhibit ciliary activity in oyster gill tissues. Enzyme abnormalities, including increased serum glutathione reductase activity, increased meconium disaccharidase activity and reduced plasma arginine esterase activity have also been reported. It is probable that all of these abnormalities are secondary to a more basic process.

**CLINICAL MANIFESTATIONS.** Most infants with cystic fibrosis appear to be normal during the neonatal period. However, an occasional affected infant will have meconium ileus (see page 363). When this is present the diagnosis of cystic fibrosis is almost certain. Occasionally excessive sweating is evident in the neonate. The sweat will contain increased electrolyte quantities. This sweat may be noted to have a "salty taste" by the mother when she kisses the infant. Respiratory infections may also

*TABLE 63–1. Risks of Producing a Child with Cystic Fibrosis (CF)\**

| One Parent | Other Parent | Risk of Cystic Fibrosis in Each Pregnancy |
|---|---|---|
| With no CF history | With no CF history | 1:1600 |
| With no CF history | With 1st cousin having CF | 1:320 |
| With no CF history | With aunt or uncle having CF | 1:240 |
| With no CF history | With sib having CF | 1:120 |
| With no CF history | With CF child by previous marriage | 1:80 |
| With no CF history | With parent having CF | 1:80 |
| With no CF history | Has CF | 1:40 |
| With sib having CF | With sib having CF | 1:9 |
| With CF child | With CF child | 1:4 |

\*Based on prevalence of cystic fibrosis of 1:1600 in the Caucasian population, & its mode of inheritance being autosomal recessive with complete penetrance. (From Bowman, B. H., and Mangos, J. A., N. Engl. J. Med. *294*:937, 1976.)

present during the first days of life, with the most consistent feature being hyperinflation of the chest. Failure to gain weight and hypoproteinemia may become evident in the weeks after birth. Bulky and fatty stools, usually the first signs of the deficiency of pancreatic enzymes, may be noted during the early months of life. Hypoprothrombinemia, from failure to absorb vitamin K, can lead to a hemorrhagic diathesis, and Dolan and Gibson have recommended performing tests for cystic fibrosis on all infants who present with vitamin K deficiency. Prolonged obstructive jaundice may also be an early manifestation of the disease.

**DIAGNOSIS.** The collection of sweat by iontophoresis for analysis of $Na^+$ and $Cl^-$, or measurement of electrical conductivity which depends on the concentrations of these ions, is the definitve diagnostic test. It may be difficult to collect a sufficient amount of sweat from infants in the first weeks of life for these chemical assays, though in expert hands this is usually possible. If an infant has an affected sibling or any signs or symptoms suggesting cystic fibrosis, sweat analysis is essential before making the diagnosis.

The application of an electrode directly to the skin to measure electrical conductivity has recently been used as a screening test in newborns. However, this method has been found to result in many "false positives" and consequently would seem to be unsuitable for routine newborn screening. The most recent newborn screening test to be used is that for albumin in meconium extracts. Owing to reduced amounts of pancreatic proteolytic enzymes, meconium of affected newborns will usually contain markedly increased albumin. However, many conditions including prematurity may result in increased meconium albumin. Conversely, the meconium from an occasional infant with cystic fibrosis many contain normal or only slightly increased albumin concentrations. Thus, this method also would seem to lack the specificity necessary for routine newborn screening. If a simple and efficient test for newborn screening were available the potential benefits of early therapy and family counseling might render routine newborn screening for cystic fibrosis a worthwhile procedure.

**TREATMENT.** No consensus exists on how vigorous one should be in treating the asymptomatic infant with cystic fibrosis. Most would agree on a normal diet and the addition of water-soluble vitamins. The prompt identification and treatment of pulmonary infections is imperative and probably preferable to chemoprophylaxis. Some hold that the initial staphylococcal pneumonia is so harmful that antibiotics should be given daily in an attempt to prevent it. Others advocate the use of mist tents overnight to moisten pulmonary secretions. We are not impressed with the evidence supporting this approach to prophylaxis. Pancreatic supplements are recommended as tolerated.

**PROGNOSIS.** Each year the prognosis for this disease improves, in part because of wider recognition and detection of milder cases, and in part, no doubt, related to therapy. Many afflicted individuals are now adults, and some of the females are parents. Sterility in the males is very common. The severity of the disease varies greatly between siblings; hence prognostication about the life span of an affected infant is unwise.

## REFERENCES

Antonowicz, I., Ishida, S., and Shwachman, H.: Studies in meconium: Disaccharidase activities in meconium from cystic fibrosis patients and controls. Pediatrics 56:782, 1975.

Bodian, M.: Fibrocystic Disease of the Pancreas: A Congenital Disorder of Mucus Production. London, Heinemann, 1952.

Bowman, B. H., and Mangos, J. A.: Current concepts in genetics: Cystic fibrosis. N. Engl. J. Med. *294:*937, 1976.

Brown, D. M., Reynolds, J. W., et al.: The use and mode of action of ethacrynic acid in nephrogenic diabetes insipidus. Pediatrics 37:447, 1966.

Craig, J. M., Haddad, H., and Shwachman, H.: The pathological changes in the liver and cystic fibrosis of the pancreas. Am. J. Dis. Child. 93:357, 1957.

Danes, B. S., and Bearn, A. G.: Oyster ciliary inhibition by cystic fibrosis culture medium. J. Exp. Med. *136:*1313, 1972.

Denning, C. R., Sommers, S. C., and Quigley, H. J.: Infertility in male patients with cystic fibrosis. Pediatrics *41:*7, 1968.

diSant'Agnese, P. A., and Talamo, R. C.: Medical progress: Pathogenesis and physiopathology of cystic fibrosis of the pancreas. N. Engl. J. Med. *227:*1287, 1343, 1399, 1967.

Dolan, T. F., and Gibson, L. E.: Possibility of cystic fibrosis in infants with vitamin K deficiency (Letter). J. Pediatr. 77:515, 1970.

Flax, L. J., and Gersh, J.: Congenital renal tubular dysfunction (nephrogenic diabetes insipidus): Report of a case complicated by calcifications in the renal pedicle. A.M.A. J. Dis. Child. 89:602, 1955.

Goyer, R. A.: Ethanolamine phosphate excretion in a family with hypophosphatasia. Arch. Dis. Child. 38:205, 1963.

Kopito, L., and Shwachman, H.: Studies in cystic fibrosis: Determination of sweat electrolytes in situ with direct reading electrodes. Pediatrics 43:794, 1969.

LaBranche, H. G., and Jefferson, R. N.: Congenital myasthenia gravis. Pediatrics 4:16, 1949.

Mangos, J. A., and Talamo, R. C. (Eds.): Fundamental Problems of Cystic Fibrosis and Related Diseases. New York, Intercontinental Medical Books Corp., 1973.

McPartlin, J. F., Dickson, J. A. S., and Swain, V. A. J.: Meconium ileus — Immediate and long term survival. Arch. Dis. Child. 47:252, 1972.

Namba, T., Brown, S. B., and Grob, D.: Neonatal myasthenia gravis: Report of two cases and review of the literature. Pediatrics 45:488, 1970.

Oppenheimer, E. H., and Esterly, J. R.: Hepatic changes in young infants with cystic fibrosis: Possible relation to focal biliary cirrhosis. J. Pediatr. 86:683, 1975.

Raine, D. N., and Roy, I.: A salt-losing syndrome in infancy: Pseudohypoadrenocorticism. Arch. Dis. Child. 37:548, 1962.

Rao, G. J. S., and Nadler, H. L.: Arginine esterase in cystic fibrosis of the pancreas. Pediatr. Res. 8:684, 1974.

Rathbun, J. C.: "Hypophosphatasia"; a new developmental anomaly. Am. J. Dis. Child. 75:822, 1948.

Robinson, P. G., and Elliott, R. B.: Cystic fibrosis screening in the newborn. Arch. Dis. Childh. 51:301, 1976.

Shapiro, B. L., Smith, Q. T., and Warwick, W. J.: Serum glutathione reductase and cystic fibrosis. Pediatr. Res. 9:885, 1975.

Schlesinger, B., Luder, J., and Bodian, M.: Rickets with alkaline phosphatase deficiency: An osteoblastic dysplasia. Arch. Dis. Child. 30:265, 1955.

Scriver, C. R., and Cameron, T.: Pseudohypophosphatasia. N. Engl. J. Med. 281:604, 1969.

Shwachman, H., Kulczycki, L. L., and Khaw, K.-T.: Studies in cystic fibrosis. A report of sixty-five patients over 17 years of age. Pediatrics. 36:689, 1965.

Sobel, E. H., Clark, L. C., et al.: Rickets: Deficiency of "alkaline" phosphatase activity and premature loss of teeth in childhood. Pediatrics 11:309, 1953.

Teng, P., and Osserman, K. E.: Studies in myasthenia gravis: Neonatal and juvenile types. J. Mt. Sinai Hosp. N.Y. 23:711, 1956.

Waring, A. J., Kajdi, L., and Tappan, V.: A congenital defect of water metabolism. Am. J. Dis. Child. 69:323, 1945.

# VIII

## Disorders of Blood,
## Blood Vessels and
## Lymphatics

# 64

# BLEEDING DISORDERS IN THE NEWBORN INFANT

*By Bertil Glader*

## PHYSIOLOGY OF NORMAL HEMOSTASIS

Normal hemostasis is a complicated process involving vascular integrity, platelets and coagulation proteins (Fig. 64–1). Bleeding disorders can be due to abnormalities in any one of these parameters. Hemorrhage caused by vascular problems (anatomical or physiological) may be responsible for some of the serious bleeding episodes (pulmonary and CNS) seen in premature infants. Unfortunately, the pathophysiology of vascular-related bleeding is poorly understood. The major defects discussed in this chapter are directly related to abnormalities in platelets and coagulation proteins.

Platelets are activated following exposure to subendothelial collagen of the severed blood vessel. In the presence of collagen, platelets release several hemostatic factors including serotonin, adenosine diphosphate (ADP) and platelet membrane lipid (platelet factor 3). Serotonin enhances vasoconstriction. Platelet factor 3 is utilized in the clotting scheme (see below). Re-

leased ADP causes platelets to reversibly aggregate into clumps, thus forming the primary or loose hemostatic plug. In conditions associated with thrombocytopenia or abnormal platelet function (unable to release cellular components), formation of the primary hemostatic plug will be defective. The production of a firm, definitive hemostatic plug depends on normal plasma coagulation in addition to platelets and vasoconstriction. This process requires the sequential activation of a series of clotting proteins, the end result of which is the formation of a fibrin clot. As seen in Fig. 64–1, there are two different pathways for initiating coagulation. The "intrinsic pathway" is stimulated when factor XII reacts with subendothelial collagen. Following this, sequential interaction with other factors (XI, IX, VIII and platelet factor 3) results in the activation of factor X. The "extrinsic" pathway is stimulated when injured tissues release a tissue thromboplastin which reacts with factor VII to activate factor X. Thus the intrinsic and extrinsic pathways activate factor X via different reactions, but beyond this step the clotting pathways are

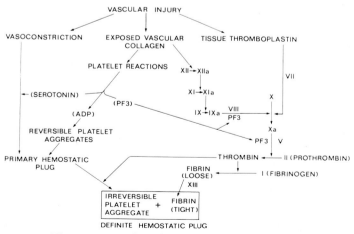

*Figure 64–1.* Physiology of normal hemostasis.

*TABLE 64–1.* *Blood Clotting Factors*

| Number | Synonyms |
|--------|----------|
| I | Fibrinogen |
| II | Prothrombin |
| III | Thromboplastin |
| IV | Calcium |
| V | Proaccelerin (labile factor) |
| VI | Activated factor V (term not used) |
| VII | Proconvertin (stable factor) |
| VIII | Antihemophiliac factor (AHF) |
| IX | Plasma thromboplastin component (PTC) Christmas factor |
| X | Stuart-Prower factor |
| XI | Plasma thromboplastin antecedent (PTA) |
| XII | Hageman factor, contact factor |
| XIII | Fibrin stabilizing factor |

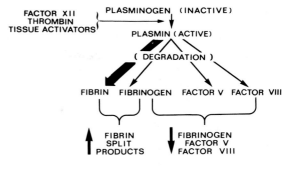

*Figure 64–2.* Physiology of fibrinolysis.

identical. Activated factor X, factor V and platelet factor 3 together convert prothrombin (factor II) into thrombin. Thrombin is a proteolytic enzyme which converts fibrinogen (factor I) into a loose fibrin clot. Factor XIII (fibrin stabilizing factor) then converts the friable clot into tight fibrin polymers. The definitive hemostatic plug consists of irreversible platelet aggregates and tight fibrin polymers. Irreversible platelet clumps are formed when thrombin reacts with reversible platelet aggregates. This brief summary indicates how the vasculature, platelets and coagulation proteins are separately and interdependently involved in normal hemostasis.

A group of physiologic clot-limiting controls react in parallel with the coagulation process. These regulating reactions are very important because plasma contains sufficient coagulant potential to convert the entire blood volume into one large thrombus once coagulation is activated. Most of these limiting controls are poorly characterized.

1. Antithrombins are proteins that neutralize the action of thrombin. When thrombin production is excessive, however, antithrombins may be consumed, thus leading to increased clotting. Neonates are relatively deficient in antithrombin III.

2. Fibrinolysis is characterized by the conversion of plasminogen, an inactive plasma protein, to plasmin, an active protein. The proteolytic activity of plasmin breaks down fibrin deposited at sites of vessel injury. In addition, plasmin degrades factors V, VIII and fibrinogen. The degradation products of fibrin and fibrinogen are known as fibrin split products (FSP's). Fibrinolysis is stimulated by many of the same factors that activate coagulation. Under normal conditions this is a beneficial process which limits the extent of fibrin deposition and maintains vascular patency. In certain pathological conditions, however, persistent activation of clotting and fibrinolysis can deplete factors V, VIII and fibrinogen, and thereby lead to bleeding. In addition, markedly increased fibrin split products enhance the hemorrhagic tendency directly by inhibiting the normal conversion of fibrinogen to fibrin.

## GENERAL APPROACH TO THE BLEEDING INFANT

**MEDICAL HISTORY AND PHYSICAL EXAMINATION.** Evaluation of any bleeding infant requires historical information regarding outcome of previous pregnancies, family bleeding problems, maternal illnesses (especially infections), drug administration (maternal and neonatal), and documentation that vitamin K was given at birth. Simple observations on physical examination (localized versus diffuse bleeding; healthy or sick infant) have tremendous importance for classifying hemorrhagic disorders. Normal infants frequently have petechiae over presenting parts secondary to venous congestion and the trauma of delivery. These petechiae are seen shortly after birth but gradually disappear and are not associated with bleeding. Infants with isolated platelet disorders generally appear healthy except for progressive petechiae, ecchymoses and/or mucosal bleeding. Hemorrhages due to vitamin K deficiency or inherited coagulation defects characteristically occur in apparently healthy children with large ecchymoses or localized bleeding (large cephalohematomas, umbilical cord bleeding or gastrointestinal hemorrhage). Bleeding due to disseminated intravascular coagulation (DIC) or liver injury generally is seen in sick infants with diffuse bleeding from several sites.

**LABORATORY EVALUATION OF BLEEDING INFANT.** The etiology of hemorrhage frequently can be identified by simple diagnostic tests. A differential diagnosis based on the platelet count, prothrombin time (PT) and partial thromboplastin time (PTT) is presented in Table 64–2.

1. PLATELET COUNT. In emergency situations, or when quantitative platelet counts cannot be obtained, a reliable estimate of the platelet count can be made by examining the peripheral blood smear. The average number of platelets per high-power field is determined after observing several fields under the microscope. This number multiplied by 15,000 is a valid estimate of the platelet count. For example, if 50 platelets are seen after examining 20 high-power fields, there is an average of 2.5 platelets per field, and the approximate platelet count is 37,500 (2.5 multiplied by 15,000). The peripheral blood smear also should include an evaluation of platelet size. Thrombocytopenia associated with normal-sized platelets generally reflects a bone marrow production defect, whereas the presence of large platelets indicates rapid production and destruction of circulating platelets.

The platelet count in term and healthy premature neonates is the same as in older children. Previously it was thought that prematures had significantly lower platelet counts than normal term infants. In part this was due to the fact that many laboratories included all premature infants in establishing their normal values. It is now generally agreed, however, that healthy prematures have platelet counts in the same range as term infants and older children. A corollary of this is that sick prema-

*TABLE 64–2. Differential Diagnosis of Bleeding in the Neonate*

| Clinical Evaluation | Laboratory Studies | | | Likely Diagnosis |
|---|---|---|---|---|
| | Platelets | PT | PTT | |
| "Sick" | ↓ | ↑ | ↑ | DIC |
| | ↓ | N | N | Platelet consumption (infection, necrotizing enterocolitis, renal vein thrombosis) |
| | N | ↑ | ↑ | Liver disease |
| | N | N | N | Compromised vascular integrity (associated with hypoxia, prematurity, acidosis, hyperosmolality) |
| "Healthy" | ↓ | N | N | Immune thrombocytopenia<br>Occult infection or thrombosis<br>Bone marrow hypoplasia (rare) |
| | N | ↑ | ↑ | Hemorrhagic disease of newborn (vitamin K deficiency) |
| | N | N | ↑ | Hereditary clotting factor deficiencies |
| | N | N | N | Bleeding due to local factors (trauma, anatomic abnormalities)<br>Qualitative platelet abnormalities (rare)<br>Factor XIII deficiency (rare) |

ture infants frequently have low platelet counts. A platelet count less than 100,000 is definitely abnormal.

2. BLEEDING TIME. This functional test measures the quality and quantity of platelets and their interaction with the vasculature. This procedure has its major value in bleeding patients with normal platelet counts and coagulation studies. A prolonged bleeding time is seen in von Willebrand's disease and functional platelet disorders. Since abnormal results are seen when the platelet count is less than 100,000, this test should not be done in patients with significant thrombocytopenia. The bleeding time in normal term and premature infants is the same as in older children.

3. PROTHROMBIN TIME AND PARTIAL THROMBOPLASTIN TIME. These two tests should be used as the initial coagulation screening procedures in any bleeding infant:

*Prothrombin Time (PT).* This test measures the extrinsic activation of factor X by factor VII, as well as the remainder of the coagulation scheme (factors V, II and fibrinogen).

*Partial Thromboplastin Time (PTT).* This test measures the intrinsic pathway (activation of factor X by factors XII, XI, IX and VIII), as well as the final coagulation reactions (V, II and fibrinogen). Most laboratories use an activated partial thromboplastin time (APTT). This test is similar to the PTT except material is added to

hasten the activation of factor XII, and thereby speed up the overall reaction.

Two important variables must be considered when collecting venous blood for neonatal coagulation studies. First, the ratio of blood to anticoagulant (3.8 per cent sodium citrate) should be 19:1 (Koepke, Rodgers, and Ollivier). The usual ratio (9:1) may give spurious results in neonates with hematocrits over 60 per cent. Second, blood should not be drawn from heparinized catheters, since even minute amounts of this anticoagulant can prolong the PTT.

Neonates have decreased levels of certain clotting factors, particularly those dependent on vitamin K (Table 64–3). Consequently, the PT and PTT in healthy term infants are slightly prolonged compared to that seen in older children. These physiological factor deficiencies are exaggerated in premature infants, and thus the PT and PTT in prematures may be even slightly more prolonged. It is important to emphasize that the differences in clotting parameters between older children and infants are physiologically normal. Any questionable abnormality must be compared to these "normal" neonatal values. Furthermore, each individual hospital must establish its own normal values, since slight modifications in blood collection or assay methods exist between different laboratories.

**TABLE 64–3.** *Coagulation Profile of Newborn Infants**

|  | *Normal Children* | *Term Infants* | *Premature Infants* |
|---|---|---|---|
| Platelet count | 200,000–400,000 | 200,000–400,000 | 150,000–350,000 |
| Bleeding time (BT) | 2.5–5.5 min | 2.5–5.5 min | 2.5–5.5 min |
| Prothrombin time (PT) | 12–14 sec | 13–20 sec | 13–21 sec |
| Partial thromboplastin time (PTT) | 37–50 sec | 45–65 sec | 45–75 sec |
| Activated partial thromboplastin time (APTT) | 25–35 sec | 30–45 sec | 35–55 sec |
| *Clotting Factors* |  |  |  |
| Normal | All Factors | Fibrinogen V, VIII, XII, XIII | Fibrinogen V, VIII, XII, XIII |
| Slightly decreased | — | II, VII, IX, X, XI | XI |
| Moderately decreased | — | — | II, VII, IX, X |

Data based on normal values published by Hathaway, W. E. (Semin. Hematol. *12:*175–188, 1975) and on normal values at Children's Hospital Medical Center, Boston, Mass.

4. FIBRINOGEN DETERMINATION. This factor is measured when attempting to differentiate DIC or liver disease from other clotting abnormalities. Reduced fibrinogen synthesis occurs in liver disease. Increased degradation of fibrinogen is seen in DIC.

5. FIBRIN SPLIT PRODUCTS (FSP's). These degradation products of fibrin and fibrinogen are increased in patients with DIC. Increased levels occasionally are seen in liver disease, possibly due to decreased clearance of FSP's. Since DIC frequently coexists with liver disease, it is often difficult to distinguish these two entities. Fibrin split products are not increased in normal infants when blood samples are properly collected.

6. APT TEST. This simple test distinguishes gastrointestinal blood loss due to neonatal hemorrhage or swallowed maternal blood.

    a. Mix 1 volume of stool or vomitus with 5 volumes of water.

    b. Centrifuge mixture, and separate clear pink supernatant (hemolysate).

    c. Add 1 ml 1 per cent NaOH to 4 ml hemolysate. Mix and observe color change after 2 minutes. Hemoglobin A changes from pink to yellow-brown color (this indicates maternal blood). Hemoglobin F resists denaturation and remains pink (this indicates fetal blood).

Approximately 30 per cent of all episodes of gastrointestinal bleeding are due to swallowed maternal blood (Sherman and Clatworthy). In those cases in which blood loss is neonatal in origin, less than 25 per cent of infants have detectable platelet or coagulation abnormalities. Presumably, gastrointestinal blood loss in most infants is due to abnormalities of the GI tract.

## BLOOD COMPONENTS USED IN THERAPY OF BLEEDING INFANTS

PLATELET TRANSFUSIONS. A unit of platelets is defined as that number of platelets obtained from one unit of blood. Depending upon available equipment, 1 to 6 units can be processed from a donor at any one time. Platelets are suspended in plasma, approximately 1 unit of platelets in 15 to 30 milliliters of plasma. The smaller volume is used for neonatal platelet therapy. In order to prevent red blood cell injury, platelets are suspended in AB negative plasma if the donor blood type is different from the recipient's. Platelets do not contain the Rh antigen, but virtually all platelet concentrates contain some RBC's. Rh negative infants, therefore, are given platelets from Rh negative donors. If emergency conditions require that Rh negative girls be given platelets from an Rh positive donor, anti-Rh immune serum should be given to protect against red blood cell isoimmunization. In cases of neonatal isoimmune thrombocytopenia, maternal platelets are obtained, washed free of antibody and resuspended in AB negative plasma. As a rule of thumb, the administration of 1 unit of fresh platelets per 5 kilograms of body weight elevates the platelet count over 100,000. Subsequently, the platelet count should decline slowly over 4 to 6 days. Failure to sustain a platelet increase indicates platelet incompatibility due to sensitization or increased platelet destruction (sepsis, DIC, anti-platelet antibody).

FRESH FROZEN PLASMA. Plasma that is frozen and stored immediately after separation contains adequate concentrations of all clotting factors. Fresh frozen plasma (10 ml/Kg) given every 12 hours provides adequate hemostasis for most causes of bleeding due to lack of factors. One unit of clotting factor is defined as that concentration present in 1 milliliter of normal pooled plasma. Whenever coagulation factors and platelets are given at the same time, the volume of platelet suspension (essentially all plasma) must be accounted for in calculating plasma therapy.

CLOTTING FACTOR CONCENTRATES. Patients with factor VIII deficiency (classical hemophilia) or factor IX deficiency (Christmas disease) occasionally require very high factor levels in cases of severe bleeding. In order to avoid problems with fluid volume overload, concentrated factor preparations should be employed. The factor VIII concentrate we use (Method Four) contains approximately 30 factor VIII units per ml. Factor IX concentrates (Konyne, Proplex) contain about 17 factor IX units per ml. In addition, factor IX concentrates contain increased amounts of factors II, VII, and X.

## HEMORRHAGIC DISEASE OF THE NEWBORN

The American Academy of Pediatrics has defined this disorder as any bleeding problem due to vitamin K deficiency and decreased activity of factors II, VII, IX and X. These clotting proteins are synthesized and stored in the liver until activated by vitamin K. Newborn infants are capable of normal factor synthesis, but because they are relatively vitamin K deficient, coagulant activity of these factors is decreased. Normally, vitamin K is obtained from the diet and from intestinal bacterial synthesis. Neonates, however, get variable amounts of dietary vitamin K during the first few days of life, and the intestine is not colonized with bacteria at birth. Therefore, as maternally derived vitamin stores are depleted during the first day of life, vitamin K deficiency actually becomes worse, clotting studies become more abnormal and significant bleeding episodes can occur between 24 and 72 hours of age.

Several years ago it was demonstrated that neonatal hemorrhagic disease could be prevented by institution of early feedings with cow's milk (Sanford et al.). This effect was due to the significantly higher vitamin K content of cow's milk compared to breast milk (Dam et al.). Neonatal hemorrhagic disease is extremely unusual today, since vitamin K is given routinely to infants at birth (see below). When bleeding does occur, it is generally because someone has failed to administer the vitamin. Rarely, hemorrhagic disease is seen in children born to epileptic mothers under treatment with Dilantin or phenobarbital (Mountain et al.). These drugs can interfere with vitamin K, and thereby cause abnormal clotting studies, extremely low factor levels and bleeding at birth. Infants born to mothers receiving coumarin compounds (vitamin K antagonists) also can bleed, because these drugs cross the placenta and aggravate normal vitamin K-dependent factor deficiencies. Heparin does not cross the placenta.

Therefore, in those maternal conditions which require anticoagulation, heparin should be substituted for coumarin a few days prior to delivery (Hirsh et al.). Heparin also should be used instead of coumarin in the first trimester of pregnancy, since coumarin compounds have been associated with teratogenic effects (Fillmore and McDevitt).

Hemorrhage due to vitamin K deficiency characteristically occurs in otherwise healthy thriving infants. Bleeding may be localized to one area (frequently gastrointestinal) or there may be diffuse ecchymoses. In cases of classical vitamin K deficiency, hemorrhage generally is seen after the first 24 hours of age. In contrast, bleeding secondary to maternal drugs such as phenobarbital, Dilantin and coumarin derivatives frequently occurs within the first 24 hours of life. The following laboratory test results suggest vitamin K deficiency in a bleeding infant: a normal platelet count, a prolonged PTT and a prolonged PT. Bleeding infants who fit this criterion should be given vitamin K (1 mg intravenously). The PT and PTT will begin to normalize after a 4-hour period, and clinical bleeding will cease if the abnormality is due to vitamin K deficiency. Failure to note improvement in bleeding and clotting tests after giving vitamin K suggests another diagnosis, such as liver disease or isolated factor deficiency. Life-threatening hemorrhages due to vitamin K deficiency are unusual but if they occur fresh frozen plasma (10 ml/Kg) should be given in addition to vitamin K.

In most centers, prophylactic vitamin K (0.5 to 1.0 mg) is given intramuscularly at the time of delivery or when the infant enters the nursery. The natural or fat soluble form of vitamin K (Aqua-Mephyton) is safe and nontoxic. High concentrations of some water soluble analogues (Menadione), however, may cause hemolysis, hyperbilirubinemia and kernicterus (Lucey and Dolan). The minimal dose of vitamin K which prevents the fall in PT and bleeding is 0.025 mg; higher concentrations have no more beneficial effect (Aballi and DeLamerens). Nevertheless, we continue to give doses which are in large excess of the minimum requirement. Previously it was thought that premature infants did not respond to vitamin K. Aballi and his co-workers, however, have demonstrated that healthy prematures do respond, although sick prematures may manifest a less than optimal change in clotting studies. It is our policy to administer vitamin K (0.5 mg) once each week to ill prematures and infants receiving total parenteral alimentation. Vitamin K given to mothers during labor has been proven to be effective in preventing neonatal bleeding, although one is never quite certain how much actually crosses the placenta. It is more rational to administer vitamin K at the time of birth, since the response to the vitamin is rapid and bleeding rarely occurs in the first 24 hours of life. Infants of mothers receiving antiseizure medications are an exception to this rule, for these neonates can bleed during the first 24 hours. In these cases, vitamin K should be given during labor in order to prevent any bleeding secondary to the trauma of delivery. Following birth, vitamin K should be given as usual to the neonate.

CASE 64–1

A 3000 gram male infant was born to a healthy gravida 1, para 1 mother after an uneventful 40 week gestation. Apgar score at birth was 9. Physical examination was normal. Breast feedings were started at 18 hours of age. On the second day of life a bruise appeared over the right buttock. Several bloody stools were noted on the third day. There were no other abnormalities. No petechiae were seen. An Apt test on the stool samples indicated the source of blood was from the infant rather than of maternal origin. The prothrombin time and partial thromboplastin time were markedly prolonged. Examination of the peripheral blood smear indicated that the platelet count was greater than 200,000. The infant was given 1 mg of vitamin K intravenously. After 5 hours no gastrointestinal bleeding was evident and the PT and PTT had decreased to nearly normal levels. The subsequent clinical course was uneventful.

COMMENT.   This is a classic case of neonatal hemorrhagic disease due to vitamin K deficiency: delayed onset of bleeding, gastrointestinal hemorrhage, normal platelet count, abnormal coagulation studies and a definite clinical and laboratory response to vitamin K administration. Although there was no apparent cause of bleeding, a check of the medical record indicated that vitamin K had not been given at birth. At the time this child entered the nursery, most of the medical personnel were actively administering to two other critically ill infants. In the midst of this confusion the infant under discussion failed to receive Vitamin K.

## HEREDITARY CLOTTING FACTOR DEFICIENCIES

Infants with hereditary clotting factor deficiencies usually are healthy and do not bleed. When hemorrhage does occur, it most commonly is manifested by local blood loss, such as gastrointestinal hemorrhage, bleeding from circumcision or umbilical stump and large cephalohematomas. The PTT and PT usually are prolonged, but the platelet count is normal. Neither bleeding nor abnormal coagulation studies respond to vitamin K. Diagnosis of most factor deficiencies can be made in the newborn period, since coagulation proteins do not cross the placenta (Cade et al.). In some cases the specific diagnosis is obscured by physiologic factor deficiencies, but virtually all hereditary clotting defects can be detected by 4 months of age.

### FACTOR VIII DEFICIENCY (CLASSICAL HEMOPHILIA, HEMOPHILIA A)

Classical hemophilia is a sex-linked disorder characterized by decreased activity of factor VIII or antihemophilic factor (AHF). Production of normal factor VIII activity is controlled by two separate genes, one autosomal and the other sex-linked. The autosomal gene regulates production of factor VIII protein, whereas the sex-linked gene regulates coagulant activity of factor VIII protein. Classical hemophilia, a sex-linked disorder, is characterized by normal amounts of factor VIII protein with markedly diminished factor VIII coagulant activity (Ratnoff). Von Willebrand's disease (see below) is an autosomal disorder characterized by decreased AHF protein and coagulant activity.

The spectrum of hemorrhagic problems in hemophiliac children is well known to most physicians. For unknown reasons, however, severe neonatal bleeding due to factor VIII deficiency is unusual. Hemorrhage which does occur generally follows traumatic procedures. In a retrospective study, Strauss and Baehner observed that less than 40 per cent of hemophiliacs hemorrhaged following circumcision, and in most cases hemorrhage was very mild. One explanation for this minimal bleeding may be that tissue injury liberates thromboplastin, and thereby activates the extrinsic pathway (which bypasses factor VIII). The severe muscle and joint hemorrhages characteristic of hemophilia in older children do not begin until infants start to crawl and walk.

Classically, hemophilia occurs in male children; females rarely are affected. There is no problem making this diagnosis in the newborn period, since neonatal factor VIII levels are the same as in older children. Although the platelet count and PT are normal, the PTT is prolonged. A specific factor assay should be done if possible because similar values are seen in deficiencies of factors IX, XI and XII. In the absence of a factor assay, however, most laboratories can make a presumptive diagnosis by modifying the PTT test. Factor VIII is absent from normal serum but is present in plasma. Therefore, if the patient's plasma is mixed with equal amounts of normal serum or plasma, the abnormal PTT will be corrected by plasma but not by serum. This result is very suggestive of factor VIII deficiency. Nevertheless, a specific factor VIII determination is ultimately necessary to confirm the diagnosis. Knowledge of the factor level also can be of prognostic significance. Children with severe hemophilia have less than 1 per cent normal factor VIII activity, whereas cases of mild to moderate disease are characterized by 1 to 20 per cent factor VIII levels.

In the absence of bleeding no specific therapy is necessary. Mild bleeding from circumcision or umbilical stump usually can be corrected by local measures such as topical thrombin or Gelfoam. Nonabsorbable substances should not be used, because bleeding may start again when the material is removed. In those cases in which bleeding is more severe, factor VIII must be given to raise the plasma concentration to 20 per cent of normal. One factor VIII unit administered per kilogram of body weight elevates the plasma concentration 2 per cent. Thus, to achieve a level that is 20 per cent of normal requires 10 factor VIII units per kilogram of body weight, or 30 factor VIII units for a 3 Kg infant. This can be achieved by 30 ml of plasma, since 1 factor VIII unit is by definition equal to that activity in 1 ml of normal plasma. Alternatively, commercial concentrates which provide factor VIII in a much smaller volume (Method Four, approximately 30 factor VIII units per ml) can be used to avoid volume overload problems. Factor VIII concentrates should be used whenever possible, especially in conjunction with surgery or with those rare life-threatening hemorrhages in which factor VIII levels of 50 to 100 per cent of normal are required. The in vivo half-life of factor VIII is relatively short, thus infusions need to be repeated every 12 hours until bleeding is under control.

## VON WILLEBRAND'S DISEASE

This common autosomal dominant disorder is characterized by abnormal platelet function and decreased factor VIII levels. In contrast to classical hemophilia, both factor VIII coagulant activity and factor VIII protein are reduced (Ratnoff). The platelet defect in von Willebrand's disease is due to decreased levels of this protein, since normal platelet function requires interaction with factor VIII. This explanation is supported by the clinical observation that plasma transfusions, even plasma from classical hemophiliacs, can correct the platelet abnormality (i.e., bleeding time) in von Willebrand's disease. In addition, plasma infusions correct the defect in factor VIII coagulant activity. Factor VIII replacement in hemophiliacs results in a transient increase in factor VIII coagulant activity (half-life of 12 hours). In von Willebrand's disease, however, a single factor VIII infusion produces an increase in factor VIII activity that is sustained for several days. Presumably the patient with von Willebrand's disease can generate the coagulant component of the factor VIII molecule once the protein factor is present.

Little is known about the neonatal course of children with von Willebrand's disease. In older children, bleeding is milder than in classical hemophilia, and most often is characterized by severe epistaxis. Occasionally, severe hemorrhage may occur after trauma or surgery. The diagnosis of this disorder can be difficult, since coagulation studies are not always abnormal. In some cases the PTT is prolonged, but this is not an invariable finding. Factor VIII levels of 20 to 50 per cent of normal usually are seen. The concentration of factor VIII protein also is 20 to 50 per cent of normal. One of the most useful diagnostic tests is that of bleeding time. Mild cases are characterized by a mildly abnormal bleeding time, and these children rarely have significant hemorrhagic manifestations. In severe cases of von Willebrand's disease, however, the bleeding time is prolonged. Soon it will be possible for many laboratories to make a more definitive diagnosis by separately measuring factor VIII coagulant activity and protein level. Treatment of a bleeding neonate suspected of having von Willebrand's disease (usually on the basis of family history) is similar to that of the infant with classical hemophilia, with the major difference that only one factor VIII infusion is required to provide adequate hemostasis. Platelet transfusions are not needed, since the platelet defect is corrected by administration of factor VIII.

### FACTOR IX DEFICIENCY (CHRISTMAS DISEASE, HEMOPHILIA B)

Although it is less common than classical hemophilia, factor IX deficiency accounts for 15 per cent of all cases of hemophilia. This disorder is also sex-linked, and the clinical manifestations are indistinguishable from those of factor VIII deficiency. Coagulation studies are the same as for infants with factor VIII deficiency: normal platelets, normal PT and prolonged PTT. In contrast to factor VIII deficiency, however, the PTT is normalized by mixing normal plasma or serum with the patient's plasma (factor IX present in plasma and serum). Definitive diagnosis requires a specific factor assay, preferably done after 2 months of age.

When excess bleeding is present in a child thought to have Christmas disease, fresh frozen plasma should be given. One unit of factor IX increases plasma IX activity 1 per cent. For minor bleeding 10 ml per Kg of body weight every 12 hours provides adequate hemostasis. With severe bleeding or in conjunction with surgery factor IX activity should be increased to 40 to 50 per cent of normal. Commercial factor IX concentrates are used to achieve these high levels.

### FACTOR XI DEFICIENCY (HEMOPHILIA C)

This autosomal recessive factor deficiency occurs primarily in Jewish families. Bleeding is rarely a serious problem, because the factor is not completely absent from plasma. It is difficult to make a specific diagnosis in neonates, since factor XI levels remain low for the first several months of life. Factor therapy rarely is required, even for surgical procedures. In a bleeding patient thought to have factor XI deficiency, fresh frozen plasma (10 ml/Kg) should be given.

### FACTOR XIII DEFICIENCY

Factor XIII (fibrin stabilizing factor) deficiency is characterized by delayed bleeding from the umbilical stump. Deficiency of this factor results in an inability to form stable fibrin polymers, and thus a very friable clot is produced. Between 24 and 48 hours after a period of apparent adequate hemostasis, the clot begins to ooze. The screening coagulation tests (platelet count, PT, PTT) are all normal. Diagnosis requires both a high index of suspicion and definitive laboratory tests. Normal fibrin clots are not dissolved by reagents such as 5M urea or monochloroacetic acid, whereas the friable clot produced in factor XIII deficient plasma is rapidly broken down by these agents. Fibrin stabilizing factor is present in plasma, and should be administered if there is significant bleeding.

## MISCELLANEOUS FACTOR DEFICIENCIES

Hereditary deficiencies of virtually all other clotting factors have been described. These are extremely rare, and significant neonatal bleeding associated with these deficiencies is even more infrequent. Diagnosis of individual factor deficiencies is suggested by unexplained abnormalities in coagulation tests, but specific factor assays are required for confirmation. As in factor IX deficiency, diagnosis of the other vitamin K-dependent factors cannot be made with certainty until the infant is 2 months of age. Fresh frozen plasma should be given for serious hemorrhage in any bleeding neonate thought to have a factor deficiency.

## INTRAVASCULAR COAGULATION SYNDROMES

The intravascular coagulation syndromes are caused by inappropriate activation of the clotting process. These events are inappropriate in that coagulation is stimulated by factors other than bleeding. Intravascular coagulation is not a disease; it is a response to local or systemic pathology. Frequently, however, the effects of accelerated coagulation are more severe than the initiating causes.

### DISSEMINATED INTRAVASCULAR COAGULATION (DIC)

Several years ago the term "secondary hemorrhagic disease" was applied to sick infants with severe bleeding not related to vitamin K deficiency. It is now apparent that this syndrome includes many infants with disseminated intravascular coagulation. Disseminated intravascular coagulation is caused by widespread activation of the clotting mechanism, brought about by a variety of systemic problems. The clinical effects of accelerated coagulation are thrombosis and bleeding. Thrombotic manifestations are due to diffuse intravascular fibrin deposition. Bleeding occurs for two reasons. 1) During accelerated coagulation, certain clotting factors (II, V, VIII and fibrinogen) are consumed at a faster rate than they are synthesized. 2) Persistent

**TABLE 64–4.** *Disseminated Intravascular Coagulation*

*Clinical Diagnosis*
Sick infant
Usually diffuse petechiae/bleeding
Rarely diffuse thrombosis (skin necrosis)

*Laboratory Diagnosis*
Decreased platelets
Prolonged PT and PTT
Decreased factors V, VIII and fibrinogen
Increased fibrin split products
Microangiopathic RBC changes

*Therapy*
1. Vigorous treatment of underlying condition (correction of hypoxia, acidosis and hypovolemia; antibiotics)
2. Plasma and platelet infusions
3. If serious bleeding continues—
   (a) consider exchange transfusion with fresh blood
   (b) continue plasma and platelet infusions as required
4. If clinical presentation mainly thrombotic—
   (a) administer heparin intravenously
   (b) after heparinization, give plasma and platelets

stimulation of clotting activates fibrinolysis, and fibrin split products are produced. These fibrin degradation products contribute to hemorrhage by inhibiting the normal conversion of fibrinogen to fibrin.

DIC is associated with a variety of conditions in the newborn period: shock, sepsis, acidosis, hypoxia, hypothermia, abruptio placentae and retention of a dead twin fetus. Unlike bleeding caused by lack of vitamin K or inherited factor deficiencies, DIC occurs in sick infants. Commonly these neonates are premature and are thus most likely to suffer from the problems known to cause DIC. The severity of DIC is generally related to the duration of the activating stimulus. Subsequent coagulation abnormalities are less severe in cases of acute and self-limited activation, such as transient hypothermia or abruptio placentae, than in those conditions associated with more prolonged disease, such as sepsis or respiratory distress syndrome. Some infants have no clinical manifestations of DIC in spite of marked laboratory abnormalities. In most cases, however, there is diffuse bleeding characterized by petechiae, oozing from venipuncture sites and gastrointestinal hemorrhages. In a small number of infants the clinical picture is dominated by thrombosis (gangrenous necrosis of skin).

The laboratory diagnosis of DIC is characterized by several distinct abnormalities: 1) Invariably there is thrombocytopenia due to increased platelet utilization. 2) The PT and PTT are prolonged owing to factor depletion. 3) Fibrinogen usually is decreased. If facilities are available for the measurement of factors V and VIII, their levels will also be found to be decreased. 4) Fibrin split products are increased because of enhanced fibrinolysis. 5) Microangiopathic red blood cell changes (cell fragments, distorted cells) are seen on the peripheral blood smear. Fragment formation is presumably due to RBC interaction with fibrin deposited on the vascular wall.

There is general agreement that successful management of infants with DIC depends on effective removal of conditions activating coagulation. Thus, the most important therapeutic considerations must be directed at associated infection, hypoxia, acidosis, hypotension and other physiologic abnormalities. Beyond this observation there is little consensus regarding the proper management of infants with DIC.

Most commonly, DIC is characterized by diffuse cutaneous bleeding. In these infants, our initial approach is to replace platelets and clotting factors with fresh frozen plasma. Occasionally, this is all that is necessary, particularly in neonates who are not very ill and who have minimally abnormal clotting studies. If bleeding persists after plasma and platelet replacement, we proceed with an exchange transfusion using citrated fresh whole blood. This procedure provides clotting factors and platelets, but it also may remove fibrin split products and some of the toxic factors causing DIC. In addition, adult red blood cells deliver oxygen more readily than do neonatal red blood cells (see Chapter 64), and this may reduce tissue damage from hypoxia. Gross and Melhorn have reported the beneficial effects of exchange transfusion in several infants with DIC. In some of these neonates, exchange transfusion corrected bleeding and coagulation prob-

lems before the associated conditions (sepsis, respiratory distress) were under control.

We occasionally see infants with DIC manifested by gangrenous necrosis of the skin (black fingers and toes). Rarely, DIC produces kidney necrosis caused by the thrombosis of large renal vessels. Teleologically, these conditions are due to a relative increase in fibrin deposition compared to factor depletion (i.e., clotting greater than fibrinolysis). Therefore, anticoagulation is a logical therapeutic modality in children with thrombotic problems. Intravenous heparin (10–15 mg/kg/hr) is given continuously for a total duration of 2 to 3 days. Once heparin has been started, platelet and plasma transfusions can be given. It is important that platelets and plasma be replaced after heparin, otherwise one merely provides substrate for more thrombus formation.

It should be pointed out that some centers employ heparin in cases of DIC in which there is bleeding without thrombotic manifestations. This therapeutic approach is based on the assumption that hemorrhage is due in part to depletion of clotting factors. Thus, heparin transiently interferes with normal coagulation and allows these factors to regenerate. There are several reports that heparin has corrected the laboratory abnormalities in DIC. The studies of Corrigan and Jordan, however, clearly demonstrate that heparin has no effect on the overall mortality from DIC.

CASE 64–2

A 1090 gram female infant was born by spontaneous delivery after 31 weeks' gestation. At birth the child was well, but by 5 hours of age respiratory distress developed, with frequent apneic episodes. At 15 hours of age bleeding from the umbilical catheter and skin was noted. Vitamin K had been given at birth. Laboratory studies revealed a markedly prolonged PT and PTT. The platelet count was 32,000. Fibrinogen was less than 100 mg per 100 ml. Fibrin split products were markedly elevated. The infant was transfused with fresh frozen plasma and platelets, but bleeding continued unabated. Intravenous heparin (15 mg/kg/hr) was started, and more platelets and factors were given. At 26 hours of age the infant died. Autopsy revealed hemorrhage into the cerebral ventricles and lungs.

COMMENT. This child was born at a time when we believed in early heparinization for DIC. Nowadays we rarely anticoagulate bleeding infants, mainly because there is little proof that it is efficacious. Furthermore, we are never certain whether fatal hemorrhages are due to DIC or to heparin therapy. Our current approach to cases like this would be to perform an exchange transfusion after the initial failure. In view of the child's gestational age and respiratory disease, one could argue that exchange transfusion should be the initial therapy once DIC is diagnosed.

### LOCALIZED INTRAVASCULAR COAGULATION

Specific organ pathology can lead to deposition of fibrin and platelets. Generally these effects are limited to localized thrombosis in the area of activation, although depletion of platelets and coagulation factors occasionally is seen. The hemolytic-uremic syndrome (HUS) is an example of localized intravascular coagulation. This disorder generally occurs in children less than 2 years of age and rarely may be seen in neonates. HUS is characterized by local deposition of fibrin and platelets within the renal vasculature. In most cases there is thrombocytopenia, but consumption of clotting factors occurs infrequently. Bleeding usually is due to decreased platelets. Intravascular fibrin interacts with red blood cells, forming distorted red blood cells or schistocytes (fragments, helmet cells). These cells are fragile and are rapidly destroyed, thus producing hemolytic anemia. Renal failure is the major clinical problem in HUS, and most therapeutic efforts are directed toward the management of this process (early peritoneal dialysis). If systemic bleeding occurs, platelets and fresh frozen plasma should be given as needed. Heparinization has not been demonstrated to be beneficial.

Localized intravascular coagulation is seen in a variety of other conditions: renal vein thrombosis, portal vein thrombosis, necrotizing enterocolitis, and large hemangiomas (section on thrombocytopenia).

### BLEEDING ASSOCIATED WITH LIVER DISEASE

Since the liver produces all clotting factors with the exception of factor VIII, it is not surprising that bleeding is a main clinical manifestation of serious liver disease. Neonatal bleeding due to liver injury generally occurs in sick infants following hypoxia or hypotension. The characteristics of this type of bleeding are very similar to those of DIC, and frequently DIC is associated with liver disease. The PT and PTT are both prolonged, and there is no significant change following vitamin K administration. The platelet count may be normal or decreased, depending on whether there is associated DIC or significant portal hypertension. Fibrin split products may be increased, owing to decreased hepatic clearance, even in the absence of DIC. A normal factor VIII level is the only feature of liver disease that distinguishes this syndrome from DIC.

Therapy for bleeding due to liver disease is largely factor replacement (10 ml plasma/kg/12 hr). Platelets are given if there is significant thrombocytopenia.

CASE 64–3

A female infant weighing 1810 gm was born to a healthy mother after 33 weeks' gestation. Shortly after birth, respirations became labored, with grunting and cyanosis. Chest x-ray was characteristic of hyaline membrane disease. Blood gases revealed the following: pH 7.26, $P_{CO_2}$ 39.6 mm Hg, and $P_{O_2}$ 30 mm Hg. The child was given assisted ventilation with a Bennett respirator and oxygen. Over the next 4 days her clinical status improved somewhat. On the fourth day, however, there was bleeding from the umbilical catheter, and a large ecchymosis was noted on the right leg. There were no petechiae or other physical abnormalities. The platelet count was 165,000 but the PT and PTT were both markedly prolonged. Vitamin K (1.0 mg) given intravenously had no effect on the bleeding or clotting studies. The fibrinogen level was less than 100 mg per 100 ml. Fibrin split products were slightly increased. There was no alteration in RBC morphology. The child was given plasma infusions over the next three days. Clotting studies improved and there was no further bleeding. At the same time the infant's respiratory status improved considerably.

**COMMENT.** In view of the relatively normal platelet count, this child's bleeding was probably due to liver disease rather than DIC. Presumably liver injury was due to hypoxia during the course of respiratory disease. Fresh frozen plasma and improvement in respiratory status resulted in cessation of all bleeding. It should be pointed out, however, that this is an atypical case of bleeding associated with liver disease. In most cases the patients are refractory to therapy and the prognosis is grave.

## BLEEDING DUE TO PLATELET ABNORMALITIES

Platelet related bleeding usually is due to thrombocytopenia, although hereditary and acquired platelet dysfunction are seen rarely. Bleeding due to platelet disturbances generally is petechial and superficial (skin and mucosa) in contrast to the large ecchymoses and muscle hemorrhages seen in coagulation disturbances. The major causes of neonatal thrombocytopenia include 1) DIC (discussed above), 2) immune reactions and 3) infection. In the absence of DIC, the PTT and PT usually are normal.

### ISOIMMUNE THROMBOCYTOPENIA

This condition is analogous to erythroblastosis due to ABO and Rh incompatibility. The infant's platelets contain an antigen which is lacking on maternal platelets. During pregnancy, fetal platelets enter the maternal circulation and stimulate antibody production against fetal platelet antigens (Harrington et al.). Maternal platelets are not affected. Although the antibody is specific for one of several platelet antigens, 50 per cent of cases are due to $Pl^{A1}$ antigens (mother is $Pl^{A1}$ negative, infant is $Pl^{A1}$ positive) (Shulman).

Children with isoimmune thrombocyto-

penia manifest increasing petechiae and mucosal bleeding during the first 48 hours of life (Pearson et al.). Generally this is the only symptom in an otherwise healthy neonate. The platelet count is decreased and may be as low as 2000. Platelets appear very large on the peripheral blood smear. Coagulation studies are normal. This disorder is suspected when isolated thrombocytopenia is seen in a thriving infant whose mother is healthy and has a normal platelet count. Definitive diagnosis requires demonstration of a neonatal platelet antigen which is lacking on maternal platelets. This can only be done in a specialized platelet laboratory.

Studies reported several years ago suggested a 10 to 15 per cent mortality with this disorder, with death usually due to CNS hemorrhage. In most cases, however, infants with neonatal isoimmune thrombocytopenia do not have serious bleeding, particularly if the platelet count is greater than 20,000. The platelet count remains low until the neonate clears maternal antibody, generally within a period of 4 to 8 weeks. In spite of this persistent thrombocytopenia, significant bleeding is seen only in the first few days of life.

Our policy is to treat all children who have platelet counts of less than 30,000, even in the absence of overt bleeding. The mainstay of therapy is transfusion of maternal platelets which have been washed and resuspended in AB-negative plasma. Random donor platelets are of little value in cases due to $Pl^{A1}$ sensitivity since 97 per cent of donors will be $Pl^{A1}$ positive. In the absence of facilities to separate platelets, a unit of maternal whole blood can be removed and transported to the closest institution that can fractionate blood. In this way platelets are provided for the infant, and red blood cells can be reinfused into the mother. In most cases, a single transfusion of maternal platelets produces a sustained elevation in the neonatal platelet count. Recently, however, we observed a clearly documented case of isoimmune thrombocytopenia (mother $Pl^{A1}$ negative, infant $Pl^{A1}$ positive) which required three separate platelet transfusions in order to elevate the peripheral platelet count. This delayed response most probably was due to the fact that this infant also was infected.

Neonates with significant bleeding or with very low platelet counts also are given hydrocortisone (10 mg every 12 hours, intravenously) until the response to maternal platelets can be assessed. The efficacy of steroid therapy in thrombocytopenias has never been clearly established but there is a general impression that these drugs increase the platelet count. In any event, it is our belief that a short course of steroids to bleeding but otherwise healthy infants is not significantly deleterious. When maternal platelets are not immediately available to treat severe hemorrhage, steroids and random donor platelets should be given. The survival time of these platelets is short, although they may be transiently functional before being coated with antibody and removed from the circulation. Exchange transfusion prior to giving random donor platelets has been advocated in order to partially remove circulating antibody.

Isoimmune thrombocytopenia differs from Rh disease in that 50 per cent of all cases occur in the first pregnancy (Shulman). Furthermore, once this entity has occurred, there is a 70 to 85 per cent probability of recurrence in subsequent pregnancies. There is at present no satisfactory assay that can detect whether an infant will be born with thrombocytopenia. Maternal anti-platelet antibody titers have been followed but have been of little prognostic value. Our approach to high risk pregnancies (i.e., previous history of isoimmune thrombocytopenia) is as follows: 1) Maternal platelets are removed the day before delivery. 2) Delivery is by elective cesarean section in order to prevent serious neonatal bleeding during passage through the birth canal. 3) Maternal platelets are transfused immediately after birth if the infant is thrombocytopenic. With this approach we have successfully avoided any major complications in thrombocytopenic infants.

CASE 64–4

A 3200 gm male infant was born to a gravida 1, para 1 mother after an uneventful pregnancy. At the time of birth the infant's physical examination was entirely normal except for a few petechiae over his chest. The infant did well until 16 hours of age, at which time he passed a grossly bloody stool. (Apt test revealed blood to be of neonatal origin.) At this time more petechiae were noted over his abdomen and shoulders. A CBC revealed the following: Hgb 16 gm/100 ml, WBC 16,000, platelet count 4500. The PT and PTT were normal. Skin, nose, throat and blood cultures were obtained, although there was no obvious infection. The mother's platelet count was 290,000, and further examination into her past medical history revealed nothing to explain her infant's thrombocytopenia. The child was given 1 unit of random donor platelets from the blood bank. His platelet count increased to 28,000 1 hour after the transfusion and was down to 6000 6 hours later. During this interval the infant had several bloody stools, but otherwise he appeared to be thriving. A unit of blood was obtained from the infant's mother, and platelets were separated. One hour after the neonate was transfused with maternal platelets, the platelet count was 120,000, and 6 hours later it was 102,000. During the remainder of the neonatal course there was no more bleeding. All previous cultures were negative. At 7 days of age the child's platelet count was 14,000. He was given another unit of maternal platelets and sent home.

COMMENT. Although platelet typing was not done on this particular child and his parents, the clinical history is classic for isoimmune thrombocytopenia. Two features of this management deserve further comment. 1) Steroids were not given with the initial platelet transfusion, although it was apparent the child probably had some form of immune thrombocytopenia. Currently we add steroids early in the therapy until we can assess the bleeding response to platelet transfusions. This is certainly a controversial area, and obviously this child did well without steroids. 2) At the time of discharge the infant was given another unit of maternal platelets. Bleeding beyond the first week of life, regardless of the platelet count, is extremely rare in isoimmune thrombocytopenia. However, since maternal platelet transfusions are relatively innocuous and potentially protective, we currently continue this practice.

## IMMUNE THROMBOCYTOPENIA SECONDARY TO MATERNAL DISEASE

In contrast to isoimmune thrombocytopenia, the antiplatelet antibody here is directed against maternal platelets. The neonate is affected to the extent that the antibody crosses the placenta and injures fetal platelets. The reasons for decreased platelets in the mother are as varied as the causes of adult immune thrombocytopenia (idiopathic, systemic lupus erythematosus, etc.). The likelihood that thrombocytopenia will develop in a child will be determined in large part by the state of the maternal disease (Goodhue and Evans). If the mother had ITP in the past but now has a normal platelet count the probability that her infant will develop thrombocytopenia is low. On the other hand, if the mother has evidence of active disease, or a low platelet count, it is likely (50 to 85 per cent) that the neonate will have thrombocytopenia. It should be noted that some splenectomized women with a history of ITP have normal platelet counts but continue to have high titers of antiplatelet antibodies. These individuals also have a high risk of bearing infants with thrombocytopenia.

These neonates are clinically identical to those with isoimmune thrombocytopenia. Rarely, an infant of a mother with lupus erythematosus will transiently develop the total symptoms of SLE, including thrombocytopenia, malar rash and L-E cells in the peripheral blood (Nathan and Snapper). Generally, however, these thrombocytopenic infants are healthy and thriving. The clinical course also is similar to the isoimmune disorder, although the platelet count may remain low for a longer period of time (up to 12 weeks). The prognosis usually is good, and significant bleeding beyond the first few days of life is most unusual.

Steroids are given to infants with platelet counts less than 20,000, or if there is any evidence of bleeding. Initial therapy is with hydrocortisone (10 mg intravenously every 12 hours). If for any reason steroids are required beyond 2 or 3 days (evidence of bleeding or platelets persistently less than 10,000) oral prednisone (1 mg/kg daily) is used for a maximum period of 3 weeks. In contrast to isoimmune thrombocytopenia, platelet transfusions have little part in the management of these patients. The maternal antiplatelet antibody usually is directed against a "public antigen" which is shared by maternal and neonatal platelets. Thus, random donor platelets are removed rapidly by the reticuloendothelial system. Nevertheless, in the presence of life-threatening hemorrhage, platelet transfusions should be given. Occasionally, incompatible platelets may be utilized for hemostasis before they are destroyed by antibody (i.e., delayed antigen-antibody reaction). Rarely, platelet responsiveness to random donor platelet transfusions may appear after previous failures to achieve an increased platelet count. Presumably, this is due to "soaking up" of antibodies by previous platelet transfusions. In severely bleeding infants refractory to steroids and random donor platelets, exchange transfusion followed by administration of platelets is indicated.

## IMMUNE THROMBOCYTOPENIA DUE TO DRUG-INDUCED MATERNAL THROMBOCYTOPENIA

Certain drugs (quinine, quinidine, sulfonamides, digitoxin) given to mothers can cause both maternal and neonatal thrombocytopenia on an immune basis (Mauer, DeVaux and Lahey). An antibody to the drug is produced by the mother. This antibody reacts with the drug, and the drug-antibody complex then attaches to the platelets (innocent bystanders), resulting in the removal of coated platelets from the circulation. The neonate is affected to the extent that drug and antibody cross the placenta into the fetal circulation. These children are clinically indistinguishable from other neonates with thrombocytopenia due to maternal disease. Significant bleeding is rare, but if it occurs platelet transfusions are indicated. This form of neonatal thrombocytopenia clears rapidly, the rate limiting factor being the neonatal clearance of drug. Once drug is removed from the neonate, platelet counts will increase even though the antibody may persist for several weeks.

## THROMBOCYTOPENIA ASSOCIATED WITH INFECTION

Thrombocytopenia frequently accompanies infection. The most commonly implicated infections are bacterial sepsis, cytomegalic inclusion disease, toxoplasmosis, syphilis, rubella and generalized herpes simplex. These infants may be relatively asymptomatic or severely ill. Rarely is thrombocytopenia the only abnormality, and in most cases it is not the major problem. Occasionally, however, significant bleeding may occur. Hepatosplenomegaly is a common clinical finding not seen in the other neonatal thrombocytopenias.

The mechanism of thrombocytopenia is multifactorial: 1) Many infections are associated with DIC, a common cause of decreased platelets. 2) Megakaryocyte platelet production may be inhibited directly by causative agents or their metabolites. 3) Reticuloendothelial hyperplasia associated with infection may lead to platelet sequestration. 4) Infectious agents may react with circulating platelets (similar to platelet + antibody) and thereby lead to their sequestration and removal.

In the absence of DIC, thrombocytopenia rarely is severe enough to cause serious bleeding. The major therapeutic effort must be directed to the underlying infection. Steroids are of no value. If serious bleeding does occur, platelet transfusions are indicated.

## THROMBOCYTOPENIA ASSOCIATED WITH GIANT HEMANGIOMAS

Hemangiomas commonly appear in the neonatal period, grow during the first few months of life and then begin to recede in size. Rarely, large superficial hemangiomas are associated with thrombocytopenia and bleeding (Kasabach and Merritt). Studies with $^{51}$chromium-labeled platelets have demonstrated that thrombocytopenia is due to sequestration and destruction of platelets within the vascular tumor (Kontras et al.). In addition, recent reports have indicated decreased levels of factors V, VIII and fibrinogen in many patients, thus suggesting that localized intravascular coagulation also occurs in these lesions.

Hemorrhage most commonly occurs after several weeks of age when the tumors are largest. Occasionally, however, bleeding is seen earlier, and at least 50 per cent of hemorrhagic angiomas initially bleed during the first month of life. Angiomas of the placenta (chorioangiomas) also can cause neonatal thrombocytopenia. Bleeding hemangiomas characteristically darken in

color, enlarge and become firm to palpation. Petechiae may appear around the periphery of the hemangioma as well as at distant sites. Systemic bleeding secondary to thrombocytopenia and/or depletion of clotting factors may occur. In some cases, however, the major clinical problems are not due to blood loss but rather are secondary to compression of vital structures (i.e., airway obstruction) as bleeding occurs into the hemangioma.

In the absence of symptoms, the best therapy for large hemangiomas is benign neglect, since almost all lesions regress spontaneously with time. Furthermore, most modes of therapeutic intervention produce serious side effects (scarring after surgery, bone growth retardation following radiation). No treatment is indicated for isolated thrombocytopenia in the absence of bleeding. If symptomatic hemorrhage occurs, platelets and fresh frozen plasma should be given as needed. In addition, attempts should be made to eradicate the angioma. The initial and most conservative approach is to attempt shrinkage of the tumor, using steroids (prednisone, 20 mg/day for 2 weeks) (Fost and Esterly). In those angiomas refractory to steroids, x-ray therapy may be useful. Radiation occasionally produces a rapid reduction in tumor size, and therefore this modality is most useful when enlarging hemangiomas cause compression of vital structures (Duncan and Halnan). We occasionally resort to surgical excision in situations that do not respond to steroids or radiation. Surgery should be done under cover of platelets and fresh frozen plasma, but even with these precautions, blood loss is usually excessive. It is difficult to remove the entire hemangioma surgically, but frequently the immediate threat to life can be decreased. The major complication in surviving patients is disfigurement brought about by the extensive surgery involved in tumor removal.

## THROMBOCYTOPENIA DUE TO BONE MARROW HYPOPLASIA

Thrombocytopenia due to decreased platelet production is usually associated with other congenital abnormalities or evidence of systemic disease. The diagnosis of a production defect is suggested by a decreased quantity of normal sized platelets on peripheral blood smear. Examination of the bone marrow is mandatory in cases of suspected marrow failure in order to rule out aplasia, leukemia or other neoplasms. Bleeding episodes are treated with platelet transfusions.

MEGAKARYOCYTE HYPOPLASIA AND BILATERAL ABSENCE OF RADII. Several cases of these two isolated congenital abnormalities have been reported (Hall et al.). These infants frequently manifest a leukemoid reaction (markedly elevated leukocyte count with many immature forms) in the peripheral blood.

FANCONI'S HYPOPLASTIC ANEMIA. This syndrome usually becomes apparent later in childhood, at which time there is pancytopenia (anemia, neutropenia, thrombocytopenia). In rare instances thrombocytopenia during infancy may be the initial manifestation of this disorder. Invariably, most patients have one or more congenital abnormalities, such as short stature, renal deformities, skeletal defects, hyperpigmentation and microphthalmia.

CONGENITAL LEUKEMIA. Bleeding due to thrombocytopenia may be the presenting sign of congenital leukemia (Chapter 111).

THROMBOCYTOPENIA SECONDARY TO MATERNAL DRUG INGESTION. Although the maternal ingestion of thiazides was previously considered to be a relatively common cause of neonatal thrombocytopenia, the general consensus now is that this is an extremely rare cause, if it exists at all (Merenstein, O'Loughlin and Plunket). It is difficult to document maternal drug ingestion as a cause of neonatal megakaryocyte failure when maternal platelets are not affected. In this category of thrombocytopenia the physician must rely upon a diagnosis of exclusion, since it is much more important not to overlook other, more subtle, causes of decreased platelet production.

DECREASED PLATELET PRODUCTION ASSOCIATED WITH INFECTION. This group (discussed above) is mentioned here only to emphasize that the thrombocytopenia of infection can be caused by suppression of normal megakaryocyte production. Pre-

sumably, this is the mechanism of thrombocytopenia that occurs in some cases of rubella.

## HEREDITARY THROMBOCYTOPENIAS

WISKOTT–ALDRICH SYNDROME. Thrombocytopenia, eczema and frequent infections due to immunologic defects characterize this disorder (Baldini). In rare instances, bleeding in the neonatal period may be the initial manifestation. Thrombocytopenia is due to an intrinsic platelet defect leading to decreased platelet survival. Unlike the large platelets seen in other thrombocytopenias characterized by a decreased life-span, those in the Wiskott–Aldrich syndrome are much smaller than normal (microplatelets). This is a sex-linked disorder affecting male children. The prognosis is poor, and children die of severe infections during the first years of life.

MISCELLANEOUS HEREDITARY THROMBOCYTOPENIAS. This group includes several poorly understood thrombocytopenias caused by either decreased platelet life-span or decreased platelet production. Family members frequently manifest thrombocytopenia. Serious neonatal bleeding problems are unusual.

HEMORRHAGE DUE TO PLATELET DYSFUNCTION. Platelet function can be assessed in vivo by the bleeding time or in vitro by observing platelet aggregation in response to known stimulants (ADP, thrombin, collagen). Neonatal platelet aggregation reportedly is abnormal, but this must not be of major significance, since the bleeding time of infants and older children is the same. Nevertheless, abnormal platelet function is suspected in any bleeding infant whose platelets are adequate and in whom coagulation studies are normal. In rare instances, hereditary disorders of platelet function (Glanzmann's thrombasthenia) may present with bleeding in the newborn period. A more important fact, however, is that neonates frequently acquire platelet dysfunction secondary to drug exposure.

Aspirin is known to cause abnormal platelet function. (Acetylation of platelet membrane by ASA inhibits release of platelet ADP and thereby prevents platelet aggregation.) In some individuals this results in bleeding. Several studies have demonstrated that aspirin taken by mothers within 2 or 3 days of delivery produces both maternal and neonatal platelet dysfunction (Corby and Schulman, Bleyer and Breckenridge). Furthermore, some infants with aspirin-induced platelet dysfunction have had suspicious hemorrhages (large cephalohematomas). Other drugs also have been implicated in neonatal platelet abnormalities. Corby and Schulman observed decreased platelet aggregation in neonates born to mothers given Demerol and Phenergan prior to delivery. No effect on maternal platelet function was noted.

A bleeding time should be done on any infant with a suspected platelet defect. Patients with von Willebrand's disease may present in a similar way, although the PTT usually is abnormal. Transfusion of random donor platelets is the treatment of choice for bleeding due to platelet dysfunction. Circulating drugs will not affect the function of transfused platelets over a short period of time.

## HEMOSTATIC ABNORMALITIES ASSOCIATED WITH SERIOUS LOCAL HEMORRHAGE

We have become relatively sophisticated in our understanding of normal hemostasis, and many major bleeding problems are currently being studied at the molecular level. The pathophysiology of the most serious neonatal bleeding problems, however, remains to be defined. These major pulmonary and central nervous system hemorrhages are discussed elsewhere in this text. The point to be emphasized here is that fatal bleeding episodes in neonates are not necessarily due to coagulation or platelet abnormalities. Massive pulmonary hemorrhage is occasionally associated with laboratory evidence of DIC or liver injury, but usually no hemostatic abnormality is detected. Similarly, coagulation abnormalities (liver injury, DIC) often are seen with the respiratory distress syndrome, and frequently children with RDS have intraventricular hemorrhages. Clotting defects,

however, are seen in only a small number of these infants with CNS hemorrhages. In most cases of intraventricular hemorrhage, local vascular factors must be important, since there often is no bleeding outside the CNS.

## REFERENCES

*General and Neonatal Hemostasis*

Bleyer, W. A., Hakami, N., and Shepart, T. H.: The development of hemostasis in the human fetus and newborn infant. J. Pediatr. 79:838, 1971.

Chessells, J. M., and Hardisty, R. M.: Bleeding problems in the newborn infant. Progress in hemostasis and thrombosis. 2:333–361, 1974.

Craig, W. S.: On real and apparent external bleeding in the newborn. Arch. Dis. Child. 36:575, 1961.

Fogel, B. J., Arias, D., and Kung, F.: Platelet counts in healthy premature infants. J. Pediatr. 73:108, 1968.

Hathaway, W. E.: The bleeding newborn. Semin. Hematol. 12:175, 1975.

Jensen, A. H., Josso, F., Zamet, P., Monset-Couchard, M., and Minkowski, A.: Evolution of blood clotting factor levels in premature infants during the first 10 days of life: A study of 96 cases with comparison between clinical status and blood clotting factor levels. Pediat. Res. 7:638, 1973.

Koepke, J. A., Rodgers, J. L., and Ollivier, M. J.: Pre-instrumental variables in coagulation testing. Am. J. Clin. Pathol. 64:591, 1975.

Oski, F. A., and Naiman, J. L.: Hematologic Problems in the Newborn. Philadelphia, W. B. Saunders Co., 1972.

Sell, E. J., and Corrigan, J. J., Jr.: Platelet counts, fibrinogen concentrations, and factor V and factor VIII levels in healthy infants according to gestational age. J. Pediatr. 82:1028, 1973.

Sherman, N. J., and Clatworthy, H. W., Jr.: Gastro-intestinal bleeding in neonates: A study of 94 cases. Surgery 62:614, 1967.

*Hemorrhagic Disease of the Newborn*

Aballi, A. J., and DeLamerens, S.: Coagulation changes in neonatal period and early infancy. Ped. Clin. North Am. 9:785, 1962.

Aballi, A. J., Lopez Banus, V., DeLamerens, S., and Rozengvaig, S.: Coagulation studies in the newborn period. I. Alterations of thromboplastin generation and effects of vitamin K on full-term and premature infants. Am. J. Dis. Child. 94:594, 1957.

Committee on Nutrition, American Academy of Pediatrics: Vitamin K compounds and the water-soluble analogues: Use in therapy and prophylaxis in pediatrics. Pediatrics 28:501, 1961.

Dam, H., Glavind, J., Larsen, H., and Plum, P.: Investigations into the cause of physiological hypoprothrombinemia in newborn children. IV. The vitamin K content of woman's milk and cow's milk. Acta Med. Scand. 112:210, 1942.

Fillmore, S. J., and McDevitt, E.: Effects of coumarin compounds on the fetus. Ann. Intern. Med. 73:731, 1970.

Gellis, S. S., and Lyon, R. A.: The influence of diet of the newborn infant on the prothrombin index. J. Pediatr. *19*:495, 1941.

Hilgartner, M. W., Solomon, G. E., and Kutt, H.: Diphenylhydantoin induced coagulation abnormalities. Pediatr. Res. *5*:408, 1971.

Hirsh, J., Cade, J. F., and O'Sullivan, E. F.: Clinical experience with anticoagulant therapy during pregnancy. Br. Med. J. *1*:270, 1970.

Lucey, J. F., and Dolan, R. G.: Hyperbilirubinemia of newborn infants associated with the parenteral administration of a vitamin K analogue to the mothers. Pediatrics *23*:553, 1959.

Mountain, K. R., Hirsh, J., and Gallus, A. S.: Neonatal coagulation defect due to anticonvulsant drug treatment in pregnancy. Lancet *1*:265, 1970.

Nammacher, M. A., Willemin, M., Hartmann, R. R., and Gaston, L. W.: Vitamin K deficiency in infants beyond the neonatal period. J. Pediatr. *76*:547, 1970.

Sanford, H. M., Gesteyer, T. H., and Wyat, L.: The substances involved in the coagulation of blood of the newborn. Am. J. Dis. Child. *43*:58, 1932.

Townsend, C. W.: The hemorrhagic disease of the newborn. Arch. Pediatr. *11*:559, 1894.

*Hereditary Clotting Factor Deficiencies*

Abildgaard, C. F.: Current concepts in the management of hemophilia. Semin. Hematol. *12*:223, 1975.

Baehner, R. L., and Strauss, H. S.: Hemophilia in the first year of life. N. Engl. J. Med. *275*:524, 1966.

Britten, A. F. H.: Congenital deficiency of factor XIII (fibrin-stabilizing factor). Am. J. Med. *43*:751, 1967.

Cade, J. F., Hirsh, J., and Martin, M.: Placental barrier to coagulation factors: Its relevance to the coagulation defect at birth and to haemorrhage in the newborn. Br. Med. J. *1*:281, 1969.

Donaldson, V. H., and Kisker, C. T.: Blood coagulation in hemostasis. *In* Nathan, D. G. and Oski, F. A. (Eds.): Hematology of Infancy and Childhood. Philadelphia, W. B. Saunders Co., 1974, pp. 561–610.

Hartmann, J. R., Howell, D. A., and Diamond, L. K.: Disorders of blood coagulation during the first weeks of life. A.M.A. J. Dis. Child. *90*:594, 1955.

Ratnoff, O. D.: The molecular basis of hereditary clotting disorders. *In* Spaet., T. (Ed.): Progress in Hemostasis and Thrombosis. Vol. 1. New York, Grune & Stratton, 1972, pp. 39–74.

Weiss, H. J.: Von Willebrand's disease. *In* Williams, W. J., et al. (eds.): Hematology. New York, McGraw-Hill Book Co., 1972.

*Intravascular Coagulation Syndromes*

Abildgaard, C. F.: Recognition and treatment of intravascular coagulation. J. Pediatr. *74*:163, 1969.

Altstatt, L. B., Dennis, L. H., Sundell, H., Malan, A., Harrison, V., Hedvall, G., Eichelberger, J., Fogel, B., and Stahlman, M.: Disseminated intravascular coagulation and hyaline membrane disease. Biol. Neonate *19*:227, 1971.

Chessells, J. M., and Wigglesworth, J. S.: Secondary haemorrhagic disease of the newborn. Arch. Dis. Child. *45*:539, 1970.

Chessells, J. M., and Wigglesworth, J. S.: Haemostatic failure in babies with rhesus isoimmunization. Arch. Dis. Child. *46*:38, 1971.

Chessells, J. M., and Wigglesworth, J. S.: Coagulation studies in preterm infants with respiratory distress and intracranial haemorrhage. Arch. Dis. Child. *47*:564, 1972.

Corrigan, J. J., and Jordan, C. M.: Heparin therapy in septicemia with disseminated intravascular coagulation. N. Engl. J. Med. *283*:778, 1970.

Deykin, D.: The clinical challenge of disseminated intravascular coagulation. N. Engl. J. Med. *283*:636, 1970.

Du, J. N. H., Briggs, J. N., and Young, G.: Disseminated intravascular coagulopathy in hyaline membrane disease: Massive thrombosis following umbilical artery catheterization. Pediatrics *45*:287, 1970.

Glaun, B. P., Weinberg, E. G., and Malan, A. F.: Peripheral gangrene in a newborn. Arch. Dis. Child. *46*:105, 1971.

Gross, S., and Melhorn, D. K.: Exchange transfusion with citrated whole blood for disseminated intravascular coagulation. J. Pediatr. *78*:415, 1971.

Hathaway, W. E., Mull, M. M., and Pechet, G. S.: Disseminated intravascular coagulation in the newborn. Pediatrics *43*:233, 1969.

Karpatkin, M., Sacker, I., and Ackerman, N.: Respiratory distress syndrome and disseminated intravascular coagulation in two siblings. Lancet *1*:102, 1972.

Lowry, M. F., Mann, J. R., Abrams, L. D., and Chance, G. W.: Thrombectomy for renal venous thrombosis in infant of diabetic mother. Br. Med. J. *3*:687, 1970.

Markarian, M., Cohen, R. J., and Milbauer, B.: Disseminated intravascular coagulation in a neonate treated with heparin. J. Pediatr. *78*:74, 1971.

Roberts, J. T., Davies, A. J., and Bloom, A. L.: Coagulation studies in massive pulmonary hemorrhage of the newborn. J. Clin. Pathol. *19*:334, 1966.

Rowe, S., and Avery, M. E.: Massive pulmonary hemorrhage in the newborn. II. Clinical considerations. J. Pediatr. *69*:12, 1966.

*Platelet Disorders*

Adner, M. M., Fisch, G. R., Starobin, S. G., and Aster, R. H.: Use of "compatible" platelet transfusions in treatment of congenital isoimmune thrombocytopenic purpura. N. Eng. J. Med. *280*:244, 1969.

Anthony, B., and Krivit, W.: Neonatal thrombocytopenic purpura. Pediatrics *30*:776, 1962.

Baldini, M.: Idiopathic thrombocytopenic purpura. N. Engl. J. Med. *274*:1245, 1302, 1360, 1966.

Bleyer, W. A., and Breckenridge, R. T.: Studies in the detection of adverse drug reactions in the newborn. II. The effects of prenatal aspirin on newborn hemostasis. J.A.M.A. *213*:2049, 1970.

Chessells, J. M., and Wigglesworth, J. S.: Haemostatic failure in babies with rhesus isoimmunization. Arch. Dis. Child. *46*:38, 1971.

Corby, D. G., and Schulman, I.: The effects of antenatal drug administration on aggregation of platelets of newborn infants. J. Pediatr. *79*:307, 1971.

Corrigan, J. J.: Thrombocytopenia: A laboratory sign of septicemia in infants and children. J. Pediatr. *85*:219, 1974.

Duncan, W., and Halnan, K. E.: Giant hemangioma with thrombocytopenia. Clin. Radiol. *15*:224, 1964.

Fost, N. C., and Esterly, N. B.: Successful treatment of juvenile hemangiomas with prednisone. J. Pediatr. *72*:351, 1968.

Goodhue, P. A., and Evans, T. S.: Idiopathic thrombocytopenic purpura in pregnancy. Obstet. Gynecol. Surg. *18*:671, 1963.

Hall, J. G., Levin, J., Kuhn, J. P., Ottenheimer, E. J., Van Berkum, K. A. P., and McKusick, V. A.: Thrombocytopenia with absent radius. Medicine 48:411, 1969.

Harrington, W. J., Sprague, C. C., Minnich, V., Moore, C. V., Aulvin, R. C., and Dubach, R.: Immunologic mechanisms in idiopathic and neonatal thrombocytopenic purpura. Ann. Int. Med. 38:433, 1953.

Kasabach, H. H., and Merritt, K. K.: Capillary hemangioma with extensive purpura. Report of a case. Am. J. Dis. Child. 59:1063, 1940.

Kontras, S. B., Green, O. C., King, L., and Duran, R. J.: Giant hemangioma with thrombocytopenia; case report with survival and sequestration studies of platelets labeled with chromium 51. Am. J. Dis. Child. 105:188, 1963.

Mauer, A. M., DeVaux, L. O., and Lahey, M. E.: Neonatal and maternal thrombocytopenic purpura due to quinine. Pediatrics 19:84, 1957.

McIntosh, S., O'Brien, R. T., Schwartz, A. D., and Pearson, H. A.: Neonatal isoimmune purpura: Response to platelet infusions. J. Pediatr. 82:1020, 1973.

Merenstein, G. B., O'Loughlin, E. P., and Plunket, D. C.: Effects of maternal thiazides on platelet counts of newborn infants. J. Pediatr. 76:766, 1970.

Nathan, D. J., and Snapper, I.: Simultaneous placental transfer of factors responsible for L.E. cell formation and thrombocytopenia. Am. J. Med. 25:647, 1958.

Pearson, H. A., Shulman, N. R., Marder, V. J., and Cone, T. E., Jr.: Isoimmune neonatal thrombocytopenic purpura. Clinical and therapeutic considerations. Blood 23:154, 1964.

Schulman, I.: Clinical Disorders of the Platelets. In Nathan, D. G., and Oski, F. A. (Eds.): Hematology of Infancy and Childhood. Philadelphia, W. B. Saunders Co., 1974, pp. 639–654.

Seip, M.: Systemic lupus erythematosus in pregnancy with haemolytic anaemia, leucopenia and thrombocytopenia in the mother and her newborn infant. Arch. Dis. Child. 35:364, 1960.

Shulman, N. R.: Immunoreactions involving platelets. I. A steric and kinetic model for formation of a complex from a human antibody, quinidine as a haptene, and platelets; and for fixation of complement by the complex. J. Exper. Med. 107:665, 1958.

Shulman, N. R., Marder, V. J., Hiller, M. C., and Collier, E. M.: Platelet and leukocyte isoantigens and their antibodies: Serologic, physiologic and clinical studies. Progr. Hematol. 4:222, 1964.

Stuart, M. J.: Inherited defects of platelet function. Semin. Hematol. 12:233, 1975.

# NEONATAL LEUKOCYTE DISORDERS

# 65

*By Bertil Glader*

Leukocytes have a central role in host defense against infection. The pathophysiology of lymphocyte disorders is discussed in the section on Immunology (Chapter 84). This chapter is mainly concerned with disorders of blood neutrophils. Many infants with granulocyte abnormalities have clinical problems in the newborn period. In most cases, however, the diagnosis of specific neutrophil disorders occurs after repeated infectious episodes, generally a few weeks to months after birth.

## NORMAL GRANULOCYTE PHYSIOLOGY

Development of myeloid cells into circulating neutrophils takes 6 to 10 days (Fig. 65–1). Approximately one-third of bone marrow myeloid cells are in some phase of cell division (blasts, promyelocytes, myelocytes), while the remaining, more differentiated cells (metamyelocytes, bands, mature granulocytes) are maintained in a storage pool. Myeloid cells continue to mature in this storage pool, although they can be released if needed in the periphery. After release from the bone marrow, neutrophils are equally distributed between circulating cells and granulocytes marginated on the vascular wall. The peripheral blood count measures only circulating cells. Granulocytes remain in the circulation for less than 24 hours before being mobilized into peripheral tissues. It is here that neutrophils begin their major function, phagocytosis of bacteria.

| COMPARTMENT | RELATIVE SIZE | TIME | FUNCTION |
|---|---|---|---|
| BONE MARROW | 20-30 | 6-10d | 1/3 PRODUCTION (BLASTS → MYELOCYTES)<br>2/3 STORAGE (METAMYELOCYTES → MATURE NEUTROPHILES) |
| ↓ VASCULAR | 1 | <1d | 1/2 CIRCULATING (MEASURED BY WBC COUNT)<br>1/2 MARGINATED ON VASCULAR WALL |
| ↓ TISSUE | ? | ? | PHAGOCYTOSIS |

*Figure 65–1.*    Neutrophil life cycle.

The term phagocytosis includes several independent but related processes: chemotaxis, opsonization, ingestion and intracellular killing (Fig. 65–2). *Chemotaxis* is the directed movement of neutrophils to areas of injury or bacterial infection. This is a metabolically dependent response of granulocytes to chemoattractants in peripheral tissues. Factors known to stimulate leukocyte migration include soluble bacterial products, complement components and antigen-antibody complexes. In vivo, chemotaxis is assessed by sequential observation of cell migration into an abraded area of skin pretreated with chemoattractants such as DPT or typhoid vaccine (Rebuck skin window). Under these conditions granulocytes initially appear within 3 to 6 hours, but by 12 hours monocytes predominate. In vitro, chemotaxis is evaluated by measuring the rate at which granulocytes traverse a filter that separates cells and chemotactically active material (Boyden chamber). This method is useful in determining what substances have chemotactic activity, but it is of questionable validity when used to compare chemotactic function of different granulocytes. Leukocyte migration through filters is a measure of several cell properties in addition to chemotactic responsiveness.

*Opsonization* is the process whereby bacteria are made more "edible" for phagocytes. The granulocyte ingestion of bacteria normally is a very slow process unless the bacterial membrane surface is first modified by various serum proteins. There are three fundamental modes of opsonization. 1) Increased concentrations of specific antibody alone rarely can prepare bacteria for ingestion. 2) More commonly, opsonization follows the reaction of small amounts of antibody with complement proteins. 3) Opsonization can also occur by bacterial complement fixation in the presence of properdin proteins. This properdin-dependent or "alternate" pathway is important, since it does not require antibody.

*Ingestion* is an active metabolic process in which the neutrophil membrane surrounds opsonized bacteria and forms an internalized vacuole or phagosome. This ingestion-related movement (as well as chemotaxis itself) is probably dependent

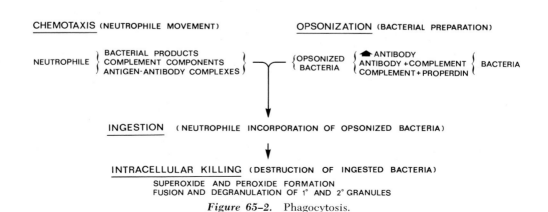

*Figure 65–2.*    Phagocytosis.

on contractile proteins. It has been suggested that reversible polymerization and depolymerization of neutrophil "actin" is responsible for this active motion.

*Intracellular killing* is the last stage of phagocytosis. One of the essential reactions in this process is the generation of superoxide and hydrogen peroxide in the area of the phagosome. The specificity and intracellular location of the enzyme responsible for this reaction are not definitely known. An equally important process is the fusion of neutrophilic granules with the phagosome, following which digestive enzymes are thrust upon the enclosed bacteria. Neutrophils contain two types of granules. Primary granules are first noted in young myeloid cells (promyelocytes), and contain several hydrolytic enzymes including myeloperoxidase. This enzyme potentiates the bactericidal effect of hydrogen peroxide. The secondary or specific granules develop in older cells (late myelocytes). These secondary lysosomal structures contain alkaline phosphatase in addition to other hydrolytic enzymes.

## GRANULOCYTE PHYSIOLOGY IN NEONATES

In older infants and children, the total and differential leukocyte count can be used to diagnose infection and distinguish between bacterial and viral processes. During the neonatal period, wide variations in the quantity and distribution of leukocytes limit the utility of these simple laboratory measurements. The total white blood cell (WBC) count shortly after birth ranges from 10,000 to 30,000 per $\mu$L, owing mainly to an increase in neutrophils, bands and metamyelocytes (Table 65–1). Occasionally, younger myeloid forms are seen also, particularly in premature infants. During the first week of life, the WBC count decreases (6000 to 15,000 per $\mu$L), immature myeloid cells disappear and neutrophils decrease to a level that equals the number of lymphocytes. In view of these marked changes, most physicians ignore neonatal WBC counts in the diagnosis of infection. Xanthou, however, has noted that the absolute neutrophil count (4000 to 7000 per $\mu$L) actually is quite stable in healthy infants after 72 hours of age. Furthermore, she observed that neonates with suspected or proved infection (after 3 days of age) manifested significant qualitative or quantitative neutrophil changes, or both. The absolute granulocyte count either was elevated above 7000/$\mu$L, or there was an increased number of circulating immature myeloid cells. Further studies are needed in order to determine if these observations can be of value in the diagnosis of neonatal sepsis. It has been found that the sedimentation rate often increases with neonatal infection, but this also needs further evaluation (Adler). Much has been written about the histochemical nitroblue tetrazolium dye reduction test as an indicator of bacterial infection in older children and infants. It is now clear that this test is nonspecific, and whether altered NBT reduction has clinical signifi-

**TABLE 65–1.** *Leukocyte Values in Term and Premature Infants ($10^3$ Cells/$\mu$L)*

| Age (hrs) | Total WBC | Neutrophils | Bands/Metas | Lymphocytes | Monocytes | Eosinophils |
|---|---|---|---|---|---|---|
| *Term infants* | | | | | | |
| 0 | 10.0–26.0 | 5.0–13.0 | 0.4–1.8 | 3.5–8.5 | 0.7–1.5 | 0.2–2.0 |
| 12 | 13.5–31.0 | 9.0–18.0 | 0.4–2.0 | 3.0–7.0 | 1.0–2.0 | 0.2–2.0 |
| 72 | 5.0–14.5 | 2.0–7.0 | 0.2–0.4 | 2.0–5.0 | 0.5–1.0 | 0.2–1.0 |
| 144 | 6.0–14.5 | 2.0–6.0 | 0.2–0.5 | 3.0–6.0 | 0.7–1.2 | 0.2–0.8 |
| *Premature infants* | | | | | | |
| 0 | 5.0–19.0 | 2.0–9.0 | 0.2–2.4 | 2.5–6.0 | 0.3–1.0 | 0.1–0.7 |
| 12 | 5.0–21.0 | 3.0–11.0 | 0.2–2.4 | 1.5–5.0 | 0.3–1.3 | 0.1–1.1 |
| 72 | 5.0–14.0 | 3.0–7.0 | 0.2–0.6 | 1.5–4.0 | 0.3–1.2 | 0.2–1.1 |
| 144 | 5.5–17.5 | 2.0–7.0 | 0.2–0.5 | 2.5–7.5 | 0.5–1.5 | 0.3–1.2 |

Data modified from Xanthou, Arch. Dis. Child., 45, 242–249, 1970.

cance on the presence or absence of infection is unclear. *In summary, the best criteria for the diagnosis of infection remains appropriate cultures and good clinical judgment, with a high index of suspicion.*

Each stage of phagocytosis has been examined in neonatal granulocytes. The in vivo movement of neutrophils to an area of inflammation is normal, although there is a delay in the subsequent appearance of mononuclear cells. The clinical significance of this is not known. In vitro studies (Boyden chamber) suggest that chemotaxis is decreased in neonatal granulocytes. For reasons discussed above, however, it is not clear whether this reflects abnormal chemotaxis or is merely a reflection of some other physical property regulating neonatal neutrophil movement. Decreased opsonic activity of neonatal serum is one phagocytic abnormality on which there is general agreement. This may be due to decreased IgM, low complement levels (C3) or defects in the properdin pathway. Approximately 15 per cent of neonates are severely deficient in certain properdin proteins (p. 769). Once bacteria are opsonized, neonatal granulocytes are capable of normal ingestion and intracellular killing.

## NEUTROPENIC DISORDERS

Neutropenia is defined as an absolute granulocyte count less than 1500 cells per $\mu$L. This may occur as a transient or chronic process. The general mechanisms of neutropenia are the same as those that produce anemia and thrombocytopenia: decreased production and increased destruction or utilization. Viral infections are the most common cause of transient neutropenia, presumably due to suppression of normal myeloid production. This form of neutropenia is of little consequence. Bone marrow aplasia or neoplasia also can present as neutropenia, and for this reason bone marrow examinations are mandatory in all noninfected children with unexplained persistent neutropenia. Formerly we thought that a paucity of bone marrow myeloid precursors characterized production defects while myeloid hyperplasia was seen in granulocytopenias due to increased

peripheral destruction. Unfortunately there are too many exceptions to this generalization, and we now consider the bone marrow as diagnostically useful, only in those neutropenias due to aplasia or neoplastic invasion.

The spectrum of clinical severity in neutropenic children is extremely variable. Most children have no clinical problems, some manifest frequent infections of moderate severity, and a few develop serious life-threatening infections. The difference between children with mild or severe disease is related to the capacity for neutrophils to be mobilized at sites of infection, and this probably is a function of the absolute neutrophil count. Severe infections are unusual with consistent mean granulocyte levels greater than 500 cells per $\mu$L. At lower neutrophil levels, however, the frequency and severity of infections increase dramatically. The degree of monocytosis may be important also, since these macrophages can partially compensate for the loss of neutrophil phagocytic function.

In the absence of infection no treatment for neutropenic children is indicated. Steroids have no role in the management of these disorders. If infection is present, however, vigorous antibiotic therapy with bactericidal drugs is indicated. In some children with severe neutropenia, and frequent life-threatening infections with one particular organism, prophylactic antibiotic therapy may be indicated. There are many inherent difficulties with this approach, but unfortunately there are few therapeutic alternatives for some of these

---

**TABLE 65–2.  *Diagnostic Evaluation of Infants with Persistent Neutropenia***

1. *Bone marrow examination*
     To rule out leukemia, neoplasm and aplastic anemia
2. *Maternal neutrophil counts*
     To rule out maternal disease or drugs
3. *Neutrophil counts on family members*
     To rule out hereditary neutropenia
4. *Anti-neutrophil antibody determination*
     To rule out immune neutropenia
5. *Repeat neutrophil counts on baby (2 times per week for 1 month)*
     To rule out cyclic neutropenia

children. Granulocyte transfusions are effective in sepsis associated with leukemia and aplastic anemia, but have not yet been systematically used in neonatal sepsis. The remainder of this section summarizes the more common neutropenic syndromes.

## ISOIMMUNE NEUTROPENIA

This disorder is the neutrophil equivalent of isoimmune thrombocytopenia and isoimmune anemia (ABO and Rh incompatibility). Fetal granulocytes possess an antigen not present on maternal neutrophils and maternal sensitization results in antibody production against fetal granulocytes. Maternal neutrophils are not affected. The measurement of neutrophil antibodies is more difficult than the detection of antibodies in other isoimmune disorders. Consequently these assays are done only in specialized laboratories. The clinical significance of anti-granulocyte antibodies is not completely understood, since 20 to 25 per cent of all multiparous women have anti-neutrophil antibodies, yet neutropenia rarely is seen in these infants. The prognosis for infants with isoimmune neutropenia is very good, and severe infections are unusual. The granulocytopenia resolves as soon as the infant clears maternal antibody (6 to 12 weeks). An increase in the neutrophil count after this period of time also helps differentiate this isoimmune disorder from other nonimmune causes of neutropenia.

## NEUTROPENIA ASSOCIATED WITH MATERNAL DISEASE

Antibodies that cause maternal neutropenia may passively cross the placenta and secondarily injure fetal granulocytes. Rare cases of maternal idiopathic neutropenia have been associated with neonatal granulocytopenia. Similarly, maternal lupus erythematosus has been implicated as a cause of immune neonatal neutropenia. In association with maternal systemic disease, however, anemia and thrombocytopenia frequently are present, and usually are more important than any coexistent neutropenia.

## IDIOPATHIC CONGENITAL NEUTROPENIA

This diverse group includes a number of poorly understood granulocytopenias that can occur as isolated entities or associated with other abnormalities. The most severe syndrome in this group is *congenital agranulocytosis*. Clinically this profound neutropenia is characterized by the neonatal onset of fulminant infections and early death. The bone marrow manifests marked myeloid hypoplasia, although rarely there are adequate early myeloid precursors. Some cases are familial. A rare and unusual variant of this disorder is known as *reticular dysgenesis*. Infants with this syndrome have no circulating neutrophils or lymphocytes. Similarly, the bone marrow contains no myeloid or lymphoid elements. All children reported with reticular dysgenesis have died within the first few weeks of life. Thymic atrophy and lymphocyte depletion of lymph nodes have been noted on autopsy.

In contrast to these severe idiopathic neutropenias, there is a large group of infants and children with benign granulocytopenia. These disorders are benign in that infections are not life-threatening and some children may be completely asymptomatic. Rarely do these children have serious neonatal infections. In most cases, the bone marrow contains myeloid precursors, and the granulocytopenia is not as low as in the severe syndromes. Chronic granulocytopenia may be the only abnormality, or there may be additional clinical features: pancreatic insufficiency, inborn errors of metabolism or immunoglobulin abnormalities. *Cyclic neutropenia* is another variant, characterized by a fluctuating granulocyte count that cycles every 21 days. At the nadir of this neutropenia, there frequently is an increased incidence of fevers and mild infections (stomatitis, gingivitis).

## NEUTROPENIA SECONDARY TO DRUGS

Many drugs have been implicated in the etiology of neutropenia. Phenothiazines, antithyroid medications and certain antibiotics (chloramphenicol, sulfonamides) have gained the most notoriety. A current up-to-date list of drugs associated with neutropenia can be obtained from the Registry on

Blood Dyscrasias of the Council on Drugs of the American Medical Association. Drugs should be considered in the etiology of any obscure neutropenia.

### NEUTROPENIA DUE TO LEUKEMIA AND OTHER NEOPLASMS

Neutropenia in these conditions is secondary to invasion and destruction of normal bone marrow elements. In contrast to that in adults, chronic neutropenia in children rarely converts to leukemia.

# DISORDERS OF LEUKOCYTE FUNCTION

Recurrent bacterial infections can occur in the presence of adequate numbers of circulating and bone marrow neutrophils. Most commonly, these infections are due to decreased serum opsonic activity caused by a lack of specific antibody (i.e., hypogammaglobulinemic states). Occasionally, abnormal granulocyte function itself is responsible. The diagnosis of neutrophil dysfunction syndromes rarely is made in the newborn period, although these infants frequently are infected. Some of these functional disorders are outlined below.

### LAZY LEUKOCYTE SYNDROME

This rare condition is characterized by recurrent fevers, frequent mild infections and neutropenia. In contrast to most other neutropenias, however, the bone marrow contains normal numbers of all myeloid cells. The main functional defect in this disorder thus may be due to abnormal membrane deformability, which limits granulocyte release from the bone marrow. This is supported by the observation that neutrophils released into the circulation do not migrate normally in response to chemotactic stimulants in vitro (Boyden chamber). Serum opsonic activity, neutrophil ingestion and intracellular killing are normal. The prognosis for children with this disorder is good.

### NEUTROPHIL MUSCULAR DYSTROPHY

Another neutrophil mobility defect recently has been described (Boxer, Hedley-Whyte, and Stossel).

CASE 65–1

A 5-month-old male infant with recurrent infections of the skin, abdominal wall and gastrointestinal tract was admitted to the Childrens Hospital Medical Center. The infant's total leukocyte count was elevated (17,000–133,000), and most of the cells were mature granulocytes. In spite of marked neutrophilia, pus never formed at sites of infection. Biopsies of infected areas contained necrotic tissue, histiocytes and lymphocytes, but no granulocytes. It was of particular interest that pus was formed following therapeutic granulocyte transfusions. Neutrophil chemotaxis was abnormal in vitro (Boyden chamber) and in vivo (Rebuck skin window). Granulocyte ingestion also was abnormal. The other stages of phagocytosis were intact. The child's clinical condition deteriorated in spite of vigorous antibiotic therapy and granulocyte transfusions. A bone marrow transplant was attempted, but was unsuccessful, and the patient died.

COMMENT. The unique motility defect in these granulocytes was attributed to an abnormality of neutrophil actin. The cell content of actin was normal, but the protein was qualitatively abnormal in that it manifested poor polymerization in vitro. As stated in the section on neutrophil physiology, reversible polymerization of actin is probably responsible for granulocyte movement associated with chemotaxis and ingestion.

### CHRONIC GRANULOMATOUS DISEASE (CGD)

This rare hereditary disorder is characterized by recurrent granulomatous infections involving lymph nodes, skin, viscera and bones. After the first few months of age hepatosplenomegaly is present. The peripheral blood neutrophil count and bone marrow are entirely normal. Chemotaxis is normal, ingestion is intact, and there are no opsonic defects. The fundamental abnormality in this condition is an inability of neutrophils to kill certain ingested bacteria

(Holmes, Page and Good). Pathologically, the persistence of viable intracellular bacteria stimulates granulomata formation in tissues to which neutrophils are transported. The molecular basis for decreased intracellular killing is not completely understood, although it is related to reduced hydrogen peroxide production in the phagosome. When CGD granulocytes ingest latex particles coated with an enzyme which generates peroxide, the intracellular killing defect is corrected. This finding partially explains the spectrum of clinical infections in children with CGD. Severe problems commonly are due to staphylococcus aureus, although infections also occur with Klebsiella, E. coli, Serratia marcescens, and Candida albicans. Each of these microorganisms contains catalase, an enzyme potentially capable of destroying whatever small amounts of peroxide are formed in the phagosome. Infections with organisms lacking catalase are not a clinical problem; presumably the trivial amount of peroxide present in CGD neutrophils is bactericidal for these agents. CGD is diagnosed by observing granulocyte inability to kill catalase-positive organisms or by failure of NBT reduction in circulating neutrophils. NBT dye reduction correlates with intracellular peroxide formation, and thus the diagnosis of CGD is one situation in which this screening test is useful. The clinical course of children with CGD is quite variable. No specific therapy is available to correct the intracellular lesion. In view of the predominance of staphylococcal infections, however, our patients currently are maintained on prophylactic dicloxacillin. There is no controlled datum to evaluate the efficacy of this therapy, but it is our impression that the frequency and intensity of infections is less. Chronic granulomatous disease is classically a sex-linked disorder affecting male children, although some cases may be autosomal recessive. In accord with the Lyon hypothesis, female carriers have both normal and abnormal neutrophils, and this is seen most clearly when the NBT slide test is performed. Clinically, female CGD carriers manifest no increased evidence of infection.

## CHEDIAK-HIGASHI SYNDROME

This autosomal recessive disorder is characterized by oculocutaneous albinism, photophobia and recurrent infections. During the course of disease hepatosplenomegaly also develops. Most patients ultimately die from infection, although death is occasionally due to a lymphoma-like illness. Thrombocytopenia is frequently present. Anemia is rare. The total white blood cell count can be normal, but neutropenia is common in severe cases. The pathognomonic laboratory finding is the presence of large granules in granulocytes and lymphocytes. Within neutrophils, these giant lysosomal structures contain peroxidase activity, and thus represent abnormal primary granules. It has been observed that these giant lysosomes fail to degranulate their contents into phagocytic vacuoles at a normal rate, and intracellular killing of certain bacteria also is abnormal. In spite of these interesting findings, however, increased susceptibility to infections is correlated best with the degree of neutropenia. The relationship of granule abnormalities to rare malignant transformation is unknown.

## REFERENCES

*Normal Granulocyte Physiology*

Athens, J. W., Raab, S. O., Haab, O. P., Mauer, A. M., Ashenbrucker, H., Cartwright, G. E., and Wintrobe, M. M.: Leukokinetic studies. III. The distribution of granulocytes in the blood of normal subjects. J. Clin. Invest. *40*:159, 1961.

Boggs, D. R.: The kinetics of neutrophilic leukocytes in health and disease. Semin. Hematol. *4*:359, 1967.

Klebanoff, S. J.: Antimicrobial mechanisms in neutrophilic polymorphonuclear leukocytes. Semin. Hematol. *12*:117, 1975.

Keller, H. U., Hess, M. W., and Cotlier, H.: Physiology of chemotaxis and random motility. Semin. Hematol. *12*:47, 1975.

Rebuck, J. W., and Crowley, J. H.: A method of studying leukocyte function in vivo. Ann. N.Y. Acad. Sci. *59*:757, 1951.

Stossel, T. P.: Phagocytosis. N. Eng. J. Med. *290*:717, 1974.

*Granulocyte Physiology in Neonates*

Adler, S. M., and Denton, R. L.: Erythrocyte sedimentation rate in the newborn period. J. Pediatr. *86*:942, 1975.

Gregory, J., and Hey, E.: Blood neutrophil response to

bacterial infection in the first month of life. Arch. Dis. Child. *47*:747, 1972.

Miller, M. E.: Chemotactic function in the human neonate: Humoral and cellular aspects. Pediat. Res. *5*:492, 1971.

Miller, M. E.: Phagocytosis in the newborn infant: Humoral and cellular factors. J. Pediatr. *74*:255, 1969.

Nathan, D. G.: NBT reduction by human phagocytes. N. Engl. J. Med. *290*:280, 1974.

Steigbigel, R. T., Johnson, P. K., and Remmington, J. S.: The nitroblue tetrazolium reduction test versus conventional hematology in the diagnosis of bacterial infection. N. Engl. J. Med. *290*:235, 1974.

Xanthou, M.: Leukocyte blood picture in healthy full-term and premature babies during neonatal period. Arch. Dis. Child. *45*:242, 1970.

Xanthou, M., Tsomides, K., Nicolopoulos, D., and Matsaniotis, N.: Leukocyte blood picture in newborn babies during and after exchange transfusion. Pediat. Res. *6*:59, 1972.

*Neutropenic Disorders*

Ackerman, B. D.: Dysgammaglobulinemia: Report of a case with a family history of a congenital gamma globulin disorder. Pediatrics *34*:211, 1964.

de Vaal, O. M., and Seynhaeve, V.: Reticular dysgenesia. Lancet *2*:1123, 1959.

Gitlin, D., Vawter, G., and Craig, J. M.: Thymic alymphoplasia and congenital aleukocytosis. Pediatrics *33*:184, 1964.

Good, R. A., and Zak, S. J.: Disturbances in gamma globulin synthesis as "experiments of nature." Pediatrics *18*:109, 1956.

Hanson, J. W., and Smith, D. W.: The fetal hydantoin syndrome. J. Pediatr. *87*:285, 1975.

Huguley, C. M., Jr.: Drug-induced blood dyscrasias. II. Agranulocytosis. J.A.M.A. *188*:817, 1964.

Kauder, E., and Mauer, A. M.: Neutropenias of childhood. J. Pediatr. *69*:147, 1966.

Kostmann, R.: Infantile genetic agranulocytosis (agranulocytosis infantilis hereditaria). A new recessive lethal disease in man. Acta Paediat. (Suppl. 105) *45*:1, 1956.

Lalezari, P., Nussbaum, M., Gelman, S., and Spaet, T. H.: Neonatal neutropenia due to maternal isoimmunization. Blood *15*:236, 1960.

Page, A. R., and Good, R. A.: Studies on cyclic neutropenia. A clinical and experimental investigation. A.M.A. J. Dis. Child. *94*:623, 1957.

Payne, R.: Neonatal neutropenia and leukoagglutinins. Pediatrics *33*:194, 1964.

Shwachman, H., Diamond, L. K., Oski, F. A., and Khaw, K-T.: The syndrome of pancreatic insufficiency and bone marrow dysfunction. J. Pediatr. *65*:645, 1964.

*Disorders of Leukocyte Function*

Baehner, R. L., and Johnston, R. B., Jr.: Chronic granulomatous disease: Correlation between pathogenesis and clinical findings. Pediatrics *48*:730, 1971.

Baehner, R. L., Nathan, D. G., and Karnovsky, M. L.: Correction of the metabolic deficiencies in the leukocytes of patients with chronic granulomatous disease. J. Clin. Invest. *49*:860, 1970.

Blume, R. S., and Wolff, S. M.: The Chediak-Higashi syndrome: Studies in four patients and a review of the literature. Medicine *51*:247, 1972.

Boxer, L. A., Hedley-Whyte, E. T., and Stossel, T. P.: Neutrophil actin dysfunction and abnormal neutrophil behavior. N. Engl. J. Med. *291*:1093, 1974.

Holmes, B., Page, A. R., and Good, R. A.: Studies of the metabolic activity of leukocytes from patients with a genetic abnormality of phagocyte function. J. Clin. Invest. *46*:1422, 1967.

Johnston, R. B., Jr., and Baehner, R. L.: Improvement of leukocyte bactericidal activity in chronic granulomatous disease. J. Clin. Invest. *49*:860, 1970.

Klebanoff, S. J.: Intraleukocytic microbicidal defects. Ann. Rev. Med. *22*:39, 1971.

Miller, M. E.: Pathology of chemotaxis and random mobility. Semin. Hematol. *12*:59, 1975.

Miller, M. E., Oski, F. A., and Harris, H. B.: Lazy-leukocyte syndrome. A new disorder of neutrophil function. Lancet *1*:665, 1971.

Quie, P. G.: Pathology of bactericidal power of neutrophils. Semin. Hematol. *12*:143, 1975.

# 66 ERYTHROCYTE DISORDERS IN INFANCY

*By Bertil Glader*

## NORMAL ERYTHROCYTE PHYSIOLOGY IN THE FETUS AND NEONATE

### FETAL ERYTHROPOIESIS

Fetal erythropoiesis occurs in three different sites: yolk sac, liver and bone marrow. Yolk sac formation of RBC's is maximal between the second and tenth weeks of gestation. The liver is a major site of erythropoiesis between the tenth and twenty-sixth weeks of gestation. Myeloid or bone marrow production of red blood cells begins around the eighteenth week, and by the thirtieth week of fetal life, bone marrow is the major erythropoietic organ. At birth, almost all RBC's are produced in the bone marrow, although a low level of hepatic erythropoiesis persists through the first few days of life. Sites of fetal erythropoiesis are occasionally reactivated in older patients with hematologic disorders such as myelofibrosis, aplastic anemia or severe hemolytic anemia.

Red blood cell production in extrauterine life is controlled in part by erythropoietin, a humoral erythropoietic stimulating factor (ESF) produced by the kidney. The role of erythropoietin in the developing fetus has not been completely defined. Current thoughts are that ESF does not influence yolk sac or hepatic erythropoiesis, but it may partially regulate myeloid RBC production (Finne and Halvorsen). Erythropoietic stimulating factor is detected in fetal blood and amniotic fluid during the last trimester of pregnancy. The concentration of this hormone increases directly with the period of gestation, and thus, erythropoietin levels in term neonates are significantly higher than in premature infants. This difference may reflect some degree of fetal hypoxia during late intrauterine life. Increased ESF titers also are seen in placental dysfunction, fetal anemia and maternal hypoxia (Finne). Fetal RBC formation is not influenced by maternal erythropoietin, since transfusion-induced maternal polycythemia (decreased maternal ESF levels) has no effect on fetal erythropoiesis (Jacobson, Marks and Gaston). Maternal nutritional status also is not a significant factor in the regulation of fetal erythropoiesis, since iron, folate and vitamin $B_{12}$ are trapped by the fetus irrespective of maternal stores. Most studies have demonstrated that women with severe iron deficiency bear children with normal total body hemoglobin content (Lanzkowsky).

Hemoglobin, hematocrit and RBC count increase throughout fetal life (Table 66–1). Extremely large RBC's (MCV 180) with an increased hemoglobin content (MCH 60) are produced early in fetal life. The size and hemoglobin content of these cells decrease throughout gestation, but the concentration of hemoglobin (MCHC) does not change significantly. Even at birth, the MCV and MCH are larger than those seen in older children and adults. Many nucleated RBC's and reticulocytes are present early in gestation, and the percentage of these cells also decreases as the fetus ages.

Hemoglobin production increases markedly during the last trimester of pregnancy. The actual hemoglobin concentration increases, but more importantly, body weight, blood volume and total body hemoglobin triple in size during this period. Fetal iron accumulation parallels the increase in total body hemoglobin content. The neonatal iron endowment at birth, therefore, is directly related to total body hemoglobin content and length of gestation. Term infants have more iron than prematures.

## RBC Physiology at Birth

In utero, fetal blood (umbilical vein) is approximately 50 per cent saturated with oxygen. This relative hypoxia may be responsible for the increased content of erythropoietin and signs of active erythropoiesis (nucleated RBC's, increased reticu-

### TABLE 66–1. *Mean Erythrocyte Values During Gestation*

| Age (weeks) | Hemoglobin (gm/100 ml) | RBC (cells/ul) | MCV ($\mu^3$) | MCH ($\gamma\gamma$) | MCHC (%) | Nucleated RBC's (% of RBC's) | Reticulocytes (% of RBC's) |
|---|---|---|---|---|---|---|---|
| 12 | 9.0 | 1.5 | 180 | 60 | 34 | 6.5 | 40 |
| 16 | 10.0 | 2.0 | 140 | 45 | 33 | 3.0 | 18 |
| 20 | 11.0 | 2.5 | 135 | 44 | 33 | 1.0 | 15 |
| 24 | 14.0 | 3.5 | 123 | 38 | 31 | 1.0 | 7 |
| 28 | 14.5 | 4.0 | 120 | 40 | 31 | 0.5 | 7 |
| 34 | 15.0 | 4.4 | 118 | 38 | 32 | 0.2 | 6 |
| 40 | 17.0 | 5.1 | 110 | 34 | 31 | 0.1 | 5 |

(Data from Oski, F. A., and Naiman, J. L.: Hematologic Problems in the Newborn, W. B. Saunders Company, 1972.)

locytes) seen in neonates at birth. When lungs become the source of oxygen, hemoglobin-$O_2$ saturation increases to 95 per cent, and erythropoiesis decreases. Within 72 hours of age, erythropoietin is undetectable, nucleated RBC's disappear and reticulocytes decrease to less than 1 per cent.

The concentration of hemoglobin during the first few hours of life increases to values greater than those seen in cord blood. This is a relative increase due to a reduction in plasma volume (Gairdner et al.) and an absolute increase due to placental blood transfusion (Usher, Shepard and Lind). The umbilical vein remains patent long after umbilical arteries have constricted, and thus transfusion of placental blood occurs when neonates are held at a level below the placenta. The placenta contains approximately 100 ml of fetal blood (30 per cent of the infant's blood volume). Approximately 25 per cent of placental blood enters the neonate within 15 seconds of birth, and by 1 minute, 50 per cent is transfused. The time of cord clamping is thus a direct determinant of neonatal blood volume. The blood volume of term infants (mean of 85 ml per kg) varies considerably (50 to 100 ml per kg) because of different degrees of placental transfusion (Usher, Shepard and Lind). These differences are readily apparent when the effects of early versus delayed cord clamping are compared at 72 hours of age: 82.3 ml per kg (early clamping) versus 92.6 ml per kg (delayed clamping). These changes are largely due to differences in RBC mass (early clamping 31 ml per kg, delayed clamping 49 ml per kg). The blood volume of premature infants (89 to 105 ml per kg) is slightly greater than that of term infants, but in large part this is due to an increased plasma volume (Usher and Lind). The RBC mass of premature infants is the same as in term neonates.

## FETAL AND NEONATAL HEMOGLOBIN FUNCTION

A variety of different hemoglobins are present during fetal and neonatal life (see discussion under Hemoglobinopathies). Fetal hemoglobin (Hgb F) is the major hemoglobin in utero, while hemoglobin A is the normal hemoglobin of extrauterine life. Both are present in the same cell, but the relative proportion of each varies with gestational and postnatal age. One major difference between hemoglobins A and F is related to oxygen transport.

The transport of oxygen to peripheral tissues is regulated by several factors including blood oxygen capacity, cardiac output and hemoglobin-oxygen affinity. 1) Oxygen capacity is a direct function of hemoglobin concentration (1 gm hemoglobin combines with 1.34 ml oxygen). 2) Compensatory changes in cardiac output can maintain normal $O_2$ delivery under conditions in which oxygen capacity is significantly reduced. 3) The oxygen affinity of hemoglobin also influences oxygen delivery to tissues. Hemoglobin A is 95 per cent saturated at arterial oxygen tensions (100 mm Hg), but this decreases to 70 to 75 per cent saturation at a venous $P_{O_2}$ of 40 mm Hg. The difference in $O_2$ content at arterial and venous oxygen tensions reflects the amount of oxygen that can be released. Changes in hemoglobin affinity for oxygen can influence $O_2$ delivery (Fig. 66–1). At any given $P_{O_2}$, more oxygen is bound to hemoglobin when oxygen affinity is increased. Stated in physiologic terms, increased hemoglobin-oxygen affinity reduces oxygen delivery, while decreased hemoglobin-oxygen affinity increases oxygen release to peripheral tissues.

The oxygen affinity of hemoglobin A in solution is greater than that for hemoglobin F. Paradoxically, however, whole blood from normal children (Hgb A) has a lower oxygen affinity than neonatal blood (Hgb F) (Allen, Wyman and Smith). This difference is related to an intermediate of RBC metabolism known as 2,3-diphosphoglycerate (2,3-DPG). This organic phosphate compound interacts with hemoglobin A to decrease its affinity for oxygen, and thereby enhance $O_2$ release. Fetal hemoglobin does not interact with 2,3-DPG to any significant extent (Bauer, Ludwig and Ludwig); consequently, cells containing hemoglobin F have a higher oxygen affinity than those containing hemoglobin A.

The increased oxygen affinity of fetal RBC's is obviously advantageous for extracting oxygen from maternal blood within

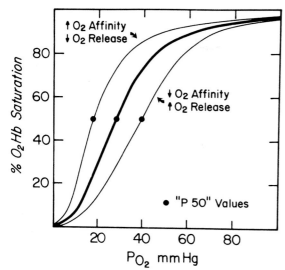

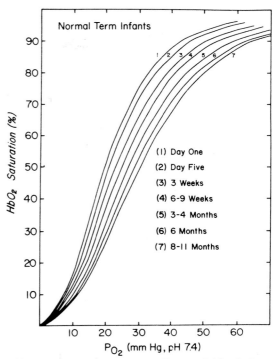

**Figure 66–1.** The oxygen dissociation curve of normal adult hemoglobin (dark line). The per cent oxygen saturation (ordinate) is plotted for arterial oxygen tensions between 0 and 100 mm Hg (abscissa). As the curve shifts to the right, more oxygen is released at any given $P_{O_2}$. Conversely, as the curve shifts to the left, more oxygen is retained on hemoglobin at any given $P_{O_2}$. The "P 50" refers to that $P_{O_2}$ where hemoglobin is 50 per cent saturated with oxygen. This term is useful in comparing the oxygen affinity of different hemoglobins. (Oski, F. A., and Delivoria-Papadopoulos, M.: J. Pediatr. 77:941, 1970.)

**Figure 66–2.** The oxygen affinity of blood from term infants at birth and at different postnatal ages. The gradual rightward shift of the oxygen saturation curve indicates increased oxygen release from hemoglobin as infants get older. This decreased oxygen affinity is due to a decrease in hemoglobin F and an increase in hemoglobin A. (Oski, F. A., and Delivoria-Papadopoulos, M.: J. Pediatr. 77:941, 1970.)

the placenta. A few months after birth, however, infant blood acquires the same oxygen affinity as that of older children (Fig. 66–2). The postnatal decrease in $O_2$ affinity is due to a reduction in hemoglobin F and an increase in hemoglobin A (which interacts with 2,3-DPG). It is an interesting fact that oxygen delivery (the difference in arterial and venous $O_2$ content) actually increases while oxygen capacity (hemoglobin concentration) decreases during the first weeks of life (Fig. 66–3). This enhanced delivery is largely a reflection of the decreased oxygen affinity of infant blood (Delivoria-Papadopoulos and coworkers). The oxygen affinity of blood from premature infants is higher than that of term infants, and the normal postnatal changes (decrease in oxygen affinity, increase in oxygen delivery) occur much more gradually in prematures (Fig. 66–3).

## GENERAL APPROACH TO ANEMIC INFANTS

**MEDICAL HISTORY AND PHYSICAL EXAMINATION.** The etiology of anemia frequently can be ascertained by medical history and physical examination. Particular importance is given to family history (anemia, cholelithiasis, unexplained jaundice, splenomegaly), maternal medical history (especially infections) and obstetrical history (previous pregnancies, length of gestation, method and difficulty of delivery). The age at which anemia becomes manifest also is of diagnostic importance. Significant anemia at birth invariably is due to blood loss or isoimmune hemolysis. After 24 hours, internal hemorrhages and other

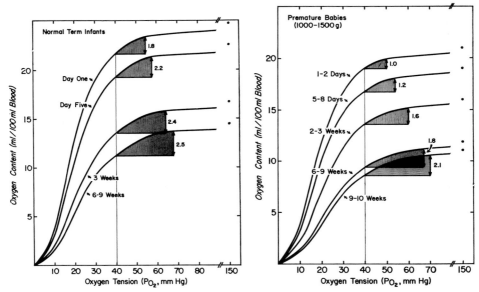

**Figure 66–3.**   Oxygen delivery in normal term and premature infants. Oxygen content (a function of total hemoglobin) is on the ordinate. Oxygen tension is on the abscissa. Oxygen delivery is measured by the difference in oxygen content at arterial (100 mm Hg) and venous (40 mm Hg) oxygen tensions. For both term and premature infants, oxygen delivery (shaded areas) increases with age. This occurs in spite of a decrease in oxygen content. (Delivoria-Papadopoulos, M., Roncevic, N. P., and Oski, F. A.: Pediatr. Res. 5:235, 1971.)

causes of hemolysis become manifest. Anemia that appears several weeks after birth can be caused by a variety of conditions including abnormalities in the synthesis of hemoglobin-beta chains, hypoplastic RBC disorders and the physiologic anemia of infancy or prematurity.

Infants with chronic blood loss anemia may appear pale, without other evidence of clinical distress. Acute blood loss can produce hypovolemic shock and a clinical state similar to severe neonatal asphyxia. Neonates with hemolytic anemia frequently show a greater than expected degree of icterus. In addition, hemolysis often is associated with hepatosplenomegaly, and in cases due to congenital infection other stigmata may be present.

**LABORATORY EVALUATION OF ANEMIA.** A simple classification of neonatal anemia based on physical examination and simple laboratory tests is presented in Table 66–2.

RBC COUNT, HEMOGLOBIN, HEMATOCRIT AND RBC INDICES.   Red blood cell values during the neonatal period are more variable than at any other time of life. The diagnosis of anemia must therefore be made in terms of "normal" values appropriate for an infant's gestational and postnatal age. The mean cord blood hemoglobin of healthy term infants ranges between 14 and 20 gm per 100 ml (Table 66–3). Shortly after birth, however, hemoglobin concentration increases. This increase is both relative (owing to a reduction of plasma volume) and absolute (owing to placental RBC transfusion). Failure of hemoglobin to increase during the first few hours of life may be the initial sign of hemorrhagic anemia. RBC values at the end of the first week are virtually identical to those seen at birth. Anemia during the first week of life is thus defined as any hemoglobin less than 14 gm per 100 ml. A significant hemoglobin decrease during this time, although within the normal range, is suspicious of hemorrhage or hemolysis. For example, a 14.5 gm hemoglobin at 7 days of age is abnormal for a term infant whose hemoglobin was 18.5 gm at birth. A slight hemoglobin reduction

TABLE 66–2. *Differential Approach to Anemia in Newborn Period*

| Hemoglobin | Reticulocytes | Bilirubin | Coombs Test | Clinical Considerations |
|---|---|---|---|---|
| Decreased | Normal/decreased | Normal | Negative | Physiologic anemia of infancy/prematurity Hypoplastic anemia |
| Decreased | Normal/increased | Normal | Negative | Hemorrhagic anemia |
| Decreased | Normal/increased | Increased | Positive | Immune-mediated hemolysis |
| Decreased | Normal/increased | Increased | Negative | Acquired or hereditary RBC defects Enclosed hemorrhage with resorption of blood Coombs negative ABO incompatibility |

normally occurs in premature infants during the first week. Beyond the first week, however, the hemoglobin concentration decreases in both term and premature infants (see Physiologic Anemia of Infancy and Prematurity).

The electronic equipment currently used for blood counts also gives statistical information regarding erythrocyte size (mean corpuscular volume [MCV]) and hemoglobin content (mean corpuscular hemoglobin [MCH]). The normal MCV ($\mu\mu$) in older children ranges from 85 to 95. Mean corpuscular volumes less than 80 are considered microcytic, while those over 100 indicate macrocytosis. Normal infant RBC's are large (MCV 105 to 125), and not until 8 to 10 weeks of age does cell size approach that of older children. Neonatal microcytosis is defined as an MCV less than 95 at

birth. The RBC hemoglobin content of neonatal cells (MCH 35 to 38) is greater than that seen in older children (MCH 30 to 33). Neonatal hypochromia is defined as an MCH less than 34. Hypochromia and microcytosis generally occur together, and invariably these abnormalities are due to hemoglobin production defects. Neonatal hypochromic microcytosis is seen with iron deficiency (chronic blood loss, late anemia of prematurity) and thalassemia disorders (alpha and gamma thalassemias).

The site at which blood is obtained is important, since peripheral stasis leads to higher hemoglobin concentrations in capillary blood compared to simultaneously obtained central venous samples. This difference can be minimized by warming an extremity to obtain "arteriolized capillary blood" (Oh and Lind). In the face of acute

TABLE 66–3. *RBC Values in Term and Premature Infants During First Week of Life*

| | Hgb (gm/100 ml) | Hct (%) | Reticulocytes (%) | Nucleated RBC's (cells/1000 RBC's) |
|---|---|---|---|---|
| *Term* | | | | |
| Cord blood | 17.0 (14–20) | 53.0 (45–61) | <7% | <1.00 |
| Day 1 | 18.4 | 58.0 | <7% | <0.40 |
| Day 3 | 17.8 | 55.0 | <3% | <0.01 |
| Day 7 | 17.0 | 54.0 | <1% | 0 |
| *Premature (less than 1500 gm)* | | | | |
| Cord blood | 16.0 (13.0–18.5) | 49 | <10% | <3.00 |
| Day 7 | 14.8 | 45 | <3% | <0.01 |

hemorrhage, however, central venous samples must be obtained because of marked peripheral vasoconstriction.

RETICULOCYTE COUNT. The normal reticulocyte count of children and older infants is 1 to 2 per cent. The reticulocyte count in term infants ranges between 3 to 7 per cent at birth, but this decreases to 1 to 3 per cent by 4 days and to less than 1 per cent by 7 days of age (Table 66–3). In prematures, reticulocyte values at birth are higher (6 to 10 per cent), and may remain elevated for a longer period of time. Nucleated red blood cells are seen in newborn infants, but they generally disappear by the third day of life in term infants, and in 7 to 10 days in premature infants. The persistence of reticulocytosis or nucleated RBC's suggests the possibility of hemorrhage or hemolysis. Hypoxia, in the absence of anemia, also can be associated with increased release of reticulocytes and nucleated RBC's.

PERIPHERAL BLOOD SMEAR. Examination of the peripheral blood smear is an invaluable aid in the diagnosis of anemia. In particular, the smear is evaluated for alterations in the size and shape of RBC's as well as abnormalities in leukocytes and platelets. Erythrocytes of older children are approximately the size of a small lymphocyte nucleus, while those of neonates are slightly larger. Red blood cell hemoglobinization (e.g., hypochromia) is estimated by observing the area of central pallor, which is one third the diameter of normal RBC's, and over one half the diameter of hypochromic cells. Spherocytes are detected by the complete absence of central pallor. The degree of reticulocytosis can be estimated, since these cells are larger and have a bluish coloration (due to RNA) when viewed in the blood smear. In order to obtain good peripheral smears in neonates, high hematocrit blood should be diluted (1:1) in saline.

SERUM BILIRUBIN. Bilirubin is a normal breakdown product of hemoglobin (Chapter 69). In cases of hemolytic anemia (increased RBC destruction) bilirubin levels are increased to above normal neonatal levels. Hyperbilirubinemia is not seen with anemia caused by external hemorrhage, although resorption of blood from large enclosed hemorrhages can produce icterus.

HAPTOGLOBIN. This glycoprotein binds free hemoglobin, and the hemoglobin-haptoglobin complex is cleared from the circulation. Decreased serum haptoglobin is a sign of hemolysis in older children, but it is not a useful measurement in neonates, since haptoglobin is normally decreased at this time of life.

COOMBS TEST. The vast majority of neonatal hemolytic anemias are due to isoimmunization. The Coombs test detects the presence of antibody on RBC's (direct Coombs) or in the plasma (indirect Coombs). The problems and validity of these tests are discussed elsewhere in this text (Chapter 71). The Coombs test is mentioned here to emphasize that one must search diligently to rule out an isoimmune disorder before embarking on a more esoteric workup of hemolysis.

BLOOD TRANSFUSIONS IN THE TREATMENT OF ANEMIA. A hemoglobin of 15 gm per 100 ml corresponds to an RBC mass of 30 ml per kg. This implies that a transfusion of 2 ml RBC per kg will increase the hemoglobin concentration 1 gm per 100 ml. Packed RBC's (hematocrit approximately 67 per cent) contain 2 ml of RBC per 3 ml packed RBC. Whole blood (hematocrit approximately 33 per cent) contains 2 ml RBC per 6 ml whole blood. Thus, the transfusion of 3 ml packed RBC per kg or 6 ml whole blood per kg will increase hemoglobin concentration 1 gm per 100 ml.

*Example:* A 3.5 kg infant with a hemoglobin of 6.5 gm per 100 ml is to be transfused to a hemoglobin of 12.0 gm per 100 ml. The difference between the desired and present hemoglobin is 5.5 gm per 100 ml. The volume of packed RBC's to be administered is 58 ml (3.5 kg × 5.5 gm per 100 ml hemoglobin difference × 3 ml packed RBC per kg). Alternatively, 116 ml whole blood will produce the same hemoglobin increase.

Whenever possible, packed RBC's should be used in order to avoid fluid volume overload. Whole blood, however, is the therapy of choice for large acute hemorrhages, since this blood loss usually is associated with hypovolemia (see discussion under Hemorrhagic Anemia). Infants with hemolytic disorders occasionally need RBC replacement therapy, although exchange transfusions are usually required if there is significant hyperbilirubinemia. The principles of exchange transfusion are the same as those employed in isoimmune hemolytic disease (Chapter 71).

Blood currently available in most blood banks is anticoagulated with acid-citrate-dextrose (ACD) or citrate-phosphate-dextrose (CPD). The use of CPD blood is preferred for several reasons. 1) The pH of CPD blood is less acidic than ACD blood. 2) The level of 2,3-DPG is maintained better in CPD, and therefore oxygen delivery of these RBC's presumably is greater. 3) Red blood cell potassium loss is less in CPD stored blood, and this decreases the risk of hyperkalemia when older bank blood is transfused. These advantages of CPD blood are only relative and therefore the freshest blood available should be used in sick neonates. It should also be noted that blood stored over 48 hours contains very few platelets, and occasionally the replacement of large blood losses with "old blood" can lead to thrombocytopenia and persistent bleeding. The use of fresh blood and platelet supplements can prevent this complication.

Heparinized blood is often used for neonatal exchange transfusions in order to obviate problems with acid-base balance and hypocalcemia (due to calcium binding by citrate). Heparinized blood is also used during surgery requiring extracorporeal circulation. Unfortunately, however, the viability of heparinized RBC's decreases rapidly during storage, and therefore this blood must be used shortly after collection. In order to minimize the economic and logistic problems of providing this form of blood, the Children's Hospital Medical Center Transfusion Service converts CPD blood (less than 5 days old) into heparinized blood. This is accomplished by adding heparin and calcium gluconate to CPD blood (for details see Kevy).

Graft-versus-host (GVH) disease rarely follows intrauterine blood transfusions for severe erythroblastosis (Naiman et al., and Parkman et al.). This is presumably due to transfusion of viable lymphocytes into immunologically incompetent fetuses. There is no current evidence that direct or exchange transfusion of neonates leads to GVH disease. Theoretically, however, some small premature infants (30 to 32 weeks' gestation) may be unable to reject foreign lymphocytes in transfused blood. For this reason, blood should be radiated (5000 rads to destroy lymphocytes) before administering to small prematures (see Immunology section, Chapter 84).

## HEMORRHAGIC ANEMIA

Anemia frequently follows fetal blood loss, bleeding from obstetrical complications and internal hemorrhages associated with birth trauma. The clinical presentation of anemia depends on the magnitude and acuteness of blood loss.

Infants with anemia subsequent to moderate hemorrhage or chronic blood loss are generally asymptomatic. The only physical findings are pallor of the skin and mucous membranes. Laboratory studies can range from a mild normochromic-normocytic anemia (hemoglobin 9 to 12 gm per 100 ml) to a more severe hypochromic-microcytic anemia (hemoglobin 5 to 7 gm per 100 ml). The only therapy required for asymptomatic children is iron (2 mg elemental iron per kg, t.i.d. for 3 months). RBC replacement is indicated only if there is evidence of clinical distress (tachycardia, tachypnea, irritability, feeding difficulties). In most cases, raising the hemoglobin to 10 to 12 gm per 100 ml will remove all signs and symptoms due to anemia. Since severely anemic infants are frequently in incipient heart failure, however, these children should be transfused very slowly (2 ml per kg per hr). If signs of congestive heart failure appear, a rapid-acting diuretic (furosemide, 1 mg per kg intravenously) should be given before proceeding with the transfusion. An alternative approach is to exchange transfuse severely anemic infants with packed RBC's for anemic whole blood. This increases the hemoglobin concentration without the danger of increasing blood volume and precipitating congestive heart failure.

Infants who rapidly lose large volumes of blood appear in acute distress (pallor, tachycardia, tachypnea, weak pulses, hypotension and shock). This presentation is distinct from that seen in neonatal respiratory asphyxia (slow respirations with intercostal retractions, bradycardia and pallor with cyanosis). The clinical response to assisted ventilation and oxygen is also different: infants with respiratory problems manifest a marked improvement, while there is little change in anemic neonates. Cyanosis is not a feature of severe anemia because the hemoglobin concentration is too low (clinical cyanosis indicates at least 5 gm per 100 ml of deoxygenated hemoglobin). The hemoglobin concentration immediately after an acute hemorrhage may be normal, since the initial response to acute volume depletion is vasoconstriction. A decreased hemoglobin may not be seen until the plasma volume has re-expanded several hours later. In view of these hemodynamic considerations, it is apparent that the diagnosis of acute hemorrhagic anemia is based largely on physical findings and evidence of blood loss. It is important to recognize these clinical features, for immediate therapy is required. Treatment is directed at rapid expansion of the vascular space (20 ml fluid per kg). The ideal fluid is cross-matched and type-specific whole blood, although this is usually not available in most emergency situations. Uncross-matched group O, Rh negative blood can be given as an alternative. If no blood is available, other plasma expanders (plasma, saline with albumin, dextran) should be given. An additional 10 ml per kg of whole blood should be administered as soon as it is available. This procedure usually improves the clinical status of infants with hypovolemia due to fetal blood loss. Neonates with serious internal hemorrhages, on the other hand, generally show a poor response.

## Fetal Hemorrhage

Fetomaternal Hemorrhage. Significant bleeding into the maternal circulation occurs in approximately 8 per cent of all pregnancies, and thus represents one of the most common forms of fetal bleeding. Small amounts of fetal blood are lost in most cases, but in 1 per cent of pregnancies fetal blood loss may be up to 40 ml of blood (Cohen et al.). Fetomaternal hemorrhage occasionally fol-

**TABLE 66–4.   *Hemorrhagic Anemia in Neonates***

*Fetal hemorrhage*
  Spontaneous fetomaternal hemorrhage
  Hemorrhage following amniocentesis
  Twin-twin transfusion

*Placental hemorrhage*
  Placenta previa
  Abruptio placentae
  Multilobed placenta (vasa previa)
  Velamentous insertion of cord
  Placental incision during cesarean section

*Umbilical cord bleeding*
  Rupture of umbilical cord with precipitous delivery
  Rupture of short or entangled cord

*Postpartum hemorrhage*
  Bleeding from umbilicus
  Cephalohematomas, scalp hemorrhages
  Hepatic rupture, splenic rupture
  Retroperitoneal hemorrhages

lows amniocentesis and placental injury (Zipursky et al.) although anemia is seen only following unsuccessful amniocentesis or where there is evidence of a bloody tap (Woo Wang et al.). For this reason, infants born to mothers who have had amniocentesis should be observed closely for signs of anemia. The effects of anemia due to fetomaternal hemorrhages are quite variable. Large acute hemorrhages can produce hypovolemic shock (Raye, Gutberlet and Stahlman), while slower, more chronic blood loss results in hypochromic microcytic anemia due to iron deficiency (Pearson and Diamond). Some infants with severe chronic anemia (hemoglobin as low as 4 to 6 gm per 100 ml) may have minimal symptoms. An examination of the maternal blood smear for the presence of fetal cells (Kleihauer-Betke preparation) is necessary in any infant with suspected fetomaternal hemorrhage. (For details of this procedure see Oski and Naiman, Hematologic Disorders of the Newborn, W. B. Saunders Co., 1972, page 63.) This test is based on the principle that hemoglobin A is eluted from RBC's at an acid pH, while hemoglobin F is not affected by these conditions. Consequently, when alcohol-fixed and acid-treated RBC's are stained with eosin, those containing hemoglobin A are colorless, while those containing hemoglobin F (fetal RBC's) appear normally colored (Table 66–5). Approximately 50 ml of fetal blood must be lost to produce significant neonatal anemia. This volume is greater than 1 per cent of the maternal blood volume, and therefore fetal cells within the maternal circulation may be detected quite readily. This test is not valid when there is coexistence of maternal hemoglobinopathies with increased hemoglobin F levels. In addition, fetal-maternal ABO incompatibility may cause rapid removal of fetal RBC's, and thus obscure any significant hemorrhage. For this reason it is important to examine maternal blood as soon as anemia due to fetal hemorrhage is suspected.

TWIN-TWIN TRANSFUSION. Transfusion of blood from one homozygous twin to another can result in anemia in the donor twin and polycythemia in the recipient. Significant hemorrhage is seen only in monochorionic monozygous twins (approximately 70 per cent of all monozygous twins). In approximately 15 per cent of these pregnancies there is a twin to twin transfusion (Rausen, Seki and Straus). Bleeding occurs because of vascular anastomosis in monochorionic placentas. The anemic donor twin is usually smaller than the polycythemic recipient. Polyhydramnios is frequently seen in the recipient twin and oligohydramnios is seen in the donor. Twin to twin transfusions should be suspected when the hemoglobin concentration of identical twins differs by more than 5 gm per 100 ml.

## PLACENTAL BLOOD LOSS

Placental bleeding during pregnancy is quite common, but in most cases hemorrhage is from the maternal aspect of the placenta. In placenta previa, however, the thin placenta overlying the cervical os frequently results in fetal blood loss. The vascular communications between multilobular placental lobes are also very fragile and are easily subjected to trauma during delivery. Vasa previa is the condition in which one of these connecting vessels overlies the cervical os and thus is prone to rupture during delivery. The perinatal death rate in vasa previa may be greater than 50 per cent. Abruptio placentae generally causes fetal anoxia and death, although surviving infants can be severely anemic. Bleeding also follows inadvertent placental incision during cesarean sections (Montague and Krevans), and thus the placenta should be inspected for injury following all cesarean sections.

## UMBILICAL CORD BLEEDING

The normal umbilical cord is resistant to minor trauma and does not bleed. The umbilical cord of dysmature infants, however, is weak and liable to rupture and hemorrhage (Raye, Gutberlet and Stahlman). In cases of precipitous delivery, a rapid increase in cord tension can rupture the fetal aspect of the cord and cause serious acute blood loss. Short or entangled umbilical cords and abnormalities of umbilical blood vessels (velamentous insertions into the placenta) are also liable to rupture and hemorrhage. Bleeding from injured umbilical cords is rapid, but generally ceases after a short period of time, owing to arterial constriction. The umbilical cord should always be inspected for abnormalities or signs of injury, particularly after unattended, precipitous deliveries.

### CASE 66–1

A 2950 gm white male infant was born by vaginal delivery to a gravida 1, para 0, white

**TABLE 66–5.** *Comparative Clinical Findings in Neonatal Respiratory Distress and Acute Hemorrhage*

|  | *Neonatal Asphyxia* | *Acute Blood Loss* |
|---|---|---|
| Heart rate | Decreased | Increased |
| Respiratory rate | Decreased | Increased |
| Intercostal retractions | Present | Absent |
| Skin color | Pallor with cyanosis | Pallor without cyanosis |
| Response to oxygen and assisted ventilation | Marked improvement | No significant change |

female at 38 weeks' gestation. Vaginal bleeding was excessive at the time of delivery, and inspection of the cord and placenta revealed a velamentous insertion of umbilical vessels into the placenta. The infant's Apgar score was 7, although he was pale and manifested moderate tachycardia and tachypnea. There were no intercostal retractions or cyanosis. Spleen and liver were not palpable. The hemoglobin concentration of blood from the umbilical vein was 13.4 gm per 100 ml. Bilirubin was 2.3. The infant was transfused with 60 ml of type-specific whole blood, following which his color improved and cardiac and respiratory status returned to normal. Eight hours after the blood transfusion, the infant's hemoglobin was 14.4 gm per 100 ml. The subsequent clinical course was unremarkable and no further transfusions were required.

COMMENT. Physical findings and a history of excessive bleeding at birth suggested some degree of blood loss. The nearly normal hemoglobin concentration at birth probably was due to immediate vasoconstriction associated with loss of blood volume. Transfusion with whole blood certainly improved the infant's clinical state, although the increase in hemoglobin was less than expected. A 60 ml transfusion of whole blood (20 ml per kg) should increase hemoglobin concentration around 3 gm per 100 ml. Failure to see this increase presumably was due to the initial vasoconstriction and subsequent vascular expansion following whole blood transfusion. This case clearly demonstrates the dramatic response to blood transfusion given to neonates with moderate but self-limited blood loss.

### POSTPARTUM HEMORRHAGE

Hemorrhagic anemia due to internal bleeding is occasionally associated with birth trauma. Characteristically, internal hemorrhages are asymptomatic during the first 24 to 48 hours of life, signs and symptoms of anemia developing after this time. Cephalhematomas can be sufficiently large to cause anemia and hyperbilirubinemia, owing to the resorption of blood (Leonard and Anthony). Scalp hemorrhages ("hemorrhagic caput") also can produce severe anemia (Pachman). These hemorrhages are

frequently more extensive than cephalhematomas, since bleeding is not limited by periosteum. Adrenal and kidney hemorrhages occasionally follow difficult breech deliveries. Splenic rupture and hemorrhage occur most commonly in association with splenomegaly, as in erythroblastosis fetalis (Philipsborn et al.). Hepatic hemorrhages are generally subcapsular and may be asymptomatic. Rupture of the hepatic capsule results in hemoperitoneum and hypovolemic shock. Hepatic hemorrhages are suspected when a previously healthy infant goes into shock with clinical manifestations of an increasing right upper quadrant abdominal mass, shifting dullness on percussion and evidence of free fluid on abdominal x-rays. In contrast to neonates with acute blood loss due to fetomaternal or umbilical vessel bleeding, the clinical response to blood replacement is generally poor in infants with hepatic hemorrhage. Exploratory laparotomy is usually required for confirmation of diagnosis and possible repair of the hemorrhagic site.

### HEMOLYTIC ANEMIA

Red blood cells from children and adults normally circulate for 100 to 120 days. Erythrocyte survival in neonates is somewhat shorter: 70 to 90 days in term infants, 50 to 80 days in prematures (Pearson). Hemolytic anemia is the clinical consequence of RBC abnormalities leading to shorter than normal erythrocyte survival. The precise mechanism of cell destruction is not known, although membrane deformability is thought to be an important determinant (LaCelle). Erythrocytes are 7 to 8 micrometers wide, while the vascular diameter in some areas of the microcirculation may be less than 3. Consequently, RBC's must deform their membrane and intracellular contents in order to pass through these narrow channels. This is no problem for normal RBC's. Abnormalities in RBC metabolism, hemoglobin, or cell shape, however, all lead to decreased RBC membrane deformability. The consequence of this decreased membrane flexibility is RBC sequestration and removal by reticuloendothelial cells of the spleen and liver.

In older infants and children, the usual

*TABLE 66–6. Hemolytic Anemia During the Newborn Period*

*Immune*
   Isoimmune: Rh and ABO incompatibility
   Maternal immune disease: Autoimmune hemolytic anemia, systemic lupus erythematosus
   Drug induced: Penicillin

*Acquired RBC disorders*
   Infection: CID, toxoplasmosis, syphilis, bacterial sepsis
   Disseminated and localized intravascular coagulation, respiratory distress syndrome

*Hereditary RBC disorders*
   Membrane defects: Hereditary spherocytosis, hereditary elliptocytosis
   Enzyme abnormalities: G6PD, pyruvate kinase
   Hemoglobinopathies: Alpha thalassemia syndromes, gamma/beta thalassemia

response to increased RBC destruction is enhanced erythropoiesis, and there may be little or no anemia if the rate of production matches the accelerated rate of destruction. In these cases of well-compensated hemolysis, the major manifestations are due to increased erythrocyte destruction (hyperbilirubinemia) and augmented erythropoiesis (reticulocytosis). During the early neonatal period, however, increased oxygen carrying capacity of blood (see Physiologic Anemia of Infancy) may obviate any compensatory erythropoietic activity in cases of mild hemolysis. Consequently, hyperbilirubinemia in excess of normal neonatal levels may be the only apparent manifestation of hemolysis. In most cases of significant hemolysis, however, some degree of reticulocytosis usually is present. The degree of hyperbilirubinemia and reticulocytosis obviously must be interpreted in terms of values appropriate for gestational and postgestational age. The major complication of hemolysis in neonates is hyperbilirubinemia, and therapeutic efforts are aimed at preventing kernicterus. Phototherapy can be employed in cases of mild hemolysis, although more severe disease may require exchange transfusion. Occasionally, symptomatic anemia necessitates RBC transfusions.

## IMMUNE HEMOLYSIS

ISOIMMUNE HEMOLYTIC DISEASE. Hemolytic anemia due to ABO and Rh in-compatibility is the most common cause of hemolysis in newborn infants.

IMMUNE HEMOLYSIS SECONDARY TO MATERNAL DISEASE. Maternal autoimmune hemolytic anemia can be associated with Coombs-positive hemolytic anemia in neonates (Bauman and Rubin). Neonates are affected to the extent that maternal antibodies cross the placenta and attack fetal RBC's, but in most instances hemolysis is minimal and transient. Steroids (prednisone 2 mg per kg) may decrease the hemolytic rate in more severe cases.

Infants born to mothers with systemic lupus erythematosus may transiently manifest hemolytic anemia as well as neutropenia and thrombocytopenia. The status of maternal health (anemia, thrombocytopenia, renal disease) will suggest this as the etiology of neonatal hemolysis.

DRUG-INDUCED IMMUNE HEMOLYSIS. Immunologically mediated hemolysis due to drugs has been documented in older children and adults. One common offending drug is penicillin. In these cases, penicillin combines with the RBC membrane, forming a hapten that elicits antibody production to the drug-RBC complex. No hemolysis occurs in the absence of penicillin even in the presence of antipenicillin antibody. The direct Coombs test is occasionally negative although the indirect Coombs test (detection of serum antibody) is positive if RBC's are first preincubated with penicillin. Hemolytic anemia has been described in a neonate given penicillin, presumably owing to the transplacental transfer of maternal antipenicillin antibodies (Clayton et al.). Hemolysis ceases once the drug is removed.

## ACQUIRED HEMOLYTIC DISEASE

INFECTION. Cytomegalic inclusion disease, toxoplasmosis, syphilis and bacterial sepsis all can be associated with hemolytic anemia. In most of these conditions some degree of thrombocytopenia also exists. Generally there is hepatosplenomegaly. In cases of bacterial sepsis, both the direct and indirect bilirubin may be elevated. The mechanism of hemolysis is not clearly defined, but it may be related to RBC sequestration in the presence of marked reticuloendothelial hyperplasia associated with infection. Documentation of infection as the cause of hemolysis is made by the presence of other clinical and laboratory stigmata of neonatal infections. Hemolysis due to infections may present early in the neonatal period, or it can be delayed for several weeks.

DISSEMINATED INTRAVASCULAR COAGULATION. This coagulation abnormality is discussed in detail elsewhere (p. 574). The hemolytic component of this disorder is secondary to the deposition of fibrin within the vascular walls. When erythrocytes interact with fibrin, fragments of RBC's are broken off, producing fragile, deformed red blood cells, or schistocytes. These cells are relatively rigid and thus incapable of normal deformation within the microcirculation. The hemolytic-uremic syndrome (p. 579) represents a localized form of intravascular coagulation that is characterized by thrombocytopenia, renal disease and hemolytic anemia. Hemolysis is characterized by RBC fragmentation, presumably for the reasons discussed above. Hemolytic anemia is also seen with the respiratory distress syndrome (Inall et al.). Whether hemolysis in these cases is due to DIC, infection or acid-base disturbances is not known.

### HEREDITARY RBC DISORDERS

MEMBRANE DEFECTS. Several RBC membrane abnormalities are associated with hemolytic anemia: stomatocytosis, elliptocytosis, desiccytosis and spherocytosis. Aside from hereditary spherocytosis (HS) these disorders are relatively uncommon.

### Hereditary Spherocytosis

This is an autosomal dominant disorder manifested by the presence of spherocytic RBC's. Spherocytes are characterized by a decreased membrane surface area to volume ratio. The volume (MCV) of HS red blood cells is relatively normal, and thus it is thought that spherocytes result from a decrease in membrane surface area. In fact, it has been established that HS erythrocytes lose membrane lipid during their life span. Spherocytes in vitro are susceptible to osmotic lysis (i.e., the release of hemoglobin when RBC's swell in hypotonic salt solutions). It is unlikely that this is an important hemolytic mechanism in vivo (Crosby and Conrad). More likely, the rigid membrane properties of spherocytes lead to splenic sequestration and hemolysis.

The clinical manifestations of hereditary spherocytosis include mild to moderate hemolysis with reticulocytosis, hyperbilirubinemia and marked splenomegaly. This is usually a well-compensated process with little or no anemia. There is a neonatal history of hemolysis and hyperbilirubinemia in approximately 50 per cent of all cases (Stamey and Diamond).

The diagnosis of HS is suspected when there is laboratory evidence of hemolysis and presence of spherocytes on the peripheral blood smear. The incubated osmotic fragility test (24 hours, 37° C) indicates that the RBC's are osmotically more fragile. This incubated osmotic fragility is most useful in bringing out the membrane defect in severe cases of HS in which few if any circulating spherocytes may be present. This paradox is due to the fact that severely affected spherocytes are rapidly removed by the spleen and do not circulate. A Coombs test and blood typing are essential in any case of spherocytosis, since the clinical and laboratory presentation of HS is similar to that seen in ABO incompatibility. Unfortunately, however, the Coombs test in ABO incompatibility is occasionally negative, thus obscuring the correct diagnosis. Examination of family members for spherocytes may be useful in these cases, although no family history of hereditary spherocytosis is found in 25 per cent of patients. Alternatively, definitive diagnosis can be deferred until maternal antibody is cleared by the neonate (after 4 months). Persistence of spherocytes at this time indicates hereditary spherocytosis.

The important hemolytic role of the spleen in HS in manifested by the rapid decrease in bilirubin and reticulocytes following splenectomy. Spherocytes persist following surgery, but the survival of these cells is normal once the spleen is removed. There is no question regarding the efficacy of splenectomy in reducing hemolysis in cases of HS. Nevertheless, we defer surgery until 5 years of age, since young splenectomized children have an increased susceptibility to overwhelming pneumococcal and *H. influenzae* sepsis (Diamond). The risk of these serious infections reportedly is decreased after 5 years of age. The most important aspect of therapy in the neonatal period is prevention of kernicterus (phototherapy, exchange transfusion). Packed RBC's should be given if there is significant anemia without hyperbilirubinemia. Survival of transfused cells is normal unless there is significant hypersplenism. Folic acid (1 mg per day) should be administered prophylactically to prevent folate-induced erythroid hypoplasia.

CASE 66–2

A 15-month-old female infant was evaluated for severe chronic hemolytic anemia. This was the first child born to a gravida 1, para 0, white female after an uneventful pregnancy and delivery. Shortly after birth the infant was noted to be icteric, and a spleen tip was easily palpable 1 to 2 cm below the left costal margin. The remainder of the physical examination was normal. At 36 hours of age, the bilirubin concentration was 16 mg per 100 ml, hemoglobin was 12 gm per 100 ml and reticulocytes were 15 per cent. Maternal blood type was O-positive, while that of the infant was A-positive. Direct and indirect Coombs tests were negative. The peripheral blood smear revealed marked variation in RBC size and shapes, but there was no predominant cell shape. An osmotic fragility test on a *fresh* blood sample was within normal limits. There was no evidence of G6PD or PK deficiency. RBC indices were normal. Hemoglobin F was 70 per cent and no abnormal hemoglobins were seen on hemoglobin electrophoresis. The infant's parents were both hematologically normal. The infant was exchange transfused with O-positive blood.

At 5 weeks of age, she again was noted to be anemic (hemoglobin 6 gm per 100 ml, reticulocytes 9 per cent, total bilirubin 2.3). Physical examination was remarkable for a palpable spleen 3 to 4 cm below the left costal margin. The child was transfused with packed RBC's.

The infant's hemolytic anemia persisted during the next 14 months, and RBC transfusions were required at 6 to 8 week intervals. Repeat laboratory evaluation at 15 months was unchanged from previous studies with one exception. The *incubated* osmotic fragility was abnormal, with a large population of osmotically fragile RBC's. Rare spherocytes were seen on the peripheral blood smear. The patient subsequently underwent splenectomy, and 6 weeks after surgery hemolysis had markedly diminished: hemoglobin increased to 12 gm per 100 ml, reticulocytes decreased to 1.2 per cent and numerous spherocytes were present in the peripheral blood. The child was placed on prophylactic penicillin in view of her risk for developing sepsis.

COMMENT. This is a case of severe hereditary spherocytosis with several unusual features. 1) Spherocytosis was not a characteristic feature of the peripheral blood until after splenectomy. Prior to surgery these cells were rapidly removed from the circulation. 2) The initial negative osmotic fragility test points out the fallibility of testing fresh blood rather than blood which has been incubated (37°C for 24 hours) in order to bring out the membrane defect. 3) Transfusion-dependent HS is very unusual, but it does occur. The decision to remove her spleen was based on splenomegaly with transfusion-dependent hemolytic anemia. The rapid cessation of hemolysis following surgery indicates that splenectomy was the proper decision.

### Hereditary Elliptocytosis

Normal individuals may have up to 15 per cent elliptical cells, but patients with this autosomal dominant disorder have 25–75 per cent elliptical RBC's in the peripheral blood. Approximately 0.04 per cent of people in the United States are affected by this abnormality, but only a small fraction (12 per cent) of individuals with elliptocytosis ever have significant hemolytic anemia (Penfold and Lipscomb). The mechanism of hemolysis is not known, and no biochemical abnormality has been demonstrated. In those rare cases in which both parents manifest elliptocytosis, significant hemolytic anemia may occur in the newborn period (Neilson and Strunk). The clinical features of this disorder are extremely variable. Elliptocytosis is usually an incidental finding in an otherwise healthy child. In other cases, the disorder may be characterized by splenomegaly, anemia and jaundice, all of which can occur in neonates. Elliptocytosis associated with hemolysis has a clinical course very similar to that of hereditary spherocytosis.

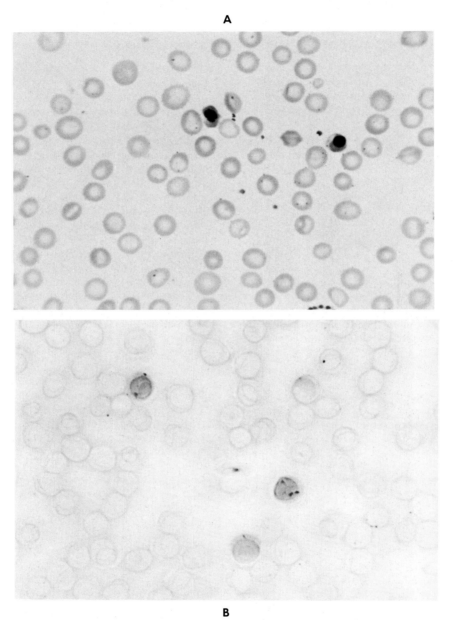

**Figure 66–4.**  *A*, Hypochromic-microcytic RBC's secondary to chronic fetal blood loss. *B*, Fetal RBC's in the maternal blood after a fetomaternal hemorrhage (acid-elution technique). *C*, Hereditary spherocytosis. *D*, Hereditary elliptocytosis. *E*, G6PD deficient RBC's during acute hemolytic episode. *F*, Heinz bodies in patient with G6PD deficient hemolysis (stained with supravital dye).

*(Illustration continued on opposite page.)*

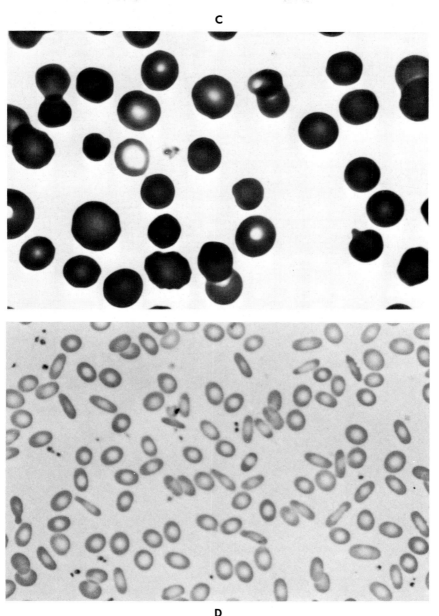

**Figure 66–4.** *Continued*

*(Illustration continued on following page.)*

**E**

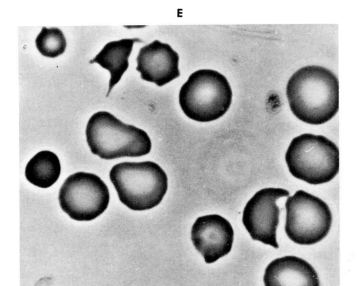

**F**

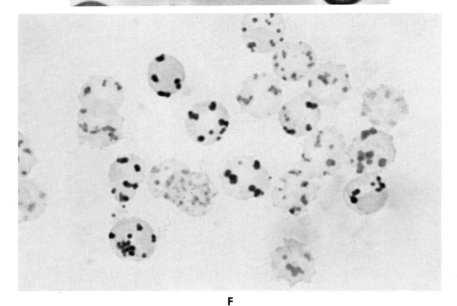

*Figure 66–4.   Continued*

### RBC Enzyme Abnormalities

Hemolysis has been reported in association with several erythrocyte enzyme deficiencies, but only two of these are of major clinical significance: Glucose-6-phosphate dehydrogenase (G6PD) deficiency, and pyruvate kinase (PK) deficiency.

### Glucose-6-Phosphate Dehydrogenase Deficiency

This RBC enzyme deficiency affects millions of people throughout the world, with the highest frequency occurring in Mediterranean countries, Africa and China (Beutler). Approximately 10 per cent of

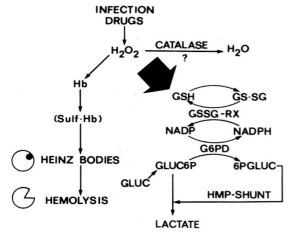

*Figure 66–5.* G6PD Hemolysis — pathophysiology.

Blacks in the United States are G6PD deficient. Generally this is a mild hemolytic disorder, although it can cause life-threatening anemia in certain individuals. Hemolysis occurs because enzyme deficient RBC's are unable to defend against the external oxidant stresses associated with infection and the administration of certain drugs (Fig. 66–5). Generation of hydrogen peroxide near or within RBC's is the common denominator of all oxidants, and the intracellular accumulation of peroxide leads to an oxidative assault on the RBC membrane, enzymes and hemoglobin. The oxidant attack on hemoglobin results in globin degradation (Heinz bodies), and this

in turn produces membrane injury leading to decreased deformability and hemolysis. Normal RBC's contain reduced glutathione (GSH), a sulfhydryl-containing tripeptide which functions as an intracellular gendarme that degrades peroxide and protects other cell proteins from oxidant injury. In order to sustain this protection, intracellular levels of GSH must be maintained. G6PD is one of the vital enzymes required for GSH regeneration. In G6PD deficient RBC's there is a limited capacity to sustain GSH, and thus these cells are vulnerable to oxidant injury and hemolysis.

The severity of hemolysis in G6PD deficiency is obviously related to the magnitude of the oxidant stress, but two other variables also are important: racial origin and sex. As erythrocytes age G6PD activity decreases, but in normal individuals the lowest activity in older RBC's is more than sufficient to protect against oxidant injury (Fig. 66–6). The defect in Black G6PD deficients is due to instability of the enzyme: G6PD activity in young cells is normal, but that in older cells is severely deficient. This is in accord with the clinical observation that hemolysis in Black G6PD deficients is self-limited, affecting only older cells in which the enzyme has decayed below a critical threshold. The abnormality in G6PD deficient Caucasians is due to even greater enzyme instability, and RBC's of all ages are affected. Consequently, hemolysis in Caucasian deficients can be severe, and result in the de-

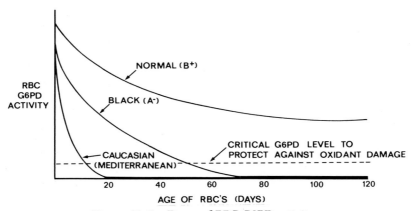

*Figure 66–6.* Decay of RBC-G6PD activity.

struction of the entire circulating RBC mass. Rare cases of death due to G6PD deficiency have been reported in these patients. Manifestations of the Chinese G6PD variant are similar to that seen in Caucasians. Favism is an idiopathic reaction resulting in massive and rapid hemolysis of G6PD deficient RBC's after eating or inhaling pollen of the fava bean. The mechanism of this reaction is unknown, although it is seen only in Caucasians and Orientals.

Glucose-6-phosphate dehydrogenase deficiency is a sex-linked disorder that causes hemolysis primarily in males. Females are variably affected, since they possess one normal X-chromosome in addition to the X-chromosome bearing the G6PD deficient gene (Fig. 66–7). In accord with the Lyon hypothesis, however, only one X-chromosome is active in a given cell line, since the other chromosome is randomly inactivated early in embryonic life (Lyon). As a consequence of this, G6PD deficient females are affected to the extent that they have Lyonized to the abnormal chromosome. A female with 50 per cent of normal G6PD activity has 50 per cent normal RBC's and 50 per cent G6PD deficient cells. The deficient cells are as vulnerable to hemolysis as deficient male RBC's.

A few Caucasian variants of G6PD deficiency are associated with chronic non-spherocytic hemolytic anemia in the absence of obvious oxidant stresses. In most cases, however, G6PD deficient individuals are not anemic and hemolysis is seen only with infection and drugs. It should be emphasized that infection (bacterial and viral) is the most common cause of hemolysis. Hepatosplenomegaly is unusual.

The diagnosis of G6PD deficiency is suggested by Coombs negative hemolytic anemia associated with drugs or infection. Special stains of the peripheral blood (brilliant cresyl blue) may reveal Heinz bodies during hemolytic episodes. Cells that look as if a "bite" had been removed (due to splenic removal of Heinz bodies) occasionally are seen on the routine peripheral blood smear. Specific diagnosis of G6PD deficiency can be made with commercially available screening kits. Unfortunately, most of these tests are relatively insensitive, and false negatives frequently are obtained if abnormal RBC's have been removed by hemolysis. This is not a problem in male Caucasians, but it certainly is a factor in diagnosing some female Caucasians and most Blacks. In these cases more sensitive tests can be employed (Fairbanks and Fernandez) or family members can be studied. If the propositus is male, his mother should also be affected, while an affected female can have a mother or father with G6PD deficiency. Alternatively, one can wait until the hemolytic crisis is over and re-evaluate the patient at a time his RBC mass has been repopulated with cells of all ages (approximately 8 to 12 weeks).

Hemolysis due to G6PD deficiency is well documented in the newborn period. The usual causal factors (drugs and infection) can be responsible, although in many cases there is no obvious oxidant threat. It is generally agreed that term Black infants with G6PD deficiency manifest no increased incidence or severity of hemolysis and hyperbilirubinemia (O'Flynn and Hsia). In premature Black infants with G6PD deficiency, however, hyperbilirubinemia has been reported but significant hemolysis is rare (Eshaghpour et al.). Severe hemolysis and hyperbilirubinemia are seen only in Caucasians and Orientals with G6PD deficiency. In one study from

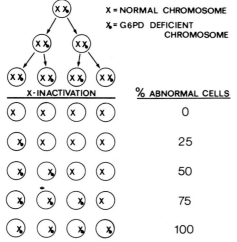

*Figure 66–7.* Lyon hypothesis of G6PD deficiency.

Greece (Doxiadis et al.), approximately 30 per cent of all exchange transfusions for hyperbilirubinemia were done in G6PD deficient infants with no evidence of isoimmune hemolytic anemia.

Therapy for hemolysis due to G6PD deficiency is as follows: 1) Prevent kernicterus by managing hyperbilirubinemia with phototherapy and/or exchange transfusion. 2) Replace RBC's if there is significant anemia. Transfused cells will survive normally. 3) Attempt to remove all potential oxidants. Treat infections and avoid all possible offending drugs. 4) Folic acid (1 mg per day) should be given to those rare individuals with chronic nonspherocytic hemolysis. No specific therapy is required in the absence of hemolysis.

CASE 66–3 (MENTZER AND COLLIER)

A male infant weighing 2722 gm was born at 38 weeks gestation to a 30-year-old Chinese, gravida 3, para 1, aborta 1, mother. Apgar score at birth was 1. Despite intensive resuscitative measures, the infant died after 2 hours, never having established spontaneous respirations. Hemoglobin was 9.8 gm per 100 ml, and the WBC count was 7200. There was marked polychromatophilia (reticulocytosis), and numerous nucleated RBC's were seen in the peripheral smear. The infant's blood type was AB positive, mother's blood type was B positive, and the Coombs test (direct and indirect) was negative. Hemoglobin electrophoresis revealed 52 per cent hemoglobin F, 45 per cent hemoglobin A and no evidence of Bart's hemoglobin or hemoglobin H. Erythrocyte G6PD activity was decreased. The infant's mother also was G6PD deficient (heterozygote). During her pregnancy, the mother had an upper respiratory infection 4 weeks prior to delivery. Ascorbic acid (250–500 mg per day) was taken for 2 weeks as therapy for this viral infection. On at least one occasion during the last month of pregnancy, she also ate fava beans.

COMMENT. Severe hemolysis and hyperbilirubinemia are not uncommon in G6PD deficient Caucasians and Chinese. As a result of this case, however, G6PD deficiency can also be considered a cause of hydrops fetalis. The reason for the disastrous course in this neonate is not known. Infection, ascorbic acid (an intracellular oxidant) or fava bean exposure could have been responsible.

## Pyruvate Kinase Deficiency

This autosomal recessive disorder occurs throughout the world and in all ethnic groups. Although its frequency is much less than that of G6PD deficiency, several hundred cases of hemolytic anemia due to this enzyme defect have been identified (Tanaka). Pyruvate kinase is one of two key enzymatic steps during which adenosine triphosphate (ATP) can be generated in RBC's. This high energy compound has a variety of functions, including the maintenance of normal RBC deformability. It is no surprise that impaired ATP production of PK deficient cells leads to a short survival in the circulation.

Pyruvate kinase deficiency is characterized by a variable degree of anemia and hemolysis. Some children manifest a moderate chronic hemolytic anemia (hemoglobin 8 to 10 gm per 100 ml, hyperbilirubinemia, reticulocytosis and splenomegaly). In other children hemolysis is much more severe, often requiring frequent blood transfusions to maintain an adequate circulating hemoglobin. Severely affected children often benefit from splenectomy, since the spleen adds a further insult to metabolically inferior RBC's. Most children with PK deficiency have neonatal jaundice, and many require exchange transfusion. Kernicterus has been reported in PK deficient neonates.

The diagnosis of PK deficiency is considered in the presence of unexplained jaundice and a Coombs negative hemolytic anemia not related to infection or drugs. The anemia is normochromic-normocytic, hemoglobin electrophoresis is normal for age, and the maternal medical history usually is negative. The peripheral blood smear is nonspecific, although irregularly contracted and densely staining erythrocytes may be seen. Specific diagnosis requires a definitive enzyme assay for pyruvate kinase. Parents manifest biochemical heterozygosity (decreased enzyme activity) but they are not anemic and there is no hemolysis.

Treatment of PK deficiency during the newborn period is symptomatic and directed at the prevention of kernicterus (phototherapy, exchange transfusion). In the presence of severe anemia RBC transfusions should be given. Transfused cells will survive normally. Folic acid (1.0 mg per day) should be given to meet the requirements of increased RBC production. Children who require frequent RBC transfusions may benefit from splenectomy, although this decision should be deferred for several months if possible.

### HEMOLYSIS DUE TO HEMOGLOBIN DISORDERS

In order to appreciate the unique hemoglobinopathies that occur in neonates an understanding of in utero hemoglobin production is essential. Hemoglobin is a tetrameric protein consisting of 4 hemes (iron-protoporphyrins), each of which is associated with a specific globin polypeptide chain. The heme groups in all known hemoglobins are identical, although there are major differences in the various globin chains (alpha, beta, gamma, delta, epsilon and zeta). Most functional hemoglobins produced beyond early embryonic life consist of two alpha chains and two non-alpha globin chains.

*Gower 1* (zeta 2, epsilon 2) is the earliest detectable embryonic hemoglobin. Currently it is thought that zeta chains are the embryonic equivalent of alpha chains.
*Gower 2* (alpha 2, epsilon 2) is another embryonic hemoglobin present in early fetal life.
*Hemoglobin Portland* (zeta 2, gamma 2) is the embryonic equivalent of fetal hemoglobin.
*Fetal hemoglobin* (alpha 2, gamma 2) accounts for 90 to 95 per cent of all hemoglobin production, and thus it is the major hemoglobin of fetal life. This maximal synthetic rate decreases after 35 weeks gestation, and at birth fetal hemoglobin accounts for 50 to 60 per cent of hemoglobin

production. This rate continues to decrease, and at 3 months of age only 5 per cent of synthesis is due to fetal hemoglobin.

*Hemoglobin A* is the major extrauterine hemoglobin. At 20 weeks gestation Hgb A accounts for 5 to 10 per cent of hemoglobin synthesis, and this increases to 35 to 50 per cent of new hemoglobin production at birth.

The hemoglobin composition of cord blood is a reflection of past and present synthesis (Figure 66–9). The concentration of hemoglobin F is 60 to 85 per cent, while the remaining 15 to 40 per cent is due to hemoglobin A. Trace amounts of other hemoglobins are also present in cord blood. Hemoglobin $A_2$ is a minor hemoglobin (less than 3 per cent of total hemoglobin in children and adults), and it may be present in small concentrations in cord blood. Bart's hemoglobin is a tetramer of gamma chains (gamma 4) which is increased in alpha thalassemic disorders (see below). Normal cord blood contains less than 1 per cent Bart's hemoglobin.

Hemolysis is associated with quantitative and qualitative hemoglobin defects. Qualitative disorders are due to the production of abnormal globin chains (sickle cell disease). Quantitative disorders are due to decreased synthesis of normal globin chains (thalassemia syndromes). Hemoglobinopathies related to beta chain abnormalities are usually not clinically apparent in the neonatal period. On the other hand, gamma chain abnormalities may be clinically manifest in neonates, and then disappear as infants get older and beta chain synthesis increases. Alpha chain disorders are seen in both infants and children.

### Thalassemia Syndromes

This group of autosomal recessive disorders is a result of decreased synthesis of normal hemoglobin polypeptides. Decreased hemoglobin production leads to anemia characterized by small RBC's (microcytes) containing less hemoglobin per cell (hypochromia). An associated hemolytic component aggravates the magnitude of anemia. Hemolysis is a consequence of continued synthesis of the remaining globin chains (e.g., decreased beta chain production in beta thalassemia is associated

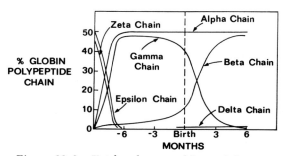

*Figure 66–8.* Fetal and neonatal hemoglobin production.

| | HEMOGLOBIN | GLOBIN POLYPEPTIDES | % IN CORD BLOOD |
|---|---|---|---|
| EMBRYONIC | GOWER - 1 | Zeta -2 , Epsilon -2 ( $\zeta_2\epsilon_2$ ) | 0 |
| | GOWER -2 | Alpha -2 , Epsilon -2 ( $\alpha_2\epsilon_2$ ) | 0 |
| | PORTLAND | Zeta -2 , Gamma -2 ( $\zeta_2\gamma_2$ ) | 0 |
| FETAL | BARTS | Gamma -4 ( $\gamma_4$ ) | <1% |
| | Hgb F | Alpha -2 , Gamma -2 ( $\alpha_2\gamma_2$ ) | 60-85 % |
| ADULT | Hgb A | Alpha -2 , Beta -2 ( $\alpha_2\beta_2$ ) | 15-40 % |
| | Hgb $A_2$ | Alpha -2 , Delta -2 ( $\alpha_2\delta_2$ ) | <1% |

*Figure 66–9.* Hemoglobin composition of cord blood.

with alpha chain accumulation in developing RBC's). The excess of unbalanced globin chains interact to form tetramers ( $\alpha_4$ , $\beta_4$ , or hemoglobin H, and $\gamma_4$ , or Bart's hemoglobin). Globin tetramers are unstable and tend to precipitate and produce cell membrane injury. The severity of injury is directly related to the instability of globin chain tetramers ( $\alpha_4 > \gamma_4 > \beta_4$ ).

ALPHA THALASSEMIA. This form of thalassemia is seen worldwide with a particularly high incidence in Asia and Africa, although it occurs in milder form in Blacks than in Orientals. Defects in alpha chain production are apparent at birth, since alpha chains constitute half the globin moiety of fetal hemoglobin. In the absence of alpha chains, gamma chain tetramers (Bart's hemoglobin) are formed. Severity of the alpha chain defect is proportional to the cord blood content of Bart's hemoglobin. The clinical and laboratory signs of alpha

thalassemia are best understood if one accepts the theory that four genes (two from each parent) regulate the normal production of alpha polypeptide chains (Table 66–7).

*Silent Carrier State.* These individuals lack one of the four genetic loci regulating alpha chain production. There are no clinical or hematologic abnormalities. Cord blood contains a slightly increased level of Bart's hemoglobin (1 to 2 per cent).

*Alpha Thalassemia Trait.* Deficiency of two determinants of alpha chain production produces a mild hypochromic microcytic anemia. There is no significant hemolysis or reticulocytosis. No therapy is required. In older children, the diagnosis is made by excluding iron deficiency, beta thalassemia trait and other causes of hypochromic microcytic anemia. In neonates, alpha thalassemia trait is manifested by a decreased MCV (less than 95) compared to normal in-

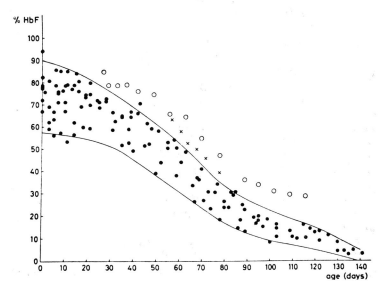

*Figure 66–10.* Decreasing concentration of fetal hemoglobin after birth. (Garby, L., Sjölin, S., and Vuille, J. C.: Acta Paediatr. *51*:245, 1962.)

**TABLE 66–7.** *Alpha Thalassemia Syndromes*

| | | Anemia | Hemolysis | $\alpha{:}\beta$ Chain Synthesis | Abnormal Hemoglobins Cord Blood | | Adult Blood |
|---|---|---|---|---|---|---|---|
| Normal | $\dfrac{\alpha/\alpha}{\alpha/\alpha}$ | None | None | 0.95–1.10 | 0–1% | $\gamma4$ | – – – |
| Silent carrier | $\dfrac{\alpha/-}{\alpha/\alpha}$ | None | None | 0.85–0.95 | 1–2% | $\gamma4$ | – – – |
| $\alpha$–Thalassemia trait | $\dfrac{-/-}{\alpha/\alpha}$ | Mild Hypochromic Microcytic | None | 0.72–0.82 | 5–6% | $\gamma4$ | – – – |
| Hemoglobin "H" disease | $\dfrac{-/-}{\alpha/-}$ | Moderate Hypochromic Microcytic | Moderate | 0.30–0.52 | 20–40% 0–5% | $\gamma4$ $\beta4$ | 20–40%  $\beta4$ |
| Homozygous $\alpha$-thalassemia ("hydrops") | $\dfrac{-/-}{-/-}$ | Severe Hypochromic Microcytic | Severe | 0 | 70–80% 15–20% 0–10% | $\gamma4$ $\beta4$ $\zeta_2\gamma_2$ | |

fants (MCV 100 to 120) (Schmaler et al.). The content of Bart's hemoglobin in cord blood is increased (5 to 6 per cent).

*Hemoglobin H Disease.* This disorder results from a deficiency of three determinants of alpha chain production. One parent has alpha thalassemia trait while the other is a silent carrier. Anemia is more severe than in alpha thalassemia trait, globin chain imbalance is greater and hemolysis may be more intense. Bart's hemoglobin accounts for 20 to 40 per cent of cord blood hemoglobin. Small amounts of hemoglobin H ($\beta_4$) also may be present. Both of these tetrameric hemoglobins are readily detected on hemoglobin electrophoresis.

*Homozygous Alpha Thalassemia ("Hydrops").* This disorder is caused by the absence of all four genetic loci for alpha chain synthesis. Both parents have alpha thalassemia trait. In the absence of alpha chains, cord blood contains Bart's hemoglobin and hemoglobin H. In addition, small amounts of hemoglobin Portland, the embryonic form of fetal hemoglobin, can be present. (In the absence of alpha chain production, zeta synthesis persists during fetal life.) Most affected infants are stillborn, although some may live for a few hours after birth. Death is due to severe anemia. The gamma and beta chain tetramers have a high oxygen affinity, which also contributes to the degree of asphyxia. These infants are hydropic at

birth, and thus are similar in appearance to neonates with severe erythroblastosis due to Rh incompatibility. Invariably there is hepatosplenomegaly. The mother has a hypochromic microcytic anemia. There is no Rh or ABO incompatibility, and the Coombs test on cord blood is negative.

BETA THALASSEMIA. This hemolytic anemia occurs throughout the world but the incidence is increased in countries surrounding the Mediterranean Sea. In the United States, it is the most common form of thalassemia seen in older children and adults. This is not specifically a neonatal problem since this disorder is due to decreased beta chain production. Infants with beta thalassemia are not anemic at birth.

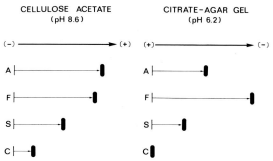

*Figure 66–11.* Migration of various hemoglobins at pH 8.6 and at pH 6.2.

Symptoms and signs first appear after 2 or 3 months of age, when the bulk of hemoglobin synthesis is due to beta chain production. The heterozygous state (thalassemia minor) is characterized by a mild hypochromic-microcytic anemia. This is a benign disorder that requires no specific therapy. These individuals have a normal life span. On the other hand, homozygous beta thalassemia (thalassemia major, or Cooley's anemia) is a severe hypochromic-microcytic anemia associated with marked hemolysis (due to accumulation of alpha chains). Most children with this disorder have a lifelong RBC transfusion requirement. Death commonly occurs before 20 years of age, usually from complications of iron overload (iron from RBC transfusions and increased intestinal absorption). Most cases of thalassemia major are diagnosed after 3 months of age, but before 1 year. A severe hemolytic anemia associated with marked hepatosplenomegaly occurs in late infancy. Hemoglobin electrophoresis indicates that almost all hemoglobin is of the fetal type, with a small amount of hemoglobin $A_2$. There is virtually no hemoglobin A.

GAMMA THALASSEMIA. The production of gamma polypeptides is regulated by four genes. The complete absence of gamma chains is incompatible with fetal life. Intermediate reduction of gamma polypeptide synthesis may produce a mild to moderate neonatal anemia characterized by a reduced percentage of fetal hemoglobin (Stamatoyannopoulos). This type of anemia resolves when significant beta chain synthesis begins.

CASE 66–4 (KAN, FORGET, AND NATHAN)

A full-term 2300 gm girl was noted to be jaundiced at 24 hours of age (bilirubin 13.7 mg). Hemoglobin was 10.4 gm per 100 ml, hematocrit 32 per cent, RBC count $3.8 \times 10^6$ $\mu$l. MCV 84 $\mu^3$, and MCH 27 pg. The reticulocyte count was 26 per cent, and there were 400 nucleated RBC's per 100 white cells. There was no Rh or ABO incompatibility, Coombs test was negative, iron and iron binding capacity were normal and there was no detectable RBC enzyme deficiency. Hemoglobin F content was 52 per cent (normal 60 to 85 per cent), and no hemoglobin Bart's was detected. The infant was transfused with packed RBC's and over the next few days nucleated RBC's disappeared, reticulocytes decreased and the hematocrit remained stable.

The infant's mother was hematologically normal, while her father had a hypochromic microcytic anemia that was diagnosed as $\beta$-thalassemia trait. At several months of age this infant was doing well, although she had a mild hypochromic microcytic anemia that clearly was due to beta thalassemia trait.

COMMENT. We frequently see neonates with severe hemolytic anemia which spontaneously disappears by several months of age, thus suggesting that some unique feature of the fetal RBC is responsible for hemolysis. This case is such an example. The presence of a hypochromic-microcytic anemia not related to iron deficiency (which occurs with chronic fetal blood loss) suggested one of the thalassemia disorders. Either alpha or gamma thalassemia could produce this degree of anemia. Alpha thalassemia was ruled out by the absence of Bart's hemoglobin in cord blood. Using very sophisticated techniques to measure the synthesis of separate globin chains, it was found that this child produced decreased amounts of gamma chains (i.e., gamma thalassemia trait). In addition, she manifested a lower than anticipated rate of beta chain synthesis (beta thalassemia trait), and thus her defect is best described as beta-gamma thalassemia. Neonatal hemolytic anemia was presumably a result of increased alpha chain accumulation in the absence of normal beta and gamma polypeptides. Hemolysis diminished as the infant got older and began to synthesize more beta chains. Her father had beta thalassemia trait, and as the patient became older she also developed the classical laboratory evidence of heterozygous beta thalassemia.

### Sickle Cell Anemia

Sickle cell anemia is caused by the production of abnormal beta globin chains. The resultant hemoglobin (alpha 2, beta-S 2) gels at low oxygen tension and thereby distorts the cell membrane forming sickled cells. Approximately 10 per cent of all Blacks in the United States are carriers of the sickle gene, and since this is an autosomal recessive disorder, one in 400 Black infants has sickle cell anemia. Individuals heterozygous for this abnormality (sickle cell trait) are asymptomatic and are not anemic. Homozygotes have sickle cell anemia and suffer from all the known vaso-occlusive and infectious problems associated with this disease. There is no anemia or sickling problem in the newborn period, since this is a beta chain abnormality. The small number of sickle cells present, however, may explain the hyperbilirubinemia occasionally seen in these neonates. The presence of sickle hemoglobin can be detected by the metabisulfite screening test ("sickle prep"). This screening procedure does not distinguish between sickle trait and sickle cell anemia, and therefore hemoglobin electrophoresis is required for definitive diagnosis. Both A and S hemoglobins are present in sickle trait while only S hemoglobin (and some fetal hemoglobin) is found in homozygous sickle cell anemia. Using conventional hemoglobin electrophoretic methods (pH 8.6, cellulose acetate) it is difficult to demonstrate the presence of small amounts of hemoglobin A when fetal hemoglobin is increased, as it is in the newborn period. It is difficult, therefore, to determine whether a newborn infant is heterozygous or homozygous for the sickle gene. By altering the conditions of electrophoresis (low pH), it is possible to separate hemoglobins A and F, and thus diagnose sickle cell disease in the newborn period (Schroeder, Jakway, and Powers).

Individuals heterozygous for the sickle gene and an additional hemoglobin abnormality may also have problems beyond the newborn period (Fig. 66–12). Heterozygosity for the sickle gene and beta thalassemia (each parent must have one defect) produces sickle-thalassemia. If one parent has hemoglobin C (another beta chain variant) while the other carries the sickle gene, there is a 25 per cent chance of offspring developing hemoglobin S-C disease. Both of these conditions (S-thalassemia, and S-C disease) manifest many of the same problems seen in sickle cell anemia, although the overall course generally is milder. These infants have no problems in the first 3 months of life.

Our approach to infants of mothers with sickle trait is as follows:

1. Whenever possible the father is evalu-

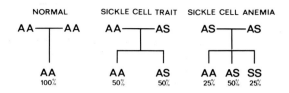

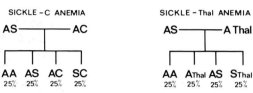

*Figure 66–12.*   Genetics of sickle cell variants.

ated for thalassemia trait (hypochromic-microcytic anemia) and hemoglobin S or C (hemoglobin electrophoresis). In the absence of these abnormalities, it is unlikely that a child will have one of the sickle syndromes.

2. Hemoglobin electrophoresis is done in the newborn period. This will reveal whether sickle hemoglobin is present. S-C disease can be detected at this time since hemoglobin F has an electrophoretic migration distinct from both S and C.

3. If hemoglobin S is detected on routine electrophoresis at birth, the procedure is repeated at a lower pH, where there is a clear resolution of hemoglobins A and F. This allows one to differentiate sickle trait from sickle cell anemia.

4. A practical alternative to (3) is to repeat the routine electrophoresis at 3 months of age. Hemoglobin F is decreased at this time and the presence of hemoglobin A easily can be detected. Waiting 3 months for a definitive diagnosis is justified medically, since the severe vaso-occlusive and infectious problems associated with sickle cell anemia are not seen before this time.

Infants born to mothers with sickle cell disease present more of a neonatal problem than those destined to develop sickle cell anemia after several months of age. It is well established that maternal morbidity and mortality are increased in pregnant women with sickle cell disease, although recent studies suggest that good obstetrical management can minimize these problems (Pritchard et al.). Nevertheless, fetal wastage and prematurity remain serious problems in these pregnancies. Approximately 35 per cent of all pregnancies end in early abortion, 17 per cent are associated with stillborns or neonatal deaths and only 48 per cent result in surviving children. Furthermore, 40 per cent of all viable infants are born premature, and 15 per cent are small for gestational age. These statistics reflect the inordinate vulnerability of the placenta to sickling. Current attempts to maintain normal placental function and decrease fetal wastage include exchange transfusion of maternal (sickle) blood for normal (hemoglobin A) blood early in the third trimester of pregnancy. It is known that this type of procedure is beneficial in other clinical conditions such as severe pulmonary sickling and central nervous system sickling. The clinical problems of neonates born to mothers with sickle cell disease (SS, S-C, S-thalassemia) are directly related to their degree of prematurity. These infants have no hematologic disease, although they will be carriers of the S, C or thalassemia gene as they begin to produce beta chains. In those cases in which the father also carries a gene for one of these hemoglobinopathies, the infant may develop hemolytic anemia at a later age.

## HYPOPLASTIC ANEMIA

Anemia due to an isolated defect in erythropoiesis is known as congenital hypoplastic anemia or the Blackfan-Diamond syndrome. Clinical manifestations of this rare idiopathic disorder generally become manifest during the first 6 months of life, although anemia is occasionally present at birth. Characteristically there is a moderate-to-severe normochromic-normocytic anemia associated with reticulocytopenia. Bilirubin is not increased. No platelet or leukocyte abnormalities are present. Bone marrow cellularity is normal to slightly decreased, but there is a striking paucity of erythroid precursors.

Corticosteroids are the backbone of therapy for children with Blackfan-Diamond anemia. In most cases, prednisone (4 mg per kg per day) produces a reticulocytosis after 1 to 2 weeks of therapy, and subsequently the steroid dose can be reduced to much lower levels. Alternate-day therapy should be used for children requiring long-term steroid administration. In most cases this will sustain a clinical remission while avoiding many of the known side effects of prolonged steroid therapy. In some cases, clinical remission can be maintained on steroid doses that are actually within the normal physiologic range of hormone production by the adrenal gland. The reason for this inordinate erythropoietic sensitivity to steroids is unknown. Packed RBC transfusions are given to symptomatic children who fail to respond to prednisone. Iron, folate and other hematinics have no role in the therapy of this disorder.

The prognosis for children who respond to steroids is very good. Nonresponders, on the other hand, generally develop hemosiderosis secondary to their lifelong RBC transfusion requirement. These children usually succumb to complications of iron storage during the second to third decade of life.

### CASE 66–5

A 2650 gm girl born after 38 weeks of gestation was noted to be pale at birth. Physical examination revealed no tachycardia, tachypnea, hepatosplenomegaly or other abnormality. Bleeding was not excessive at the time of delivery, and there was no abnormality of the placenta or umbilical cord. The following laboratory data were obtained: hemoglobin 11.4 gm per 100 ml, MCV 102, MCH 34, reticulocytes 2.4 per cent, WBC count 17,400, platelet count 230,000, bilirubin 2.8 mg per 100 ml. The mother's blood type was O-positive, while the infant's was B-positive. Coombs test was negative. A Kleihauer-Betke preparation of the maternal blood smear did not reveal RBC's with fetal hemoglobin.

At this time it was thought that anemia was due to a fetomaternal bleed, and iron therapy (2 mg Fe per kg, tid) was started. At 7 weeks, her hemoglobin had fallen to 6.8 gm per 100 ml and she was transfused with packed RBC's up to a hemoglobin of 11.5 gm per 100 ml. By 3 months of age her hemoglobin again decreased to 7.5 gm per 100 ml and the reticulocyte count was only 0.1 per cent. Bone marrow examination was normal except that erythroid precursors were virtually nonexistent. The infant was started on prednisone (4 mg per kg) and within 9 days reticulocytosis was noted. Prednisone was decreased to 0.2 mg per kg over the next 6 weeks, after which the hemoglobin was 9.2 gm per 100 ml. The steroid dose was further reduced to 0.2 mg every other day and at 7 months of age, when her hemoglobin was 11.9 gm per 100 ml, prednisone was discontinued altogether. Approximately 3 months later, hemoglobin again had decreased (7.8 gm per 100 ml) and the reticulocyte count was only 0.2 per cent. Steroids were restarted and erythropoiesis again was stimulated. Subsequently the child has been able to maintain a normal hemoglobin while on a small maintenance dose of prednisone (0.2 mg per kg, qod).

COMMENT. The initial diagnosis was thought to be anemia due to a fetomaternal blood loss. The absence of fetal cells in the maternal circulation could have been caused by ABO incompatibility between mother and child. The diagnosis of congenital hypoplastic anemia was suspected because of the lower than expected hemoglobin and also because of a failure to respond to iron therapy. This suspicion was confirmed by the absence of erythroid precursors in the marrow and the dramatic response to corticosteroids. Newborn infants normally manifest erythroid hypoplasia during the first few weeks of life, and it is frequently difficult to distinguish this from the marrow picture of congenital hypoplastic anemia. The obvious difference is that erythropoiesis resumes spontaneously in normal infants (see Physiologic Anemia of Infancy and Prematurity).

## PHYSIOLOGIC ANEMIA OF INFANCY AND PREMATURITY

At birth the mean hemoglobin of term infants (17.0 gm per 100 ml) is slightly greater than in prematures (16.0 gm per 100 ml). The hemoglobin concentration in term infants subsequently decreases to a plateau at which it remains throughout the first year of life (Table 66–8). This is known as the *physiologic anemia of infancy*. A similar process occurs in premature infants except that hemoglobin falls more rapidly and reaches a lower concentration. This is known as the *anemia of prematurity*. After 1 year of age there is little difference between the hemoglobin values of term and premature infants.

### PHYSIOLOGIC ANEMIA OF INFANCY

The hemoglobin-oxygen saturation at birth increases from 50 per cent to 95 per cent, thus producing an increase in blood oxygen content and a cessation of erythropoiesis. Subsequently, the hemoglobin concentration begins to decrease, since there is no replacement of aged RBC's as they are normally removed from the circulation. Iron from degraded RBC's is stored in tissue for future hemoglobin synthesis. The hemoglobin concentration continues

*TABLE 66–8.   Hemoglobin Changes During First Year of Life*

| Week | Term | Premature (1.2–2.5 kg) | Premature (<1.2 kg) |
|---|---|---|---|
| 0 | 17.0 (14.0–20.0) | 16.4 (13.5–19.0) | 16.0 (13.0–18.0) |
| 1 | 18.8 | 16.0 | 14.8 |
| 3 | 15.9 | 13.5 | 13.4 |
| 6 | 12.7 | 10.7 | 9.7 |
| 10 | 11.4 | 9.8 | 8.5 |
| 20 | 12.0 | 10.4 | 9.0 |
| 50 | 12.0 | 11.5 | 11.0 |
| Lowest hemoglobin (mean) | 10.3 (9.5–11.0) | 9.0 (8.0–10.0) | 7.1 (6.5–9.0) |
| Time of nadir | 6–12 Weeks | 5–10 Weeks | 4–8 Weeks |

to fall until a point is reached at which tissue oxygen needs are greater than oxygen delivery. This occurs sometime between 6 and 12 weeks of age, when hemoglobin has reached a level of 9.5 to 11.0 gm per 100 ml. Erythropoiesis resumes at this time, and iron previously stored in reticuloendothelial tissues is utilized for hemoglobin synthesis. These stores provide normal term infants with sufficient iron for hemoglobin synthesis until 20 weeks of age. It is unnecessary to administer iron during this period, since it will not prevent the physiologic decrease in hemoglobin. Any iron that is given will be added to stores for future use. It must be emphasized that this physiologic hemoglobin decrease does not represent "anemia" in the true sense of the term. Rather, it is a reflection of the excess oxygen delivery relative to tissue $O_2$ needs. There is no hematological problem and no therapy is required.

## ANEMIA OF PREMATURITY

The magnitude of anemia in prematures is directly related to birth weight, and in large measure it is an exaggeration of the physiologic anemia of infancy. The anemia of prematurity, however, differs in several respects from that seen in term infants.

1. The hemoglobin nadir is reached at an earlier age (4 to 8 weeks). Presumably this is due to the relatively decreased RBC survival of premature infants compared to term neonates (Pearson).

2. The hemoglobin nadir is lower in prematures (6.5 to 9.0 gm per 100 ml) compared to term infants (9.5 to 11.0 gm per 100 ml). This difference may be a function of decreased tissue oxygen requirements, because premature infants consume less oxygen (ml $O_2$ per kg per min) than term neonates (Mestyan et al.). In accord with this concept erythropoietin is produced by term infants at hemoglobins of 10 to 11 gm per 100 ml, while no erythropoietin is detected in prematures at significantly lower hemoglobin concentrations (Buchanan and Schwartz, McIntosh). It is unlikely that this merely represents blunted erythropoietin responsiveness, for hypoxic prematures with respiratory or cardiac disease readily generate increased erythropoietin levels.

The lower hemoglobin concentrations seen in premature infants may thus represent a physiological state of balanced oxygen delivery and oxygen needs. This is supported by the clinical observation that many premature infants with hemoglobin levels of 6 to 7 gm per 100 ml are quite healthy, with no evidence of cardiac or respiratory distress.

3. Although the hemoglobin concentration of premature and term infants is similar at birth, the total body hemoglobin (and iron) content is significantly less in prematures. Consequently, iron depletion occurs earlier in prematures than in term infants. Most prematures are endowed with sufficient iron to maintain hemoglobin synthesis for 10 to 14 weeks. Iron administered before this time is stored for later use, but it does not influence the rate or level of the physiological decrease in hemoglobin (Schulman). In fact, iron given to prematures during the first weeks of life may actually aggravate the anemia of prematurity (see discussion of vitamin E, below). After 2 months of age, however, iron supplements must be given in order to maintain hemoglobin synthesis and to prevent iron deficiency (the late anemia of prematurity). Iron is given as ferrous sulfate (2 mg of elemental iron per kg per day for a period of 6 months). This amount of iron is met by currently available iron-fortified formulas.

4. *Role of vitamin E deficiency.* Vitamin E is an antiperoxidant compound vital to the integrity of erythrocytes. Red blood cells are susceptible to membrane injury and hemolysis in the absence of this vitamin (Fig. 66–13). Three factors are integrally related to the pathophysiology of this hemolysis: lipid composition of RBC membrane, catalysts of lipid peroxidation and vitamin E. 1) Lipid composition of erythrocytes is influenced by the quality of lipids in plasma and diet. An increase in dietary polyunsaturated fatty acids (PUFA) increases RBC membrane PUFA content. 2) Unsaturated bonds in PUFA undergo oxidation with the formation of free radicals and lipid peroxides. High concentrations of oxygen and certain heavy metals (iron) catalyze this reaction. Once free radicals and lipid peroxides are formed, these compounds further catalyze the peroxidation of

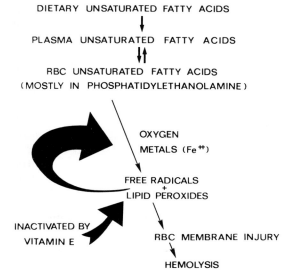

DIETARY UNSATURATED FATTY ACIDS

PLASMA UNSATURATED FATTY ACIDS

RBC UNSATURATED FATTY ACIDS
(MOSTLY IN PHOSPHATIDYLETHANOLAMINE)

OXYGEN
METALS (Fe$^{++}$)

FREE RADICALS
+
LIPID PEROXIDES

INACTIVATED BY
VITAMIN E

RBC MEMBRANE INJURY

HEMOLYSIS

*Figure 66–13.* Hemolysis of vitamin E deficient erythrocytes.

**TABLE 66–9.  *Vitamin E Responsive Hemolytic Anemia in Premature Infants***

|  | Pretreatment | Post-treatment |
|---|---|---|
| Vitamin E (mg/dl) | $0.25 \pm 0.15$ | $0.95 \pm 0.23$ |
| $H_2O_2$ Hemolysis (%) | $80 \pm 14$ | $8 \pm 10$ |
| Hgb (gm/100 ml) | $7.6 \pm 1.1$ | $9.8 \pm 0.8$ |
| Reticulocytes (%) | $8.2 \pm 2.9$ | $3.0 \pm 1.5$ |

*Vitamin E dependent hemolytic anemia in premature infants ($1480 \pm 205$ gm) diagnosed at 6 to 11 weeks of age. Infants were treated with 270 to 1094 international units (IU) of vitamin E. The mean response to treatment was seen in 10 days. (Data from Oski, F. A., and Barness, L. A.: J. Pediatr. 70:211, 1967.)

PUFA (a chain reaction). 3) Vitamin E inactivates lipid peroxides and thereby inhibits further lipid peroxidation. The requirement for vitamin E is increased when dietary PUFA are increased or in the presence of excessive catalytic activity from $O_2$ or metals. Lipid peroxides produce RBC membrane injury and hemolysis in the absence of adequate vitamin E.

Premature infants are endowed with significantly less vitamin E than term neonates. This deficiency state persists for 2 to 3 months, at which time their intestinal absorption of vitamin E becomes similar to that of term infants. Hemolytic anemia occurring in premature infants (less than 1500 gm) at 6 to 10 weeks of age is one known consequence of vitamin E deficiency (Oski and Barness, Ritchie and co-workers). This anemia is characterized by decreased hemoglobin, reticulocytosis, reduced vitamin E levels and increased RBC peroxide hemolysis (a measure of RBC vitamin E content). Signs of hemolytic anemia rapidly disappear following vitamin E administration (Table 66–9).

This observation suggests that the anemia of prematurity may in part be due to vitamin E deficiency. Oski and Barness demonstrated that premature infants given daily vitamin E (15 IU per day) had higher hemoglobins and lower reticulocytes than a control group not given the vitamin (Table 66–10). Similar results have been reported in several elegant studies by Melhorn and Gross. Thus it appears that vitamin E deficiency may contribute to the *magnitude* of anemia in prematurity.

Since iron catalyzes the peroxidation of PUFA in vitro, Melhorn and Gross questioned whether iron therapy aggravated the anemia of prematurity. After 6 weeks of age, they observed lower hemoglobins and higher reticulocytes in neonates given iron (8 mg per kg per day) compared to infants given no additional supplements. Because this study was done in prematures receiving therapeutic, rather than prophylactic, iron dosages, Williams and her co-workers re-examined this problem in neonates given artificial formulas fortified with iron (approximately 10 to 15 mg iron per liter formula or 3 to 4 mg iron per day). The results of this limited but provocative study emphasize the importance of dietary fatty acid composition in addition to iron content (Table 66–11). Infants fed formulas low in linoleic acid (similar to breast milk) manifested the same hemoglobin and reticulocyte count, with or without added iron. Neonates fed with formulas containing an increased content of linoleic acid (with or without iron) demonstrated a positive peroxide hemolysis test, thus indicating a state of relative vitamin E deficiency. Reticulocytosis and decreased hemoglobins, however, were seen only in neonates fed formulas with both increased linoleic acid and iron.

**TABLE 66–10.** *Effect of Supplemental Vitamin E on Anemia of Prematurity*[*]

|  | Control | Vitamin E (15 IU/day) |
|---|---|---|
| Birth weight | 1176 ± 182 Gm | 1278 ± 180 Gm |
| *6–8 Weeks of age* |  |  |
| Vitamin E (mg/100 ml) | 0.22 ± 0.10 | 1.00 ± 0.25 |
| $H_2O_2$ hemolysis (%) | 66 ± 21 | 9 ± 9 |
| Lowest Hgb (Gm/100 ml) | 7.7 ± 1.5 | 9.2 ± 1.3 |
| Highest reticulocytes (%) | 6.7 ± 2.5 | 3.1 ± 0.7 |

[*]Premature infants were given prophylactic vitamin E (15 international units per day) and the vitamin E level, peroxide hemolysis, hemoglobin concentration and reticulocyte count were measured after 6 to 8 weeks. These values were compared to a group of control infants not given vitamin E supplements. (Data from Oski, F. A., and Barness, L. A.: J. Pediatr. 79:211, 1967.)

In summary, the anemia of prematurity can be separated into early and late phases. The two components of the early anemia are due to 1) an aggravation of the normal physiologic anemia of infancy (not preventable), and 2) a low grade of hemolysis due to vitamin E deficiency (preventable). The late phase of anemia occurs at 3 to 4 months after erythropoiesis resumes and iron stores are depleted (preventable).

On the basis of our current concepts of anemia in prematures, an ideal physiological approach to the nutritional management of these infants can be devised.

1. Vitamin E (25 IU or 0.5 ml of Aquason E) should be given daily until 8 to 10 weeks of age. There is no known toxic effect of vitamin E given in these dosages to premature infants.
2. Formulas similar to mother's milk (low in linoleic acid) should be used in order to maintain a low content of RBC polyunsaturated fatty acids. Currently this is satisfied by all commercially available formula preparations.
3. During the first 2 months, iron supplements are not needed. In fact, iron should be avoided, since this metal may enhance lipid peroxidation.
4. After 2 months of age, iron supplements (2 mg per kg per day) must be given in order to prevent the late anemia of prematurity.

## POLYCYTHEMIA

An increased hematocrit may reflect a relatively decreased plasma volume or an absolute increase in RBC mass. True polycythemia is due to an increased RBC mass.

Polycythemia in older children is seen with arterial hypoxemia (cyanotic heart disease, pulmonary disorders), tumors (renal, hepatic, cerebellar) and abnormal hemoglo-

**TABLE 66–11.** *Influence of Iron Supplementation on Anemia of Prematurity*[*]

| *Formula* | (1) | (2) | (3) | (4) |
|---|---|---|---|---|
| Linoleic acid content | 12.8% | 12.8% | 32.4% | 32.4% |
| Vitamin E (IU/liter) | 10 | 10 | 10 | 10 |
| Iron (mg/liter) | 0 | 13.3 | 0 | 12.0 |
| *5 Weeks* |  |  |  |  |
| Peroxide hemolysis (%) | 1.8 ± 4.7 | 3.2 ± 2.2 | 62.2 ± 26.0 | 53.0 ± 35.5 |
| Hemoglobin (gm/100 ml) | 10.4 ± 1.8 | 9.6 ± 0.6 | 10.6 ± 1.5 | 8.1 ± 1.3 |
| Reticulocytes (%) | 2.7 ± 1.3 | 1.8 ± 1.5 | 2.3 ± 1.1 | 5.2 ± 2.5 |

[*]Premature infants were fed formulas containing low (1,2) or high (3,4) linoleic acid content, and with (2,4) or without (1,3) added iron. All formulas contained low supplements of vitamin E. The peroxide hemolysis, hemoglobin and reticulocyte count were measured after 5 weeks. (Data obtained from Williams, M. L., et al.: N. Engl. J. Med. 292:887, 1975.)

bins (increased oxygen affinity). Polycythemia vera or primary erythrocytosis is rare. Neonatal polycythemia is generally due to fetal hypertransfusion or to one of the placental dysfunction syndromes. Hypertransfusion occurs with delayed umbilical cord clamping (see RBC Physiology at Birth) or maternal blood loss into the fetal circulation (Michael and Mauer). In addition, twin to twin transfusions can produce polycythemia in one infant (usually the larger) and anemia in the other twin (Sacks). Neonatal polycythemia occasionally is associated with toxemia, placenta previa, postmaturity and small for gestational age infants (Humbert et al.). It is thought that the increased RBC mass associated with these placental insufficiency syndromes reflects fetal hypoxia and increased erythropoietin production. Recently, however, Oh and his co-workers have suggested an additional mechanism to explain hypoxia-induced polycythemia. They observed that acute maternal (and fetal) hypoxia increased the fetal RBC mass by augmenting the fraction of placental blood transfused into the fetus.

Blood viscosity increases at hematocrits greater than 60 per cent, and this in turn leads to a reduction of blood flow (Fig. 66–14). Oxygen transport, which is determined by hemoglobin (oxygen content) and blood flow, is maximal in the normal hematocrit range. At low hematocrits, oxygen transport is decreased because of limited oxygen capacity, while at higher hematocrits, decreased oxygen transport is due to reduced blood flow. These changes are further modified when the effects of normovolemia and hypervolemia are compared. Hypervolemia is advantageous, since this distends the vasculature, decreases peripheral resistance and thereby increases blood flow and oxygen transport at any given hematocrit. These physiologic concepts are of therapeutic importance, since most cases of polycythemia are associated with an increased blood volume (i.e., hypervolemia).

Most polycythemic infants are asymptomatic. The physical examination is normal except for a plethoric appearance and occasionally cyanosis. Cyanosis is due to relative stasis of high hematocrit blood. Symptoms of hyperviscosity may occasionally be present: respiratory distress, convulsions, congestive heart failure, priapism and renal vein thrombosis. Hyperbilirubinemia is common, because an elevated RBC mass increases the bilirubin load to the liver (1 gm hemoglobin produces 34 mg bilirubin). Hypoglycemia and hypocalcemia are also associated with neonatal polycythemia.

The diagnosis of neonatal polycythemia is not as clear cut as that of anemia. Certainly most infants are polycythemic if adult or childhood criteria of polycythemia are applied. In neonates, however, polycythemia is defined as a hemoglobin greater than 22 gm per 100 ml, or a hematocrit greater than 65 per cent. The etiology of polycythemia can often be ascertained by history (twin pregnancy, delayed cord clamping) or physical examination (small for gestational age infant). In many cases, however, there is no apparent cause.

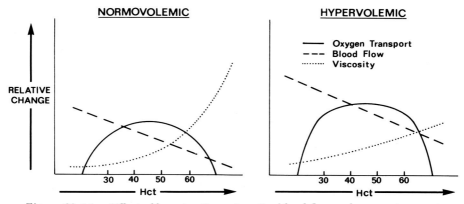

*Figure 66–14.* Effect of hematocrit on viscosity, blood flow and oxygen transport.

It is our policy to decrease the RBC mass of all infants with symptomatic polycythemia: respiratory difficulties, CNS symptomatology, congestive heart failure. Whenever possible, partial exchange transfusion with fresh plasma is preferred over simple phlebotomy, since oxygen transport is better in the face of hypervolemia. If signs of congestive heart failure persist following hematocrit reduction, diuretics and digitalization are indicated. The general principles for the partial exchange have been outlined by Oski and Naiman:

$$\text{Volume of blood exchanged for plasma} =$$
$$\text{Blood volume} \times \frac{\text{Observed Hct} - \text{Desired Hct}}{\text{Observed Hct}}$$

Assume blood value of 100 ml per kg. Desired Hct is 60 per cent, since viscosity is relatively normal at this level. Exchange should be done in 10 ml volumes.

Example: A 3 kg dyspneic infant with an 80 per cent hematocrit requires a partial exchange.

$$\text{Blood volume} = 3 \text{ kg} \times 100 \text{ ml/kg} = 300 \text{ ml}$$
$$\frac{\text{Observed Hct} - \text{Desired Hct}}{\text{Observed Hct}} = \frac{80-60}{80} = 0.25$$

Therefore, volume of exchange = 300 ml × 0.25 = 75 ml.

The treatment of asymptomatic neonates with polycythemia is not as clearly defined. In view of the frequency of hyperbilirubinemia, our current approach is to do a "prophylactic" partial exchange in neonates with hematocrits greater than 75 per cent. Close monitoring for signs of hypoglycemia and hypocalcemia is necessary in all polycythemic infants.

***TABLE 66–12.** Etiology of Neonatal Polycythemia*

| |
| --- |
| Placental hypertransfusion |
|    Delayed cord clamping |
|    Twin-twin transfusion |
|    Maternal-fetal transfusion |
| |
| Placental insufficiency syndromes |
|    Small for gestational age infants |
|    Toxemia |
|    Postmaturity |
|    Placenta previa |

CASE 66–6

A gravida 2, para 1, white female delivered a 2950 gm male infant following a normal pregnancy, labor and delivery. At birth the child had an Apgar score of 6. Physical examination revealed a cyanotic infant with a grade III/VI systolic heart murmur. The liver edge was palpable 2 cm below the right costal margin, and the spleen tip was palpable. Chest X-ray revealed a markedly enlarged heart with increased pulmonary vascular markings. The hemoglobin was 26 gm per 100 ml and the hematocrit was 79 per cent. There were no other hematologic abnormalities. The child was partially exchanged with plasma and the post-exchange hematocrit was 62 per cent. Subsequently the child's color improved, heart murmur disappeared and there were no remaining signs of congestive heart failure.

**COMMENT.** The clinical findings in this infant were initially very suspicious of organic heart disease. All cardiac signs cleared rapidly once polycythemia was recognized and treated, thus indicating that the cardiac effects were secondary to polycythemia-induced hyperviscosity. This series of events is distinct from that seen in older children with cyanotic heart disease and polycythemia. The increased RBC mass in these infants represents a compensatory adjustment by which adequate oxygen transport is maintained in the presence of arterial hypoxemia. Consequently, phlebotomy of RBC's from these patients can produce an acute hypoxic insult. During the newborn period, however, infants with cyanotic heart disease are not polycythemic (Gatti et al.), and it is extremely unlikely that neonatal polycythemia is due to underlying organic heart disease.

## METHEMOGLOBINEMIA

Hemoglobin iron is normally in the reduced or ferrous ($Fe^{++}$) state. Methemoglobin is an oxidized derivative of hemoglobin in which iron is in the ferric ($Fe^{+++}$) state. In contrast to ferrohemoglobin, ferrihemoglobin (methemoglobin) does not complex with oxygen. Significant methemoglobinemia, therefore, reduces blood oxygen capacity and transport.

In vivo small amounts of hemoglobin are

continually being oxidized by endogenous agents including oxygen itself (auto-oxidation). Normally, however, less than 1 per cent of hemoglobin is methemoglobin, because RBC's can reduce the relatively low levels of ferrihemoglobin that are formed:

1. *NADH-methemoglobin reductase* is the enzyme that catalyzes the reduction of methemoglobin under physiologic conditions. Hereditary deficiency of this enzyme produces methemoglobinemia. NADH (dihydronicotinamide adenine dinucleotide) is a required cofactor produced by metabolic reactions.

2. *NADPH-methemoglobin reductase* by itself is unable to reduce methemoglobin to any significant extent. Individuals lacking this enzyme do not have methemoglobinemia. In the presence of certain redox compounds (e.g., methylene blue), however, this enzyme rapidly reduces methemoglobin to ferrohemoglobin. Thus, this enzyme is important in the treatment of methemoglobinemia with methylene blue. NADPH (dihydronicotinamide adenine dinucleotide phosphate) is a required cofactor that is generated by cell metabolism. G6PD is one of the main sites of NADPH production in RBC's.

3. *Reduced glutathione (GSH)* can directly and nonenzymatically reduce ferrihemoglobin. Quantitatively, this reaction is less important than NADH-methemoglobin reductase.

An increased methemoglobin concentration is caused by disruption of the delicate balance between oxidation and reduction of hemoglobin iron. Two forms of methemoglobinemia are seen: acquired or toxic methemoglobinemia (common), and congenital methemoglobinemia (rare).

*Acquired methemoglobinemia* occurs in normal individuals exposed to increased concentrations of chemicals that oxidize hemoglobin iron. During the first weeks of life neonates are particularly susceptible to this form of methemoglobinemia: 1) Fetal hemoglobin is more readily oxidized to the ferric state than is hemoglobin A (Martin and Huisman). 2) Neonates are transiently deficient in NADH-methemoglobin reductase activity (Ross), a deficiency that persists for the first 3 or 4 months of life (Bartos and Desforges). One class of chemicals that will readily oxidize hemoglobin iron includes nitrite and nitrate compounds. Nitrite is the active agent. Nitrates are converted to nitrites by intestinal bacteria. Neonates given "well water" with an increased nitrate con-

tent occasionally develop methemoglobinemia (Comly). Also, the feeding of vegetable preparations with high levels of nitrate (cabbage, spinach, beets, occasionally carrots) can produce methemoglobinemia in infants (Keating et al.). Aniline derivatives constitute another class of chemicals that will oxidize hemoglobin, and methemoglobinemia has been caused in neonates by marking nursery diapers with aniline dyes. Drugs administered prior to delivery can also produce methemoglobinemia in mothers and newborn infants. Prilocaine, a local anesthetic used for obstetrical purposes, is such an agent (Climie et al.). It should be noted that most agents capable of oxidizing hemoglobin will, in fact, produce methemoglobin in normal individuals if the concentration of oxidant chemical is sufficiently high. Increased infant susceptibility to these chemicals during the first weeks of life is relative to fetal hemoglobin content and the degree of NADH-methemoglobin reductase deficiency.

*Congenital methemoglobinemia* can be due to inherited hemoglobin or enzyme abnormalities. 1) *Hemoglobin M disorders* are rare autosomal dominant defects brought about by amino acid substitutions in the normal globin chain. As a result of these substitutions, heme iron is more stable in the ferric than the ferrous state. The normal methemoglobin reductive capacity cannot compensate for this instability of ferrous heme. M hemoglobins can be caused by alpha or beta chain defects, but only alpha chain abnormalities are present in the newborn period. Heterozygotes have increased methemoglobin levels and some degree of cyanosis but otherwise are asymptomatic. No therapy is indicated (and none is possible). The homozygous state is obviously incompatible with life. 2) *NADH-methemoglobin reductase deficiency* is a rare autosomal recessive disorder in which the rate of ferrihemoglobin reduction is markedly reduced. Heterozygotes are asymptomatic and do not have methemoglobinemia unless challenged by toxic agents. Homozygote deficients generally have 15 to 40 per cent methemoglobin levels. These patients are cyanotic but otherwise asymptomatic.

The cardinal clinical manifestation of methemoglobinemia is cyanosis without evidence of cardiac or respiratory disease (normal physical examination, chest x-ray, EKG, and arterial $Po_2$). Cyanosis may be present at birth (suggesting hereditary methemoglobinemia) or may suddenly appear in an otherwise asymptomatic infant (suggesting toxic or acquired methemoglobinemia). Blood appears dark in color but, in contrast to deoxygenated blood, mixing with air does not change the color to bright red. This is the basis of a simple screening test to detect methemoglobin (Harley and Celermajer): A drop of blood is placed on filter paper and then allowed to dry while the filter paper is waved in air. Blood that is not saturated with oxygen turns red, while methemoglobin remains brown. This test detects levels of ferrihemoglobin greater than 10 per cent of total hemoglobin. Most laboratories can quantitatively measure methemoglobin concentrations using spectrophotometric techniques (Evelyn and Malloy). Cyanosis is apparent at

**TABLE 66–13.** *Approach to Infants with Cyanosis and Methemoglobinemia*

---

*Cyanosis associated with respiratory and cardiac findings*
  Blood turns red when mixed with air
  Decreased arterial $Po_2$
  Consider pulmonary, cardiac or CNS disease

*Cyanosis with or without respiratory and cardiac findings*
  Blood turns red when mixed with air
  Normal arterial $Po_2$
  Consider polycythemia syndromes (αOCBC)

*Cyanosis without respiratory or cardiac findings*
  Blood remains dark after mixing with air
  Arterial $Po_2$ normal
  Consider methemoglobinemia syndromes:
  A. Rapid clearing of methemoglobin following methylene blue
    (1) Consider toxic methemoglobinemia (look for environmental oxidants)
    (2) Consider NADH-methemoglobin reductase deficiency (do enzyme assay)
  B. Reappearance of methemoglobinemia after initial response to methylene blue
    (1) Consider NADH-methemoglobin reductase deficiency
  C. No change in methemoglobin following methylene blue
    (1) Consider hemoglobin M disorders (do hemoglobin electrophoresis)
    (2) Consider associated G6PD deficiency (do enzyme assay)

---

methemoglobin levels of 1.5 gm per 100 ml (10 per cent of total hemoglobin). Symptoms due to decreased oxygen transport are generally not apparent until 30 to 40 per cent of hemoglobin is oxidized to methemoglobin. Levels greater than 70 per cent are incompatible with life. Methemoglobinemia is not associated with anemia, hemolysis or other hematologic abnormalities.

Neonates with greater than 15 to 20 per cent methemoglobin are treated with methylene blue (1 mg per kg as a 1 per cent solution in normal saline). The response to methylene blue is both therapeutic and diagnostic. A rapid decrease in methemoglobin occurs within 1 to 2 hours if the cause of methemoglobin is due to an acquired toxic agent or a deficiency of NADH-methemoglobin reductase. Failure to note improvement following methylene blue suggests one of the M hemoglobins, and this can be confirmed by hemoglobin electrophoresis. Decreased NADPH generation (i.e., G6PD deficiency) also produces a less than optimal response to methylene blue. (It should be pointed out that G6PD deficiency per se is not a *cause* of methemoglobinemia but rather it may cause a poor response to methylene blue.) A reappearance of methemoglobinemia after an initial response to methylene blue suggests a deficiency of NADH-methemoglobin reductase, although the persistence of an occult oxidant must be kept in mind. The diagnosis of NADH-methemoglobin reductase deficiency requires an enzyme assay, which is done in specialized hematology laboratories. Most infants with hereditary methemoglobinemia are asymptomatic and require no therapy. In older children, therapy is occasionally given for cosmetic reasons to decrease cyanosis. This is readily accomplished with daily oral administration of ascorbic acid or methylene blue. Methylene blue will produce blue urine, but this is harmless.

## REFERENCES

*Normal Erythrocyte Physiology in the Fetus and Neonate*
Allen, D. W., Wyman, J., and Smith, G. A.: The oxygen equilibrium of fetal and adult hemoglobin. J. Biol. Chem. *203*:81, 1953.

Bauer, C., Ludwig, I., and Ludwig, M.: Different effects of 2,3-diphosphoglycerate and adenosine triphosphate on oxygen affinity of adult and fetal hemoglobin. Life Sci. 7:1339, 1968.

Delivoria-Papadopoulos, M., Roncevic, N. P., and Oski, F. A.: Postnatal changes in oxygen transport of term, premature, and sick infants: The role of red cell 2,3-diphosphoglycerate and adult hemoglobin. Pediatr. Res. 5:235, 1971.

Finne, P. H.: Erythropoietin levels in cord blood as an indicator of intrauterine hypoxia. Acta Paediatr. Scand. 55:478, 1966.

Finne, P. H., and Halvorsen, S.: Regulation of erythropoiesis in the fetus and newborn. Arch. Dis. Child. 47:683, 1972.

Gairdner, D., Marks, J., Roscoe, J. D., and Brettell, R. O.: The fluid shift from the vascular compartment immediately after birth. Arch. Dis. Child. 33:489, 1958.

Jacobson, L. O., Marks, E. K., and Gaston, E. O.: Studies on erythropoiesis. XII. The effect of transfusion-induced polycythemia in the mother on the fetus. Blood 14:644, 1959.

Lanzkowsky, P.: The influence of maternal iron deficiency on the haemoglobin of the infant. Arch. Dis. Child. 36:205, 1961.

Oski, F. A., and Delivoria-Papadopoulos, M.: The red cell, 2,3-diphosphoglycerate, and tissue oxygen release. J. Pediatr. 77:941, 1970.

Usher, R., and Lind, J.: Blood volume of the newborn premature infant. Acta Paediatr. Scand. 54:419, 1965.

Usher, R., Shepard, M., and Lind, J.: The blood volume of the newborn infant and placental transfusion. Acta Paediatr. Scand. 52:497, 1963.

*General Approach to Anemic Infants*

Gill, F. M., and Schwartz, E.: Anemia in early infancy. Pediatr. Clin. North Am. 19:841, 1972.

Kevy, S. V.: The storage of erythrocytes. *In* Nathan, D. G., and Oski, F. A. (Eds.): Hematology of Infancy and Childhood. Philadelphia, W. B. Saunders Co., 1974, p. 860.

Matoth, Y., Zaizor, R., and Varsano, I.: Postnatal changes in some red cell parameters. Acta Paediatr. Scand. 60:317, 1971.

Naiman, J. L., Punett, H. H., Lischner, H. W., Destine, M. L., and Arey, J. B.: Possible graft-versus-host reaction after intrauterine transfusion for Rh erythroblastosis fetalis. N. Engl. J. Med. 281:697, 1969.

Oh, W., and Lind, J.: Venous and capillary hematocrit in newborn infants and placental transfusion. Acta Paediatr. Scand. 55:38, 1966.

Parkman, R., Mosier, D., Umansky, I., Cochran, W., Carpenter, C. B., and Rosen, F. S.: Graft-versus-host disease after intrauterine and exchange transfusions for hemolytic disease of the newborn. N. Engl. J. Med. 290:359, 1974.

Schwartz, A. D.: Differential diagnosis of neonatal anemia. Paediatrician 3:107, 1974.

Seip, M.: The reticulocyte level and erythrocyte production judged from reticulocyte studies in newborn infants during the first week of life. Acta Paediatr. Scand. 44:355, 1955.

*Hemorrhagic Anemia*

Cohen, F., Zuelzer, W. W., Gustafson, D. C., and Evans, M. M.: Mechanisms of isoimmunization. I. The transplacental passage of fetal erythrocytes in homo-specific pregnancies. Blood 23:621, 1964.

Grobbelaar, B. G., and Dunning, E. K.: A method of calculating the volume of transplacental foetomaternal haemorrhage. Brit. J. Haematol. 17:231, 1969.

Kirkman, H. N., and Riley, H. D.: Posthemorrhagic anemia and shock in the newborn due to hemorrhage during delivery: A report of 8 cases. Pediatrics 24:92, 1959.

Kirkman, H. N., and Riley, H. D.: Posthemorrhagic anemia and shock in the newborn. A review. Pediatrics 24:97, 1959.

Leape, L. L., and Bordy, M. D.: Neonatal rupture of the spleen. Report of a case successfully treated after spontaneous cessation of hemorrhage. Pediatrics 47:101, 1971.

Leonard, S., and Anthony, B.: Giant cephalohematoma of newborn. Am. J. Dis. Child. 101:170, 1961.

Montague, A. C. W., and Krevans, J. R.: Transplacental hemorrhage in cesarean section. Amer. J. Obstet. Gynecol. 95:1115, 1966.

Pachman, D. J.: Massive hemorrhage in the scalp of the newborn infant. Hemorrhagic caput succedaneum. Pediatrics 29:907, 1962.

Pearson, H. A., and Diamond, L. K.: Fetomaternal transfusion. Am. J. Dis. Child. 97:267, 1959.

Phillipsborn, H. F., Traisman, H. S., and Greer, D.: Rupture of the spleen: A complication of erythroblastosis fetalis. N. Engl. J. Med. 252:159, 1955.

Ratten, G. J.: Spontaneous haematoma of the umbilical cord. Austral. New Zeal. J. Obstet. Gynecol. 9:125, 1969.

Rausen, A. R., Seki, M., and Strauss, L.: Twin transfusion syndrome. A review of 19 cases studied at one institution. J. Pediatr. 66:613, 1965.

Raye, J. R., Gutberlet, R. L., and Stahlman, M.: Symptomatic posthemorrhagic anemia in the newborn. Pediatr. Clinics North Am. 17:401, 1970.

Sacks, M. O.: Occurrence of anemia and polycythemia in phenotypically dissimilar single ovum human twins. Pediatrics 24:604, 1959.

Schwartz, J., Surchin, H., Lupu, H., and Cooperberg, A. A.: Severe hypochromic anemia in a newborn due to fetal-maternal transfusion. Can. Med. Assoc. J. 95:369, 1966.

Siddall, R. S., and West, R. H.: Incision of placenta at cesarean section: A cause of fetal anemia. Am. J. Obstet. Gynecol. 63:425, 1952.

Woo Wang, M. Y. F., McCutcheon, E., and Desforges, J. F.: Fetomaternal hemorrhage from diagnostic transabdominal amniocentesis. Am. J. Obstet. Gynecol. 97:1123, 1967.

Zipursky, A., Pollock, J., Chown, B., and Israels, L. G.: Transplacental fetal maternal hemorrhage after placental injury during delivery or amniocentesis. Lancet 2:493, 1963.

*Hemolytic Anemia*

Austin, R. F., and Desforges, J. F.: Hereditary elliptocytosis: An unusual presentation of hemolysis in the newborn associated with transient morphologic abnormalities. Pediatrics 44:196, 1969.

Bard, H.: The postnatal decline of hemoglobin F synthesis in normal full-term infants. J. Clin. Invest. 55:395, 1975.

Baumann, R., and Rubin, H.: Autoimmune hemolytic anemia during pregnancy with hemolytic disease in the newborn. Blood *41*:293, 1973.

Beutler, E.: Abnormalities of the hexosemonophosphate shunt. Semin. Hematol. 8:311, 1971.

Clayton, E. M., Hyun, B. H., Palumbo, V. N., and Dean, V. M.: Penicillin induced positive Coombs' test in a newborn. Am. J. Clin. Pathol. 52:370, 1969.

Crosby, W. H., and Conrad, M. E.: Hereditary spherocytosis: Observations on hemolytic mechanisms and iron metabolism. Blood *15*:662, 1960.

Diamond, L. K.: Splenectomy in childhood and the hazard of overwhelming infection. Pediatrics *43*:886, 1969.

Doxiadis, S. A., and Valaes, T.: The clinical picture of glucose-6-phosphate dehydrogenase deficiency in early infancy. Arch. Dis. Child. *39*:545, 1964.

Eshaghpour, E., Oski, F. A., and Williams, M.: The relationship of erythrocyte glucose-6-phosphate dehydrogenase deficiency to hyperbilirubinemia in Negro premature infants. J. Pediatr. *70*:595, 1967.

Fairbanks, V. F., and Fernandez, M. N.: The identification of metabolic errors associated with hemolytic anemia. J.A.M.A. *208*:316, 1969.

Forget, B. G., and Kan, Y. W.: Thalassemia and the genetics of hemoglobin. *In* Nathan, D. G., and Oski, F. A. (Eds.): Hematology of Infancy and Childhood. Philadelphia, W. B. Saunders Co., 1974, p. 450.

Friedman, S., Atwater, J., Gill, F. M., and Schwartz, E.: α-Thalassemia in Negro infants. Pediatr. Res. 8:955, 1974.

Glader, B. E., Fortier, N., Albala, M. M., and Nathan, D. G.: Congenital hemolytic anemia associated with dehydrated erythrocytes and increased potassium loss. N. Engl. J. Med. *291*:491, 1974.

Glader, B. E., and Nathan, D. G.: Haemolysis due to pyruvate kinase deficiency and other glycolytic enzymopathies. Clin. Haematol. *4*:123, 1975.

Gross, G. P., and Hathaway, W. E.: Fetal erythrocyte deformability. Pediatr. Res. 6:593, 1972.

Kan, Y. W., Allen, A., and Lowenstein, L.: Hydrops fetalis with alpha thalassemia. N. Engl. J. Med. *276*:18, 1967.

Kan, Y. W., Forget, B. G., and Nathan, D. G.: Gamma-beta thalassemia: A cause of hemolytic disease of the newborn. N. Engl. J. Med. *286*:129, 1972.

Kan, Y. W., Schwartz, E., and Nathan, D. G.: Globin chain synthesis in the alpha thalassemia syndromes. J. Clin. Invest. *47*:2515, 1969.

Krueger, H. C., and Burgert, E. O., Jr.: Hereditary spherocytosis in 100 children. Mayo Clin. Proc. *41*:821, 1966.

LaCelle, P. L.: Alteration of membrane deformability in hemolytic anemias. Semin. Hematol. 7:355, 1970.

Lyon, M. F.: Gene action in the X-chromosome of the mouse. Nature *190*:372, 1961.

Mentzer, W. C., Jr., and Collier, E.: Hydrops fetalis associated with erythrocyte G-6-PD deficiency and maternal ingestion of fava beans and ascorbic acid. J. Pediatr. 86:565, 1975.

Miller, D. R., Rickles, F. R., Lichtman, M. A., LaCelle, P. L., Bates, J., and Weed, R. I.: A new variant of hereditary hemolytic anemia with stomatocytosis and erythrocyte cation abnormality. Blood 38:184, 1971.

Milner, P. F.: The sickling disorders. Clin. Haematol. 3:289, 1974.

Nathan, D. G., and Pearson, H. A.: Sickle cell syndromes and hemoglobin C disease. In Nathan, D. G., and Oski, F. A. (Eds.): Hematology of Infancy and Childhood. Philadelphia, W. B. Saunders Co., 1974, p. 419.

Nielson, J. A., and Strunk, K. W.: Homozygous hereditary elliptocytosis as a cause of hemolytic anemia in infancy. Scand. J. Haematol. 5:486, 1968.

O'Flynn, M. E. D., and Hsia, D. Y.: Serum bilirubin levels and glucose-6-phosphate dehydrogenase deficiency in newborn American Negroes. J. Pediatr. 63:160, 1963.

Oski, F. A., and Diamond, L. K.: Erythrocyte pyruvate kinase deficiency resulting in congenital nonspherocytic hemolytic anemia. N. Engl. J. Med. 269:763, 1963.

Pearson, H. A.: Life-span of the fetal red blood cell. J. Pediatr. 70:166, 1967.

Pearson, H. A., Shanklin, D. R., and Brodine, C. R.: Alpha-thalassemia as a cause of nonimmunologic hydrops. Am. J. Dis. Child. *109*:168, 1965.

Penfold, J. B., and Lipscomb, J. M.: Elliptocytosis in man, associated with hereditary hemorrhagic telangiectasia. Quart. J. Med. *12*:157, 1943.

Pritchard, J. A., Scott, D. E., Whalley, P. J., Cunningham, F. G., and Mason, R. A.: The effects of maternal sickle cell hemoglobinopathies and sickle cell trait on reproductive performance. Am. J. Obstet. Gynecol. *117*:662, 1973.

Schmaier, A. H., Maurer, H. M., Johnston, C. L., and Scott, R. B.: Alpha thalassemia screening in neonates by mean corpuscular volume and mean corpuscular hemoglobin determination. J. Pediatr. 83:794, 1973.

Schroeder, W. A., Jakway, J., and Powers, D.: Detection of hemoglobins S and C at birth: A rapid screening procedure by column chromatography. J. Lab. Clin. Med. 82:303, 1973.

Stamatoyannopoulos, G.: Gamma-thalassemia. Lancet 2:192, 1971.

Stamey, C. C., and Diamond, L. K.: Congenital hemolytic anemia in the newborn. Am. J. Dis. Child. *94*:616, 1957.

Trucco, J. T., and Brown, A. K.: Neonatal manifestations of hereditary spherocytosis. Am. J. Dis. Child. *113*:263, 1967.

Valaes, T., Karaklis, A., Stravrakakis, D., Bavela-Stravrakakis, K., Perakis, A., and Doxiadis, S. A.: Incidence and mechanism of neonatal jaundice related to glucose-6-phosphate dehydrogenase deficiency. Pediatr. Res. 3:448, 1969.

Wasi, P., Na-Nakorn, S., and Pootrakul, S.: The α-thalassaemias. Clin. Haematol. 3:383, 1974.

Zarkowsky, H. S., Oski, F. A., Sha'afi, R., Shohet, S. B., and Nathan, D. G.: Congenital hemolytic anemia with high sodium, low potassium red cells. I. Studies of membrane permeability. N. Engl. J. Med. 278:573, 1968.

*Hypoplastic Anemia*

Diamond, L. K., Allen, D. M., and Magill, F. B.: Congenital (erythroid) hypoplastic anemia. Am. J. Dis. Child. *102*:149, 1961.

Diamond, L. K., and Blackfan, K. D.: Hypoplastic anemia. Am. J. Dis. Child. 56:464, 1938.

Hughes, D. W. O.: Hypoplastic anemia in infancy and childhood. Arch. Dis. Child. 36:349, 1961.

Pearson, H. A., and Cone, T. E.: Congenital hypoplastic anemia. Pediatrics 19:192, 1957.

*Physiologic Anemia of Infancy and Prematurity*

Buchanan, G. R., and Schwartz, A. D.: Impaired erythropoietin response in anemic premature infants. Blood 44:347, 1974.

Dallman, P. R.: Iron, vitamin E, and folate in the preterm infant. J. Pediatr. 85:742, 1974.

Delivoria-Papadopoulos, M., Roncevic, N. P., and Oski, F. A.: Postnatal changes in oxygen transport of term, premature, and sick infants: The role of red cell 2,3-diphosphoglycerate and adult hemoglobin. Pediatr. Res. 5:235, 1971.

Gross, S., and Milhorn, D. K.: Vitamin E dependent anemia in the premature infant. III. Comparative hemoglobin, vitamin E, and erythrocyte phospholipid responses following absorption of either water-soluble or fat-soluble d-alpha tocopherol. J. Pediatr. 85:753, 1974.

Halvorsen, S., and Finne, P. H.: Erythropoietin production in the human fetus and newborn. Ann. N.Y. Acad. Sci. 149:576, 1968.

McIntosh, S.: Erythropoietin excretion in the premature infant. J. Pediatr. 86:202, 1975.

Melhorn, D. K., and Gross, S.: Vitamin E-dependent anemia in the premature infant I. Effects of large doses of medicinal iron. J. Pediatr. 79:569, 1971.

Melhorn, D. K., and Gross, S.: Vitamin E-dependent anemia in the premature infant II. Relationships between gestational age and absorption of vitamin E. J. Pediatr. 79:581, 1971.

Mestyan, J., Fekete, M., Bata, G., and Jarai, I.: The basal metabolic rate of premature infants. Biol. Neonatol. 7:11, 1964.

O'Brien, R. T., and Pearson, H. A.: Physiologic anemia of the newborn infant. J. Pediatr. 79:132, 1971.

Oski, F. A., and Barness, L. A.: Vitamin E deficiency: A previously unrecognized cause of hemolytic anemia in the premature infant. J. Pediatr. 70:211, 1967.

Pearson, H. A.: Life-span of the fetal red blood cell. J. Pediatr. 70:166, 1967.

Ritchie, J. H., Fish, M. B., McMasters, V., and Grossman, M.: Edema and hemolytic anemia in premature infants. N. Engl. J. Med. 279:1185, 1968.

Schulman, I.: The anemia of prematurity. J. Pediatr. 54:663, 1959.

Shojania, A. M., and Gross, S.: Folic acid deficiency and prematurity. J. Pediatr. 64:323, 1964.

Stockman, J. A., III: Anemia of prematurity. Semin. Hematol. 12:163, 1975.

Stoutenborough, K. A., Sutherland, J. M., Meineke, H. A., and Light, I. J.: Erythropoietin levels in cord blood of control infants and infants with respiratory distress syndrome. Acta Paediatr. Scand. 58:121, 1969.

Williams, M. L., Shott, R. J., O'Neal, P. L., and Oski, F. A.: Role of dietary iron and fat on vitamin E deficiency anemia of infancy. N. Engl. J. Med. 292:887, 1975.

*Polycythemia*

Baum, R.: Viscous forces in neonatal polycythemia. J. Pediatr. 69:975, 1966.

Danks, D. M., and Stevens, L. H.: Neonatal respiratory distress associated with a high hematocrit reading. Lancet 2:499, 1964.

Gatti, R. A., Muster, A. J., Cole, R. B., and Paul, M. H.: Neonatal polycythemia with transient cyanosis and cardiorespiratory abnormalities. J. Pediatr. 69:1063, 1966.

Gross, G. P., Hathaway, W. E., and McGaughey, H. R.: Hyperviscosity in the neonate. J. Pediatr. 82:1004, 1973.

Humbert, J. R., Abelson, H., Hathaway, W. E., and Battaglia, F. C.: Polycythemia in small for gestational age infants. J. Pediatr. 75:812, 1969.

Kontras, S. B.: Polycythemia and hyperviscosity syndromes in infants and children. Pediatr. Clin. North Am. 19:919, 1972.

Michael, A. F., Jr., and Mauer, A. M.: Maternal-fetal transfusion as a cause of plethora in the neonatal period. Pediatrics 28:458, 1961.

Minkowski, A.: Acute cardiac failure in connection with neonatal polycythemia (in monovular and single newborn infants). Biol. Neonatol. 4:61, 1962.

Oh, W., Omori, K., Emmanouilides, G. C., and Phelps, D. L.: Placenta to lamb fetus transfusion in utero during acute hypoxia. Am. J. Obstet. Gynecol. 122:316, 1975.

Sacks, M. O.: Occurrence of anemia and polycythemia in phenotypically dissimilar single-ovum human twins. Pediatrics 24:604, 1959.

Stone, H. O., Thompson, H. K., Jr., and Schmidt-Nielsen, K.: Influence of erythrocytes on blood viscosity. Am. J. Physiol. 214:913, 1968.

Wood, J. L.: Plethora in the newborn infant associated with cyanosis and convulsions. J. Pediatr. 54:143, 1959.

*Methemoglobinemia*

Bartos, H. R., and Desforges, J. F.: Erythrocyte DPNH dependent diaphorase levels in infants. Pediatrics 37:991, 1966.

Climie, C. R., McLean, S., Starmer, G. A., and Thomas, J.: Methaemoglobinaemia in mother and foetus following continuous epidermal analgesia with prilocaine. Br. J. Anaesth., 39:155, 1967.

Comly, H. R.: Cyanosis in infants caused by nitrates in well water. J.A.M.A. 129:112, 1945.

Evelyn, K. A., and Malloy, H. T.: Microdetermination of oxyhemoglobin, methemoglobin, and sulfhemoglobin in a single sample of blood. J. Biol. Chem. 126:655, 1938.

Farmer, M. B., Lehmann, H., and Raine, D. N.: Two unrelated patients with congenital cyanosis due to haemoglobinopathy M. Lancet 2:786, 1964.

Fisch, R. O., Berglund, E. B., Bridge, A. G., Finley, P. R., and Raile, R.: Methemoglobinemia in a hospital nursery. A search for causative factors. J.A.M.A. 185:124, 1963.

Gerald, P. S.: The electrophoretic and spectroscopic characterization of hemoglobin M. Blood 12:936, 1958.

Harley, J. D., and Celermajer, J. M.: Neonatal methaemoglobinaemia and the "red-brown" screening test. Lancet 2:1223, 1970.

Jaffe, E. R., and Hsieh, H-S.: DPNH-Methemoglobin reductase deficiency and hereditary methemoglobinemia. Semin. Hematol. 8:417, 1971.

Lees, M. H., and Jolly, J.: Severe congenital methaemoglobinaemia in an infant. Lancet 2:1147, 1957.

Lo, S. S., Hitzig, W. H., and Martin, H. R.: Hereditary methemoglobinemia due to diaphorase deficiency. Acta Haematol. *43*:177, 1970.

Martin, H., and Huisman, T. H. J.: Formation of ferrihaemoglobin of isolated human haemoglobin types by sodium nitrite. Nature *200*:898, 1963.

Nurse, D. S.: Congenital methaemoglobinaemia. Med. J. Austr. *47*:692, 1960.

Quie, P. G., Fisch, R. O., and Raile, R.: Methemoglobinemia and hemolytic anemia in normal newborns and normal prematures. Lancet *82*:428, 1962.

Ross, J. D.: Deficient activity of DPNH-dependent

methemoglobin diaphorase in cord blood erythrocytes. Blood *21*:51, 1963.

Shearer, L. A., Goldsmith, J. R., Young, C., Kearns, O. A., and Tamplin, B. R.: Methemoglobin levels in infants in an area with high nitrate water supply. Am. J. Pub. Health *62*:1174, 1972.

Smith, R. P., and Olson, M. V.: Drug-induced methemoglobinemia. Semin. Hematol. *10*:253, 1973.

Vigil, J., Warburton, S., Haynes, W. S., and Kaiser, L. R.: Nitrates in municipal water supply cause methemoglobinemia in infants. Pub. Health Rep. *80*:1119, 1965.

# THE COLLAGEN DISEASES                   67

## PERIARTERITIS NODOSA

**INCIDENCE.** Periarteritis nodosa is uncommon in the pediatric age group. Approximately 110 cases had been reported in infants and children below 15 years of age up to 1954. By 1963 20 cases had been described which involved infants within the first year of life, and only four of these manifested their first symptoms within the first month.

**ETIOLOGY AND PATHOLOGY.** Rich demonstrated that periarteritis nodosa is a hypersensitivity reaction. In 1942 he recorded eight cases in which the typical clinical and pathologic picture followed large doses of either sulfonamide or animal serum. The following year he was able, with Gregory, to reproduce the characteristic changes in rabbits by massive injections of foreign serum. The identity of the offending allergen is by no means always obvious.

Many arteries, usually small or medium-sized, contain scattered nodular enlargements. Those of the heart, kidneys and adrenals are favorite sites for the lesions, but any others may take part in the disorder. One sees intimal thickening, focal inflammation involving the media, going on to necrosis, fibrosis and aneurysmal dilatation. Inflammatory cells include polymorphonuclears, lymphocytes and plasma cells. The elastic fibers become disrupted.

In between the nodules the arteries may be thickened, their lumens narrowed for long distances. Intravascular thrombosis is seen in many places.

**DIAGNOSIS.** At present it is almost impossible to arrive at the correct diagnosis during very early life unless an artery in the subcutaneous tissue is involved and a nodule can be palpated and removed for histologic examination. The four neonatal cases reported have presented in entirely different fashions.

Wilmer's Case II was an infant who began to vomit on the eighth day, had dyspnea on the tenth day and died in shock the same day with signs of extensive pneumonic consolidation without fever.

His urine contained blood. The lungs and kidneys were sites of extensive hemorrhage. His blood contained an abundance of platelets.

Wilmer's Case I was an infant who became ill on the twenty-fifth day, having been perfectly well until then. The earliest signs were a blotchy eruption and puffy eyelids. On the thirty-fourth day he had a petechial eruption, fever, diarrhea and vomiting of bright blood. He was anemic, and his peripheral blood contained no platelets. He died after a right-sided convulsion. Autopsy showed a huge adrenal hemorrhage in addition to periarteritis nodosa.

The case of Liban et al. was entirely different. This infant had vomited, failed to gain and had suffered episodes of fever since birth. At 3 weeks she became cyanotic, and crepitant rales were heard in her lungs, but x-ray film of the chest was said to have been normal. At 6 weeks she was undernourished, dehydrated and cyanotic. Coarse rales were present throughout her lungs, and there was now a loud systolic murmur. Diarrhea and vomiting followed. By 4 months she had gained no weight, cyanosis was deeper, the liver was enlarged, and x-ray film showed slight enlargement of the heart. By 8½ months she was marantic, dyspneic and deeply cyanotic, the lungs were full of moist rales, the liver and spleen were enlarged, but the heart murmur had disappeared. Electrocardiogram showed right-sided heart strain. X-ray film of the chest now showed a greatly enlarged heart and round, well-defined shadows throughout both lung fields (Fig. 67–1). She died 10 days later. The pulmonary and coronary arteries were those most intensively and extensively involved in the periarteritic process in this infant.

The infant of Roberts and Fetterman became ill at 5 weeks of age with fever, upper respiratory tract infection and a macular rash with central clearing of many macules. Hemorrhagic ulceration of the buccal mucosa followed, then pericardial effusion and heart failure and finally evidences of arterial thrombosis of one arm and one leg. There was leukocytosis with granulocytosis, but no eosinophilia, and the urine contained a few red and white blood cells and granular casts. The systolic blood pressure rose to 160 in the right arm, 200 in the right leg. Muscle biopsies revealed nothing abnormal.

This great diversity of clinical manifestations is to be expected in this disorder, and the task of diagnosis is clearly an almost impossible one in the neonate.

Onset with fever and a macular rash, persistence of fever, the development of hypertension and abnormal urinary sediment, and enlargement of the heart with electrocardiographic evidences of myocardial ischemia should arouse strong suspicions of the diagnosis, and sudden drop of blood pressure in one limb is strongly confirmatory. Eosinophilia and thrombocytopenia occur, but by no means invariably.

**TREATMENT.** Corticosteroids should be given in the hope of suppressing the disease. The prognosis is poor even with the best supportive therapy.

## SYSTEMIC LUPUS ERYTHEMATOSUS (SLE)

Strictly speaking SLE is not a neonatal disorder, although infants born to affected mothers can have clinical manifestations of SLE. These features include the characteristic malar rash, anemia, leukopenia,

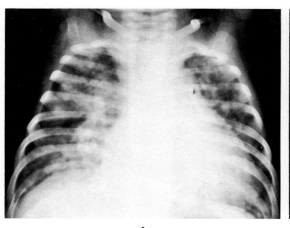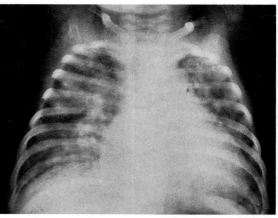

**A**                                                            **B**

*Figure 67–1.* Periarteritis nodosa. *A,* Anteroposterior view of chest taken when the infant was 7½ months old. A previous film taken at the age of 6 weeks had been read as showing a "heart of normal shape; hilar markings increased." The original legend on this one reads, "Slight cardiac enlargement; prominent vascular shadows in the lungs." *B,* Similar projection made at the age of 8½ months, 10 days before death. Now the legend reads, "Heart enlarged in all directions; round, well-defined shadows scattered in both lung fields, particularly near the right hilum; confluent, patchy and hazy shadows in both lung fields. On fluoroscopy, no hilar pulsations were noted." (Liban, E., Shamir, Z., and Schorr, S.: J. Dis. Child. 88:210, 1954. From Hadassah University Hospital, Jerusalem, Israel. Photographs reproduced with the kind permission of the senior author.)

thrombocytopenia and/or a positive "L-E Prep." It is presumably the transplacental passage of maternal globulins that is responsible for these abnormalities. In virtually all cases, these neonatal features of SLE are transient and require no specific treatment.

## REFERENCES

Garsenstein, N., Pollak, V. E., and Kark, R. M.: Systemic lupus erythematosus and pregnancy. N. Engl. J. Med. 267:165, 1962.

Liban, E., Shamir, Z., and Schorr, S.: Periarteritis nodosa in a 9-month old infant. A.M.A. J. Dis. Child. 88:210, 1954.

Mijer, F., and Olsen, R. N.: Transplacental passage of the L.E. factor. J. Pediat. 52:690, 1958.

Nathan, D. J., and Snapper, I.: Simultaneous placental transfer of factors responsible for L. E. cell formation and thrombocytopenia. Am. J. Med. 25:647, 1958.

Rich, A. R.: The role of hypersensitivity in periarteritis nodosa as indicated by 7 cases developing during serum sickness and sulfonamide therapy. Bull. Johns Hopkins Hosp. 71:123, 1942.

Rich, A. R., and Gregory, J. E.: Experimental demonstration that periarteritis nodosa is a manifestation of hypersensitivity. Bull. Johns Hopkins Hosp. 72:65, 1943.

Roberts, F. B., and Fetterman, G. H.: Polyarteritis nodosa in infancy. J. Pediatr. 63:519, 1963.

Seip, M.: Systemic lupus erythematosus in pregnancy with haemolytic anaemia, leucopenia and thrombocytopenia in the mother and her newborn infant. Arch. Dis. Child. 35:364, 1960.

Wilmer, H. A.: Two cases of periarteritis nodosa occurring in the first month of life. Bull. Johns Hopkins Hosp. 77:275, 1945.

# IDIOPATHIC HEREDITARY LYMPHEDEMA

# 68

Milroy's disease is the eponym for this disorder in common usage in this country. Nonne described it in 1891, under the title "elephantiasis congenita hereditaria," one year earlier than Milroy. It is marked by firm edema of one or more extremities.

**INCIDENCE.** Over 50 cases have been reported to date. In 17 years eight examples were observed in the Toronto Hospital for Sick Children.

**ETIOLOGY AND PATHOGENESIS.** A familial pattern indicating that it is transmitted as a nonsex-linked recessive can be discovered in most instances.

McKendry et al. injected Patent Blue V dye into the first interdigital web of limbs with lymphedema and of the opposite limbs as normal controls. On the normal side blue-green streaks appeared soon over the dorsum of the foot and ankle, spread upward in the line of the long saphenous vein, reaching the groin in about 20 minutes. Dissection showed lymph channels and glands stained blue-green. Dye then spread upward until the skin of the entire body was discolored. Dye similarly injected on the affected side remained *in situ,* never ascending even as far as the foot. Tissue examined histologically revealed a mass of dilated lymph channels indistinguishable from lymphangioma. The disorder appears to result from failure of communication between peripheral lymph channels and more centrally placed ones.

Rarely lymphedema of one or more extremities coexists with manifestations of lymphatic channel blockage in other areas, such as chylothorax and chylous ascites.

**DIAGNOSIS.** Edema of one or several extremities is often noted at birth, although later onset at any time during infancy or childhood is not uncommon. The leg is involved much more often than the arm. Originally only the foot may be affected, but swelling may then extend gradually to the knee or hip. The affected limb may reach a large size, fully justifying the descriptive term "elephantiasis." The tissues feel firmer than those of truly edematous extremities, and deep pressure produces little or no pitting.

There is no pain or tenderness or loss of motility except for some awkwardness dependent upon excessive size. The limbs are subject to repeated bouts of an erysipeloid-like infection, with fever, local redness, heat and increased swelling. These are self-limited, lasting 2 to 7 days.

In the newborn, Milroy's disease must be differentiated from generalized edema of all kinds. This is simple enough, since the swelling in Milroy's disease is never universal and symmetrical even though

both feet or both hands may be involved. Nor does the edema pit so deeply. The same differences are found in Turner's disease, and other characteristic anomalies are encountered in this syndrome. Localized lymphangiomas or hemangiomas should cause no confusion.

**TREATMENT.** Several operative procedures have been devised with the object of diverting lymph drainage to deeper channels. The most widely used has been the Kondoleon operation, in which long strips of skin and subcutaneous tissue are excised from the entire length of the lymphedematous extremity. This approach to the prob-

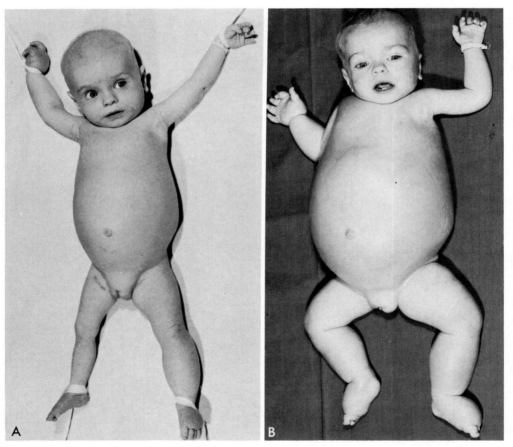

*Figure 68–1. A,* Infant 12 months of age with swelling of the right arm and left leg and some abdominal protuberance. *B,* At 15 months of age. In addition to swelling of the right arm and left leg, there is extreme abdominal enlargement and some generalized edema. (Reprinted from Pediatrics *19:*21, 1957, with the kind permission of Dr. J. B. J. McKendry.)

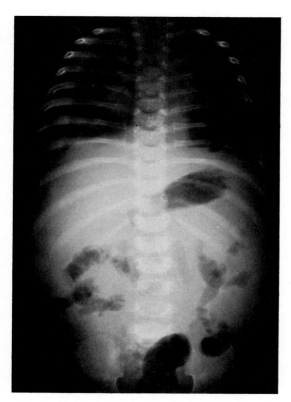

*Figure 68–2.* X-ray photograph of patient shown in Figure 68–1, made at age of 4½ months, showing pleural and abdominal effusions.

lem not only is deforming but also is seldom effective.

In a few well documented cases cortisone or prednisone has successfully reduced the swelling, and small running doses have maintained the improvement. Panos reports an example of such a cure with prednisone, utilizing doses of 30 mg a day for one week, 25 mg a day for another week, and so on gradually down to 5 mg a day as a maintenance dose.

### CASE 68–1

(This case is abstracted from McKendry, Lindsay and Gerstein. We are indebted to Dr. J. B. J. McKendry, of Toronto, Canada, for permission. It is their Case 4.)

A 7 pound 15 ounce (3600 gm) female infant was the second child born to her mother. The family history was negative from the standpoint of the infant's illness. No details of pregnancy or labor are given. At birth firm edema of the left leg was noted, and while the infant was still in the delivery room the right forearm and hand were seen to swell (Fig. 68–1). During her nursery stay she ate and behaved normally, and swellings remained unchanged.

At 2 months eczema developed. At 3 months the area involved by edema increased somewhat, and by 5 months the face was swollen, and ascites and right hydrothorax had developed (Fig. 68–2). From 1 year on there was dyspnea with gross abdominal swelling only partially relieved by periodic paracenteses. She died at 15 months after 3 weeks of intractable asthmatic bronchitis. A total of 22 aspirations of fluid had been performed, amounting to 10,500 cc of ascitic and pleural fluid!

Injection of 0.8 cc of 11 per cent Patent Blue V dye into the first web space of each foot showed no upward movement of the dye on the lymphedematous side, but rapid spread of the dye on the nonedematous side. It reached the groin in 20 minutes, the pleura in 30 minutes, then colored the whole body surface. After 60 minutes an abdominal paracentesis revealed colored chyle.

The case was studied intensively during 10 admissions to hospital. The details of blood and body fluid chemistry will not be reviewed here.

At autopsy death appeared to have been caused by bronchopneumonia. The thoracic duct was intact and patent, although unstained by dye instilled into the stomach before death. There were many dilated lymphatic channels resembling hemolymphangiomas, suggesting widespread multiple peripheral obstructions to lymph flow, most notable in the clinically edematous limbs. "The fluid in thoracic and abdominal cavities may also represent a back pressure phenomenon of parietal and visceral lymphatics rather than small breaks in the thoracic duct which we were unable to demonstrate."

A case almost identical to this one was presented in a clinicopathologic conference at the Alexandria Hospital by Drs. Colin MacRae and Elson B. Helang. In this one, congenital absence of the thoracic duct was discovered at autopsy.

These two cases differ in some important respects from the one reported by Morphis et al. In this infant innumerable lymphangiomas were discovered, involving all the bones examined, the posterior mediastinum and the spleen. Chylous fluid was found not only in the pleural cavities, but also within the bone marrow, and prominently dilated lymphatic channels were seen in other viscera. This generalized lymphangioma appears to represent an entity different from the prior ones.

# REFERENCES

MacRae, C., and Helang, E. B.: Clinicopathological Conference, Alexandria Hospital, Mar. 11, 1966. Personal Communication.

McKendry, J. B. J., Lindsay, W. K., and Gerstein, M. C.: Congenital defects of the lymphatics in infancy. Pediatrics 19:21, 1957.

Milroy, W. A.: Chronic hereditary edema: Milroy's disease. J.A.M.A. 91:1172, 1928.

Morphis, L. G., Arcinus, E. L., and Krause, J. R.: Generalized lymphangioma in infancy with chylothorax. Pediatrics 46:566, 1970.

Nonne, U.: Vier Fälle von Elephantiasis congenita hereditaria. Arch. Path. Anat. 125:189, 1891.

Panos, T. C.: Prednisone in the management of idiopathic hereditary lymphedema (Milroy's disease). J.A.M.A. 161:1475, 1956.

# IX

## Jaundice

# 69

# GENERAL CONSIDERATIONS
*Revised by Frank Oski*

Jaundice results when bilirubin accumulates in the blood. By adult standards, virtually every newborn infant develops jaundice as defined as a serum concentration of unconjugated bilirubin in excess of 2 mg per 100 ml. Approximately 5 to 10 per cent of all infants weighing more than 2500 gm at birth achieve bilirubin values in excess of 10 mg per 100 ml during the first week of life, and 25 per cent of infants weighing less than 2500 gm exceed this value.

Bilirubin is derived from the breakdown of heme. Heme is an essential component of all oxygen-dependent electron transport systems in mitochondria and in microsomes, so that virtually all cells of the body are a potential source of bilirubin. Under usual circumstances, however, the chief source of this pigment originates from the destruction of hemoglobin within the erythrocyte. The catabolism of 1 gm of hemoglobin results in the production of 34 mg of bilirubin. A second major source of heme breakdown products is derived from the degradation of heme proteins of hepatic cells. The normal newborn produces 8.5 ± 2.3 mg bilirubin per kg per day, which is more than double the bilirubin production of 3.6 mg per kg per day observed in the normal adult. About two to three times more bilirubin is derived from nonerythrocyte sources in newborns than in adults.

Jaundice may result from a number of major causes. These include 1) an increased breakdown of heme; 2) defective uptake and transport of bilirubin within the liver cells; 3) impaired conjugation within the hepatic microsomes; 4) defective excretion of the bilirubin; and 5) increased reabsorption of the pigment from the intestinal tract. In many infants more than one factor may operate to produce hyperbilirubinemia.

## BILIRUBIN FORMATION AND EXCRETION

The destruction of circulating red cells accounts for 80 to 90 per cent of the daily bilirubin production in the adult and for about 75 per cent in the newborn infant. Red cells are removed from the circulation by the reticuloendothelial system, the hemoglobin is catabolized and the heme is converted to bilirubin. During this process of hemoglobin catabolism, the iron is salvaged and retained by the body for reutilization. The globin moiety of hemoglobin is converted into its component amino acids and also reutilized.

The conversion of heme to bilirubin takes place in the entire reticuloendothelial system. Recent observations have led to a better understanding of the enzymatic mechanisms that mediate the conversion of heme to bile pigments. Tenhunen and Marver have demonstrated that the critical enzyme in this process is heme oxygenase, which is found in the microsomal fraction of a variety of tissues. Its action is to cleave the methene bridge of the heme molecule, converting the ringed tetrapyrrole to the linear tetrapyrrole, biliverdin. In this process the carbon atom at this bridge is converted to carbon monoxide. The formation of carbon monoxide from heme is essentially equimolar in man, one mole of carbon monoxide being produced from the degradation of one mole of heme. For this reason the measurement of carbon monoxide production rates or carboxyhemoglobin levels within the blood have proved useful in documenting increased heme breakdown as a cause of hyperbilirubinemia.

The biliverdin produced by the action of heme oxygenase is then rapidly reduced to bilirubin by a second enzyme, biliverdin reductase, which is also present in the soluble fraction of these same cells. The yellow bilirubin molecule then leaves its cell of origin and enters the plasma, is complexed with albumin, and is transported to the liver for eventual conjugation and excretion.

Bilirubin has long been noted to exist in two different forms in serum. In 1913 van den Bergh differentiated them on the basis of their reaction with diazotized sulfanilic acid as direct and indirect-reacting bilirubin. The indirect-reacting form was soluble in chloroform and lipid, but not in aqueous solutions at physiologic pH. Claireaux et al. noted that it was the indirect type which was responsible for kernicterus, and the level of indirect-reacting bilirubin remains the essential measurement in the consideration of the likelihood of toxicity. It was subsequently shown that the bilirubin-binding capacity of serum albumin, which is related to the concentration of albumin, is another consideration in the risk of kernicterus. In vitro 1 mole of albumin binds 2M of bilirubin, or 1 gm of albumin at pH 7.4 binds 15 mg of bilirubin. Albumin-bound bilirubin does not penetrate the brain cells.

The difference between the two bilirubins was discovered simultaneously by Schmid in the United States, Talafant in Czechoslovakia and Billing and Lathe in England in 1956. The direct-reacting bilirubin is a diglucuronide, having been conjugated with glucuronic acid. The reaction can take place in vitro in the presence of liver microsomes as a source of the enzyme glucuronyl transferase. This major advance in understanding of bilirubin metabolism led to numerous studies which have enhanced knowledge of physiologic jaundice of infancy, Crigler-Najjar jaundice and the role of drugs in exaggerating jaundice at many ages.

Presumably most of the conjugation of bilirubin occurs in the liver; however, other tissues, such as kidney and intestinal mucosa, have the capacity to do so in vitro. Other modes of conjugation also occur, including formation of bilirubin sulfate, and an alkali-labile fraction as well.

The steps in hepatic uptake, conjugation and excretion, studied with tritiated bilirubin in rats by Bernstein et al., are thought to include binding of unconjugated bilirubin in the cytoplasm of the liver cell to a protein other than albumin, perhaps glucuronyl transferase. The bound bilirubin is then transferred to the endoplasmic reticulum where conjugation occurs. Since no significant storage of conjugated bilirubin has been found in the hepatic cell, it is thought that once conjugated it is rapidly excreted.

Two mechanisms have been suggested to explain the liver's ability to rapidly and selectively transfer bilirubin from the plasma into the hepatocyte. First, these cells may possess unique receptors capable of binding organic anions such as bilirubin. These receptors presumably would have a much greater affinity for bilirubin than does serum albumin. The precise role of the liver cell membrane in bilirubin metabolism and particularly its role in the newborn still awaits clarification. Once the bilirubin gets within the liver cell, it is bound to two hepatic proteins, named Y and Z by Arias and associates. These protein carriers then transport the unconjugated bilirubin to the endoplasmic reticulum for conjugation. It has been proposed that transient deficiencies of these carrier proteins in the newborn may be one of the factors in the genesis of hyperbilirubinemia.

Defective uptake of bilirubin by the liver cells is a possible explanation for hyperbilirubinemia, and is thought to be the basis of the defect in Gilbert's disease, since in vitro assays of glucuronide excretion of other substances is not impaired in that condition. The role of enzymes for bilirubin transport in infants remains to be elucidated.

Defective canalicular excretion or mechanical block in the biliary tract are of course well recognized in infancy and will be considered in more detail under biliary atresia.

Finally, another explanation for prolongation and exaggeration of hyperbilirubinemia in intestinal obstruction is the presence of a significant enterohepatic recirculation of bilirubin. When bilirubin diglucuronide accumulates in the small bowel, it is capable of degradation to bilirubin through the action of beta glucuronidase in the bowel wall. The unconjugated fraction can then be absorbed into the circulation. When the intestinal tract contains bacterial flora, the conjugated bilirubin is rapidly oxidized to urobilin and not reabsorbed.

## AMNIOTIC FLUID BILIRUBIN

Bilirubin is found in the amniotic fluid in normal pregnancies as early as the twelfth week, and increases from 16 to 30 weeks. Thereafter it decreases, so that normally by 36 weeks there is little left. In isoimmunized pregnancies, there is a characteristic peak in the spectral absorption curve of amniotic fluid at 450 m$\mu$, which has been widely used to diagnose the extent of the isoimmunization of the fetus. Several pigments in addition to bilirubin are in normal amniotic fluid, including coproporphyrin III, biliverdin, and urobilinogen. The source of these pigments remains unknown.

## BILIRUBIN EXCRETION IN THE FETUS

In the fetus, the elimination of bilirubin must be largely across the placenta, which requires that it remain in a nonpolar or unconjugated form. Studies in guinea pigs by Schenker et al. have shown that when labelled unconjugated bilirubin was injected into the fetus, it was present in the maternal bile within 15 minutes. In contrast, almost no movement of conjugated bilirubin could be demonstrated. Similar observations have been reported in the rhesus monkey by Lester et al. in 1963.

We shall discuss the subject under a mixed clinical-physiopathologic classification, as follows:

I. Physiologic icterus of the newborn
II. Hemolytic icterus
    A. Hemolytic disease of the newborn
        1. Due to Rh incompatibility
        2. Due to ABO incompatibility
        3. Due to other rare incompatibilities
        4. Due to hemolytic anemias of other kinds
    B. Kernicterus
III. Obstructive jaundice
    A. Congenital atresia of the bile ducts
        1. Extrahepatic
        2. Intrahepatic
    B. Choledochal cyst and pseudocholedochal cyst
    C. Obstructive jaundice of obscure origin (neonatal giant-cell hepatitis)
IV. Miscellaneous causes of jaundice
    A. Other infections
    B. Toxic hepatitis
    C. Congenital familial nonhemolytic jaundice
    D. With pyloric stenosis
    E. With cystic fibrosis
    F. With enzyme deficiencies
    G. Cirrhosis of the liver

## REFERENCES

Bernstein, L. H., Ezzer, J. B., Gartner, L., and Arias, I. M.: Hepatic intracellular distribution of tritium-labelled unconjugated and conjugated bilirubin in normal and Gunn rats. J. Clin. Invest. 45:1194, 1966.

Brown, A. K.: Bilirubin metabolism in the developing liver. *In* Assali, N. (Ed.): *Biology of Gestation.* Vol. II. New York, Academic Press, 1968.

Claireaux, A. E., Cole, P. G., and Lathe, G. H.: Icterus of the brain in the newborn. Lancet 2:1226, 1953.

Lester, R., and Schmid, R.: Intestinal absorption of bile pigments. I. The enterohepatic circulation of bilirubin in the rat. J. Clin. Invest. 42:736, 1963.

Levi, A. J., Gatmaitan, Z., and Arias, I. M.: Two hepatic cytoplasmic protein fractions, Y and Z, and their possible role in the hepatic uptake of bilirubin, sulfobromophthalein and other anions. J. Clin. Invest. 48:2156, 1969.

Maisels, M. J.: Bilirubin. On understanding and influencing its metabolism in the newborn infant. Pediatr. Clin. North Am. 19:447, 1972.

Schenker, S., Dawlser, N., and Schmid, R.: Bilirubin metabolism in the fetus. J. Clin. Invest. 43:32, 1964.

Sherlock, S.: *Diseases of the Liver and Biliary System.* Oxford, Blackwell Scientific Publications, 1968.

Tenhunen, R., and Marver, H. S.: The enzymatic conversion of heme to bilirubin by microsomal heme oxygenase. Proc. Natl. Acad. Sci. U.S.A. 61:748, 1968.

# PHYSIOLOGIC ICTERUS (JAUNDICE) OF THE NEWBORN

## 70

*Revised by Frank Oski*

**DEFINITION.** Measuring the bilirubin content of blood reveals that all newborns, mature as well as immature, have levels for several days after the first day of life that are above those considered normal at any other period of life (Fig. 70–1). The term "physiologic jaundice" should be confined to those infants in whom no pathologic process is responsible for accelerated red cell breakdown, impaired conjugation or excretion of bilirubin by the liver, or increased bilirubin reabsorption from the intestinal tract. Physiologic jaundice should not manifest itself during the first 24 hours of life. Bilirubin values should not exceed 12 mg per 100 ml in full-term infants or 15 mg per 100 ml in premature infants during the first week of life.

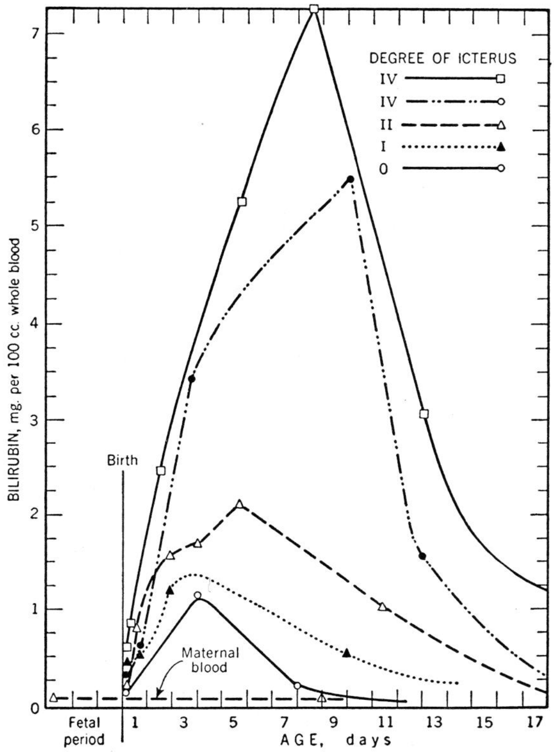

**ETIOLOGY.** A voluminous literature has accumulated dealing with the pathogenesis of icterus neonatorum. Many theories have been advanced, some of which now strike us as bizarre. Virchow, as early as 1847, first suggested excessive destruction of red blood cells in the first week of life as the basic cause. Mollison demonstrated by transfusion experiments that erythrocytes of newborns break down twice as rapidly as do those of adults. Alton Goldbloom and Gottlieb laid great stress upon increased osmotic fragility of the red cells of umbilical cord blood, whereas Hsia, Gellis, and Richard Goldbloom demonstrated beyond question that a proportion of the newborn's erythrocytes showed increased mechanical fragility. Ylppö, in 1913, proposed the theory that functional immaturity of the liver prevented its excreting all the bilirubin formed, permitting some to be returned to the circulating blood. Most students of the problem have concluded that increased blood destruction plays a role in physiologic jaundice of the newborn by increasing the load of bilirubin the liver must dispose of, but that the hepatic immaturity of the neonate is primarily responsible for hyperbilirubinemia. Weech's Béla Schick lecture for 1947 had rendered this conclusion practically inescapable. It is now generally appreciated that more than one mechanism is responsible for the hyperbilirubinemia that occurs during the newborn period. Some of these mechanisms, which act in concert to produce elevations in bilirubin level, are listed in Table 70–1.

**DIAGNOSIS.** One may assume that jaundice is physiologic if it does not appear

*Figure 70–1.* Course of neonatal bilirubinemia as recorded by Ylppö in Ztschr. f. Kinderh., Vol. 9.

precociously, that is, before 24 hours of age, and if it does not last beyond the fourteenth day of life. It almost never produces symptoms, but some sleepiness and anorexia in those infants in whom the serum bilirubin level rises above 8 mg per 100 ml may be attributable to it.

**LABORATORY INVESTIGATIONS.** Red and white blood cell counts, reticulocyte counts, and coagulation indices remain normal. The urine contains no bile or excess of urobilin. Bilirubin content of the blood rises to its height on the second to the fourth day, reaching its maximum early when cord bilirubin had been low, late when it had been high, and falls to normal between the seventh and fourteenth days in the full-term infant. It reaches the apogee about the eighth day in the premature infant and falls to normal roughly a week later. Bilirubin is of the indirect type. Liver function tests reveal no abnormalities except those consistent with the state of maturity of the infant.

Kramer has recalled to our attention an observation made long ago, that there is a head-to-foot advancement of jaundice with increasing bilirubin levels. If the feet and hands, including the palms and soles, are icteric, the serum level is almost certainly greater than 15 mg per 100 ml.

A great deal of attention has been paid in the last few years to standardization of the method for assaying bilirubin in the blood serum because of discrepancies in results from various hospital laboratories. The Committee on Fetus and Newborn of the American Academy of Pediatrics, William A. Silverman, Chairman, has laid down specific recommendations for making up an acceptable standard.

**TREATMENT.** Probably few subjects have promoted more controversy than that of the indications for exchange transfusion in instances of physiologic jaundice. In recent years our own ideas have been influenced by some significant new studies. There is little doubt that the risk of neurologic damage at a given level of serum bilirubin is affected by the weight of the infant and the concomitance of asphyxia or respiratory distress. The interaction of prematurity, a low Apgar score, and the level of indirect-reacting bilirubin was clearly shown in the results of the collaborative project of the National Institutes of Health, reported by Boggs et al. For infants of less than 2000 gm, with a 5-minute Apgar score of less than 7, 50 per cent had some mental and motor impairment at bilirubins of 10 or under. Seventy per cent had impairment at bilirubins of 16 and over. Regrettably from

**TABLE 70–1.**  *Possible Factors Involved in Producing "Physiologic Jaundice"*

| Factor | Clinical Correlate |
|---|---|
| 1. Increased bilirubin load to liver cell.<br> Newborns have increased blood volume, erythrocytes with a reduced lifespan, increased ineffective erythropoiesis, and increased bilirubin reabsorption from gut | Bilirubin levels tend to be higher in infants with polycythemia or delayed cord clamping. Infants with reduced bowel motility tend to have higher bilirubin levels |
| 2. Defective uptake of bilirubin from the plasma<br> Decreased Y protein | Caloric deprivation may reduce formation of hepatic binding proteins. Decreased caloric intake results in higher bilirubin levels |
| 3. Defective bilirubin conjugation<br> Decreased UDP glucuronyl transferase activity | UDP glucuronyl transferase activity decreased with inadequate caloric intake. Enzyme may be inhibited by factors in some mother's breast milk. Hypothyroidism reduces enzyme activity |
| 4. Defective bilirubin excretion | Congenital infections |
| 5. Inadequate hepatic perfusion | May occur with hypoxia or in patients with congenital heart disease. Both situations associated with increased incidence of hyperbilirubinemia |

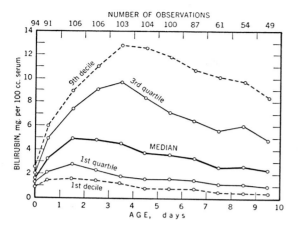

**Figure 70–2.** Course of neonatal bilirubinemia as recorded by L. T. Davidson, K. K. Merritt, and A. A. Weech: Am. J. Dis. Child. *61*:958, 1941.

the aspect of therapy, there was no single level of bilirubin below which a good outcome was assured. Another factor in the risk of kernicterus is thought to be the level of the serum albumin. Bilirubin bound to albumin is less likely to penetrate cells and cause kernicterus. The administration of albumin to an infant with hyperbilirubinemia will cause a rise in the serum bilirubin, presumably by back diffusion from extravascular tissue spaces. The degree of saturation of available albumin with bilirubin can be measured in several ways; for practical purposes Odell proposes use of the bilirubin-to-total-protein ratio; when it exceeds 3.7, he finds that the risk of central nervous system damage increases. In practice it is sometimes convenient to measure total serum solids, calculate serum proteins, and divide the total bilirubin value by that number. Since serum proteins may be very low in premature infants, those criteria for exchange may lead to the procedure when the bilirubin is 12 to 14 mg per 100 ml.

Other forms of therapy include the use of blue light to reduce levels of serum bilirubin. Although the effect of light on the level of serum bilirubin was noted by Cremer et al. and Franklin in England in 1958, and studied extensively by Ferreira and others in Brazil in the early 1960's, the extensive controlled studies of Lucey and colleagues published in 1968 brought the

significance of this' form of therapy to the attention of American pediatricians. Apparently light, either natural or cool blue fluorescent, converts the bilirubin to less toxic metabolites. The long-term fate of those infants treated by light needs to be known for assurance of the safety of this form of therapy. Its efficacy in lowering the serum bilirubin is beyond question. One rational approach to the management of the newborn infant with hyperbilirubinemia suggested by Maisels is depicted in Table 70–2.

Another approach to therapy is the treatment of infants with phenobarbital to increase the ability of the liver to excrete bilirubin. Stern et al. have shown that infants given 10 mg per kilogram per day of phenobarbital will have lower levels of bilirubin by the fourth or fifth day of life, and an increased ability to excrete bilirubin. The indications for the use of phenobarbital therapy are ill defined as are its short-term and long-term side effects. It does not act rapidly to lower serum bilirubin levels and is less effective in infants of low birth weight.

## PROLONGED PHYSIOLOGIC (?) HYPERBILIRUBINEMIA

Infants in whom asymptomatic jaundice persists through the third week or longer, and who manifest none of the abnormal signs or laboratory evidences indicative of disease, present puzzling problems. We are beginning to be able to explain some of the examples in this catchall group.

Newman and Gross found that prolonged jaundice was more common in breast-fed than in artificially fed newborns. They were able furthermore to accelerate fall in serum bilirubin concentrations by substituting cow's milk formulas for some or all of the breast milk feedings. They attribute delay in resolution of jaundice to the presence in the breast milk of some mothers of pregnane-3, alpha-2, beta diol, a hormone which interferes with bilirubin excretion. Unfortunately, this observation has been widely misinterpreted to mean that prolonged jaundice is usually related to human milk. The relationship may exist,

**TABLE 70–2.** *Guidelines for the Management of Hyperbilirubinemia as a Function of Age, Birth Weight and Bilirubin Level*

| *Serum* Indirect Bilirubin (*mg/100 ml*) | *<24 hr* | | *24–48 hr* | | *49–72 hr* | | *>72 hr* | |
|---|---|---|---|---|---|---|---|---|
| | *<2500 gm* | *>2500 gm* | *<2500 gm* | *>2500 gm* | *<2500 gm* | *>2500 gm* | *<2500 gm* | *>2500 gm* |
| 0–5 | 0 | | 0 | | 0 | | 0 | |
| 5.1–10 | Phototherapy if hemolysis present | | 0 | | 0 | | 0 | |
| 10.1–14.9 | Exchange if hemolysis | | Phototherapy | | Phototherapy | | Phototherapy | |
| 15–19.9 | Exchange transfusion | | Exchange transfusion | | Phototherapy | | Phototherapy | |
| 20 or more | Exchange transfusion | | Exchange transfusion | | Exchange transfusion | | Exchange transfusion | |

In the presence of any of the following, the infant should be treated as if the bilirubin level were in the next higher category:
Perinatal asphyxia
Five minute Apgar of less than 7
Respiratory distress syndrome
Metabolic acidosis (pH below 7.25)
Serum protein of 5.0 gm/100 ml or less
Birth weight of less than 1500 gm
Signs of central nervous system deterioration

but it is extremely rare, and has not been demonstrated to affect bilirubin levels in the first 4 days of life as noted by Dahms et al. at Cornell.

Another subgroup recently separated has

been that of red-cell enzyme deficiencies. Since these are not physiologic, they are described more fully in their proper place (pp. 610–614).

The figures that we have quoted have been largely based upon determinations made upon European and American babies. Brown and Boon point out that in Chinese, Indian and Malay full-term newborns the median bilirubin values reach considerably higher levels and persist longer than they do in British babies born in Singapore. The first two-week bilirubin curves of these Asiatic full-term infants resembled closely those of the British premature newborns.

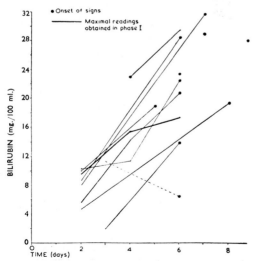

**Figure 70–3.** Serum bilirubin levels in babies with kernicterus. (Meyer, T. C.: Arch. Dis. Child. *31:*75, 1956.)

### REFERENCES

Behrman, R. E.: Preliminary report of the committee on phototherapy in the newborn infant. J. Pediatr. 84:135, 1974.

Bengtsson, B., and Verneholt, J.: A follow-up study of hyperbilirubinemia in healthy full-term infants without isoimmunization. Acta Paediat. Scand. 63:70, 1974.

Bernstein, L. H., Ezzer, J. B., Gartner, L., and Arias, I. M.: Hepatic intracellular distribution of tritium-labelled unconjugated and conjugated bilirubin in normal and Gunn rats. J. Clin. Invest 45:1194, 1966.

Boggs, T. R., Hardy, J. B., and Frazier, T. M.: Correlations of neonatal serum total bilirubin concentrations and developmental status at age eight months. J. Pediatr. 71:553, 1967.

Brown, A. K.: Bilirubin metaboli..m in the developing liver. *In* Assali, N. (Ed.): *Biology of Gestation.* New York, Academic Press, 1968, Vol. II, p. 355.

Brown, W. R., and Boon, W. H.: Ethnic group differences in plasma bilirubin levels of full-term healthy Singapore newborns. Pediatrics 36:745, 1965.

Chalmers, I., Campbell, H., and Turnbull, A. C.: Use of oxytocin and incidence of neonatal jaundice. Br. Med. J. 2:116, 1975.

Cremer, R. J., Perryman, P. W., and Richards, P. H.: Influence of light on the hyperbilirubinemia of infants. Lancet 1:1094, 1958.

Dahm, B. B., Krauss, A. N., Gartner, L. M., Klain, D. B., Soodalter, B. A., and Auld, P. A. M.: Breast feeding and serum bilirubin values during the first 4 days of life. J. Pediatr. 83:1049, 1973.

Davidson, L. T., Merritt, K. K., and Weech, A. A.: Hyperbilirubinemia in newborn. Am. J. Dis. Child. 61:958, 1941.

Desmonts, G., and Couvreur, J.: Congenital toxoplasmosis, a prospective study of 378 pregnancies. N. Engl. J. Med. 290:1110, 1974.

Ferreira, H. C., Berezin, A., Barbieri, D., and Larrubia, N. M.: Superillumination in the treatment of hyperbilirubinemia in the newborn. Rev. Ass. Med. Brasil 6:201, 1960.

Franklin, A. W.: Influence of light on the hyperbilirubinemia of infants. Lancet 1:1227, 1958.

Goldbloom, A., and Gottlieb, R.: Icterus neonatorum. Am. J. Dis. Child. 38:57, 1929.

Hsia, D. Y.-Y., Goldbloom, R. B., and Gellis, S. S.: Studies of the mechanical fragility of erythrocytes. III. Relation to physiologic jaundice of the newborn infant. Pediatrics 13:24, 1954.

Kaplan, E., Herz, F., Scheye, E., and Robinson, L. D., Jr.: Phototherapy in ABO hemolytic disease of the newborn infant. J. Pediatr. 79:911, 1971.

Kramer, L. I.: Advancement of dermal icterus in the jaundiced newborn. Am. J. Dis. Child. 118:454, 1969.

Lucey, J., Ferreiro, M., and Hewitt, J.: Prevention of hyperbilirubinemia of prematurity by phototherapy. Pediatrics 41:1047, 1968.

Maisels, J. M.: Bilirubin. Pediat. Clin. North Am. 19:447, 1972.

McKay, R. J.: Current status of use of exchange transfusion in newborn infants. Pediatrics 33:763, 1964.

Meyer, T. C.: A study of serum bilirubin levels in relation to kernicterus and prematurity. Arch. Dis. Child. 31:75, 1956.

Mollison, P. L.: The survival of transferred erythrocytes in haemolytic disease of the newborn. Arch. Dis. Child. 18:161, 1943.

Newman, A. J., and Gross, S.: Hyperbilirubinemia in breast-fed infants. Pediatrics 32:995, 1963.

Odell, G. B., Cohen, S. N., and Kelly, P. C.: Studies in kernicterus. II. The determination of the saturation of serum albumin with bilirubin. J. Pediatr. 74:214, 1969.

Saigal, S., O'Neill, A., Surainder, Y., Chua, L., and Usher, P.: Placental transfusion and hyperbilirubinemia in prematures. Pediatrics 49:406, 1972.

Shennon, A. T.: The effect of phototherapy on the hyperbilirubinemia of Rh incompatibility. Pediatrics 54:417, 1974.

Silverman, W. A.; Chairman, Committee on Fetus and Newborn, The American Academy of Pediatrics: Recommendations on a uniform bilirubin standard. Pediatrics 31:878, 1963.

Stern, L., Khanna, N. N., Pharm, G. L., and Yaffe, S. J.: Effect of phenobarbital on hyperbilirubinemia and glucuronide formation in newborns. Am. J. Dis. Child. 120:26, 1970.

Thoene, J. G., Talbert, J. L., Subramanian, S., and Odell, G. B.: Use of the hand refractometer in determining total serum proteins of infants and children. J. Pediatr. 71:413, 1967.

Virchow, cited by A. Goldbloom and R. Gottlieb: Icterus neonatorum. Am. J. Dis. Child. 38:57, 1929.

Voldes, O. S., Maurer, H. M., Shumway, C. N., Draper, D. A., and Hossaini, A. A.: Controlled clinical trial of phenobarbital and/or light in reducing neonatal hyperbilirubinemia in a predominantly Negro population. J. Pediatr. 79:1015, 1971.

Weech, A. A.: The genesis of physiologic hyperbilirubinemia. Advances Pediat. 2:346, 1947.

Ylppö, A.: Icterus neonatorum. Ergabnisse d. Ges. Med. 5:222, 1924.

# 71

# HEMOLYTIC DISEASE OF THE NEWBORN

*Revised by Frank Oski*

## HEMOLYTIC DISEASE DUE TO RH INCOMPATIBILITY

The term "hemolytic disease of the newborn" has largely replaced the older name "erythroblastosis fetalis." This is so for two reasons: first because an excess of circulating nucleated red blood cells is encountered in a number of diverse situations, and further because erythroblastosis is one of the less important diagnostic features of the disase. The general term "hemolytic disease of the newborn," followed by a qualifying phrase denoting etiology, seems far preferable.

**INCIDENCE.** Next to icterus neonatorum the most common cause of jaundice in the newborn is hemolytic disease due to Rh incompatibility. Approximately 15 per cent of all Caucasians are Rh negative, 85 per cent Rh positive. The chances of two Rh-negative persons mating are very small; hence more than four of five marriages of Rh-negative females take place with Rh-positive males. This amounts to about one out of eight of all the marriages in this country. The over-all incidence of Rh positivity of fetuses resulting from these matings is 65 per cent. Fortunately not all these fetuses have hemolytic disease. If they did, one out of every 10 babies born would suffer from it. As it is, for not completely understood reasons, only one out of 20-odd Rh-incompatible matings, hence one out of approximately 200 to 250 over-all matings in the United States, gives rise to an infant with hemolytic disease of the newborn. The disorder is much less common among black and brown races than among whites.

**PATHOLOGY.** Some of the pathologic changes are the end-results of blood destruction and regeneration, some of jaundice and liver damage. Other alterations found in the most severe examples cannot be explained so simply. Results of excessive blood destruction and regeneration include splenomegaly and hepatomegaly, widespread extramedullary hematopoiesis and hemosiderin deposition. Fetal anemia plays an important role in the production of hydrops fetalis, or universal edema of the newborn, perhaps through fetal cardiac failure, although hypoproteinemia and capillary damage may be contributing factors. Yellow staining of tissues is not present at birth, but becomes more and more intense after a few days. Of outstanding significance in this category is staining of basal nuclei and other areas of the brain, so-called kernicterus (see p. 659). The liver may show widespread plugging of canaliculi with inspissated bile and beginning fibrosis in the portal areas. Less easily explained organic alterations are cardiac enlargement, not necessarily due to anemia, and hyperplasia of the islands of Langerhans like that seen in infants of diabetic mothers. Hemorrhage into the pulmonary tissues and elsewhere is not an uncommon terminal finding for which no certain explanation is at hand.

These findings are limited to cases of extreme severity. Milder ones may show little more than slight enlargement of the spleen and evidences of blood regeneration, while those of intermediate grade may manifest some alterations but not others.

**ETIOLOGY AND PATHOGENESIS.** Hemolytic disease of the newborn is essentially a disease caused by transfer of incompatible erythrocytes from fetal to the maternal circulation. Antibodies manufactured by the mother then pass back across the placenta to the fetus, where the hemolytic process is set in motion. This may be so severe as to cause intrauterine death, usually with anemia and edema, or mild enough to permit gestation to proceed to term, when a continuation of hemolysis brings about increasing anemia and jaundice and their sequelae.

Erythrocyte blood groups are determined by the presence of antigenic material on the surface of the red cell membrane. The Rh blood groups represent many different types of antigens. The most important of these antigens in terms of clinical significance is the D or $Rh_0$ antigen. The presence of this antigen on the red cell membrane results in the cell being identified as "Rh-positive" and its absence results in it being labelled "Rh-negative." There are two other major groups of antigens related to the D antigen. They are referred to as the Cc and Ee antigens. These three antigens appear to be the product of a single gene. The frequency of three in these genes in a Caucasian population is as follows: CDe, 0.41; cde, 0.39; cDE, 0.14. Other genes such as Cde, or cDe, are less frequent. These estimates are for single genes and since chromosomes are paired it means that the antigens of a red cell will be determined by two Rh genes.

Although antibodies directed against blood groups A and B normally develop in individuals whose red cells do not possess these antigens ("naturally occurring isohemagglutinins"), exposure to Rh positive cells must occur in a Rh-negative individual before antibodies are produced. Naturally occurring isohemagglutinins of the anti-A or anti-B variety are generally of IgM class and do not cross the placenta from mother to fetus. Antibodies produced as a result of antigenic stimulation are of both the IgM and IgG variety. Antibodies of the IgG variety do cross the placenta and result in erythrocyte sensitization.

Serologic reactions between antibodies and red cells are in large part determined by the molecular nature of the antibody, IgG or IgM. IgM antibodies are capable of producing agglutination of red cells suspended in saline and are referred to as "complete antibodies." IgG antibodies will not produce agglutination under such circumstances and are referred to as "incomplete antibodies."

The red cell coated with an IgG antibody can be identified and agglutination can occur if these cells are treated with an anti IgG antibody (the Coombs' reaction), or if the sensitized cells are suspended in albumin or treated with enzymes such as papain, which reduce the cell surface charge, and allow for agglutination to occur.

The development of hemolytic disease by an Rh-positive fetus of an Rh-negative mother can be readily explained. Rh positive cells must gain entry into the circulation of an Rh negative individual. This entry usually occurs during the course of pregnancy, but it is now recognized that the first contact, or sensitizing event, may have occurred when the Rh negative mother was herself a fetus. Entry of her mother's Rh positive erythrocytes may have sensitized her, which serves to explain why some Rh negative mothers appear sensitized during their first pregnancy. One stands on less solid ground in attempting to explain why 20 infants with such a set-up do not have disease, while only one does. Several factors are involved in this apparent discrepancy. It is not certain that fetal blood seeps into the maternal circulation in all pregnancies. If it does, and if the isoimmunologic blood groups also differ, such fetal blood as does cross the placental barrier may be destroyed so rapidly that Rh sensitization does not take place. Or fetal antigen may cross the placental barrier and enter the maternal circulation, but still not call forth in many mothers the expected response of antibody formation.

Some of the different clinical pictures of the disease may be explained by the time the antigen-antibody reaction begins. If it starts several months before term, and is severe, blood destruction produces profound anemia. The resulting excess of bilirubin is almost entirely taken care of by the placental and maternal circulations; hence jaundice and liver damage do not follow. (There are exceptions to this general rule, that is, some severely affected fetuses are born with high bilirubin levels in their cord blood, 25 to 50 per cent of which may be direct-reacting.) Instead, anemia leads to heart failure, and universal edema supervenes. When on the other hand, the hemolytic process is initiated later, reaching its height just before or at term, anemia at birth is not so severe, and the newborn must handle the excess of bilirubin with his own immature liver. The premature infant stands in double jeopardy in view of his handicap with respect to the conjugation of bilirubin. An amount of hemolysis which might be innocuous to a full-term infant may raise the premature infant's serum bilirubin level to dangerous heights.

**DIAGNOSIS.** The Rh-positive infant born of an Rh-negative sensitized mother may have no illness whatsoever. Fifteen to 20 per cent fall into this category. The rest have disease in which jaundice, anemia and edema are the outstanding signs, commingled in varying proportions.

In a mild case the condition at birth is quite satisfactory. Jaundice makes its appearance earlier than is to be expected in physiologic icterus, within the first 24 to 36 hours, and becomes moderately intense. The spleen may become palpable, the liver somewhat enlarged. After about the fourth day jaundice begins to subside, along with the hepatosplenomegaly, and moderate pallor becomes noticeable. This persists for a number of weeks.

When the disease is more severe, jaundice may be obvious at birth in yellow discoloration of the cord and skin, but this is rare, or it appears within a few hours. It rapidly becomes more and more intense, until a deep greenish-yellow hue is attained by the third or fourth day. The entire body, but especially the extremities, may be puffy and edematous to the touch. The spleen and liver become very large. Feedings are taken poorly and may be regurgitated. The infant appears critically sick. Pallor of the mucous membranes becomes obvious. The heart enlarges, its sounds become "wooly," and it may rapidly fail. Respirations become rapid and labored, and bloody material may issue from the mouth, suggesting either heart failure or pulmonary hemorrhage, or both. On the third or fourth day, or a bit later, retraction of the head, stiffening spells, rolling of the eyes downward or frank convulsions may indicate that kernicterus has supervened.

Rarely edema is the predominant sign. The fetus is grotesquely puffed and waterlogged, the serous cavities overfilled with transudate, the abdomen distended and flat to percussion. There is severe anemia and cardiac enlargement, but no jaundice. Infants with hydrops fetalis, or universal edema of the newborn, ordinarily are stillborn, but may be live-born. A few have been saved by prompt heroic action. Almost equally rarely is anemia the principal symptom, at times the only one. These infants show pallor and little or no jaundice. Their hearts may enlarge and fail.

## HYDROPS FETALIS FROM OTHER CAUSES

The recognition that hydrops fetalis is often associated with isoimmunization has contributed to the failure to recognize that the same clinical picture may result from other causes.

It should be remembered that infants may be born hydropic because of congenital cardiac defects, polycystic kidneys and other renal defects or congenital syphilis. A list of other recognized causes of hydrops fetalis is presented in Table 71–1.

**TABLE 71–1.   *Causes of Hydrops Fetalis***

Severe chronic anemia in utero
   Isoimmunization
   Homozygous alpha-thalassemia
   G6PD deficiency with maternal drug ingestion
Cardiac failure
   Severe congenital heart disease
   Premature closure of foramen ovale
   Large arteriovenous malformation
   Prolonged supraventricular tachycardia
Hypoproteinemia
   Renal disease (congenital nephrosis, renal vein
      thrombosis)
   Congenital hepatitis
Intrauterine infections
   Syphilis
   Toxoplasmosis
   Cytomegalovirus
Miscellaneous
   Maternal diabetes mellitus
   Umbilical or chorionic vein thrombosis
   Fetal neuroblastomatosis
   Chagas' disease
   Achondroplasia
   Cystic adenomatoid malformation of the lung
   Pulmonary lymphangiectasia
   Choriocarcinoma in situ
   Congenital Gaucher's disease
   Urethral atresia
   Placental chorioangioma

LABORATORY INVESTIGATIONS. The hemoglobin content of the cord blood varies from normal to moderately reduced in most cases, but may be exceedingly low in a few. Hemoglobin generally falls within the first week and remains low in untreated cases for 6 to 8 weeks, after which it slowly rises. The degree of fall varies with the severity of the particular case. After transfusion hemoglobin rises to more normal levels, but it almost invariably falls again to remain at about 8 to 10 gm per 100 ml for the first 6 to 8 weeks of life.

A technical problem arises in the first day of life in terms of the site of sampling for hemoglobin and hematocrit determinations. Acrocyanosis can result in higher hemoglobin values in capillary blood from a heel than those in venous blood. Moe reports the average capillary hemoglobin at birth is 19.4 gm, and cord hemoglobin 15.7 gm. Corresponding values for hematocrit are 65.3 in capillary blood and 51.7 in cord blood.

The red blood cell count follows the same general curve as does hemoglobin content. Nucleated red cells are consistently increased in number at birth, a fact which gave the disease its first name. Their number roughly approximates the severity of the case. Counts of 25 to 100 or more per 100 white blood cells are not unusual. They disappear from the circulation within a few days. Reticulocytes are also increased in number, and their percentage may be used as one of the better prognostic criteria. There is usually moderate leukocytosis with increased polymorphonuclear percentage. Platelets may fall to low levels. This, coupled with physiologic lengthening of prothrombin conversion time expected on the second and third days, possibly increased by liver damage, may account for the bleeding phenomena observed. In severely ill infants, laboratory evidence of disseminated intravascular coagulation can usually be demonstrated.

The urine shows an excess of urobilinogen consistent with exaggerated hemolysis. Bile appears in the urine later only if the "inspissated bile syndrome" supervenes.

In all but the mildest cases the cord blood bilirubin is found to be above 3 mg per 100 ml. Depending upon severity, its rise may be slow or rapid. It may never exceed 8 or 10 mg on the second or third day, tapering off to normal by the eighth or tenth day, or it may rise sharply to dangerous heights by the twenty-fourth hour. If treatment is withheld, it may continue to rise for several more days, attaining levels not reached in any other condition. The largest part of the total bilirubin content is of the indirect type. Any shift of this proportion toward a preponderance of the direct type suggests that a complication or sequela has supervened.

In babies who are severely jaundiced at birth with bilirubin levels in the range of 15 to 25 mg per 100 ml, much of the pigment is usually of the conjugated-direct reacting variety. Cornblath et al. have reported two of these, one of whom died and was autopsied. His liver showed evidences of severe damage.

In medically sophisticated communities the Rh status of the mother and father and the presence or absence of circulating Rh antibodies are known before delivery. If they are not, these facts must be determined immediately when a baby is noted to be jaundiced within the first 24 hours. In addition, studies of the baby's blood should be accomplished to ascertain 1) his Rh group, 2) presence of Rh antibody attached to erythrocytes (direct Coombs test), and 3) presence or absence of freely circulating antibodies.

Several recent studies have verified the fact that many erythroblastotic infants suffer from significant hypoglycemia. This correlates with the hyperplasia of the islets of Langerhans so often found in those babies who die. In explanation From et al. demonstrated marked elevation of serum immunoreactive insulin in 12 infants with erythroblastosis fetalis over the levels found in 14 normal neonates.

TREATMENT. Chronologically, the first decision to be made is whether or not the fetus in jeopardy should be delivered before awaiting termination of pregnancy. Two criteria were utilized in the past in arriving at this decision: the mother's history with respect to previous delivery of erythroblastotic infants and the curve of the mother's Rh antibody titer.

In 1950 Vaughan, Allen and Diamond reported that if the mother had not previously delivered a baby with erythroblastosis fetalis and if she had never received a transfusion of Rh-positive blood, the resulting infant was considerably more apt to be free of disease or to recover if hemolytic disease developed than if either of these events had taken place. Good results, no clinical disease or recovery, occurred in 74 per cent in the first instance, about 40 per cent in the latter, whereas death, kernicterus or stillbirth accounted for 26 versus 60 per cent in the two groups, respectively. Although many exceptions to this rule have been noted by all observers, it remains a satisfactory generalization from the statistical point of view.

The same authors showed the deleterious effects upon the subsequently born infants of high titers of antibody in the maternal blood. A highest titer in bovine albumin of 1:64 or more proved ominous in their experience, 10 per cent of the resulting infants dying and 35 per cent developing kernicterus. Again numerous exceptions have been noted, but again the generalization is of use.

For a few years there was a strong tendency to induce premature delivery in cases which fulfilled these two criteria. It was soon realized that prematurity itself added an appreciable hazard, and the practice fell into disrepute. The pendulum is again swinging cautiously toward decision in favor of induction of labor or cesarean section in the face of a high maternal titer and bad history. The decision is reinforced by the discovery of hydramnios, by diminution in fetal activity, and by either a sharp rise or a sharp fall in maternal antibody titer late in pregnancy.

Boggs has made a very strong case in favor of interruption of pregnancy in selected "high risk" and "intermediate risk" cases. He defines the first simply as a pregnancy of a mother who has given birth previously to a stillborn infant because of erythroblastosis fetalis or to a hydropic fetus. The second refers to a pregnancy subsequent to the delivery of a live erythroblastotic fetus who was not hydropic. With interruption before the due date his survival rate was considerably higher

than without. He advises that one never interrupt pregnancy before 34 weeks, that "high-risk" pregnancies be terminated at 34 to 35 weeks, "intermediate" ones at 36 to 37 weeks, low-risk ones at 38 weeks. He leaves the choice of method of interruption to the judgment of the obstetrician. We are in agreement with the first two recommendations.

Obstetricians have long been aware of the discoloration of the amniotic fluid in association with isoimmunization, but it was not until 1952 that Bevis carried out a systematic study of the phenomenon and described the spectral absorption curve of the pigments. Late in 1961, Liley refined the analysis and related the height of the 450 $m\mu$ "bulge" on spectral absorption to the likelihood of fetal death from hemolytic disease. Since then amniotic fluid spectrophotometry has come into wide clinical use to determine the health of the fetus and the possible need for fetal transfusion or early delivery.

Serial measurements of optical density allow designation of the risk to the infant of allowing the pregnancy to proceed. When dangerous levels of pigment are detected, intrauterine transfusion may provide enough red cells to allow the fetus to survive in utero. Some infants have been transfused as early as 21 weeks and then every 3 to 4 weeks thereafter. The survival of some infants is doubtless attributable to the fetal transfusions. The procedure of instillation of red cells into the fetal peritoneal cavity is not without hazard, however. Occasionally the needle pierces the thorax or the liver rather than the peritoneal cavity. Other times, labor ensues as a result of the manipulation of the uterus.

Lucey summarizes the experience with fetal transfusion succinctly as follows: "The best candidate for fetal transfusion is from 28 to 32 weeks of age, has a high Zone II or low Zone III $\Delta$OD 450 (rising or not) decreasing on successive amniocenteses), and does not have hydrops fetalis." The procedure "has a low mortality risk for the mother, about a 5 per cent mortality for the fetus, and appears to decrease the perinatal mortality from erythroblastosis fetalis by about 50 per cent."

The next decision to be made is whether

exchange transfusion should be carried out immediately after delivery. This is based upon clinical or hematologic grounds supplemented by the known facts of the mother's previous pregnancies. If the infant is born jaundiced or pale, or both, if there is obvious edema or if the spleen and liver are greatly enlarged, exchange transfusion will be performed immediately. Should the clinical condition at birth be satisfactory, one will await the results of blood tests. A negative direct Coombs test result rules out Rh sensitization. If the direct Coombs test result is positive, a cord blood hemoglobin of less than 11 gm per 100 ml in full-term infants, less than 14 gm in premature infants, is generally considered adequate reason for proceeding with exchange transfusion. So is a cord bilirubin content of more than 4 mg per 100 ml.

The borderline cases in which the clinical condition is good, the Coombs test result positive, but hemoglobin above these figures and bilirubin below 4 mg cause the most perplexity. A bad maternal history with respect to prior pregnancies argues in favor of active treatment.

In infants in whom exchange transfusion is not felt to be immediately indicated, phototherapy should be instituted. Phototherapy has been shown to reduce the need for repeat exchange transfusions in infants with Rh incompatibility and to reduce the need for initial exchange transfusion in infants with ABO incompatibility.

Babies in the doubtful category should be watched closely for any change in clinical condition, and blood studies should be performed every 4 to 6 hours. Anorexia, vomiting, lethargy, signs of cerebral irritation, a rapidly rising curve of bilirubin or a rapidly falling hemoglobin level should swing the balance in favor of therapeutic intervention. It is difficult to designate set limits for these factors beyond which transfusion should be done. We know that the danger point for bilirubin content is about 15 to 20 mg per 100 ml and that above this level kernicterus becomes a possible and frightening complication. One should intervene if it exceeds 6 mg per 100 ml in the first 6 hours, 10 mg in the first 12 hours or 20 mg. at any time in a term infant. A useful guide for infants of low birth weight,

when indices of serum bilirubin binding capacity are not clinically available, is to perform an exchange transfusion when the bilirubin level reaches the infant's birth weight divided by 100. Specifically, an infant of 900 grams would be exchanged at a bilirubin of 9 mg per 100 ml, while an infant of 1400 grams would be exchanged at a bilirubin of 14 mg per 100 ml. The gradient of the rise gives a fair indication of the height that will be achieved, although this is far from certain. A rising bilirubin concentration in the order of 0.75 to 1.0 mg per hour is considered by many to be an indication for exchange transfusion.

A low and rapidly falling hemoglobin level, if accompanied by rapidly rising bilirubin, calls for action. If bilirubin remains at a low level while hemoglobin falls quickly, a rare but not unheard of situation, the much less arduous treatment of simple transfusion may be given. The particular virtue of exchange tranfusion is reduction of bilirubin concentration, but Oski and Naiman remind us that severe anemia, with actual or imminent heart failure, is an equally valid indication. In these infants the added burden of 40 or 50 ml of blood may be fatal, whereas cautious replacement, guided by venous pressure determinations, of several hundred milliliters of anemic blood by packed red blood cells may be lifesaving.

Second, third and at times a larger number of exchange transfusions may have to be performed. Normally there is a "rebound" after the end of a transfusion caused by the binding of extravascular tissue bilirubin to the fresh, nonbilirubin-laden albumin which has replaced the infant's bound albumin. If the "rebound" level exceeds 20 mg per 100 ml and remains at that level or rises after 8 to 12 hours, re-exchange is in order. Wishingrad and Elegant reported two favorable results after five and eight replacement transfusions in two very sick newborns.

Odell has made a strong case for the greater efficacy in reduction of bilirubin levels by the injection of salt-free albumin, 1.0 gm per kilogram of body weight, 2 to 4 hours prior to the exchange transfusion. He was able to remove an average of 40 per cent more bilirubin after such "priming" than without it, and feels fairly sure that the need for subsequent exchange transfusions was lessened. He warns that it should not be used in severely anemic or edematous children, since blood volume is increased by albumin injections. Ruys and van Gelderen condemn the procedure on this ground, but Odell has demonstrated its safety amply. Waters and Porter advocate, not priming, but replacement of 25 or 50 ml of donor plasma with 25 ml (6.25 gm) or 50 ml (12.5 gm) of salt-free human albumin prior to exchange.

**PROGNOSIS.** The high mortality rates and high incidence of kernicterus so usual in the 1940's have been reduced gratifyingly by the more general utilization of exchange transfusion. Several clinics can boast of results comparable to those of Diamond and of Arnold et al. The latter group achieved a survival rate of 97.5 per cent, with but one case of kernicterus discovered among 217 survivors. There still remains an appreciable percentage of fetal deaths in the last months of pregnancy with which we must learn to deal more successfully. Early induction of labor or cesarean section probably saves a few infants. Fetal transfusion in the proper hands certainly saves a few more.

The outlook for premature infants with hemolytic disease of the newborn is graver than it is for mature infants. Hsia and Gellis showed that the former demonstrate a higher late bilirubin rise than do the latter. Black-Schaffer et al. argue, with credibility, that the essential difference may lie in the immaturity of the premature infant's hepatic function which permits hyperbilirubinemia to reach higher levels for the same rate of hemolysis. *All premature infants with a positive direct Coombs test result should be given an exchange transfusion.*

**DANGERS OF EXCHANGE TRANSFUSION.** The hazards of exsanguination transfusion begin with induction of heart failure by overrapid introduction of blood. It is wise to determine venous pressure periodically throughout the procedure and to remove more blood than is infused if this figure rises above 60 mm of water. Trevor Wright found that infants were not distressed unless umbilical vein pressure exceeded

12 cm of blood. Overcooling of the heart has been blamed for cardiac arrest. Donor blood must be warmed throughout the operation. Depletion of serum calcium by citrate added to donor blood has caused tetany with convulsions and occasionally death. One milliliter of 10 per cent calcium gluconate should be injected after each 100 ml has been exchanged (one half as much in premature infants), and care should be taken to carry out this injection slowly.

Many of the hazards of exchange transfusion are summarized in Table 71–2. Most of these hazards can be avoided by careful attention to detail, appropriate warming of the infant during the procedure, and constant monitoring of the heart. The use of blood, anticoagulated with citrate-phosphate-dextrose (CPD), and less than 5 days of age will also reduce biochemical side effects. With experienced personnel and a non-hydropic infant, the mortality of an exchange transfusion should be less than 1 per cent.

More recently the danger of inducing high potassium levels, especially hazardous when serum calcium is low, has been pointed out. The serum potassium concentration of these infants is often high to begin with. If one then uses banked blood which has been stored for more than 2 or 3 days, one may introduce an excess of potassium with which the infant's kidneys cannot cope. It is possible that a number of the sudden deaths which have occurred during exsanguination transfusion have resulted from hyperkalemia. The best preventive is to insist upon fresh blood. Calcium given as recommended above is of help. Campbell's suggestion that one give insulin routinely warrants further investigation. Serum potassium determinations performed serially throughout the procedure would be of tremendous help, but in many hospitals this would not be feasible. Periodic electrocardiographic tracings can be taken more easily and should be almost equally informative in this regard.

Exhaustive studies on the electrolyte changes during exchange transfusion have cast doubt upon the probability that most deaths during or shortly after exchange transfusion have been caused by the factors mentioned. Inordinately high citrate levels

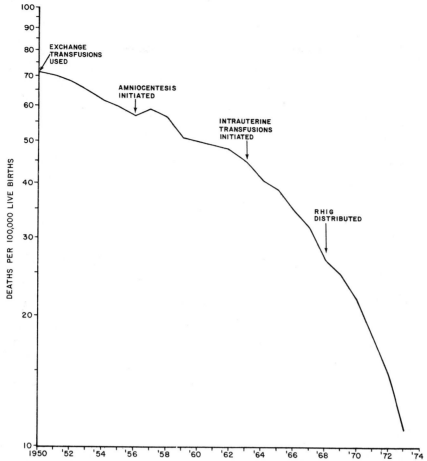

*Figure 71–1.* Infant death rates for hemolytic disease of the newborn, United States, 1950–1973. (From Center for Disease Control: Rh Hemolytic Disease Surveillance, Annual Report. June 1975.)

are given consideration. Van Praagh is concerned with the acidity of stored blood increased by the addition of citrate solution and its hazard in lowering the pH of the recipient's blood. Many sudden deaths are still not explainable.

Significant changes in acid-base balance occur if citrated blood is used for the exchange. The pH of the donor blood is usually about 6.0 to 8.0, and during an exchange the ·blood in the infant will be about 7.20 to 7.30, depending on the condition at the start of the procedure. In the few

hours after exchange, as citrate is metabolized to bicarbonate, the infant will be relatively alkaline, sometimes with a pH of 7.50 to 7.60. Heparized blood or THAM added to the donor blood obviates this problem, but introduces another, namely a hemorrhagic tendency or hypoglycemia.

Infants who survive the critical first week may be expected to become moderately anemic within the following week or two. This results from a continuation of hemolysis by the antibodies left behind in the infant's tissues. It is impossible to remove

*TABLE 71–2. Potential Hazards of Exchange Transfusion*

| | |
|---|---|
| Vascular | Embolization with air or clots |
| | Thrombosis of portal vein |
| | Hemorrhagic infarction of the colon |
| Cardiac | Cardiac arrhythmias and shock if more than 10 per cent of blood volume is removed acutely |
| | Volume overload |
| | Cardiac arrest |
| Metabolic | Hyperkalemia |
| | Hypernatremia |
| | Hypocalcemia |
| | Hypomagnesemia |
| | Acidosis—temporary |
| | Rebound alkalosis |
| | Hypoglycemia—post-exchange |
| Coagulation | Overheparinization |
| | Thrombocytopenia |
| Infections | Bacteremia |
| | Hepatitis |
| | Malaria |
| | Cytomegalovirus infection |
| Miscellaneous | Mechanical injury to donor cells |
| | Thermal injury to donor cells if overwarmed in heating coil |
| | Hypothermia |
| | Graft versus host reaction if transfusion occurs in unsuspected immunoincompetent recipient |

them all by exchange transfusion. Coupled with this is the fact that the bone marrow at this age is normally in an aregenerative phase. Finally regeneration of erythrocytes may be further retarded by the transfusion. This anemia is not responsive to iron. Further transfusion should be avoided, since it may again postpone red cell regeneration, until the hemoglobin content falls below 7.0 to 8.0 gm per 100 ml.

Babies who are known to be sensitized, whose direct Coombs test result is positive, but who do not become ill within their normal nursery sojourn are too often discharged as well, and given no further thought. This is reprehensible, since many of these infants will have delayed anemia. Hemoglobins in this group may fall to levels low enough to warrant one or two simple transfusions. *Iron will neither prevent nor cure this form of anemia.*

Those babies who survive kernicterus must be observed closely for evidence of permanent brain damage. These will appear in the majority.

**PREVENTION OF ISOIMMUNIZATION.** It is of course a source of great satisfaction to be able to add a section entitled Prevention to a description of a disease. Rarely in the history of medicine has a single generation witnessed the original description of a disease and then seen the evolution of precise means of diagnosis and insight into pathogenesis, followed by an effective although cumbersome form of therapy and then a means of prevention. It is surely equally satisfying to reflect that these advances were made by systematic study and inductive reasoning rather than pure chance.

The first hint of a means of prevention dates from 1943, shortly after the discovery of the Rh factor, when Levine reported that ABO incompatibility protects against Rh sensitization, presumably by destruction of any ABO incompatible fetal red cells entering the maternal circulation. The possibility then emerged of destruction of fetal cells by injection of anti-D serum into the mother at the time of initial sensitization. The obvious problem was to know when the mother was first sensitized, and if it would occur all at once or in multiple stages through gestation. Clinical evidence suggested that the first incompatible pregnancy was the one that sensitized, and that sensitization must occur near the time of delivery, since antibodies were rarely demonstrable during that pregnancy, but could be found in the early weeks of the next incompatible pregnancy.

A major advance in the quest of a means of prevention came with the advent of a very sensitive and specific test for the presence of fetal erythrocytes in the maternal circulation. The Kleihauer technique of acid elution met the criteria of sensitivity. It was shown by Finn et al. on male volunteers that as little as 1 ml of fetal blood injected into their circulations could be detected, and that quantitation between 1 and 10 ml was possible. The application of these techniques to study of Rh-negative women supported the thesis that sensitization usually occurs at delivery of the first Rh-positive child. Later these same investigators showed that immunization of the

Rh-negative males after injection of Rh-positive cells could be prevented by administration of high anti-D titer serum.

The availability of high titer anti-D IgG prepared from Rh immune plasma has made it possible to treat hundreds of women after delivery of the first child, and follow-up through subsequent pregnancies has confirmed the high order of protection available. Freda and colleagues, who first studied IgG preparations, recommend 1 to 5 ml of gamma a-globulin within 36 hours of delivery.

It is fortunate that the protective antibodies may be given within 72 hours of delivery with good effect. As little as 300 $\mu$g of anti-D IgG in a single intramuscular dose is adequate. As greater experience accumulates, doubtless other patterns of protection will emerge. Some advocate use of the anti-D antibodies at 34 weeks' gestation in Rh-negative primigravidas, because some women are sensitized before delivery.

## HEMOLYTIC DISEASE DUE TO ABO INCOMPATIBILITY

In 1944 Halbrecht coined the term "icterus praecox" to denote the development of jaundice within the first 24 hours of life, before one expects physiologic icterus to become manifest. He noted that most of these infants belonged to a blood group which differed from that of their mothers and concluded that there existed a cause-and-effect relation between jaundice and heterospecificity.

**INCIDENCE.** Halbrecht discovered 90 cases of icterus praecox among 16,000 babies, one per 180 births. This figure approximates the 1:200 to 250 who develop Rh erythroblastosis. Nevertheless, approximately 25 per cent of all pregnancies are heterospecific, as opposed to 12 per cent which are Rh-incompatible, which means that only one of 45 heterospecific infants, contrasted with one of 20 Rh-incompatible ones, gets into trouble because of non-matching maternal and fetal blood. Since most ABO incompatibles who do become jaundiced manifest no illness beyond the mild jaundice which clears rapidly and spontaneously, it is clear that this form is considerably less important clinically than Rh incompatiblity. Ordinarily the fetus must be protected against the harmful effects of heterospecificity by mechanisms not yet completely understood.

For reasons not at all understood, girls are more likely to be affected than are boys, by a ratio of 3:1 (Grundbacher).

**ETIOLOGY.** When hemolysis of fetal blood does occur in the course of heterospecific pregnancy, its pathogenesis differs from that of Rh erythroblastosis in one main regard. Prior sensitization is not required, since group O mothers already possess a and b agglutinins, which may traverse the placental barrier and come in contact with the infant's A or B erythrocytes. It is evident that under these circumstances firstborns should be in as great jeopardy as those of later rank, and Halbrecht's observations confirm this presupposition. Thirty of his 90 cases of icterus praecox occurred in infants of primigravidae. But Chan et al. believe that firstborns affected by "natural" antibodies become less severely ill than babies of later rank in whom "natural" antibodies are supplemented by those the mother elaborates in response to her infant's red blood cells or secretions, so-called immune antibodies. Other observers disagree with this conclusion.

Zuelzer and Kaplan carried out a searching investigation of the clinical, hematologic and serologic aspects of the entire problem of heterospecific pregnancies, and Zuelzer has clarified their findings in a monograph on the subject. What follows is a brief condensation of their data and conclusions.

There are three combinations that might cause trouble for the fetus. These are mother A-infant B, mother B-infant A and mother O-infant A, B or AB. In actuality only the mother O-infant A or B situation, with rare exceptions, leads to hemolytic disease. The offending antigen is almost always A, and what is more, A of the specific subgroup $A_1$. In Grundbacher's experience with 47 affected infants, 45 were of the blood type $A_1$ and only two were $A_2$. There were no B's. Since in all heterospecific pregnancies of this nature A antigen is present in the fetus and anti-A agglutinin circulates in the mother's serum, one must explain why the babies resulting from all such matings do not have hemolytic disease. Two possible answers present themselves. Either most fetuses have protective mechanisms or only a few mothers elaborate abnormal antibodies, "immune" antibodies as opposed to the "natural" ones always present.

A potent protective mechanism in all probability is the presence of A or B substance in tissue cells of all persons of those groups as well as in the body fluids of the "secretors." There is some evidence to indicate that this substance in placental cells neutralizes much of the maternal agglutinin before it can enter the fetal circulation, although again there is not complete agreement on this point. A second protection resides in the fact that fetal and neonatal A antigen is relatively weak, thus providing "some protection against maternal antibodies that have crossed the placental barrier, a suggestion previously put forward by Tovey" (Grundbacher). A third suggestion is that even though some hemolysis takes place, the livers of most infants are capable of excreting the small additional load of bilirubin.

It has become clear that an excess of maternal antibody as demonstrated by unusually high titers of anti-A or anti-B in maternal or fetal circulation is not the deciding factor between hemolytic disease or its absence. And it is surely true that the antibodies discovered in hemolytic disease do indeed differ from "natural" antibodies in several respects. Why some mothers produce "immune" antibodies and others do not has not been explained. The fact may have nothing at all to do with heterospecific pregnancy, since "dangerous universal donors," i.e. group O persons who have "immune" antibodies, have been recognized for many years.

**DIAGNOSIS.** Infants with icterus praecox due to hemolytic disease caused by heterospecific pregnancy exhibit jaundice within the first 36 hours of life. Generally these infants do not become ill. They do not have anemia, and the liver and spleen do not enlarge. Jaundice disappears in 3 to 7 days.

Rarely, however, the disease assumes greater severity, and every gradation described for Rh hemolytic disease may be encountered. Cases with more severe jaundice, anemia and hepatosplenomegaly are seen. In some the hyperbilirubinemia reaches dangerous heights from the point of view of the development of kernicterus. One rarely sees an infant severely anemic at birth, in threatened or actual heart failure or in true shock. Even babies with fullblown hydrops fetalis have been born, exactly as in Rh hemolytic disease.

**LABORATORY FINDINGS.** Hemoglobin and red blood cell count are usually normal, although in severe cases they may be depressed to extremely low levels. In the moderately symptomatic case hemoglobin levels of approximately 12.0 gm. are usual. Stained smear shows an unusual number of spherocytes and nucleated erythrocytes in moderate numbers. Reticulocytosis and polychromasia are conspicuous.

Serum bilirubin is slightly higher than the average in most cases. In the series of Hsia and Gellis bilirubin was high at birth in all 21 cases, rose sharply in the first 3 days and reached levels in eight of the 21 that were high enough to warrant exchange transfusion. These cases were selectively severe and are not representative of the entire group.

Almost always the mother will belong to blood group O, the infant to A.

In the infant's serum the direct Coombs test result is generally negative, and if positive is only weakly so. The indirect Coombs test result, using adult red cells of the same group as the infant's, is almost always positive, making it one of the more useful laboratory tests for verifying the diagnosis.

In maternal serum, demonstration of "immune" antibody by the original Witebsky technique, or a modification of this test, is most informative. This consists in neutralizing "natural" antibodies by exposure to A or B substance, thereafter proving its ability still to agglutinate the infant's cells or adult cells of the same group.

Kaplan et al. have added one more test to our armamentarium. The activity of erythrocyte cholinesterase is sharply diminished in the red blood cells of newborn infants with ABO hemolytic disease. This is not true for Rh hemolytic disease or for other disorders producing jaundice in newborns.

**DIFFERENTIAL DIAGNOSIS.** Kaplan et al. lay down these criteria for distinguishing ABO hemolytic disease. The disease is suspected if 1) icterus appears within 24 hours, 2) serum bilirubin level exceeds 12 mg per 100 ml in the first 72 hours, or 3) ABO disease had developed in a prior sibling. The suspicion is strengthened if 1) spherocytes are found and 2) if reticulocytes exceed 12 per cent. The suspicion is rendered a virtual certainty if one of these serologic abnormalities is found: 1) positive direct Coombs test result, 2) positive indirect Coombs test result using infant's serum and adult red blood cells of the same type, or 3) positive eluate test result using similar red blood cells and eluate of the infant's serum. To this list may now be added 4) diminution of erythrocyte acetylcholinesterase activity in the infant's red blood cells.

**TREATMENT.** Most cases require no treatment at all. Hyperbilirubinemia probably should be managed in the same way it is handled no matter what its cause. Zuelzer suggests that one may have a bit more leeway in the use of exchange transfusion in ABO disease than in Rh disease. This may well be true, but until we learn more about differences between hyperbilirubinemias of Rh and ABO origin we believe they should be handled in the same manner.

The rare case demonstrating severe anemia or hydrops fetalis at birth should also be treated by exchange transfusion.

## HEMOLYTIC DISEASE DUE TO RARE BLOOD GROUP INCOMPATIBILITIES

A few antigens other than A, B, C, D, E and F have been reported upon occasion to produce a clinical picture similar to that described in the preceding sections. Baker et al. described such a case in which the father and the infant were Duffy-positive (Fy$^a$), the mother Duffy-negative. Anti-Duffy antibody was demonstrated in the mother's blood *post partum*. The mother

had been sensitized either by her first infant, who was normal, or by transfusions given after this delivery. Her second pregnancy resulted in an anencephalic fetus, her third in a 6-month stillbirth. The fourth baby had icterus praecox, his bilirubin level rising to 21 mg at 76 hours, at which time exchange transfusion was performed. Direct Coombs test result was weakly positive.

Other antigens responsible for neonatal hemolytic disease are the so-called hR, or little c, d or e, of which little c is the most common cause of disease—although it too is rare—Kell, Duffy and a few others. We shall not go into details about these unusual variants, since their differentiation is entirely a matter for the special laboratory. One should only remember that babies born with these abnormal antigens are (or may be) Rh-negative, but that their direct Coombs test results are strongly positive. Discovery of an infant, therefore, who is born with evidences of hemolytic disease of the newborn, who has a positive direct Coombs test result, but is Rh-negative, calls for thorough hematologic investigation with respect to the less common antigens.

## HEMOLYTIC DISEASE DUE TO CONGENITALLY ABNORMAL ERYTHROCYTES

Congenital defects of the erythrocyte manifest themselves in the newborn period and simulate hemolytic disease of the newborn that is caused by isoimmunization. The most common of these is red cell glucose-6-phosphate dehydrogenase deficiency. Hereditary spherocytosis also may produce intense hyperbilirubinemia during this period of life. The intrinsic defects of the red cell associated with either anemia or jaundice in the neonatal period are described in detail in Chapter 66.

### REFERENCES

Anders, D., Kinderman, G., and Pfeifer, V.: Metastasizing fetal neuroblastoma with involvement of the placenta simulating fetal erythroblastosis. J. Pediatr. 82:50, 1973.

Arnold, D. P., Witebsky, E., Selkirk, G. H., and Alford, K. M.: Clinical and serological experiences in treating hemolytic disease of the newborn. J. Pediatr. *46*:520, 1955.

Ascari, W. Q., Allen, A. F., Baker, W. J., and Pollack, W.: Rh₀(D) immune globulin (human): Evaluation in women at risk of immunization. J.A.M.A. *205*:1, 1968.

Baker, J. B., Grewar, D., Lewis, M., Ayukawa, H., and Chown, B.: Haemolytic disease of the newborn due to anti-Duffy (Fyᵃ). Arch. Dis. Child. *31*:298, 1956.

Bevis, D. C. A.: Antenatal prediction of hemolytic disease of newborn. Lancet *1*:395, 1952.

Bevis, D. C. A.: Composition of liquor amnii in haemolytic disease of newborn. J. Obstet. Gynaec. Brit. Cmwlth. *60*:244, 1953.

Black-Schaffer, B., Kambe, S., Furuta, M., and Moloney, W. C.: Neonatal jaundice and kernicterus. A.M.A. J. Dis. Child. *87*:737, 1954.

Boggs, T. R.: Survival rates in Rh sensitizations; 140 interrupted versus 141 uninterrupted pregnancies. Pediatrics *33*:758, 1964.

Boggs, T. R., and Abelson, N. M.: Early and reliable guide in the prognosis and management of hemolytic disease of the newborn. A.M.A. J. Dis. Child. *88*:506, 1954.

Campbell, W. A. B.: Potassium levels in exchange transfusion. Arch. Dis. Child. *30*:513, 1955.

Chan, A. C., Chung, F., and Keitel, H. G.: ABO hemolytic disease: Serologic diagnosis with the two stage direct antiglobulin test by means of fresh serum J. Pediatr. *61*:405, 1962.

Cohen, F., Zuelzer, W. W., Gustafson, D. C., and Evans, M. M.: Mechanisms of isoimmunization. I. The transplacental passage of fetal erythrocytes in nonspecific pregnancies. Blood *23*:621, 1964.

Cornblath, M., Kramer, I., and Kelly, A. B.: Rh isoimmunization associated with regurgitation jaundice beginning in utero. Sinai Hosp. J. *4*:124, 1955.

Day, R. L., and Haines, M. S.: Intelligence quotients of children recovered from erythroblastosis fetalis since the introduction of exchange transfusion. Pediatrics *13*:333, 1954.

Dunn, H. G.: Hemolytic disease of the newobrn due to ABO incompatibility. A.M.A. J. Dis. Child. *85*:655, 1953.

Farquhar, J. W., and Smith, H.: Clinical and Biochemical changes during exchange transfusion. Arch. Dis. Child. *33*:142, 1958.

Finn, R., Harper, D. T., Stallings, S. A., and Krevans, J. R.: Transplacental hemorrhage. Transfusion *3*:114, 1963.

Freda, V. J., Gorman, J. G., and Pollack, W.: Suppression of the primary Rh immune response with passive Rh IgG immunoglobulin. N. Engl. J. Med. *277*:1022, 1967.

Freda, V. J., Gorman, J. G., Pollack, W., and Bowe, E.: Current concepts: Prevention of Rh hemolytic disease. N. Engl. J. Med. *292*:1014, 1975.

From, G. L. A., Driscoll, S. G., and Steinke, J.: Serum insulin in newborn infants with erythroblastosis. Pediatrics *44*:549, 1969.

Ginsburg, S. J., and Groll, M.: Hydrops fetalis due to infantile Gaucher's disease. J. Pediatr. *82*:1046, 1973.

Gottschalk, W., and Abramson, D.: Placental edema and fetal hydrops: A case of congenital cystic adenomatoid malformation of the lung. Obstet. Gynecol. *10*:626, 1957.

Grundbacher, F. J.: ABO hemolytic disease of the newborn: A family study with emphasis on the strength of the A antigen. Pediatrics *35*:916, 1965.

Grundorfer, J.: Latent hemolytic disease of the newborn infant: The variable quantitative relationship between the amount of maternal Rh antibodies and the extent of damage of the Rh-positive infant. J. Pediatr. *40*:172, 1952.

Halbrecht, I.: Icterus; further studies on its frequency, etiology, prognosis and the blood chemistry of the cord blood. J. Pediatr. *39*:185, 1951.

Halbrecht, I., Brzoza, M., and Lahav, M.: Studies on fetal liver functions in homo- and heterospecific pregnancies, with special reference to icterus praecox of the newborn. J. Pediatr. *52*:701, 1958.

Hsia, D. Y.-Y., and Gellis, S. S.: Studies on erythroblastosis due to ABO incompatibility. Pediatrics *13*:503, 1954.

Jim, R. T. S., and Chen, F. K.: Hyperbilirubinemia due to glucose-6-phosphate dehydrogenase deficiency in a newborn Chinese infant. Pediatrics *31*:1046, 1963.

Kaplan, E., Herz, F., and Hsu, K. S.: Erythrocyte cholinesterase activity in ABO hemolytic disease of the newborn. Pediatrics *33*:205, 1964.

Kelsall, G. A., Vos, G. H., Kirk, R. L., and Shield, J. W.: The evaluation of cord-blood hemoglobin, reticulocyte percentage and maternal antigobulin titer in the prognosis of hemolytic disease of the newborn (erythroblastosis fetalis). Pediatrics *20*:221, 1957.

Levine, P.: The pathogenesis of erythroblastosis fetalis (a review). J. Pediatr. *23*:656, 1943.

Liley, A. W.: Liquor amnii analysis in the management of the pregnancy complicated by Rhesus sensitization. Am. J. Obstet. Gynecol. *82*:1358, 1961.

Lucey, J. F.: Current indications and results of fetal transfusions. Pediatrics *41*:139, 1968.

Miller, G., McCoord, A. B., Joos, H. A., and Clausen, S. W.: Studies of serum electrolyte changes during exchange transfusion. Pediatrics *13*:412, 1954.

Moe, P. J.: Umbilical cord blood and capillary blood in the evaluation of anemia in erythroblastosis fetalis Acta Pediat. Scand. *56*:391, 1967.

Naiman, J. L.: Current management of hemolytic disease of the newborn. J. Pediatr. *80*:1049, 1972.

Odell, G., Cohen, S. N., and Gordes, E. H.: Administration of albumin in the management of hyperbilirubinemia by exchange transfusion. Pediatrics *30*:613, 1962.

Orzalesi, M., Gloria, F., Lucarelli, P., and Bottino, E.: ABO incompatiblity: Relationship between direct Coombs' test positivity and neonatal jaundice. Pediatrics *51*:288, 1973.

Oski, F. A., and Naiman, J. L.: Hematologic Problems in the Newborn. Philadelphia, W. B. Saunders Company, 1966.

Parkman, R., Mosier, D., Umansky, I., Cochran, W., Carpenter, C. B., and Rosen, F. S.: Graft-versus-host disease after intrauterine and exchange transfusions for hemolytic disease of the newborn. N. Engl. J. Med. *290*:359, 1974.

Pierson, W. E., Barrett, C. T., and Oliver, T. K.: The

effect of buffered and non-buffered ACD blood on electrolyte and acid-base homeostasis during exchange transfusion. Pediatrics 41:802, 1968.

Polacek, K.: The clinical assessment of haemolytic disease of the newborn. Arch. Dis. Child. 30:217, 1955.

Pomerance, H. H., and Salerno, L. J.: A survey of the Rh problem in a mixed racial group. J. Pediatr. 38:349, 1951.

Raivio, K. O., and Isterlund, K.: Hypoglycemia and hyperinsulinemia associated with erythroblastosis fetalis. Pediatrics 43:217, 1969.

Ruys, J. H., and van Gelderen, H. H.: Administration of albumin in exchange transfusions. J. Pediatr. 61:413, 1962.

Sacks, M. S., Spurling, C. L., Bross, I. D. J., and Jahn, E. F.: Study of the influence of sex of donor on survival of erythroblastotic infants treated by exchange transfusion. Pediatrics 6:772, 1950.

Sweet, L., Reid, W. D., and Roberton, N. R. C.: Hydrops fetalis in association with chorioangioma of the placenta. J. Pediat., 82:91, 1973.

Taylor, W. C., Grisdale, L. C., and Stewart, A. G.: Unexplained death from exchange transfusion. J. Pediatr. 52:694, 1958.

van Praagh, R.: Causes of death in infants with hemo-lytic disease of the newborn (erythroblastosis fetalis). Pediatrics 28:223, 1961.

Vaughan, V. C., III, Allen, F. H., Jr., and Diamond, L. K.: Erythroblastosis fetalis. Pediatrics 6:173, 1950.

Ward, F. A.: The Rhesus factor. Tyds. vir Geneesk. December 26, 1965.

Waters, W. J., and Porter, E.: Indications for exchange transfusion based upon the role of albumin in the treatment of hemolytic disease of the newborn. Pediatrics 33:749, 1964.

Weldon, V. V., and Odell, G. B.: Mortality risk of exchange transfusion. Pediatrics 41:797, 1968.

Wiener, A. S.: Elements of blood group nomenclature with special reference to Rh-Hr blood types. J.A.M.A. 199:131, 1967.

Wishingrad, I., and Elegant, L. D.: Multiple replacement transfusions in two infants with Rh erythroblastosis. Pediatrics 28:331, 1961.

Wright, T.: A new technique in exchange transfusion. Arch. Dis. Child. 36:400, 1961.

Zuelzer, W. W., and Cohen, F.: ABO hemolytic disease and heterospecific pregnancy. Pediat. Clin. North Am. 4:405, 1957.

Zuelzer, W. W., and Kaplan, E.: ABO heterospecific pregnancy and hemolytic disease. A.M.A. J. Dis. Child. 88:158, 307, 1954.

# KERNICTERUS

*Revised by Frank Oski*

# 72

Kernicterus literally means nuclear jaundice. It is a term first applied by Schmorl in 1904 to the postmortem finding of yellow staining of basal ganglia in infants who died during or shortly after an attack of severe jaundice. The diagnosis can be made now with reasonable certainty during life, the prognosis is bad, and treatment, after the disorder has become established, is not often helpful. On the other hand, kernicterus can be prevented almost completely.

**PATHOLOGY.** The basal nuclei, globus pallidus, putamen and caudate nucleus are most intensely affected, but cerebellar and bulbar nuclei as well as white and gray matter of the cerebral hemispheres may also be involved. Deep yellow staining by bile is all that is seen in the acute stage, but widespread destructive changes become obvious in these areas if the infant survives this stage.

**PATHOGENESIS.** The close connection between kernicterus and systemic jaundice has never been doubted. There was some question earlier whether hyperbilirubinemia alone was sufficient cause, or whether other factors had to be operative simultaneously. Some thought that brain tissue had to be damaged, as perhaps by the antigen-antibody reaction of Rh incompatibility, before it could be stained and further harmed by the circulating bilirubin. This proved to be highly unlikely since kernicterus of identical characteristics was seen to follow not only the blood group incompatibilities but the hemolysis of spherocytosis, the nonspherocytic anemias, sepsis neonatorum and the nonobstructive and nonhemolytic jaundice of Crigler-Najjar disease. (See p. 673.) Even more intriguing was the observation that kernicterus may complicate physiologic jaundice, rarely, to be sure, in the full-term infant, but not uncommonly in the premature infant.

As more and more careful studies upon bilirubin levels of newborns were completed, it became increasingly apparent why premature infants suffer kernicterus so much oftener than mature ones and why kernicterus strikes them later than it does full-term infants. We shall quote one of the earlier excellent studies, that reported by Meyer, of the Birmingham group of students of the problem. Bilirubin concentration curves for infants in each 500-gm birth-weight group from less than 1500 gm to more than 3500 gm showed a startling elevation for each successively smaller group over the next larger one (Fig. 72–1). In full-term infants the curve agreed closely with that of Weech and co-workers; that is, a level of approximately 3 to 4 mg per 100 ml was reached on the second day, after which it fell steadily. In the smallest premature babies, less than 1500 gm birth weight, the mean bilirubin concentration was approximately 5 mg on the second day, more than 8 mg on the fourth day and over 10 mg on the sixth day. In 20 infants levels of over 18 mg were attained, and 12 of these had kernicterus. In all the various

studies this bilirubin concentration of 18 to 20 mg per 100 ml appeared until recently to be the critical point below which kernicterus was unlikely to develop and above which it became highly probable.

Fascinating exceptions to this general rule have been reported. Silverman and Harris et al. found that premature infants given sulfisoxazole and penicillin prophylactically suffered kernicterus much more frequently than did those not taking these drugs. What is more, kernicterus appeared in them when their bilirubin concentrations were below the so-called critical level. They concluded that sulfisoxazole was the drug at fault. Odell and Cohen have explained this seeming paradox by demonstrating that some sulfonamides and a number of other organic substances compete successfully with bilirubin for binding sites upon serum albumin. When sulfisoxazole is given, its serum concentration rises and that of bilirubin falls proportionately. Bilirubin released from its albumin bonds diffuses into tissues and causes cellular damage.

Many other exceptions have since been encountered. Stern and Denton saw six infants die of kernicterus, whose maximum bilirubins were below 18 in two, and below 19 in two more. The authors concluded that asphyxia, acidosis and hypercapnia were involved in the occurrence of kernicterus in these babies. Gartner et al. found kernicterus post mortem in nine of 14 autopsied low birth weight infants whose peak bilirubin concentrations ranged from 9.4 to 15.6 mg per 100 ml. All of them had had low Apgar scores at birth and developed the respiratory distress syndrome.

This matter has been discussed in the section on prematurity (Chap. 4), but since it is of such great importance and since it has bearing on mature babies as well, it merits a brief summarization here.

One certainty is that the bilirubin which damages nerve cells is of the indirect-reacting type. Another is that one cannot assign a safe maximum level with assurance. Many newborns survive levels of 30 or more with no apparent damage. Many others develop kernicterus whose maximum levels fall far below the 20 mg per

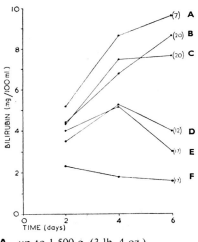

A—up to 1,500 g. (3 lb. 4 oz.).
B—1,500-2,000 g. (3 lb. 4 oz.-4 lb. 6 oz.).
C—2,000-2,500 g. (4 lb. 6 oz.-5 lb. 8 oz.).
D—2,500-3,000 g. (5 lb. 8 oz.-6 lb. 10 oz.).
E—3,000-3,500 g. (6 lb. 10 oz.-7 lb. 10 oz.).
F—over 3,500 g. (7 lb. 10 oz.).

*Figure 72–1.* Average serum bilirubin levels in 93 babies. (Meyer, T. C.: Arch. Dis. Child. *31*:75, 1956.)

100 ml so long accepted as the limit of safety.

The reasons for this are many. Most of them have to do with the concentration and the bilirubin binding ability of the infant's serum albumin. Albumin forms a bond with indirect-reacting bilirubin, and the combination is innocuous. Total albumin content is therefore of the utmost importance. Levels of 3.0 gm per 100 ml or more (usually found when that of the total serum protein is 5.5 or more) seem to offer protection to the brain when bilirubin concentrations are below 18 to 20 per cent. Lower levels, which small prematures may possess, permit too much unbound bilirubin to diffuse into the tissues.

Other matters of importance are those deviations from normal which do not permit albumin binding or which force the albumin to release its bonded bilirubin. Sulfadiazine has already been mentioned, and other drugs taken by the mother or the infant, such as salicylates, may have the same effect. A number of students of this problem have implicated asphyxia, acidosis and hypercapnia with certainty, and hypoglycemia almost as surely.

Large doses of vitamin K or its analogues favor the development of hyperbilirubinemia. Vitamin $K_1$ (Phytonadione) seems considerably safer in this regard than do some of its synthetic analogues (Mephyton, AquaMephyton, Synkayvite).

**DIAGNOSIS.** The disorder develops in jaundiced infants between the third and eighth days of life, rarely later. In full-term infants with Rh or ABO erythroblastosis it is apt to appear on the third or fourth day, in premature infants on the fourth to tenth day. In infants with familial hyperbilirubinemia of the Crigler-Najjar type it appears usually in the second to fifth week of life, but may occur as late as adolescence. Sucking ceases, vomiting appears, the facies loses expression, the head retracts. Oculogyric movements make their appearance, and the infant becomes flaccid or rigid, with opisthotonos. Cyanotic spells, muscle twitchings or convulsions may precede death, or recovery may take place gradually. Very mild attacks may be missed unless watched for closely. They may be evidenced only by a day or two of lethargy

and a tendency for the eyes to roll downward (the setting sun sign). Only months later may one be certain that these signs had indeed indicated kernicterus.

Stern and Denton pointed out that only two of their six kernicteric infants, all small prematures, manifested these signs. The other four died within 12 hours of the first of a series of apneic spells, with no other symptoms whatsoever.

There is no laboratory test other than the high level of indirect-reacting bilirubin in the blood which is confirmatory of the diagnosis. Bilirubin may be present in measurable amounts in the cerebrospinal fluid of deeply jaundiced infants, but the degree of its concentration in this location bears no relation to the presence or absence of kernicterus. It appears rather to be related to the amount of protein which the spinal

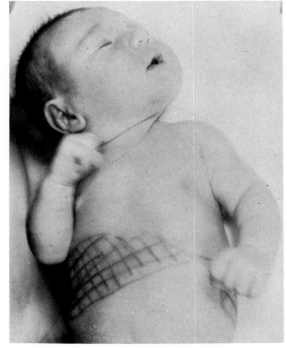

*Figure 72–2.* Infant with severe hemolytic disease of the newborn in whom kernicterus has developed. Note the enlarged liver and spleen. The posture is typical of athetosis, the head turned sharply to one side, one arm rigidly extended, the other just as rigidly flexed. Movements were characteristically writhing.

fluid contains, the bilirubin being bound to the albumin as it is in serum.

**PROGNOSIS.** Kernicterus is an exceedingly serious disorder. Among full-term infants who acquire it, half die promptly, whereas three quarters of affected premature infants die in the active stage. Those who succumb should be accounted the fortunate ones, for it becomes increasingly clear that athetosis, deafness and mental defect are in store for the majority of the survivors. Zuelzer and Kaplan diagnosed kernicterus four times among 38 ABO-incompatible infants with deep jaundice. Two died promptly, a third died at 6 months, and the fourth was grossly retarded at 8 months. One more of the group, undiagnosed in the neonatal period, demonstrated ataxia, athetosis and mental retardation later in life. Crosse and her collaborators followed the 16 survivors of their 60 kernicteric prematures. At the age of 1 year the 13 who could be examined were all retarded. Hearing was impaired in seven, speech delayed in all. Three were already rigid, six were having "stiffening spells," four oculogyric crises. Retrospective studies done in schools for cerebral spastics have been revealing. Asher and Schonell, to quote but one, found among 368 such children 55 athetotics; 19 of these had had hemolytic disease of the newborn, and 12 more had had severe jaundice in the neonatal period for other reasons. Among the 313 nonathetoid spastics, only seven gave such a history. The association of athetosis with deafness makes the retrospective diagnosis of neonatal kernicterus likely, although this combination is also frequent among children who survived fetal rubella.

Mental retardation without motor defect may follow untreated or incompletely treated hyperbilirubinemia of the newborn, according to Day and his collaborators. They found highly significant differences between the I.Q.'s of untreated newborns with hemolytic disease of the newborn, who recovered without motor defect, and their "normal" siblings.

**TREATMENT.** Once kernicterus has become established, treatment is of little avail. (Diamond, whose opinion on any point in this field cannot be disregarded, disagrees with this statement. He believes that exchange transfusion helps the early cases.) The truly successful treatment is preventive. This can be accomplished in nearly all cases if one remains constantly alert to the danger, not only in infants with hemolytic disease, but also in any newborn with jaundice and, particularly, in premature infants with jaundice. Exchange transfusion must be performed on any newborn infant with hemolytic disease due to blood group incompatibility and other hemolytic processes whose bilirubin level reaches 20 mg. per 100 ml or if the shape of the bilirubin curve makes it likely that this level will be reached. McKay in 1964 concluded that the allowable level for healthy premature infants is 23 to 25, for healthy full-term infants 28 to 30 mg per 100 ml; but if they are sick in any way, these limits drop to 18 to 22 and 20 to 24 mg. A good many of us would now make the levels for sick babies, especially those with asphyxia or respiratory distress, a great deal lower than these. A working guideline proposed by Maisels is shown in Figure 70–2. Transfusion must be repeated if, after the initial fall, bilirubin concentration rises much above the pretransfusion level, or if it persists at that level for many hours.

In Odell's hands the use of salt-free albumin (1 hour or so prior to exchange transfusion, 1.0 gm per kilogram) has been free of hazard and apparently quite effective in reducing the number of repeat exchange transfusions required. The indication is a blood serum albumin concentration of less than 3.0 gm per 100 ml.

Since overdoses of vitamin K have been implicated as a factor in excessive hemolysis, and since overdosage has been shown to serve no useful purpose, it is recommended that vitamin $K_1$ be used, 0.5 to 1.0 mg intramuscularly, limited to one dose when used prophylactically, and repeated daily for two or three days when indicated for treatment.

Sulfisoxazole for the prophylaxis or treatment of infection in the newborn premature is definitely contraindicated.

The efficacy of exchange transfusion in preventing kernicterus can no longer be doubted. As a single example, Arnold et al. reported just one case of kernicterus among the last 217 newborns given exchange transfusion. The results of Diamond and his group have been equally striking.

## REFERENCES

Arnold, D. P., Witebsky, E., Selkirk, G. H., and Alford, K. M.: Clinical and serological experience in treating hemolytic disease of the newborn. J. Pediatr. 46:520, 1955.

Asher, P., and Schonell, F. E.: Survey of 400 cases of cerebral palsy in childhood. Arch. Dis. Child. 25:360, 1950.

Crosse, V. M., Meyer, T. C., and Gerrard, J. W.: Kernicterus and prematurity. Arch. Dis. Child. 30:501, 1955.

Day, R.: Kernicterus: Further observations on the toxicity of heme pigments. Pediatrics 17:925, 1956.

Day, R., and Johnson, L.: Kernicterus. In: Progress in Hematology, Vol. II. New York, Grune and Stratton, 1959.

Gartner, L. M., Snyder, R. N., Chabon, R. S., and Bernstein, J.: Kernicterus: High incidence in premature infants with low serum bilirubin concentrations. Pediatrics 45:906, 1970.

Harris, R. C., Lucey, J. F., and Maclean, J. R.: Kernicterus in premature infants associated with low concentrations of bilirubin in the plasma. Pediatrics 21:875, 1958.

Johnson, L., Garcia, M. L., Figuèroa, E., and Sarmiento, F.: Kernicterus in rats lacking glucuronyl transferase. A.M.A. J. Dis. Child. 101:322, 1961.

Johnson, L., Sarmiento, F., Blanc, W. A., and Day, R.: Kernicterus in rats with an inherited deficiency of glucuronyl transferase. A.M.A. J. Dis. Child., 97:591, 1959.

Lending, M.: The relationship of hypercapnia to the production of kernicterus. Proc. Soc. Ped. Res. Seattle, Wash., 1964, p. 33.

Lucey, J. F., Hibbard, E., et al.: Kernicterus in asphyxiated newborn rhesus monkeys. Exp. Neurol. 9:43, 1964.

McKay, R. J.: Current status of use of exchange transfusion in newborn infants. Pediatrics 33:763, 1964.

Meyer, T. C.: A study of serum bilirubin levels in relation to kernicterus and prematurity. Arch. Dis. Child. 31:75, 1956.

Najjar, V. A.: The metabolism of bilirubin. Pediatrics 10:1, 1952.

Odell, G. B., and Cohen, S.: The effect of pH on the protein binding of bilirubin. Am. J. Dis. Child. 105:525, 1960.

Stern, L., and Denton, R. L.: Kernicterus in small premature infants. Pediatrics 35:483, 1965.

Weech, A. A.: The genesis of physiologic hyperbilirubinemia. In Advances in Pediatrics. New York, Interscience Publishers, Inc., 1947, Vol. 2.

Zuelzer, W. W., and Kaplan, E.: ABO Heterospecific pregnancy and hemolytic disease: A study of normal and pathological variants. IV. Pathological variants. A.M.A. J. Dis. Child. 88:319, 1954.

# OBSTRUCTIVE JAUNDICE

*Revised by Frank Oski*

# 73

## CONGENITAL ATRESIA OF THE BILE DUCTS

In the last several years we have witnessed a major reorientation in our thinking with respect to the entity termed congenital atresia of the bile ducts. In the past, the clinician attempted to distinguish hepatitis from atresia by a variety of diagnostic procedures, and deferred operative intervention for several months in hopes that patients with hepatitis would get better, while assuming that little or nothing could be done for infants with anatomic abnormalities.

There is now a growing consensus that neonatal hepatitis and biliary atresia may be opposite ends of a single spectrum of disease and that the pathologic process observed is dynamic and ever changing. The pathologic picture observed depends on the time of the intrauterine insult, the nature of the insult and the age at which the infant is examined.

Loose and ambiguous use of the term biliary atresia has led to confusion concerning the approach to therapy. Only surgical exploration, an operative cholangiogram if a gallbladder is present, a careful dissection of the porta hepatis and microscopic examination of liver tissue can enable one to classify the patient's disease into intrahepatic or extrahepatic biliary obstruction with or without atresia.

With this information in hand, the following diagnostic classification can be made:

1. Complete intrahepatic biliary atresia
   a. Normal extrahepatic biliary system
   b. Hypoplastic extrahepatic biliary system
   c. Complete extrahepatic biliary atresia
2. Complete extrahepatic biliary atresia
   a. Normal number of intrahepatic ducts
   b. Decreased number of intrahepatic ducts
3. Hypoplasia of the extrahepatic biliary trees
   a. Normal numbers of intrahepatic ducts
   b. Decreased numbers of intrahepatic ducts

Such a classification is essential now that it has become apparent due to the pioneering work of Kasai and the recent success of Lilly that infants with functioning intrahepatic ducts may benefit from surgical procedures that employ a variety of anastomotic techniques that result in adequate biliary drainage. Patients without intrahepatic ducts cannot be salvaged. Intrahepatic ducts may disappear over a period of several months in the presence of complete extrahepatic obstruction; thus early surgical intervention is necessary in order to produce benefit.

**INCIDENCE.** Holmes, in 1916, based his conclusion concerning operability upon 112 cases reported until then. By 1951 Ahrens et al. stated that 264 cases of extrahepatic duct atresia plus 10 of the intrahepatic form were discoverable in the literature. Thaler and Gellis have studied carefully 135 cases admitted to one hospital in a 10-year period. The disorder is not rare, nor is it common.

**PATHOLOGY.** Almost any conceivable pattern of absence or atresia of one or more of the components of the biliary outflow tract has been encountered. All the extrahepatic ducts may be absent or, rarely, all the intrahepatic ducts. The hepatic, cystic or common duct may be atretic. The gallbladder may be absent or hypoplastic or it may have no connection with the liver or the duodenum. Stenosis rather than complete atresia may be found.

The liver shows all gradations of damage ranging from biliary stasis to advanced biliary cirrhosis, depending upon the length of time the particular infant survives. This is discussed in greater detail in the paragraph headed Liver Biopsy. The spleen enlarges as portal hypertension advances. The bones may become rachitic or osteoporotic because of defective absorption of vitamin D and of calcium. In advanced cases foci of destruction of skeletal muscle may be discovered after careful search. Weinberg et al. correlate this lesion with prolonged deprivation of vitamin E.

**ETIOLOGY.** There is little evidence that congenital biliary atresia is familial or hereditary. One must presume that it results from some noxious process that affects adversely the development of the bile duct system early in gestation. Congenital rubella and cytomegalovirus infections have been associated with biliary atresia. The final pattern evolves from two distinct portions of the liver anlage, the larger cranial part forming parenchyma plus hepatic and common ducts, the small caudal part eventuating in gallbladder and cystic duct. These two must accomplish juncture secondarily. Congenital defects of many kinds are the end-results of imperfections in this complex evolution.

**DIAGNOSIS.** The prime sign of congenital biliary atresia is persistent jaundice. Many times the icterus appears to be a continuation of physiologic icterus of the newborn, and one begins to suspect serious trouble only when the color fails to fade at the expected time. In other cases jaundice is not noted until 1, 2 or even 3 or more weeks have passed, after which it persists and deepens. A story dating the onset of jaundice after 6 weeks of age is good evidence, after 4 weeks fair evidence, that the disorder is something other than atresia. Surprisingly enough, jaundice appears often to be variable in intensity, alternately deepening and lightening. Just because one would expect complete atresia to give rise to jaundice steadily increasing in intensity, such variability tends to mislead. The second diagnostic sign is absence of bile in the stools. Some infants oblige by passing the typical clay-colored stools from the fourth or fifth day on. In other instances confusion arises because stools fail to become absolutely white for several weeks or months, or because some are clay-colored while others contain a tinge of brown or green. The usual explanation advanced for this latter phenomenon is that heavily jaundiced intestinal epithelial cells may be sloughed off and incorporated in the bulk of the stool. The effect of these two factors, variability in intensity of jaundice and delay and variability in absoluteness of acholia in stools, is to cast doubt upon the congenital origin and completeness of the obstruction. One can only warn that not too much weight be assigned to these red herrings. Within these limitations jaundice and acholic stools constitute the pathognomonic signs. Jaundice steadily increases in depth to its maximum, ultimately imparting to the infant a deep yellow color, due to bilirubin, mixed with a greenish discoloration, due to biliverdin. The liver soon becomes large and excessively firm. In the first few months the baby does not appear or act as though he is ill. Venous dilatation appears over the surface of the protuberant abdomen, greatest over its upper half, and ascites develops. The spleen enlarges.

Fat-soluble vitamins are poorly absorbed in the absence of bile salts from the intestine, but deficiencies in vitamins A, D and K do not become manifest until after the neonatal period. Vitamin E deficiency may be demonstrated by laboratory tests, and the absorption of an orally administered dose of Aquasol E has been proposed as a simple test to distinguish hepatitis from biliary atresia.

Blood is normal in the neonatal period. Hemoglobin content and red and white blood cell counts fall within the usual range, and there is no excess of nucleated erythrocytes or reticulocytes. The urine contains bile in large quantities, but no urobilinogen. By 4 to 6 weeks of age most patients are anemic with elevations in their reticulocyte counts.

Serum bilirubin becomes elevated by the end of the first week and gradually rises to a maximum, where it remains throughout life with fluctuations. Much of the bilirubin is of the direct type.

Liver function tests may indicate liver damage, but not until considerably later in life after cirrhotic alterations have begun to develop.

Blood cholesterol level tends to rise gradually pari passu with increasing liver damage. This never happens as early as the neonatal period.

Several transaminating enzymes have been measured in the sera of infants with persistent jaundice. Serum glutamic oxalacetic transaminase (SGOT) is found normally in adult blood in amounts of activity ranging from 8 to 40 units per milliliter of serum per minute, in normal newborns from 13 to 120. Glutamic pyruvic transaminase (SGPT) is present in adult serum in the range from 5 to 35 units, in newborn serum from 12 to 90 units (Kove et al.). In bile duct atresia the activities of these enzymes may increase to levels of 500 to 700 units, whereas in hepatitis this figure may rise as high as more than 1000. Unfortunately there is a good deal of overlapping in these two conditions. Recent studies of serum aminopeptidase suggest that activity of this enzyme may permit sharper differentiation, but these results await confirmation.

A promising diagnostic aid is the measurement of serum $\alpha$-fetoprotein. Zeltzer and co-workers found this to be elevated in 10 of 11 patients with neonatal hepatitis and in only 1 of 6 infants with biliary atresia.

Thaler and Gellis make a strong case for the rose bengal I[131] excretion test as the most reliable, although still not perfect, diagnostic test of biliary atresia. Excretion of less than 10 per cent of the dye in the stool was found in all his extrahepatic obstructions, whereas in his cases of hepatitis the average was 32 per cent. Nevertheless 20 per cent of these latter cases were obstructed also, with less than 10 per cent of the dye excreted.

In an infant with persistent jaundice and apparent biliary obstruction, efforts should be made by 6 to 8 weeks of age to determine the precise etiology. In addition to conventional measurements of liver enzymes, diagnostic procedures should include one or more of the following in an attempt to determine if obstruction is present: I[131] rose bengal excretion test, oral vitamin E absorption test, duodenal intubation and analysis for bile acids. If the tests are equivocal or indicate the presence of obstruction, surgery should be performed in an attempt to establish a precise diagnosis and possibly correct or ameliorate the problem. Surgery should be performed by a surgeon familiar with the problem and capable of performing an anastomosis if indicated. At the time of exploratory laparotomy, a cholangiogram should be obtained as well as a liver biopsy.

**LIVER BIOPSY.** There has been some alteration in the thinking of neonatal pathologists about the pictures which characterize biliary atresia versus the other causes of persistent neonatal jaundice with a high proportion of direct-reacting bilirubin. Brough and Bernstein believe, as had several others before them, that bile duct and ductular proliferation is its most reliable sign. The second is hypertrophic changes in hepatic artery branches. Bile plugs in dilated ducts, fibrosis, largely portal, inflammatory changes and giant-cell transformation are seen, but in less than one-half of the examples. These findings contrast with those of neonatal hepatitis, in which hepatocellular damage and inflammation, mostly portal infiltration with mononuclear cells, are the outstanding signs. Giant-cell transformation is far from universal in them, and duct proliferation is seen, but rarely (see Fig. 74–1).

**TREATMENT.** The results of Kasai and Lilly indicate that in approximately 25 per cent of infants, sustained postoperative biliary drainage can be achieved following a successful anastomosis. For success, an infant must have functioning intrahepatic ducts. Surgical success has not been achieved in children operated upon after 4 months of age. It has been the common practice to defer surgery until 4 months of age because of the observations of Thaler and Gellis regarding the ill effects of laparotomy and cholecystangiography upon those infants who turn out not to have congenital atresia. Sixty per cent of their babies subjected to surgery died or developed disturbed liver function later, while only 10 per cent of those not operated upon ended up this badly. It would appear that with improved anesthetic techniques and pre- and postoperative care, these risks can be reduced for the child with hepatitis, and

more infants with biliary atresia may be salvaged. Danks and associates demonstrated that approximately 50 per cent of their infants with extrahepatic biliary atresia were potentially correctable.

Other surgical maneuvers have been attempted with few successes. Norris and Rothman found both hepatic ducts patent and bile-containing, but the gallbladder, cystic duct and common duct atretic. They cut the hepatic ducts and sutured the opened duodenal wall about their proximal stumps, with ultimate success. Attempts to imbed a wedge of raw, freshly cut liver into the duodenum have met with failure.

If anastomosis proves to be impossible, one is left with the tasks of keeping the infant comfortable, in as good nutritional state as possible and free of vitamin deficiencies. Fat-soluble vitamins should be given in the water-miscible form. Drisdol with vitamin A is superior to oily preparations. Vitamin $K_1$ may be indicated later in the course. It is possible that added tocopherol may avert some muscle damage due to vitamin E deficiency. The distressing itching which is a feature in some infants may prove to be unresponsive to all forms of sedative and antihistaminic therapy. Treatment with cholestyramine is worthy of trial even though Lottsfeldt et al. believe that this anion exchange resin will be ineffective in cases of complete biliary obstruction.

**PROGNOSIS.** Death will supervene in all cases of biliary atresia which cannot be surgically converted. An occasional infant upon whom this diagnosis has been made may suddenly and spontaneously be relieved of his jaundice after many months. This does not mean that atresia is reversible, but that diagnosis has been incorrect. Errors of this sort have been made even after careful exploration in reputable clinics. One must therefore qualify one's grave prognosis to the parents by pointing out that this slim possibility exists. Most deaths will be caused by hepatic failure or by the bleeding of portal hypertension and will occur between 6 months and 2 years of age. A few children live years longer. Kernicterus does not complicate biliary atresia. This is because much of the

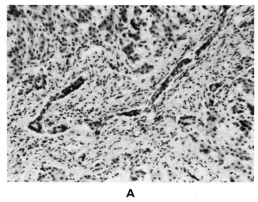

A

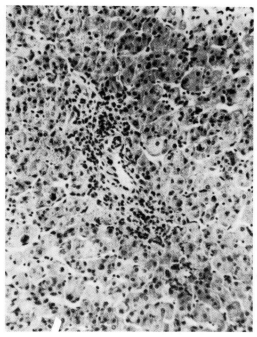

B

*Figure 73–1.* *A,* Bile duct proliferation and portal fibrosis in an infant with obstruction of the common duct by a plug of inspissated secretions. (Original magnification, 200×.) *B,* Hepatitis with moderate portal inflammation; hepatocellular changes are mild, and multinucleated cells are few. (Original magnification, 200×.) (Brough, A. J., and Bernstein, J.: Pediatrics. *43*:519, 1969.)

accumulated bilirubin is of the direct kind, and dangerous levels of indirect hyperbilirubinemia are not reached.

## ATRESIA OF THE INTRAHEPATIC BILE DUCTS

This extraordinary variant of the biliary atresia group has been studied most carefully and described most completely by Ahrens, Harris and MacMahon. Its clinical course differs in some particulars from that of atresia of extrahepatic ducts.

**INCIDENCE.** Only 10 cases had been reported until 1951, when 264 cases of extrahepatic atresia had appeared in the literature. Danks and Bodian found among 110 cases of neonatal obstructive jaundice: seven of intrahepatic atresia versus 58 of the extrahepatic variety and 45 of neonatal hepatitis. It is therefore extremely infrequent.

**PATHOLOGY.** Characteristic is the absence of bile ducts of any size within the liver substance. Bile capillaries are present within each lobule, and these often are dilated and contain plugs of inspissated bile. Extrahepatic ducts are usually absent also, but in three of the 10 early reported cases the extrahepatic duct system seemed perfectly normal. No remnants of compressed, chronically inflamed or fibrosed ducts are found. Nor is pericholangiolitis discoverable. Fibrosis is minimal, and cirrhosis is extremely slow to develop and seldom attains the degree it does when atresia is extrahepatic. Ahrens et al. believe that this slow development of cirrhosis stems from the absence of intrahepatic ducts, which cannot therefore produce liver injury by distention, backflow of bile and periductal inflammation.

**DIAGNOSIS.** The chief difference in the clinical course between intrahepatic and extrahepatic atresia lies in the slowness of advance of the disease in the former as opposed to the latter. Jaundice appears at the same time and is equally persistent, but the liver enlarges much more slowly and does not become so hard and nodular. The nutritional state remains fairly good, and the life span is long. Infants with intrahepatic atresia show a great tendency to cutaneous xanthomatosis. This sign does not develop before 18 months of age, usually later, and it may be more apparent in this group because of their increased life expectancy. Xanthomas appear and disappear with fluctuations in the serum lipid content.

**LABORATORY INVESTIGATIONS.** The blood, stool and urine findings are exactly the same as those in extrahepatic atresia. Blood lipid content gradually increases over the course of months or years of biliary obstruction of any type.

**TREATMENT.** No specific treatment is available. Cholestyramine is more likely to produce lowering of the bilirubin level and subsidence of itching in this form of jaundice than in the extrahepatic obstructive variety.

**PROGNOSIS.** As has been indicated, the life span of patients with this variety of biliary atresia appears to be considerably longer than that of those in the extrahepatic group. Patients living 10 years or more have been observed. The ultimate prognosis is grave.

## CHOLEDOCHAL CYST

Cystic dilatation of the common duct results from congenital defect of the duct wall, a mucosal valve or abnormal course of the duct through the duodenal wall. The dilatation is confined to the common duct itself and does not involve the hepatic or cystic ducts or the gallbladder. It may reach the size of an orange or larger.

**INCIDENCE.** Over 200 cases have been reported in all age groups, but it is an extreme rarity for choledochal cyst to become symptomatic and to be diagnosed within the neonatal period. In Brough and Bernstein's experience with 39 proved cases of obstructive lesions causing persistent neonatal jaundice, 36 were extrahepatic atresias, one was an obstructive bile plug and two were choledochal cysts.

**DIAGNOSIS.** In older persons a triad consisting of jaundice, abdominal pain and an upper abdominal tumor suggests the diagnosis strongly. In the neonatal period the mass is not necessarily large enough to

palpate, but it may be huge, filling the entire abdomen. This was true in the last example we saw. Pain is not prominent or easy to localize. When a cystic mass is felt within the abdomen in the presence of jaundice, the possibility must be entertained seriously. Wide fluctuations in the depth of the jaundice are highly suggestive. In the final analysis differential diagnosis can be made only by cholecystography or by direct observation after laparotomy.

**LABORATORY INVESTIGATIONS.** Since jaundice results from blockage by the expanding cyst of entry of bile into the duodenum, the findings will be those of obstructive jaundice. Stools become acholic, the urine contains bile but no urobilin and the serum bilirubin level rises, a large proportion of the total bilirubin being direct. Biopsy of the liver will reveal a picture indistinguishable from that of extrahepatic atresia.

**TREATMENT.** After the cyst has been visualized by cholecystography or by exploratory laparotomy its wall should be anastomosed to that of the duodenum.

**PROGNOSIS.** Cholecystoduodenostomy should result in cure. Again, if operative intervention is delayed, irreversible liver damage may occur.

## PSEUDOCHOLEDOCHAL CYST

Whereas choledochal cyst results from a congenital defect of the common duct, pseudocholedochal cyst is an iatrogenic disorder which follows injury to the common duct at operation.

Only one case has been observed originating in the neonatal period. This case, reported by Smith and Seeley, is of sufficient interest to be abstracted briefly.

A previously normal male infant began to vomit at three weeks and was operated upon for pyloric stenosis shortly thereafter. Ten days after the Fredet-Ramstedt operation had been performed, vomiting, diarrhea, anorexia and low-grade fever appeared. Thirty-six hours later jaundice was noted, and the stools became white, the urine dark. After 3 weeks the abdomen was greatly distended. Paracentesis yielded 1000 cc of amber fluid. The fluid promptly reappeared, and two further taps were done. On admission at 14 weeks the presumed diagnosis was cirrhosis of the liver with ascites. The infant was pale and emaciated, and the abdomen was distended and covered with dilated veins. Icterus had disappeared, the liver was not enlarged, but the spleen was palpable. X-ray film showed a large soft tissue density almost filling the right side of the abdomen. At operation a cyst was seen whose friable wall was inadvertently ruptured, releasing 550 cc of dark green fluid. The fibrous wall was adherent to the small and large bowel, peritoneum and liver. A transected common duct was found. This was ligated, and cholecystogastrostomy was performed. Convalescence was uneventful.

## REFERENCES

Ahrens, E. H., Harris, R. C., and MacMahon, H. E.: Atresia of the intrahepatic bile ducts. Pediatrics 8:628, 1951.

Bennett, D. E.: Problems in neonatal obstructive jaundice. Pediatrics 33:735, 1964.

Bernstein, J., Braylan, R., and Brough, A. J.: Bile plug syndrome: A correctible cause of obstructive jaundice in infants. Pediatrics 43:273, 1969.

Brough, A. J., and Bernstein, J.: Liver biopsy in the diagnosis of infantile obstructive jaundice. Pediatrics 43:519, 1969.

Bruton, O. C., Metzger, J. F., and Sprinz, H.: Experience with needle biopsy of the liver in infants and children. Pediatrics 16:836, 1955.

Danks, D., and Bodian, M.: A genetic study of neonatal obstructive jaundice. Arch. Dis. Child. 38:378, 1963.

Danks, D., Campbell, P. E., Clarke, A. M., Jones, P. G., and Solomon, J. R.: Extrahepatic biliary atresia. The frequency of potentially operable cases. Am. J. Dis. Child. 128:684, 1974.

Dickinson, E. H., and Spencer, F. C.: Choledochal cyst: Report of a case with unusual features. J. Pediatr. 41:462, 1952.

Farber, S., and Craig, J. M.: Clinical pathological conference: Jaundice and pruritus from birth. J. Pediatr. 51:584, 1957.

Holmes, J. B.: Congenital obliteration of the bile ducts: Diagnosis and suggestions for treatment. Am. J. Dis. Child. 11:405, 1916.

Kasai, M., Kimura, S., Asakura, Y., Suzuki, H., Taira, Y., and Onashi, E.: Surgical treatment of biliary atresia. J. Pediatr. Surg. 3:665, 1968.

Kasai, M., Watanabe, I., and Ohi, R.: Follow-up studies of long-term survivors after hepatic portoenterostomy for "noncorrectable" biliary atresia. J. Pediatr. Surg. 10:173, 1975.

Kaye, K., Koop, C., et al.: Needle biopsy of the liver. J. Dis. Child. 98:699, 1959.

Koop, C. E.: Biliary atresia and the Kasai operation. Pediatrics 55:9, 1975.

Kove, S., Goldstein, S., and Wróbleski, F.: Serum transaminase activity in neonatal period: Valuable aid in differential diagnosis of jaundice in the newborn infant. J.A.M.A. 168:860, 1958.

Lilly, J. R.: The Japanese operation for biliary atresia: Remedy or mischief? Pediatrics 55:12, 1975.

Lottsfeldt, F. I., Krivit, W., Aust, J. B., and Carey, J. B., Jr.: Cholestyramine therapy in intrahepatic biliary cirrhosis. N. Engl. J. Med. 269:186, 1963.

Melhorn, D. K., Gross, S., and Izant, R. J., Jr.: The red cell hydrogen peroxide hemolysis test and vitamin E absorption in the differential diagnosis of jaundice in infancy. J. Pediat. 81:1082, 1972.

Norris, W. J., and Rothman, P. E.: Congenital obliteration of the bile ducts; report of a case treated successfully by anastomosis of hepatic ducts to duodenum. A.M.A. J. Dis. Child. 81:681, 1951.

O'Donohoe, N. V.: Obstructive jaundice in haemolytic disease of the newborn treated with magnesium sulphate. Arch. Dis. Child. 30:234, 1955.

Smith, A. G., and Seeley, S. F.: Pseudocholedochal cyst. Pediatrics 12:536, 1953.

Swenson, O., and Fisher, J. H.: Surgical aspects of liver disease. Pediatrics 16:135, 1955.

Thaler, M. M., and Gellis, S. S.: Studies in neonatal hepatitis. Am. J. Dis. Child. 116:257, 262, 271, 280, 1968.

Walker, W. A., Krivit, W., and Sharp, H. L.: Needle biopsy of the liver in infancy and childhood: A safe diagnostic aid in liver disease. Pediatrics 40:946, 1967.

Weinberg, T., Gordon, H. H., Oppenheimer, E. H., and Nitowsky, H. M.: Myopathy in association with tocopherol deficiency in cases of congenital biliary atresia and cystic fibrosis of the pancreas. Am. J. Path. 34:565, 1958.

Whitten, W. W., and Adie, G. C.: Congenital biliary atresia. J. Pediatr. 40:539, 1952.

Zeltzer, P. M., Neerhout, R. C., Fonkalsrud, E. W., and Stiehm, E. R.: Differentiation between neonatal hepatitis and biliary atresia by measuring serum-alpha-protein. Lancet 1:373, 1974.

# 74

# PROLONGED OBSTRUCTIVE JAUNDICE OF UNCERTAIN ETIOLOGY (NEONATAL GIANT-CELL HEPATITIS)

*Revised by Frank Oski*

Between one third and one half of infants with persistent obstructive jaundice do not have primary biliary atresia. Although, as previously indicated, biliary atresia and neonatal hepatitis may be different behaviors of the same disease process, in many instances an entity defined as neonatal hepatitis can be recognized as distinct in its pathologic picture and clinical course. The distinctive pathologic picture is the presence of a cholestatic inflammatory process. Giant cell transformation is present but significant bile duct proliferation is absent. Biopsy specimens may demonstrate disorganized lobular architecture, fibrosis, round cell infiltration and extramedullary hematopoiesis.

**INCIDENCE.** This disorder cannot be considered rare, being observed in two or three patients per year in most large children's hospitals. Milder forms of this entity are much more common and may occur in great numbers during certain viral epidemics such as rubella.

**ETIOLOGY.** Neonatal hepatitis has multiple etiologies. Viral agents recognized to produce the disease include rubella, cytomegalovirus, herpes simplex, Coxsackie and the hepatitis B virus. Hepatitis may also be observed in infants born with congenital infections due to toxoplasmosis and syphilis. In addition, a clinical picture indistinguishable from that observed with infectious agents may be seen in some infants with severe hemolytic disease or galactosemia. In many instances, an etiologic agent is not determined. Familial cases do occur, and in such patients the disease appears to carry a much worse prognosis.

Mothers who are carriers of the hepatitis B antigen, formerly known as the virus of serum hepatitis, may transmit this virus transplacentally. Stevens and associates were able to demonstrate such an occurrence in approximately 20 per cent of pregnancies in which mothers were known carriers. Such infants rarely demonstrate any neonatal evidence of hepatic disease. Many infants born of mothers carrying the hepatitis B antigen will themselves become antigen positive postnatally, either as a result of virus acquisition during the birth process or because of close maternal-infant contact during the first few weeks of life. Kattamis and co-workers were able to demonstrate the presence of hepatitis B antigen in the sera of 10 of 23 infants with hepatitis in whom clinical manifestations of disease appeared between 2 and 4 months of age. Kohler and colleagues were able to prevent the acquisition of hepatitis B antigen by infants of carrier mothers by the administration of gamma globulin high in hepatitis B antibody to babies during the first week of life.

Hsia et al. have presented statistical data which suggest that some cases of this disease might be hereditary, dependent upon a single autosomal gene defect. Danks and Bodian's examination of this question yielded equivocal results. In Scott's fascinating family an apparently healthy mother gave birth to three infants who became jaundiced at 1 month, 7 days and 4 months, respectively, and to two other infants who never became ill. Since homologous serum hepatitis has an incubation period of 60 to 150 days, this situation might be explained by virus crossing the placenta of a carrier mother at different times during gestation, or not crossing at all in the course of two of her pregnancies, or by Hsia's hypothesis.

Lawson and Boggs reviewed 23 patients with neonatal hepatitis and found two classes of patients: familial, five patients, and sporadic, eighteen patients. The patients with the familial form of the disease had significantly more serious morbidity and higher mortality rates than those with the sporadic form, independent of any form of surgical procedures.

**PATHOLOGY.** The microscopic pictures of the livers of these children have been discussed, along with those of children suffering from congenital extrahepatic duct atresias (p. 663). In the majority, but not all, the distinction can be made by the histological pattern.

**DIAGNOSIS.** Jaundice is the primary sign of neonatal hepatitis. It has been observed at birth, but usually it becomes apparent days or weeks after birth. Onset more than 4 weeks after birth probably, after 6 weeks surely, makes this diagnosis more likely than that of biliary atresia, if one can trust the informant. Abdominal distention and increasing size of the liver appear with or soon after the jaundice. Later, with advancing cirrhosis, the liver may shrink in size and become hard. At this stage splenomegaly becomes prominent, and ascites may develop. Fever is usually absent. These infants, in contrast to those with biliary atresia, may appear ill, eat poorly and vomit. Stools become acholic within the first few weeks, but this sign may be intermittent. If intermittence is striking, it may be considered a strong, but not absolute, indicator of the absence of congenital atresia. The urine becomes dark concomitant with the disappearance of color from the stool.

Fletcher et al. reported an extraordinary, and we believe unique, case of an infant with neonatal hepatitis who was born with massive ascites. He was greatly improved by exchange transfusion and, thanks to excellent supportive care, made a complete recovery after 7 weeks of being very ill indeed.

In many instances the clinical differentiation of hepatitis from biliary atresia is not possible with absolute certainty.

**LABORATORY EXAMINATION.** The differentiation between obstructive jaundice on the basis of hepatocellular disease due to neonatal hepatitis and that due to obstruction of the extrahepatic biliary tree is very difficult in many instances. This is because hepatitis often produces prolonged and essentially complete obstruction of the passage of bile from the liver into the gastrointestinal tract. Certain diagnostic procedures, however, may aid in making a distinction.

A gradually rising serum bilirubin level suggests atresia, while an irregularly declining serum bilirubin suggests hepatitis.

The presence of a serum that is positive for alpha fetoprotein suggests the diagnosis of neonatal hepatitis.

The radioactive rose bengal test may also aid in diagnosis. Patients with obstructive jaundice who have patent bile ducts excrete 5 to 20 per cent of the injected dye in their stools, while those with biliary atresia excrete 8 per cent or less (in 72 hours).

The fat-soluble vitamin E is poorly absorbed when bile salts do not reach the small intestine. Measurement of vitamin E absorption as described by Lubin and coworkers or by Melhorn and associates is a simple procedure which correlates nicely with the results of rose bengal testing and the pathologic picture found at laparotomy.

Javid has proposed that analysis of the type of bile acid retention may also serve to distinguish atresia from hepatitis.

Administration of phenobarbital or cholestyramine increases the rose bengal excretion and lowers the serum bilirubin and bile salts in many patients with intrahepatic obstruction.

Recovery of a viral agent or serologic demonstration of an infection with rubella, hepatitis B virus, cytomegalovirus or toxoplasmosis strongly suggests the presence of neonatal hepatitis, although some of these agents may be observed in the presence of a pathologic picture of biliary atresia.

Many infants will ultimately require surgical exploration, cholangiography and liver biopsy so that the etiology of the persistent jaundice may be determined. Before such procedures are performed, other diseases that may produce liver diseases must also be excluded. These include alpha-1-

antitrypsin deficiency, galactosemia, tyrosinemia and cystic fibrosis.

It is now the general consensus that operative diagnosis should not be postponed beyond 2 months of age so that those patients with correctable forms of biliary atresia can be cured.

**PROGNOSIS.**   The form of neonatal hepatitis that follows, or is simultaneous with, hemolytic diseases of the newborn, the so-called inspissated bile syndrome, carries an excellent prognosis. All of Hsia's 23 patients reported in 1952 made complete recoveries. Sixty per cent of Thaler and Gellis' patients who did not have hemolytic disease, on the other hand, either died or suffered cirrhosis of the liver and portal hypertension if they had been laparotomized, whereas only 10 per cent did as badly if they had not been explored. In contrast, Lawson observed that five of nine patients with non-familial forms of neonatal hepatitis were well despite surgery. In those without surgery the prognosis was the same with 6 of 9 being well at follow-up. Dr. Gellis has (in 1975) revised his recommendation to deeper exploration in light of success with newer operative approaches, and advocates exploration "much earlier than four months."

**TREATMENT.**   No uniformly effective treatment is currently available for the management of patients with hepatitis. Steroids produce erratic results.

# REFERENCES

See also References to Chapter 72 (p. 663).

Alper, C. A. and Johnson, A. M.: Alpha-1-antitrypsin deficiency and disease. Pediatrics 46:837–840, 1970.

Bellin, L., and Bailit, I. W.: Congenital cirrhosis of the liver associated with infectious hepatitis of pregnancy. J. Pediatr. 40:60, 1952.

Bruton, O. C., Metzger, J. F., and Sprinz, H.: Experience with needle biopsy in infants and children. Pediatrics 16:836, 1955.

Capps, R. B., et al.: Infectious hepatitis in infants and small children. The clinical and laboratory picture with special reference to the nonicteric form. A.M.A. J. Dis. Child. 89:701, 1955.

Danks, D., and Bodian, M.: A genetic study of neonatal obstructive jaundice. Arch. Dis. Child. 38:378, 1963.

Dunn, P.: Obstructive jaundice and hemolytic disease of the newborn. Arch. Dis. Child. 38:596, 1963.

Fletcher, C. B., Eakin, E. L., and Rothman, P. E.: Fetal ascites — liver giant-cell transformation. Am. J. Dis. Child. 108:554, 1964.

Gellis, S. S.: Biliary atresia. Pediatrics 55:8, 1975.

Gellis, S. S., Craig, J. M., and Hsia, D. Y.-Y.: Prolonged obstructive jaundice in infancy. IV. Neonatal hepatitis. A.M.A. J. Dis. Child. 88:285, 1954.

Harris, R. C., Andersen, D. H., and Day, R. L.: Obstructive jaundice in infants with normal biliary tree. Pediatrics 13:293, 1954.

Hsia, D. Y.-Y., Boggs, J. D., Driscoll, S. G., and Gellis, S. S.: Prolonged obstructive jaundice in infancy. V. The genetic component in neonatal hepatitis. A.M.A. J. Dis. Child. 95:485, 1958.

Hsia, D. Y.-Y., Patterson, P., Allen, F. H., Jr., Diamond, L. K., and Gellis, S. S.: Prolonged obstructive jaundice in infancy. Pediatrics 10:243, 1952.

Kattamis, C. A., Demetrios, D., and Matsaniotis, M.: Australia antigen and neonatal hepatitis syndrome. Pediatrics 54:157, 1974.

Kohler, P. F., Dubois, R. S., Merrill, D. A., and Bowes, W. A.: Prevention of chronic neonatal hepatitis B virus infection with antibody to the hepatitis B surface antigen. N. Engl. J. Med. 291:1378, 1974.

Landing, B. H.: Considerations of the pathogenesis of neonatal hepatitis, biliary atresia and choledochal cyst — the concept of infantile obstructive cholangiopathy. In Bill, A. H., and Kasai, M. (eds.): Progress in Pediatric Surgery. Baltimore, University Park Press. 1974, Vol. 2, pp. 113–139.

Lawson, E. E., and Boggs, J. D.: Long term follow-up of neonatal hepatitis: Safety and value of surgical exploration. Pediatrics 53:650, 1974.

Lightwood, R. C.: Proc. 15th Ann. Meeting, British Paediatric Assn. Arch. Dis. Child. 18:156, 1943.

Lightwood, R. C., and Bodian, M.: Biliary obstruction associated with icterus gravis neonatorum. Arch. Dis. Child. 21:209, 1946.

Lubin, B. H., Baehner, R. L., Schwartz, E., Shohet, S., and Nathan, D. G.: Red cell peroxide hemolysis test in differential diagnosis of obstructive jaundice in the newborn period. Pediatrics 48:562, 1971.

Rich, A. R.: Pathogenesis of forms of jaundice. Bull. Johns Hopkins Hosp. 47:338, 1930.

Scott, R. B., Wilkins, W., and Kessler, A.: Viral hepatitis in early infancy. Pediatrics 13:447, 1954.

Stevens, C. E., Beasley, R. P., Tseu, J., and Lee, W. C.: Vertical transmission of hepatitis B antigen in Taiwan. N. Engl. J. Med. 292:771, 1975.

Stokes, J., Jr., Wolman, I. J., Blanchard, M. S., and Farquhar, J. D.: Virus hepatitis in the newborn: Clinical features, epidemiology, and pathology. A.M.A. J. Dis. Child. 82:2137, 1951.

Talamo, R. C., and Feingold, M.: Infantile cirrhosis with hereditary alpha-1-antitrypsin deficiency. Am. J. Dis. Child. 25:845–847, 1973.

Watkins, J. B.: Bile acid metabolism and fat absorption in newborn infants. Pediatr. Clin. North Am. 21:501–512, 1974.

Weller, T., and Hanshaw, J. B.: Virologic and clinical observations on cytomegalic inclusion disease. N. Engl. J. Med. 266:1233, 1962.

# JAUNDICE OF OTHER VARIETIES

*Revised by Frank Oski*

# 75

## JAUNDICE DUE TO OTHER INFECTIONS

Jaundice is not uncommonly associated with *sepsis neonatorum, congenital syphilis, generalized herpes simplex infection, Weil's disease, congenital toxoplasmosis* and *cytomegalic disease*. All these have been discussed in detail in their appropriate places.

The jaundice may be caused by an accumulation of both conjugated and unconjugated bilirubin. When increased quantities of conjugated bilirubin are present, the physician should be particularly suspicious that infection may be present. It has been estimated that jaundice alone may be the initial manifestation of infection in approximately 10 per cent of infants.

Since 1963 a striking association has been noted between urinary tract infections due mainly to *E. coli* and jaundice. Seeler and Hahn in 1969 were able to report on 11 such cases they had themselves seen over a period of only 11 months in one hospital. Seven of these were diagnosed within the first 28 days of life. In only two was the percentage of direct to total bilirubin as low as 9, and these two were the youngest of the babies, 7 and 9 days of age. In the rest the direct fraction ranged from 24 to 60 per cent of the total. All recovered after appropriate antibiotic treatment. The possibility that there exist pyelopathic strains of *E. coli* is being considered seriously.

## JAUNDICE DUE TO TOXIC SUBSTANCES

Accidental poisoning with hepatotoxic substances such as arsenic, phosphorus and chloroform is no problem in the neonate. A rare cause of liver damage is a metabolite of galactose, probably galactose-1-phosphate, which accumulates in many organs in congenital galactosemia. Jaundice is a symptom of this disorder, but it is usually mild, appearing about the fourth day of life and seldom lasting more than a week. Only rarely, in the hyperacute form, does jaundice appear earlier and become intense (p. 534).

## CONGENITAL FAMILIAL NONHEMOLYTIC JAUNDICE

By the title above Crigler and Najjar reported an extraordinary variety of icterus beginning shortly after birth.

**INCIDENCE.** Crigler and Najjar described seven patients in whom the diagnosis was assured and eight more in whom it seemed probable in retrospect. All 15 derived from the same pair of forebears. The disorder is an extreme rarity.

**ETIOLOGY AND PATHOGENESIS.** The three families whose children were studied were related. Twelve of the 15 affected or probably affected infants were third-generation descendants of a consanguineous marriage. Both males and females are liable. It appears to be transmitted as an autosomal recessive.

At autopsy kernicterus was found in most cases. The livers showed no pathologic alterations except bile thrombi in the canaliculi. No obstructive lesions were found. In vivo and post mortem no evidences of increased hemolysis or of infection were discovered. The authors concluded that this is primarily a physiologic rather than a pathologic disorder of the liver. By now it has been shown conclusively that these patients are born with a lack or deficiency of the enzyme glucuronyl transferase.

Day and Johnson and their collaborators have studied intensively the Gunn strain of rats. These extraordinary animals carry an autosomal genetic defect leading to deficiency of glucuronyl transferase. Heterozygotes are comparatively normal, but homozygotes exhibit a Crigler-Najjar syndrome almost identical with the disease as it affects human beings. These observers have taught us much about the pathogenesis of kernicterus by their studies of this species.

**DIAGNOSIS.** All the cases yield the same monotonous history. Jaundice appears on the second day, increases to a high level, 10 to 44 mg of bilirubin per 100 ml of serum, and remains there. The liver and spleen do not enlarge, and anemia is not prominent. Many die of kernicterus. The bilirubin is almost entirely indirect-reacting. No increased hemolysis, infection or biliary obstruction can be demonstrated.

**TREATMENT.** Until recently nothing other than exchange transfusion could be offered these children. In 1966 Yaffe and his co-workers were able to reduce the level of bilirubin in one of these babies by the use of phenobarbital, to the point at which jaundice disappeared. They were able to keep up this effect for many months. They concluded that this "may represent the first therapeutic application of enzyme induction."

In 1969 Arias et al. showed that phenobarbital does not succeed in reducing bilirubin levels in all these apparently similar children. But in those recalcitrant to phenobarbital, phototherapy is effective,

again for a long period of time. Two simultaneous reports in 1969 have amply verified this finding. It appears that "this hepatic disorder occurs in two forms which appear phenotypically homogeneous but are genotypically heterogeneous. Patients whose defects are transmitted as an autosomal recessive . . . do not show a decrease in serum bilirubin levels when phenobarbital is administered. In contrast, patients whose serum bilirubin concentrations decrease during phenobarbital therapy appear to inherit their abnormality as an autosomal dominant character" (Crigler, 1969).

Some of the features that distinguish these two forms of the disease are listed in Table 75-1.

## THE BILE-PLUG SYNDROME

It has been suspected for many years that obstructive jaundice can be caused by plugs in the extrahepatic bile ducts. Bernstein et al. have converted this suspicion into a certainty by demonstrating such plugs in two infants, one becoming jaundiced as early as the sixth day, one as late as 7 weeks of age. This second baby was saved after demonstration by cholangiogram of obstruction in the distal end of the common duct, and the removal of an impacted mass of dark, granular, bile-colored material.

**TABLE 75–1.** *Features that Distinguish the Two Forms of Crigler-Najjar Syndrome*

|  | Type I | Type II |
|---|---|---|
| Onset of jaundice | At birth | From birth to 10 years |
| Life expectancy | Death in infancy | Adult survival |
| Bilirubin (mg/dl) levels | 17 to 43 (M = 27) | 6 to 22 (M = 13) |
| Kernicterus | Usual | None |
| Bile |  |  |
|    Color | Colorless | Normal |
|    Bilirubin glucuronide | Trace | Abundant |
| Urinary urobilinogen | Decreased | Decreased |
| Menthol glucuronide excretion | Decreased | Decreased |
| Hepatic glucuronyl transferase activity | Decreased | Decreased |
| Oral cholecystogram | Normal | Normal |
| Liver biopsy | Normal | Normal |
| BSP excretion | Normal | Normal |
| Phenobarbital effect on: |  |  |
|    Bilirubin concentration | None | Marked reduction |
|    Transferase activity | None | Increased |
|    Fecal urobilinogen | None | Increased |
| Inheritance | Autosomal recessive | Autosomal dominant |

## JAUNDICE ASSOCIATED WITH HYPERTROPHIC PYLORIC STENOSIS

Martin and Siebenthal first reported two cases of jaundice in association with hypertrophic stenosis. They were unable to find any similar records in the literature, nor have we encountered any.

**COMMENT.** Since the original report by Martin and Siebenthal, others have also noted this association. It has been estimated to occur with a frequency ranging from 2.6 to 17 per cent. Numerous theories have been proposed to explain this relationship but, as yet, no single explanation appears to explain the phenomenon. Martin and Siebenthal originally proposed that the pyloric tumor produced a direct obstruction of the common bile duct. This hypothesis did not explain the fact that the jaundice is generally a result of the accumulation of unconjugated bilirubin. In many instances the pyloric tumors have not been large enough to produce obstruction. Others have proposed that the jaundice is a result of inadequate caloric intake, dehydration, or gastric hypersecretion of gastrin. It has been proposed that gastrin may inhibit bilirubin conjugation.

A similar unconjugated hyperbilirubinemia may be observed in infants with other forms of high intestinal obstruction.

## JAUNDICE IN CYSTIC FIBROSIS OF THE PANCREAS

Gatzimos and Jowitt called attention to the previously unrecognized association of jaundice with mucoviscidosis. They pointed out that although pathologic changes in the liver, varying from fatty metamorphosis to biliary cirrhosis, have been seen frequently at biopsy and autopsy, jaundice has been regarded as an unusual symptom.

They described the clinical, blood chemical and pathologic findings in four cases in which jaundice was a prominent sign.

Case 1 was the only newborn in the series and the only one in whom jaundice appeared in the neonatal period. She was brought to the Indiana University Medical Center on her fourth day of life, having had no bowel movements since birth. A sibling had died of a similar condition some years before. Examination showed icterus, abdominal distention and increased bowel sounds. Total serum bilirubin was 8.3 mg per 100 ml; the van den Bergh reaction was direct.

Operation revealed meconium ileus; the meconium was evacuated, and she seemed improved. Distention recurred, however, within a few days. A second operation was performed, but she went downhill and died 16 days after admission. During this time total bilirubin had risen to 17.8 mg per 100 ml of serum.

Autopsy showed the bile ducts to be grossly patent. Under the microscope much mucus was seen in the intrahepatic biliary ducts, bile plugs in the intercellular canaliculi and bile ducts, fatty metamorphosis and congestion.

In the older infants the same picture was seen plus varying degrees of biliary fibrosis.

The authors conclude: "It is possible that the pathogenesis of the liver lesion is a primary obstruction of the intrahepatic biliary ducts by the viscid mucus, with a resultant ductal hyperplasia, liver cell atrophy and biliary fibrosis."

Talamo and Hendren reported another such case, the fourth now described in a newborn, who had bilirubinemia with elevation of the direct fraction on the day of birth. Both levels rose until the fourth week, and then cleared completely. On the second day, anastomosis to bypass atresia of the jejunum caused by intrauterine volvulus and irrigation of the distal bowel filled with inspissated meconium had been carried out. These authors too felt that the initial event accounting for the jaundice had been inspissation of viscid material in bile ductules. Taylor and Qaqundah proposed a similar explanation in their patient.

## JAUNDICE IN CONGENITAL MALROTATION

Jaundice in the newborn with congenital malrotation of the intestine was first described in 1963. More recently Porto reviewed the 50 cases of malrotation seen in his hospital since 1955, 38 of whom were newborns. In seven of these with no other possible reason for jaundice, hyperbilirubinemia was noted. Two required exchange transfusion. The direct fraction in only one was as high as 37 per cent of the total; in the rest it ranged from 4 to 13 per cent.

## JAUNDICE ASSOCIATED WITH HYPOTHYROIDISM

Somehow the concomitance of jaundice and hypothyroidism, so well documented by Akerrén in 1954, has been too often overlooked. The case of Eden and Weinstein is a good example. As the authors point out quite correctly, the ultimate mental capacity of the hypothyroid child may well depend upon the time the diagnosis is made and treatment is begun. In the later example of McGillivray et al. the answer was arrived at somewhat earlier.

According to Crigler, "a deficiency of thyroid hormones presumably accounts for decreased glucuronide conjugation of bilirubin in the hypothyroid infant."

## JAUNDICE ASSOCIATED WITH THE TRISOMY 17-18 SYNDROME

We have mentioned elsewhere the extraordinary discovery of Alpert et al. of seven examples of neonatal hepatitis and biliary atresia among 19 autopsied cases of the 17-18 trisomy syndrome. The authors believed that "the biliary atresia . . . may be the end result of a hepatitis involving not only the parenchyma but the biliary epithelium as well, analogous to the process observed in neonatal rubella hepatitis."

The nature of this unexpected association remains unclear.

## NEONATAL CIRRHOSIS OF THE LIVER

Typical nodular Laennec's cirrhosis, with fibrosis limited to the portal regions, is not seen in the very young infant. A disease resembling adult cirrhosis clinically, but with fibrosis distributed more broadly, is encountered. In addition, biliary cirrhosis resulting from obstruction to the outflow of bile is encountered, but more than 1 month is needed for this clinical or pathologic picture to develop fully.

**INCIDENCE.** Cirrhosis of the liver is not exceedingly rare in the total pediatric age group. Craig et al. were able to find 98 cases in a 30-year period in the Children's Hospital of Boston. It is rare in the neonatal period, however, Thaler having discovered only 24 examples in very young infants in a 23-year period in the Toronto Hospital for Sick Children.

**ETIOLOGY.** Most cirrhosis in children develops after long-continued obstruction to outflow of bile. Congenital atresia accounts for a good many of these, while a few follow cystic fibrosis, choledochal cyst or other obstructions. Erythroblastosis and galactosemia account for a few. A substantial minority appears to follow neonatal giant-cell or viral hepatitis. According to Thaler and Gellis, cirrhosis does not become apparent before the age of 1 year in these children. It developed in about 50 per cent of their infants with hepatitis who continued to exhibit liver abnormalities for this length of time.

We are concerned here with the small number of infants who are sick at birth or who become sick within the first few weeks of life with an illness which resembles cirrhosis from the start, which is rapidly progressive and terminates within a few months, and in whose livers the alterations of full-blown cirrhosis are seen at biopsy or autopsy. Most observers have considered these to be examples of rapidly progressive fetal or neonatal hepatitis, but Thaler's observations cast considerable doubt upon this assumption. He does not attempt to offer an alternative theory of pathogenesis.

**DIAGNOSIS.** Thaler's description of 24 babies with neonatal cirrhosis deserves summarization. Most of these babies were of low birth weight; almost all were male (20/24). In eight the disease was apparent at birth; the latest onset was at 9 weeks.

The presenting sign in most was gastrointestinal upset with vomiting and diarrhea. They failed to gain or lost weight. Jaundice followed, with light stool and dark urine in the majority. The temperature was not elevated. Convulsions, abdominal distention or peripheral edema was noted in a few. The liver became enlarged in most, the spleen in about one third. The course was rapidly progressive, anemia, hypoproteinemia, ascites, edema and deepening jaundice ensuing. Terminal hemorrhagic manifestations were frequent. None survived longer than 6 months after the onset.

**LABORATORY FINDINGS.** Most showed leukocytosis. Half had a hemolytic form of anemia. The serum bilirubin level was elevated, with direct-reacting bilirubin comprising 35 to 40 per cent of the total. Total serum proteins were low but gamma globulins were relatively increased.

Urines all contained bile; some contained an excess of urobilinogen, some none.

**BIOPSY AND AUTOPSY FINDINGS.** Ascites was present in all. The livers were large and finely or coarsely granular. Spleens were large. In the liver were widespread fibrosis, mostly periportal, distortion of hepatic plates, vacuolization of cells, distended central veins, ductal hyperplasia. *Only rarely were giant cells seen.* There was no necrosis and no evidence of acute inflammation.

These livers and those of neonatal giant-cell hepatitis seem strikingly different from the outset.

**TREATMENT.** In the very small number of operable cases biliary cirrhosis may be ameliorated or cured by a suitable bypass procedure. Nothing other than supportive therapy can be offered to patients with the other varieties of cirrhosis.

## NEONATAL HEPATIC NECROSIS

Ruebner et al. encountered four cases of virtually total hepatic necrosis and one of massive necrosis in newborn infants. Only two of these infants presented with jaundice, but all developed severe bleeding from many sites. The pathologic changes in their livers resembled those of acute yellow atrophy in older individuals. The authors were unable to assign any cause for this unusual condition.

## PORTAL HYPERTENSION

The syndrome of portal hypertension is divisible into the intrahepatic form, associated with cirrhosis of the liver, and the extrahepatic form, caused by congenital narrowing or thrombosis of the portal, superior mesenteric or splenic vein. It consists of splenomegaly, the development of varices over the abdomen and within esophagus or rectum, anemia, leukopenia and thrombocytopenia. It is usually signalized by hematemesis or tarry stools.

Portal hypertension does not become manifest in the neonate. It merits the attention of neonatologists because so many cases have their origin in the neonatal period. Hsia and Gellis could elicit histories of infection at that time in 12 of their 21 examples of the extrahepatic form. Shaldon and Sherlock report a similar experience. There seems little doubt that these infections result in pylephlebitis, with compromise of the portal circulation. Oski et al. have seen three examples of portal hypertension in infants 7 months, 9 months and 13 months of age in whom portal vein trauma was almost surely the causative factor. In two of them difficult, prolonged exchange transfusions had been performed soon after birth, while in the third a catheter had been allowed to indwell in the umbilical vein for a number of days in order to supply parenteral fluids. They recommend therefore that umbilical vein catheters not be left in place longer than absolutely needed, that if umbilical infection is present or if difficulty is encountered during insertion of the catheter, some other site for transfusion should be used.

## REFERENCES

Akerrén, Y.: Prolonged jaundice in the newborn associated with congenital myxedema, a syndrome of practical importance. Acta Paediat. *43*:411, 1954.

Alpert, L. I., Strauss, L., and Hirschhorn, K.: Neonatal hepatitis and biliary atresia associated with trisomy 17–18 syndrome. N. Engl. J. Med., *280*:16, 1969.

Arias, I. M.: Inheritable and congenital hyperbilirubinemia. N. Engl. J. Med. *285*:1416, 1971.

Arias, I. M., Gartner, L. M., et al.: Chronic nonhemolytic unconjugated hyperbilirubinemia with glucuronyl transferase deficiency. Am. J. Med. *47*:395, 1969.

Bernstein, J., Braylan, R., and Brough, A. J.: Bile-plug

syndrome: A correctable cause of obstructive jaundice in infants. Pediatrics *43*:273, 1969.

Brown, A. K., and Cevik, M.: Hemolysis and jaundice in a newborn following maternal treatment with sulfamethoxypyridazine (Kynex). Pediatrics *36*:742, 1965.

Collins, D. L.: Neonatal hepatitis, including a case associated with neonatal hepatitis during pregnancy. Canad. Med. Assoc. J. *75*:832, 1956.

Craig, J. M., Gellis, S. S., and Hsia, D. Y.-Y.: Cirrhosis of the liver in infants and children. A.M.A. J. Dis. Child. *90*:299, 1955.

Crigler, J. F., Jr.: Phenobarbital, hormones and bilirubin. Johns Hopkins Med. J. *125*:245, 1969.

Crigler, J. F., Jr., and Najjar, V. A.: Congenital familial non-hemolytic jaundice with kernicterus. Pediatrics *10*:169, 1952.

Eden, A. N., and Weinstein, V.: Neonatal jaundice and cretinism. N.Y. State J. Med. *64*:2914, 1964.

Flatz, G., et al.: Glucose-6-phosphate dehydrogenase deficiency and neonatal jaundice. Arch. Dis. Child. *38*:566, 1963.

Gatzimos, C. D., and Jowitt, R. H.: Jaundice in mucoviscidosis (fibrocystic disease of pancreas). A.M.A. J. Dis. Child. *89*:182, 1955.

Gorodischer, R., Levy, G., et al.: Congenital non-obstructive nonhemolytic jaundice: Effect of phototherapy. N. Engl. J. Med. *282*:375, 1970.

Hsia, D. Y.-Y., and Gellis, S. S.: Portal hypertension in infants and children. A.M.A. J. Dis. Child. *90*:290, 1955.

Jim, R. T. S., and Chu, F. K.: Hyperbilirubinemia due to glucose-6-phosphate dehydrogenase deficiency in a newborn Chinese infant. Pediatrics *31*:1046, 1963.

Johnson, L., Sarmiento, F., Blanc, W. C., and Day, R.: Kernicterus in rats with an inherited deficiency of glucuronyl transferase. A.M.A. J. Dis. Child. *97*:591, 1959; *101*:322, 1961.

Martin, J. W., and Siebenthal, B. J.: Jaundice due to hypertrophic pyloric stenosis. J. Pediatr. *47*:95, 1955.

McGillivray, M. H., Crawford, J. D., and Robey, J. S.: Congenital hypothyroidism and prolonged neonatal hyperbilirubinemia. Pediatrics *40*:283, 1967.

Oppenheimer, E. H., and Esterly, J. R.: Hepatic changes in young infants with cystic fibrosis: possible relation to focal biliary cirrhosis. J. Pediatr. *86*:683, 1975.

Oski, F. A., Allen, D. M., and Diamond, L. K.: Portal hypertension—a complication of umbilical vein catheterization. Pediatrics *31*:297, 1963.

Porto, S. O.: Jaundice in congenital malrotation of the intestine. Am. J. Dis. Child. *117*:684, 1969.

Rooney, J. C., Hill, D. J., and Danks, D. M.: Jaundice associated with bacterial infections in the newborn. Am. J. Dis. Child., *122*:39, 1971.

Ruebner, B. H., Bhagavan, B. S., et al.: Neonatal hepatic necrosis. Pediatrics *43*:963, 1969.

Schärli, A., Sieber, W. K., and Kiesewetter, W. B.: Hypertrophic pyloric stenosis at the Children's Hospital of Pittsburgh from 1912 to 1967. J. Pediatr. Surg. *4*:108, 1969.

Seeler, R. A., and Hahn, K.: Jaundice in urinary tract infection in infancy. Am. J. Dis. Child. *118*:553, 1969.

Shaldon, S., and Sherlock, S.: Obstruction to the extrahepatic portal circulation in children. Lancet *1*:63, 1962.

Still, W. J. S.: Familial hepatic cirrhosis. Arch. Dis. Child. *30*:354, 1955.

Talamo, R. C., and Hendren, W. H.: Prolonged obstructive jaundice: Report of a case with meconium ileus and jejunal atresia. Am. J. Dis. Child. *115*:74, 1968.

Taylor, W. F., and Qaqundah, B. Y.: Neonatal jaundice associated with cystic fibrosis. Am. J. Dis. Child. *123*:161, 1972.

Thaler, M. M.: Fatal neonatal cirrhosis: Entity or end result? Pediatrics *33*:721, 1964.

Weller, T. H., and Hanshaw, J. B.: Virologic and clinical observations on cytomegalic inclusion disease. N. Engl. J. Med. *266*:1233, 1962.

Yaffe, S. J., Levy, G., et al.: Enhancement of glucuronide conjugating capacity in a hyperbilirubinemic infant due to apparent enzyme induction by phenobarbital. N. Engl. J. Med. *275*:1461, 1966.

# 76

# DIFFERENTIAL DIAGNOSIS OF JAUNDICE

*Revised by Frank Oski*

An attempt should be made to establish the etiology of jaundice in all infants in whom the bilirubin level exceeds 5 mg per 100 ml during the first day of life or 10 mg per 100 ml at any time during the newborn period.

The initial diagnostic attempt should be to determine if the jaundice is a result of an increased production of bilirubin, an impairment of bilirubin conjugation, an increased reabsorption of bilirubin from the intestinal tract or a combination of all three of these factors.

A history of the pregnancy and delivery, the time jaundice was initially noted, the infant's history and physical examination and selected laboratory tests in both the mother and infant will generally enable the physician to arrive at a correct presumptive diagnosis. The salient aspects of the history, physical examination and laboratory tests are described in Table 76–1.

Jaundice that appears within the first 24 hours of life is usually the result of increased production of bilirubin as a result of a hemolytic process. In general, the more severe hemolytic anemias will be manifested by early jaundice rather than by late appearance of pallor. Rh incompatibility or ABO incompatibility are the most common causes of hemolytic disease associated with jaundice during the first day of life. Other congenital defects of red cell metabolism may also be associated with jaundice during this period and must be considered in the differential diagnosis of an infant with an unexplained hemolytic anemia. In some instances, jaundice associated with severe infection may appear during the first day. Some features that are useful in distinguishing ABO, Rh and infectious origins of jaundice are described in Table 76–2. If infection is responsible, cytomegalic inclusion disease is the most likely possibility, toxoplasmosis ranks next, and neonatal hepatitis is a possibility. In some epidemic years rubella will lead the list. A few bacterial septicemias manifest jaundice within the first day. Physical examination supplies a few valuable differentiating points.

If the newborn is jaundiced, but neither sick nor pale, is not covered with petechiae and ecchymoses, and has little or no enlargement of the spleen or liver, ABO or mild Rh hemolytic disease is the best bet. If he looks very sick, he may have either severe hemolytic disease or nonbacterial infection. Skin hemorrhages and a large liver and spleen speak strongly for the latter.

Further diagnostic studies may have to be postponed and transfusion started at this point if the infant is in shock or is obviously very anemic. The first blood withdrawn will then be subjected to a number of tests. The mother's and father's blood may also have to be investigated.

Studies that should be undertaken include the following:

1. Infant's hemoglobin, serum bilirubin and its partition, red blood cell count, number of spherocytes, nucleated red blood cell number, reticulocyte percentage, white cell count and differential platelet count, direct and indirect Coombs test results, infant's and parents' isoimmunologic and Rh grouping.

2. If Rh is positive and direct Coombs test result is strongly positive, search for circulating Rh antibodies.

3. If Rh is negative and direct Coombs test result is strongly positive, search for rare antigens (hR, Kell, Duffy, and so on).

4. If Rh is negative and direct Coombs test result is negative or weakly positive, and if infant belongs to group A or B and mother to group O, do an indirect Coombs test and search for circulating anti-A or anti-B antibodies. Presence and number of spherocytes are of the utmost importance. Follow this with the Witebsky test.

5. If no blood group incompatibility exists and this observation is confirmed by negativity of both Coombs test results, perform blood culture, urine sediment study for cytomegalic inclusion cells and virus culture, complement fixation and dye tests for this disease, for toxoplasmosis and for rubella. These latter should be done with mother's serum as well. The infant's IgM concentration and the presence or absence of IgM's against specific diseases will be extremely helpful.

These results may be interpreted by the data in Table 76–2. The qualifications are pointed out in footnotes.

This oversimplification points out a few important differential points. Infections are as likely to produce erythroblastosis as is hemolytic disease. Only ABO disease induces spherocytosis, aside, of course, from hereditary spherocytosis. With rare exceptions thrombocytopenia with jaundice this early means infection. The standard pattern for ABO disease is infant A, mother O,

**TABLE 76–1.  *Data Collection in the Diagnosis of Neonatal Jaundice***

| Information | Significance |
|---|---|
| *Family History* | |
| Parent or sibling with history of jaundice or anemia | Suggests hereditary hemolytic anemia such as hereditary spherocytosis |
| Previous sibling with neonatal jaundice | Suggests hemolytic disease due to ABO or Rh isoimmunization |
| History of liver disease in siblings or disorders such as cystic fibrosis, galactosemia, tyrosinemia, hypermethioninemia, Crigler-Najjar syndrome or alpha-1-antitrypsin deficiency | All associated with neonatal hyperbilirubinemia |
| *Maternal History* | |
| Unexplained illness during pregnancy | Consider congenital infections such as rubella, cytomegalovirus, toxoplasmosis, Herpes, syphilis, or hepatitis |
| Diabetes mellitus | Increased incidence of jaundice among infants of diabetic mothers |
| Drug ingestion during pregnancy | Ingestion of sulfonamides, nitrofurantoins, anti-malarials may initiate hemolysis in G-6-PD deficient infant. |
| *History of Labor and Delivery* | |
| Vacuum extraction | Increased incidence of cephalohematoma and jaundice |
| Oxytocin induced labor | Increased incidence of hyperbilirubinemia |
| Delayed cord clamping | Increased incidence of hyperbilirubinemia among polycythemic infants |
| Apgar score | Increased incidence of jaundice in asphyxiated infants |
| *Infant's History* | |
| Delayed passage of meconium or infrequent stools | Increased enterohepatic circulation of bilirubin. Consider intestinal atresia, annular pancreas, Hirschsprung's disease, meconium plug, drug induced ileus (hexamethonium) |
| Caloric intake | Inadequate caloric intake results in delay in bilirubin conjugation |
| Vomiting | Suspect sepsis, galactosemia, or pyloric stenosis; all associated with hyperbilirubinemia. |
| *Infant's Physical Exam* | |
| Small for gestational age | Infants frequently polycythemic and jaundiced |
| Head size | Microcephaly seen with intrauterine infections associated with jaundice |
| Cephalohematoma | Entrapped hemorrhage associated with hyper-bilirubinemia |

*(Table continued on opposite page.)*

direct Coombs test result negative or weakly positive, indirect Coombs test results positive. If direct bilirubin in the blood exceeds 2.0 mg per 100 ml in this age group, infection is probably present. Exceptions to this rule exist. A strongly positive direct Coombs test result and absent ABO or Rh incompatibility call for studies directed toward other rare blood group incompatibilities.

Jaundice beginning during the second or third day is probably physiologic. If, however, the infant appears ill, if the liver or spleen is enlarged, if urobilin or bile ap-pears in excess in the urine or if conjugated bilirubin is found in the blood, other explanations should be sought.

Jaundice first appearing at 4 days or later cannot be due to hemolytic disease of the newborn. Sepsis neonatorum must now be considered seriously, as well as hereditary spherocytosis and its congeners. Intranatally or postnatally acquired virus infection (cytomegalic disease, generalized herpes simplex) must be thought of as well as the bacterial infections. Nor can neonatal hepatitis be ignored, since its onset may take place at any time from birth to 4 months.

**TABLE 76-1.** *Data Collection in the Diagnosis of Neonatal Jaundice* — Continued

| Information | Significance |
| --- | --- |
| Pallor | Suspect hemolytic anemia |
| Petechiae | Suspect congenital infection, overwhelming sepsis or severe hemolytic disease as cause of jaundice |
| Appearance of umbilical stump | Omphalitis and sepsis may produce jaundice |
| Hepatosplenomegaly | Suspect hemolytic anemia or congenital infection |
| Optic fundi | Chorioretinitis suggests congenital infection as cause of jaundice |
| Umbilical hernia | Consider hypothyroidism |
| Congenital anomalies | Jaundice occurs with increased frequency among infants with trisomic conditions |

*Laboratory Data*

| | |
| --- | --- |
| **Maternal** | |
| Blood group and indirect Coombs test | Necessary for evaluation of possible ABO or Rh incompatibility |
| Serology | Rule out congenital syphilis |
| **Infant** | |
| Hemoglobin | Anemia suggests hemolytic disease or large entrapped hemorrhage. Hemoglobin above 22 gm/100 ml associated with increased incidence of jaundice |
| Reticulocyte count | Elevation suggests hemolytic disease |
| Red cell morphology | Spherocytes suggest ABO incompatibility or hereditary spherocytosis. Red cell fragmentation seen in disseminated intravascular coagulation |
| Platelet count | Thrombocytopenia suggests infection |
| White cell count | Total white cell count less than 5000/mm$^3$ or increase in band forms to greater than 2000/mm$^3$ suggests infection |
| Sedimentation rate | Values in excess of 5 during the first 48 hours indicate infection or ABO incompatibility |
| Direct bilirubin | Elevation suggests infection or severe Rh incompatibility |
| Immunoglobulin M | Elevation indicates infection |
| Blood group and direct and indirect Coombs test | Required to rule out hemolytic disease as a result of isoimmunization |
| Carboxyhemoglobin level | Elevated in infants with hemolytic disease or entrapped hemorrhage |
| Urinalysis | Presence of reducing substance suggests diagnosis of galactosemia |

Repeated blood, urine, nose and throat cultures are now in order, as well as fragility tests, virus cultures and complement-fixation studies.

Icterus that persists beyond the usual duration of physiologic jaundice may be hemolytic, functional or obstructive. If hemolytic, it may be the result of persistent sepsis, of pyelonephritis, of hereditary erythrocyte malformation or, very rarely indeed, of congenital hemoglobin disorders or erythrocyte enzyme defects. The morphology of the red cells, their osmotic fragility, electrophoretic studies, enzyme studies and repeated blood cultures should differentiate this group.

If bilirubinemia is pronounced, and the serum bilirubin is almost entirely of the indirect type, yet there is no evidence of increased hemolysis (reticulocytosis, normoblastosis and erythroblastosis in the blood, increased urobilin in the stool or urine), one should think first of events that can predispose to hepatic recirculation of bilirubin absorbed from the intestine, and, if this is not the cause, of hypothyroidism.

### TABLE 76–2.   *Laboratory Tests in Jaundice that Begins Within the First 24 Hours*

| Disease Process | Blood Smear | | | Infant's Erythrocytes | | | Infant's Bilirubin | | Antibodies | | | | Special Tests for Infection |
|---|---|---|---|---|---|---|---|---|---|---|---|---|---|
| | Sphero-cytes | Erythro-blasts | Reduced Platelets | Group O | Rh-Positive | Direct Coombs | Direct | In-direct | Indirect Coombs | A or B | Rh | Witebsky | |
| ABO hemolytic disease | + | + | Rarely and later | Never° | 0 or + | Rarely and weak | No >2.0 mg. % | + | + | + | 0 | + | 0 |
| Rh hemolytic disease | 0 | + | Rarely and later | ± | +† | + and strong | Rarely > 2.0 mg. % | + | + | 0 | + | 0 | 0 |
| Infection | 0 | + | + often | ± | 0 | 0 | + | + | 0 | 0 | 0 | 0 | +†‡ |

° The infant's blood group is usually A.

† In hR (little c, d or e) sensitization and those caused by other rare antigens, the Rh will be negative.

‡ In toxoplasmosis Sabin's dye test becomes positive early, while complement fixation becomes positive later. At this stage dye tests should be positive in the mother and infant, complement fixation only in the mother. If cytomegalic inclusion disease is the cause, the urinary sediment should show inclusion bodies and should yield the virus upon culture. Specific IgM tests are highly desirable.

Then one is justified in thinking seriously of congenital familial nonhemolytic jaundice.

Persistent obstructive jaundice is a sign that causes much diagnostic perplexity. Its characteristics include a high proportion of direct-reacting bilirubin in the serum (usually 35 per cent or more of the total), diminished or absent bilirubin and urobilin in stools and increased bile in the urine. Diagnostic possibilities include (1) anatomic obstructions (atresia of bile ducts, bile duct plug, choledochus or pseudocholedochus cyst or, rarely, cystic fibrosis, hypertrophic pyloric stenosis, intestinal atresia or malrotation of the intestine); (2) neonatal hepatitis (following erythroblastosis fetalis, congenital or acquired hemolytic anemia, or with no known underlying disease); and (3) neonatal cirrhosis of the liver. Clinically there are few differentiating features between these. A fair one is that infants with bile duct atresia do not appear ill during the neonatal period. They eat well and gain fairly well at first. Nor are those infants ill who have obstructive jaundice which follows hemolytic disease. Those with hepatitis, and especially those with cirrhosis, look and act sick, eat poorly and may have fever and may vomit often. Infants with hemolytic disease of the newborn will usually have gone through a stage of nonobstructive jaundice within the first week of life, and the obstructive episode will either have followed directly on its heels or will have appeared a few days or weeks after subsidence of the first. The knowledge that hemolytic disease had been manifest earlier makes the diagnosis of inspissated bile syndrome secondary to this disorder simple. If one does not have this knowledge, retrospective tests as described above will still be diagnostic.

Liver function tests are of little differentiating value. Unfortunately flocculation and turbidity tests seldom become positive in newborns except in neonatal cirrhosis of the liver. The rose bengal excretion test may be of greater use, since the dye is well excreted in a large number of the hepatitis group, but poorly in the atresias. Serum transaminase activities have some differential diagnostic value.

It is wise to move slowly with these infants, especially if they appear ill. With watchful waiting a fair proportion of them will improve and ultimately recover. If no improvement has occurred by the end of the first month, punch biopsy of the liver may be performed. If the microscopic picture then suggests atresia rather than hepatitis, exploratory laparotomy is in order. This must be done as quickly and nontraumatically as possible. Then if obstruction to the hepatic or common duct is visualized in the x-ray films, careful exploration and, possibly, a definite shunting procedure should be attempted.

## REFERENCES

Adler, S. M., and Denton, R. L.: The erythrocyte sedimentation rate period. J. Pediatr. 86:942, 1975.

Alden, E. R.., et al.: Carboxyhemoglobin determination in evaluating neonatal jaundice. Am. J. Dis. Child. 127:214, 1974.

# X

# Disorders of the Head, Spine and Nervous System

# 77

# NEUROLOGIC ASSESSMENT OF THE NEWBORN INFANT

*By William E. Bell*

The formation and maturation of the nervous system compose a complex process, which is little influenced by the event of birth except that the birth process and early postnatal period represent a time of particular risk to the morphology and continued development of the newborn infant. The brain is not simply small in size but must be considered immature compared to that of its adult counterpart, both biochemically and histologically, with many changes yet to occur in the ensuing months and years. Neurologic function is decidedly related to degree of nervous system maturation, a fact clearly exhibited by the functional differences between the small premature infant and the intact neonate born at term. For those patterns of infant and child development, as well as intellect, to unfold in a normal sequence, it is necessary that maturation of the brain, from closure of the neural tube to final myelination of the frontal association fibers, proceed unhampered and in orderly fashion.

In early fetal life the surface of the brain is smooth until approximately 24 weeks, when fissuring of the cerebral hemispheres first appears. At birth, the brain of the term infant shows all primary and secondary fissures and sulci but the tertiary sulci are only partly developed. The four major lobes are clearly distinguishable at birth, although the frontal and temporal poles are relatively short compared to those of the older child.

Migration of neuroblasts from the ependymal and subependymal regions of the lateral ventricles to the region of the future cerebral cortex occurs between the third and seventh fetal months. By the time of birth, the cerebral cortex exhibits lamination similar to that of the adult brain, although, on gross observation of the sectioned brain, the demarcation between cortical gray matter and underlying white matter is not yet distinct. Nissl bodies are not yet present in cortical neurons, except in certain Betz cells in the motor cortex. The cerebellum in the newborn is notable for its striking external granular cell layer composed of eight to 12 rows of densely packed cells, which gradually disappear during the first postnatal year. Myelin, elaborated from proliferating oligodendrocytes, appears in the brain in various places at different times. Certain brain stem pathways acquire myelin early in gestation but even at birth, the cerebral white matter, including the corticospinal tracts and the optic nerves, are poorly myelinated.

The brain of the term newborn infant weighs 330 to 350 grams, only a quarter of that of the average adult brain but accounting for approximately 10 per cent of the total body weight at birth. In contrast, the brain of the average adult represents only about 1.5 to 2 per cent of the total body weight. Within the first year, the brain enlarges to a weight of approximately 950 grams. This rapid growth during the first postnatal year is largely the result of continued myelination and tremendous elaboration of dendritic processes, thus establishing the neuronal connections necessary for the complex behavior characteristic of the infant and child.

## NEUROLOGIC EXAMINATION

Neurologic examination of the newborn infant is an observational art that requires a certain degree of knowledge of the variations of neonatal behavior, a considerable degree of patience and a conservative attitude regarding the significance and the predictive value of certain deviations of performance that can be influenced by many systemic and environmental factors. A single examination may suffice to document the presence of neurologic integrity in a newborn or may be adequate when signs of disease are obvious and definite. When signs are marginal or only suggestively abnormal, however, a second examination or even daily evaluations will yield more reliable information on the nature of the problem. Many of our present concepts of neurologic and behavioral function of the newborn infant are derived from the detailed and astute observations of André-Thomas, Saint-Anne Dargassies, and Illingworth.

Neurologic examination of the newborn child should begin with an adequate period of observation, first before removal of the clothing and then in more detail with the infant completely undressed. Ideally, the baby should be awake, not crying, not cool or exposed to a cold environment and approximately two hours should have elapsed since its last feeding. General aspects to be noted because of their possible association with neurologic function include the respiratory rate and rhythm, cutaneous abnormalities such as plethora, jaundice or evidence of sepsis and the presence of external minor anomalies, especially of the hands, feet, external ears, eyes or genitalia.

Important components of the infant's behavior to be observed include the state of wakefulness or alertness, the resting posture the child assumes in the supine and prone positions, the capability of the child to perform similar but not necessarily symmetrical movements of the limbs on the two sides and the character of the cry. The posture of the normal term infant in the prone position is one of partial flexion of the arms and legs, with legs adducted so that the thighs are maintained under the abdomen. When awake, the baby on his abdomen is able to rotate the head from side to side and temporarily elevate it from the surface of the crib. The awake neonate lying on his back will exhibit purposeless, poorly coordinated limb movements, usually consisting of alternating flexion and extension in reciprocal fashion on the two sides. Minimal or absent motor activity, or strikingly asymmetrical motor activity in which one arm or one side of the body is little moved, is clearly suggestive of neuro-

logic dysfunction. Eye movements are difficult to assess during the first few days after birth. Discrete following movements are not expected at this time, but an alert infant often appears to fixate on the examiner's face, and some degree of conjugate ocular activity is usually seen. Abrupt, transient horizontal nystagmus is commonly present in the newborn, especially on movement of the child, and should not be judged to be abnormal. The newborn infant will blink when a bright light is shined in his eyes, will show head turning toward a diffuse light (Goldie and Hopkins), will reveal pupillary reactions to light stimulation and may blink to a loud noise. The cry of an intact newborn is a vigorous and reasonably sustained one, easily elicited by flicking the bottom of the foot or sometimes by eliciting the Moro response. A high-pitched shrill cry, a cry which on repeated observations on different examinations is weak and unsustained or an inability to provoke a cry are indicators of probable neurologic abnormalities.

Muscle tone is evaluated by passive movement of various parts of the body, ideally with the infant awake and not crying. Since limb tone, like various reflexes, is influenced or altered by tonic neck reflexes, it is important to have the child's head in a neutral position when these assessments are made. The normal term infant is physiologically "hypertonic" with a certain degree of resistance being present to extension at the elbow and the knee. Muscle tone should be symmetrical when one side is compared to the other. Muscle tone may be diminished in various degrees, providing an important sign for diagnostic analysis but by itself it is without localizing implications. Absolute flaccidity, the ultimate in muscle hypotonicity, is most often encountered in the child who is comatose, in which case the prognosis depends on the cause of coma. Flaccidity in the awake term infant can occur under a variety of circumstances, including traumatic insults to the upper portion of the spinal cord, disease of the spinal anterior horn cells or abnormalities of the neuromuscular junction or muscles.

Certain deep tendon reflexes can be elicited in the neonate but have limited value except when definitely asymmetrical reactions are elicited. The triceps jerk and ankle jerk cannot usually be obtained during the period of flexor tone predominance. The knee jerk is moderately brisk and is often associated with adduction of the opposite thigh. Unsustained ankle clonus of three to four beats is common in the days immediately after birth and does not represent an abnormal finding. The plantar response to stimulation of the lateral surface of the sole of the foot is a much discussed phenomenon but of limited usefulness in the clinical assessment of the newborn. The claim that all newborn and young infants have Babinski signs is an overstatement in need of qualification. Although it is true that extension of the great toe is often part of the response to plantar stimulation in early infancy, this normal response is usually quite different from the slow, tonic extension associated with fanning of the other toes seen in the 3- or 4-month-old with spastic lower limbs. The normal response to plantar stimulation is frequently a quick withdrawal with flexion of the knee and prompt but unsustained extension of the great toe. Hogan and Milligan have shown that the first, and most important, response to stroking of the sole of the newborn's foot is a flexor reaction of the great toe, which may then be followed by other movements.

Examination of the head of a newborn infant should include observation and description of its shape, measurement in centimeters of the occipitofrontal circumference, palpation and estimation of degree of separation of sutures, and palpation and measurement of the size of the anterior fontanel. Care must be used in determining the head circumference, and the same landmarks should be used with each estimate. A disposable paper tape is preferred to a metal one and should extend around the head from a point approximately 1 centimeter above the supraorbital margin anteriorly to the farthest point on the occiput posteriorly. In some instances, auscultation of the head and attempt at transillumination are additional useful procedures. The status of the cranial sutures and anterior fontanel, especially on serial examinations over the course of weeks or months, is one of the most reliable indicators of conditions that include increased intracranial pressure or those that have interfered with continued normal brain growth. The anterior fontanel is best evaluated with the infant quiet and held in the sitting position. The range of normal fontanel size and the conditions that retard fontanel closure have been reviewed by Popich and Smith. In addition to primary neurologic conditions in which increased intracranial pressure is present, a tense fontanel in infancy occurs in some cases with cardiac failure. An unusual finding on examination of the head is a parietal bony defect along the sagittal suture, located approximately 2 centimeters anterior to the posterior fontanel. This is referred to as a third fontanel but is not in fact a fontanel in that it is not located at the junction of the parietal and adjacent bones. This bony defect results from failure of completion of ossification in the parasagittal parietal region and has been identified especially in infants with Down's syndrome and the congenital rubella syndrome (Tan, and Chemke and Robinson).

A notable aspect of the neurologic assessment of the newborn infant pertains to the normal but temporary presence of a group of reactions known as "neonatal reflexes." These aspects of newborn function are generally attributed to mechanisms at the brain-stem level that can be provoked by the appropriate stimulus because of the relative lack of cerebral inhibition. Because of this, it has sometimes been assumed that the cerebral hemispheres are essentially nonfunctional in the newborn period. Logic and keen observation would suggest otherwise, even though the influence of cerebral function on behavior is less in the newborn period than later in infancy and during childhood (Robinson). Vision and hearing are present at the moment of birth, and voluntary smiling can sometimes be observed between 2 and 4 weeks after birth. In the absence of proved data one way or the other, it would be prudent not to discount the possibility of learning at a certain level, even in the newborn period.

From the clinical standpoint the Moro response is the best known and most useful of the various neonatal reflexes. It can be elicited in a number of ways, such as abrupt but gentle hyperextension of the neck by allowing the head to fall backward, or by abrupt release of both hands, having pulled the child up slightly from the supine position. The response consists of sudden abduction of the proximal portions of the arms, extension at the elbows and opening of the fists with abduction of the fingers (Parmelee). Normal infants frequently cry immediately after the response is provoked. The Moro response gradually diminishes, to disappear by 3 to 4 months of age, or even later in prematurely born infants. Its persistence significantly beyond its expected date of disappearance or its absence or diminished intensity in the first few weeks of life represents abnormalities indicative of neurologic dysfunction. Marked and persistent asymmetry of the response occurs with brachial plexus stretch injuries, clavicular fractures or conditions associated with hemiparesis. Grasp reaction, rooting and sucking reflexes, placing reaction and stepping response are additional characteristics of the normal newborn infant which persist for 1 to 3 months and whose presence adds to the probability of neurologic integrity. The Babkin reflex is a curious and poorly understood response in which pressure by the thumbs of the examiner on the palms of both hands of the infant results in opening of the mouth. It can be elicited in many newborn infants, normal or abnormal, except in those lethargic or in coma. It is present in premature infants, even as early as 26 weeks' gestation (Parmelee).

Interpretation of neurologic findings in the premature infant is more difficult because guidelines are less well established, function varies to a degree depending on body weight, and a higher percentage are affected with illness of a respiratory or other type. Small premature infants show less evidence of alertness or wakefulness than do their term counterparts, and exhibit considerably less spontaneous motor activity. The motor activity observed is often brief in duration and jerky in character. The infant born at 26 to 30 weeks' gestation is usually either limp or moderately hypotonic and lies with limbs in an extended position. At a gestational age of 34 weeks, the lying posture is "frog-like," with legs partially flexed and abducted at the hips and partially flexed at the knees. Some resistance to passive movement of the extremities can be appreciated at this time but less than is expected in the term infant. Hypotonia in the upper limbs in the premature baby can be demonstrated by the scarf sign, performed by holding the infant's right hand and extending the arm, then carrying the arm across the neck of the child toward the opposite side. In the hypotonic infant the arm covers the neck like a scarf, while in the term infant normal muscle tone limits the range of motion at the shoulder. Pupillary reflexes to light appear after approximately 30 weeks, and head turning to light occurs somewhere between 32 and 36 weeks of gestational age. Rooting and sucking reflexes are usually difficult to elicit in infants of less than 30 weeks of gestation. The Moro response likewise is either poorly established or is absent before 29 to 30 weeks.

## ASSESSMENT OF GESTATIONAL AGE

When it is recognized that infants of low birth weight can be small because of short gestation (premature infant) or because of retardation of intrauterine growth (small-for-dates infant), methods of distinguishing the two on the basis of clinical assessment became important. External characteristics, including skin texture and color, peripheral edema, lanugo, nipple formation, breast size, external ear form and firmness and external genitalia, correlate with gestational age to some extent but are less than entirely precise (Farr et al., Dubowitz et al). With the awareness that neurologic function correlates more closely to gestational age than to body weight at birth, investigators developed complex methods of assessment of neurologic findings, as additional ways of arriving at gestational age. The system devised by Robinson (Table 77–1) utilizes five reflex responses, including pupillary reaction, traction response, glabellar tap, neck-righting, and head-turning to diffuse light. Gestational age can be

TABLE 77–1.   *Reflexes of Value in Assessing Gestational Age**

| Reflex | Stimulus | Positive Response | Gestation (wk.) if Reflex is | |
|---|---|---|---|---|
| | | | Absent | Present |
| Pupil reaction | Light | Pupil contraction | <31 | 29 or more |
| Traction | Pull up by wrists from supine | Flexion of neck or arms | <36 | 33 or more |
| Glabellar tap | Tap on glabella | Blink | <34 | 32 or more |
| Neck-righting | Rotation of head | Trunk follows | <37 | 34 or more |
| Head-turning | Diffuse light from one side | Head-turning to light | Doubtful | 32 or more |

*Robinson, R. J.: Arch. Dis. Child. *41*:437, 1966.
Note: Twenty-nine weeks means 203 days after the first day of the last menstrual period. If there is a conflict between two results, the reflex placed higher in the table is more likely to give the true gestational age.

roughly estimated by these observations, since pupillary reaction to light develops from 29 to 31 weeks of gestation, glabellar tap reflex from 32 to 34 weeks, traction response from 33 to 36 weeks, neck-righting reflex from 34 to 37 weeks, and head-turning to diffuse light from 32 to 36 weeks. The method developed by Amiel-Tison is largely dependent on the gradual increase of muscle tone which occurs progressively with increasing gestational age (Fig. 77–1). An additional method to differentiate the low birth weight infant or short gestation from the

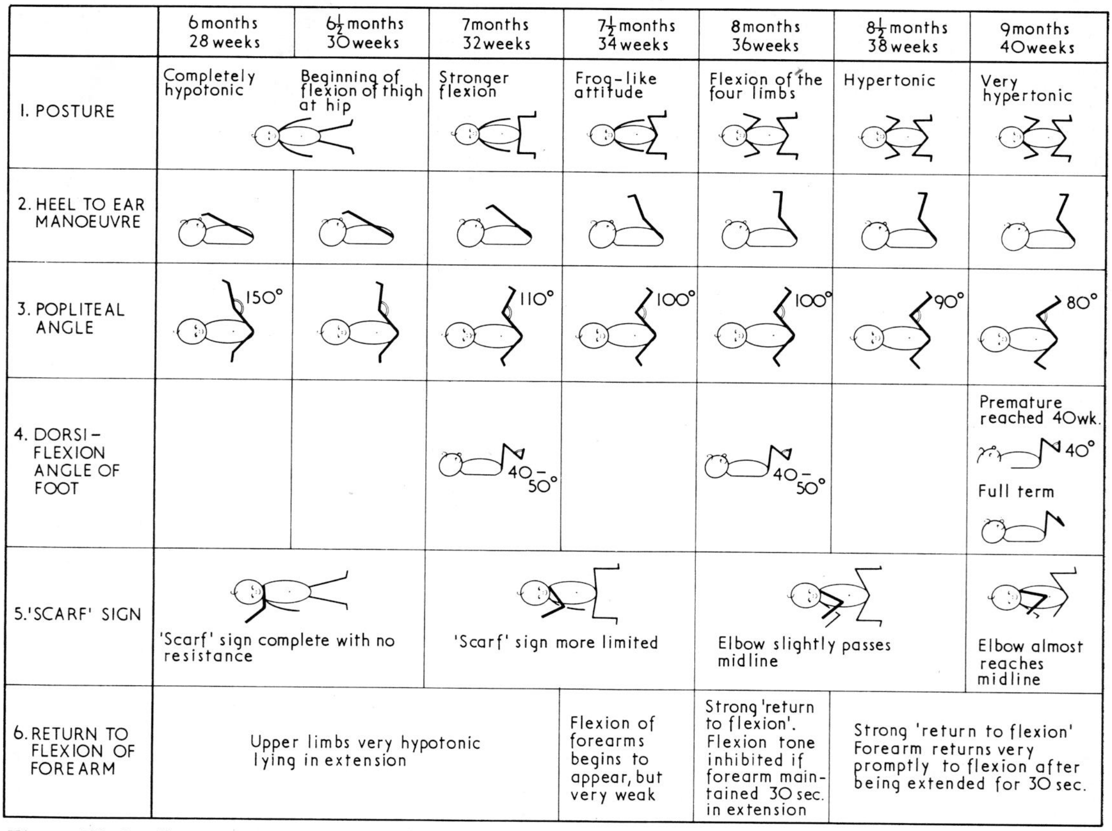

*Figure 77–1.*   Passive tone. Increase of tone with maturity illustrated by means of six clinical tests. (Amiel-Tison, C.: Arch. Dis. Child. *43*:89, 1968.)

small-for-dates infant is on the basis of ulnar nerve motor conduction velocity (Schulte et al., Moosa and Dubowitz, Dubowitz et al.). The mean conduction velocity for the ulnar nerve of the term newborn infant is approximately 30 meters per second and is progressively slower with progressively shorter gestational ages. Electroencephalographic methods have also been used to judge gestational age by determination of the latency of photo-evoked responses from the occipital cortex (Engel and Butler). Infants of a conceptual age of 40 weeks were found to have a mean latency of the response to photic stimulation of approximately 153 milliseconds, at 38 weeks the latency was 169 milliseconds, at 36 weeks 203 milliseconds, at 32 weeks 221 milliseconds, and at 29 weeks 230 milliseconds.

## SKULL X-RAYS

X-rays of the skull of the newborn child should be obtained when the head is abnormally large or small in comparison with the expected normal range for body weight, when there are abnormalities of its shape not explained by molding secondary to the delivery process, when the possibility of fracture exists on the basis of the presence of a cephalhematoma or a traumatic delivery, or in the presence of findings suggestive of an intrauterine acquired infection. Skull films are also indicated in neonates who exhibit certain neurologic abnormalities not readily explained on the basis of perinatal hypoxia or cardiorespiratory disturbances. Their value in the determination of the presence of increased intracranial pressure in the newborn is limited, however, and should not be assumed to be as reliable as clinical examination, including such methods as palpation of the sutures and anterior fontanel, and transillumination of the skull (Fig. 77–2).

Pathologic calcification within the brain parenchyma is an unusual roentgenographic finding in the infant, but its presence strongly suggests a congenital infection. The absence of calcification by no means excludes the possibility of intrauterine infection, and, in fact, most infected infants do not have evidence of cerebral calcification. Periventricular calcification, especially with microcephaly, is suggestive of cytomegalovirus infection acquired in utero, while more diffuse mineral deposition can be seen with congenital toxoplasmosis.

## LUMBAR PUNCTURE

The method of performance of lumbar puncture and cerebrospinal fluid examination in the newborn infant is similar to that in the older child. The procedure is quite

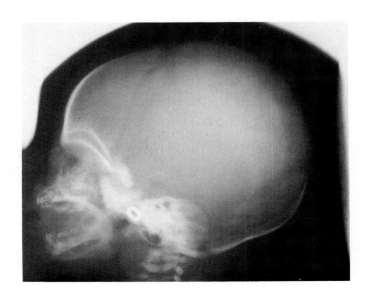

*Figure 77–2.* Skull x-ray, normal 2-day-old infant. Lateral projection. The calvarium is poorly mineralized compared with that of the older child, resulting in less striking contrast between sutures and adjacent bone.

safe, because the spinal cord in the term infant at birth terminates at approximately the level of the second lumbar vertebral body and because the patent cranial sutures and open fontanels diminish the possibility of internal herniations in conditions with increased intracranial pressure. The procedure can be done with the infant in either the sitting or lateral recumbent position. A short, 22-gauge needle, with or without a stylet, is preferred by most. Concern has been raised that a penetrating needle without a stylet might possibly introduce epithelial fragments into the subarachnoid space which later might give rise to intraspinal epidermoid tumors (Shaywitz). This remains speculative, has not yet been proved, and perhaps is more applicable to the child who might require multiple spinal taps. Points to remember in the performance of the procedure are the short distance from the skin surface to the subarachnoid space, especially in the premature child, and the absolute requirement to maintain the tip of the needle in the midline as it is directed through the soft tissues towards the subarachnoid space. The slightest deviation of the plane of the needle is likely to result in an unsuccessful tap. By far the most important reason for cerebrospinal fluid examination in the newborn child is to determine the presence or absence of infection. In some instances the procedure can be diagnostically useful to document the presence of intracranial hemorrhage.

Measurement of the pressure of cerebrospinal fluid is entirely unreliable in the crying, struggling infant and is best not attempted when these circumstances prevail. The time required and manipulation of the needle by attaching the manometer increase the risk of dislodging the tip from the subarachnoid space, thus eliminating the opportunity to obtain a CSF specimen uncontaminated by blood. When coma or lack of response to needle penetration prevails, an opening pressure can often be obtained, after a small quantity of fluid is captured for cell count and culture.

In the normal term infant, the cerebrospinal fluid is usually crystal clear, while variable degrees of xanthochromia are more often seen in the premature baby.

Xanthochromia is caused by the presence of approximately 400 to 500 red blood cells per cubic millimeter, or secondary to hyperbilirubinemia. Studies have shown that there is not a direct relationship between the levels of serum and spinal fluid bilirubin in the newborn child, probably reflecting the individual variations in the blood-CSF and blood-brain barriers (Stempfel and Zetterström). A number of red blood cells and up to 10 white blood cells per mm$^3$ can be accepted as insignificant in the first few days after birth. White cells are largely mononuclear in type although two or three neutrophils per mm$^3$ can be present in the absence of infection. The range of the cerebrospinal fluid protein value is far greater in the intact newborn infant than in the older child. In the full term infant, levels between 45 and 100 mg per 100 ml can be considered normal while in the premature baby, a protein content of up to 180 mg per 100 ml can occur without evident neurologic disease (Otila, and Bauer et al.). The CSF protein concentration bears a roughly inverse relationship to weight of the premature child and thus is probably a function of degree of maturity of vascular permeability and the blood-CSF barrier (Arnhold and Zetterström).

The cerebrospinal fluid alterations associated with bacterial meningitis in the newborn period are generally similar to those at any other age. The protein value is commonly much higher than is usually the case in the older child with meningitis, probably indicative of the greater necrotizing effect of bacterial infection on the immature brain. It is important to recognize that it is possible, although unusual, for a child to have meningitis even though the cerebrospinal fluid is clear to gross observation, contains few cells, and has a normal glucose content. For this reason, Gram stain and appropriate cultures should be made on every spinal fluid specimen obtained from the neonate, regardless of the other findings.

## SUBDURAL TAPS

Transfontanel subdural tap is a reasonably safe procedure if proper precautions are taken. The hair should be shaved well beyond the site of the needle penetration, and the scalp should be properly cleansed with the appropriate substances. After application of a sterilizing agent to the skin, it should be allowed to dry or wiped dry before insertion of the needle. The site chosen for the tap should be as close to the junction of the fontanel with the coronal suture as possible to avoid injury to the midline superior sagittal sinus.

Subdural taps are done in the newborn period to identify the presence of blood in the subdural space or the existence of effusions complicating bacterial meningitis. Both sides should be tapped, even if localizing signs on examination suggest the possibility of fluid collection on one side. The procedure should be preceded by transillumination of the head.

Transfontanel ventricular taps are only occasionally indicated in the newborn infant and should be done or directed by a person experienced with the procedure. Ventricular tap is sometimes warranted in the child with a tense, bulging fontanel believed to have an intraventricular hemorrhage in whom subdural taps are negative. Ventricular taps may also be indicated for the intraventricular instillation of antibiotics in certain cases of purulent meningitis.

## TRANSILLUMINATION

Transillumination of the head is a valuable technique which incurs no expense and is entirely safe, but which requires that the examiner recognize and be familiar with normal variations, especially in the low birth weight infant. The examiner should use the same three-battery-powered flashlight for all examinations, so that the intensity of illumination remains constant. The room must be entirely darkened and a brief period of time to become adapted to the dark should be taken before making the evaluation. The light, with a soft rubber adapter, must be placed flush with the head of the child. The glow of light extends 2 to 2.5 cm from the rim of the light source in the frontal region of the term infant and even farther in the premature child. Abnormal transillumination occurs when subdural ef-

fusions are present and in the child with hydranencephaly. In infants with the Dandy-Walker syndrome it may also be positive over the posterior fossa.

## ELECTROENCEPHALOGRAPHY

In the older infant or child the electroencephalogram, when interpreted by a competent individual, is a valuable diagnostic tool. It provides aid in the confirmation of a convulsive disorder, in the localization of a supratentorial mass lesion or in adding evidence of the absence of structural brain disease in the presence of certain symptoms or signs. Even in the patient with a mature nervous system, however, one must recognize the limitations of electroencephalography, that minor deviations from normal need not be of clinical significance and that the results of an electroencephalogram must be used in conjunction with the historical data, the physical findings and the information accumulated from other studies.

In the newborn period the electroencephalogram has even greater restrictions on its clinical applicability, in part because of the limited ability of the immature cerebral cortex to produce recordable electrical potentials. The electroencephalogram of the premature infant is characterized by discontinuous and disorganized activity which gradually becomes synergistic over the two hemispheres with increasing gestational age (Dreyfus-Brisac). Before the twenty-sixth week of gestational age, the recording is irregular, with bursts of up to one-per-second waves alternating with periods of near electrical silence lasting several seconds. Beyond 28 weeks, bursts become more regular and some intermittent fast activity begins to emerge (Engel). In the full-term infant, the electroencephalogram reveals low voltage activity, generally less than 50 microvolts, with occasional three-to-five-per-second waves of slightly higher voltage than the general background (Anderson and Gibbs, Rosen and Satran). Kellaway has stated that when abnormal focal discharges are found in the early weeks after birth, they tend to be localized in the areas of maximal neuronal development, chiefly the primary projection areas. He found the occipital region to account for approximately 75 per cent of all foci seen in early infancy and most of the remainder to arise from the rolandic region.

The value of the electroencephalogram in the neonate with convulsions does not parallel that of the procedure in older children. This is the result of two factors: the electrophysiologic differences in the immature compared with the more mature nervous system and the much higher frequency with which neonatal seizures are caused by identifiable metabolic or infectious diseases, or secondary to perinatal cerebral insults. The interictal EEG of the newborn may be normal, may reveal a localized electrical focus of sharp or spike activity, or may show independent foci originating in one or, more often, both cerebral hemispheres. The characteristic hypsarrhythmic pattern associated with infantile spasms does not occur in the newborn period and is rarely seen prior to 3 months of age. A single electroencephalogram in the convulsing neonate usually adds little to the immediate management of the problem, although Rose and Lombroso have found the procedure to have some prognostic implications. Among their series, neonates with seizures and a normal EEG had an 86 per cent chance of normal development, whereas those with a distinctly abnormal record had only a 7 per cent chance of subsequent normal development.

## COMPUTED TOMOGRAPHY

Computed tomography (C.T.) is useful in newborn patients in whom the diagnosis of intraventricular hemorrhage is suspected. Fresh hemorrhage has specific density measurements by C.T. This technique permits the diagnosis of hemorrhage to be confirmed with obvious advantages in the determination of prognosis and management. At the same time, the cerebrospinal fluid spaces can be assessed, excluding or confirming severe dysgenetic, degenerative or hydrocephalic disease.

## REFERENCES

Amiel-Tison, C.: Neurological evaluation of the maturity of newborn infants. Arch. Dis. Child. *43*:89, 1968.

Anderson, E., and Gibbs, E.: The normal and abnormal electroencephalogram of the neonate. Clin. Electroencephalography *1*:30, 1970.

André-Thomas, Chesni, Y., and Saint-Anne Dargassies, S.: The neurological examination of the infant. Little Club Clinics in Developmental Medicine No. 1, 1960.

Arnhold, R. G., and Zetterström, R.: Proteins in the cerebrospinal fluid in the newborn. Pediatrics *21*:279, 1958.

Bauer, C. H., New, M. I., and Miller, J. H.: Cerebrospinal fluid protein values of premature infants. J. Pediatr. *66*:1017, 1965.

Chemke, J., and Robinson, A.: The third fontanelle. J. Pediatr. *75*:617, 1969.

Dreyfus-Brisac, C.: The electroencephalogram of the premature infant. World Neurology *3*:5, 1962.

Dubowitz, L. M. S., Dubowitz, V., and Goldberg, C.: Clinical assessment of gestational age in the newborn infant. J. Pediatr. *77*:1, 1970.

Dubowitz, V., Whittaker, G. F., Brown, B. H., and Robinson, A.: Nerve conduction velocity—an index of neurological maturity of the newborn infant. Develop. Med. Child Neurol. *10*:741, 1968.

Engel, R.: Maturational changes and abnormalities in the newborn electroencephalogram. Dev. Med. Child Neurol. *7*:498, 1965.

Engel, R., and Butler, B. V.: Appraisal of conceptual age of newborn infants by electroencephalographic methods. J. Pediatr. *63*:386, 1963.

Farr, V., Mitchell, R. G., Neligan, G. A., and Parkin, J. M.: The definition of some external characteristics used in the assessment of gestational age in the newborn infant. Dev. Med. Child Neurol. *8*:507, 1966.

Goldie, L., and Hopkins, I. J.: Head turning towards diffuse light in the neurological examination of newborn infants. Brain *87*:665, 1964.

Hogan, G. R., and Milligan, J. E.: The plantar reflex of the newborn. N. Engl. J. Med. *285*:502, 1971.

Illingworth, R. S.: An introduction to developmental assessment in the first year. Little Club Clinics in Developmental Medicine No. 3, 1962.

Kellaway, P.: Electroencephalographic characteristics of the newly born. *In* Kay, J. K. (Ed.): Physical Diagnosis of the Newly Born. Forty-sixth Ross Conference on Pediatric Research, Columbus, Ohio, 1964, p. 86.

Moosa, A., and Dubowitz, V.: Assessment of gestational age in newborn infants: Nerve conduction velocity versus maturity score. Dev. Med. Child Neurol. *14*:290, 1972.

Otila, E.: Studies on the cerebrospinal fluid in premature infants. Acta Paediat. (Suppl. 35)*8*:1–100, 1948.

Parmelee, A. H., Jr.: A critical evaluation of the Moro reflex. Pediatrics *33*:773, 1964.

Parmelee, A. H., Jr.: The hand-mouth reflex of Babkin in premature infants. Pediatrics *31*:734, 1963.

Popich, G. A., and Smith, D. W.: Fontanels: Range of normal size. J. Pediatr. *80*:749, 1972.

Robinson, R.: Cerebral function in the newborn. Dev. Med. Child Neurol. 8:561, 1966.

Robinson, R. J.: Assessment of gestational age by neurological examination. Arch. Dis. Child. *41*:437, 1966.

Rose, A. L., and Lombroso, C. T.: Neonatal seizure states. A study of clinical, pathological, and electroencephalographic features in 137 full-term babies with a long-term follow-up. Pediatrics *45*:404, 1970.

Rosen, M. G., and Satran, R.: The neonatal electroencephalogram. Am. J. Dis. Child. *111*:133, 1966.

Saint-Anne Dargassies, S.: La maturation neurologique du prématuré. Etud. Neonatal. *4*:71, 1955.

Saint-Anne Dargassies, S.: Neurodevelopmental symptoms during the first year of life. Dev. Med. Child Neurol. *14*:235, 1972.

Sarff, L. D., Platt, L. H., and McCracken, G. H., Jr.: Cerebrospinal fluid evaluation in neonates. Comparison of high risk infants with and without meningitis. J. Pediatr. 88:473, 1976.

Schulte, F. J., Michaelis, R., Linke, I., and Nolte, R.: Motor nerve conduction velocity in term, preterm, and small-for-dates newborn infants. Pediatrics 42:17, 1968.

Shaywitz, B. A.: Epidermoid spinal cord tumors and previous lumbar punctures. J. Pediatr. 80:638, 1972.

Stempfel, R., and Zetterström, R.: Concentration of bilirubin in cerebrospinal fluid in hemolytic disease of the newborn. Pediatrics 16:184–193, 1955.

Tan, K. L.: The third fontanelle. Acta Paediat. Scand. 60:329, 1971.

# PERINATAL TRAUMA TO THE HEAD AND TO CRANIAL AND PERIPHERAL NERVES

# 78

*By William E. Bell*

## MOLDING OF THE HEAD

The fetal head is occasionally asymmetrically shaped as a result of unusual pressures upon it while still within the uterus as well as by the pressures sustained during delivery.

Parmelee, in 1931, reported upon molding of the face and head caused by the bizarre positions the fetus may assume within the uterus. He maintained that distorted faces are not infrequently encountered at birth, in which the lower jaw is asymmetrical, one side is straightened out or concave and the opposite side is normally convex. A rounded depression is often seen under the angle of the jaw on the flattened side extending backward to the mastoid region. There may be mild or severe malocclusion. He believed that the deformity arose from the fetal position; that is, extreme flexion of the neck plus rotation of the head to one side so that the shoulder pressed constantly upon the jaw of that side (Fig. 78–1). Commonly there is no disability, and the deformity disappears within a few months. Parmelee did include one case in which facial palsy seemed to stem from pressure upon the facial nerve in the region of the stylomastoid process.

Parmelee mentioned having seen a uterine fibroid cause a similar depression of the fetal face and skull. Barr described another in which cesarean section had to be performed because the head failed to descend after two hours of labor. The infant's head lay pillowed upon a large fibroid. A deep depression deformed almost the entire left side of the skull. X-ray study showed no fracture. The skull regained its normal shape within a few weeks, but by the end of the first year the infant was observed to be severely retarded.

When the head is large, the outlet rigid and labor prolonged, a situation often pertaining in primiparity, the newborn infant's head may appear misshapen immediately after birth. The sutures override one another, the fontanels are tiny or obliterated and the soft tissues overlying the skull may be soft and boggy because of caput succedaneum. Very severe molding of the

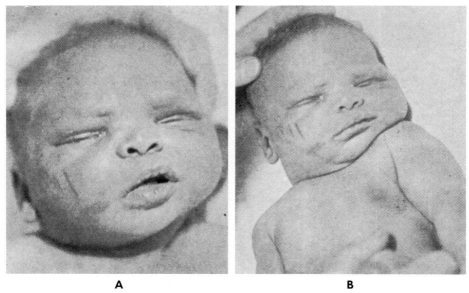

**A**                                                                          **B**

*Figure 78–1.* *A*, Asymmetry of the jaws; deep impression of the shoulder under and anterior to the left ear and a concavity of the mandible to the left of the chin. The infant was the mother's twenty-third. *B*, Reproduction of probable intrauterine posture. (Parmelee, A. H.: Am. J. Dis. Child. *42*:1155, 1931.)

head is tolerated by most infants, but in some it is associated with laceration of intracranial venous structures, giving rise to subdural hematomas.

In caput, the hemorrhage and edema are situated beneath the aponeurosis, external to the periosteum (Fig. 78–2). In rare instances, so much blood is sequestered in this location that anemia develops, possibly of sufficient severity that life is endangered. Pachman has reported such a case (Fig. 78–2*C*) and Van der Horst has described 10 cases of severe exsanguinating cephalhematoma which he encountered among African children. Nine of these were of the subaponeurotic variety, one subperiosteal. Kozinn et al. reported three cases, pointing out that massive scalp hemorrhage may indicate an underlying coagulation defect such as hemophilia or hemorrhagic disease of the newborn.

## CEPHALHEMATOMA

Cephalhematoma is best known as a usually benign traumatic subperiosteal hemorrhage in the parietal region of the newborn infant. An identical lesion, how-

ever, can occur in the older infant or child following head trauma. In the neonate, it is not invariably inconsequential and on rare occasions can be the source of significant problems. Some authors restrict the term cephalhematoma to subperiosteal hemorrhages while others include subperiosteal bleeding as well as the less frequent subgaleal, or subaponeurotic, neonatal scalp hemorrhages. The former, which are restricted in their location by suture lines they cannot extend across, are rarely associated with sufficient blood loss to be life-threatening. In contrast, subgaleal hemorrhage in the neonate is unlimited by suture lines and can involve the entire scalp bilaterally and extend into the soft tissues of the neck and face, producing marked swelling of the forehead and closure of the eyelids. Extensive blood loss in such cases usually, but not always, represents a complication of some form of coagulation defect, such as vitamin K deficiency hemorrhagic disease of the newborn (Robinson and Rossiter).

The most important factors associated with the occurrence of subperiosteal cephalhematomas in the newborn infant include forceps delivery, primiparity and large size of the infant. Vaginal delivery is

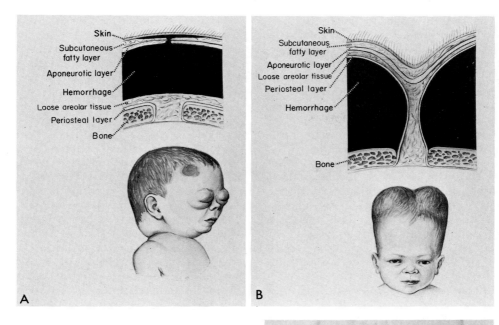

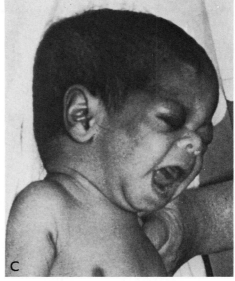

*Figure 78–2.* *A*, Location of edema and hemorrhage in caput succedaneum. *B*, Location of hemorrhage in cephalhematoma. *C*, Patient with massive hemorrhagic caput succedaneum, whose hemoglobin level fell to 2.2 gm per 100 ml by the age of 48 hours. (Reprinted with the permission of Daniel J. Pachman, M.D., of the University of Illinois Pediatric Department. The photograph, but not the diagrammatic sketches, appeared in Pediatrics, 29:907, 1962.)

not necessarily a prerequisite for the occurrence of this lesion, however, since cephalhematomas have been observed in infants born by cesarean section. The incidence of neonatal cephalhematoma has varied somewhat in different studies but most have found it to occur in 1.5 to 2.5 per cent of births (Zelson et al., Kendall and Woloshin). The great majority are parietal in location and, as noted above, are confined to the parietal region on the affected side by the periosteal attachment at the suture line. Approximately 15 per cent are bilateral and are often asymmetrical in size. Rarely, a cephalhematoma is found in the occipital region in midline location, where it can easily be confused with an encephalocele until spontaneous resolution begins. Linear skull fracture underlying a parietal cephalhematoma is found in some cases but is probably less common currently than is generally believed. In 1952, Kendall and Woloshin reported the presence of underlying fractures in 25 per cent of a series of 69 cephalhematomas. More recently, Zelson et al. found fractures in only 5.4 per cent of 111 infants with cephalhematomas and postulated that the reduced incidence reflected the much less common use of forceps for delivery in the past decade.

The cephalhematoma in the newborn appears in the form of a firm, localized mass which does not transilluminate. Within a few days after birth, change in the consistency of the clotted blood gives rise to a sharp, palpable ridge or crater edge near the periphery that can be confused with fracture by the inexperienced examiner. Depending on the size of the lesion, a cephalhematoma is usually gradually absorbed over periods of from 2 to 8 weeks.

**COMPLICATIONS.** In many patients, roentgenographic examination will reveal hyperostosis of the outer table of the skull which persists for several months after clinical evidence of the lesion has disappeared. Much less often there is persistent thickening of the parietal calvarium at the site of the original lesion, at times with widening of the diploic space, or cystic defects in the region. In some cases, calcium deposition within the clot occurs in a surprisingly short period of time and can be visualized roentgenographically.

Cephalhematomas of large volume can be associated with anemia or, more often, hyperbilirubinemia, as a consequence of absorption of the blood products (Kozinn et al.). An infrequent but dangerous complication is abscess formation within a cephalhematoma in a septic newborn infant or secondary to contamination during attempted needle aspiration of the lesion (Burry and Hellerstein, Lee and Berg). The increasing use of fetal scalp monitoring during labor and delivery might also conceivably predispose to the occurrence of infection by contiguous spread to a cephalhematoma. Suppuration within a cephalhematoma may be associated with obvious signs of localized infection or can remain surprisingly silent during progression of the lesion. It should be suspected whenever there is rapid enlargement of the mass several days after birth, the development of cutaneous erythema over the lesion or otherwise unexplained fever and leukocytosis. An infected cephalhematoma may be complicated by osteomyelitis of the underlying skull or by meningitis, either associated with sepsis or secondary to intracranial extension through an adjacent skull fracture or a cranial suture (Levy et al., Ellis et al.). Diagnosis is established by needle aspiration whenever an infected cephalhematoma is suspected.

**TREATMENT.** Management of a cephalhematoma in the newborn infant is fundamentally conservative but should include the obtaining of skull films to determine the presence or absence of an underlying fracture, and periodic checks of the hemoglobin and serum bilirubin, the latter if the child becomes jaundiced. Needle aspiration of the uncomplicated cephalhematoma is not indicated, since spontaneous resolution is expected and because of the hazard of bacterial contamination by needle penetration. Underlying skull fractures do not create a management problem and need no specific therapy unless there is significant depression of bone fragments.

The primary indication for aspiration is clinical evidence of suppuration within the cephalhematoma. If purulent material is found by aspiration, serious consideration should be given to more complete drainage by surgical incision. The identification of infection in the lesion warrants blood culture and spinal fluid examination, in addition to the appropriate antibiotic regimen depending on the most likely causative organism.

# SKULL FRACTURES IN THE NEWBORN INFANT

The skull of the infant at birth is less mineralized than it is later in childhood and also is more pliable because of the patency of the cranial sutures. For these reasons, there can be considerable distortion of the infant's head shape in utero and during the birth process without injury to the skull itself. Fractures can occur, however, and may be acquired in utero, during labor or secondary to the application of forceps.

Intrauterine fracture of the infant's skull is usually the result of compression of the skull against the promontory of the sacrum (Alexander and Davis) and can complicate a traumatic event to the mother's abdomen or pelvis, or can occur secondary to the forces of uterine contraction.

Most skull fractures identified in the neonate are parietal or frontal in location and linear in type (Chasler). Some are associated with an overlying cephalhematoma. Simple linear fractures appear on x-ray as lines of decreased density and may be seen only in one view. Such nondisplaced fractures are considered to be benign lesions that are expected to heal spontaneously and need no therapeutic measures. Depressed skull fractures in the newborn infant can occur in the conventional form in which there is a complete disruption of the bony margin at the fracture site with inward displacement of some portion of the bone. A more characteristic depressed skull injury acquired in utero or during the process of labor is inward buckling of one parietal bone, much like an indentation of a ping-pong ball (Fig. 78–3). A break in the continuity of the bone may not be present or may be evident over only a

short length at the margin of the depression. This form of depressed skull injury is best seen in the anteroposterior or posteroanterior views of the skull and sometimes is not apparent at all on the lateral skull views. Depressed skull fractures acquired before or during the birth process are usually considered to be lesions that should be corrected. Non-surgical methods of elevation of depressed fractures have been successful in some cases (Raynor and Parsa, Schrager) but operative correction is required for most.

## FACIAL NERVE PARALYSIS

The seventh cranial nerve is a mixed nerve whose motor branches supply the muscles of facial expression with the exception of the levator palpebrae superioris. In addition, the motor fibers of the facial nerve innervate the platysma, stapedius, posterior belly of the digastricus and the stylohyoid muscles. The motor nucleus of the facial nerve is located in the tegmentum of the pons. That part of the facial nucleus sending fibers to the lower part of the face receives its supranuclear innerva-

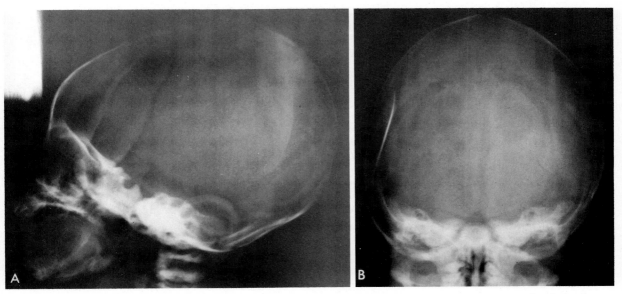

*Figure 78–3.* *A* and *B*. Lateral and AP skull x-rays of 1-day-old infant. Depressed skull injury is visualized clearly on the AP view as a linear streak of increased density. Such injuries are the result of inward buckling of the poorly mineralized skull of the newborn infant. The actual break in the continuity of the bone is present over a short distance only.

tion from the contralateral cerebral cortex, while the portion of the facial nucleus supplying the upper part of the facial musculature receives bilateral cortical innervation. As a result, facial palsy resulting from a lesion of the opposite cerebral hemisphere characteristically involves mainly the lower two thirds of the face, with relative sparing of the eyelid and forehead. Injury to the motor nucleus or the facial nerve itself more likely will cause variable degrees of weakness of all portions of the muscles of facial expression on the ipsilateral side. Facial palsy caused by a supranuclear lesion is referred to as a central facial palsy, while that secondary to damage of the nucleus or the facial nerve is called peripheral facial paresis or paralysis.

Congenital facial palsy is usually unilateral and is of the peripheral type in the majority of cases. Central facial weakness due to an acute lesion of the opposite cerebral hemisphere is infrequently seen in the newborn infant and is usually accompanied by a motor deficit of the arm or leg on the same side of the body. The incidence of congenital facial paralysis is not clearly established and has been reported to be between 0.25 per cent and 6.4 per cent (McHugh et al., Hepner) of live births. It is generally believed that unilateral facial weakness noted at birth is the result of compression of the facial nerve, although the precise site of injury and time of occurrence have been a subject of debate. Trauma to the nerve distal to its emergence from the stylomastoid foramen by forceps application has been regarded as one important cause, but Hepner found the incidence of facial palsy to be the same in infants born with and without the use of forceps. He assumed that pressure on the maternal sacrum during labor was responsible for most cases of unilateral facial paralysis in the newborn infant. Parmelee proposed that some cases were the result of intrauterine posture of the fetal head in which marked flexion and rotation of the head resulted in compression of the mandible and lateral neck against the shoulder with associated compression of the peripheral portion of the facial nerve. Involvement of the seventh nerve as it traverses the facial canal within the mastoid is proba-

bly unusual but has been reported (McHugh). The term Bell's palsy, or idiopathic facial palsy, is not applicable to the congenital form of peripheral facial paralysis, although Bell's palsy has been noted in infants as young as 4 to 8 weeks of age (McLellan and Parrino, Fishbein et al.).

Unilateral, congenital facial weakness is most obvious when the infant cries, at which time there is lack of complete eyelid closure along with lack of normal lower facial muscle contraction on the paretic side. Experience with electrodiagnostic tests is limited in infants with congenital facial paresis as compared to older children and adults with acquired facial nerve deficits. The facial nerve excitability test in some instances can, however, distinguish complete from partial denervation, thus providing some possible prognostic information (McHugh et al.). The percentage of infants who recover is unknown. The general belief is that the prognosis for recovery in infants with congenital facial palsy secondary to facial nerve compression is favorable, although some are left with permanent deficits. Treatment is conservative, since spontaneous improvement is expected in most. Were it known that the site of compression of the facial nerve was within its bony canal and should improvement not occur within the first weeks after birth, surgical decompression with the aid of the operating microscope would be a consideration (McHugh).

## CONGENITAL HYPOPLASIA OF THE DEPRESSOR ANGULI ORIS MUSCLE

In recent years, there has been recognition of a syndrome with localized facial weakness in which the lower lip on one side fails to be depressed on crying, resulting in an "asymmetric crying facies" (Nelson and Eng, Papadatos et al.). It is now believed that this localized muscle deficit is the result of congenital hypoplasia of the depressor anguli oris muscle, whose normal function is to draw the lower corner of the lip downward and evert it. The resulting facial symmetry when the child cries is often misinterpreted by the parents, who may assume the normal side of the face is the abnormal one because they observe the lower lip on the intact side to be pulled down. The abnormal side is, in fact, the side on which the lower lip remains unaltered in position when crying occurs. The cosmetic significance of this minor anomaly lessens as the child gets older, probably largely because the older child is engaged in crying far less than in infancy.

Localized facial paresis causing an asymmetric crying facies can occur in isolated fashion; however, observations have revealed a variable association with other anomalies. Of 44 infants with this syndrome, Pape and Pickering found 27 to have major anomalies of the skeletal, genitourinary, respiratory or cardiovascular systems. A much lower incidence of associated defects was reported by Perlman and Reisner, who found two patients with significant anomalies out of 41 with the localized facial defect. The disorder most strongly associated with this facial defect is congenital cardiac disease, an observation made by Cayler in 1967. The most commonly associated cardiac defect has been ventricular septal defect, but other cardiac lesions have also been described. The term "cardiofacial syndrome" has been applied to such cases.

### BILATERAL CONGENITAL FACIAL PARALYSIS

Bilateral, nontraumatic, congenital facial paralysis without other cranial nerve defects is exceedingly rare. Considerable feeding difficulties in infancy result, and the related poor sucking ability leads to slow weight gain. The infant's face is expressionless, and the eyes do not close when crying. Little is known regarding the site of the pathology in such cases but agenesis of the seventh nerve nuclei in the pons has been postulated (Bonar and Owens). A similar facial appearance is seen in the newborn infant who manifests myotonic dystrophy, although here the apparent facial diplegia is a muscular disorder rather than one caused by dysfunction of the seventh nerves or their nuclei. The infant with facial weakness associated with myotonic dystrophy can be recognized because of the commonly associated findings such as diffuse decrease in muscle tone, foot deformities and presence of the disease in its

more characteristic form in one parent, usually the mother.

A more widely recognized form of congenital facial diplegia is that associated with bilateral abducens paralysis, known as the Mobius syndrome. Other defects can also occur in the child with Mobius syndrome, including other lower cranial nerve deficits, hypoplasia of the pectoralis muscles, talipes varus or equinovarus foot deformity, or mental retardation. Congenital paralysis of the sixth and seventh cranial nerves in these cases is usually attributed to aplasia of the corresponding cranial nerve nuclei, although some have a supranuclear origin or can be secondary to primary hypoplasia of the involved musculature.

### BRACHIAL PLEXUS PALSY

Traction, stretch or avulsion injuries during birth to part or all of the brachial plexus are potentially serious from the functional standpoint. In most instances, the injury and resulting limb weakness is unilateral, with the right arm being affected approximately twice as often as the left. Rarely, the disorder is bilateral giving rise to serious disabilities if recovery does not occur. The incidence of this type of birth injury has not been well documented but it is generally agreed that it has decreased considerably in recent decades with improved obstetrical techniques. In one series extending from 1932 to 1962, brachial plexus palsy was found in 0.38 per 1000 live births (Adler et al.).

**ETIOLOGY.** The two factors most consistently associated with birth injury to the brachial plexus are excessive weight of the child and complications of the labor and delivery process. Prolonged and difficult labor accompanied by heavy sedation of the mother resulting in a relaxed, large infant represent a combination of factors which increase the vulnerability of the child to this lesion. Breech delivery occurred in 9 per cent of the series of 123 patients described by Adler and colleagues, thus being a less important factor than the size of the infant.

**CLINICAL FEATURES.** Trauma to the brachial plexus during the delivery process occurs with variable degrees of severity. Involvement predominantly of the fifth and sixth cervical rootlets is referred to as Erb-Duchenne palsy, while injury mainly to the seventh and eighth cervical and first thoracic rootlets is termed Klumpke's paralysis. In other cases, virtually all the nerve rootlets of the brachial plexus are affected, resulting in a total brachial plexus paralysis (Fig. 78–4).

Stretch injury at the upper portion of the brachial plexus during birth is the most common form of this disorder, in which there is weakness or paralysis of the deltoid, serratus anterior, biceps, teres major, brachioradialis and supinator muscles. Weakness of these muscles, which are innervated by the fifth and sixth cervical roots, results in the characteristic clinical picture in which the affected arm is in a position of tight adduction and internal rotation at the shoulder, in addition to extension and pronation at the elbow. Added involvement of the seventh cervical root causes weakness of the extensors of the wrist and fingers leading to a flexion deformity of the hand due to sustained contraction of the flexor muscles supplied by the median nerve. Denervation of the serratus anterior, rhomboids and other periscapular muscles adds to the motor disability around the shoulder and produces winging of the scapula. Infrequently, the rootlets forming the phrenic nerve are also involved, in which case, the diaphragm is elevated and is relatively immobile.

Klumpke's paralysis, or birth injury to the lower brachial plexus, is much less common than the above and is characterized by weakness of the flexors and extensors of the wrist and of the intrinsic hand musculature. Horner's syndrome on the same side coexists in some cases, owing to damage of the first thoracic rootlet. In other cases, all rootlets composing the brachial plexus are affected, giving rise to a flaccid, functionless limb at birth when the injury is severe. Still others reveal evidence of involvement of all or most of the rootlets of the brachial plexus in the days immediately after birth but soon demonstrate recovery of hand function, leaving a pattern compatible with Erb-Duchenne upper brachial plexus palsy.

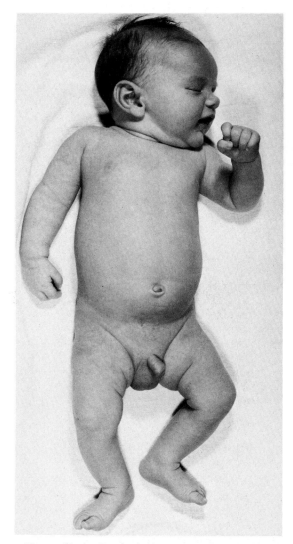

*Figure 78–4.* Brachial plexus stretch paralysis affecting the right arm. Child was the result of a difficult vertex delivery, birth weight was 4350 grams. In addition to the paresis of the right arm, he had Horner's syndrome on the right side. The right arm is virtually immobile and is held in a position of adduction and partial internal rotation.

In addition to the characteristic posture assumed by the denervated arm, the muscle weakness can be demonstrated by the asymmetrical response provoked by eliciting the Moro reflex and by the lack of limb movement when the infant is made to cry. Sensory deficits are most likely present in the distribution corresponding to the affected cervical roots but are usually difficult to demonstrate when the plexus is only partially injured. Clavicular fractures, fractures of the proximal portion of the humerus and dislocation of the shoulder (Babbit and Cassidy) are the orthopedic complications sometimes observed in the neonate or young infant with a brachial plexus palsy. It is also important to remember that abnormalities of labor and delivery that predispose to brachial plexus birth trauma can be associated with cerebral or spinal cord injuries, in which case recognition in the neonatal period is rendered more difficult.

**PROGNOSIS.** Probability of recovery is difficult to predict in the immediate newborn period, although the child with a partial plexus lesion who shows definite improvement of motor function by 1 to 2 weeks after birth will probably recover completely or with only minor deficits. When no improvement has occurred by 6 months of age, the likelihood of a permanent and significant deficit is high. The limb permanently denervated from birth is weak or paralyzed and does not grow in a normal fashion as the child ages. Skeletal growth is affected as well as other soft tissues, with the final result being an arm that is abnormally small in circumference and strikingly short in length. The infant with Horner's syndrome at birth caused by a lower plexus lesion may later in childhood exhibit heterochromia iridis, with the lighter colored iris being on the side with ptosis and miosis.

Among 20 infants followed for 6 months by Eng, six had recovered with minimal deficits, 11 showed fair recovery but with persistence of some degree of motor disability, and three retained severe abnormalities.

**MANAGEMENT.** Treatment should be started early to prevent joint contractures but is best delayed for 7 to 10 days after birth because one may assume that edema of the damaged rootlets is present immediately after birth. X-rays of the chest and of the shoulder joint and proximal humerus are obtained to exclude fractures and diaphragm paralysis. The parents are instructed in the method to perform gentle passive movement of the shoulder, elbow, wrist and small joints of the hand. When appropriate, supportive splints can be designed to maintain the wrist, thumb and fingers in proper alignment. The "Statue-of-Liberty" splint used in past years is no longer advised because it enhances contracture about the shoulder and can predispose to shoulder joint damage. Reconstructive orthopedic surgery is indicated in certain instances to improve function of the permanently affected arm and hand, but is not usually performed until 4 years of age or later.

## SCIATIC NERVE PALSY

The sciatic nerve is ordinarily not susceptible to birth injury; however, it can be damaged in the infant by injection of materials or drugs into the umbilical artery or by misplaced gluteal injections. Injuries to the sciatic nerve can result in either temporary or permanent deficits, and may be of variable degrees of severity. In some cases, weakness of dorsiflexion of the foot along with sensory loss on the dorsal surface of the foot are the only obvious deficits. More severe injuries are associated with extensive weakness and eventual atrophy of all muscle groups below the knee, in addition to weakness of the hamstring muscles on the affected side.

Ischemic sciatic neuropathy in the infant has been described following injections into the umbilical artery (Mills, San Agustin et al.) and secondary to accidental intra-arterial injection of drugs administered to the region of the buttocks (Knowles). Sciatic nerve involvement in such cases has been attributed to spasm or occlusion of the inferior gluteal artery. Motor and sensory deficits corresponding to the innervation supplied by the sciatic nerve are accompanied by signs of vascular insufficiency in the region of the buttocks and throughout the affected lower limb. Improvement usually follows the insult but permanent sequelae, including weakness and atrophy, are not uncommon.

Direct trauma to the sciatic nerve can result from misplaced gluteal injections of antibiotics or other substances (Gilles and Matson, Scheinberg and Allensworth,

Combes et al.). The young infant, and especially the premature one, is particularly susceptible to this type of nerve injury, mainly because of the much smaller size of the gluteal musculature. Early recognition of this complication of intramuscular injection is important to allow physical therapy and other measures to minimize joint contractures. Gilles and Matson advise surgical resection of the damaged nerve segment if clinical improvement does not occur within 6 months following the injury.

## REFERENCES

Alder, J. B., and Patterson, R. L., Jr.: Erb's palsy. Long-term results of treatment in eighty-eight cases. J. Bone Jt. Surg. 49-A:1052, 1967.

Alexander, E., Jr., and Davis, C. H., Jr.: Intra-uterine fracture of the infant's skull. J. Neurosurg. 30:446, 1969.

Babbitt, D. P., and Cassidy, R. H.: Obstetrical paralysis and dislocation of the shoulder in infancy. J. Bone Jt. Surg. 50-A:1447, 1968.

Barr, S. J.: Unusual pressure effect of a fibroid. J. Obstet. Gynaec. Brit. Emp. 59:529, 1952.

Bonar, B. E., and Owens, R. W.: Bilateral congenital facial paralysis. Am. J. Dis. Child. 38:1256, 1929.

Burry, V. F., and Hellerstein, S.: Septicemia and subperiosteal cephalhematomas. J. Pediatr. 69:1133, 1966.

Cayler, G. G.: An "epidemic" of congenital facial paresis and heart disease. Pediatrics 40:666, 1967.

Cayler, G. G.: Cardiofacial syndrome. Congenital heart disease and facial weakness, a hitherto unrecognized association. Arch. Dis. Child. 44:69, 1969.

Chasler, C. N.: The newborn skull. The diagnosis of fracture. Am. J. Roentgenol. 100:92, 1967.

Combes, M. A., Clark, W. K., Gregory, C. F., and James, J. A.: Sciatic nerve injury in infants. Recognition and prevention of impairment resulting from intragluteal injections. J.A.M.A. 173:1336, 1960.

Ellis, S. S., Montgomery, J. R., Wagner, M., and Hill, R. M.: Osteomyelitis complicating neonatal cephalhematoma. Am. J. Dis. Child. 127:100, 1974.

Eng, G. D.: Brachial plexus palsy in newborn infants. Pediatrics 48:18, 1971.

Fishbein, J. F., Shadravan, I., Hebert, L., and Funes, R.: Idiopathic Bell palsy in a 2-month-old child. Am. J. Dis. Child. 128:112, 1974.

Gilles, F. H., and Matson, D. D.: Sciatic nerve injury following misplaced gluteal injection. J. Pediatr. 76:247, 1970.

Hepner, W. R., Jr.: Some observations on facial paresis in the newborn infant: Etiology and incidence. Pediatrics 8:494, 1951.

Kendall, N., and Woloshin, H.: Cephalhematoma associated with fracture of the skull. J. Pediatr. 41:125, 1952.

Knowles, J. A.: Accidental intra-arterial injection of penicillin. Am. J. Dis. Child. 111:552, 1966.

Kozinn, P. J., Ritz, N. D., Moss, A. H., and Kaufman, A.: Masive hemorrhage — scalps of newborn infants. Am. J. Dis. Child. 108:413, 1964.

Lee, Y., and Berg, R. B.: Cephalhematoma infected with Bacteroides. Am. J. Dis. Child. 121:77, 1971.

Levy, H. L., O'Connor, J. F., and Ingall, D.: Bacteremia, infected cephalhematoma, and osteomyelitis of the skull in a newborn. Am. J. Dis. Child. 114:649, 1967.

McHugh, H. E.: Facial paralysis in birth injury and skull fractures. Arch. Otolaryngol. 78:443, 1963.

McHugh, H. E., Sowden, K. A., and Levitt, M. N.: Facial paralysis and muscle agenesis in the newborn. Arch. Otolaryngol. 89:131, 1969.

McLellan, M. S., and Parrino, C. S.: Bell's palsy at 1 month 4 days of age. Am. J. Dis. Child. 117:729, 1969.

Mills, W. G.: A new neonatal syndrome. Br. Med. J. 2:464, 1949.

Nelson, K. B., and Eng, G. C.: Congenital hypoplasia of the depressor anguli oris muscle: Differentiation from congenital facial palsy. J. Pediatr. 81:16, 1972.

Pachman, D. J.: Massive hemorrhage into the scalp of the newborn infant. Hemorrhagic caput succedaneum. Pediatrics 29:907, 1962.

Papadatos, C., Alexiou, D., Nicolopoulos, H., Mikropoulos, H., and Hadzigeorgiou, E.: Congenital hypoplasia of depressor anguli oris muscle. Arch. Dis. Child. 49:927, 1974.

Pape, K. E., and Pickering, D.: Asymmetric crying facies: An index of other congenital anomalies. J. Pediatr. 81:21, 1972.

Parmelee, A. H.: Molding due to intra-uterine posture. Facial paralysis probably due to such molding. Am. J. Dis. Child. 42:1155, 1931.

Perlman, M., and Reisner, S. H.: Asymmetric crying facies and congenital anomalies. Arch. Dis. Child. 48:627, 1973.

Raynor, R., and Parsa, M.: Nonsurgical elevation of depressed skull fracture in an infant. J. Pediatr. 72:262, 1968.

Robinson, R. J., and Rossiter, M. A.: Massive subaponeurotic hemorrhage in babies of African origin. Arch. Dis. Child. 43:684, 1968.

San Agustin, M., Nitowsky, H. M., and Borden, J. N.: Neonatal sciatic palsy after umbilical vessel injection. J. Pediatr. 60:408, 1962.

Scheinberg, L., and Allensworth, M.: Sciatic neuropathy in infants related to antibiotic injections. Pediatrics 19:261, 1957.

Schrager, G. O.: Elevation of depressed skull fracture with a breast pump. J. Pediatr. 77:300, 1970.

Van der Horst, R. L.: Exsanguinating cephalhematoma in African newborn infants. Arch. Dis. Child. 38:280, 1963.

Zelson, C., Lee, S. J., and Pearl, M.: The incidence of skull fractures underlying cephalhematomas in newborn infants. J. Pediatr. 85:371, 1974.

# PERINATAL INSULTS TO THE BRAIN AND SPINAL CORD

# 79

*By William E. Bell*

## INTRODUCTION

Transient or permanent cerebral dysfunction secondary to factors related to labor, delivery or the immediate neonatal period can occur under a wide variety of circumstances and has received many designations, such as birth injury, cerebral birth trauma, perinatal brain damage and perinatal cerebral hypoxia. No single term has been found to be adequately descriptive or etiologically correct, partly because of the multifactorial nature of the pathogenesis of many of the neurologic insults incurred at this critical time. While designations such as cerebral birth injury or birth trauma are reasonably acceptable, they can be erroneously equated with mechanical injury or trauma and assumed to be secondary to factors entirely controllable by the physician in charge of the labor and delivery. A descriptive phrase loosely used as an explanation to the child's parents can result in the leveling of unwarranted criticism of the attending obstetrician. It is not that mechanical injuries to the brain do not occur during the birth process, but that they are far outnumbered by disturbances due to fetal oxygenation, cerebral arterial perfusion and cerebral venous drainage. Most of the adverse events during labor that lead to fetal distress and cerebral dysfunction are secondary to impaired transplacental diffusion of oxygen from mother to fetus, whereas the most common neonatal disturbance that produces neurologic deficits is respiratory disease, especially hyaline membrane disease in the premature infant. Conversely, the great majority of perinatal insults to the spinal cord, cranial nerves or peripheral nerve rootlets are mechanical in origin.

The development of fetal distress, and thus the possibility of neurologic injury, often occurs without forewarning. Certain maternal conditions, however, predispose the infant to problems during labor and delivery and should be recognized as increased risk situations. Maternal diabetes or hypertension, infection of many types, blood group incompatibility, chronic renal disease, pre-eclampsia or eclampsia, prolonged rupture of membranes and the so-called placental insufficiency syndrome with prolonged gestation are all associated with an enhanced possibility of fetal distress.

Specific events during parturition that can lead to fetal distress and neurologic insults include dystocia due to cephalopelvic disproportion or abnormal fetal positions or presentations. Maternal hypoxia, hypotension, and pathologically increased intrauterine pressure associated with precipitous labor are additional conditions in which transplacental perfusion of the fetus may be jeopardized. Abruptio placentae and placenta previa increase fetal risk by a diminution of maternal-fetal exchange and acute fetal blood loss. Prolapse of the umbilical cord, especially in association with transverse or breech fetal positions, is a readily identifiable factor that may restrict fetal oxygenation, and intrauterine mechanical compression of the cord is a cause of an unknown number of cases of fetal distress. Knots in the cord or looping of the cord around the infant's neck are sometimes incriminated as events producing clinical distress but are generally believed to be rare causes. Abnormal insertion of the umbilical cord upon the placenta, such as velamentous insertion, can be complicated by mechanical compression leading to fetal asphyxia or laceration of vessels during labor producing severe fetal blood loss.

Drug-induced fetal or neonatal respiratory depression from inhalation anesthetics, barbiturates, narcotics or phenothiazines administered to the mother during labor has become less frequent with improved obstetrical techniques. Magnesium administered to the eclamptic mother for control of hypertension will cross the placenta to the fetus and can result in severe respiratory and neurologic depression (Lipsitz, Lipsitz and English). Caudal anesthesia of the mother in labor has also been followed by adverse fetal effects in cases of accidental injection of the local anesthetic into the fetal scalp or superior sagittal sinus (Sinclair et al.). The infant affected in this manner is limp at birth, with bradycardia and apnea, and with convulsions occurring soon after birth.

Respiratory disturbances, especially hyaline membrane disease in the premature infant, represent the most common of the numerous conditions in the immediate postnatal period that can compromise cerebral function. Pulmonary infections, congenital anomalies affecting ventilatory function and certain types of congenital cardiac disease can also result in neuropathologic changes in the neonate. Important metabolic aberrations that contribute to structural and functional deficits of the brain with the above disorders include hypoglycemia and hyperviscosity (Gross et al., Wood).

## NEUROPATHOLOGIC PATTERNS

Developmental and maturational changes of the brain are reflected by differences in the neuropathology of anoxic-ischemic insults at different stages. As a result, the topographic and microscopic cerebral abnormalities produced by such injuries are different in the premature than they are in the full term infant, and in both as compared to anoxic-ischemic lesions acquired by the adult. While there has been and continues to be debate and dispute about the pathogenesis of certain types of perinatal insults to the brain, the accumulated information now allows a certain degree of interpretation of the relationship of birth weight, type of injury and localization of pathology to the clinical and neuropathologic pattern of the various types of "cerebral palsy" as seen in the older child. Recognizing that different forms of injury to the nervous system can occur together and

that a certain degree of overlap is to be expected, the perinatal and early postnatal neurologic insults can be categorized into four patterns (Towbin). The first is cerebral periventricular damage, predominantly infarctional in type, with or without periventricular or intraventricular hemorrhage. This is the pattern characteristically seen in the premature child asphyxiated during parturition or in the neonatal period. Hemorrhage may be mild or localized, or extend massively into the lateral ventricles. Bleeding is explained by the structurally immature characteristics of the periventricular germinal matrix, damaged by infarction and hypoxia, and does not have as its origin mechanical trauma. Survivors with neurologic sequelae are usually classified as having the cerebral diplegic type of cerebral palsy with spastic defects that affect the lower extremities more than the upper but without significant dyskinesis.

The second form of perinatal cerebral insult is gray matter hypoxic-ischemic damage, which is observed in the term infant and which affects the actively proliferating cerebral cortex and certain subcortical nuclear areas, such as the thalamus and the basal ganglia. Hemorrhagic lesions in the involved regions are much less characteristic in the term infant than in the premature child. These perinatal gray matter injuries are the forerunners of the chronic lesions of the older child termed ulegyria, or atrophic cortical sclerosis, and status marmoratus, which refers to hypermyelination in areas with neuronal depletion. The clinical correlates in those with persisting neurologic deficits include the athetoid or dystonic types of cerebral palsy, with variable grades of spasticity, and often with seizures and mental retardation.

The third type of perinatal injury is spinal cord damage, sometimes associated with brain stem involvement. This insult is primarily mechanical and is clearly associated with longitudinal traction during breech extraction, or, less commonly, with rotational forces during a difficult vertex delivery. The fourth pattern of perinatally acquired neurologic disease is also the result of mechanical trauma, and is especially related to mechanisms of labor which result in excessive molding and distortion of the fetal head, giving rise to bleeding into the subdural spaces. Supratentorial subdural hematomas usually result from stretch injuries of venous channels extending from the cortical surface to the major dural sinuses, while posterior fossa subdural bleeding is more likely to have as its origin tentorial tears. Subdural hemorrhage in either location giving rise to clinical neurologic signs in the neonatal period is not common but is important because of the availability of treatment.

# PERINATAL ASPHYXIA

The term asphyxia refers to a condition in which there is hypoxia associated with carbon dioxide retention. When such conditions prevail during parturition or in the newborn period, oxygen deficit and increased carbon dioxide tension are usually compounded by acidosis, systemic hypotension or shock, and sometimes other derangements such as hypoglycemia, consumption coagulopathy or blood loss. Hypoxia and carbon dioxide retention provoke cerebral vasodilatation and edema, while cerebral perfusion may be reduced by diminished myocardial contractility secondary to hypoxia and acidosis. Thus, the pathogenesis of the neuropathologic alterations of this group of disorders which occur during or just after the birth process are complex and multifactorial in many instances. Observations in humans have shown that the type of cerebral pathology secondary to asphyxiating insults differs in premature infants from term born infants, while experiments with monkeys have revealed that the degree of pathologic alterations is related to the severity and duration of the anoxic-ischemic insult (Windle). In the premature child whose cerebral damage is a result of uteroplacental dysfunction during the birth process, or ventilatory insufficiency after birth, the predominant lesions are located in the periventricular germinal matrix, with or without hemorrhage in the area or extending into the lateral ventricles (Banker). In the full-term child, lesions are more striking in the cortical and deep nuclear gray matter, and in the subcortical white matter.

## PERIVENTRICULAR LEUKOMALACIA AND INTRAVENTRICULAR HEMORRHAGE

Periventricular damage, often with hemorrhage, has long been recognized to be the characteristic type of asphyxia-induced pathologic change in the premature child. The explanation for these lesions has been a topic of wide debate, with some investigators assuming an anoxic origin, others favoring their origin on the basis of thrombosis of the vein of Galen (Schwartz) and still others postulating arterial ischemia and ischemic infarction as the primary underlying cause.

The designation of periventricular leukomalacia was applied in 1962 by Banker and Larroche and served as the impetus for continued study of the process. The majority of infants affected with this condition are of low birth weight and have sustained episodes of anoxia, usually with bradycardia, apnea or cardiac arrest requiring resuscitation. The pathologic characteristics of periventricular leukomalacia on gross observation include foci of white matter necrosis, bilaterally present but not always symmetrical, located in the corona radiata just anterior to the lateral ventricles (Fig. 79–1). Microscopically, the early lesions are those of areas of coagulation necrosis with loss of normal architecture and homogeneity of the tissue. At the margins of the zones of necrosis, injury to axons produces so-called retraction balls, a histologic reaction demonstrable with silver stains.

In some cases complicated by hyperbilirubinemia in the early postnatal period, the zones of periventricular necrosis are stained with bilirubin, which can be seen grossly. Hemorrhages in the areas of periventricular necrosis vary from microscopic perivascular collections of blood to massive extravasions of blood into the white matter bilaterally and extending into the lateral ventricles.

Although the pathogenesis of periventricular leukomalacia and associated hemorrhagic lesions in the premature child remains speculative, the prominent infarctional characteristic of the lesions would seem most compatible with a disturbance of arterial supply to the affected regions (Banker and Larroche, Armstrong and Norman). The periventricular sub-

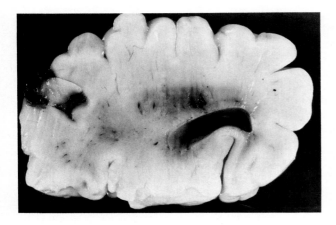

*Figure 79–1.* Periventricular leukomalacia. Prematurely born child with perinatal asphyxia. There is hemorrhagic softening of the cerebral white matter adjacent to the lateral ventricle.

ependymal germinal matrix is a region of special vulnerability to certain insults during fetal life or in the immediate postnatal period of the prematurely born child. In early fetal life, it represents the site of origin of primitive cellular elements which eventually migrate to establish the laminated cerebral cortex. As depletion of the subependymal cell population occurs with advancing fetal age, the germinal matrix remains as a highly vascularized region, notable for numerous thin-walled, delicate veins, which drain into the deep galenic venous system. The arterial supply to this region has been shown by DeReuck to be from ventriculopedal branches of deep penetrating arteries and ventriculofugal branches of the choroidal arteries. The region of periventricular tissue between these two arterial systems represent end zones, or so-called "water-shed" areas, located a few millimeters from the ventricular wall. This border zone has been considered an area of least resistance from the standpoint of arterial supply. The most plausible explanation for periventricular leukomalacia is that the infarctional lesions are the result of localized failure of arterial perfusion of this vulnerable region (Armstrong and Norman, DeReuck et al.).

A common accompaniment of deep white matter lesions in the asphyxiated newborn premature infant is a variable degree of hemorrhage, either within the involved parenchymal regions or extending into the lateral ventricular system (Cole et al., Ross et al., Fedrick and Butler). Bleeding in this situation is not traumatic but most likely is initiated in the infarcted subependymal region once circulation is restored (Fig. 79–2). Factors related to the origin of bleeding probably include the thin-walled character of the subependymal matrix terminal veins, hypoxic-ischemic injury to the venous walls and increased venous pressure secondary to the effects of hypoxia and acidosis on the heart. When hemorrhage is extensive, it ruptures through the necrotic ependyma and can totally occupy both lateral ventricles. Thrombocytopenia or consumption coagulopathy have been regarded as contributing factors by some authors but are probably not primary precipitating causes (Armstrong and Norman,

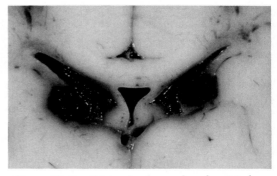

*Figure 79–2.* Bilateral subependymal matrix hemorrhage in a premature newborn infant. There is extensive intraventricular spread of bleeding in addition to periventricular leukomalacia in the form of hemorrhagic softening extending out from the angles of the lateral ventricles.

Chessells and Wigglesworth, Anderson et al.).

**CLINICAL ASPECTS.** The degree of functional abnormality of the newborn infant secondary to asphyxia incurred during the labor and delivery process naturally depends on the severity of the insult and the period of time it lasts. Fetal distress during parturition is assumed by the presence of bradycardia or tachycardia, or by the presence of meconium-contaminated amniotic fluid. The recent development of more sophisticated methods of fetal monitoring has added further dimensions to our ability to assess the fetal state during labor. After birth, the infant subjected to perinatal hypoxia but without mechanical injury can be expected to show certain alterations of muscle tone and alertness that are different with increasing degrees of oxygen deprivation (Brown et al.). The very mildly affected infant may have essentially normal muscle tone but be "jittery" with tactile stimulation and exhibit irritability and some degree of feeding difficulty. Seizures are not common in this group but can occur. A greater hypoxic insult gives rise to more definite signs, which include irritability, vomiting, increased muscle tone, excessive clonus and a high pitched, poorly sustained cry. Tremulousness, especially that provoked by abrupt change of limb position or tactile stimulation, can closely resemble clonic seizural activity and is frequently confused with it. The severely asphyxiated newborn infant is markedly hypotonic to flaccid, exhibits little spontaneous limb movement and frequently has recurrent seizures. Such a child does not cry on painful stimulation and has minimal, if any, Moro or grasp reactions, and absent sucking and swallowing responses. The respiratory pattern is likely to be irregular, sometimes complicated by apneic episodes with bradycardia. Apnea can also sometimes be triggered by handling the child. The pupils are more often pin-point than dilated, and blink response to light is absent. In addition to convulsions, the clinical course of the child with an insult of this magnitude can be complicated by hypothermia, aspiration pneumonia, hypoglycemia, hypocalcemia, hypermagnesemia (Engel and Elin) and hyponatremia secondary to inappropriate antidiuretic hormone secretion (Feldman et al.). The type of neurologic signs recorded in the newborn period are of some predictive value in that complete recovery is expected in the mildly affected child whereas death or lasting sequelae is customary in the severely damaged infant who is flaccid and comatose, and who has repeated convulsions for several days after birth. In those falling between those two grades of severity, predictions are best deferred until the passage of time clarifies the outcome.

The premature infant with massive intraventricular hemorrhage usually has hyaline membrane disease with signs primarily those of respiratory insufficiency for the first 24 to 48 hours after birth. Precipitous deterioration indicative of the occurrence of intracranial bleeding is usually observed on the second or third day after birth (Tsiantos et al.). Clinical signs are superimposed on previously existent manifestations of respiratory insufficiency and include sudden cardiovascular collapse, convulsions and loss of pupillary reactions. Bulging of the anterior fontanel and hyperpyrexia have been considered common findings in the infant with intraventricular hemorrhage but are by no means always present (Pomerance and Richardson, Tsiantos et al.).

## BIRTH INJURIES OF THE SPINAL CORD

Spinal cord injury during the labor or delivery process is probably the most underestimated form of birth damage to the central nervous system. Severe insults result in apnea at birth, with a significant mortality in the neonatal period. The spinal canal and cord are frequently not examined at necropsy in such cases, and thus damage to this area is often overlooked. Even in those who survive, mild injuries to the lower cervical and upper thoracic spinal cord with attendant spastic paraparesis can easily be confused with the similar constellation of findings characteristic of the cerebral diplegic form of cerebral palsy occurring in the prematurely born infant.

The concept of spinal cord birth injury was popularized in the 1920's by the writings of Crothers, Crothers and Putnam, and Ford. The incidence of the disorder was considerably greater at that time, and has subsequently diminished with improved obstetrical techniques. Abnormal intrauterine presentations and breech extraction remain the most common obstetrical factors associated with spinal cord birth trauma, although it can occur with vertex deliveries. It is estimated that approximately 75 per cent of cases occur in infants delivered in the breech position (Stern and Rand).

**CLINICAL ASPECTS.** In general, the site of spinal cord injury in breech-born infants is usually the lower cervical or upper thoracic region, while in vertex presentations it is more often the upper cervical region. The neurologic signs depend on both the localization of the spinal cord trauma and its severity. When the lesion is lower cervical or upper thoracic, the infant at birth exhibits a weak cry, scaphoid chest and protuberant abdomen. The lower limbs are flaccid and reveal either absent movements or paretic motor activity. Degree of involvement of the arms varies, and in some cases markedly asymmetrical weakness is observed. In others, persistent function of the biceps with paralyzed triceps muscles results in the characteristic posture of the arms flexed at the elbows. A sensory level to pinprick, sometimes asymmetrical, can usually be identified at the segment indicative of the upper level of the spinal cord lesion. Pin sensation is best assessed by observing facial expression during the test, since abrupt movement of the limb may represent a spinal reflex response. Distention of the bladder frequently occurs later in the first day of life. Flaccidity and areflexia persist in some infants, but in others after weeks or months the tone in the affected limbs becomes enhanced and hyperreflexia with clonus and pathologic toe signs supervene.

The child with an upper cervical cord birth injury is more likely to be apneic at birth, in addition to having flaccid paralysis of all four extremities. Respiratory insufficiency at this time can complicate the process, both diagnostically and prognostically, by the addition of a cerebral insult to the already present cervical cord damage (Towbin).

Pathologically, cord injuries vary in degree from those with small focal hemorrhages, to gross hemorrhagic necrosis, to frank and complete transection of the cord. Subarachnoid bleeding, meningeal laceration, and injury or avulsion of spinal nerve rootlets may accompany the spinal cord insult. Towbin has emphasized the importance of spinal epidural hemorrhage sometimes present in cases with birth trauma to the spinal cord. In severe cases associated brain stem lesions also occur.

**DIAGNOSIS.** The possibility of traumatic myelomalacia at birth should be suspected in the infant with flaccid limbs with a sensory level, especially in whom the facial appearance is that of wakefulness or alertness. A difficult breech extraction or other abnormal intrauterine fetal position is an important suggestive point but is not always the case. Lumbar puncture will usually show bloody or xanthochromic fluid with a partial or complete block on the Queckenstedt test. Pantopaque myelography will localize the site of the lesion and usually reveals a complete spinal block at the level of the lesion. The procedure, however, is not usually indicated when the diagnosis is certain.

**PATHOGENESIS.** Spinal cord injury associated with breech delivery is primarily the result of excessive longitudinal traction which occurs when force is applied to the legs or hips while the head is held tightly within the uterus. Although the vertebral column can be stretched considerably in the neonate, the spinal cord itself cannot be elongated without damage to its parenchyma (Leventhal). Intrauterine hyperextension of the neck in breech presentation represents a particular hazard to the spinal cord, as does any torsional force applied to the fetus during the birth process (Abroms et al., Bresnan and Abroms). While the main force causing cord trauma with breech presentation is longitudinal traction, the chief factor with cephalic delivery is probably excessive torsion or rotation. Hypotonia secondary to intrauterine asphyxia has been proposed as a possible factor increasing the risk of cord injury (DeSouza and Davis).

MANAGEMENT. In some cases the immediate problem is respiratory support. Treatment of the spinal cord lesion itself is conservative since surgery has little to offer. Physical therapy measures are begun as soon as the infant stabilizes and the diagnosis is certain. Bladder dysfunction must be dealt with, and in some infants nasogastric tube feeding is required. Respiratory infection creates a continuous threat to the child with intercostal muscle weakness and is a common cause of death among infants who survive the first few days after birth.

CASE 79-1

A white male infant was delivered 1 week before the expected date of confinement and weighed at birth 5 pounds 4 ounces (2380 gm). Delivery was complicated by double footling breech presentation and by wrapping of the cord about the neck. During extraction a "snap" was heard and was commented upon. He cried immediately and breathed spontaneously. General vigor seemed poor, activity less than average, cry weak. At 2 days "muscle tone seemed poor, especially in the lower extremities." At 6 weeks of age the legs were again noted to be of diminished tone and the cry weak, but the infant had done moderately well with respect to feeding and gaining. At 10 weeks he was examined carefully for the first time. He was poorly developed and nourished and cried a great deal. He lay with arms flexed and wrists extended, legs limply assuming the frog position. There were atrophy of the hands and flexor muscles of the forearms, early contracture at the elbows and diminished biceps and triceps reflexes. The chest was poorly developed and showed no intercostal activity, but only diaphragmatic breathing motion. The abdomen was full, and the muscles offered little resistance to deep palpation. In the legs, although limp, the deep tendon reflexes were increased and there was crossed adductor response. Anal sphincter tone was poor, and urine dribbled.

Spinal tap on the third day yielded fluid which was grossly bloody, and was probably traumatic. At 2½ weeks the fluid contained 60 crenated red blood cells per cubic millimeter, but at 3 months it contained 105 mg of protein per 100 ml, and pressure responses revealed complete spinal block. There was no evidence of sweating of the lower limbs after prolonged exposure to the heat lamp. A laminectomy was performed, and complete disruption of the cord from the seventh cervical to the first thoracic level was found. He died 4 days after the operation.

## SUBDURAL HEMATOMA

Bleeding into the subdural space of sufficient quantity to result in clinical manifestations can be provoked by mechanical forces associated with the birth process. Most subdural hemorrhages are supratentorial and bilateral in location, but they can also occur in the posterior fossa. Subdural hematomas originating during labor or delivery are frequently associated with complications that result in excessive molding of the fetal head. The source of bleeding is generally believed to be secondary to laceration or rupture of bridging veins which extend from the cortical surface to the superior sagittal sinus, or from venous disruption associated with tentorial laceration (Chase). Excessive size of the infant, prematurity and breech delivery, and difficult forceps extraction are factors that predispose to the possible occurrence of this type of intracranial hemorrhage. Certain pre-existent diseases of the child, such as osteogenesis imperfecta, increase the risk of subdural bleeding because of lack of normal protective mechanisms.

Acute subdural hematomas over the cerebral convexities giving rise to clinical signs in the newborn period are quite infrequent, and only a limited number have been reported (Schipke et al., Natelson and Sayers). Signs indicative of acute subdural collections of blood are variable but include pallor, lethargy, irritability, vomiting, convulsions, poor Moro response and bulging of the anterior fontanel. The diagnosis is confirmed by transfontanel subdural taps which also represent the initiation of treatment. Brisk bleeding into the subdural spaces of sufficient quantity to produce immediate signs of increased pressure can deplete the blood volume and cause distress on this basis. Blood administration may be necessary in such cases.

The better known and more widely recognized form of infantile subdural hematoma is that which is usually identified a few months after birth and which is manifested by progressive head enlargement, seizures, developmental delay, and anemia in some. History or evidence of postnatal trauma is frequently absent in these infants, and in past years most were assumed to have acquired the lesions by birth trauma. Although injury during parturition can account for a certain number of chronic subdural hematomas in infancy, many, if not most, are probably the result of physical trauma of one type or another after birth. Long bone and chest x-rays will place some in the category of the battered child syndrome. Evidence of recent bleeding from the appearance of fluid obtained when subdural taps are done, or the presence of retinal hemorrhages in the child over two months of age, should not be ascribed to birth trauma. Regardless of etiology, infantile subdural hematomas are managed by transfontanel subdural taps at daily intervals until the quantity of fluid has diminished considerably or is no longer obtainable (McLaurin et al.). When fluid collections cannot be eliminated by this method, a subdural-to-peritoneal shunt (Moyes et al.) or other type of shunt is indicated.

Acute subdural hematoma in the posterior fossa of the newborn infant is an unusual disorder which can be recognized with a high index of suspicion but is likely to prove fatal if not identified and removed. The large child is more often affected than the small one, and complications of labor and delivery resulting in excessive molding of the head have been described in a number of the reported cases. Hemorrhage into the posterior fossa in the neonate is generally believed to emanate from tentorial tears that extend into the lateral or straight sinus, or laceration of the vein of Galen. Rupture of bridging veins from the cerebellum to the lateral sinus or vein of Galen can also be caused by mechanical stress at birth leading to subdural hemorrhage (Gilles and Shillito).

Clinical signs of a subtentorial hematoma in the neonate make their appearance early, often from 1 to several days after birth. Irritability, lethargy, vomiting, high-pitched cry and hypotonia are common early manifestations of this lesion, and are sometimes associated with pallor or respiratory distress when the volume of blood loss has been significant (Pitlyk et al.). As the mass enlarges, the fourth ventricle is displaced forward and soon becomes obstructed, giving rise to ventricular distention proximal to the site of obstruction and manifested by progressive signs of increased intracranial pressure. The anterior fontanel is tense, sutures are increasingly spread, and the head circumference rapidly enlarges. Nystagmus, when observed, is likely to be the only specific sign of cerebellar dysfunction.

The first diagnostic considerations in the newborn infant with the above-described signs are usually either supratentorial subdural hematomas or hydrocephalus secondary to subarachnoid bleeding induced by a traumatic delivery. Transfontanel subdural taps exclude the former possibility, and the severity of signs plus the rapid development of pressure manifestations should raise doubt as to the latter. In almost all cases of neonatal posterior fossa hemorrhage, cerebrospinal fluid examination shows bloody fluid with a xanthochromic supernatant and a very high protein content. Although lumbar puncture in such cases is not desirable because of the potential hazard, it is likely to be done before the diagnosis is suspected. Ventricular tap reveals similar findings in addition to a significant elevation of the opening pressure. Ventriculography is the most definitive diagnostic method in that a posterior fossa mass is revealed by the presence of anterior displacement and obstruction of the fourth ventricle.

A posterior fossa subdural hematoma in the neonate can be surgically evacuated, with the outcome being dependent on the degree of cerebellar contusion that has occurred. It is not uncommon that communicating hydrocephalus will complicate the post-craniectomy course, requiring an eventual bypass shunt procedure (Carter and Pittman).

## INTRACRANIAL HEMORRHAGE IN THE NEWBORN INFANT

Although certain types of intracranial hemorrhage have been discussed above, the total spectrum is herein placed in perspective. Asphyxia and mechanical trauma account for the vast majority of hemorrhagic intracranial lesions that occur during the birth process or in the newborn infant. Intracranial bleeding of one type or another is commonly found at autopsy when death occurs in the neonatal period, although it is not always a major causative factor accounting for demise of the child. In a series of 393 postmortem examinations of neonates with various diseases, Gröntoft identified macroscopic intracranial hemorrhage in 120. Bleeding may develop in the subarachnoid space, the subdural spaces, within the lateral ventricles or simultaneously within more than one of these regions. Significant epidural hemorrhage in the newborn is quite rare, as is a large collection of blood in a localized area within the parenchyma of the brain. When parenchymal bleeding does occur, it is usually in the form of multiple petechial lesions or hemorrhage within a venous infarction.

Subarachnoid bleeding is more often observed in the premature infant than in the full term child and can have its origin from either asphyxia or mechanical injuries. Blood in the subarachnoid space is of no great consequence in the newborn from the standpoint of acute signs. Neurologic findings that are present usually reflect the associated cerebral insult incurred by the same factor that caused subarachnoid bleeding. Neonatal subarachnoid hemorrhage is an important cause of communicating hydrocephalus (Lorber and Bhat, Larroche), a complication that must be watched for by the appropriate methods of examination in the weeks following birth.

Subpial hemorrhage refers to a collection of blood dissecting beneath the pia and is an uncommon form of intracranial bleeding that has been described in premature infants with respiratory distress (Friede). This may be bilateral or unilateral and can cause localized disturbance of cortical function. Acute subdural hematomas, previously discussed, are also unusual in the neonatal period but are important because of their accessibility to treatment measures. Subdural hemorrhages, either above the tentorium or in the posterior fossa, are the result of mechanical forces during labor or delivery which cause undue distortion of the shape of the head. Intraventricular hemorrhage is a much more common lesion, and is found predominantly in the prematurely born infant whose early hours after birth are complicated by respiratory distress. The primary site of bleeding is in the periventricular subependymal matrix with subsequent extension into the lateral ventricular system. Asphyxia, shock and increased venous pressure are the primary pathogenetic factors giving rise to this type of intracranial bleeding. The initial lesion in the periventricular germinal matrix is most likely ischemic infarction with hemorrhage representing a secondary process in the infarcted region.

Intracranial hemorrhage from neoplastic or congenital vascular anomalies in the newborn period or in early infancy is rare but has been described. Intraventricular hemorrhage can emanate from small hemangiomata of the choroid plexus (Doe et al.). Subarachnoid and parenchymal bleeds have been reported in early infancy from aneurysms or arteriovenous malformations but are decidedly unusual (Pickering et al., Garcia-Chavez and Moossy, Beatty). Aneurysms of the vein of Galen in the newborn can bleed but usually cause clinical signs on the basis of obstructive hydrocephalus and high output cardiac failure. Intraventricular bleeding in early infancy can arise from a papilloma of the choroid plexus, but the most customary syndrome produced by this unusual tumor is rapid and progressive head enlargement.

## DIFFERENTIAL DIAGNOSIS OF PERINATAL CEREBRAL INSULTS

Abnormalities of neurologic function in the newborn infant caused by perinatal asphyxial or mechanical insults are differentiated from other conditions with similar manifestations by knowledge of the events during labor and delivery, and appropriate laboratory studies such as blood glucose, urea nitrogen, electrolytes, lumbar puncture and x-rays of the chest. In the small premature infant, especially one with respiratory distress or cardiac failure, the significance and cause of clinical functional abnormalities in regard to alertness or neurologic signs are usually difficult to assess in the early postnatal period. Passage of time and serial evaluations are frequently required to ascertain whether significant neurologic deficits are present.

Recurrent apneic spells in the premature infant pose a very difficult problem in regard to their relationship to neurologic function. The pathogenesis of this phenomenon is poorly understood despite its common occurrence. The occurrence of apneic episodes in an infant with a markedly irregular respiratory pattern usually suggests structural brain disease due to asphyxia, hemorrhage or a major anomaly of the central nervous system. Recurrent apnea in the premature newborn with tachypnea secondary to hyaline membrane disease is much more frequent, and in this situation, apnea can possibly be explained on the basis of medullary "immaturity," or may be associated with other factors, such as blood gas abnormalities, increase in the environmental temperature, electrolyte disturbances or sepsis. Its presence does not necessarily imply significant morphologic brain disease. Apneic episodes in infants beyond the immediate newborn period can be seizural manifestations which respond to anticonvulsant treatment, but this is probably infrequent. Recurrent apnea is sometimes the first manifestation of sepsis or meningitis, but here again, the pathogenesis is unclear.

Convulsions in the newborn infant are commonly observed in association with other signs compatible with intracranial injury acquired during labor and delivery. This represents the single most common cause of neonatal seizures in most centers, but should only be accepted after other possible causes amenable to direct treatment are excluded. Hypoglycemia, hypocalcemia, hypomagnesemia and sepsis or meningitis are primary and immediate considerations because of the need for specific therapy. Convulsions in the newborn can also occur with congenital cerebral anomalies, intrauterine acquired infections, certain aminoacidurias and disturbances of pyridoxine metabolism; they can also be secondary to maternal intake of narcotics, barbiturates or other drugs.

Hypotonia in the neonatal period is seen in many conditions, including those with perinatal insults to the brain and spinal cord. Hypotonia with certain other disorders, such as mongolism or other trisomic states, glycogen storage disease or cyanotic congenital heart disease, are readily recognized by the associated physical and biochemical abnormalities. Myotonic dystrophy can be manifested in the newborn period, particularly when the disease is transmitted from the affected mother (Dyken and Harper). The symptomatic infant with this disorder reveals severe decrease in muscle tone, poor sucking and swallowing ability and some degree of respiratory difficulty. Talipes equinovarus or other joint deformities, and bilateral facial paresis with ptosis are common additional findings in the newborn infant. The subsequent identification of mental retardation is frequent in children who exhibit clinical signs of myotonic dystrophy in the early postnatal period. Percussion myotonia cannot be demonstrated in the affected infant but diagnosis can be made on the basis of the physical signs and the presence of the disease in the mother. Familial dysautonomia, although rare, is another disorder characterized by decreased muscle tone, sucking and swallowing dysfunction and respiratory difficulty in the newborn and early infant period. Such children may be assumed to have brain disease, either prenatally or perinatally induced, until the subsequent findings clarify the nature of the problem. Familial dysautonomia is rarely diagnosed in the newborn period (Geltzer et al.), although diagnosis is possible if the consideration is entertained. Diagnostic methods include the instillation of 2.5 per cent methacholine in the conjunctival sac, which produces pupillary constriction in the infant with this disease but no response in the normal child. Urine content of homovanillic acid is elevated while that of vanillylmandelic acid is decreased. Intradermal injection of histamine in the child with familial dysautonomia produces a wheal but without the associated axon flare that occurs in normal individuals.

Other causes of neonatal hypotonia that

can be confused with cerebral insults acquired during the birth process include disorders of the anterior horn cells, neuromuscular junction or muscles. Werdnig-Hoffman's disease is usually identified a few months after birth but can result in abnormalities in the immediate newborn period. Hypotonia is accompanied by hyporeflexia, muscle atrophy and fasciculations of the tongue. Infants with this disease retain a normal degree of mental alertness, awareness and prompt response to painful stimuli, features which set it apart from most cerebral insults which are manifested by decreased muscle tone. Neonatal myasthenia gravis is a rare disease which can be suspected by the presence of the disease in the mother. The infant with this disease exhibits diffuse muscle weakness without atrophy. Diagnosis is confirmed by temporary improvement following an intravenous injection of edrophonium or intramuscular injection of prostigmine hydrochloride. Congenital myopathies are rare causes of hypotonia in the newborn period. Like Werdnig-Hoffmann's disease, they are diagnosed by special procedures, such as electromyography and examination of muscle biopsy.

## THE CONCEPT OF "CEREBRAL PALSY"

The multiple definitions that have been proposed for "cerebral palsy" reflect the heterogeneous nature of the disorders included. In 1861, William Little emphasized the important relationship between prematurity or perinatal asphyxia and the subsequent occurrence of spastic disabilities, with or without other neurologic deficits. Had the term "cerebral palsy" been restricted to those non-progressive neurologic conditions associated with prematurity or with origin secondary to insults during or immediately after the birth process, it would have represented a diagnostic concept of considerable usefulness, even if not entirely correct from the anatomical standpoint. Instead, "cerebral palsy" came to be the subject of varied definition, with most claiming it to include any non-progressive

disturbance of motor control whose origin is an intracranial insult before birth, during birth or in the early years after birth (MacKeith et al., Minear, Malamud et al., Brandt). Crothers and Paine aptly summarized the concept of "cerebral palsy" by stating that the term does not designate a disease in the usual medical sense but is a useful administrative designation which refers to persons handicapped by motor disorders due to non-progressive abnormalities of the brain which occur early in life.

Applying the above definition, which thus includes a complex group of etiologic causes, the incidence of "cerebral palsy" has been estimated at between one and two per thousand births (Bobath, Griffiths and Barrett, Asher and Schonell). Authors designed elaborate classifications of the conditions, most of which were on the basis of the type of abnormality of tone exhibited by the patient. Recognized patterns have included 1) the spastic type, 2) the athetoid or dystonic type, 3) the ataxic type, 4) the atonic type, and 5) those with mixed forms. Subclassifications have also been constructed; for example, the spastic type is subdivided into the spastic diplegic form, the spastic quadriplegic form, the spastic hemiplegic type and so on.

To a certain degree, the type and distribution of tone abnormality correlates with an etiologic cause, although considerable overlap exists. The spastic diplegic type of "cerebral palsy" usually, but not always, is seen in the product of a premature birth complicated by perinatal or neonatal asphyxia (Berenberg and Ong). The corresponding pathologic changes are usually deep seated, especially in the periventricular white matter. Athetoid or dystonic types are commonly the result of neonatal asphyxiating injuries sustained by the full-term child or secondary to kernicterus due to uncontrolled hyperbilirubinemia. Pathologic abnormalities in this group tend to involve the cortical region and deep nuclear gray matter, and, in kernicterus, the globus pallidus, subthalamic nucleus, the hippocampus and various cranial nerve nuclei. The ataxic type of "cerebral palsy" is probably not determined by perinatal injuries but in most instances represents the clinical manifestation of cerebellar malformations. The alleged atonic type remains a somewhat mysterious concept, perhaps partially explained by the natural history of certain of the above described patterns. It is widely recognized that, although the pathologic processes associated with these conditions are stable or non-progressive, the clinical picture is a gradually changing one from birth up to two or more years thereafter. Athetosis is not commonly recognized before the infant reaches 12 to 18 months, and less commonly may not even evolve until later in the first decade (Hanson et al.). Marked hypotonia, the "atonic" phase, accompanied by developmental retardation precedes the appearance of spastic diplegia or spastic quadriplegia by several months (Byers, Ingram).

It is not proposed that yet another definition be considered, but from the practical medical standpoint, this author finds the diagnosis of "cerebral palsy" useful only in those conditions in which motor deficits stem from injury to the brain during the birth process or immediately thereafter, or in the premature infant who presumably sustains injury at the same time. The infant with neurologic damage resulting from intrauterine-acquired cytomegalovirus infection is more appropriately diagnosed as having congenital cytomegalovirus infection. The morbid condition in a two-year-old child who sustains head injury followed by a non-progressive hemiparesis is more logically labeled post-traumatic encephalopathy manifested by spastic hemiparesis, seizures and so on. Likewise, in the child with neurologic and intellectual disabilities based on anomalous formation of the brain of unknown cause the disorder is more correctly classified as congenital cerebral malformation, etiology undetermined. This diagnostic method is better comprehended by the parents of neurologically damaged children and enhances the meaning of epidemiologic data among the various diagnostic categories. Although the diagnostic use of the term "cerebral palsy" in this fashion does not entirely comply with the current definition, its merit is that it gives a certain degree of specificity to the term and decreases confusion among physicians in the various medical specialties, including the pediatrician, the orthopedist and the neurosurgeon.

## REFERENCES

Abroms, I. F., Bresnan, M. J., Zuckerman, J. E., Fischer, E. G., and Strand, R.: Cervical cord injuries secondary to hyperextension of the head in breech presentations. Obstet. Gynecol. *41*:369, 1973.

Anderson, J. M., Brown, J. K., and Cockburn, F.: On the role of disseminated intravascular coagulation in the pathology of birth asphyxia. Develop. Med. Child Neurol. *16*:581, 1974.

Armstrong, D., and Norman, M. G.: Periventricular leukomalacia in neonates. Arch. Dis. Child. *49*:367, 1974.

Asher, P., and Schonell, F. E.: A survey of 400 cases of cerebral palsy in childhood. Arch. Dis. Child. *25*:260, 1950.

Banker, B. Q.: The neuropathological effects of anoxia and hypoglycemia in the newborn. Develop. Med. Child Neurol. *9*:544, 1967.

Banker, B. Q., and Larroche, J-C.: Periventricular leukomalacia of infant. Arch. Neurol. *7*:386, 1962.

Beatty, R. A.: Surgical treatment of a ruptured intracerebral arteriovenous malformation in a newborn. Pediatrics *53*:571, 1974.

Berenberg, W., and Ong, B. H.: Cerebral spastic paraplegia and prematurity. Pediatrics *33*:496, 1964.

Bobath, K.: The neuropathology of cerebral palsy and its importance in treatment and diagnosis. Cerebral Palsy Bull. *8*:13, 1959.

Brandt, S.: Some remarks on terminology and classification. Cerebral Palsy Bull. *5*:43, 1959.

Bresnan, M. J., and Abroms, I. F.: Neonatal spinal cord transection secondary to intrauterine hyperextension of the neck in breech presentation. J. Pediatr. *84*:734, 1974.

Brown, J. K., Purvis, R. J., Forfar, J. O., and Cockburn, F.: Neurological aspects of perinatal asphyxia. Develop. Med. Child Neurol. *16*:567, 1974.

Byers, R. K.: Evolution of hemiplegias in infancy. Am. J. Dis. Child. *61*:915, 1941.

Carter, L. P., and Pittman, H. W.: Posterior fossa subdural hematoma of the newborn. J. Neurosurg. *34*:423, 1971.

Chase, W. H.: An anatomical study of subdural hemorrhage associated with tentorial splitting in the newborn. Surg. Gynecol. Obstet. *51*:31, 1930.

Chessells, J. M., and Wigglesworth, J. S.: Coagulation studies in preterm infant with respiratory distress and intracranial hemorrhage. Arch. Dis. Child. *47*:564, 1972.

Cole, V. A., Durbin, G. M., Olaffson, A., Reynolds, E. O. R., Rivers, R. P. A., and Smith, J. F.: Pathogenesis of intraventricular hemorrhage in newborn infants. Arch. Dis. Child. *29*:722, 1974.

Crothers, B.: Injury to the spinal cord in breech extractions as an important cause of foetal death and of paraplegia in childhood. Am. J. Med. Sci. *165*:94, 1923.

Crothers, B., and Paine, R. S.: The Natural History of

Cerebral Palsy. Cambridge, Harvard University Press, 1959.

Crothers, B., and Putnam, M. C.: Obstetrical injuries of the spinal cord. Medicine 6:41, 1927.

De Reuck, J.: The human periventricular arterial blood supply and the anatomy of cerebral infarctions. Europ. Neurol. 5:321, 1971.

De Reuck, J., Chattha, A. S., and Richardson, E. P., Jr.: Pathogenesis and evolution of periventricular leukomalacia in infancy. Arch. Neurol. 27:229, 1972.

DeSouza, S. W., and Davis, J. A.: Spinal cord damage in a newborn infant. Arch. Dis. Child. 49:70, 1974.

Doe, F. D., Shuangshoti, S., and Netsky, M. G.: Cryptic hemangioma of the choroid plexus. Neurology 22:1232, 1972.

Dyken, P. R., and Harper, P. S.: Congenital dystrophica myotonica. Neurology 23:465. 1973.

Engel, R. R., and Elin, R. J.: Hypermagnesemia from birth asphyxia. J. Pediatr. 77:631, 1970.

Fedrick, J., and Butler, N. R.: Certain causes of neonatal death. II. Intraventricular hemorrhage. Biol. Neonate 15:257, 1970.

Feldman, W., Drummond, K. N., and Klein, M.: Hyponatremia following asphyxia neonatorum. Acta Paediat. Scand. 59:52, 1970.

Ford, F. R.: Breech delivery in its possible relation to injury of the spinal cord with special reference to infantile paraplegia. Arch. Neurol. Psychiat. 14:742, 1925.

Friede, R. L.: Subpial hemorrhage in infants. J. Neuropath. Exper. Neurol. 31:548, 1972.

Garcia-Chavez, C., and Moosey, J.: Cerebral artery aneurysm in infancy. Association with agenesis of the corpus callosum. J. Neuropath. Exper. Neurol. 24:492, 1965.

Geltzer, A. I., Gluck, L., Talner, N. S., and Polesky, H. F.: Familial dysautonomia. Studies in a newborn infant. N. Engl. J. Med. 271:436, 1964.

Gilles, F. H., and Shillito, J., Jr.: Infantile hydrocephalus: Retrocerebellar subdural hematoma. J. Pediatr. 76:529, 1970.

Gontoft, O.: Intracranial hemorrhage and blood-brain barrier problems in the newborn. Acta Pathol. Microbiol. Scand. Suppl. 100, 1–109, 1954.

Griffiths, M. I., and Barrett, N. M.: Cerebral palsy in Birmingham. Develop. Med. Child Neurol. 9:33, 1967.

Gross, G. P., Hathaway, W. E., and McGaughey, H. R.: Hyperviscosity in the neonate. J. Pediatr. 82:1004, 1973.

Hanson, R. A., Berenberg, W., and Byers, R. K.: Changing motor pattern in cerebral palsy. Develop. Med. Child Neurol. 12:309, 1970.

Ingram, T. T. S.: The neurology of cerebral palsy. Arch. Dis. Child. 41:337, 1966.

Larroche, J-C.: Post-hemorrhagic hydrocephalus in infancy. Anatomical study. Biol. Neonate 20:287, 1972.

Leventhal, H. R.: Birth injuries of the spinal cord. J. Pediatr. 56:447, 1960.

Lipsitz, P. J.: The clinical and biochemical effects of excess magnesium in the newborn. Pediatrics 47:501, 1971.

Lipsitz, P. J., and English, I. C.: Hypermagnesemia in the newborn infant. Pediatrics 40:856, 1967.

Little, W. J.: On the influence of abnormal parturition, difficult labors, premature birth, and asphyxia neonatorum on the mental and physical condition of the child, especially in relation to deformities. Trans. Obstet. Soc. London 3:293, 1861.

Lorber, J., and Bhat, U. S.: Posthemorrhagic hydrocephalus. Arch. Dis. Child. 49:751, 1974.

MacKeith, R. C., Mackenzie, I. C. K., and Polani, P. E.: Definition of cerebral palsy. Cerebral Palsy Bull. 5:23, 1959.

Malamud, N., Itabashi, H. H., Castor, J., and Messinger, H. B.: An etiologic and diagnostic study of cerebral palsy. J. Pediatr. 65:270, 1964.

McLaurin, R. L., Isaacs, E., and Lewis, H. P.: Results in nonoperative treatment in 15 cases of infantile subdural hematoma. J. Neurosurg. 34:753, 1971.

Minear, W. L.: A classification of cerebral palsy. Pediatrics 18:841, 1956.

Moyes, P. D., Thompson, G. B., and Cluff, J. W.: Subdural peritoneal shunts in the treatment of subdural effusions in infants. J. Neurosurg. 23:584, 1965.

Natelson, S. E., and Sayers, M. P.: The fate of children sustaining severe head trauma during birth. Pediatrics 51:169, 1973.

Pickering, L. K., Hogan, G. R., and Gilbert, E. F.: Aneurysm of the posterior inferior cerebellar artery. Am. J. Dis. Child. 119:155, 1970.

Pitlyk, P. J., Miller, R. H., and Stayura, L. A.: Subdural hematoma of the posterior fossa: Report of a case. Pediatrics 40:536, 1967.

Pomerance, J. J., and Richardson, C. J.: Hyperpyrexia as a sign of intraventricular hemorrhage in the neonate. Am. J. Dis. Child. 126:854, 1973.

Ross, J. J., and Dimmette, R. M.: Subependymal cerebral hemorrhage in infancy. Am. J. Dis. Child. 110:531, 1965.

Schipke, R., Riege, D., and Scoville, W. B.: Acute subdural hemorrhage at birth. Pediatrics 14:468, 1954.

Schwartz, P.: Birth Injuries of the Newborn: Morphology, Pathogenesis, Clinical Pathology, and Prevention. New York, Hafner Publishing Co., 1961.

Sinclair, J. C., Fox, H. A., Lentz, J. F., Fuld, G. L., and Murphy, J.: Intoxication of the fetus by a local anesthetic. A newly recognized complication of maternal caudal anesthesia. N. Engl. J. Med. 273:1173, 1965.

Stern, W. E., and Rand, R. W.: Birth injuries to the spinal cord. Am. J. Obstet. Gynecol. 78:498, 1959.

Towbin, A.: Central nervous system damage in the human fetus and newborn infant. Am. J. Dis. Child. 119:529, 1970.

Towbin, A.: Latent spinal cord and brain stem injury in newborn infants. Develop. Med. Child. Neurol. 11:54, 1969.

Towbin, A.: Spinal cord and brain stem injury at birth. Arch. Pathol. 77:620, 1964.

Tsiantos, A., Victorin, L., Relier, J. P., Dyer, N., Sundell, H., Brill, A. B., and Stahlman, M.: Intracranial hemorrhage in the prematurely born infant. J. Pediatr. 85:854, 1974.

Windle, W. F.: An experimental approach to prevention or reduction of the brain damage of birth asphyxia. Develop. Med. Child Neurol. 8:129, 1966.

Wood, J. L.: Plethora, in the newborn infant associated with cyanosis and convulsions. J. Pediatr. 54:143, 1959.

# 80

# ABNORMALITIES IN SIZE AND SHAPE OF THE HEAD

*By William E. Bell*

## INTRODUCTION

Disturbances of the size or shape of the head in the neonate are commonly observed due to minor, transient problems and less frequently to a more serious disorder. Examination of the head, which is an important part of the physical examination of every newborn infant, should not be limited to observation alone. The head should be inspected, palpated and measured with every examination, and in some infants should be percussed, auscultated, transilluminated and x-rayed. Roentgenograms of the skull of the newborn infant are of greatest value in the demonstration of intracranial calcification or fractures of the skull but are less reliable indicators of the significance of suture spread or of abnormalities of the anterior fontanel than are the fingers of an experienced clinician.

The most common causes of deviation of the head shape in the newborn period are cephalhematoma and molding secondary to the effects of the birth process. The calvarium of the premature infant is customarily smaller in circumference than that of his term-born counterpart and is also notable for its elongation in the anteroposterior direction. In craniosynostosis the configuration of the head is determined by which suture or sutures are closed and the condition is recognized by the characteristic appearance and palpatory findings along with x-ray demonstration of cranial sutural fusion.

Definite abnormalities of head size in the neonate represent potentially more serious conditions. The microcephalic infant presents an abnormally small head which, by measurement in centimeters, is smaller than two standard deviations from the mean. Because of the considerable variation in head circumference soon after birth, depending on length of gestation and birth weight, it is prudent to defer the diagnosis of microcephaly except in obvious situations until the passage of time has clarified the situation.

There are many causes of abnormal head enlargement in the newborn period, all of which are incorporated under the nonspecific term macrocephaly, meaning large head. Thus, macrocephaly may be the result of hydrocephalus due to one of many causes, hydranencephaly, subdural effusions or hematomas, or a large brain. Megalencephaly refers to abnormal enlargement of the brain, which may occur in a number of syndromes. Hydrocephalus implies pathologic ventricular enlargement, which, in the vast majority of cases, results from obstruction of cerebrospinal fluid flow at some point along its pathways. Most cases in newborn children are caused by congenital anomalies of the aqueduct of Sylvius or by meningeal inflammation. It is important to remember, however, that certain unusual causes of hydrocephalus can be amenable to direct surgical attack, such as those resulting from paracollicular arachnoid cyst, posterior fossa subdural hematoma, posterior fossa tumor, or papilloma of the choroid plexus.

## ANENCEPHALY

Anencephaly is a lethal malformation in which the vault of the skull is absent and the exposed brain is amorphous. Between 75 and 80 per cent of these infants are stillborn and the remainder succumb within hours or a few days after birth. The etiology of this grotesque anomaly is unknown, although epidemiologic studies suggest a familial predisposition, at least to a certain extent. In the United States anencephaly has been found in 0.5 to 2 per 1000 births, while in Ireland the prevalence rate is as high as 5.9 per 1000 births (Alter, Nakano, Coffey and Jessop). Most investigators have favored non-closure of the neural tube in early embryonic life as the cause of this defect, but others have provided evidence of damage to or reopening of the prosencephalon after closure (Padget, Toop et al.).

Anencephaly occurs two to four times more often in girls than in boys. A high percentage of these babies are premature, and associated polyhydramnios is not uncommon. The cranial defect is associated with open spinal cord anomalies in 10 to 20 per cent of cases. In addition to the grossly anomalous character of the cerebral hemispheres, the hypothalamus is quite malformed, and the cerebellum is usually rudimentary or absent. Brain stem tissue is identifiable. The internal carotid arteries are hypoplastic, a condition probably secondary to the lack of normal brain formation (Vogel). The anterior lobe of the pituitary gland is present in the anencephalic infant but the adrenal glands are abnormally small.

Diagnosis of anencephaly is obvious at the moment of birth. The liveborn infant is clothed and fed in the customary fashion until natural death occurs. Of great interest is the recent identification of an increased content of alpha-fetoprotein in amniotic fluid in the fetus with anencephaly or other open neural tube defects, allowing prenatal diagnosis between 12 and 16 weeks of gestation (Milunsky and Alpert, Brock and Sutcliffe). Alpha-fetoprotein, which accounts for the majority of fetal serum globulin, is synthesized by normal embryonal liver cells and the yolk sac. It is uncertain how it gains entrance into the amniotic fluid in the presence of open neural tube defects but its high content at a certain stage of pregnancy represents a useful diagnostic tool. Because the recurrence risk for parents who have had one anencephalic child is approximately 5 per cent (Carter and Roberts), amniocentesis for alpha-fetoprotein determination is indicated in such women during subsequent pregnancies. This, unfortunately, allows prenatal detection of only a minority of anencephalic fetuses. The possible hazards of amniocentesis do not allow its routine performance in all pregnancies, but the recent findings

of alpha-fetoprotein in maternal serum in affected pregnancies may result in a widescale detection method (Wald et al., Brock et al.).

## MICROCEPHALY

Strictly translated microcephaly refers to abnormally small head size, but the term also implies disease of the brain and eventual mental retardation. For this reason, the clinician should be careful not to use this diagnosis in the newborn period unless the findings unequivocally indicate its presence. The microcephalic child not only has an abnormally small head circumference compared to body length and weight, but the rate of head growth over the first few postnatal weeks or months is likewise abnormal. Thus, serial head measurements demonstrating lack of normal head enlargement are usually more reliable than a single determination.

Definition of microcephaly is less than entirely precise but usually refers to an occipitofrontal head circumference smaller than two standard deviations from the mean. The expected normal head circumferences at birth and in the first few weeks can be obtained for term infants from the graphs compiled by Nellhaus, and those for premature infants from the data collected by Lubchenco and colleagues. Strict adherence to head size and postnatal age only can be misleading, for inferences relative to intellectual skills cannot be drawn from these criteria, since children with head circumferences below two standard deviations are by no means always mentally retarded (Avery et al., Martin). A child with "measurement microcephaly" who is of small stature because of familial factors or growth retardation secondary to malabsorption or cardiac disease is, therefore, not necessarily in the same category from the standpoint of C.N.S. function as one with microcephaly resulting from organic brain disease.

Microcephaly has been variously classified, with some authors using the ambiguous term "true" while others have attempted to categorize the condition into primary and secondary types. Probably the most accurate etiologic classification of microcephaly includes genetic and acquired types, although in many cases there is neither a family history of similar problems or an event prenatally or later to account for damage to the brain. Certain neonates with microcephaly—some if not most being genetically determined—are obviously abnormal at birth in regard to a distinctly small head size, confirmed roentgenographically (Fig. 80–1), and characteristic facial and cranial configuration. Their rounded heads with small or absent anterior fontanel and recessed or sloped forehead indicative of the shallow anterior cranial fossa readily identify them as infants with severe morphologic cerebral abnormalities. In some, signs of neurologic dysfunction such as hypotonicity, hypertonicity or an abnormal cry are immediately present, while others function surprisingly normally for the first few months after birth. The type of pathology found in infants of this sort varies, but abnormalities of the gross configuration of the brain are usual.

Lissencephaly is near total or total absence of cerebral convolutions (agyria), reminiscent of the fetal brain during the second to fourth months of gestation (Miller).

Pachygyria appears to represent a developmental arrest of maturation and cell migration at a slightly later stage, with the result being abnormally broad, flat cerebral convolutions with a thick cerebral cortex. The ventricular system is usually mildly enlarged, and other anomalies, such as areas of gray matter heterotopia, are usually present in these types of malformed brains.

Polymicrogyria is more often associated with hydrocephalus than microcephaly and is characterized by either localized or generalized excessive and small cerebral convolutions. Whether microgyria is associated with an arrest of neuronal migration or is a result of an insult to the post-migratory cortex has not been entirely clarified (Richman et al.).

Microcephaly is present in infants with certain chromosomal disturbances, such as trisomy 13–15 and trisomy 17–18. The best known intrauterine acquired causes are transplacentally transmitted infections such as rubella, cytomegalovirus disease and toxoplasmosis. Maternal phenylketonuria with serum phenylalanine levels over 15 mg. per 100 ml during pregnancy is a cause of microcephaly and intrauterine growth failure (Fisch et al., Frankenburg et al.). Maternal irradiation exposure (Plummer) and certain drugs can possibly lead to brain damage and microcephaly. Perinatal hypoxic-ischemic insults lead to neurologic dysfunction in the neonatal period and may result in microcephaly which becomes apparent months later. Early postnatal cerebral insults, such as infection, head trauma or severe hypoxic episodes, likewise dis-

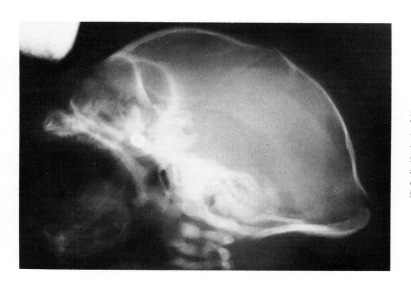

*Figure 80–1.* Microcephaly, skull x-ray, lateral projection. Three-day-old child with birth weight of 4120 grams. The calvarium is decidedly small for the facial structures. The cranial sutures are patent and the skull is more densely mineralized than is usual for this age.

turb subsequent brain growth, leading to microcephaly.

## CRANIOSYNOSTOSIS

Craniosynostosis (craniostenosis) is a disorder in which premature closure of one or more cranial sutures results in a disturbance of the shape and configuration of the skull. In many instances, premature fusion of the sutures is the only evident abnormality the child exhibits; in others, craniosynostosis and other associated anomalies represent an identifiable syndrome, often genetically determined. These "primary" forms of premature cranial suture closure are in contrast to conditions in which early suture closure is a passive process resulting from lack of normal brain growth. This is observed in the infant with microcephaly and can occur subsequent to successful shunt procedures for advanced hydrocephalus. Abnormally rapid suture closure in early infancy can also occur in association with certain metabolic disturbances, most notable being the rachitic disorders and idiopathic hypercalcemia (Reilly et al.).

The etiology of primary craniosynostosis is not known. Most cases unassociated with other anomalies are sporadic, although repeated occurrence within a family has been described. Craniosynostosis consistently associated with certain other anomalies, such as Crouzon's disease or Apert's syndrome, may appear in sporadic fashion but are generally regarded to be inherited disorders. An explanation for the type of deformity of the head resulting from premature closure of one or other cranial sutures was proposed by Virchow in 1851. He observed that inhibition of normal growth of the skull occurred in a direction perpendicular to the suture that is prematurely fused, resulting in compensatory enlargement in a direction parallel to the unyielding suture. The time at which cranial sutures normally achieve functional closure is quite variable but abnormal sutural diastasis is commonly observed in children up to 10 or 12 years of age suffering increased intracranial pressure. The metopic suture differs from the other major sutures in that closure normally occurs in the first year of life. Trigonocephaly, therefore, occurs only when fu-

sion of the metopic suture takes place in fetal or very early postnatal life. In general, the most overt cranial deformities are the result of prenatal suture closure, regardless of which suture or sutures are affected (Ingraham et al.). Since the brain reaches approximately 80 per cent of the adult weight by 3 to 4 years of age, individual suture closure at this time is a matter of little consequence.

CLINICAL ASPECTS. Certain types of craniosynostosis, such as sagittal suture synostosis, are more common in males than females. Isolated closure of the sagittal suture, the most common variety of the disease, is the one least often associated with other defects. Premature closure of the coronal sutures can likewise occur as the only apparent abnormality but is more often associated with other congenital anomalies. Oxycephaly secondary to multiple cranial suture fusion represents the least common form of the condition and is the most severe type because of the resulting restriction of cerebral growth and subsequent increased intracranial pressure.

The newborn infant with sagittal craniosynostosis presents with an elongated but narrow head, often with a small or absent anterior fontanel (Figs. 80–2 and 80–3). The forehead is usually considerably more broad than the occipital region. A palpable ridge is present, especially over the posterior portion of the fused suture. Although the sagittal suture may be closed along its total length, it is important to recognize that suture closure over even a short segment will effectively limit growth of the skull perpendicular to the entire length of that suture. In the absence of other anomalies, the infant with scaphalocephaly secondary to sagittal synostosis is not expected to have abnormal neurologic signs or signs of increased pressure. The signs are only those of distortion of head shape, since compensatory growth through other sutures permits normal brain growth. The problem is generally considered to be primarily cosmetic; however, examples are not rare of older children with uncorrected sagittal synostosis who subsequently developed visual disturbances or increased intracranial pressure (Andersson and Gomez, Anderson and Geiger).

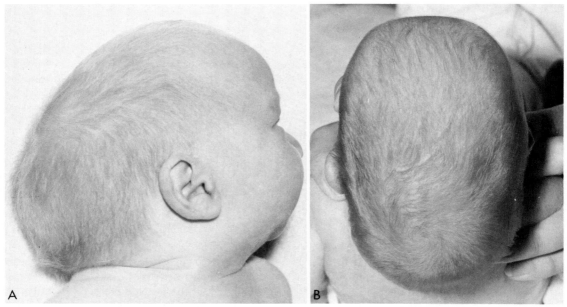

***Figure 80–2.*** Three-week-old infant with sagittal craniosynostosis. *A,* Lateral view demonstrates the elongated head shape with tapering in the occipital region. Except for the abnormal configuration of the head, the child is developmentally normal for age. *B,* Vertex view reveals the characteristic long, narrow shape of the calvarium with premature closure of the sagittal suture.

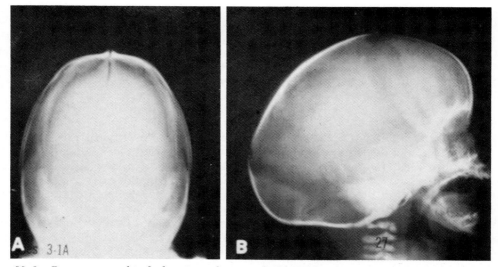

***Figure 80–3.*** Roentgenographic findings in a three-week-old child with sagittal craniosynostosis. *A,* Occipital view reveals the narrow configuration of the skull with "heaping up" of bone along the fused sagittal suture. *B,* Lateral view demonstrates the scaphalocephalic shape of the skull with hyperostosis of the closed sagittal suture. The coronal and lambdoidal sutures are more separated than normal. (Hope, J. W., Spitz, E. B., and Slade, H. W.: Radiology 65:183, 1955.)

Bilateral coronal synostosis results in a brachycephalic head shape in which the skull is broad anteriorly but shortened in the anteroposterior direction and with elevation of the skull in the region anterior to the fontanel (Fig. 80–4). The forehead is broad and flattened, usually with a "pinched" appearance just above and lateral to the eyebrows. The eyes appear wide-set and, in some cases proptosis is present. Palpable ridges are sometimes present over fused coronal sutures but are rarely as definite as the ridging over a closed sagittal suture. Bilateral coronal craniosynostosis is frequently associated with other anomalies and is the most common type of sutural closure in children with familial craniosynostosis, including Crouzon's disease or Apert's syndrome. Unilateral coronal synostosis gives rise to an asymmetrical cranial deformity called plagiocephaly. The forehead adjacent to the fused coronal suture is flattened or indented, the eyebrow is elevated and the homolateral eye appears prominent. The ocular prominence results from the associated involvement of the orbit, which is shallower and more oblique than is normally the case.

Prenatal or early postnatal fusion of the metopic suture leads to a narrow, triangular shape to the forehead, which has a palpable and visible ridge betraying the underlying closed suture. The orbits are oval-shaped and the eyes are abnormally closely approximated, a condition referred to as hypotelorism. The keel-shaped, angulated forehead of the infant with trigonocephaly is best observed by viewing the head from the vertex. Metopic suture synostosis occurs either in isolated fashion without other defects, or associated with other, often significant, anomalies (Anderson et al.). One associated pattern is the presence of midline facial clefts and arhinencephaly, or absence of the olfactory nerves and other parts of the rhinencephalon, in addition to a single anterior lateral ventricle with hypoplasia or absence of the corpus callosum (Currarino et al.). The child with trigonocephaly and associated cerebral defects is expected to reveal early developmental retardation and eventual mental retardation.

Premature closure of the lambdoid su-

tures alone is very rare but can occur on occasion with sagittal synostosis or with total cranial suture fusion. Oxycephaly, or total suture synostosis, is an infrequent but se-

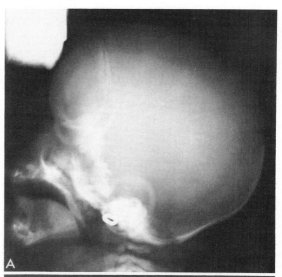

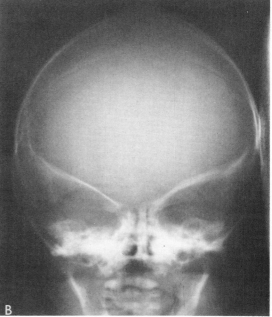

*Figure 80–4.* Roentgenographic findings in a newborn infant with bilateral coronal craniosynostosis. *A,* Lateral view of the skull shows the short anteroposterior diameter and hyperostosis along both fused coronal sutures. *B,* The PA view of the skull demonstrates the elevated and oblique position of the sphenoid ridge on either side.

vere form of craniosynostosis, and is the only type of the disease in which the head circumference of the child may be significantly reduced. Inability of the brain to expand causes increased pressure symptoms and signs, both clinical and roentgenographic. Growth of the skull in such infants occurs in regions of least resistance, with the result being bilateral bulging of the temporal squama just about the ears and striking prominence at the bregma. Thinning of the calvarium and deeply convolutional markings are seen on x-ray examination in such cases. Visual loss, retardation and seizures may later complicate this disorder, owing to the effects of chronic increased pressure on the immature brain.

In certain cases premature cranial suture closure is part of a spectrum of anomalies giving rise to identifiable syndromes with eponymic designations. Crouzon's disease, or craniofacial dysostosis, is commonly inherited on a dominant basis, although some cases occur in the absence of a family history. Clinical features include cranial deformity, usually due to coronal synostosis, but other sutures may also be affected. In rare instances, all cranial sutures are fused at birth in the child with Crouzon's disease, leading to gross disturbances of the face and head and severe effects of increased pressure (Shiller). Facial abnormalities that are constantly present include a "parrot's beak" deformity of the nose, maxillary hypoplasia, protrusion of the mandible and exophthalmos, often associated with divergent strabismus (Dodge et al.). Untreated patients are susceptible to a variety of problems secondary to intracranial hypertension or compression of the orbital contents and optic nerves. A bizarre but rare disorder with features somewhat similar to those of Crouzon's disease is referred to as Kleeblattschädel, or cloverleaf skull (Angle at et., Feingold et al.). Intrauterine synostosis of multiple or all cranial sutures in concert with hydrocephalus accounts for the grotesque characteristics of the child with this severe malformation. At birth, the infant exhibits advanced exophthalmos, hypertelorism, bulging in the areas of the closed anterior fontanel and the squamosal sutures, and downward displacement of the ears. In some cases, facial bone deformities are similar to those of Crouzon's disease, suggesting a possible relationship of Kleeblattschädel to heredictary craniofacial dysostosis (Hall et al.). The anomaly has also been associated with the skeletal changes of thanatophoric dwarfism (Partington et al.), and with other anomalies.

Apert's syndrome, or acrocephalosyndactyly, occurs in either sporadic or familial fashion and has been claimed to be related to increased paternal age. The pattern of suture closure varies to some degree but bilateral coronal synostosis is by far the most common (Fig. 80–5). Syndactylism of the hands and feet is the distinguishing feature of this disorder, although other anomalies may also be found. Choanal atresia or stenosis has been observed in some and can create airway problems during certain diagnostic studies unless recognized. Related syndromes have received a variety of designations, such as Carpenter's syndrome and Chotzen's syndrome, depending on the combined anomalies (Table 80–1).

**DIAGNOSIS.** Craniosynostosis in the newborn or young infant is usually suspected on the basis of an abnormality of the shape of the head. The distinctive palpable and sometimes visible ridge over the prematurely closed suture is an additional aid in identification of the condition. Roentgenographic examination is confirmatory in most instances but can be misleading unless one is familiar with the possible radiographic variations. For example, trigonocephaly may be obvious from the appearance of the child and the presence of a distinctive ridge, even though the metopic suture may appear patent on radiographic examination. The metopic suture is best observed by x-ray examination using a modified Water's view or the submental-vertex view. Hyperostosis and "heaping up" of a synostosed suture, in addition to the configuration of the skull generally, are the usual most dependable x-ray findings indicative of craniosynostosis. Unaffected sutures are often disproportionately separated, reflecting compensatory effects allowing brain growth.

Several conditions must be differentiated from craniosynostosis in the newborn and

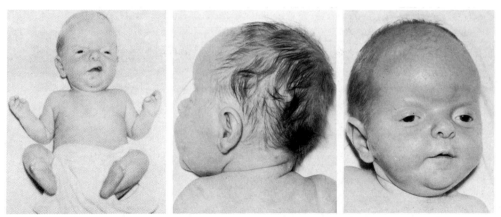

**Figure 80–5.** Apert's syndrome (acrocephalosyndactyly). Bilateral coronal synostosis results in a brachycephalic head shape with "high" forehead and shortened AP diameter of the skull. Note the bilateral syndactyly.

young infant. The infant's head is frequently asymmetrical because of postural effects, a condition especially likely to occur when the child lies with its head turned in one direction. This is seen with torticollis and also in developmentally retarded children who remain relatively immobile longer than normal. The result is unilateral occipital flattening, usually with some degree of flattening of the forehead on the opposite side. A small or absent anterior fontanel in the first few weeks after birth raises concern regarding either the rate of brain growth or the patency of sutures. This anomaly can occur as a normal variation or can be the result of an accessory bone arising from a separate ossification center in the anterior fontanel. This is called an anterior fontanel bone (Girdany and Blank) and is of no clinical significance. The size and shape of the head is normal in such infants, and sutures are patent radiographically. Microcephaly is the most commonly discussed differential diagnostic consideration with craniosynostosis but is usually easily differentiated on the basis of physical examination of the child and x-ray examination of the skull. Whereas the size of the head is abnormally small in the microcephalic child, it is the configuration that is disturbed in most cases of craniosynostosis. Microcephaly is characterized on skull x-rays by a relatively thick calvarium in many instances, without convolutional markings and with sutures that are approximated or overlapped but without bony fusion, at least in the newborn period.

**TREATMENT.** Debate has long existed about the advisability of surgical correction for craniosynostosis, the optimal time of its performance, the age at which it is no longer beneficial, and whether it is totally for cosmetic reasons or if it is important in some cases to prevent visual loss, mental retardation or other neurologic deficits. To some degree, the confusion is attributed to observations made years ago when craniosynostosis and microcephaly were not clearly separated prior to attempts at surgical intervention. Although more recently certain authors have doubted the benefits of surgical treatment of craniosynostosis (Hemple, Freeman and Borkowf), the consensus of current opinion is that properly performed linear craniectomy is of definite value if done sufficiently early (Shillito and Matson, Anderson and Geiger, Andersson and Gomes).

For the best cosmetic results, surgical treatment of craniosynostosis is usually recommended when the infant is between 4 and 8 weeks of age. Severe cases with total suture fusion and secondary increased intracranial pressure are often attacked even earlier. When surgery has not been done for either sagittal, metopic or coronal syn-

**TABLE 80–1.   *Classification of Premature Cranial Suture Closure***

I. "Simple" craniosynostosis
   A. Scaphocephaly—premature closure of the sagittal suture
   B. Brachycephaly—premature closure of the coronal sutures
   C. Oxycephaly—premature closure of all cranial sutures
   D. Trigonocephaly—premature closure of the metopic suture
   E. Plagiocephaly—premature closure of one coronal or lambdoidal suture
II. Craniosynostosis with associated anomalies
   A. Crouzon's disease (craniofacial dysostosis). Premature closure of coronal or other sutures, beaked nose, maxillary hypoplasia, prognathism, exophthalmos
   B. Kleeblattschädel (cloverleaf skull). Multiple cranial suture synostosis with hydrocephalus. Facial dysostosis and long bone anomalies in some cases
   C. Apert's syndrome (acrocephalosyndactyly). Premature closure of coronal or other sutures, syndactylism
   D. Carpenter's syndrome (acrocephalopolysyndactyly). Acrocephaly, peculiar facies, brachysyndactyly of fingers, polysyndactyly of toes, mental retardation, other anomalies
   E. Chotzen's syndrome. Acrocephalosyndactyly with hypertelorism, ptosis, mental retardation
   F. Pfeiffer syndrome. Acrocephalosyndactyly with broad thumbs and great toes, normal intellect
   G. Trigonocephaly with hypotelorism, arhinencephaly
III. Secondary craniosynostosis
   A. Following shunts for hydrocephalus
   B. Early, passive sutural closure with microcephaly
   C. Associated with metabolic disease (rickets, idiopathic hypercalcemia of infancy, hypophosphatasia)

ostosis by age 12 to 18 months, it is not likely that much can be achieved cosmetically. It is unclear whether surgery beyond 1 year of age is indicated because of the possible future compromise of vision or development of increased pressure, but in some cases it is a consideration.

The accepted procedure for sagittal synostosis is bilateral parasagittal craniectomies and lining of the bony margins with some inert substance to prevent refusion of the edges. The procedure for a fused metopic suture is linear craniectomy through the suture itself in addition to establish-

ment of horizontal incisions of the frontal bone across each supraorbital region from the temporal end of the coronal suture to the midline, to allow expansion of the frontal bones. Fused coronal sutures are likewise attacked directly with bony excision at the site of the closed suture. When multiple synostosis is present, surgical correction is often staged, with the procedures done a week or more apart.

## MEGALENCEPHALY

Megalencephaly is a disorder in which the head is enlarged because of abnormal enlargement of the brain. It occurs under a wide variety of circumstances, sometimes present at birth but often not becoming evident until later in infancy. Megalencephaly is familial in some instances and can occur with or without other associated anomalies (Riley and Smith). Although it is frequently accompanied by developmental and mental retardation, hypotonia or convulsions, it can occur in the absence of any evident neurologic deficit. In the newborn or young infant, megalencephaly is difficult to differentiate from hydrocephalus by the clinical findings. Signs of increased intracranial pressure are not present, cranial sutures are not abnormally separated and the anterior fontanel is soft although frequently large. Ultrasound studies are needed in some cases in which the head continues to enlarge at a disproportionate rate. The ventricles in megalencephaly are normal in size or only slightly enlarged, while in hydrocephalus considerable ventricular expansion is expected. The recently developed technique of computerized axial tomography provides a safe and non-invasive method of determining lateral ventricular size. This procedure also is a useful tool in the diagnostic evaluation of the infant with an enlarged head. In the infant with head enlargement, demonstration of normal ventricles by this method usually eliminates the need for the more formidable air ventriculography study.

Megalencephaly occurs in several recognized syndromes, most of which are more applicable to the older infant or child than to the neonate. In the later stages of Tay-Sachs disease and Alexander's disease the brain often is significantly enlarged. In some cases of neurofibromatosis, head enlargement is explained on the basis of a large brain. In the newborn infant, megalencephaly may be associated with achondroplasia, cerebral gigantism or the degenerative disorder referred to as Canavan's disease. The Russell-Silver syndrome is a form of intrauterine growth retardation in which an abnormally large head is notably associated with a low birth weight (Szalay, Fuleihan et al.) (Fig. 80–6). The striking discrepancy between head size and body size of children with this disorder raises the consideration of hydrocephalus but the large head is the result of a relatively large brain. Other features often observed with the Russell-Silver syndrome include limb asymmetry, triangular shape of the face and elevated urinary gonadotropins.

# HYDROCEPHALUS

The term hydrocephalus encompasses a group of conditions associated with ventricular enlargement which, in most cases, is secondary to obstruction of the normal egress and flow of cerebrospinal fluid from its points of origin to its sites of absorption. In this context, hydrocephalus implies the presence of an increased quantity of cerebrospinal fluid under increased pressure, the latter being present either intermittently or persistently, and either currently or at some time in the past. Abnormal enlargement of the head often occurs when hydrocephalus begins prenatally, in the newborn period or in early childhood, but does not occur when the onset is in later childhood or the adult years.

Our current stage of knowledge indicates that in the vast majority of instances, hydrocephalus in humans results from obstruc-

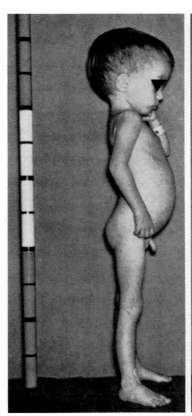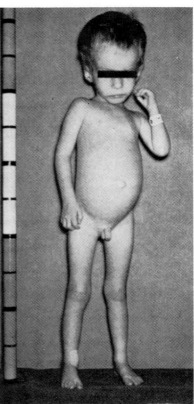

*Figure 80–6.* Abnormally large head compared to body size in a child with the Russell-Silver syndrome. Such children are often erroneously suspected of having hydrocephalus but can be identified appropriately by the low birth weight for gestational age and the characteristic facial features. Striking limb asymmetry is often present. (Szalay, G. C.: J. Pediatr. 63:622, 1963.)

tion at some point along the cerebrospinal fluid pathways. For this reason, the time-honored reference to intraventricular obstruction as "obstructive" hydrocephalus must be revised. Since virtually all hydrocephalus is obstructive, designations such as intraventricular obstructive (or non-communicating) and extraventricular obstructive (or communicating) convey greater meaning and avoid the confusion engendered by terms otherwise commonly used. Intraventricular obstructive, or non-communicating, hydrocephalus is most likely to be caused by abnormalities where the pathways are most narrow, including the aqueduct of Sylvius, the fourth ventricle or the foramina of Monro. Developmental anomalies, especially of the aqueduct, neoplasms, cystic lesions, aneurysms or ependymal changes secondary to infection or hemorrhage are the commonest causes of blocks within the ventricular system that lead to hydrocephalus.

Extraventricular obstructive hydrocephalus is synonymous with communicating hydrocephalus, an acceptable term that implies free communication of the ventricular system with the cervical subarachnoid space and to the region of the basilar cisterns. The term indicates that the obstruction is at some point distal to the outlet foramina of the fourth ventricle, usually at the level of the basilar cisterns, or within the arachnoid over the surface of the brain, or at the presumed absorptive site, the arachnoid villi.

The only recognized exception to the rule that hydrocephalus results from obstruction either within or without the ventricular system occurs with the rare choroid plexus papilloma. Ventricular enlargement in infants with this tumor is attributed to cerebrospinal fluid secretion from the lesion in excess of the systems' absorptive capabilities (Matson and Crofton). Although in many or even most cases, communicating hydrocephalus in patients with choroid plexus papillomas results from excessive fluid formation, hemorrhage from the lesion also may cause a basilar or arachnoid villi block, thus adding another causative factor (Laurence et al.).

**ETIOLOGIC AND PATHOLOGIC CONSIDERATIONS.** In a significant number of hy-drocephalic infants, lesions are identified which account for the condition even though their cause is unknown (Table 80–2). For example, neoplasms within the posterior fossa or of the choroid plexus, arachnoid cysts or aneurysms of the vein of Galen produce hydrocephalus by obvious mechanisms, although the etiology of the primary abnormality is not explainable. A posterior fossa subdural hematoma in the newborn results in fourth ventricle obstruction by compression and has its origin from hemorrhage secondary to head trauma. In a like manner, acquired hydrocephalus, usually of the communicating type, frequently is etiologically related to a preceding subarachnoid hemorrhage or meningeal infection. Intracranial bleeding may accompany birth trauma or be delayed for several days after perinatal hypoxia (Lourie and Berne). In either instance, block at the level of the basilar cisterns can lead to communicating hydrocephalus. By far the most common type of congenital hydrocephalus is that associated with other major anomalies, including meningomyelocele and encephalocele. Among 558 infants with hydrocephalus reviewed by Lorber

---

**TABLE 80–2.   *Classification and Types of Hydrocephalus***

Noncommunicating (intraventricular obstructive)
  1. Maldevelopments of the aqueduct
     stenosis
     forking ("atresia")
     septum
     gliosis
  2. Obstruction due to mass lesions (neoplasm, cyst, hematoma, aneurysm of the vein of Galen)
  3. Obstruction secondary to exudate, hemorrhage or parasites
  4. Obstruction of the fourth ventricle outlet foramina (Dandy-Walker, arachnoiditis)
Communicating (extraventricular obstructive)
  1. Postinfectious, posthemorrhagic or developmental adhesions of basilar cisterns or surface subarachnoid space
  2. Arachnoid villi obstruction by erythrocytes
  3. Communicating hydrocephalus with the Arnold-Chiari malformation
  4. Developmental failure of arachnoid villi (presumptive)
  5. Hypovitaminosis A (experimental animals)
Communicating hydrocephalus due to excessive cerebrospinal fluid formation (choroid plexus papilloma)

and Bassi, 478 had spina bifida cystica. Of the remainder, 67 with congenital hydrocephalus had no obvious cause and 41 were infants with acquired hydrocephalus secondary to hemorrhage or meningitis early in infancy. Hydrocephalus associated with meningomyelocele is often caused by aqueductal obstruction, although some are of the communicating type with disturbance of subarachnoid flow perhaps being secondary to the Arnold-Chiari malformation. Lorber (1961) found that 80 per cent of newborn infants with meningomyeloceles had associated hydrocephalus. Infants with lumbar myeloceles with paraplegia had a 96 per cent incidence of hydrocephalus. Hydrocephalus was usually demonstrable in the newborn period, and surgical repair of the meningomyelocele did not appear to influence the development or progression of hydrocephalus. In many babies in this series, Lorber demonstrated the presence of hydrocephalus even though the head circumference was normal.

Excluding the above categories of hydrocephalus secondary to an obvious compressive lesion, the etiology of many cases of congenital hydrocephalus or those appearing in early infancy remains unidentified. Infections, including toxoplasmosis, cytomegalovirus disease and syphilis, account for congenital hydrocephalus in a relatively small proportion of cases. Another small percentage of infants with hydrocephalus due to aqueductal stenosis inherit the disease as a sex-linked recessive trait (Bickers and Adams, Edwards et al., Needleman and Root). Except for the clustering of males within a family and the occasional maldevelopment of thumbs (Edwards et al., Warren et al.), this form of hydrocephalus is not distinguishable from many other types in the neonate. Genetic factors in congenital hydrocephalus otherwise remain speculative. Among siblings of patients with primary congenital hydrocephalus without spine defects, the incidence of anencephaly and spina bifida cystica has been estimated to be five times higher than expected in the general population (Lorber and De). The empirical risk of a major congenital malformation in subsequent offspring following birth of a child with congenital hydrocephalus is approximately 1 in 25 (Lorber and De).

The most common site of intraventricular obstruction in infants with congenital hydrocephalus is within the aqueduct. The underlying pathology may be one of several types, separable in most instances only by histologic examination. Forking ("atresia") of the aqueduct consists of a nonpatent system in which the aqueduct at various levels consists of multiple channels lined by ependyma which may or may not communicate with one another and which are separated by neural tissue. This lesion may occur as an isolated abnormality causing hydrocephalus or may be associated with other anomalies, especially meningomyelocele and the Arnold-Chiari malformation.

In stenosis of the aqueduct, the aqueduct is histologically normal but abnormally small in caliber. There is an absence of excessive subependymal glia or other evidence of an inflammatory reaction. Little is known of the origin of this disorder. It may represent a form of hydrocephalus which is slowly progressive or which may even remain silent until later in childhood. Gliosis of the aqueduct also has defied explanation as to its origin and may give rise to hydrocephalus in older children or even adults. The aqueduct is narrowed or occluded by overgrowth of subependymal glia, while the ependymal lining may be replaced by gliosis. No definite relation to preceding infection has been established in such cases. Neuroglial septum is another rare obstructive lesion of the aqueduct.

Of considerable interest in regard to the aqueductal lesions described above is the recent discovery of experimental viral infections as a cause of structural abnormalities of the aqueduct. Intracerebral injection of polyoma virus in rodents has produced hydrocephalus, but with a marked inflammatory reaction unlike the aqueductal lesions presumed to be maldevelopments (Li and Jahnes, Holtz et al.). Experimental hydrocephalus has also been produced in suckling hamsters by the inoculation of reovirus type I (Margolis and Kilham). Hydrocephalus due to aqueductal stenosis without inflammatory changes was induced in hamsters by intracerebral injection of mumps virus (Johnson and Johnson). Fluorescent antibody staining indicated that virus growth was limited to the ependymal cells in these animals. Timmons and Johnson subsequently described a child with mumps encephalitis followed by recovery but with manifestations of hydrocephalus developing almost 2 years later. Narrowing of the aqueduct was demonstrated by air encephalography and was presumed to be a sequela of the previous viral illness. Findings such as these suggest the possibility of intrauterine viral infection as a cause of some cases of congenital hydrocephalus with aqueductal occlusion.

The Dandy-Walker syndrome is an unusual form of hydrocephalus in the newborn infant. Although head enlargement with this condition may be obvious at birth, in some cases it does not become apparent until months later. Speculation continues in regard to the pathogenesis of this type of malformation, but most authors believe it is the result of prenatal lack of development or atresia of the outlet foramina of Luschka and Magendie. The end result is marked cystic distention of the fourth ventricle with lateral displacement of the cerebellar hemispheres. The vermis of the cerebellum is hypoplastic, being represented only by a thin sheet of tissue roofing the distended fourth ventricle. Other cerebral anomalies are seen in some cases, and include agenesis of the corpus callosum and porencephaly. The Dandy-Walker syndrome is suspected clinically in the infant with head enlargement in whom the greatest degree of enlargement is from the region of the external ears to the occiput. Diagnosis becomes more probable when an abnormal degree of transillumination is observed over the region of the posterior fossa but not elsewhere. X-rays of the skull of the older child with the Dandy-Walker syndrome reveal the characteristic elevated position of the transverse sinuses and the torcula but these structures cannot be visualized in the newborn infant.

**CLINICAL ASPECTS.** Symptoms and signs observed vary depending upon the age of the child, the acuteness of onset and the rapidity of progression. In the newborn period and in early infancy, there is a wide variation of clinical manifestations, depending in part on the rapidity of progression of the illness. Occasionally, the head of the hydrocephalic infant is so large at term that normal birth is impossible unless the head is decompressed by insertion of a needle into the ventricle. Most feel that birth by cesarean section is not justified because of dystocia due to fetal head enlargement. As a generalization, infants with intraventricular obstructive hydrocephalus show more rapid progression of head enlargement and other clinical signs than do those with communicating hydrocephalus. In some instances, the baby shows no abnormality of behavior, feeds well and progresses adequately in motor skills, with the only sign that a medical problem exists being the abnormally rapid rate of growth of the head. More often, the infant with congenital hydrocephalus is irritable, feeds poorly, has recurrent vomiting and shows inadequate weight gain. Seizures are not common in infants with hydrocephalus, and papilledema is infrequent, even in those with marked head enlargement. If the condition proceeds unarrested, optic atrophy may eventually develop. The infant with hydrocephalus resulting from aqueductal obstruction from compression by an aneurysm of the great vein of Galen may show signs largely due to high output cardiac failure. Heart failure in the absence of evidence of internal cardiac anomalies plus a loud bruit over the scalp are the clinical findings that suggest this unusual condition.

Developmental motor skills are occasionally delayed but some hydrocephalic infants progress in a remarkably normal fashion during the first year. Hydrocephalus of mild degree does not account for profound developmental delay by 6 to 12 months of age unless the retardation is due to the disorder that caused the hydrocephalus. As hydrocephalus progresses, the disproportion between head size and size of the facial structures becomes more apparent. Distention of scalp veins and enlargement and bulging of the anterior fontanel reflect elevated intracranial pressure. Increased muscle tone and hyperreflexia in the lower limbs have been attributed to stretching of fibers arising in the parasagittal area that must project around the angle of the lateral ventricle to enter the internal capsule en route to supply the legs (Yakovlev). These fibers could be affected earlier, with progressive ventricular enlargement, than the descending fibers to the upper limbs, which arise more laterally on the motor strip. Late signs in hydrocephalic infants include distortion of the orbital structures causing the "setting sun" sign and the "cerebral cry," characterized by its brevity and high-pitched, shrill quality. A variety of ocular signs can occur in the infant with congenital hydrocephalus, although lack of cooperation and irritability make analysis difficult. Internal strabismus is occasionally observed and limited vertical gaze may be present. Horizontal nystagmus also may be evident.

**DIAGNOSIS.** The most important aspect of the physical examination of an infant who is believed to have hydrocephalus is accurate measurement of the occipitofrontal circumference of the head. A single measurement is useful and may strongly point towards the existence of some form of disease state; however, serial determinations at periodic intervals with results plotted on a graph are often of greater value. Rate of change, especially precipitous change, of head size is frequently more informative than the results of any one particular measurement.

Transillumination of the skull should be performed whenever hydrocephalus is considered (Shurtleff). The procedure is performed in a darkened room, and the observer should delay until he is adequately dark adapted. A three-battery-powered flashlight with a soft rubber adapter that will permit sealed contact with the infant's scalp is sufficient. In the normal infant, extension of the glow beyond the rim of the light source does not occur more than 2.5 cm in the frontal region or 1 cm in the occipital region (Dodge and Porter). Abnormalities of transillumination in hydrocephalus indicate that the cerebral mantle is less than 1 cm in depth. In addition to advanced hydrocephalus or "hydranencephaly," abnormal transillumination may be observed in infants with subdural effusions, scalp edema or porencephaly. Arachnoid cysts over the convexity of the brain

may also be demonstrable by transillumination (Anderson and Landing). An infant with the Dandy-Walker syndrome may exhibit abnormal transillumination adjacent to the dilated fourth ventricle. Care must be taken not to overinterpret the findings with small premature infants, because of the extreme thinness of the skull overlying the subarachnoid space characteristic of such infants (Horner et al.).

A transfontanel tap of the lateral ventricle as an isolated procedure in an infant with an abnormally large head is usually not indicated, although exceptions do exist. As a general rule, if one is sufficiently concerned to do a ventricular tap, the child probably needs air ventriculography. Repeated needle passage through brain tissue may result in porencephalic cyst formation at the needle tract site secondary to damage to the parenchyma of the brain (Lorber and Emery). Rapid head enlargement in the infant of a few weeks of age who appears disproportionately ill may warrant examination of the ventricular fluid to eliminate the possibility of meningitis. Regardless of the circumstances, performance of ventricular taps should be done only by one knowledgeable and skillful at the procedure and only under aseptic conditions. During the study, the subdural spaces should be inspected to exclude fluid collections therein as a cause of infantile head enlargement.

Radiologic examination of the skull of the newborn or infant with hydrocephalus reveals enlarged head size and suture spread in most instances. The posterior fossa frequently is relatively small in those with hydrocephalus due to congenital aqueductal obstruction and is impressively enlarged when hydrocephalus is related to the Dandy-Walker syndrome. Congenital hydrocephalus secondary to toxoplasmosis may be associated with multiple and diffuse intracranial calcification. The infant with a meningomyelocele frequently has a honeycombed appearance to the calvarium, referred to as craniolacuna or lückenschadel. This pattern is temporary and does not resemble the increased digital markings observed in older children with increased intracranial pressure.

Definitive diagnosis, localization of the

site of obstruction and exclusion of a mass or compressive lesion are largely dependent on contrast procedures (Fig. 80–7). Each case must be individualized to determine which procedure, or combination of procedures, offers the most useful information with the lowest possible risk. Infants with marked head enlargement are usually studied with air ventriculography using sufficient air to exclude a choroid plexus papilloma but not so much that predisposes to collapse of the thinned cerebral mantle and massive intracranial bleeding. Proper positioning of the infant will permit movement of air into the third ventricle and aqueduct, the site of frequent obstructive lesions. When air does not visualize this region, 2 ml of Pantopaque may be injected into the lateral ventricle and subsequently moved to the aqueduct to demonstrate the precise level of obstruction. Positive contrast material should be resorted to only when necessary because of possible adverse effects on the ependyma.

Angiography is of greatest value when hydrocephalus is believed to be due to an aneurysm of the vein of Galen suspected from a cranial bruit plus high-output car-

diac failure. Angiographic features of aqueductal stenosis have been described by Huang et al. and include evidence of hydrocephalus such as bowing of the pericallosal artery and stretching, with depression of the posterior cerebral artery on the lateral view. The internal cerebral vein is flattened and depressed and its tributary vessels are elongated. In the posterior circulation, the superior cerebellar artery is displaced downward, while structures in the lower portion of the posterior fossa remain unaffected. Carotid angiography may also be required to distinguish the infant with so-called "hydranencephaly" and hugely dilated ventricular spaces from the infant with positive transillumination of the skull due to massive subdural collections of fluid, possibly secondary to intrauterine ventricular rupture.

In 1964, DiChiro reported a scanning technique for evaluation of the CSF dynamics, utilizing the intrathecal injection of radioiodinated serum albumin ($^{131}$RISA). The procedure has been called cisternography; however, isotope encephalography would seem to be more descriptive and subject to less misinterpretation. Various

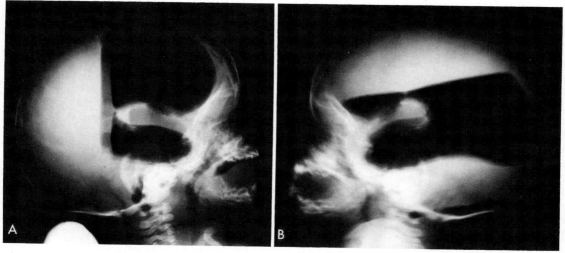

*Figure 80–7.* Congenital hydrocephalus, communicating (extraventricular obstructive) in type. Air ventriculogram. *A,* Brow up, lateral view reveals the markedly distended anterior portions of the frontal and temporal horns. Air is visualized in the distal part of the fourth ventricle extending through the foramen magnum, indicating that intraventricular obstruction is not present. *B,* Hanging head, lateral view. This projection allows the intraventricular air to move to visualize the posterior and inferior portions of the ventricular system. The aqueduct and fourth ventricle can sometimes be demonstrated by this method but did not occur in this case. Air in the occipital region is in the cisterna magna, indicating communication from the lateral ventricles to the outlet foramina of the fourth ventricle.

radiopharmaceuticals have been used for this purpose, and injection sites have included the lumbar theca, cisterna magna and the lateral ventricle. [131]RISA administered into the lumbar subarachnoid space remains the preferred approach by most investigators. Movement or position of the patient following lumbar injection does not seem to affect dispersion of the radiopharmaceutical. Following the instillation of the radioactive material into the lumbar subarachnoid space, scans of the head are made at periodic intervals, for example, at 2, 6, 24 and 72 hours. In the normal individual, radioactivity is detected in the basilar cisterns by 2 hours, in the sylvian fissures by 6 hours, and over the convexity of the brain by 12 to 24 hours after injection. Radioactivity is largely dissipated by 48 hours and ventricular collection of the radioactive material does not occur in the normal individual.

Although isotope encephalography has many useful purposes, it is of greatest value in patients with communicating hydrocephalus. In this condition, isotope injected into the lumbar subarachnoid space can be demonstrated within the enlarged ventricles, where it is retained in large quantity for 48 to 72 hours. When ventricular enlargement is secondary to primary cerebral atrophy, the isotope flow pattern follows normal pathways and lateral ventricular isotope collection either does not occur or is minimal.

In intraventricular obstructive hydrocephalus, no isotope enters the ventricular system after lumbar injection, and the flow pattern is normal unless an associated extraventricular block is present. The patency of a ventriculoatrial shunt can be assessed by intraventricular injection of the isotope (Glasauer et al.). Adequate shunt function is indicated by isotope movement in the ventricular fluid toward the shunt, followed by its rapid clearing from the ventricles. Shunt failure leads to prolonged ventricular stasis of radioactivity. In general, isotope encephalography has its greatest value in older individuals with so-called "occult" hydrocephalus and is of limited usefulness in the early infant period.

Computerized axial tomography utilizing the EMI scanner, a new diagnostic x-ray method of measuring the transmission of photons through tissue, has been developed in Great Britain by Ambrose and Hounsfield. The procedure is rapid and safe, and records cranial and intracranial structures of different densities, thus reliably demonstrating the size and configuration of the lateral ventricular system. The greatest value of the technique in the infant age group is in assessment of head enlargement and the visualization of the presence or absence of hydrocephalus (Fig. 80–8). When ventricular enlargement is demonstrated, the site of obstruction remains to be outlined by other methods. In certain instances, however, more hazardous air contrast studies can be eliminated when the EMI scan reveals normal ventricles in the infant suspected of hydrocephalus on the basis of borderline head enlargement.

**TREATMENT.** Despite remarkable advances in the comprehension of the physiology and pathology of hydrocephalus, our ability to provide consistently successful

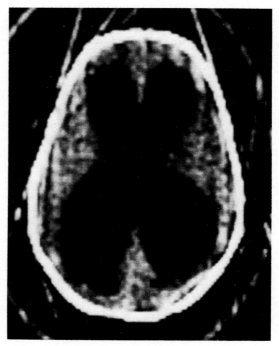

*Figure 80–8.* Computerized axial tomography (EMI scan). Advanced hydrocephalus in a 2-month-old infant. Horizontal plane with frontal portion of the skull at the top. The skull is dense white and the lateral ventricles, which are almost symmetrically distended, are black.

treatment has not yet been achieved. Medical therapy has offered relatively little, and the multiplicity of surgical procedures that have been developed stand in evidence of the lack of complete acceptance of any single approach. Although an attitude of total pessimism is unwarranted, the currently available surgical treatment of the infant with progressive hydrocephalus must be recognized to be less than ideal and to be characterized by a variety of potential frustrating and perplexing complications.

The desirability of surgical treatment for congenital hydrocephalus in which the cause cannot be removed requires consideration of the expected benefits from treatment compared to the natural course of the illness. Laurence and Coates (1962) studied 182 untreated cases collected over 20 years and found that 89 (48 per cent) had died and 81 (44 per cent) were considered to have arrested spontaneously. Of the "arrested" group, 38 per cent were judged to have IQ's of 85 or above. Yashon (1963) reported 58 patients with unoperated infantile hydrocephalus, 23 of whom had a fatal outcome. Of the survivors, 31 were considered "arrested." The concept of spontaneous arrest of infantile hydrocephalus, however, is subject to varied meanings depending on how the term is defined and what methods are used to demonstrate its occurrence. To have significance, arrest of hydrocephalus should mean that further growth of the head does not occur, at least until the rest of the body has caught up with the head size from the relative standpoint. Furthermore, arrest of the process should allow restoration of the ventricular size toward normal with re-establishment of the cerebral mantle. Assigning the designation of "arrested hydrocephalus" to a neurologically devastated child whose head has reached enormous proportions but then ceases to grow is artificial, is probably in error and dilutes the potential meaning of "significant arrest." If reasonably rigid criteria are adhered to, spontaneous and permanent arrest of progressive hydrocephalus in infancy appears to be an infrequent event (Foltz and Shurtleff, Lorber and Zachary). When comparing the outcome of untreated infantile hydrocephalus patients with those managed surgically, there is little doubt that the results are better in the treated group, in which the immediate success rate for control of hydrocephalus is in the range of 70 per cent (Yashon).

When surgical treatment of the infant or child with progressive hydrocephalus is necessary, the method selected depends on many factors, including the site of the obstruction, certain characteristics of the ventricular fluid and the experience with different procedures of the surgeon doing the operation. In some cases, procedures of a temporary nature are indicated when it is suspected that the more conventional shunt operations will be unsuccessful. For example, a child recovering from meningitis or subarachnoid hemorrhage complicated by communicating hydrocephalus can be maintained by the use of a ventriculostomy reservoir until a more permanent shunt can be inserted (Rickham and Penn). The high-protein-containing ventricular fluid often present in such cases will likely block the valves of the more permanent shunts, requiring repeated revisions. Regardless, treatment of infantile hydrocephalus must be assumed to be surgical in most cases because medical measures have not been adequate.

Surgical treatment of progressive hydrocephalus in infancy has included either the so-called "physiologic" operations of third ventriculostomy or choroid plexectomy, or the more commonly used shunting procedures. The first widely recognized shunting procedure for hydrocephalus was developed by Torkildsen in 1939 and is known as ventriculocisternostomy. The Torkildsen shunt drains fluid from one lateral ventricle to the cisterna magna, and thus its use is restricted to hydrocephalus of the non-communicating type. It remains of value for the older child or adult with an obstructive process in the posterior fossa but, for technical reasons, is not applicable to the infant. Shunts from the ventricle or spinal subarachnoid space to almost every conceivable body cavity have subsequently been designed. Most have now been abandoned except for the occasional use of a subarachnoid-ureteral shunt, the frequent use of the ventriculoperitoneal shunt, and the most popular ventriculoatrial (vascular) shunt.

Ventriculoperitoneal shunts are applicable to either communicating or non-communicating hydrocephalus but are plagued by the predisposition of the peritoneal end of the device to become repeatedly obstructed (Scott et al., Jackson and Snodgrass). Except for the need for periodic revision, the peritoneal shunts are far less often beset by late complications than are the vascular shunts. Numerous modifications have improved the outlook of the ventriculoperitoneal shunt, and some now prefer it to the ventriculoatrial shunt even though the need for revision remains great (Hammon).

Nulsen and Spitz introduced the Holter valve in 1952, and Pudenz et al. followed with the Heyer valve in 1957. In 1964, the Hakim valve was added as an additional system for vascular shunting. The development of these unidirectional valves paved the way for the use of the vascular system as a site for CSF shunting from the lateral ventricle. Until 1963, Scarff was able to find reports on 345 cases of hydrocephalus treated with ventriculoatrial shunts, with an operative mortality of 2 to 3 per cent and with an initial arrest of the process in 65 per cent. One of the major problems with all types of shunts used in the treatment of hydrocephalus has been obstruction of the catheter. This problem has been of special importance when the shunt is inserted in the small infant in whom linear growth eventually results in retraction of the distal end of the tube from its position in the right atrium. It is generally recognized that placement of the end of the tube or retraction of the end into the neck vessels will be followed by nonfunction within a short period of time. For this reason, periodic revision and lengthening of the tube is recommended by some. Bacterial infection with colonization of the valve remains the most important complication of vascular shunts, and is one of the main reasons why many now prefer peritoneal shunting in the newborn infant.

## "HYDRANENCEPHALY"

Cruveilhier is generally credited with the first description of what is now referred to as "hydranencephaly" although Crome and Sylvester claimed it had been recognized before. Spielmeyer subsequently introduced the term hydranencephaly.

Hydranencephaly is a purely descriptive designation which indicates that abnormal transillumination is observed if the patient is in the newborn or infant age group and is associated with enormous ventricular enlargement with little or no cerebral mantle (Fig. 80–9). The basal ganglia, brain stem and cerebellum are present in such patients but may reveal a variety of morphologic abnormalities. The causes, which are multiple, include any severe encephaloclastic insult that occurs in the prenatal period, during the birth process or even postnatally. A small number of such cases probably result from a severe developmental anomaly in which normal formation of the cerebral mantle has not occurred (Yakovlov and Wadsworth). Thus, hydranencephaly should not be considered a diagnostic entity but the end result of one of many destructive processes of the cerebrum. An additional source of confusion in previously reported cases has been the lack of differentiation of infants who exhibit abnormal transillumination because of profound ventricular distention, or "hydranencephaly," from those in whom the location of the massive fluid collection is in the subdural spaces. Although the clinical signs may be similar, this group is likely to show fewer physical abnormalities and to live longer, and may be assumed, from transfontanel air studies, to have "hydranencephaly" unless angiography or pneumoencephalography is performed. The cause of the fluid collections external to the brain is unknown and in the past was referred to as "external" hydrocephalus.

Many types of injuries to the immature brain have been suggested as causes of near-total to total cerebral hemisphere destruction, several of which have been well documented. Courville has emphasized the pathology of successive gradations of oxygen deprivation extending from minimal laminar cortical neuronal changes to virtual total hemisphere destruction from severe insults. Carotid vascular insufficiency has been suggested by some authors because of the sparing of portions of the inferior

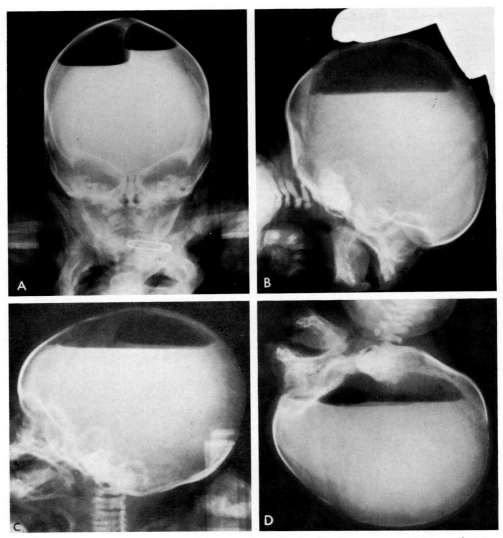

*Figure 80–9.* Hydranencephaly. Air ventriculography with the head in various positions showing virtual absence of the cerebral mantle. The head size is abnormally large for the facial structures, a finding in such children that usually indicates obstruction from one cause or another within the aqueduct.

temporal and occipital lobes. Muir commented that the carotid arteries were often hypoplastic in these patients but pointed out that involution of the vessels could be a secondary effect due to cerebral absence rather than as a causative factor. Lindenberg and Swanson described five infants with postnatal, acquired disorders in whom bilateral hemisphere destruction was attributed to arterial compression at the base of the skull from severe

brain swelling. In two cases, acute bacterial meningitis was the initiating illness, possibly also a factor leading to necrotizing cerebral changes.

The question of whether far-advanced hydrocephalus without an additional process affecting the brain can lead to the pattern referred to as "hydranencephaly" remains unanswered. Halsey et al. (1971) considered the possibility but could find no documented example. Many reported cases with encephaloclastic insults to the cerebral parenchyma have exhibited associated hydrocephalus, the latter most likely accelerating the injurious effect of the primary insult to the brain. That intraventricular or basilar cistern block should occur in such cases is not surprising, as rapid cerebral dissolution yields considerable foreign material into the ventricular system. Those who develop an obstructive factor, or hydrocephalus, are probably those with progressive head enlargement. The absence of associated hydrocephalus in patients with severe encephaloclastic insults gives rise to a picture with positive transillumination but with lack of head enlargement, and subsequently, an abnormally small head.

The clinical manifestations observed in infants with marked ventricular enlargement permitting transillumination are variable. Although children with these disorders may appear intact to the mother, careful examination by one familiar with neurologic activity of the neonate will reveal abnormalities in most. Abnormalities usually recognized include excessive sleepiness, or irritability manifested by continuous crying during the waking state. Feeding problems are usual, often because of lethargy and poor sucking ability. Tremulousness of limbs and increased muscle tone are frequently observed along with enhanced deep tendon reflexes. Nystagmus may be excessive, and optic atrophy is common. The normal neonatal reflexes, such as the grasp, Moro and stepping reflexes, can usually be elicited but become abnormal because of their persistence beyond the expected time of disappearance (Halsey et al., 1968). If the child survives beyond 2 or 3 months, expected developmental landmarks are not achieved and the evidence of spasticity becomes more apparent. Autonomic dysfunction is sometimes manifested by wide swings in body temperature, in part related to the environmental temperature (Appenzeller et al.). In most of these infants, electroencephalography reveals markedly depressed voltages or even a virtually flat tracing. Ventricular fluid may be clear and with a normal protein content, or xanthochromic with a marked increase in protein, again depending on the cause of the process.

Many infants with these disorders characterized by severe cerebral destruction die early in infancy while a few survive for remarkably long periods of time. Of 28 children with "hydranencephaly" reviewed by Hunziker, only nine survived beyond 3 months of age.

## CRANIUM BIFIDUM WITH ENCEPHALOCELE

Cranium bifidum, a congenital defect of the skull, is located at or near the midline in most cases and is analogous to the vertebral defect in spina bifida. It need not be, but almost always is, accompanied by protrusion of meningeal tissue, meningeal tissue containing glial elements, or variable amounts of brain tissue. These cranial defects with tissue herniations have been classified in various and complex fashion (Emery and Kalhan). A practical and simple classification is to consider those lesions containing only meningeal tissue or meningeal tissue and glial elements to be cranial meningoceles, and those harboring components of brain to be cranial encephaloceles. The incidence of the latter significantly exceeds that of the former. Approximately 75 to 80 per cent occur in the occipital region, and the remainder are parietal, frontonasal, intranasal or in the nasopharyngeal region.

CLINICAL ASPECTS. Cranium bifidum with occipital encephalocele affects girls more than boys (Guthkelch). Although the cranial lesion may be the only abnormality, a significant number of cases will be associated with other defects, such as meningomyelocele, midline facial clefts, deformities of the extremities or congenital heart disease. Unless the encephalocele is small and covered by hair it is readily apparent at birth in the form of a soft, round, midline mass which is usually partially or totally covered by skin and which varies in size from a centimeter in diameter up to two or three times the circumference of the infant's head (Fig. 80–10). The head size of the neonate with occipital encephalocele is normal in some cases; however, in others microcephaly is present initially, and hydrocephalus subsequently develops.

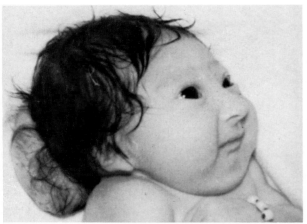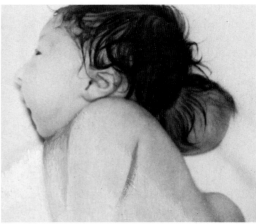

*Figure 80–10.* Occipital meningoencephalocele. The sloping forehead and small head circumference are evident, although progressive ventricular enlargement often subsequently occurs in such children.

A frontonasal encephalocele presents as a rounded mass at the base of the nose, usually associated with widening of the nasal root and separation of the eyes. Basal encephaloceles, including the intranasal and nasopharyngeal types, differ from the above, more common, types in that there is no visible external mass, and thus diagnosis is not usually established until later in childhood or even until adulthood (Pollock et al.). The intranasal (transethmoidal) encephalocele is accompanied by a widened nasal root and increased intraocular distance but does not ordinarily become symptomatic until the occurrence of nasal obstruction, epistaxis or recurrent episodes of bacterial meningitis (Blumenfeld and Skolnik). Less common types of basal encephaloceles are located in the nasopharynx, sphenoid sinus or posterior orbit, and likewise are not usually identified in the infant age group (Pollock et al.).

**DIAGNOSIS.** Occipital and parietal encephaloceles are quickly identified in the newborn infant by the character of the lesion and the common but not invariable roentgenographic demonstration of the associated skull defect (Fig. 80–11). Transillumination of the lesion is of some diagnostic value in certain cases, and ventriculography before and after surgical repair provides information about associated cerebral anomalies and the presence and degree of hydrocephalus.

Frontonasal encephalocele must be differentiated from the so-called nasal "glioma" and dermoids or teratomas in the same region. Pulsation of the mass is suggestive of an encephalocele but is not usually present. Bulging of the lesion with temporary bilateral jugular vein compression also would suggest its communication with the subarachnoid space but this sign is also not entirely reliable. In many in-

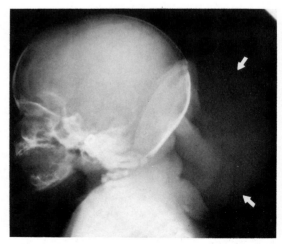

*Figure 80–11.* Occipital meningoencephalocele, lateral skull x-ray. The large extracranial sac containing meningeal and brain tissue is outlined by white arrows. Surgical excision of the lesion was followed by progressive hydrocephalus which required a shunting procedure.

stances a precise diagnosis is not available until histologic examination following surgical removal. Intranasal encephalocele should be suspected when an intranasal mass is identified in the child or adult who has a broad nasal bridge and wide-set eyes. It should also be considered in any child who has unexplained recurrent meningitis. This lesion is occasionally biopsied, the preoperative assumption being that it represents a polyp. Specimens obtained from the nasal cavity by biopsy should be submitted for histologic examination, because if not diagnosed, a biopsied encephalocele is likely to lead to cerebrospinal fluid rhinorrhea and subsequent meningitis. Appropriate x-rays, and especially tomography, are of great importance in the diagnosis of basal encephaloceles, regardless of their location (Pollock et al.).

**TREATMENT.** Whenever possible, an encephalocele should be surgically removed early in life. Hydrocephalus complicates surgical repair in a significant number of cases and is handled by some form of shunt procedure when it occurs. Certain cases must be managed conservatively when the head is distinctly small and the sac contains large amounts of brain tissue, especially if the contained brain includes brain stem or cervical spinal cord elements. Prognosis that the infant will survive, that hydrocephalus will not develop or that mental retardation will not eventually appear is far better for those with meningoceles and considerably worse when the lesion contains brain tissue (Lorber, Mealey et al.).

## CASE HISTORIES

### CASE 80–1

(Abstracted with the permission of Dr. R. M. N. Crosby of Baltimore.)

A white female infant was born at the Hospital for Women of Maryland after a normal pregnancy and labor. The mother had had three prior miscarriages. The baby breathed and cried spontaneously. She had a 3- to 4-cm occipital encephalocele, which was pedunculated and completely covered by skin. On the sixth day this was surgically removed. The sac contained meninges and heterotopic neural tissue. Thereafter, the head began to enlarge. Air study showed no filling of the fourth ventricle or aqueduct of Sylvius. At 18 days, operative cure was attempted, but the operation had to be cut

short because of anesthetic difficulties. Nevertheless, a small hole was torn in the anterior third ventricle prior to hasty closure. The head circumference diminished in the next 11 days from 35.5 to 34.0 cm. After 1 month at home the head again began to enlarge. A third ventriculostomy was done, and this too was unsuccessful. At the age of 3 months a ventriculoureterostomy was performed and was followed by arrest of hydrocephalus. At 6 months the head circumference was 44 cm; the fontanel was 3 cm across and was depressed. She was found to be developmentally normal at this time. At 11 months she was obese, could sit and vocalized a great deal and her head measured only 45 cm. At 1 year meningitis developed, which responded to antibiotic therapy. She had been receiving the usual addition of 1 gm of salt in her diet ever since the shunt had been made. At last report she was a normal, intelligent 2 year old.

**COMMENT.** This example indicates the need for optimism and perseverance despite recurrent complications of therapeutic efforts. This baby was terribly important to the parents, whose three prior products of conception had been miscarried. The encephalocele was removed, and the subsequent hydrocephalus, in this instance probably a part of the original congenital malformation rather than a sequela, was treated vigorously. The result has repaid many times over the anguish of the baby's early months.

### CASE 80–2

A white female infant weighed 6 pounds 12 ounces (3060 gm) at birth. Length was 49.5 cm, head circumference 34.3 cm. A marble-sized swelling was noted to the nasal side of the canthus of the right eye, which felt firm but cystic. The right side of the nose seemed obstructed. A tentative diagnosis of dermoid cyst was entertained. The swelling did not change in size, but at 4 months there was a polyp-like mass high in the right nasal cavity from which seeped a watery discharge. At this time an x-ray film of the skull showed "just to the right of the midline in the region of the glabella a faint linear translucency approximately 3 mm wide by 5 mm long, extending laterally and downward from the midline. This may represent defect of the bone structure." Biopsy of the nasal mass revealed "normal nervous tissue." At the age of 5 months a right frontal craniotomy was done and a slender stalk could be seen extending from the inferior medial surface of the frontal pole through the cranial defect. This was divided, and the bony defect was plugged with bone wax. Nasal discharge ceased, and the external mass did not change, but the nasal mass shrank somewhat at first. At 17 months the nasal and external masses were resected. When last seen at 5 years of age, the infant was completely well and normal in all respects.

**COMMENT.** This frontobasal encephalocele presented as a cystic mass between the root of the nose and the eye and, later, as a polyp-like mass high in the nose on the same side. X-ray film showed the bone defect through which the stalk emerged. Fortunately it consisted only of meninges and heterotopic neural tissue, so that its removal was attended by no loss in function.

# REFERENCES

Alter, M.: Anencephalus, hydrocephalus, and spina bifida. Arch. Neurol. 7:411, 1962.

Anderson, F. M., and Geiger, L.: Craniosynostosis. A survey of 204 cases. J. Neurosurg. 22:229, 1965.

Anderson, F. M., and Landing, B. H.: Cerebral arachnoid cysts in infants. J. Pediatr. 69:88, 1966.

Anderson, F. M., Gwinn, J. L., and Todt, J. C.: Trigonocephaly. Identity and surgical treatment. J. Neurosurg. 19:723, 1962.

Andersson, H., and Gomes, S. P.: Craniosynostosis. Review of the literature and indications for surgery. Acta Pediat. Scand. 57:47, 1968.

Angle, C. R., McIntire, M. S., and Moore, R. C.: Cloverleaf skull: Kleeblattschädel-deformity syndrome. Am. J. Dis. Child. 114:198, 1967.

Appenzeller, O., Snyder, R., and Kornfeld, M.: Autonomic failure in hydrencephaly. J. Neurol. Neurosurg. Psychiat. 33:532, 1970.

Avery, G. B., Meneses, L., and Lodge, A.: The clinical significance of "measurement microcephaly." Am. J. Dis. Child. 123:214, 1972.

Bickers, D. S., and Adams, R. D.: Hereditary stenosis of the aqueduct of Sylvius as a cause of hydrocephalus. Brain 72:246, 1949.

Blumenfeld, R., and Skolnik, E. M.: Intranasal encephaloceles. Arch. Otolaryngol. 82:527, 1965.

Brock, D. J. H., Bolton, A. E., and Scrimgeour, J. B.: Prenatal diagnosis of spina bifida and anencephaly through maternal plasma-alpha-fetoprotein measurement. Lancet 1:765, 1974.

Brock, D. J. H., and Sutcliffe, R. G.: Alpha-fetoprotein in the antenatal diagnosis of anencephaly and spina bifida. Lancet 2:197, 1972.

Carter, C. O., and Roberts, J. A. F.: The risk of recurrence after two children with central nervous system malformations. Lancet 1:306, 1967.

Coffey, V. P., and Jessop, W. J. E.: A study of 137 cases of anencephaly. Brit. J. Prev. Soc. Med. 11:174, 1957.

Courville, C. B.: Etiology and pathogenesis of laminar cortical necrosis. Arch. Neurol. Psychiat. 79:7, 1958.

Crome, L., and Sylvester, P. E.: Hydranencephaly (hydrencephaly). Arch. Dis. Child. 33:235, 1958.

Cruveilhier, J.: Anatomie Pathologique du Corps Humain. Vol. 2, Paris, Bailliere, 1929.

Currarino, G., and Silverman, F. N.: Orbital hypotelorism, arhinencephaly, and trigonocephaly. Radiology 74:206, 1960.

DiChiro, G.: New radiographic and isotopic procedures in neurosurgical diagnosis. J.A.M.A. 188:524, 1964.

Dodge, H. W., Wood, M. W., and Kennedy, R. L. J.: Craniofacial dysostosis: Crouzon's disease. Pediatrics 23:98, 1959.

Dodge, P. R., and Porter, P.: Demonstration of intracranial pathology by transillumination. Arch. Neurol. 5:594, 1961.

Edwards, J. H., Norman, R. M., and Roberts, J. M.: Sex-linked hydrocephalus: report of a family with 15 affected members. Arch. Dis. Child. 36:481, 1961.

Emery, J. L., and Kalhan, S. C.: The pathology of exencephalus. Develop. Med. Child Neurol. 12:(Suppl.) 22:51, 1970.

Feingold, M., O'Connor, J. F., Berkman, M., and Darling, D. B.: Kleeblattschädel syndrome. Am. J. Dis. Child. 118:589, 1969.

Fisch, R. O., Doeden, D., Lansky, L. L., and Anderson, J. A.: Maternal phenylketonuria. Detrimental effects on embryogenesis and fetal development. Am. J. Dis. Child. 118:847, 1969.

Foltz, E. L., and Shurtleff, D. B.: Five-year comparative study of hydrocephalus in children with and without operation (113 cases). J. Neurosurg. 20:1064, 1963.

Frankenburg, W. K., Duncan, B. R., Coffelt, R. W., Koch, R., Coldwell, J. G., and Son, C. D.: Maternal phenylketonuria: Implications for growth and development. J. Pediatr. 73:560, 1968.

Freeman, J. M., and Borkowf, S.: Craniostenosis. Review of the literature and report of thirty-four cases. Pediatrics 30:57, 1962.

Fuleihan, D. S., Der Kaloustian, V. M., and Najjar, S. S.: The Russell-Silver syndrome. Report of three siblings. J. Pediatr. 78:654, 1971.

Girdany, B. R., and Blank, E.: Anterior fontanel bone. Am. J. Roentgenol. 95:148, 1965.

Glasauer, F. E., Alker, G. J., Jr., and Leslie, E. B.: Isotope cisternography and ventriculography. Evaluation of hydrocephalus in children. Am. J. Dis. Child. 120:109, 1970.

Guthkelch, A. N.: Occipital cranium bifidum. Arch. Dis. Child. 45:104, 1970.

Hall, B. D., Smith, D. W., and Shiller, J. G.: Kleeblattschädel (cloverleaf) syndrome: Severe form of Crouzon's disease? J. Pediatr. 80:526, 1972.

Halsey, J. H., Jr., Allen, N., and Chamberlin, H. R.: Chronic decerebrate state in infancy. Neurologic observations in long surviving cases of hydranencephaly. Arch. Neurol. 19:339, 1968.

Halsey, J. H., Jr., Allen, N., and Chamberlin, H. R.: The morphogenesis of hydranencephaly. J. Neurol. Sci. 12:187, 1971.

Hammon, W. H.: Evaluation and use of the ventriculo-peritoneal shunt in hydrocephalus. J. Neurosurg. 34:792, 1971.

Hemple, D. J., Harris, L. E., Svien, H. J., and Holman, C. B.: Craniosynostosis involving the sagittal suture only: Guilt by association? J. Pediatr. 58:342, 1961.

Holtz, A., Borman, G., and Li, C. P.: Hydrocephalus in mice infected with polyoma virus. Proc. Soc. Exper. Biol. Med. 121:1196, 1966.

Horner, F. A., Webb, N. C., Jr., and Welch, K.: Diag-

nosis of collection of subdural fluid by transillumination. (Abstr.) Am. J. Dis. Child. 96:594, 1958.

Huang, Y. P., Wolf, B. S., Antin, S. P., Okudera, T.,
and Kim, I. H.: Angiographic features of aqueductal
stenosis. Am. J. Roentgenol. 104:90, 1968.

Hunziker, K.: Uber einen fall von Hydranencephalie.
Mschr. Psychiat. Neurol. 114:129, 1974.

Ingraham, F. E., Alexander, E., and Matson, D. D.:
Clinical studies in craniosynostosis: Analysis of fifty
cases and description of a method of surgical treatment. Surgery 24:518, 1948.

Jackson, I. J., and Snodgrass, W.: Peritoneal shunts in
the treatment of hydrocephalus, 4 year study of 62
patients. J. Neurosurg. 12:216, 1955.

Johnson, R. T., and Johnson, K. P.: Hydrocephalus following viral infection. The pathology of aqueductal
stenosis developing after experimental mumps virus
infection. J. Neuropath. Exper. Neurol. 27:591,
1968.

Laurence, K. M., and Coates, S.: The natural history of
hydrocephalus. Detailed analysis of 182 unoperated
cases. Arch. Dis. Child. 37:345, 1962.

Laurence, K. M., Hoare, R. D., and Till, K.: The diagnosis of the choroid plexus papilloma of the lateral
ventricle. Brain 84:628, 1961.

Li, C. P., and Jahnes, W. G.: Hydrocephalus in suckling mice inoculated with SE polyoma virus. Virology 9:489, 1959.

Lindenberg, R., and Swanson, P. D.: "Infantile hydranencephaly"—a report of five cases of infarction
of both cerebral hemispheres in infancy. Brain
90:839, 1967.

Lorber, J.: Systematic ventriculographic studies in infants born with meningomyelocele and encephalocele. The incidence and development of hydrocephalus. Arch. Dis. Child. 36:381, 1961.

Lorber, J.: The prognosis of occipital encephalocele.
Develop. Med. Child Neurol. 9:(Suppl. 12):75,
1967.

Lorber, J., and Bassi, U.: The etiology of neonatal
hydrocephalus. Develop. Med. Child Neurol. 7:289,
1965.

Lorber, J., and De, N. C.: Family history of congenital
hydrocephalus. Develop. Med. Child Neurol.
12:(Suppl. 22) 94, 1970.

Lorber, J., and Emery, J. L.: Intracerebral cysts complicating ventricular needling in hydrocephalic infants. A clinico-pathologic study. Develop. Med.
Child Neurol. 6:125, 1964.

Lorber, J., and Zachary, R. B.: Primary congenital
hydrocephalus. Arch. Dis. Child. 43:516, 1968.

Lourie, H., and Berne, A. S.: A contribution on the etiology and pathogenesis of congenital communicating hydrocephalus. Neurology 15:815, 1965.

Lubchenco, L. O., Hansman, C., and Boyd, E.: Intrauterine growth in length and head circumference as
estimated from live births at gestational ages from
26 to 42 weeks. Pediatrics 37:403, 1966.

Margolis, G., and Kilham, L.: Experimental virus-in-
duced hydrocephalus. J. Neurosurg. 31:1, 1969.

Martin, H. P.: Microcephaly and mental retardation.
Am. J. Dis. Child. 119:128, 1970.

Matson, D. D., and Crofton, F. D. L.: Papilloma of the
choroid plexus in childhood. J. Neurosurg. 17:1002,
1960.

Mealey, J., Jr., Dzenitis, A. J., and Hockey, A. A.: The

prognosis of encephaloceles. J. Neurosurg. 32:209,
1970.

Miller, J. Q.: Lissencephaly in 2 siblings. Neurology
13:841, 1963.

Milunsky, A., and Alpert, E.: The value of alpha-fetoprotein in the prenatal diagnosis of neural tube
defects. J. Pediatr. 84:889, 1974.

Muir, C. S.: Hydranencephaly and allied disorders.
Arch. Dis. Child. 34:231, 1959.

Nakano, K. K.: Anencephaly: A review. Develop.
Med. Child Neurol. 15:383, 1973.

Needleman, H. L., and Root, A. W.: Sex-linked hydrocephalus. Pediatrics 31:396, 1963.

Nellhaus, G.: Head circumference from birth to eighteen years. Pediatrics 41:106, 1968.

Nulsen, F. E., and Spitz, E. B.: Treatment of hydrocephalus by direct shunt from ventricle to jugular
vein. Surg. Forum 2:399, 1952.

Padget, D. H.: Neuroschisis and human embryonic
maldevelopment. J. Neuropath. Exper. Neurol.
29:192, 1970.

Partington, M. W., Gonzales-Crussi, F., Khakee, S. G.,
and Wollin, D. G.: Cloverleaf skull and thanatophoric dwarfism. Arch. Dis. Child. 47:656, 1971.

Plummer, G.: Anomalies occurring in children exposed in utero to the atomic bomb in Hiroshima.
Pediatrics 10:687, 1952.

Pollock, J. A., Newton, T. H., and Hoyt, W. F.: Trans-
sphenoidal and transethmoidal encephaloceles. Radiology 90:442, 1968.

Pudenz, R. H., Russell, F. E., Hurd, A. H., and Shel-
den, C. H.: Ventriculo-auriculostomy. A technique
for shunting cerebrospinal fluid into the right auri-
cle. J. Neurosurg. 14:171, 1957.

Reilly, B. J., Leeming, J. M., and Fraser, D.: Craniosynostosis in the rachitic spectrum. J. Pediatr.
64:396, 1964.

Richman, D. P., Stewart, R. M., and Caviness, V. S.,
Jr.: Cerebral microgyria in a 27-week fetus: An
architectonic and topographic analysis. J. Neuropath. Exper. Neurol. 33:374, 1974.

Rickham, P. P., and Penn, I. A.: The place of the ventriculostomy reservoir in the treatment of myelo-
meningocoeles and hydrocephalus. Develop. Med.
Child Neurol. 7:296, 1965.

Riley, H. D., Jr., and Smith, W. R.: Macrocephaly,
pseudopapilledema and multiple hemangiomata.
Pediatrics 26:293, 1960.

Scarff, J. E.: Treatment of hydrocephalus: An historical and critical review of methods and results. J.
Neurol. Neurosurg. Psychiat. 26:1, 1963.

Scott, M., Wycis, H. T., Murtagh, F., and Reyes, U.:
Observations on ventricular and lumbar subarach-
noid peritoneal shunts in hydrocephalus in infants.
J. Neurosurg. 12:165, 1955.

Shiller, J. G.: Craniofacial dysostosis of Crouzon. Pediatrics 23:107, 1959.

Shillito, J., Jr., and Matson, D. D.: Craniostenosis: A
review of 519 surgical patients. Pediatrics 41:229,
1968.

Shurtleff, D. B.: Transillumination of skull in infants
and children. Am. J. Dis. Child. 107:14, 1964.

Spielmeyer, W.: Ein Hydranencephales zwillingspaar.
Arch. Psychiat. Nervenkr. 39:807, 1904-1905.

Szalay, G. C.: Pseudohydrocephalus in dwarfs: The
Russell dwarf. J. Pediatr. 63:622, 1963.

Timmons, G. D., and Johnson, K. P.: Aqueductal stenosis and hydrocephalus after mumps encephalitis. N. Engl. J. Med. *283*:1505, 1970.

Toop, J., Webb, J. N., and Emery, A. E. H.: Muscle differentiation in anencephaly. Develop. Med. Child Neurol. *15*:164, 1973.

Torkildsen, A.: A new palliative operation in cases of inoperative occlusion of the Sylvian aqueduct. Acta Chir. Scand. *82*:117, 1939.

Virchow, R.: Ueber den Cretinismus, namentlich in franken, und uber pathologische Schadelformen. Verh. phys-med. Ges Wurzburg *2*:230, 1851.

Vogel, F. S.: The anatomic character of the vascular anomalies associated with anencephaly, with consideration of the role of abnormal angiogenesis in the pathogenesis of cerebral malformation. Am. J. Path. *39*:163, 1961.

Wald, N. J., Brock, D. J. H., and Bonnar, J.: Prenatal diagnosis of spina bifida and anencephaly by maternal serum-alpha-fetoprotein measurement. Lancet *1*:765, 1974.

Warren, M. C., Lu, A. T., and Ziering, W. H.: Sex-linked hydrocephalus with aqueductal stenosis. J. Pediatr. *63*:1104, 1963.

Yakovlev, P. I.: Paraplegias of hydrocephalus (clinical note and interpretation). Am. J. Ment. Defic. *51*:561, 1947.

Yakovlev, P., and Wadsworth, R. C.: Schizencephalies. A study of the congenital clefts in the cerebral mantle. Part I. J. Neuropath. Exper. Neurol. *5*:116, 1946.

Yashon, D.: Prognosis in infantile hydrocephalus. J. Neurosurg. *20*:105, 1963.

Yashon, D., Jane, J. A., and Sugar, O.: The course of severe untreated infantile hydrocephalus. J. Neurosurg. *23*:509, 1965.

# 81

# SEIZURES IN THE NEWBORN INFANT

*By William E. Bell*

Seizures in the newborn infant differ from those in the older child in that an etiologic cause can be identified with much greater frequency in the very young. In most instances, the possible underlying cause, rather than the danger of the seizure itself, represents a medically emergent situation. Another difference in seizures in the neonate compared to those in his older counterpart is the spectrum of clinical patterns observed. The newborn infant rarely exhibits a convulsion manifested by an initial tonic phase followed by generalized clonic movements, and can exhibit neither petit mal nor psychomotor seizures, such as occur later in childhood. The most common type of seizure in the newborn infant has been referred to as "fragmentary" (Rose and Lombroso) or multifocal clonic (Volpe), consisting of asymmetrical clonic jerking or shifting clonic movements which migrate from limb to limb in nonordered fashion. Strictly focal seizures involving one or both limbs on one side of the body are also common and occur with generalized cerebral insults, including metabolic disturbances.

Generalized tonic seizures resembling episodes of decerebrate rigidity can also occur in the neonate. An irregular respiratory pattern, an ocular deviation, or pupillary abnormalities will usually accompany the postural disturbance of this seizure type, which often reflects severe underlying brain disease with poor prognostic implications. Other seizure manifestations in the neonate, and especially in the premature newborn infant, are much more subtle than the above and it is difficult to recognize that they are seizural. Abrupt changes in the respiratory pattern or even apneic spells are examples, but are usually associated with deviation of the eyes, transient nystagmus, chewing-like movements or brief twitching of the distal parts of an extremity.

Episodic disturbances that must be differentiated from convulsive activity in the newborn child include "jitteriness," which differs from seizures in its tendency to be provoked or enhanced by tactile stimulation and its precipitation by placing body parts in certain positions. The intensely spastic infant may be erroneously assumed to be convulsing when clonus is provoked by certain exogenous stimuli. Such movements in the hypertonic child can usually be promptly stopped by altering the limb position, a maneuver not usually effective when movements are seizural in type.

Comments regarding prognosis of the infant with seizures have little meaning unless one considers etiologic subgroups. In other words, the eventual outcome is heavily determined by the nature of the underlying brain disease or systemic disorder that causes the child to convulse. Seizures due to hypocalcemia beginning 5 to 10 days after birth in an otherwise normal infant should have an excellent outcome, but seizure in an asphyxiated premature baby with intraventricular bleeding is likely to be followed by significant sequelae, and possibly death. Rose and Lombroso showed that the electroencephalogram can provide some prognostic information, regardless of the cause of neonatal seizures. In their study, neonates with seizures with a normal EEG had an 86 per cent chance of normal development by age 4 years, while those with significant EEG abnormalities of certain types had only a 7 per cent chance of normal development.

**ETIOLOGIC FACTORS.** Although there are many possible causes of seizures in the newborn infant, most cases are the result of one of a relatively few disorders (Table 81-1). The most common identifiable causes include anoxic-ischemic encephalopathy secondary to perinatal complications, hypocalcemia, hypoglycemia and infections of various types (Freeman). The single most common explanation for neonatal seizures in past years was some form of cerebral injury associated with the labor and delivery process. In recent years, certain series have revealed that metabolic disturbances, especially hypocalcemia, represent the most frequent etiologic factor. In a significant percentage of cases in which seizures occur in the neonatal period no definite etiologic factors become evident and the cause remains undetermined.

Perinatal complications associated with hypoxic and ischemic insults to the brain are much more important than traumatic injuries in the production of seizures in the newborn infant. Seizures are most com-

**TABLE 81–1.  Etiologic Factors in Neonatal Seizures**

| |
|---|
| Perinatal injuries |
| Metabolic |
|   Hypocalcemia |
|   Hypoglycemia |
|   Hypomagnesemia |
|   Hyponatremia, hypernatremia |
|   Aminoacidurias |
|   Pyridoxine dependency |
|   Hyperviscosity |
|   Hyperbilirubinemia |
| Infection |
|   Bacterial sepsis — meningitis |
|   Neonatal tetanus |
|   Encephalitis |
|     Herpes simplex |
|     Cytomegalovirus |
|     Rubella |
|     Coxsackie, ECHO |
|     Toxoplasmosis |
| Developmental anomalies |
|   Congenital cerebral malformations |
|   Sturge-Weber syndrome |
|   Incontinentia pigmenti |
| Drug related |
|   Drug withdrawal |
|     Narcotics |
|     Alcohol |
|     Barbiturates |
|   Mepivacaine injection into fetal scalp |
| Familial neonatal seizures |
| Congenital cerebral neoplasms |

mon in the first 2 or 3 days after birth in this group and are usually associated with other interictal abnormalities such as "jitteriness," hypertonicity, hypotonicity or lethargy. Seizures in the infant with a congenital cerebral malformation may be difficult to distinguish diagnostically from those caused by perinatal damage, partly because infants with cerebral anomalies sometimes exhibit distress during or just after delivery. Numerous types of malformations of the brain may be associated with neonatal seizures. Diagnosis is suspected on the basis of abnormalities of the head size or the presence of other, evident anomalies.

There are numerous metabolic disorders that give rise to seizures in the newborn infant, the most frequent being hypocalcemia. Hypocalcemia of "early onset," occurring during the first 2 or 3 days after birth, is observed in the infant of low birth weight for gestational age, associated with perinatal complications, in infants of diabetic mothers, and in a variety of other stress situations. The reduced serum calcium in such infants may cause or contribute to the occurrence of convulsions; however, in some infants, correction of the calcium deficit does not alleviate the neurologic abnormalities. Hypocalcemia of "late onset" occurs late in the first week or early in the second week after birth and is usually attributed to the phosphate load in feedings in the presence of relative parathyroid and renal immaturity. Seizures due to this are rapidly abolished by elevation of the serum calcium level. It is important to remember that neonatal hypocalcemia that proves to be resistant to therapy may be secondary to maternal hyperparathyroidism (Mizrahi and Gold, Hartenstein and Gardner), idiopathic neonatal hypoparathyroidism (Smith and Zike) or the DiGeorge syndrome, in which congenital absence of the parathyroid and thymus glands is associated with other anomalies (Kretschmer et al.). Another curious and poorly understood disorder occurs in neonatal hypocalcemia that responds poorly to supplemental calcium: the reduction of this ion secondary to primary hypomagnesemia (Paunier et al., Vainsel et al.). Tetany, convulsions and hypocalcemia characterize this condition; however, the reduced serum calcium cannot be successfully corrected until the deficiency of serum magnesium is eliminated (Davis et al.). Seizures may occur in the neonatal period with this disorder but can be delayed in onset for several months after birth.

Neonatal hypoglycemia is another important metabolic cause of seizures as well as other abnormal neurologic signs. Hypoglycemia in the neonate is diagnosed when glucose levels are less than 30 mg per 100 ml in the full term infant and less than 20 mg per 100 ml in the premature child. The infant of a diabetic mother, the infant stressed during parturition or in the newborn period and the newborn infant with hyperviscosity are all susceptible to hypoglycemia, which may precipitate convulsions. Organic hyperinsulinism caused by such lesions as islet cell hyperplasia or islet cell

tumors have been described in the neonate but are rare. Additional metabolic causes of neonatal seizures include hyponatremia, hypernatremia, various aminoacidurias and polycythemia with hyperviscosity (Gross et al., Wood). Hyponatremia in the newborn infant can be caused by excessive administration of salt-free fluids to the mother during labor or to the child after birth. It may also occur as the result of inappropriate secretion of antidiuretic hormone, resulting in water retention, or increased salt loss secondary to diarrhea. Neonatal hypernatremia has followed accidental substitution of salt for sugar in infant feedings and has occurred with severe diarrhea. A number of genetically determined aminoacidurias are associated with neonatal seizures but those with hyperammonemia and metabolic acidosis are the most widely recognized (Berenberg and Kang, Kang et al.).

Although vitamin $B_6$, or pyridoxine, dependency is a more rare metabolic defect which causes neonatal or even intrauterine seizures (Begsovec et al.), it is important because of the availability of treatment. Infants with this familial inborn metabolic error require far more pyridoxine than the normal child and exhibit neonatal difficulties when it is not provided (Scriver, Waldinger and Berg). Respiratory dysfunction, neuromuscular hyperirritability, and convulsions which can lead to death unless treatment is instituted are the clinical hallmarks of this disorder.

Seizures are common events in newborn infants who have infections of various types, the most important being bacterial meningitis. Because of this possibility, lumbar puncture and cerebrospinal fluid examination are warranted whenever unexplained seizures occur in the young infant. Other infectious illnesses that may be associated with neonatal seizures are congenital rubella, cytomegalovirus encephalitis, toxoplasmosis and disseminated infection with herpes simplex or Coxsackie B viruses.

The narcotic withdrawal syndrome in newborn infants of mothers who are narcotic addicts has been recognized with increased frequency in recent years (Naeye et al.). Although convulsions are not common among these infants, they have been observed in those severely affected (Zelson et al.). Signs of neonatal withdrawal usually appear during the first or second day after birth, but in exceptional cases can be delayed for several days (Kandall and Gartner). The offspring of addicted mothers are usually prematurely born or small for gestational age. The usual withdrawal signs include irritability, tremulousness, tachypnea, vomiting or diarrhea, and fever. The more severely affected infant may have sufficient fluid loss to become dehydrated, develop hypocalcemia or exhibit frank generalized convulsions. Diagnosis might be anticipated when the mother admits to drug intake, has withdrawal symptoms herself or attempts to leave the hospital with the infant against medical advice within one day after birth.

Intoxication of the infant by accidental injection of a local anesthetic, such as mepivacaine, into the scalp during caudal anesthesia of the mother is an additional possible cause of seizures soon after birth (Sinclair et al., Rosefsky and Petersiel). Bradycardia is associated with respiratory depression, limpness, dilated pupils and convulsions soon after birth. The puncture wound, identifying the site of the injection into the fetal scalp, is visible in some cases. Gastric lavage and exchange transfusion have been recommended for this condition because of its life-threatening characteristics (Sinclair et al.).

**DIAGNOSIS AND TREATMENT.** The primary concern in the newborn infant with seizures is the immediate identification of those causes which are amenable to some specific form of treatment. Therefore, the appropriate studies must be performed to exclude hypocalcemia, hypoglycemia, hypomagnesemia, hyponatremia, sepsis and meningitis. Pyridoxine dependency can be added to this list, although it is a rare disorder. Diagnosis of seizures secondary to perinatal complications can be accepted only after the above possibilities have been eliminated by the results of the laboratory examinations. In most cases, the infant who is convulsing because of hypoxic-ischemic injuries acquired during birth can be diagnosed on the basis of the history of perinatal distress, the presence of other abnormal neurologic signs and the frequent presence of blood in the cerebrospinal fluid.

The diagnostic assessment should include a complete blood count and urinalysis, serum glucose, calcium, phosphorus, magnesium and electrolytes. A rapid estimate of the blood sugar range can be made by a Dextrostix test. If the test indicates a low serum glucose, it is advisable to administer 25 per cent glucose intravenously, after blood is obtained for glucose determination.

At a later date, further studies indicated may include blood pH, serum ammonium, and serum aminoacid determinations. Serologic tests for rubella, cytomegalovirus, toxoplasmosis and other infections may also be advisable, depending on the other laboratory findings. Blood culture and lumbar puncture for cerebrospinal fluid examination, as well as skull and chest x-rays, are additional valuable procedures. Electroencephalography is a further consideration but should not be requested until the more urgent information is obtained and management of the problem is underway. The electroencephalogram is not as important in the newborn infant with seizures as in the older child, but is useful in that group in which seizures are not explained on the basis of a readily identifiable metabolic or infectious cause.

Treatment is determined on the basis of the underlying explanation of seizures, with or without the addition of anticonvulsant medication. For example, seizure due to hypoglycemia can usually be controlled by intravenous administration of 2 to 3 ml per kg of 25 per cent glucose, followed by appropriate measures to maintain the blood glucose level. Hypocalcemic convulsions in the newborn are terminated by intravenously administered 10 per cent calcium gluconate in a dose of 2 to 5 ml, depending on the body weight of the infant. Repeated injections may be necessary, and subsequent oral feedings usually require supplemental calcium lactate or levulinate. Hypomagnesemia is corrected by cautious intravenous injection of 2 or 3 per cent magnesium sulfate in a dose of 2 to 6 ml, depending on the size of the child. When no etiologic cause is found and seizures recur, a trial dose of 50 mg of pyridoxine hydrochloride parenterally should be given. The rare pyridoxine dependency state is identified by a dramatic clinical and electroencephalographic response to this medication. Its presence requires continued oral therapy with high doses of pyridoxine.

Recurrent seizures not controlled promptly by one of the above measures warrant treatment with phenobarbital given orally or by intramuscular injection every 6 to 8 hours. The amount of phenobarbital needed to control seizures in the young infant varies from case to case but is frequently greater per kilogram than in older children. The dose range is between 3 and 8 mg per kilogram per day although amounts over 5 mg per kilogram per day will often result in sedation and subsequent feeding difficulties. A common approach is to initiate therapy with a relatively low dose, increasing it gradually as necessary to control seizures. The dose should be reduced when seizures are controlled but the child is lethargic from the drug. How long to continue treatment depends on many factors. When only one or two seizures occur in the first few days after birth, and the infant progresses normally over the next few weeks, treatment can often be terminated 4 to 8 weeks after birth.

Frequent and severe convulsions in the newborn period sometimes require more aggressive therapy than outlined above. Sodium amytal, paraldehyde, and diazepam (Valium) given intravenously have each been championed by various authors. Paraldehyde should not be used in the presence of respiratory disease, and any of the three can cause respiratory arrest if the dose given is sufficiently large. Diazepam is the most widely used preparation to control continuous, threatening seizures. In the newborn, the intravenous dose varies from 0.5 to 3 mg, which sometimes must be repeated at hourly intervals. When such drugs are used intravenously, equipment and capability for intubation and ventilatory support must be readily available should respiratory arrest occur.

## ANTICONVULSANT THERAPY OF THE MOTHER DURING PREGNANCY

The most commonly used anticonvulsants, including diphenylhydantoin, phenobarbital and primidone, have been shown to cross the placenta and gain entrance into the fetus. The concentration of phenobarbital has been found to be approximately the same in umbilical cord serum as in the serum of the mother, indicating that the fetus is exposed to the same concentration as that of the mother (Melchior et al.). The same is true for diphenylhydantoin, which is then excreted very slowly by the neonate during the first 2 days after birth (Mirkin).

Adverse effects of anticonvulsant drugs on the fetus appear to be uncommon and, for the most part, are probably related to the maternal blood level. High levels of phenobarbital or primidone in the neonate can cause neurologic and respiratory suppression and can be followed by a withdrawal reaction in the infant similar to that in maternal narcotic addiction (Martinez and Snyder).

Various anticonvulsants, but especially diphenylhydantoin, have also been incriminated as a cause of a coagulation defect in the newborn infant that is manifested by hemorrhage on the first day of life (Solomon et al., Mountain et al.). The diminished clotting factors in this disorder are similar to those in hemorrhagic disease of the newborn and, like them, can be prevented by vitamin K administration at birth.

Still another suspected danger of anticonvulsant administration during pregnancy is the possibility of teratogenicity (Speidel and Meadow, Lowe, Annegers et al.). Studies have revealed the rate of congenital malformations in offspring of treated epileptic women to be two to three times higher than in nonepileptic women. Many types of anomalies have been observed in such infants, including facial clefts, hypoplasia of the digits, congenital cardiac defects and malformations of the nervous system. The possibility of teratogenic effects, and of the other fetal effects of anticonvulsants given during pregnancy, warrants careful monitoring of serum levels of the pregnant epileptic patient.

## REFERENCES

Annegers, J. F., Elveback, L. R., Hauser, W. A., and Kurland, L. T.: Do anticonvulsants have a teratogenic effect? Arch. Neurol. 31:364, 1974.

Bejsovec, M., Kulenda, Z., and Ponca, E.: Familial intrauterine convulsions in pyridoxine dependency. Arch. Dis. Child. 42:201, 1967.

Berenberg, W., and Kang, E. S.: The congenital hyperammonemic syndrome. Develop. Med. Child Neurol. 13:355, 1971.

Davis, J. A., Harvey, D. R., and Yu, J. S.: Neonatal fits associated with hypomagnesaemia. Arch. Dis. Child. 40:286, 1973.

Freeman, J. M.: Neonatal seizures—diagnosis and management. J. Pediat. 77:701, 1970.

Gross, G. P., Hathaway, W. E., and McGaughey, H. R.: Hyperviscosity in the neonate. J. Pediatr. 82:1004, 1973.

Hartenstein, H., and Gardner, L. I.: Tetany of the newborn associated with maternal parathyroid adenoma. N. Engl. J. Med. 274:266, 1966.

Kandall, S. R., and Gartner, L. M.: Late presentation of drug withdrawal symptoms in newborns. Am. J. Dis. Child. 127:58, 1974.

Kang, E. S., Snodgrass, P. J., and Gerald, P. S.: Ornithine transcarbamylase deficiency in the newborn infant. J. Pediatr. 82:642, 1973.

Kretschmer, R., Say, B., Brown, D., and Rosen, F. S.: Congenital aplasia of the thymus gland (DiGeorge's syndrome). N. Engl. J. Med. 279:1295, 1968.

Lowe, C. R.: Congenital malformations among infants born to epileptic women. Lancet 1:9, 1973.

Martinez, G., and Snyder, R. D.: Transplacental passage of primidone. Neurology 23:381, 1973.

Melchior, J. C., Svensmark, O., and Trolle, D.: Placental transfer of phenobarbitone in epileptic women, and elimination in newborns. Lancet 2:860, 1967.

Mirkin, B. L.: Diphenylhydantoin: Placental transport, fetal localization, neonatal metabolism, and possible teratogenic effects. J. Pediatr. 78:329, 1971.

Mizrahi, A., and Gold, A. P.: Neonatal tetany secondary to maternal hyperparathyroidism. J.A.M.A. 190:155, 1964.

Mountain, K. R., Hirsh, J., and Gallus, A. S.: Neonatal coagulation defect due to anticonvulsant drug treatment in pregnancy. Lancet 1:265, 1970.

Naeye, R. L., Blanc, W., Leblanc, W., and Khatamee, M. A.: Fetal complications of maternal heroin addiction: Abnormal growth, infections, and episodes of stress. J. Pediatr. 83:1055, 1973.

Paunier, L., Radde, I. C., Kooh, S. W., Connen, P. E., and Fraser, D.: Primary hypomagnesemia with secondary hypocalcemia in an infant. Pediatrics 41:385, 1968.

Rose, A. L., and Lombroso, C. T.: Neonatal seizure states. A study of clinical, pathological, and electroencephalographic features in 137 full-term babies with a long-term follow-up. Pediatrics 45:404, 1970.

Rosefsky, J. B., and Petersiel, M. E.: Perinatal deaths associated with mepivacaine paracervical-block anesthesia in labor. N. Engl. J. Med. 278:530, 1968.

Scriver, C. R.: Vitamin B6-dependency and infantile convulsions. Pediatrics 26:62, 1960.

Sinclair, J. C., Fox, H. A., Lentz, J. F., Fuld, G. L., and Murphy, J.: Intoxication of the fetus by a local anesthetic. N. Engl. J. Med. 273:1173, 1965.

Smith, F. G., Jr., and Zike, K.: Idiopathic hypoparathyroidism in neonatal period. Am. J. Dis. Child. 105:182, 1963.

Solomon, G. E., Hilgartner, M. W., and Kutt, H.: Coagulation defects caused by diphenylhydantoin. Neurology 22:1165, 1972.

Speidel, B. D., and Meadow, S. R.: Maternal epilepsy and abnormalities of the fetus and newborn. Lancet 2:839, 1972.

Vainsel, M., Vandervelde, G., Smulders, J., Vosters, M., Hubain, P., and Loeb, H.: Tetany due to hypomagnesaemia with secondary hypocalcemia. Arch. Dis. Child. 45:254, 1970.

Volpe, J.: Neonatal seizures. N. Engl. J. Med. 289:413, 1973.

Waldinger, C., and Berg, R. B.: Signs of pyridoxine dependency manifest at birth in siblings. Pediatrics 32:161, 1963.

Wood, J. L.: Plethora in the newborn infant associated with cyanosis and convulsions. J. Pediatr. 54:143, 1959.

Zelson, C., Rubio, E., and Wasserman, E.: Neonatal narcotic addiction: 10 year observation. Pediatrics 48:178, 1971.

# MISCELLANEOUS DISORDERS OF THE INTRACRANIAL CONTENTS

# 82

*By William E. Bell*

## FOCAL INTRACRANIAL SUPPURATIVE LESIONS

Despite the frequent occurrence of bacterial sepsis and meningitis in the newborn and young infant, brain abscesses as well as other focal suppurative infections are unusual in this age group. When abscess within the cerebrum does occur in early infancy, it is usually secondary to septicemia and without the predisposing conditions that pertain in the older child or adult. Cyanotic congenital heart disease, suppurative sinusitis and otitis are not significant causes of brain abscess until after two years of age.

Abscess within the parenchyma of the brain, especially, is decidedly rare, and when present is not often suspected during life because of the nonspecific character of the clinical manifestations (Sanford, Butler et al., Munslow et al.). Vomiting, lethargy, convulsions and signs of increased intracranial pressure are the most common features of brain abscess in the young infant. Tenseness of the anterior fontanel and rapidly progressive head enlargement have been present in most reported cases in early infancy (Hoffman et al.). Fever is frequently absent, but peripheral blood leukocytosis is customary. Cerebral abscess formation in the infant is multiple in some cases, but when solitary is likely to reach enormous proportions before causing death or until the lesion is identified by special studies. In a number of cases, diagnosis during life occurred unexpectedly when the abscess was entered during attempted transcoronal ventriculography. Treatment consists of appropriate antibiotic therapy and proper drainage of the lesion by one method or another. The mortality rate is high in this age group. Progressive hydrocephalus requiring shunting is a common complication among survivors.

Subdural empyema is a more common intracranial suppurative lesion than brain abscess in early infancy (Farmer and Wise). Suppuration may be either unilateral or bilateral, and most cases complicate gram negative or staphylococcal meningitis. Either subdural empyema, epidural empyema or meningitis may also complicate an infected cephalhematoma in the newborn child. Pus in the subdural space is poorly tolerated by the young infant and is sometimes complicated by cortical vein or venous sinus thrombosis. Signs due to the lesion are usually obscured by those of meningitis, and recognition depends on the performance of transfontanel subdural taps. Subdural empyema represents a serious complication of meningitis in the infant

and is associated with a high incidence of lasting sequelae.

## INTRACRANIAL VENOUS SINUS THROMBOSIS

Thrombosis of the superior sagittal sinus or of multiple intracranial venous sinuses is a devastating insult in the infant, in part because of the cerebral damage from the disturbance of venous drainage, but also because of the other cerebral effects of the primary condition that causes it. The most widely recognized cause of dural sinus occlusion in early infancy is diarrhea with severe dehydration, especially of the hypernatremic type (Luttrell and Finberg). It may also complicate generalized sepsis or sepsis with meningitis or subdural empyema. Hyperviscosity secondary to cyanotic congenital heart disease, especially if associated with infection or dehydration, is another possible precipitating factor.

In the living infant, diagnosis of venous sinus thrombosis is difficult because the clinical signs are not specific and are usually intermixed with neurologic signs related to the underlying cause. Cerebral dysfunction in the infant with sinus thrombosis results from impairment of cortical venous drainage, with secondary cortical vein distention or occlusion giving rise to extensive hemorrhagic cerebral infarction. Bilateral signs, focal or generalized convulsions, coma, and signs of increased intracranial pressure are present in most (Yang et al.). The cerebrospinal fluid is blood-tinged or xanthochromic as the result of subarachnoid bleeding, and the protein content is significantly increased. The mortality rate in infants with major dural sinus thrombosis is high, and survivors are left with neurologic deficits of variable degree.

## CONGENITAL INTRACRANIAL ANEURYSMS AND VASCULAR MALFORMATIONS

Saccular, or "berry," aneurysms, generally considered to be the result of localized congenital defects of the media of the arterial wall, rarely give rise to clinical illness in the childhood age group. They are usually located on major vessels at the base of the brain, and give rise to symptoms and signs either by rupture with subarachnoid hemorrhage or by a mass effect with compression upon adjacent structures. Clinical manifestations in the newborn period or in early infancy caused by aneurysms of this type are exceedingly rare but have been described (Pickering et al., Shucart and Wolpert). In the few neonatal cases described, spontaneous intracranial bleeding is characterized by an abrupt onset, irritability, vomiting, decreased alertness or coma and findings indicative of sudden increase in intracranial pressure. Diagnosis before death depends upon angiographic examination.

A better known type of congenital aneurysm that can produce signs in the newborn infant is aneurysmal malformation of the great vein of Galen (Fig. 82–1). This lesion, which represents an arteriovenous shunt of large volume, usually presents in the form of high-output cardiac failure, often associated with a loud bruit audible over the head (Gomez et al., Levine et al., Montoya et al.). Thus, this is one form of neurologic disease in which the initial signs include tachypnea, tachycardia and hepatomegaly, with little else to localize the primary lesion until auscultation of the head is performed. In some cases, obstruction of the aqueduct from the adjacent lesion gives rise to hydrocephalus with rapidly progressive head enlargement. Diagnosis of this type of vascular malformation is suspected in the infant with cardiomegaly not explained on the basis of intracardiac anomalies or the presence of extracardiac arterial to venous shunts, as might occur within the liver, the lungs or the peripheral vascular system. The probability is enhanced if a loud cranial bruit is heard or if hydrocephalus coexists. Diagnosis of the lesion is proved by carotid angiography. Surgical treatment of aneurysm of the vein of Galen has been attempted (Morelli), although, when associated with cardiac failure, the lesion carries a poor prognosis in the infant.

Arteriovenous malformations in the cere-

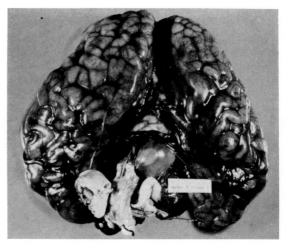

*Figure 82–1.* Aneurysm of the vein of Galen. Large, saccular mass is located just dorsal to the upper brain stem and, thus, in close proximity to the aqueduct of Sylvius. Initial clinical manifestations are caused by either aqueductal obstruction or high-output cardiac failure.

bral parenchyma only rarely produce clinical signs in the newborn or young infant but can be a source of spontaneous bleeding or seizures (Beatty). Intraventricular hemorrhage, sometimes fatal, can occur in early infancy as well as in older persons from a cryptic hemangioma of the choroid plexus (Doe et al.). Most described cases have been identified at necropsy.

## CONGENITAL BRAIN TUMORS

Although certain types of intracranial tumors are believed to arise from congenital "rests," it is decidedly unusual for abnormal signs to be present in the neonatal period. Chordomas originate from notochord remnants but rarely become symptomatic until adulthood. It has been postulated that craniopharyngiomas develop from remains of the embryonic Rathke pouch but only infrequently cause abnormal signs in the young infant (Azar-kia et al., Tabaddor et al.).

Congenital brain tumors that do give rise to neurologic abnormalities in the newborn period are often associated with abnormal head enlargement, are frequently not diagnosed until surgery or autopsy and are more likely to be of unusual histologic types than those in older children. A number of cases with cerebral teratomas have been described in newborn infants, sometimes with massive involvement of the brain by the neoplasm (Oberman, Greenhouse and Neubuerger, Finck and Antin). Meningiomas (Mendiratta et al.), medulloblastomas (Kadin et al., Papadakis et al.), and pontine gliomas (Luse and Teitelbaum) have been reported in the neonate, but have no characteristic clinical features that will aid in their recognition.

Papilloma of the choroid plexus sometimes will cause abnormal head enlargement in the early weeks of life and is an important lesion because of the possibility of its surgical removal (Matson and Crofton). Infants with this tumor are usually considered to have hydrocephalus due to the more common causes until an intraventricular mass is demonstrated by air ventriculography.

Nasal glioma is a congenital tumor composed of connective tissue and neural elements. The lesion may present extranasally, as a firm non-pulsatile mass at the base of the nose or intranasally, in which case it is easily confused with a nasal polyp (Strauss et al., Katz and Lewis). The mass is benign and is generally regarded to be a glial heterotopia and not a brain tumor in the usual sense. Differential diagnosis includes dermoid cyst, nasal polyp, and nasal encephalocele.

## CONGENITAL SCALP DEFECT

Congenital scalp defect, also known as aplasia cutis congenitalis, is an uncommon anomaly which occurs in either sex. It may occur in an otherwise normal child, it may be associated with a wide variety of other cerebral or extracranial anomalies (Fowler and Dumars, Ruiz-Maldonado and Tamayo), or it may occur in the child with trisomy 13–15. Rarely, congenital scalp defects are associated with similiar cutaneous lesions elsewhere on the body. In many cases, congenital scalp defect occurs in sporadic fashion. It has also been observed

in siblings (Hodgman et al.) and in both a parent and offspring (Johnsonbaugh et al.).

The most common location of the defect is at the vertex but, occasionally, paired lesions are found in the parietal regions. At birth, a congenital scalp defect is often ulcerated or crusted, and may appear to be infected. Over the following weeks or months the lesion becomes covered by a layer of epithelium and subsequently resembles a scarred area. The region of the defect remains devoid of hair thereafter.

In most cases, the underlying skull is intact; however, in some there are underlying skull defects of variable size which close spontaneously during the first few months after birth. Still others have associated oval or circular defects in the skull which persist into adulthood.

The pathogenesis of this anomaly has been debated for years and remains undetermined. Autosomal dominant inheritance has been suggested in certain cases. Treatment is conservative in most cases, especially in those with cerebral anomalies resulting in severe functional defects. Plastic repair has been recommended in certain instances (Kosnik and Sayers).

## CONGENITAL DERMAL SINUSES

A congenital dermal sinus is a developmental defect in which a tract lined by squamous epithelium extends inward from the surface of the skin. Since midline fusion of ectodermal and neuroectodermal tissues occurs last at the cephalic and caudal ends of the neural tube, the majority of such defects of fusion occur in the lumbosacral and suboccipital regions. Those that terminate superficially without neurologic involvement are referred to as pilonidal sinuses and are of consequence because of their susceptibility to indolent and recurrent infection. Others penetrate to the meninges or even to the fourth ventricle intracranially, or the subarachnoid space intraspinally. These lesions are of much greater importance because of the hazard of neurologic infection or because of the presence of local associated anomalies. In some cases, the termination of an intracranial or intraspinal dermal sinus is expanded to form a dermoid cyst which can cause signs by compression of adjacent tissue or by ventricular obstruction when within the fourth ventricle, by aseptic meningitis due to contamination of the cerebrospinal fluid secondary to rupture of the lesion, or by purulent meningitis or even abscess if the lesion becomes secondarily infected.

Intracranial dermal sinuses are midline lesions usually located in the suboccipital region. The sinus tract opening may be difficult to identify in this region because it is often obscured by the scalp hair. When the defect is suspected on the basis of recurrent meningitis, especially if caused by proteus or staphylococcus, it is sometimes wise to shave the hair in the occipital region to be certain of its presence or absence. A small, circular defect in the skull can be seen on x-ray in some cases; however, absence of a roentgenographic defect does not exclude the possibility. Bacterial meningitis is the most important complication of a congenital dermal sinus and is the primary reason for surgical excision. The presence of abnormal head enlargement in the infant, or signs of increased pressure in the older child with an occipital dermal sinus, usually indicates posterior fossa obstruction caused by a dermoid cyst or abscess within a cyst at the termination of the sinus.

Intraspinal dermal sinuses can be located anywhere along the midline of the spine, but most are low lumbar or lumbosacral in location. The external or surface opening is usually surrounded by thickening or discoloration of the skin. X-rays of the spine in most cases reveal spina bifida or other spinal anomalies in the region when the sinus penetrates the meninges. Widening of the spinal canal with erosion of the pedicles suggests the presence of a cystic expansion of the sinus tract and warrants myelographic examination. Congenital dermal sinuses in the spinal region are often identified only after the child has experienced one or more episodes of suppurative meningitis. Any one of several organisms can be the offender: *Escherichia coli*, staphylococcus, proteus or *Hemophilus influenzae*. Treatment, regardless of location, includes complete surgical excision of the sinus tract and also of an associated intraspinal or intracranial cystic lesion, if present.

## FAMILIAL DYSAUTONOMIA (RILEY-DAY SYNDROME)

Familial dysautonomia is a rare disorder, inherited in autosomal recessive fashion, which occurs predominantly in children of Eastern European Jewish ancestry. When first described in 1949 by Riley and colleagues, the clinical manifestations of the illness were believed to be due to dysfunction of the autonomic nervous system. Subsequent observations have suggested that the basic defect is probably related to a disturbance in the production or release of a neurohumoral transmitter substance.

Clinical signs of this condition are usually present soon after birth, although their non-specific character makes early diagnosis exceedingly difficult (Table 82–1). Diminished muscle tone, poor Moro response, difficulty with feeding because of inability to coordinate the suck and swallowing mechanisms, and respiratory distress are the usual initial abnormalities in the neonatal and early infancy period (Geltzer et al.). Other findings subsequently observed in the child with familial dysautonomia include developmental retardation, episodic fever, absent deep tendon reflexes, diminished to absent lacrimation, scoliosis, excessive sweating, episodic hypertension and relative indifference to pain stimulation. As the result of reduced pain sensation, older children frequently show the effects of recurrent traumatic lesions, such as corneal ulcerations, Charcot joints or soft tissue scars or deformities of the fingers or toes. While not a major feature, some authors have commented on the susceptibility of children with this disease to exhibit breath-holding spells in infancy (Riley and Moore). One of the most constant and valuable diagnostic signs is the reduction or absence of circumvallate papillae on the tongue, a finding usually associated with impaired taste sensation (Pearson et al.).

Certain special techniques have been developed which allow confirmation of the diagnosis of familial dysautonomia once it is suspected clinically. An abnormal response to intradermal histamine was reported by Smith and Dancis in 1963. Intracutaneous injection of 0.03 to 0.05 ml of

*TABLE 82–1.   Symptoms of Familial Dysautonomia**

| Symptom | Age at Onset or Recognition |
|---|---|
| **Autonomic nervous system:** | |
| Skin blotching | 5 hr. |
| Coldness of extremities | 5 hr. |
| Vacillation of temperature | 24 hr. |
| Incoordination of suck and swallow | 24 hr. |
| Bowel irregularities | 2 wk. |
| Labile hypertension | 1 mo. |
| Postural hypotension | 1 mo. |
| Reduced or absent tear and resulting corneal abrasions | 6 wk. |
| Drooling | – |
| **Neuromuscular system:** | |
| Diminished deep tendon reflexes | Birth |
| Hypotonia | Birth |
| Poor muscular coordination | 24 hr. |
| Small stature | 2 mo. |
| Dysarthria | – |
| Scoliosis | – |
| **Sensory disturbance:** | |
| Indifferent response to pain | Birth |
| Corneal anesthesia | 6 wk. |
| **Central nervous system:** | |
| Motor-skill retardation | 6 wk. |
| Breath holding | 2 mo. |
| Behavior disturbance | 6 mo. |
| Periodic vomiting | – |
| Mental retardation | ? |
| Convulsions | ? |
| **Biochemical studies:** | |
| Positive methacholine test | 2 wk. |
| Positive histamine test | 2 wk. |
| Elevated HVA | 3 wk. |
| Depressed VMA | 3 wk. |

*Geltzer, A. I., Gluck, L., Talner, N. S., et al.: N. Engl. J. Med., *271*:436, 1964.

histamine phosphate 1:1000 in the normal person produces a wheal, surrounded by a zone of erythema which extends from one to three cm from the borders of the wheal. The reaction is well developed within 4 to 5 minutes, persists for more than 10 minutes and is associated with local discomfort. In the patient with familial dysautonomia, the wheal is not associated with a zone of surrounding erythema and is relatively painless. The abnormal reaction is not pathognomonic of the disorder in that similar results may occur in the child with atopic dermatitis or with certain types of peripheral neuropathy.

Another test of diagnostic value is the pupillary response to instillation onto the conjunctiva of 2.5 per cent methacholine. The normal patient shows no pupillary reaction to this substance, but prompt pupillary constriction occurs in the child with familial dysautonomia, as well as in the patient with Adie's tonic pupil (Goldberg et al.).

An abnormality of catecholamine metabolism which also can be used diagnostically was demonstrated in this disease by Smith et al. in 1963. Homovanillic acid (HVA), derived from precursors of noradrenalin and adrenalin, is increased in the urine, while vanillylmandelic acid (VMA), a breakdown product of noradrenalin and adrenalin, is reduced (Gitlow et al.).

The pathology of this disease has been variously described in different reports, with some demonstrating no significant microscopic abnormalities of the nervous system (Yatsu and Zussman). Degenerative changes within the reticular formation were described by Cohen and Solomon, while focal demyelination of the posterior columns of the spinal cord was observed by Fogelson et al. Reduction in the number of unmyelinated fibers in peripheral nerve tissue was found in a child with the disease by Aguayo and colleagues. Still other authors have described decreased numbers or abnormalities of nerve cells in autonomic and dorsal root ganglia (Solitare and Cohen, Pearson et al.).

Management of the child with familial dysautonomia is conservative, and genetic advice is provided to the family. Ophthalmologic treatment includes artificial lacrimation or other measures to prevent corneal damage secondary to decreased corneal sensation and lack of normal tear production. Bethanecol (Urecholine) is a parasympathomimetic agent that may improve certain of the distressing features of this disorder but has not been extensively used to date (Axelrod et al.). Surgical procedures requiring general anesthesia carry increased risks because of the susceptibility to blood pressure fluctuations and the abnormal response of the child with this disease to hypoxia and hypercapnia

(Kritchman et al., Riley and Moore). Such procedures should be undertaken only by persons familiar with the various dangers of certain anesthetic agents and blood gas alterations in this particular condition.

## REFERENCES

Aguayo, A. J., Nair, C. P. V., and Bray, G. M.: Peripheral nerve abnormalities in the Riley-Day syndrome. Arch. Neurol. 24:106, 1971.

Axelrod, F. B., Branom, N., Becker, M., Nachtigall, R., and Dancis, J.: Treatment of familial dysautonomia with bethanecol (Urecholine). J. Pediatr. 81:573, 1972.

Azar-Kia, B., Krishnan, U. R., and Schechter, M. M.: Neonatal craniopharyngioma. J. Neurosurg. 42:91, 1975.

Beatty, R. A.: Surgical treatment of a ruptured intracerebral arteriovenous malformation in a newborn. Pediatrics 53:571, 1974.

Butler, N. R., Barrie, H., and Paine, K. W. E.: Cerebral abscess as a complication of neonatal sepsis. Arch. Dis. Child. 32:461, 1975.

Cohen, P., and Solomon, N. H.: Familial dysautonomia: Case report with autopsy. J. Pediatr. 46:663, 1955.

Doe, F. D., Shuangshoti, S., and Netsky, M. G.: Cryptic hemangioma of the choroid plexus. Neurology 22:1232, 1972.

Farmer, T. W., and Wise, G. R.: Subdural empyema in infants, children and adults. Neurology 23:254, 1973.

Finck, F. M., and Antin, R.: Intracranial teratoma of the newborn. Am. J. Dis. Child. 109:439, 1965.

Fogelson, M. H., Rorke, L. B., and Kaye, R.: Spinal cord changes in familial dysautonomia. Arch. Neurol. 17:103, 1967.

Fowler, G. W., and Dumars, K. W.: Cutis aplasia and cerebral malformation. Pediatrics 52:861, 1973.

Geltzer, A. I., Gluck, L., Talner, N. S., and Polesky, H. F.: Familial dysautonomia. Studies in the newborn infant. N. Engl. J. Med. 271:436, 1964.

Gitlow, S. E., Bertani, L. M., Wilk, E., Li, B. L., and Dziedzic, S.: Excretion of catecholamine metabolites by children with familial dysautonomia. Pediatrics 46:513, 1970.

Goldberg, M. F., Payne, J. W., and Brunt, P. W.: Ophthalmologic studies of familial dysautonomia. Arch. Ophthalmol. 80:732, 1968.

Gomez, M. R., Whitten, C. F., Nolke, A., Bernstein, J., and Meyer, J. S.: Aneurysmal malformation of the great vein of Galen causing heart failure in early infancy. Pediatrics 31:400, 1963.

Greenhouse, A. H., and Neubuerger, K. T.: Intracranial teratomata of the newborn. Arch. Neurol. 3:718, 1960.

Hodgman, J. E., Mathies, A. W., Jr., and Levan, N. E.: Congenital scalp defects in twin sisters. Am. J. Dis. Child. 110:293, 1965.

Hoffman, H. J., Hendrick, E. B., and Hiscox, J. L.: Cerebral abscess in early infancy. J. Neurosurg. 33:172, 1970.

Johnsonbaugh, R. E., Light, I. J., and Sutherland, J. M.: Congenital scalp defects in father and son. Am. J. Dis. Child. 110:297, 1965.

Kadin, M. E., Rubinstein, L. J., and Nelson, J. S.: Neonatal cerebellar medulloblastoma originating from the fetal external granular layer. J. Neuropath. Exper. Neurol. 29:583, 1970.

Katz, A., and Lewis, J. S.: Nasal gliomas. Arch. Otolaryngol. 94:351, 1971.

Kosnik, E. J., and Sayers, M. P.: Congenital scalp defects: aplasia cutis congenita. J. Neurosurg. 42:32, 1975.

Kritchman, M. M., Schwartz, H., and Papper, E. M.: Experiences with general anesthesia in patients with familial dysautonomia. J.A.M.A. 170:529, 1959.

Levine, O. R., Jameson, A. G., Nellhaus, G., and Gold, A. P.: Cardiac complications of cerebral arteriovenous fistula in infancy. Pediatrics 30:563, 1962.

Luse, S. A., and Teitelbaum, S.: Congenital glioma of brain stem. Arch. Neurol. 18:196, 1968.

Luttrell, C. N., and Finberg, L.: Hemorrhagic encephalopathy induced by hypernatremia. Arch. Neurol. Psychiat. 81:424, 1959.

Matson, D. D., and Crofton, F. D. L.: Papilloma of the choroid plexus in childhood. J. Neurosurg. 17:1002, 1960.

Mendiratta, S. S., Rosenblum, J. A., and Strobos, R. J.: Congenital meningioma. Neurology 17:914, 1967.

Montoya, G., Dohn, D. F., and Mercer, R. D.: Arteriovenous malformation of the vein of Galen as a cause of heart failure and hydrocephalus in infants. Neurology 21:1054, 1971.

Morelli, R. J.: Surgery of aneurysms of the great vein of Galen. Rocky Mountain Med. J. 65:41, 1968.

Munslow, R. A., Stovall, V. S., Price, R. D., and Kohler, C. M.: Brain abscess in infants. J. Pediatr. 51:74, 1975.

Oberman, B.: Intracranial teratoma replacing brain. Arch. Neurol. 11:423, 1964.

Papadakis, N., Millan, J., Grady, D. F., and Segerberg, L. H.: Medulloblastoma of the neonatal period and early infancy. J. Neurosurg. 34:88, 1971.

Pearson, J., Budzilovich, G., and Finegold, M. J.: Sensory, motor, and autonomic dysfunction: The nervous system in familial dysautonomia. Neurology 21:486, 1971.

Pearson, J., Finegold, M. J., and Budzilovich, G.: The tongue and taste in familial dysautonomia. Pediatrics 45:739, 1970.

Pickering, L. K., Hogan, G. R., and Gilbert, E. F.: Aneurysm of the posterior inferior cerebellar artery. Rupture in a newborn. Am. J. Dis. Child. 119:155, 1970.

Riley, C. M., Day, R. L., Greeley, D. M., and Langford, W. S.: Central autonomic dysfunction with defective lacrimation: Report of five cases. Pediatrics 3:468, 1949.

Riley, C. M., and Moore, R. H.: Familial dysautonomia differentiated from related disorders. Pediatrics 37:435, 1966.

Ruiz-Maldonado, R., and Tamayo, L.: Aplasia cutis congenita, spastic paralysis, and mental retardation. Am. J. Dis. Child. 128:699, 1974.

Sanford, H. N.: Abscess of the brain in infants under twelve months of age. Am. J. Dis. Child. 35:256, 1928.

Shucart, W. A., and Wolpert, S. A.: An aneurysm in infancy presenting with diabetes insipidus. J. Neurosurg. *37*:368, 1972.

Smith, A. A., and Dancis, J.: Response to intradermal histamine in familial dysautonomia—a diagnostic test. J. Pediatr. *63*:889, 1963.

Smith, A. A., Taylor, T., and Wortis, S. B.: Abnormal catecholamine metabolism in familial dysautonomia. N. Engl. J. Med. *268*:705, 1963.

Solitare, G. B., and Cohen, G. S.: Peripheral autonomic nervous system lesions in congenital or familial dysautonomia. Neurology *15*:321, 1965.

Strauss, R. B., Callicott, J. H., and Hargett, I. R.: Intranasal neuroglial heterotopia. Am. J. Dis. Child. *111*:317, 1966.

Tabaddor, K., Shulman, K., and Dal Canto, M. C.: Neonatal craniopharyngioma. Am. J. Dis. Child. *128*:381, 1974.

Yang, D. C., Sohn, D., and Anand, H. K.: Thrombosis of the superior longitudinal sinus during infancy. J. Pediatr. *74*:570, 1969.

Yatsu, F., and Zussman, W.: Familial dysautonomia (Riley-Day syndrome). Arch. Neurol. *10*:459, 1964.

# 83

# MISCELLANEOUS DISORDERS OF THE SPINE, SPINAL CORD, AND PERIPHERAL NERVOUS SYSTEM

*By William E. Bell*

## SPINA BIFIDA CYSTICA (MENINGOCELE, MENINGOMYELOCELE, AND LIPOMENINGOCELE)

The newborn infant with a meningomyelocele complicated by the usual motor and sensory defects of the lower extremities, the associated intracranial abnormalities and neurogenic sphincter dysfunction represents a great tragedy for the family as well as an exceedingly difficult multidisciplinary management problem for the physician. Probably no other problem in the category of infant and childhood diseases has been the source of greater dispute and heated argument than that of the optimal management of the defective child who is afflicted with spina bifida cystica.

Although the etiology and pathogenesis of these defects remain obscure, their relationship to embryologic development is reasonably clear. The central nervous system develops from infolding of a thickened area of ectoderm called the neural, or medullary, plate which gives rise to the neural groove and, subsequently, the neural tube. The process of closure of the neural tube

begins in the thoracic region and proceeds in either direction, being completed by the fourth embryonic week. With closure of the neural tube, the ectoderm and neuroectoderm become separated and the ectoderm fuses in the midline dorsally. Mesodermal tissue surrounds the neural tube, separating it from the surface ectoderm, and subsequently forms the vertebral column. The various forms of spina bifida are the end result of a disturbance of this embryonic process. Most authors have accepted the concept that these defects are produced by an undetermined insult which prevents normal fusion and closure, although an alternative theory is that the neural tube becomes ruptured after closure, secondary to increased pressure within the central canal (Gardner). The discovery of myeloschisis in a human embryo only five millimeters in length is supportive evidence for the failure of closure postulate (Lemire et al.).

**CLINICAL MANIFESTATIONS.** The most common and the least significant form of spina bifida is spina bifida occulta, a mesodermal abnormality in which there is nonfusion of the vertebral laminar arches.

Diagnosis is essentially a radiologic, the arch defect alone being without clinical significance. As an isolated defect, most are located at the first sacral or fifth lumbar vertebra. Spina bifida cystica is a laminar arch defect through which either meninges or meninges and neural elements protrude. Herniation of dura and arachnoid alone without neural components in the sac is called a meningocele. The soft, rounded mass on the back is usually skin covered although, infrequently, associated failure of ectodermal closure produces a sac covered by a delicate membrane that is susceptible to infection. Motor function in the legs is expected to be normal with this lesion unless there are other dysplastic changes of the spinal cord or brain. Meningomyeloceles (myeloceles, localized rachischisis) are 10 to 20 times more frequent than meningoceles and are of far greater consequence. The herniated sac contains meninges as well as neural tissue. Only infrequently does skin cover the lesion except in those patients in whom an associated lipoma overlies the defect, the so-called lipomeningomyelocele (Fig. 83–1).

In most cases, the defect at birth is flat, consisting of poorly organized cord tissue lying exposed on the surface at the midline and surrounded by a pink or bluish, delicate, semi-transparent membrane (Fig. 83–2). With the passage of time, fluid accumulation results in elevation of the lesion giving rise to its cystic-like appearance of variable size (Fig. 83–3). The spinal cord superior to the surface lesion is frequently malformed, the most common disturbance being hydromyelia. Although meningomyeloceles may be located anywhere along the spinal column, the most common sites are the thoracolumbar, the lumbar or the lumbosacral regions. The incidence of spina bifida cystica shows some geographic variation. In the series studied by Laurence and Tew, an incidence of just less than 4 per 1000 total births was found.

The type and degree of neurologic deficit in a child with a meningomyelocele is determined by the location and size of the lesion, a matter succinctly reviewed by Stark. A large myelocele with the upper level extending to $T_8$ vertebral level

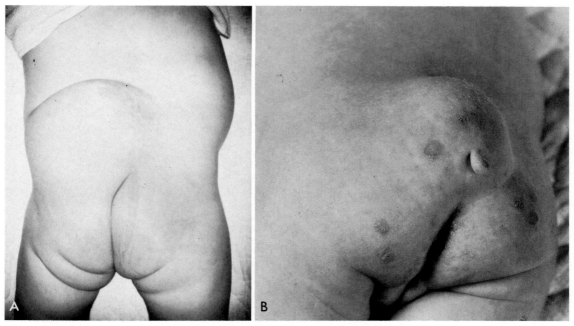

***Figure 83–1.*** Two examples of lipomeningocele. Each presents in the left buttock as a firm, well circumscribed, lobulated tumor which became tense when the infant cried. Over the surface of **B** are some macular erosions and a congenital skin tag and dimple. This last may be the pilonidal dimple displaced by the tumor.

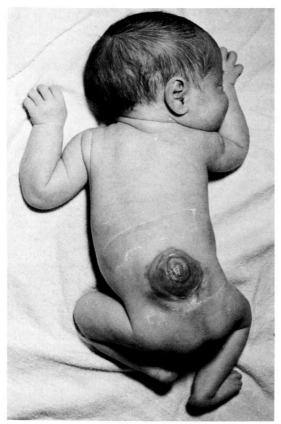

*Figure 83–2.* Lumbar meningomyelocele in a 3-day-old infant. There is moderate weakness of the proximal muscle groups and more extensive weakness of the distal musculature in the lower extremities. The lesion was flat at birth but began to elevate in the next 2 days.

the hips, and there is extension at the knees and a calcaneovarus position of the feet. Several types of foot deformity may result with lumbosacral and sacral myeloceles, the position and posture being determined by which muscles retain innervation and which are paralyzed. Regardless of the upper level of the lesion, infants with clinical evidence of denervation of muscles supplied by $S_{2-3-4}$ can be expected to have neurogenic bladder dysfunction.

Hydrocephalus only infrequently complicates spinal meningoceles but is a common complicating problem in the child with a meningomyelocele. It is generally stated that 85 to 90 per cent of infants with meningomyeloceles have hydrocephalus of one type or another. The pathogenesis of hydrocephalus in these infants has been a matter of speculation for a number of years and remains unclear to the present time. Aqueductal obstruction of one of several types accounts for ventricular enlargement in some cases (Emery), although others have extraventricular obstructive (communicating) hydrocephalus. Blockage at the foramen magnum secondary to the Arnold-Chiari malformation, thus preventing access of cerebrospinal fluid to the intracranial subarachnoid space, has been stated to be a cause of communicating hydrocephalus in these cases but is doubted by

creates denervation of the abdominal muscles bilaterally and of all groups in the lower extremities. The abdomen bulges in the flank regions, and the legs are motionless and flaccid, without significant joint deformity if the entire spinal cord below the upper level is affected. The anal sphincter is patulous, and sensation is absent to the upper limits of the midline lesion. A low lumbar meningomyelocele with sparing of function down to $L_4$ results in sustained contraction of the hip flexors, quadriceps and tibialis anterior muscles but with paralysis of the hamstrings, gastrocnemius and intrinsic musculature of the feet. The result is a striking deformity in which the lower limbs are held in flexion at

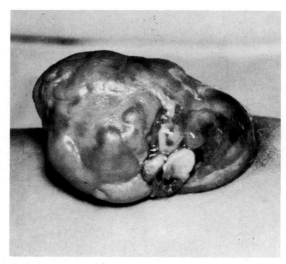

*Figure 83–3.* Closeup view of a lumbosacral myelomeningocele. The mass is covered with thin, transparent membrane. No well differentiated nervous tissue can be distinguished with assurance.

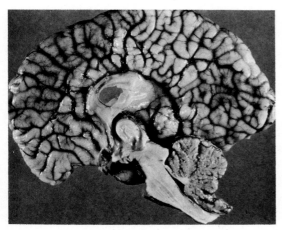

**Figure 83–4.** Arnold-Chiari malformation. Child with a thoracolumbar meningomyelocele. The Arnold-Chiari malformation consists of elongation of the lower brain stem with downward displacement of the inferior part of the vermis of the cerebellum. The tectal plate is "beaked" and the massa intermedia is enlarged. Polymicrogyria is present.

some investigators (Drummond and Donaldson). Whatever the cause, hydrocephalus of moderate degree is sometimes present in the neonate with meningomyelocele, even in the absence of abnormal suture separation or head enlargement.

The Arnold-Chiari malformation comprises a complex group of anomalies of the hindbrain that is present in many, but not all, infants with meningomyeloceles. Also known as the Chiari type II anomaly, it is composed of elongation and downward displacement of the pons and medulla, downward displacement of the cerebellar vermis, which protrudes through the foramen magnum, beak-shaped deformity of the tectal plate and enlargement of the massa intermedia (Fig. 83–4). On roentgenographic examination most infants with meningomyelocele and the Arnold-Chiari malformation exhibit a characteristic defect of the skull referred to as lückenschädel, or craniolacuna (Fig. 84–5). This peculiar, honeycombed appearance of the skull on x-ray is transient, disappearing in the early months after birth. It probably is the result of a defect in membranous bone formation and not secondary to in utero intracranial hypertension, as is often stated. Various theories have been postulated to explain the Arnold-Chiari malfor-

mation; these include traction from below due to attachment of the spinal cord at an abnormally low vertebral level, and herniation of hindbrain structures caudally secondary to hydrocephalus above. The most strongly supported theory is that the Arnold-Chiari malformation is an associated anomaly that occurs in concert with other spinal defects and originates in the embryonic period.

An interesting but somewhat usual clinical disturbance in the infant with a meningomyelocele and the Arnold-Chiari malformation is laryngeal stridor. Most reported cases have developed stridor a few weeks after birth, at a time when hydrocephalus was notably progressive. In some, stridor disappeared following shunt therapy or suboccipital craniectomy (Kirsch et al., Adeloye et al.), but in others, relief of hydrocephalus has had little influence on the respiratory difficulty (Fitzsimmons). Caudal displacement of the medulla, secondary to increased pressure above, resulting in traction on the vagus nerves has been suggested as an explanation for this disorder but without complete verification. Bilateral medullary hemorrhages involving the region of the nucleus ambiguus were found in the cases described by Morley.

**DIAGNOSIS.** The presence of a meningomyelocele in the newborn infant is obvious in most instances. The small, skin-covered lesion with minimal motor deficits

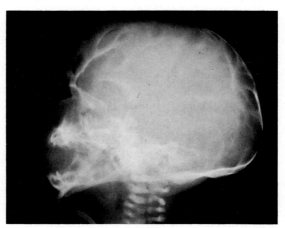

**Figure 83–5.** Lückenschädel, or craniolacuna. Honeycombed pattern of the skull in the newborn infant with meningomyelocele, and usually associated with hydrocephalus.

in the legs can present some initial diagnostic difficulties and rarely is not proven to be a defect in neural tube closure until operation is performed. More practical diagnostic issues in the infant with a meningomyelocele are whether or not hydrocephalus coexists or hydronephrosis is present. An important recent development is prenatal recognition of "open" defects in neural tube closure by the estimation of alpha-fetoprotein content in amniotic fluid. Elevated levels of alpha-fetoprotein in amniotic fluid obtained by amniocentesis between 12 and 16 weeks of pregnancy have been regarded as reliable evidence of a neural tube malformation since the report by Brock and Sutcliffe in 1973. This method has thus far been of value in mothers known to be at increased risk because of a previously affected child. Expanded antenatal detection allowing identification of the first affected child hopefully will one day be realized by extensions of this and other methods (Wald et al.) (see p. 35).

**TREATMENT.** Management of the child with a neural tube closure defect of the spinal region requires a multidisciplinary approach that involves several medical and surgical specialties. The unusual spinal meningocele, which is covered only by a delicate membrane, is surgically corrected as early as possible because of the excellent potential outcome and the danger of infection until the lesion is removed. Those that are skin covered are also surgically excised, although the timing of the procedure is much less critical. Even when the meningocele appears uncomplicated, the child should be evaluated periodically following surgery to be certain that hydrocephalus is not developing and that bladder function is normal.

Selection of methods of treatment for the child with an "open" meningomyelocele with neurologic bladder dysfunction, weakness of the legs and hydrocephalus is far more controversial, for established guidelines are available for only a small percentage. The infant who has a small lesion with minimal or mild neurologic deficits is a candidate for immediate or early surgical closure unless the sac is obviously infected or sepsis is evident. The child who has a large "open" lesion, especially if infected, total paralysis of the legs and significant head enlargement due to advanced hydrocephalus at birth has little chance of survival and virtually no possibility of eventual reasonable intellectual or motor function. This condition is ordinarily not managed surgically in view of the limited accomplishments of this approach.

The child with a meningomyelocele between these two extremes of severity poses the current dilemma with regard to management. The choice between immediate aggressive therapy, delayed and stepwise surgical therapy or totally conservative treatment should logically be partially based on the natural history of the condition. The available information about natural history has solved few problems in this country, where most affected infants receive at least partial therapy, such as antibiotics for acquired infections and shunts for hydrocephalus. In studies of infants who received no therapy except for conventional feeding and infant care, the majority, perhaps over 90 per cent, have died by 1 year of age (Hide et al., Lorber, 1972).

During the last decade, the procedure of immediate surgical closure of the spinal lesion and early shunting therapy for hydrocephalus was adopted in certain centers in Great Britain (Sharrard). This approach developed from the recognized dismal outcome among many in whom treatment was delayed and because of the belief that deterioration of motor function in the legs resulted from desiccation of the exposed neural tissue after birth. After several years' experience with immediate and aggressive surgical treatment, certain observers (Lorber, 1971) now believe a more conservative approach is warranted, with candidates for early operation selected on an individual basis. To this date, the "best" method of treatment of the infant with a meningomyelocele remains in question and the ideal solution is clearly in the areas of prevention and prenatal detection.

## DIASTEMATOMYELIA

The term diastematomyelia designates a split or cleft in a segment of the spinal cord; conventionally, however, it refers to a congenital anomaly in which the cord is transected by a bony or cartilaginous septum that extends from the posterior surface of a vertebral body to the dura or laminar arch dorsally. The etiology of this unusual malformation is unknown; however, it affects girls more than boys and is usually associated with other defects which allow identification of its presence (Perret, Dale).

Although the intraspinal defect is present at birth, neurologic signs are not usually noted until after the child begins to ambulate and a disturbance of gait becomes evident. In almost all cases, the lesion is in the lower thoracic or lumbar region and is associated with an overlying cutaneous abnormality in the form of a tuft of hair, a hemangioma or a visible and palpable lipoma. The absence of such overlying cutaneous abnormalities has been described with diastematomyelia but is quite rare (Sedzimir et al.). Except for the associated cutaneous lesions, detectable abnormalities in the newborn or early infant period are not common, but, when present, they consist of a unilateral foot deformity such as talipes varus or pes cavus, or atrophy of one lower extremity, usually with a foot deformity. In most cases, neurologic abnormalities are first observed 2 or more years after birth and include gait disturbances, limb atrophy, asymmetrical spastic signs in the lower extremities or evidence of neurogenic bladder dysfunction. Spinal cord dysfunction with diastematomyelia often appears to be progressive in childhood, although the cause of this is not clear. Progression of neurologic deficits has been attributed to differential growth rate between the vertebral column and the spinal cord, resulting in gradual downward shearing of the spinal cord by the bony spicule. This explanation has been doubted by some authors, since there is little "ascent" of the spinal cord relative to the vertebral spine after the first few months of life (Guthkelch).

Roentgenographic abnormalities in the child with diastematomyelia are striking and are usually suggestive of the diagnosis. In most cases spina bifida, hemivertebrae and other anomalies are present in the vicinity of the defect. The most consistent x-ray finding is interpedicular widening a few segments above and below the site of the bony or cartilaginous spur without erosion of pedicles. The midline septum, or spur, is roentgenographically visible in certain instances, but its absence on x-ray does not exclude the diagnosis. Myelography establishes the diagnosis in most cases in that the dye column is divided by the septum, producing a linear or circular midline defect.

Treatment is laminectomy, with removal of the median septum, which traverses the cord. Past experience has indicated that surgical treatment is not followed by recovery of limb atrophy or foot deformity but that it can usually be expected to arrest further progression of neurologic deficits.

## CONGENITAL INTRASPINAL TUMORS

Intraspinal tumors, which are infrequent in early infancy, are less likely to be intramedullary in infants than they are in older children. Because of the rare occurrence of intraspinal masses in this age group, of the difficulty in recognizing the progressive nature of the neurologic deficits and of the relatively less diagnostic value of neurogenic bladder and sensory disturbances, early identification of such lesions is often delayed. They are easily confused with, and erroneously diagnosed as, cerebral palsy, cervical cord birth injury or brachial plexus stretch palsy. Before an effective polio vaccine became available, polio was a commonly mistaken diagnosis until the progressive features became apparent.

Intraspinal lesions above the second lumbar vertebra cause signs of spinal cord dysfunction. The character of signs of cord involvement or compression are less predictable in infants than in older children. Although spastic signs are expected, the infant with a cervical or thoracic cord lesion can present with hypotonic limbs which exhibit enhanced deep stretch reflexes. Spinal rigidity, although not always present, is a finding that should suggest the possibility of some form of intraspinal mass, regardless of the age of the child. Intraspinal lesions below the second lumbar vertebra give rise to manifestations of cauda equina compression or to a combination of signs indicative of involvement of the conus medullaris and the cauda equina. Compression of the cauda equina results in hypotonic or flaccid legs, often asymmetrically so, with reflex loss and muscular atrophy in affected regions. A sensory level to pin stimulation usually indicates a spinal cord lesion but can also occur with intraspinal lesions below the termination of the spinal cord.

Although astrocytomas or ependymomas of the spinal cord can occur in infancy, they are unusual in the early infant period (Tachdjian and Matson). Signs of congenital neuroblastoma are usually those of metastatic disease, and include hepatomegaly and cutaneous nodules (Schneider et al.), but direct invasion to the intraspinal epidural space can also complicate these lesions. Direct extension from a primary adrenal tumor is likely to affect the mid-to-low thoracic cord, while that from a mediastinal neuroblastoma will involve the low cervical or upper thoracic portion of the spinal cord. Sarcomatous lesions of various types can either invade the epidural space from the retroperitoneal region or arise primarily within the spinal canal. Extramedullary compression of the spinal cord can also result from a variety of benign or malignant tumors of the vertebrae.

Probably the most frequently identified intraspinal tumor in the young infant is the intradural lipoma (Swanson and Barnett, Debowitz et al.). Most are found in the lumbar or lumbosacral region, although they can occur elsewhere. The presence of a lumbar intradural lipoma is usually signalled by the presence of an associated extradural lipomatous mass, which presents as a soft painless swelling on the midline of the low back. A cutaneous dermal sinus or hemangioma is frequently observed in the region of the superficial mass. X-rays of the spine are diagnostically revealing in most cases because of the presence of widening of the pedicles with pedicular erosion. When the intradural mass extends into the lower part of the spinal canal, hypoplasia or destructive changes of the sacrum are often visualized. Neurologic signs caused by an intradural lipoma in many cases do not develop until the child is a few years of age when unilateral or bilateral, but asymmetrical, weakness and atrophy of the legs are observed. Neurogenic bladder dysfunction is subsequently added to the picture as are variable sensory deficits, especially in the distal portions of the lower extremities and the saddle region. The neurologic abnormalities may very slowly get worse or remain stable for a number of years. In some cases, the intraspinal mass extends cephalad, to be attached to the conus medullaris. When this prevails, the physical signs may include those of dysfunction of the distal portion of the spinal cord and of the cauda equina. Signs of denervation in the infant with this lesion, when present, are usually in the form of a foot deformity and wasting of one lower limb, with associated deep reflex asymmetry. The advisability of surgical excision of the intradural lipoma is a controversial matter. Complete removal cannot usually be accomplished because of the intimate relationship between the mass and the neural elements. Partial excision is recommended when there is evidence of progressive neurologic dysfunction, although every effort must be made not to produce additional deficits from the surgical procedure itself.

Diagnosis of an intraspinal tumor of any type is on the basis of the clinical findings, appropriate x-rays of the spine and contrast myelography. The latter procedure is technically more difficult in the infant than in the older child and especially so if a lumbar puncture has been done within a few days preceding the study. For this reason, it is advisable to withhold a spinal fluid examination until the time of myelography if an intraspinal mass is suspected.

## SPINAL EPIDURAL ABSCESS

Spinal epidural suppuration is uncommon at any age in childhood but is especially rare in early infancy. Of the few reported cases in the young infant, most have been caused by *Staphylococcus aureus,* and most have resulted from hematogenous spread in the septic child. Congenital dermal sinus in the low back can be complicated by epidural abscess formation, although this is infrequent, particularly in infancy.

Because of the anatomic adherence of the dura anteriorly to the vertebral bodies, epidural suppuration involves the posterior portion of the epidural space. In the cervical region, the epidural space is exceedingly shallow but reaches a greater depth in the mid-thoracic and the low lumbar regions. For this reason, epidural abscesses are usually located below the fourth thoracic vertebra and especially in the lumbar area. Involvement in the cervical region in an infant has been described, however (Miller and Hesch).

Clinical manifestations of an epidural abscess depend somewhat on the location of the lesion, although its identification is far more difficult in infancy than in the older child. Fever, vomiting, irritability and spinal rigidity are commonly described signs (Palmer and Kelly, Aicardi and Lepintre, Rushworth and Martin). Reduced motor activity of the legs is less readily observed in the infant, and thus spinal cord or cauda equina damage is likely to become severe before the diagnosis is established in this age group. Lumbar epidural abscess gives rise to hypotonic or flaccid weakness of the lower limbs, with diminished deep reflexes, while a thoracic lesion produces cord compression and is more likely to result in spastic signs in the legs.

In lumbar epidural abscess, a lumbar puncture is likely to identify the lesion because pus is encountered before the dura is penetrated. When this happens, it is important to aspirate what one can but not to advance the needle further into the subarachnoid space. When the abscess is in the thoracic region, lumbar puncture usually reveals a limited quantity of xanthochromic, high-protein-containing fluid in the subarachnoid space, the removal of which makes contrast myelography much more difficult thereafter. For this reason, whenever a spinal epidural abscess is suspected clinically, one should be prepared to perform contrast myelography at the time of the initial lumbar puncture if the findings indicate a spinal block at a higher level. When myelography is necessary in the infant but cannot be accomplished from the lumbar position, the cisternal route is an alternative.

Treatment of spinal epidural abscess includes intravenously administered antibiotics and surgical drainage of the lesion. The prognosis is far better in early recognized cases, accounting for the disadvantage to the young infant with this disease. The greater the neurologic deficits, and the longer they persist before surgical drainage, the less degree of recovery is expected.

## MYASTHENIA GRAVIS IN THE NEWBORN INFANT

Myasthenia gravis is a disease of unknown etiology in which a defect of neuromuscular transmission produces muscle weakness. The disorder in childhood has been classified into neonatal and juvenile types. Transient neonatal myasthenia gravis occurs in infants born of mothers with the disease (Kibrick). Symptoms may be present at birth or may appear in the first day or so of life, with feeding problems manifested by poor suck and swallowing abilities being the most common early abnormalities. The infant with this disorder is hypotonic or flaccid, with a poverty of spontaneous limb movements. The neck muscles are often powerless, resulting in total lack of support of the head when the baby is pulled upward. The Moro response is sluggish or absent, and the cry is weak. When stimulated, the child may appear to be making "crying movements" of the face, but with little sound produced. Weakness of respiratory effort may result in cyanosis. Bilateral facial weakness may be evident on crying, as eye closure is incomplete or absent. External ophthalmoplegia, a common initial sign of myasthenia gravis in older persons, is much less commonly found in the neonatal form. The signs of this disease respond dramatically to appropriate doses of anticholinesterase medication, which establishes the diagnosis and initiates therapy.

Neonatal myasthenia in the infant of a myasthenic mother is a transient disorder with spontaneous disappearance of signs between 2 and 6 weeks after birth and is not expected to recur later in life. Unless recognized and treated, some myasthenic infants will die in the first few days of life. Treatment with Prostigmin (neostigmine) during this period is necessary, but one must anticipate the spontaneous resolution of the disease and stop therapy at the appropriate time to avoid cholinergic intoxication. The mother who gives birth to an infant with this condition may have overt manifestations of the disease, may be in remission or, rarely, may be in the preclinical phase of the disease and develop symptoms later. The offspring of most mothers with myasthenia gravis are unaffected; infants who develop the transient myasthenic state represent only 10 to 15 per cent of those born of myasthenic mothers (Namba et al.). The possibility should be anticipated when any mother with myasthenia gravis enters labor. Tensilon (edrophonium chloride) and parenteral Prostigmin should be available in the delivery room prior to birth of the child. If the infant is significantly weak or hypotonic or has respiratory distress, 0.5 mg of Tensilon should be injected slowly into the umbilical vein. If improvement is definite, diagnosis is established; and treatment may be initiated with an intramuscular injection of Prostigmin methylsulfate in a dose of 0.05 to 0.1 mg. Thereafter, oral Prostigmine or Mestinon (pyridostigmine bromide) should suffice.

Congenital persistent myasthenia gravis is the other neonatal form of the disease; it occurs in infants of mothers unaffected by the illness. This condition is exceedingly rare, and the manifestations are usually mild. Because of these features, congenital myasthenia gravis is difficult to recognize and diagnosis is usually delayed for months or even years. In some cases, fetal movement is described as weak by the mother. The infant's cry is weak, and feeding difficulties are usual in the first few weeks of life. Facial muscle weakness or ptosis may be noted, but external ocular palsies are less commonly found than in the older child. The disorder persists into childhood, with either spontaneous remissions or myasthenic crises being unusual (Millichap and Dodge). Variations in the pattern of neonatal myasthenia may occur, as illustrated by the case described by Greer and Schotland. The infant of a normal mother presented signs of myasthenia gravis at birth which, however, spontaneously abated at six days of age. Treatment is with Prostigmin or Mestinon; however, some cases respond only partially to these drugs. Thymectomy has been performed in early childhood for this illness (Clark and Van de Velde), but is of concern in the very young because of the possible influence on the development of normal immune mechanisms.

Neonatal myasthenia must be distinguished from other disorders that produce weakness in the newborn. To prevent needless death, the possibility of the disease should be anticipated in every baby of a myasthenic mother. Although Werdnig-Hoffman's disease in the newborn may resemble myasthenia, the presence of muscle atrophy, fasciculations of the tongue and the lack of response to cholinergic drugs in Werdnig-Hoffman's disease should distinguish the two. Respiratory distress syndromes or choanal atresia might be suggested by the respiratory difficulty in the myasthenic newborn. Appropriate studies, including chest x-ray and the passage of a nasal catheter, promptly exclude these possibilities. The difficulties in handling secretions that are experienced by the myasthenic newborn may resemble the cardinal sign of esophageal atresia. Cyanosis and tachypnea of the myasthenic infant may also be confused with congenital heart disease. The same signs, plus generalized hypotonia, might be suggestive of generalized glycogenosis until the Tensilon or Prostigmin tests clarify the diagnosis. Cerebral birth injury frequently is associated with neonatal flaccidity or hypotonia and also enters the differential diagnosis. The chief distinguishing feature is the appearance of alertness and responsiveness in the flaccid child with myasthenia as opposed to the lethargy and stupor that accompany cerebral birth insults. In the final analysis, the diagnosis of neonatal myasthenia gravis depends on consideration of the possibility in the infant with muscle weakness and respiratory problems and performance of the proper pharmacologic diagnostic test.

# CONGENITAL MYOPATHIES

Congenital muscular dystrophy has microscopic features similar to other, more common, types of muscular dystrophy. Unlike the Duchenne type which is sex linked and is first manifested by muscle weakness between 2 and 3 years of age, the rare congenital form may affect either sex. It is manifested at birth and in early infancy by hypotonia, generalized weakness, facial muscle involvement and diffuse muscle atrophy. Muscle enzymes are normal or only slightly elevated (Zellweger et al.). Death may occur at various ages after birth although evidence of progression of the muscular process is usually not distinct.

Nemaline myopathy, first described by Shy and colleagues in 1963, is a form of rod myopathy which is sometimes familial (Spiro and Kennedy) and in which the characteristic cytoplasmic inclusions originate in the Z band of skeletal muscle. Although generally considered to be a primary disease of skeletal muscle, certain authors have provided evidence that formation of nemaline structures perhaps is the result of abnormalities of innervation, especially of alpha motor neuron innervation (Karpati et al.). Like other congenital, non-progressive myopathies, nemaline myopathy in infancy is characterized by hypotonic, wasted and weak musculature. Later in childhood, dysmorphic features such as high-arched palate, scoliosis, pectus deformities and long, slender limbs are sometimes seen (Hudgson et al.).

Central core disease is another form of congenital, non-progressive myopathy, first described in 1956 (Shy and Magee). Autosomal dominant inheritance has been suggested for this rare disorder, which is characterized by hypotonia and delayed developmental landmarks in infancy. Weakness is usually mild to moderate, primarily involves proximal muscle groups and does not appear to progress with aging. The diagnostic hallmark of the disease is the microscopic appearance with hematoxylin and eosin or Gomori trichrome stained muscle of central "cores" within most of the muscle fibers. The core zones have been shown to be composed of closely packed myofibrils with absence of mito-chondria or sarcotubules (Dubowitz and Roy).

Myotubular (centronuclear) myopathy is a congenital myopathy in which the pathologic condition consists of muscle fibers which resemble fetal myotubes (Spiro et al.). This disturbance has been described by some authors as type I fiber hypotrophy with central nuclei. Diminished tone and muscle weakness are usually slowly progressive from infancy and generally involve the facial and extraocular muscles. The disorder is considered to have a sex-linked recessive mode of transmission.

Other, distinctly rare, forms of myopathy can present in early infancy with hypotonia and weakness, including the various types of the mitochondrial myopathies. These conditions have been divided into the megaconial type, associated with enlarged mitochondria, and the pleoconial type, in which there is an increase in the number of mitochondria (Shy et al.).

These disorders, as well as the rare multicore disease (Engel et al.), sarcotubular myopathy (Jerusalem et al.) and reducing body myopathy (Brooke and Neville), are all infrequent to rare causes of the "floppy infant syndrome." They are clinically suspected by the presence of hypotonia, hyporeflexia and muscular atrophy in the child in whom such findings cannot be explained on the basis of injury or disease of the brain or spinal cord. Electromyography is usually helpful in separating myopathic disorders from anterior horn cell disease, while pharmacologic tests distinguish the rare neonatal or congenital myasthenic state from primary disease of muscle. Definitive diagnosis can only be established by light and electron microscopic examination of muscle tissue.

## REFERENCES

Adeloye, A., Singh, S. P., and Odeku, E. L.: Stridor, myelomeningocele, and hydrocephalus in a child. Arch. Neurol. *23*:271, 1970.

Aicardi, J., and Lepintre, J.: Spinal epidural abscess in a 1-month-old child. Am. J. Dis. Child. *114*:665, 1967.

Brock, D. J. H., and Sutcliffe, R. G.: Alpha-fetoprotein in the antenatal diagnosis of anencephaly and spina bifida. Lancet 2:197, 1972.

Brooke, M. H., and Neville, H. E.: Reducing body myopathy. Neurology 22:829, 1972.

Clarke, R. R., and Van de Velde, R.: Congenital myasthenia gravis. A case report with thymectomy and electron microscopic study of resected thymus. Am. J. Dis. Child. 122:356, 1971.

Dale, A. J. D.: Diastematomyelia. Arch. Neurol. 20:309, 1969.

Drummond, M. B., and Donaldson, A. A.: Air, myodil and conray studies in the hydrocephalus of myelomeningocele. Develop. Med. Child. Neurol. (16:Suppl.) 32:131, 1974.

Dubowitz, V., Lorber, J., and Zachary, R. B.: Lipoma of the cauda equina. Arch. Dis. Child. 40:207, 1965.

Dubowitz, V., and Roy, S.: Central core disease of muscle: Clinical, histochemical and electron microscopic studies of an affected mother and child. Brain 93:133, 1970.

Emery, J. L.: Deformity of the aqueduct of Sylvius in children with hydrocephalus and myelomeningocele. Develop. Med. Child. Neurol. (16:Suppl.) 32:40, 1974.

Engel, A. G., Gomez, M. R., and Groover, R. V.: Multicore disease. Mayo Clin. Proc. 46:666, 1971.

Fitzsimmons, J. S.: Laryngeal stridor and respiratory obstruction associated with meningomyelocele. Arch. Dis. Child. 40:687, 1965.

Gardner, W. J.: Hydrodynamic mechanism of syringomyelia: its relationship to myelocele. J. Neurol. Neurosurg. Psychiat. 28:247, 1965.

Greer, M., and Schotland, M.: Myasthenia gravis in the newborn. Pediatrics 26:101, 1960.

Guthkelch, A. N.: Diastematomyelia with median septum. Brain 97:729, 1974.

Hide, D. W., Williams, H. P., and Ellis, H. L.: The outlook for the child with a myelomeningocele for whom early surgery was considered inadvisable. Develop. Med. Child. Neurol. 14:304, 1972.

Hudgson, P., Gardner-Medwin, D., Fulthrope, J. J., and Walton, J. N.: Nemaline myopathy. Arch. Neurol. 17:1125, 1967.

Jerusalem, F., Engel, A. G., and Gomez, M. R.: Sarcotubular myopathy. Neurology 23:897, 1973.

Karpati, G., Carpenter, S., and Andermann, F.: A new concept of childhood nemaline myopathy. Arch. Neurol. 24:291, 1971.

Kilbrick, S.: Myasthenia gravis in the newborn. Pediatrics 14:365, 1954.

Kirsch, W. M., Duncan, B. R., Black, F. O., and Stears, J. C.: Laryngeal palsy in association with myelomeningocele, hydrocephalus, and the Arnold-Chiari malformation. J. Neurosurg. 28:207, 1968.

Laurence, K. M., and Tew, B. J.: Natural history of spina bifida cystica and cranium bifidum cysticum. Arch. Dis. Child. 46:127, 1971.

Lemire, R. J., Shepard, T. H., and Alvord, E. C., Jr.: Caudal myeloschisis (lumbo-sacral spina bifida cystica) in a five millimeter (horizontal XIV) human embryo. Anat. Rec. 152:9, 1965.

Lorber, J.: Results of treatment of myelomeningocele. An analysis of 524 unselected cases, with special reference to possible selection for treatment. Develop. Med. Child Neurol. 13:279, 1971.

Lorber, J.: Spina bifida cystica. Results of treatment of 270 consecutive cases with criteria for selection for the future. Arch. Dis. Child. 47:854, 1972.

Miller, W. H., and Hesch, J. A.: Nontuberculous spinal epidural abscess. Am. J. Dis. Child. 104:269, 1962.

Millichap, J. G., and Dodge, P. R.: Diagnosis and treatment of myasthenia gravis in infancy, childhood, and adolescence. A study of 51 patients. Neurology 10:1007, 1960.

Morley, A. R.: Laryngeal stridor, Arnold-Chiari malformation and medullary haemorrhages. Develop. Med. Child Neurol. 11:471, 1969.

Namba, T., Brown, S. B., and Grob, D.: Neonatal myasthenia gravis: Report of two cases and review of the literature. Pediatrics 45:488, 1970.

Palmer, J. J., and Kelly, W. A.: Epidural abscess in a 3-week-old infant: Case report. Pediatrics 50:817, 1972.

Perret, G.: Diagnosis and treatment of diastematomyelia. Surg. Gynecol. Obstet. 105:69, 1957.

Rushworth, R. G., and Martin, P. B.: Acute spinal epidural abscess: A case in an infant with recovery. Arch. Dis. Child. 33:261, 1958.

Schneider, K. M., Becker, J. M., and Krasna, I. H.: Neonatal neuroblastoma. Pediatrics 36:359, 1965.

Sedzimir, C. B., Roberts, J. R., and Occleshaw, J. V.: Massive diastematomyelia without cutaneous dysraphism. Arch. Dis. Child. 48:400, 1973.

Sharrard, W. J. W.: Meningomyelocele: Prognosis of immediate operative closure of the sac. Proc. Roy. Soc. Med. 56:510, 1963.

Shy, G. M., Engel, W. K., Somer, J. E., and Wanko, T.: Nemaline myopathy. A new congenital myopathy. Brain 86:793, 1963.

Shy, G. M., Gonatas, N. K., and Perez, M.: Two childhood myopathies with abnormal mitochondria. I. Megaconial myopathy. II. Pleoconial myopathy. Brain 89:133, 1966.

Shy, G. M., and Magee, K. R.: A new congenital nonprogressive myopathy. Brain 79:610, 1956.

Spiro, A. J., and Kennedy, C.: Hereditary occurrence of nemaline myopathy. Arch. Neurol. 13:155, 1965.

Spiro, A. J., Shy, M., and Gonatas, N. K.: Myotubular myopathy. Arch. Neurol. 14:1, 1966.

Stark, G. D.: Neonatal assessment of the child with a myelomeningocele. Arch. Dis. Child. 46:539, 1971.

Swanson, H. S., and Barnett, J. C., Jr.: Intradural lipomas in children. Pediatrics 29:911, 1962.

Tachdjian, M. O, and Matson, D. D.: Orthopaedic aspects of intraspinal tumors in infants and children. J. Bone Joint Surg. 47-A:223, 1965.

Wald, N. J., Brock, D. J. H., and Bonnar, J.: Prenatal diagnosis of spina bifida and anencephaly by maternal serum-alpha-fetoprotein measurement. Lancet 1:765, 1974.

Zellweger, H., Afifi, A., McCormick, W. F., and Mergner, W.: Severe congenital muscular dystrophy. Am. J. Dis. Child. 114:591, 1967.

# XI

Infections

# 84

# IMMUNOLOGY

## *By Robertson Parkman*

## GENERAL CONSIDERATIONS

A consequence of the unique physiology of the neonatal immune system is that the normal infant is protected against some pathogens to which older children are susceptible, while being at risk to suffer severe infections with organisms that give little difficulty later in life (e.g., enteric gramnegative bacteria, herpes simplex virus, cytomegalovirus, Candida albicans). This chapter will deal with some of the unique aspects of the neonatal immune system and how they relate to the neonate's susceptibility to infectious disease.

The newborn infant at the time of birth passes from a relatively pathogen-free environment to one containing a great variety of pathogens—bacterial, viral, fungal or protozoan. The success of the infant in protecting himself against these pathogens depends upon the capacity of his immune system to respond. Some components of the immune system are fully functional at birth, while others have not fully matured.

## SEX DIFFERENCES IN SUSCEPTIBILITY TO INFECTIONS

Several groups have explored the problem of the apparent increased susceptibility of males as opposed to females to a great variety of infections. Washburn and his collaborators noted that the newborn male manifested this enhanced susceptibility even more than did older males. For bacterial meningitis the newborn male-to-female ratio was 1.81:1; for septicemias it was 2.02:1. The authors suggest that these differences "are consistent with the expectations of a genetic hypothesis that concerns a gene locus on the X chromosome of human beings, which is involved with the synthesis of immunoglobulins."

The defense mechanisms of the newborn

infant can be divided into cellular and humoral components (Table 84–1). Those mechanisms that require previous exposure to the specific pathogen to be effective are called immune, while those components that require no prior exposure for their effectiveness are non-immune or general.

## SPECIFIC HUMORAL IMMUNITY

### IMMUNOGLOBULINS

Immunoglobulins are the mechanisms by which specific humoral immunity is mediated. The immunoglobulin molecule is composed of four polypeptide chains: two light chains and two heavy chains. There are presently five known classes of immunoglobulins that are named according to their heavy chains, which are unique for each class: IgG, IgA, IgM, IgD and IgE. The light chains are common to all the immunoglobulin classes (Merler and Rosen).

### IgG

IgG is the predominant immunoglobulin (approximately 75 per cent) in adult life. Antibodies to viruses, bacterial toxins and the encapsulated pyogenic bacteria are almost exclusively IgG (Table 84–2). Maternal IgG molecules are actively transported across the placenta so that at birth infants have IgG levels equal to, if not slightly

TABLE 84–1. *Defense Mechanisms Against Infectious Pathogens*

|  | *Humoral Defense* | *Cellular Defense* |
|---|---|---|
| General | Complement system Properdin system | Granulocytes Monocytes Reticuloendothelial system |
| Immune | Immunoglobulins | Lymphocytes |

**TABLE 84–2.    *Antibodies Passively Acquired by the Fetus***

| Antibodies in Cord Blood Equal to or Higher than Those in Maternal Blood | Antibodies in Cord Blood Less than Those in Maternal Blood, at Times Absent |
|---|---|
| Tetanus antitoxin | Streptococcus agglutinins |
| Diphtheria antitoxin | H. influenzae antibodies |
| Smallpox hemagglutinins | Blood group isoagglutinins |
| Antistreptolysins | Shigella antibodies |
| Antistaphylolysins | Poliomyelitis antibodies |
| B. pertussis antibodies | Salmonella somatic (O) antibodies |
| Toxoplasma (complement-fixing and neutralizing) | E. coli (H and O) antibodies |
| Salmonella flagellar (H) antibodies | Rh complete antibodies |
| Rh blocking antibodies | Heterophile antibodies |

greater than, those of their normal mothers. The IgG molecule has a specific combining site that permits it to attach to the placental cells. The mechanism by which the IgG is transferred is unknown; however, there may be some selectivity based upon the fact that infants of hypergammaglobuline-mic mothers have normal IgG levels and that infants may have smallpox hemagglu-tination inhibition titers significantly greater than those of their mothers. The transplacental transfer of IgG increases with increasing gestational age, with the majority being transferred in the third tri-mester (Fig. 84–1), so that premature in-fants have decreased cord IgG levels when compared to full-term infants. Transplacen-tally derived maternal IgG is degraded by

the newborn with a half-life of three to four weeks; thus, biologically significant mater-nal IgG may be present in the infant's circulation for from 3 to 6 months, depend-ing upon the initial IgG levels, with the duration being least in premature infants (Washburn).

The full-term infant of a normal mother has a full complement of adult IgG antibod-ies; therefore, newborn infants are not susceptible to most common viral infec-tions (measles, rubella, chickenpox) until the transplacentally acquired antibody titer drops to biologically non-protective levels after the first several months. Passive an-tibody protection against the encapsulated pyogenic organisms (e.g., staphylococcus, *Hemophilus influenzae,* streptococcus, pneumococcus) is also present for the first several months. There are no passive trans-placental antibodies to the somatic an-tigens of the enteric gram-negative orga-nisms.

At birth, the synthetic rate of IgG is less than the adult rates. The lowered synthetic rate of IgG may continue for the first sev-eral months of life, so that the total serum IgG level decreases to its minimal value at 3 to 4 months, after which time the serum IgG levels begin to rise in normal children. If there is a delay in the onset of increased IgG synthesis, the period of hypogamma-globulinemia may be prolonged.

The transplacental transfer of maternal IgG may, in some cases, have a detrimental effect on the fetus or newborn. If the mother has either naturally occurring or immune IgG antibodies against red blood cell antigens, such as ABO, Rh, Kell, Le, or

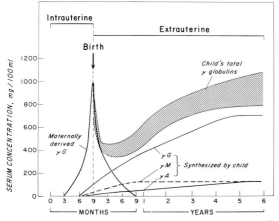

**Figure 84–1.**    Schematic representation of fetal and neonatal immunoglobulin levels. (Adapted from C. A. Janeway in Nelson, W. E., Vaughan, V. C., and McKay, R. J. (Eds.): Textbook of Pediatrics. Philadelphia, W. B. Saunders Co.)

platelet antigens present on the infant cells, such antibodies will cause the increased destruction of the red blood cells or platelets in the fetus, producing either erythroblastosis fetalis or neonatal isoimmunothrombocytopenia. Blood group A or B individuals usually produce isohemagglutinins of the IgM class, while group O individuals may produce isohemagglutinins of the IgG class. Thus, blood group A and B infants of blood group O mothers may receive naturally occurring IgG antibodies transplacentally, producing ABO-incompatible erythroblastosis. The presence of passive antibody may interfere with active immunization with certain antigens. Therefore, immunization with antigens to which the mother has IgG antibodies should not occur when the transplacental IgG is biologically present; that is, earlier for the bacterial protein antigens (DPT) and later for the systemic viral vaccines (measles and mumps) (Provenzano et al.).

### IgM

IgM represents 15 per cent of normal adult immunoglobulins. Antibodies to gram-negative enteric organisms, blood group antigens, and some viral antigens are IgM (Table 84–2). At birth, normally less than 20 to 40 mg per 100 ml of IgM is found in the cord blood. Most, if not all, neonatal IgM is produced by the infant; the synthesis of IgM by the fetus begins by 10 to 15 weeks of gestation. Neonatal IgM levels of greater than 20 mg per 100 ml are presumed to be the result of either increased antigenic stimulation in utero or placental leaks. Therefore, increased (greater than 20 mg per 100 ml) IgM levels at birth should suggest the possibility of an intrauterine infection (cytomegalovirus, toxoplasmosis, rubella or other). Usually little maternal IgM antibody is found in the fetal and neonatal circulation, so that the neonate has no passive antibody protection against the gram-negative enteric bacteria (Cohen and Norins).

### IgA

IgA comprises 10 to 15 per cent of normal adult serum immunoglobulins; however, its principal role is felt to be related to its role as the primary immunoglobulin in secretions such as nasal and gastrointestinal in which most of the IgA antibody is locally produced, with only about 10 per cent being derived from the circulatory IgA. IgA does not cross the placenta. Usually, no IgA is found in cord blood; a cord IgA of greater than 20 mg per 100 ml is most likely to be fetal in origin and is a sign, like increased IgM, of a possible intrauterine infection.

Colostrum has a very high IgA content. IgA, unlike other immunoglobulins, is resistant to the proteolytic effects of gastric acid; therefore, maternal colostric IgA may play some role in passive immunity to enterobacteria, although no firm evidence is available. Infants given oral polio vaccine whose mothers had colostric antibodies may have decreased antibody levels. Normal infants have detectable serum IgA levels by the end of the first month of life, but adult levels are not achieved until the age of 10 years (Smith, 1969).

### IgE

IgE antibodies do not cross the placenta in significant amounts. The most important biological activity of IgE immunoglobulin resides in the skin-sensitizing reaginic antibodies. Infants of mothers with significant allergic histories and symptoms do not give positive wheal-and-flare reactions to antigens to which their mothers are sensitive.

### IgD

IgD globulins have no known specific biological activity. Although little IgD is found in cord blood, 50 per cent of cord blood lymphocytes contain IgD on their cell surface.

### Immune Reactivity

Until recently, it was felt by many that the newborn infant was immunologically incompetent; that is, that the infant was incapable of specific humoral or cellular immune responses. However, it has become clear that the fetus and newborn can respond normally to a wide variety of antigens (Silverstein). Specific IgM antibody to intrauterine infections such as syphilis and rubella has been detected by 16 to 20 weeks of gestation, and IgG antibodies of fetal origin have been detected in the third trimester. After birth, the infant has his primary experience to most antigens, and antibodies to enterobacilli and skin bacteria soon appear in the circulation.

The presence of maternal IgG may decrease the newborn's response to some antigens, contributing to the previous concept of the newborn's immuno-incompetence.

## SPECIFIC CELLULAR IMMUNITY

### LYMPHOCYTE ONTOGENY

Lymphocytes can be subdivided into two classes: T or thymus-derived and B or bone marrow-derived lymphocytes (Raff). T lymphocytes in both adults and fetuses form rosettes with sheep red blood cells and are responsible for protection against fungal, most viral and some enterobacillary infections, and mediate homograft rejections. B lymphocytes are characterized by the presence of immunoglobulin on their cell surfaces and a surface receptor for the third component of the complement system (C3). Some circulating B lymphocytes after antigen exposure migrate to the lymph nodes, where they differentiate into plasma cells that synthesize much of the circulating immunoglobulins.

Whereas the newborn infant has significant passive humoral immunity in the form of transplacental maternal IgG, the infant's cellular immunity is found totally in lymphocytes of fetal origin. Immunocompetent cells capable of responding to foreign lymphocytes in the mixed lymphocyte reaction are found in the fetal liver at 5 weeks of gestational age. Prior to 8 weeks of gestation, the thymus is composed of only stromal and reticular elements (fetal thymus). After that time, lymphocytes are first found and lymphoid follicles and Hassall's corpuscles develop (adult thymus); by 12 to 14 weeks, T lymphocytes are found in the fetal spleen. By 15 to 20 weeks of gestation, the fetus has significant numbers of peripheria T lymphocytes (August et al., 1971).

Lymphocytes that stain with a fluoresceinated antiserum to IgM are first found in the fetal liver at 9 weeks and in the spleen at 11 weeks. Fetal spleen cells are capable of in vitro IgM synthesis at 11 weeks and IgG synthesis at 13 weeks. Thus, by 20 weeks of gestational age, the fetus has the capacity to respond specifically to a variety of antigenic stimuli. The fetal immune response is limited, however, by the lack of antigenic stimulation that occurs in utero.

At birth, the absolute number of T lymphocytes is increased as compared to adult levels, even though the percentage of T lymphocytes is lower than adult levels (Fig. 84–2). The number of B lymphocytes as determined by the presence of a receptor for C3 is increased at birth in both absolute number and percentage. Adult values for T and B lymphocytes are found by 2 to 3 years of age (Fleisher et al.).

Immunocompetent T lymphocytes function primarily by the release of non-specific mediators, such as migration inhibition factor (MIF) and interferon, after the specific stimulation of sensitized lymphocytes. Neonatal lymphocytes are capable of MIF production after stimulation with allogenic lymphocytes, and interferon production is normal after non-specific mitogenic stimulation.

Because of the privileged nature of the uterus, the circulating neonatal T lymphocytes are virginal; thus, the infant displays no skin test reactivity to intradermal skin testing and no in vitro production of MIF to specific antigenic stimulation. The infant's response to fungal and viral infections is in the nature of a primary rather than a secondary response. It takes 5 to 10 days for unsensitized T lymphocytes to become capable of full function. This delay in appearance of specifically immune T lymphocytes may explain the neonate's susceptibility to severe and sometimes fatal infections with viruses such as cytomegalovirus and herpes simplex. Before the infant is capable of a successful cellular immune response (5 to 10 days), death may have occurred. Thus, the normal immune responses cannot be expected to be of significant aid. The use of direct anti-viral therapy, such as ARA-A, should be considered.

The lack of sensitized lymphocytes is also the basis for the high frequency of oral

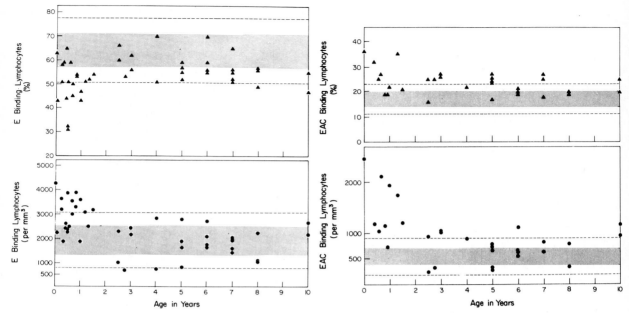

**Figure 84–2.** Scattergram demonstrating the percentage and absolute number of E-binding (T) lymphocytes (*A*) and EAC-binding lymphocytes (*B*) in infants and children. Shaded areas represent the normal adult levels ±1 S.D. (From Fleisher, T. A., et al.: Pediatrics 55:163, 1975.)

and perineal moniliasis in infants. Moreover, recurrent moniliasis with adequate drug therapy (mycostatin) should suggest a possible cellular immune defect.

Although the newborn's lymphocytes appear to be qualitatively normal, there is some evidence that they can be made partially tolerant to foreign histocompatibility antigens. Infants given exchange transfusions with *fresh* blood showed increased survival of skin grafts from the blood donors but not from random individuals (Fowler et al.).

### CASE 84–1

A 36-week-gestation female infant was born after receiving two intrauterine transfusions at 30 and 32 weeks of gestation for Rh erythroblastosis. After birth, two exchange transfusions were necessary for hyperbilirubinemia. All intrauterine and exchange transfusion bloods were from male donors. At 12 days, the infant developed hepatosplenomegaly, a skin rash, and thrombocytopenia.

Bone marrow aspiration revealed spontaneously dividing male cells, and 25 per cent of peripheral blood lymphocytes demonstrated a male karyotype. The diagnosis of graft-versushost disease was made. Although treatment with

anti-thymocyte globulin was instituted, the patient died.

**COMMENT.** The spontaneously dividing male cells were from the first of the exchange transfusions. Since the patient had no demonstrable primary immunodeficiency, it was felt that she had been made partially tolerant to certain histocompatibility antigens because of the intrauterine transfusion. Because of the partial tolerance, she was unable to reject the lymphocytes from the exchange transfusion blood, which ultimately produced graft-versushost disease. The irradiation of exchange transfusion blood with 5000 R would eliminate the possibility of graft-versus-host disease (Parkman et al., 1974).

## GENERAL HUMORAL IMMUNITY

The complement system is a series of nine serum proteins that can react in a sequential fashion with "complement-fixing" antibody that has reacted with circulating soluble antigens or the surface antigens of bacteria, cells, fungi or protozoa. The activated complement system liberates

a series of protein mediators which can 1) increase vascular permeability, 2) attract granulocytes, 3) permit phagocytosis of antibody-coated micro-organisms or 4) cause lysis and death of the organisms. People and animals that have low or absent C1, C2, C3, C4, C5, C6 and C7 have been identified. Only those individuals with a low or absent C5 and C3 have had an increased susceptibility to infections.

The fetus is capable of synthesizing all normal serum proteins, even though the concentrations of some components are decreased as compared to adult values (i.e., alpha-lipoprotein, haptoglobin, ceruloplasmin, C3 and factor B). The concentration of the third component of the complement system, C3, seems to determine the rate of phagocytosis of antibody-coated bacteria. The fixation of C3 to bacteria requires the sequential addition of C1, C4 and C2 after either IgM or IgG antibodies have interacted with the bacterial cell wall. Since the neonatal C3 level, 70 to 110 mg per 100 ml, is less than adult values of 100 to 200 mg per 100 ml, the opsonizing capacity of the neonate's serum is decreased, but the clinical importance of this decrease is not clear.

Because the neonate has very low levels of his own IgG and is only beginning to make significant IgM, another mechanism is clearly necessary for the opsonization of bacteria to which the neonate has no antibody. The properdin system provides such an opsonic mechanism. The rate of phagocytosis mediated by the properdin system is controlled by the level of factor B; since the concentration of factor B is low in most cord blood samples and absent in some, the capacity of neonatal serum to support phagocytosis by adult granulocytes of particles coated with gram-negative lipoprotein is markedly reduced and may account in some part for the increased susceptibility of neonates to gram-negative enteric infections (Stossel et al.).

## GENERAL CELLULAR IMMUNITY

### GRANULOCYTE FUNCTION

Granulocyte function in newborn infants appears to be generally normal as meas-

ured either in vitro or in vivo by cutaneous skin windows. Previous reports of phagocytic defects may have been caused by the serum defects described above rather than primary granulocytic dysfunction. The chemotactic response of neonatal granulocytes to normal stimuli may be slightly decreased.

### RETICULOENDOTHELIAL SYSTEM (RES)

The RES is composed of the fixed phagocytic cells of the spleen, liver and other body tissues. Like the circulating granulocytes and monocytes, they are responsible for the removal of circulating pathogens and foreign particles. RES phagocytosis is partially dependent upon serum factors that may be depressed in newborn serum.

The absence of a significant proportion of the RES as in congenital hyposplenia leads to an increased frequency of bacterial infections, presumably due to the decreased capacity of the RES to clear the blood stream of the opsonized bacteria (Kevy et al.).

## SPECIFIC IMMUNE DEFICIENCIES

### AGAMMAGLOBULINEMIA

Certain humans are incapable of normal immunoglobulin production (Geha et al.). The most severe deficiency is found in those patients who have X-linked agammaglobulinemia and who have an absolute absence of B lymphocytes and no significant immunoglobulin production of any class. Individuals with such a disorder suffer from recurrent infections with the encapsulated pyogenic bacteria (staphylococcus, streptococcus, pneumococcus, meningococcus, and *Hemophilus influenzae*). Since significant maternal IgG is present until at least 3 months of age, an increased incidence of bacterial infections is not seen until after that time. The diagnosis can be established at birth by the absence of circulating B lymphocytes in the infant's peripheral blood.

The common variable form of agammaglobulinemia is a sporadic disease of later onset in which B lymphocytes are present that are capable in some cases of immunoglobulin synthesis but not secretion.

In both forms of agammaglobulinemia the number and the function of the T lymphocytes is normal.

Some patients in later life can suffer from selective lack of IgG subclasses or from dysgammaglobulinemia in which decreased IgG levels are associated with increased IgM or IgA levels, or both. The onset of recurrent infections starts later in life with these syndromes, however.

## DiGeorge Syndrome

The DiGeorge syndrome is the consequence of a developmental abnormality involving the third and fourth pharyngeal pouches. The abnormalities include midline cardiac defects, absent parathyroid glands leading to neonatal tetany, an atypical facies including hypertelorism (Fig. 84–3) and high arched palate, auricular maldevelopment and absence of the thymus gland. Because of the lack of a thymus gland, significant T lymphocyte maturation does not occur, although B lymphocytes appear in normal numbers. The infants suffer from recurrent fungal infections, especially moniliasis, and the common viral illnesses may be fatal. The triad of typical facies, neonatal tetany and lymphopenia should

suggest the diagnosis. The lack of normal proliferation in response to stimulation by phytohemagglutinin is definitive proof of the diagnosis. The infant's immune defect can be corrected by the subcutaneous transplantation of a fetal thymus (August et al., 1970). Within 24 hours, immunocompetent T lymphocytes of recipient origin will appear. Any fresh blood products given to such infants should be irradiated before administration in order to eliminate the possibility of graft-versus-host disease.

## Severe Combined Immunodeficiency (Swiss Form of Agammaglobulinemia)

Severe combined immunodeficiency (SCID) is most probably a primary defect of the lymphoid stem cell. The normal maturation of the lymphoid stem cell is blocked, leading to an absence or marked decrease in both peripheral T and B lymphocytes. The child thus affected suffers from viral and fungal infections (T cell deficiency), and from infections with pyogenic bacteria (B cell deficiency). Since lymphocytes are not present to migrate normally to the thymus, the thymus does not differentiate from its fetal architecture to the adult form. The presence of a fetal thymus is the sine qua non of SCID. In questionable cases, a thymic biopsy will establish the diagnosis.

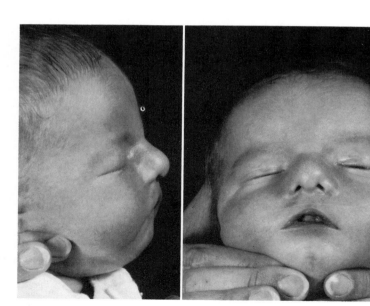

*Figure 84–3.* Typical facies of infant with DiGeorge's syndrome. Note the hypertelorism, shortened lip philtrum and lowset, notched pinnae.

The infants may be clinically well for the first one to two months before they present with recurrent diarrhea, oral moniliasis, pulmonary congestion and recurrent pyogenic infections.

The two genetic forms of the disease, the X-linked and autosomal recessive, have equal frequency leading to a male to female ratio of 3:1. Approximately 50 per cent of infants with the autosomal recessive form have a concomitant absence of normal adenosine deaminase (ADA) in their red cells and other tissues. The absence of ADA has allowed prenatal diagnosis of SCID in one case from cultured amnion cells (Hirschhorn et al.).

Infants suspected of SCID because of a positive family history should be placed in isolation at birth. A chest x-ray to determine the presence of a normal thymic shadow should be obtained, and the capacity of the infant's lymphocytes to respond to PHA and to rosette with sheep red blood cells should be determined. The absence of T lymphocytes in the presence of a previous family history establishes the diagnosis. As in the case of DiGeorge syndrome, all blood products should be irradiated with 5000 R prior to administration to infants suspected of suffering from SCID. Infants affected with SCID have been made immunologically normal by the transplantation of bone marrow from histoidentical donors. The engrafted lymphoid stem cells develop normally, and the patient develops a normal immune system, the cells of which are of donor origin (Gatti et al.).

## RECURRENT PYOGENIC INFECTIONS

Since neonates have adequate maternal IgG, recurrent infections with pyogenic bacteria cannot be due to decreased IgG levels but instead must be due to defects in the other components of the defense system; that is, other humoral factors, especially C3 and/or C5 or primary defects of the granulocytes.

The congenital absence of C3 will produce a markedly reduced rate of phagocytosis, predisposing the infant to infections. The absence of C5 has been associated with Leiner's syndrome, which improved with the infusion of fresh plasma. The C5 defect may also reduce the production of chemotactic factors necessary for granulocyte recruitment.

If the granulocytes are unable to be mobilized and to phagocytose at a normal rate, bacterial infections will start in the neonatal period in spite of adequate immunoglobulin levels.

If granulocytes are unable to kill ingested bacteria, as in the case of chronic granulomatous disease (CGD), infections will start in the neonatal period. The basic defect of CGD is still not clear (Holmes et al.).

## CONCLUSION

The newborn infant may suffer severe infections from a spectrum of pathogens that is markedly different from the organisms causing disease in older children and adults. The infant has passive antibody protection against many of the common bacterial and viral pathogens, and is thus protected. The marginal defects, however, that have been described in the neonate, including decreased serum C3 and Factor B concentrations, decreased granulocyte chemotactic activity and possible decreased RES function, may contribute to the increased incidence of enterobacillary infections that is observed. The virgin state of the infant's T lymphocytes may lengthen the time period required before the newborn cells are able to control fungal and viral infections.

## REFERENCES

Alper, C. A., Colten, H. R., Rosen, F. S., et al.: Homozygous deficiency of the third component of complement (C3) in a patient with repeated infections. Lancet 2:1179, 1972.

August, C. S., Levey, R. H., Berkel, I., et al.: Establishment of immunological competence in a child with congenital thymic aplasia by a graft of fetal thymus. Lancet *1*:1080, 1970.

August, C. S., Berkel, A. I., Driscoll, S., et al.: Onset of lymphocyte function in the developing human fetus. Pediat. Res. 5:539, 1971.

Bazaral, M., Orgel, A., and Hamburger, R. N.: IgE levels in normal infants and mothers and an inheritance hypothesis. J. Immunol. *107*:794, 1971.

Brambell, F. W. R., and Hemmings, W.: The transmission of antibodies from mother to fetus. *In* C. A. Villee (Ed.): The Placenta and Fetal Membranes. Baltimore, Williams & Wilkins, 1960, p. 71.

Brown, G., and Greaves, M. F.: Cell surface markers for human T and B lymphocytes. Eur. J. Immunol. 4:302, 1974.

Bruton, O. C.: Agammaglobulinemia. Pediatrics 9:722, 1952.

Carr, M. C., Stites, D. P., and Fudenberg, H. H.: Dissociation of responses to phytohemagglutinin and adult allogeneic lymphocytes in human fetal lymphoid tissues. Nature (New Biol.) 241:279, 1973.

Cohen, I. R., and Norins, L. C.: Antibodies of the IgG, IgM, and IgA classes in newborn and adult sera reactive with gram-negative bacteria. J. Clin. Invest. 47:1053, 1968.

Cooper, M. D., Faulk, W. P., Fudenberg, H. H., et al.: Meeting report of the Second International Workshop on Primary Immunodeficiency Diseases in Man. Clin. Immunol. and Immunopathol. 2:416, 1974.

DeKoning, J., Van Bekkum, D. W., Dicke, K. A., et al.: Transplantation of bone marrow cells and fetal thymus in an infant with lymphopenic immunological deficiency. Lancet 1:1223, 1969.

Dossett, J. H., Williams, R. C., and Quie, P. G.: Studies on interaction of bacteria, serum factors, and polymorphonuclear leucocytes in mothers and newborns. Pediatrics 44:49, 1969.

Eitzman, D. V., and Smith, R. T.: The non-specific inflammatory cycle in the neonatal infant. A.M.A. J. Dis. Child. 97:326, 1959.

Fleisher, T. A., Luckasen, J. R., Sabad, A., et al.: T and B lymphocyte sub-populations in children. Pediatrics 55:162, 1975.

Forman, M. L., and Stiehm, E. R.: Impaired opsonic activity but normal phagocytosis in low-birth-weight infants. N. Engl. J. Med. 281:926, 1969.

Fowler, R., Jr., Schubert, W. K., and West, C. D.: Acquired partial tolerance to homologous skin grafts in the human infant at birth. Ann. N.Y. Acad. Sci. 87:413, 1960.

Gatti, R. A., Allen, H. D., Meuwissen, H. J., et al.: Immunological reconstitution of sex-linked lymphopenic immunological deficiency. Lancet 2:1366, 1968.

Geha, R. S., Schneeberger, E., Merler, E., et al.: Heterogeneity of "acquired" or common variable agammaglobulinemia. N. Engl. J. Med. 291:1, 1974.

Gitlin, D., and Craig, J. M.: The thymus and other lymphoid tissues in congenital agammaglobulinemia. Pediatrics 32:517, 1963.

Gitlin, D., and Biasucci, A.: Development of gamma G, gamma A, gamma M, beta-l-c/beta-l-a, C'l esterase inhibitor, ceruloplasmin, transferrin, hemopexin, haptoglobin, fibrinogen, plasminogen, alpha-1-antitrypsin, orosomucoid, beta-lipoprotein, alpha-2-macroglobulin, and pre-albumin in the human conceptus. J. Clin. Invest. 48:1433, 1969.

Gluck, L., and Silverman, W. A.: Phagocytosis in premature infants. Pediatrics 20:951, 1957.

Graham, C. W., Saba, T. M., Lolekha, S., et al.: Deficient serum opsonic activity for macrophage function in newborn infants. Proc. Soc. Exp. Biol. Med. 143:991, 1973.

Hirschhorn, R., Berates, N., Rosen, F. S., et al.: Adenosine deaminase deficiency in a child diagnosed prenatally. Lancet 1:69, 1975.

Holmes, B., Quie, P. G., Windhorst, D. B., et al.: Fatal granulomatous disease of childhood, an inborn error of phagocytic function. Lancet 1:1225, 1966.

Janeway, C. A.: Diagnosis of hypogammaglobulinemia. J.A.M.A. 180:320, 1962.

Keller, R., Dwyer, J. E., et al.: Intestinal IgA neutralizing antibodies in newborn infants following poliovirus immunization. Pediatrics 43:330, 1969.

Kempe, C. H., and Benenson, A. S.: Vaccinia: Passive immunity in newborn infants. J. Pediatr. 42:525, 1953.

Kevy, S. V., Tefft, M., Vawter, G. F., et al.: Hereditary splenic hypoplasia. Pediatrics 42:752, 1968.

Kohler, P. F.: Maturation of the human complement system. J. Clin. Invest. 52:671, 1973.

Kretschmer, R., Say, B., et al.: Congenital aplasia of the thymus gland (DiGeorge's syndrome). N. Engl. J. Med. 279:1295, 1968.

Lawton, A. R., Self, K. S., Royal, S. A., et al.: Ontogeny of B lymphocytes in the human fetus. Clin. Immunol. and Immunopathol. 1:84, 1972.

Lepow, M. L., Warren, R. J., Gray, N., Ingram, V. G., and Robbins, F. C.: Effect of Sabin type I poliomyelitis vaccine administered by mouth to newborn infants. N. Engl. J. Med. 264:1071, 1961.

Merler, E., and Rosen, F. S.: The gamma globulins. I. Structure and synthesis of the immunoglobulins. N. Engl. J. Med. 275:480, 1966.

Miller, M. E.: Demonstration and replacement of a functional defect of the fifth component of complement in newborn serum. A major tool in the therapy of neonatal septicemia. Pediatr. Res. 5:379, 1971.

Miller, M. E.: Chemotactic function in the human neonate: Humoral and cellular aspects. Pediatr. Res. 5:487, 1971.

Miller, M. J., Sunshine, P. J., and Remington, J. S.: Quantitation of cord serum IgM as a screening procedure to detect congenital infection: Results in 5,006 infants. J. Pediatr. 75:1287, 1969.

Osborn, J. J., Dancis, J., and Julia, J. F.: Studies of the immunology of the newborn infant. I. Age and antibody production. II. Interference with active immunization by passive transplacental circulating antibody. Pediatrics 9:736, 10:328, 1952.

Osborn, J. J., Dancis, J., and Rosenberg, B. F.: Studies of the immunology of the newborn infant. III. Permeability of the placenta to maternal antibody during fetal life. Pediatrics 10:450, 1952.

Parkman, R., Mosier, D., Umansky, I., et al.: Graft-versus-host disease following intrauterine and exchange transfusions for hemolytic disease of the newborn. N. Engl. J. Med. 290:359, 1974.

Parkman, R., Gelfand, E. W., Rosen, F. S., et al.: Severe combined immunodeficiency and adenosine deaminase deficiency. N. Engl. J. Med. 292:714, 1975.

Propp, R. P., and Alper, C. A.: "C3" synthesis in the human fetus and lack of transplacental passage. Science 162:672, 1968.

Provenzano, R. W., Wetterlow, L. H., and Sullivan, C. L.: Immunization and antibody response in the newborn infant. I. Pertussis inoculation within 24 hours of birth. N. Engl. J. Med. 273:959, 1965.

Raff, M. D.: T and B lymphocytes and immune responses. Nature 242:19, 1973.

Ray, C. G.: The ontogeny of interferon production by human leukocytes. J. Pediatr. 76:94, 1970.

Rosen, F. S., and Janeway, C. A.: Immunologic competence of the newborn infant. Pediatrics 33:159, 1964.

Silverstein, A. M.: Ontogeny of the immune response. Science 144:1423, 1964.

Smith, R. T.: Development of fetal and neonatal immunological function. In N. Assali (Ed.): Biology of Gestation, Vol. II: The Fetus and Neonate. New York, Academic Press, 1968.

Smith, R. T.: Gamma A immunoglobulins and the concept of local immunity. Pediatrics 43:317, 1969.

Smith, R. T., and Eitzman, D. V.: The development of the immune response. Pediatrics 33:163, 1964.

Stiehm, E. R., Ammann, A. J., and Cherry, J. D.: Elevated cord macroglobulins in the diagnosis of intrauterine infections. N. Engl. J. Med. 275:971, 1966.

Stossel, T., Alper, C. A., and Rosen, F. S.: Serum-dependent phagocytosis of paraffin oil emulsified with bacterial lipopolysaccharide. J. Exp. Med. 137:690, 1973.

Warwick, W. J, Good, R. A., and Smith, R. T.: Failure of passive transfer of delayed hypersensitivity in the newborn human infant. J. Lab. Clin. Med. 56:139, 1960.

Washburn, T. C.: A longitudinal study of serum immunoglobulins in newborn premature infants. Bull. Johns Hopkins Hosp. 118:40, 1966.

Yeivin, R., Salzberger, M., and Olitzki, A. L.: Development of antibodies to enteric pathogens: Placental transfer of antibodies and development of immunity in childhood. Pediatrics 18:19, 1956.

# BACTERIAL AND VIRAL INFECTIONS OF THE NEWBORN

# 85

*By George H. McCracken, Jr. and Jorge B. Howard*

In this chapter we attempt to present pertinent information concerning commonly encountered bacterial infections of newborn infants. Emphasis is placed on pathogenesis, diagnosis and management, and every effort has been made to discuss recent data, particularly with regard to antimicrobial therapy. The area of perinatal infectious diseases is advancing so rapidly that it is impossible to be comprehensive, relevant and practical in a single chapter on this subject. It is hoped that the reader will be stimulated to pursue specific areas of interest through the bibliography and the recent medical literature.

## RATIONAL ANTIBIOTIC USAGE IN NEONATES

Selection of antibiotic therapy in newborn infants must depend on 1) the historical experience with infections in the nursery, 2) the susceptibility of commonly encountered bacterial pathogens and 3) familiarity with antibiotic pharmacokinetics in neonates. It is important for pediatricians to know which organisms cause disease most commonly in the nursery or intensive care unit and if antimicrobial susceptibilities of these pathogens have changed significantly within the last 6 to 12 months. For example, the kanamycin susceptibilities of *E. coli* strains isolated from neonates in some North American nurseries have changed recently (Howard and McCracken, 1975). Although significant kanamycin resistance was present in the early 1970's, this is no longer the case in nurseries where usage of this drug was restricted for several years. During this period of limited administration, R-factor mediated kanamycin-resistant *E. coli* strains disappeared, so that when the drug was used again in these units, re-emergence of resistance was not encountered. Careful monitoring of antimicrobial susceptibilities and judicious antibiotic usage in nurseries are helpful in selecting appropriate therapy and in preserving the usefulness of these drugs for a longer period of time.

The rapidly changing physiological processes characteristic of the neonatal period may profoundly affect the pharmacology of antimicrobial agents. Absorption, distribution, metabolism and excretion of drugs depend in part on the maturity and age of the infant. The dosage and frequency of administration schedule must be determined for infants of different gestational and chronological ages and cannot be extrapolated from studies of normal adults. Failure to take these physiological and metabolic changes into account when administering antibiotics to neonates may result in either ineffective or toxic drug dosages.

As a rule, a single antibiotic should be used to treat specific infections such as penicillin G for group B beta-hemolytic streptococcal disease, ampicillin for Listeria and enterococcal infections, and methicillin for penicillinase-producing staphylococci. On the other hand, combining two drugs is good medical practice when initiating therapy for systemic bacterial disease before results of cultures and susceptibility testing are available. Thus, a penicillin (either penicillin G or ampicillin) and an aminoglycoside (either kanamycin or gentamicin) are combined to treat suspected septicemia or meningitis. Once the organism has been identified and the susceptibilities determined, the single most effective drug or combination of drugs should be administered.

Although antibiotics are commonly used in an attempt to prevent infection of neonates, they are effective prophylactically *only* when directed against a single pathogen. For example, penicillin G is effective in preventing group A beta-hemolytic streptococcal infection in patients with previous rheumatic fever, and topical 1 per cent silver nitrate, tetracycline or chloramphenicol effectively prevent ophthalmia neonatorum. On the other hand, when antibiotics are used as "broad coverage" against many potential pathogens, they are rarely effective. This umbrella method of chemoprophylaxis encourages the emergence of resistant strains among previously susceptible bacteria and causes aleration of the normal bacterial flora of the gastrointestinal and respiratory tracts.

Table 85–1, Dosage Regimens for Antibiotics Commonly Used in Newborn Infants, is intended as a guide for treating neonatal bacterial diseases. Modification of these schedules may be necessary in certain specific infections and in patients with compromised hepatic or renal function.

## PATHOGENESIS OF NEONATAL INFECTIONS

Throughout pregnancy and until the membranes rupture, the infant is well pro-

**TABLE 85–1.** *Dosage Regimens for Antibiotics Commonly Used In Newborn Infants*

| Drug | Route | Daily Dosage Infants <1 Week of Age | Daily Dosage Infants 1–4 Weeks of Age |
|---|---|---|---|
| Amikacin sulfate | IM, IV | 15 mg/kg (2) | 15 mg/kg (2 or 3) |
| Ampicillin sodium°° | IV, IM | 50 mg/kg (2)° | 100 mg/kg (3) |
| Carbenicillin disodium | IV, IM | 225–300 mg/kg (3 or 4) | 400 mg/kg (4) |
| Chloramphenicol sodium succinate | IV, IM | 25 mg/kg (1) | 50 mg/kg (1 or 2) |
| Colistimethate sodium | IV, IM | 5–8 mg/kg (2 or 3) | 5–8 mg/kg (2 or 3) |
| Colistin sulfate | Oral | 15 mg/kg (4) | 15 mg/kg (4) |
| Gentamicin sulfate | IM, IV | 5 mg/kg (2) | 7.5 mg/kg (3) |
| Kanamycin sulfate | IM, IV | 15–20 mg/kg (2) | 20–30 mg/kg (2 or 3) |
| Methicillin sodium°° | IV, IM | 50–75 mg/kg (2) | 75–100 mg/kg (3 or 4) |
| Nafcillin sodium°° | IV, IM | 50 mg/kg (2) | 75–100 mg/kg (4) |
| Neomycin sulfate | Oral | 100 mg/kg (3 or 4) | 100 mg/kg (3 or 4) |
| Oxacillin sodium | IV, IM | 50 mg/kg (2) | 150–200 mg/kg (4) |
| Crystalline penicillin G potassium°° | IV, IM | 50,000 units/kg (2) | 50,000–125,000 units/kg (3) |
| Penicillin G procaine | IM | 50,000 units/kg (1) | 50,000 units/kg (1) |
| Polymyxin B sulfate | IV, IM | 3.5–5 mg/kg (2 or 3) | 3.5–5 mg/kg (2 or 3) |
| Tobramycin sulfate | IM, IV | 4 mg/kg (2) | 4 mg/kg (2 or 3) |

°Numbers in parentheses represent numbers of doses in which the daily dosage should be equally divided.
°°For meningitis, double the recommended dosage.

tected from microbes. It is usually not until delivery and in the immediate neonatal period that the infant is exposed to many organisms including aerobic and anaerobic bacteria, viruses, fungi and protozoa. (A few fetuses become infected transplacentally [see Chapter 5]. This encounter initiates colonization of the respiratory and gastrointestinal tracts. The vast majority of neonates establish their microbial flora without incident; however, an occasional infant develops disease caused by one of these organisms. The factors contributing to conversion from colonization to disease are not completely understood.

The two most common bacterial pathogens during the neonatal period are the group B beta-hemolytic streptococcus and *Escherichia coli*. These two organisms account for approximately 70 per cent of systemic neonatal bacterial diseases. Both organisms are acquired primarily from the mother during the intrapartum period. The acute septicemic form of group B streptococcal disease may be caused by any of the group B types ($B_I$, $B_{II}$ or $B_{III}$) and the specific B type causing disease is usually found also in the maternal vaginal tract. Epidemiologic studies have shown that from 5 to 30 per cent of pregnant women are vaginally colonized with group B streptococci. Approximately the same percentage of infants as mothers are asymptomatically infected with these organisms. The major infantile colonization sites are skin, nasopharynx and rectum. The group B streptococcus will persist in the nasopharynx and rectum for weeks to months, while cutaneous infection is usually lost by several weeks of age. It has been estimated that for every 100 infants colonized with group B streptococci, one infant will develop disease caused by this organism (Baker and Barrett, 1973).

Group B streptococcal meningitis is caused almost exclusively by the $B_{III}$ organisms. These organisms may be acquired from non-maternal sites. Clusters of three or four cases of meningitis caused by group B streptococci occurred in nurseries during short time periods, suggesting nosocomial acquisition.

Recent studies have shown that approximately 80 per cent of *E. coli* strains causing neonatal meningitis possess a single, specific capsular polysaccharide antigen, designated K1 (Robbins et al., 1974). This is remarkable when one considers that there are over 100 recognized K antigens associated with *E. coli* strains. By contrast, approximately 40 per cent of *E. coli* strains causing neonatal septicemia possess K1 and only 10 to 15 per cent of strains causing septicemia and urinary tract infections in adults contain this antigen.

The reason for this association between K1 antigen and *E. coli* strains causing neonatal meningitis and, to a far lesser degree, septicemia is unknown. Animal studies have demonstrated that *E. coli* possessing K1 are highly virulent for mice and that this lethal effect can be completely prevented by pretreatment of mice with minute amounts of specific K1 antibody (Robbins et al., 1974). Furthermore, outcome from neonatal meningitis is directly correlated with the presence, concentration and persistence of K1 antigen in cerebrospinal fluid and blood of these infants (McCracken et al., 1974).

Extensive epidemiologic studies have shown that approximately 20 to 30 per cent of newborn babies are colonized rectally with *E. coli* K1 (Sarff et al., 1975). Thirty to 40 per cent of infants and children have K1 organisms on rectal swab culture, as do nearly 50 per cent of women at the time of delivery. Approximately two thirds of babies born to K1 positive mothers will be colonized with the identical serotypes of *E. coli* K1. Vertical transmission of these organisms has been documented in 70 per cent of neonates with *E. coli* K1 meningitis and as the major route of neonatal gastrointestinal colonization. The colonization to disease ratio for *E. coli* K1 is similar to that observed for group B streptococci; that is, approximately 100–200:1. Nosocomial infection with *E. coli* K1 has also been observed in our premature nursery.

Although the pathogenesis of neonatal group B streptococcal and *E. coli* K1 disease has not been completely elucidated, a reasonable hypothesis can be advanced. Studies in children and adults have clearly demonstrated that protection from disease caused by pneumococci, meningococci and *Hemophilus influenzae*, type b, is afforded by specific antibody directed against the capsular polysaccharides possessed by these organisms. A lack of $B_{III}$ antibody in sera from infants and their mothers with neonatal group $B_{III}$ streptococcal disease has been documented recently (Baker and Kasper, 1976.) It is possible, but by no means proved to date, that a lack of K1 antibody in sera of neonates predisposes to *E. coli* K1 disease as well. The mouse protection studies lend credence to this contention.

Although this discussion has centered on only two organisms causing neonatal disease, there are considerable data supporting the importance of vertical transmission of other microorganisms during the intrapartum period. These include *Listeria monocytogenes,* anaerobic bacteria (Chow et al., 1974), mycoplasma (Shurin et al., 1975), chlamydia (Goscienski, 1970), trichomonas (Al-Saliki et al., 1974), *Candida albicans* (Kozinn et al., 1958) and such viruses as cytomegalovirus and *Herpesvirus hominis.* Additional studies are needed to elucidate the pathogenesis of these infections during the perinatal period.

# SEPTICEMIA

Sepsis neonatorum is a disease of infants who are less than 1 month of age, are clinically ill and have positive blood cultures. The presence of clinical manifestations distinguishes this condition from the transient bacteremia observed in some healthy neonates.

The incidence of sepsis neonatorum is approximately 1 and 4 cases per 1000 live births for full-term and premature infants, respectively. These incidence rates vary from nursery to nursery and depend upon conditions predisposing to infection.

**PREDISPOSING FACTORS.** A number of factors have been shown to dispose to neonatal bacterial diseases, and includes age and parity of the mother, prenatal care, sex of the infant, gestational age and associated congenital anomalies. Perinatal maternal complications such as abruptio placenta, placenta praevia, maternal toxemia, premature rupture of the membranes and chorioamnionitis all increase the incidence of neonatal septicemia. Congenital anomalies that cause a breakdown of anatomical barriers or of the immunologic system predispose to infection.

Septicemia seems to be more frequent in male than in female infants. A hypothesis to explain this difference is that the factors regulating immunoglobulin synthesis may be on the X chromosome; therefore, presence of two X chromosomes produces greater genetic diversity to the female's immunologic defenses.

Over the past 5 years ventilatory equipment and monitoring devices have made it possible to treat severely ill infants more effectively. However, these apparatuses have acted as fomites of relatively nonpathogenic organisms, resulting in nosocomial infection. The frequency of these infections varies and is usually sporadic. It may be difficult to recognize these opportunistic infections because of the severe underlying illness requiring intensive therapy and the frequent usage of antimicrobial agents in these infants.

**CLINICAL MANIFESTATIONS.** The early signs and symptoms of septicemia are nonspecific and are frequently recognized only by the mother or nurse. Early temperature imbalance with transient hyper- or hypothermia, tachypnea, bouts of apnea, tachycardia, lethargy, vomiting or diarrhea, and unwillingness to nipple feed may be noted. Jaundice, petechiae, seizures and hepatosplenomegaly are late signs and usually denote a poor prognosis.

Although it is tempting to recommend a workup for septicemia in all infants with non-specific clinical manifestations, this is both impractical and unnecessary in many instances. A complete history and physical examination, coupled with clinical experience, are the best guides in determining the extent of workup. If doubt exists, a blood culture should be obtained.

**ETIOLOGY.** During the past 30 years there has been a shift in the microorganisms responsible for neonatal septicemia and meningitis. In the 1930's and 1940's the predominant organism was group A beta-hemolytic streptococcus, which was replaced in the 1950's by phage group I *Staphylococcus aureus.* From the late 1950's to the present time *Escherichia coli* and group B beta-hemolytic streptococci have accounted for approximately 70 per cent of infections. The prevalence rates for a specific bacterial pathogen vary from nursery to nursery and may change rather abruptly in any one unit. Knowledge of the most commonly isolated bacteria in a nursery or intensive care unit, coupled with the antimicrobial susceptibilities of these organisms, is invaluable in treating suspected sepsis neonatorum.

STREPTOCOCCAL DISEASE. The group B streptococcus is the most common gram-positive organism causing septicemia and meningitis during the first month of life. As indicated earlier (see Pathogenesis), vertical transmission of this organism from mother to infant is the most common route of infection. Nosocomial acquisition of infection has been implicated in some nurseries and may be more common than heretofore recognized. Incidence rates for all neonatal streptococcal disease in Dallas for the period from 1969 through 1973 were 0.6 to 2.4 cases (mean, 1.4 cases) per 1000 live deliveries. The incidence rates for septicemia alone were 0.3 to 1.7 cases per 1000 deliveries (Howard and McCracken, 1974). More recently, rates of 3.1 and 4.2 cases per 1000 live deliveries have been documented in 1974 and 1975, respectively.

Group B streptococcal infection may manifest in a variety of ways ranging from asymptomatic colonization and bacteremia to septicemia, pneumonia and meningitis. The authors have treated two patients with osteomyelitis, four patients with septic arthritis, two patients with otitis media, and one patient each with facial cellulitis, ethmoiditis, scalp abscess and conjunctivitis (Howard and McCracken, 1974).

Two clinically and epidemiologically distinct forms of illness have been described (Franciosi et al., 1973). The early or acute onset type, which usually manifests in the first days of life, is characterized by a high incidence of maternal complications, especially premature labor and prolonged rupture of the amniotic membranes. These infants are usually desperately ill within hours of delivery and may exhibit unexplained apnea or tachypnea, respiratory distress with hypoxia and shock. Chest roentgenograms reveal a diffuse pulmonary infiltrate similar to that seen following aspi-

ration or may be indistinguishable from the findings characteristic of hyaline membrane disease. Colonization of the infant most likely occurs prior to or during passage through the colonized birth canal. The mortality rate is 50 to 80 per cent. Pneumonitis is the primary finding on pathologic examination, and postmortem cultures of the lung, blood and cerebrospinal fluid yield group B organisms. However, histologic evidence of meningitis is usually lacking.

The "delayed" meningitic form of disease usually presents at 1 to 12 weeks of age and is indistinguishable from the other forms of purulent meningitis. Group B streptococci are grown from cultures of blood and cerebrospinal fluid, and the mortality rate is 20 to 40 per cent. The group $B_{III}$ organism appears to be the principal offender in this condition. The pathogenesis is uncertain, but failure to culture the $B_{III}$ organism from the maternal cervix suggests that acquisition of the pathogen may be from other persons in the infant's environment.

Group A beta-hemolytic streptococcal disease is not as common now as in previous decades (Dillon, 1966). Disease caused by this organism varies from a low-grade, chronic omphalitis to fulminant septicemia and meningitis. Because of the explosive nature of this organism in nursery settings, constant surveillance for colonized infants and prompt recognition of disease are mandatory in order to avert a nursery outbreak of disease.

ENTEROCOCCAL DISEASE. The true incidence of enterococcal disease of the newborn is unknown. The organism appears to be a common contaminant of blood cultures in a significant number of infants, particularly when the blood is obtained from the femoral vessels. The importance of identifying the enterococcus as the etiologic agent in septicemia relates primarily to selection of appropriate antimicrobial therapy. In our experience ampicillin alone is satisfactory for treatment of enterococcal septicemia.

STAPHYLOCOCCAL DISEASE. In the 1950's phage group I *Staphylococcus aureus* was the most common bacterial agent causing septicemia in neonatal units. Its unique invasive properties caused disseminated disease with widespread manifestations, including neonatal mastitis, furunculosis, septic arthritis, osteomyelitis and septicemia. Because blood stream infection is usually secondary to local invasion, a careful search for the primary focus must be made in all septic babies. Microbial surveillance, intensified infection control measures and local skin care have reduced colonization and disease rates caused by the group I organism.

More recently, coagulase positive staphylococcal disease in nurseries has been caused by organisms of the phage II group (Melish and Glasgow, 1971). These organisms produce an exotoxin (exfoliatin) that causes intraepidermal cleavage through the granular cell layer due to disruption of desmosomes (Melish et al., 1972). Clinical disease may take one of several forms, which include bullous impetigo, toxic epidermal necrolysis, Ritter's disease and nonstreptococcal scarlatina. The initial finding in Ritter's disease is intense, painful erythema not unlike a severe sunburn. Over the next hours bullous formation may occur which, when ruptured, leaves a tender, weeping erythematous area. A characteristic desquamation of large epidermal sheets occurs approximately 3 to 5 days after onset of illness. A fine desquamation is commonly seen in the perioral region. Bullous impetigo has been the most common disease associated with nursery outbreaks of phage group II staphylococcal infections.

Coagulase negative staphylococci (*Staphylococcus epidermidis*) may be identified in blood cultures of babies and are frequently dismissed as contaminants. Repeated isolation of this organism from blood associated with clinical signs of septicemia should alert the physician to its pathogenic role. Coagulase negative staphylococci are frequently associated with ventriculoatrial shunt infections in patients with hydrocephalus. Eradication of infection frequently requires shunt revision and appropriate antimicrobial therapy. Approximately 20 per cent of these organisms are resistant to penicillin G, and an occasional strain will also be resistant to methicillin. Thus, it is important for the bacteriology laboratory to determine the antimicrobial susceptibilities of this organism in order to assure optimal therapy.

LISTERIA MONOCYTOGENES. The pathogenesis and clinical diseases caused by *Listeria monocytogenes* are similar to those caused by group B streptococci (Nelson, 1970). A fulminant disseminated disease may occur during the first several days of life. The pathogen may be acquired transplacentally or by aspiration at the time of vaginal delivery and multiple organ systems are involved. The infant frequently presents with hypothermia, lethargy and poor feeding. A characteristic rash consisting of small, salmon-colored papules scattered primarily on the trunk may be observed in some infants. Chest x-ray reveals a granulomatous-type infiltrate in some patients, and hepatosplenomegaly is common. Listeria serotypes Ia, Ib and IVb produce the early onset disease while serotype IVb is the predominate type in the late onset form (Albritton, Wiggins and Feeley, 1976).

A delayed form of neonatal listeriosis occurs in the second through fifth weeks of life and primarily involves the meninges. The cerebrospinal fluid white blood cell count will contain 20 to 60 per cent mononuclear cells and gram-stained smears demonstrate pleomorphic, gram variable, coccobacillary forms. These are frequently missed by the untrained observer. The bacteriologic laboratory should be forewarned of the clinical suspicion of Listeria meningitis because these microorganisms are frequently discarded as contaminants because of their tinctorial and morphological similarities with diphtheroids. Overnight refrigeration of the spinal fluid specimens will frequently enhance growth of this organism.

ESCHERICHIA COLI DISEASE. *E. coli* are the most common gram-negative bacteria causing septicemia during the neonatal period. Annual incidence rates for the past 5 years in Dallas have remained reasonably constant at 0.3 to 0.8 cases per 1000 live births (Howard and McCracken, 1974). Approximately 40 per cent of *E. coli* strains causing septicemia possess K1 capsular antigen, and strains identical to that in blood can usually be identified in the patient's nasopharynx or rectal cultures (see Pathogenesis). The clinical features of *E. coli* septicemia are generally similar to those observed in infants with disease caused by other pathogens.

*Pseudomonas septicemia* may present with a characteristic violaceous papular lesion or lesions which after several days develop central necrosis. Although this is most commonly observed in pseudomonas infection, it may also be associated with other pathogens. The neonate who receives broad spectrum antibiotics while in an environment potentially contaminated by "water-bugs" (respirators, moist oxygen, etc.) is particularly prone to disease caused by pseudomonas species or other fastidious organisms.

**DIAGNOSIS.** The diagnosis of septicemia can only be made by recovery of the organism from blood cultures. Blood should be obtained from a peripheral vein rather than from the umbilical vessels, the outer several millimeters of which are frequently colonized with bacteria. Femoral vein aspiration may result in cultures contaminated with coliform organisms from the perineum. It is frequently helpful to obtain cultures of other sites prior to initiating antimicrobial therapy. For example, percutaneous bladder aspiration of urine for culture is frequently helpful in identifying the urinary tract as the focus of infection. Nasopharyngeal, skin and rectal cultures are frequently positive in the early septicemic form of listeriosis and group B streptococcal disease but it must be remembered that colonization of these sites occurs commonly. Examination of material obtained from gastric aspiration for leukocytes and bacteria has been advocated as a means to identify infants who are at risk of developing systemic bacterial disease. It should be pointed out that the leukocytes in the infant's stomach are of maternal origin, and the bacteria observed on stained smears are probably carried from the nasopharynx to the stomach upon intubation. Thus, a history of amnionitis and examination of a pharyngeal swab smear for bacteria are as meaningful as a study of gastric aspirates. All infants with suspected septicemia should have a cerebrospinal fluid examination and culture prior to therapy.

The peripheral white blood cell count is a non-specific test that may be difficult to interpret in newborn infants because normal counts may be as high as 30,000 cells per cubic millimeter on the first day of life. Neutropenia with an increased number of band-forms is highly suggestive of bacterial disease, even in the absence of other laboratory evidence of septicemia.

Many other laboratory tests have been recommended in the evaluation of neonates with suspected bacterial diseases. The erythrocyte sedimentation rate in infected patients is usually markedly elevated above the normal range of 1 or 2 mm per 1 hour at 12 hours of age to 17 to 20 mm per 2 hours at 14 days of age. Elevated rates are not usually observed until 24 to 48 hours after clinical signs of disease first occur.

The unstimulated nitroblue tetrazolium test to differentiate viral from bacterial disease has been used in older infants and children. The test has not proved useful in diagnosing neonatal bacterial disease, because the percentage of polymorphonuclear cells with reduced dye is elevated in healthy neonates. However, recent evidence suggests that the nitroblue tetrazolium test may be significantly reduced in neonates with bacterial disease presumably due to a non-specific toxic effect on leukocytes. Elevated serum macroglobulin values are not observed early in the course of postnatally acquired bacterial disease, and an elevated IgM may reflect congenital viral infection.

**THERAPY.** Before the definitive diagnosis of septicemia is made and prior to the availability of microbial susceptibility studies, antibiotic therapy should be initiated using a combination that includes a penicillin and an aminoglycoside. The choice of antibiotics must be based on the historical experience of the nursery and the antimicrobial susceptibilities of bacteria recently isolated from both sick and healthy neonates. As initial therapy, we prefer carbenicillin or ampicillin in combination with either kanamycin or gentamicin. Ampicillin and carbenicillin are active in vitro against *Listeria monocytogenes* and enterococci as well as against many *E. coli* strains. Carbenicillin is combined with kanamycin in order to provide anti-pseudomonas activity. When the historical experience of the nursery or the physical findings suggest pseudomonas infection, carbenicillin in combination with gentamicin should be used. Because of extensive clinical experience, kanamycin is the preferred aminoglycoside for susceptible coliform bacteria. Recent studies have shown that 90 per cent or more of *E. coli* strains obtained from nurseries previously experiencing kanamycin resistance are again susceptible to this drug. Pharmacologic studies have shown that the currently recommended kanamycin dosage of 15 mg per kg per day given every 12 hours to all neonates be modified to 15 to 30 mg per kg per day in two or three divided doses, depending on the birth weight and chronologic age. Gentamicin has been used safely and effectively in the treatment of neonatal bacterial diseases. In order to retain its effectiveness, this drug should be reserved for therapy of infections caused by kanamycin-resistant coliforms and Pseudomonas species. Once the pathogen is identified and its antimicrobial susceptibilities known, the most effective and least toxic drug or combination of drugs should be used. The newer aminoglycosides tobramycin and amikacin should not be used until there is additional data available concerning long-term toxicity. The one exception to this rule is for therapy of disease caused by kanamycin and gentamicin resistant gram negative organisms.

## PURULENT MENINGITIS

The relative incidence of purulent meningitis of the newborn varies among institutions and is higher in those city hospitals where prenatal care is suboptimal and where complicated pregnancies and deliveries often result in high risk premature births. Incidence rates are approximately two to four cases per 10,000 live births and may be as high as one case per 1000 live births in some nurseries. Group B betahemolytic streptococci and *E. coli* strains account for about 70 per cent of all cases and *Listeria monocytogenes* is seen in an additional 5 per cent of infants.

Infants with group B streptococcal meningitis usually present beyond the first several days of life, and the group B$_{III}$ organism is the principal serotype encountered in these infants. The mortality is 20 to 40 per cent. Streptococcal disease occurring in the first 48 hours after delivery is usually manifested as acute respiratory distress with or without shock. Although the organism is frequently isolated from postmortem cerebrospinal fluid cultures from these infants, histologic evidence of meningeal inflammation is usually lacking (Franciosi et al., 1973).

Approximately 80 per cent of all *E. coli* causing meningitis possess K1 antigen. The 018 and 07 somatic types and H6 and H7 flagellar types are most commonly associated with K1 strains cultured from cerebrospinal fluid (Sarff et al., 1975). The presence, concentration and persistence of this capsular polysaccharide antigen in cerebrospinal fluid and blood of infants with meningitis correlate directly with outcome from disease. The current mortality rates for neonatal *E. coli* meningitis vary from 20 to 30 per cent in some centers to 50 and 60 per cent in others.

**PATHOLOGY.** The pathologic findings are similar regardless of bacterial etiology. Studies of the fulminant, early onset form of group B streptococcal disease have shown primarily a bronchopneumonia and shock without histologic evidence of meningeal involvement. The most consistent findings at necropsy of babies dying of meningitis are purulent exudate of the meninges and of the ependymal surfaces of the ventricles associated with vascular inflammation. The inflammatory response of neonates is similar to that observed in adults with meningitis, with the exception that babies have a sparsity of plasma cells and lymphocytes during the subacute stage of meningeal reaction. Hydrocephalus and a non-infectious encephalopathy can be demonstrated in approximately 50 per cent of infants dying with meningitis. Subdural effusions occur rarely in neonates. In contrast, this complication of meningitis is common in infants 3 to 12 months of age. Varying degrees of phlebitis and arteritis of intracranial vessels can be found in all infants dying of meningitis. Thrombophlebitis with occlusion of veins may occur in the subependymal zones. K1 antigen has been demonstrated in brain tissue of infants succumbing to *E. coli* K1 infection.

**CLINICAL MANIFESTATIONS.** The early signs and symptoms of neonatal meningitis are frequently indistinguishable from those of septicemia. Specific findings such as stiff neck and Kernig and Brudzinski signs are rarely found. Lethargy, feeding problems and altered temperature are the most frequent presenting complaints, and respiratory distress, vomiting, diarrhea and abdominal distention are common findings. A bulging fontanelle may be a late sign of meningitis. Seizures are observed frequently and may be caused by direct central nervous system inflammation or occur in association with hypoglycemia, hyponatremia or hypocalcemia.

**DIAGNOSIS.** Interpretation of cerebrospinal fluid cell counts in newborn infants may be difficult (Naidoo, 1968, and Sarff et al., 1976). During the first several days of life, as many as 32 white blood cells per mm$^3$ (mean, 8 cells per mm$^3$) may be found in cerebrospinal fluid of healthy or high risk, uninfected babies. Approximately 60 per cent of these cells are polymorphonuclear leukocytes. During the first week, the cell count slowly diminishes in full-term and increases in premature infants. Cell counts in the range of 0 to 10 cells per mm$^3$ are observed at 1 month of age. The cerebrospinal fluid protein concentration may be as high as 170 mg per 100 ml and the cerebrospinal fluid glucose to blood glucose percentage ratio is 44 per cent to greater than 100 per cent in both preterm and term infants. Thus, it is apparent that the total evaluation of the cerebrospinal fluid examination is necessary in order to make an early diagnosis of neonatal meningitis. Although the cerebrospinal fluid cell counts and protein and sugar concentrations from normal infants overlap with those from infants with meningitis, less than 1 per cent of babies with proved meningitis have a totally normal cerebrospinal fluid study on the initial lumbar tap (Sarff et al., 1976).

It is important to examine carefully stained smears of cerebrospinal fluid from every infant with suspected meningitis. Grossly clear fluid may contain few white blood cells and many bacteria. The stained smears from approximately 20 per cent of neonates with proved meningitis will be interpreted as showing no bacteria. As the name implies, *Listeria monocytogenes* commonly evokes a mononuclear cellular response in the cerebrospinal fluid.

Two new techniques to rapidly diagnose bacterial meningitis have recently been described. The first counter-immunoelectrophoresis (CIE), is used to detect bacterial capsular antigens in cerebrospinal fluid. Studies to date indicate that antigen can be identified in cerebrospinal fluid of approximately two thirds of infants with *E. coli* K1, *H. influenzae*, type b, and pneumococcal and meningococcal meningitis McCracken et al., 1974; Shackelford et al., 1974). If concentrated urine is examined for antigen, the diagnosis of H. influenzae and meningococcal disease can be established in most patients. Group B streptococcal antigen has also been measured in body fluids. Quantitation of antigen is helpful in the prognosis of infants with purulent meningitis.

The second method involves detection of endotoxin utilizing the limulus lysate assay. Endotoxin can be measured in cerebrospinal fluid of patients with meningitis caused by coliform bacteria, *H. influenzae*, type b, or meningococcus (Nachum et al., 1973). Both the CIE and the limulus lysate techniques take less than 1 hour to run and can be established in most hospital laboratories. If both methods are used, approximately 80 per cent of neonates with coliform meningitis can be identified within an hour of the initial lumbar tap (McCracken and Sarff, 1976).

Blood and urine cultures should be obtained from every infant with suspected meningitis.

**THERAPY.** Selection of appropriate antibiotic therapy is based in part on the achievable cerebrospinal fluid levels of these drugs in relationship to the susceptibility of the organisms causing disease. The highest cerebrospinal fluid kanamycin and gentamicin concentrations in spinal fluid are approximately 40 per cent of the peak serum levels and are only equal to or slightly greater than the minimal inhibitory concentrations for disease-causing coliforms. In contrast, cerebrospinal fluid penicillin and ampicillin concentrations may be only 10 per cent of the corresponding peak serum levels, but these values are usually 10- to 100-fold higher than the greatest minimal inhibitory concentrations for group B streptococci and *L. monocytogenes*. The ability to attain spinal fluid antimicrobial activity that is many times greater than is necessary to inhibit the pathogen may explain the rapid sterilization of spinal fluid cultures from infants with gram-positive meningitis. Delayed sterilization of cerebrospinal fluid cultures from neonates with gram-negative meningitis may likewise be due to the low inhibitory and bactericidal spinal fluid concentrations. As a result of these considerations, it may be necessary in some infants with coliform meningitis to alter the therapeutic regimens by adding a second antibiotic, by selecting a different aminoglycoside or by changing the route of administration.

At the present time, ampicillin and either gentamicin or kanamycin are recommended for initial therapy of neonatal meningitis. The dosages of ampicillin are 100 mg per kg per day in two divided doses during the first week of life and 200 mg per kg per day in three divided doses thereafter. The dosages for gentamicin and kanamycin are the same as those used for septicemia (Table 85–1). All infants should have a repeat spinal fluid examination and culture at 24 to 36 hours after initiation of therapy. If organisms are seen on methylene blue or gram-stained smears of the fluid, modification of the therapeutic regimen should be considered. The Neonatal Meningitis Cooperative Study Group was unable to demonstrate a significant improvement in morbidity and mortality rates for infants treated with intrathecal gentamicin (1 mg daily) compared with those treated with parenteral therapy only (McCracken and Mize, 1976). It is possible that larger dosages of gentamicin intrathecally (2 to 4 mg daily) may be more efficacious but there are as yet no data to support this contention. In our experience, most infants with delayed sterilization of spinal fluid have ventriculitis, and cultures of ventricular fluid yield the pathogen. These infants usually improve with adequate drainage of the ventricles and direct instillation of gentamicin into the ventricles. Thus, an alternative therapeutic approach to infants with gram-negative meningitis may be to perform a diagnostic ventricular tap on the first or second day of illness and to instill gentamicin intraventricularly if ventriculitis is documented. There are presently no data to substantiate this approach to therapy. If intrathecal or intraventricular gentamicin is used, it is advisable to monitor cerebrospinal or ventricular fluid levels in order to be certain that the drug is present in therapeutic and safe concentrations. Intrathecal or intraventricular therapy is continued until the fluid is sterile.

Once the pathogen has been identified and the susceptibility studies are available, the single drug or combination of drugs that is most effective should be used. In general, penicillin is preferred for group B streptococcal infection, ampicillin for *L. monocytogenes* and *Enterococcus*, ampicillin plus gentamicin or kanamycin for coliforms, and carbenicillin with or without gentamicin for *Pseudomonas* infections. There is no precise method for determining duration of antimicrobial therapy. A useful guide is to continue therapy for approximately 2 weeks after sterilization of cerebrospinal fluid cultures or for a minimum of 2 weeks for gram-positive meningitis and of 3 weeks for gram-negative meningitis, whichever is longest.

Attention to general supportive therapy is of utmost importance in caring for infants with meningitis. Disturbances of fluid and electrolyte balance are common, particularly in the first several days of illness when inappropriate antidiuretic hormone secretion may lead to fluid retention and hyponatremia. Ventilatory assistance is frequently necessary, and blood pressures should be carefully monitored. During the course of illness, hemoglobin and hematocrit values should be checked frequently, because infection may exaggerate and prolong the anemias of infancy, particularly in premature infants. Some authorities recommend transfusions with fresh, whole blood or frozen plasma as a means of providing non-specific factors of host resistance.

**PROGNOSIS.** The mortality in neonatal meningitis is high. The overall mortality rate is approximately 20 to 50 per cent, depending on the etiologic agent, the high risk factors predisposing the infant to illness and the ability of nursery personnel and physicians to provide general supportive care. Short and long-term sequelae of neonatal meningitis are frequent. The acute complications include communicating or noncommunicating hydrocephalus, subdural effusions, ventriculitis, deafness and blindness. Gross retardation may be obvious immediately. However, many infants will appear relatively normal at time of discharge, and only after prolonged and careful followup will perceptual difficulties, reading problems or signs of minimal brain damage become apparent. Approximatley 40 to 50 per cent of survivors will have some evidence of neurologic damage.

## ASEPTIC MENINGITIS

Aseptic meningitis is an acute nonbacterial inflammatory disease of the meninges which is caused principally by viral agents. The illness occurs frequently in older infants and children, but is uncommon in newborn infants. Disease in young infants is either sporadic or occurs in sharply defined epidemics. It is important to differentiate aseptic from bacterial meningitis of infancy because therapy and prognosis are different in the two conditions.

In young infants it is frequently difficult to clinically separate aseptic meningitis from encephalitis. The etiology of viral central nervous system disease depends in part on seasonal variation, age and immune status of the host. In older infants and children, the enteroviruses (Coxsackie B and echoviruses) account for most cases of aseptic meningitis during the summer months, whereas mumps, lymphocytic choriomeningitis and other viruses are more common during the other seasons. During epidemics of arthropod-borne encephalitis, such as those caused by St. Louis or California encephalitis virus, a mild aseptic meningitis may be seen in young infants and occasionally in neonates. The mild nature of the disease in early life may be due in part to passively transferred antibodies from immune mothers and the relatively isolated status of young infants with regard to community outbreaks. On the other hand, certain viruses appear to cause significant disease primarily in the very young, such as encephalomyocarditis caused by Coxsackie B viruses and hemorrhagic meningoencephalitis due to *Herpes-virus hominis.* In Coxsackie B disease, multiple organs including brain, myocardium, blood, kidney and liver may be involved (Eichenwald et al., 1967, and Overall and Glasgow, 1970). In one nursery outbreak, Coxsackie B5 caused aseptic meningitis only (Brightman et al., 1966). Echovirus type II-prime has been etiologically associated with a nursery epidemic of aseptic meningitis (Miller et al., 1968) and sporadic cases have been caused by echoviruses 9 and 14.

Encephalitis with or without involvement of the meninges may occur in young infants and is caused by the above mentioned viral agents as well as by the arboviruses. Involvement by the latter agents is principally by Eastern equine encephalomyelitis and Western equine encephalomyelitis. St. Louis encephalomyelitis is rare in newborn infants. Congenital infections caused by cytomegalovirus, *Herpesvirus hominis,* type 2, or rubella virus produce encephalitis in a variable percentage of infants.

**SYMPTOMS.** Poor temperature control, lethargy, diminished appetite and "failure-to-thrive" are the most common presenting symptoms. In some infants, a shock-like syndrome associated with seizures occurs. It may be difficult to differentiate this clinical illness from that of bacterial meningitis. In a small percentage of patients, an erythematous maculopapular eruption with or without petechiae may suggest a viral etiology.

**DIAGNOSIS.** Aseptic meningitis should be suspected if several infants in a nursery develop illness over a short period of time or if illness is detected in an infant during a community outbreak of aseptic meningitis. Lymphocytic choriomeningitis virus should be suspected if pet hamsters are present in the household of the patient. Although outbreaks are caused by a single viral agent, the clinical manifestations may differ among infected infants. While some infants manifest respiratory symptoms, others may have gastrointestinal illness, and all may have findings indicating involvement of the meninges. Aseptic meningitis is diagnosed in these infants by failure to demonstrate bacteria or fungi on stained smears and on cultures of cerebrospinal fluid. The cerebrospinal fluid white blood cell count is usually in the range of 50 to 200 cells per mm³, and the cells are usually mononuclear; lower counts may be confused with those observed in normal neonates (see Bacterial Meningitis). Occasionally, high counts with predominance of polymorphonuclear cells may be observed early in illness. The cerebrospinal fluid protein and sugar content are usually within normal limits, although hypoglycorrhachia may be seen in mumps or lymphocytic choriomeningitis infection. If doubt exists as to the cause of the cerebrospinal fluid pleocytosis after the initial lumbar tap, a second examination should be performed approximately 4 to 6 hours later. The absolute white blood cell count and percentage of neutrophils should significantly increase and the spinal fluid glucose to blood glucose ratio decrease if the patient has bacterial meningitis. A definitive diagnosis is made by isolation of the viral agent from cultures of throat or rectum (rarely from cerebrospinal fluid), accompanied by a significant rise in serum antibody titer to the specific agent.

At the present time, there is no specific antiviral therapy for postnatally acquired viral meningitis. Intensive supportive care is frequently necessary, with particular attention to maintenance of pH and electrolyte balance, respiratory assistance and adequate nutrition. When one or more infants develop illness in a newborn nursery, every effort should be made to define the etiology and source of infection. The affected infants should be isolated and treated as a cohort until discharge. Although the infant may appear well at discharge, several long-term followup studies have shown neurologic deficits in some infants with neonatal aseptic meningitis.

## OTITIS MEDIA

Otitis media is infrequently diagnosed in neonates because of the paucity of clinical findings and the difficulty in examining the infant's tympanic membrane (Warren and Stool, 1971). The external canal is narrow and often filled with cheesy debris. Because the healthy baby's membrane may appear thickened and dull, mobility of the drum by pneumoscopy should be used as the single most reliable indicator of middle ear infection.

Neonatal otitis media occurs commonly in premature infants and almost exclusively in bottle-fed babies. The exact incidence of this disease is unknown, but it has been estimated to occur in approximately 1 to 5 per cent of infants 0 to 6 weeks of age. The onset of illness is insidious, and the most common complaints are usually rhinorrhea, irritability and failure to thrive. Fever greater than 38° C. and tugging of the affected ear are unusual.

It is important that all neonates with suspected otitis media have needle aspiration of middle ear contents. This is because the pathogens associated with disease are different from those encountered in infants beyond the first several months of life (Bland, 1972). The material obtained from aspiration is cultured in suitable media, and a stained smear is prepared for direct visualization of bacteria. *E. coli*, *Staphylococcus aureus* and *Klebsiella pneumoniae* are causative in approximately one fifth of cases. *Diplococcus pneumoniae* and *H. influenzae* are the most frequently encountered pathogens during the first 6 weeks of life, as they are during the entire infancy period. All neonates with otitis media should be treated in the hospital with parenterally administered antibiotics Selection of initial therapy is based on results of the Gram-stained smear. If organisms are not observed, methicillin and gentamicin should be started and continued until results of cultures and susceptibility studies are available.

The importance of establishing the diagnosis and etiology of otitis media in neonates and of employing appropriate therapy cannot be overemphasized. Missed diagnosis and improper therapy may result in a chronic course of middle ear disease throughout infancy and, occasionally, in extension of infection to adjacent structures such as the mastoid or central nervous system.

## DIARRHEAL DISEASE

Diarrheal disease during the neonatal period is usually brief and self-limited.

Brief episodes of loose stools secondary to alterations of diet and feeding pattern are common in young infants. Modern sterilization practices and increased emphasis on infection control measures have significantly reduced the incidence of bacterial diarrhea in nurseries.

**ETIOLOGY AND PATHOGENESIS.** On the basis of present information, bacteria are believed to cause diarrhea by one of two mechanisms (DuPont and Hornick, 1973, and Rudoy and Nelson, 1975). The first involves colonization of the upper small bowel by an organism capable of producing enterotoxin, a bacterial exotoxin. These bacteria attach to, but do not invade, the gut wall. The enterotoxin causes stimulation of cyclic-AMP, which in turn inhibits sodium and chloride transport across the intestinal wall. As a result, these salts are lost into the lumen of the upper bowel, followed passively by water, causing a net loss of high electrolyte-containing stools. *Vibrio cholera*, some *E. coli* (almost exclusively nonenteropathogenic strains) and *Vibrio parahemolyticus* are examples of bacteria which cause diarrhea by this mechanism. The importance of recognizing this form of diarrheal disease is emphasized in a recent nursery outbreak in the Southwestern United States (Boyer et al., 1975). Severe, watery diarrhea was observed in 59 infants during a 9 month period and 7 per cent of the infants died, secondary to altered hepatic function and a hemorrhagic diathesis. An 0142/K86/H6 *E. coli* strain was responsible for this outbreak. This organism was not identified by the bacteriology laboratory as an enteropathogenic strain. By special laboratory techniques, this *E. coli* 0142 was shown to produce labile enterotoxin and was not invasive, as judged by several in vitro test systems.

The second mechanism for bacterial diarrhea involves invasion of the intestinal mucosa. Shigella dysentery is the classic example of this disease. Colonic invasion and subsequent destruction of the mucosa cause an outpouring of polymorphonuclear cells and mucus. The resultant diarrhea is usually bloody and contains mucus and pus. Salmonella species also invade the intestinal mucosa, but extensive destruction does not occur. The epithelial lining is left intact, and the organism reaches the lamina propria, where an inflammatory response is elicited.

**CLINICAL MANIFESTATIONS.** It may be difficult to differentiate the causes of diarrhea in neonates on the basis of clinical findings only (Nelson and Haltalin, 1971). As a general rule, diarrhea caused by enteropathogenic strains of *E. coli* is insidious in onset, is associated with seven to 10 green, watery stools a day, and is usually without blood or mucus. The infants do not appear acutely ill. Complications are rare and are related primarily to dehydration and electrolyte disturbances. Salmonella gastroenteritis is usually associated with five to 10 foul-smelling, loose green stools daily, which rarely contain mucus or blood. Complications are unusual and include extraintestinal foci of infection such as septicemia, osteomyelitis or septic arthritis. Shigellosis is rare in neonates but when encountered, it is an acute illness associated with a profuse, watery, non-odorous diarrhea frequently containing blood and mucus. The infants may be very toxic, and illness in a small number of patients will initially mimic meningitis or gram-negative shock. Suppurative complications are rare, but dehydration and electrolyte disturbances are common and need immediate and constant attention.

A useful procedure for differentiating enteroinvasive from enterotoxigenic diarrhea is examination of fecal material for polymorphonuclear cells. Feces from patients with dysentery show significant numbers of polymorphonuclear cells, while those from patients with enterotoxigenic disease show very few neutrophils. A mononuclear inflammatory response is said to present in stools from patients with *Salmonella typhi* disease. This test may be helpful in selecting appropriate antimicrobial therapy.

**THERAPY.** The single most important aspect of therapy for infantile diarrhea is maintenance of hydration and electrolyte balance. As a rule, parenteral solutions containing appropriate electrolytes should be administered during the time of active diarrhea and the infant should be examined and weighed frequently to insure proper rehydration and prevention of complications. Estimation of fluid loss from diarrhea and vomiting should be carefully recorded and used as a basis for replacement therapy.

The selection of an antimicrobial agent depends in part on the mechanism of diarrhea. An absorbable antibiotic such as ampicillin or chloramphenicol is indicated for disease caused by invasive bacteria, while orally administered non-absorbable drugs such as neomycin or colistin sulfate are used for non-invasive organisms which produce enterotoxin.

All nursery infants with enteropathogenic *E. coli* should receive neomycin or colistin sulfate orally, whether they are symptomatic or not. Neomycin is administered orally in a dosage of 100 mg per kg per day in three or four divided doses. Colistin sulfate is administered in a dosage of 15 to 17 mg per kg per day orally in four divided doses. The duration of therapy is 3 to 5 days. Longer periods of therapy are unnecessary and may result in neomycin-induced steatorrhea (Nelson, 1971). If enteropathogenic *E. coli* are isolated from stools of non-hospitalized, asymptomatic infants, it is usually not necessary to treat these infants with antimicrobial agents; however, they should be followed carefully.

All infants with Salmonella gastroenteritis should have blood cultures performed and be examined for development of disease at other sites, such as bones and joints. Neonates with symptomatic Salmonella infections should receive antimicrobial therapy because of the greater potential for systemic infection in these patients. Older infants and children with Salmonella gastroenteritis and asymptomatic neonates with positive stool cultures for Salmonella species should not receive antibiotics. In these patients, antimicrobial therapy may prolong gastrointestinal Salmonella carriage and does not significantly affect the clinical course of disease. When therapy is indicated in the neonate or young infant, ampicillin is the drug of choice and should be administered parenterally in a dosage of 50 to 100 mg per kg per day, divided in two or three doses. Therapy is continued for approximately 5 to 7 days.

Although shigellosis in the neonate is rare, it may be associated with significant morbidity and mortality. All neonates with symptomatic shigellosis should be treated with ampicillin in a dosage of 50 to 100 mg per kg per day, administered parenterally in two or three divided doses. Duration of therapy is approximately 5 days. In some hospitals a significant percentage of ampicillin-resistant Shigella strains have been encountered. In these centers, trimethoprim and sulfamethoxazole is the initial drug of choice. The dosage is 10 mg TMP per 50 mg SMK per kg per day in two divided doses for 5 days.

Any infant with diarrhea must be isolated from the other babies in the nursery. Surveillance of other infants in the unit and institution of infection control measures are also indicated (see Nosocomial Bacterial Disease).

## URINARY TRACT INFECTION

Improved methods for obtaining sterile specimens have made it possible to define more accurately the incidence of neonatal urinary tract infection. Utilizing bladder aspiration technique (Edelman et al., 1973), bacteriuria may be demonstrated in approximately 1 per cent of full-term infants and 3 per cent of premature infants. Urinary tract infections are more common in babies born to bacteriuric mothers and in males during the neonatal period, in contrast to the predominance of females beyond this period.

**ETIOLOGY.** *Escherichia coli* is the most common etiologic agent of urinary tract infections. Approximately 70 per cent of *E. coli* strains belong to one of eight common somatic antigen groups similar to those found in older patients. Renal parenchymal disease may be associated with one of several *E. coli* capsular types: K1, K2ac, K12 or K13 (Kaijser, 1972). Klebsiella and Pseudomonas species are encountered less frequently. Proteus species commonly cause urinary tract disease in infants with meningomyeloceles. Gram-positive bacteria, with the exception of enterococci, are rare causes of urinary tract infection.

**CLINICAL MANIFESTATIONS.** The majority of infants with significant bacteriuria are asymptomatic. When symptoms are present they are usually non-specific and include poor weight gain, altered temperature, cyanosis or gray skin color, abdominal distention, with or without vomiting, and loose stools. Jaundice, hepatomegaly and thrombocytopenia may be observed in a few infants with urinary tract infection, and these findings are associated with septicemia and/or cholestatic hepatitis in some babies. Localizing signs suggesting urinary tract involvement are unusual; when present, they usually consist of a weak urinary stream on voiding and/or an abdominal tumor from bladder distention or hydronephrosis.

DIAGNOSIS. The diagnosis of urinary tract infection is confirmed by examination and culture of urine. The results of these tests depend largely on the method of urine collection. Most pediatricians obtain urine with a sterile, plastic receptacle applied to the cleansed perineum. However, urine obtained by this method may have an elevated cell count because of recent circumcision, vaginal reflux of urine or contamination from the perineum. Neonatal asphyxia may also increase the urinary cell count. White blood cells must be differentiated from round epithelial cells, which appear in the urine in significant numbers during the early days of life. The leukocyte count varies inversely with chronologic age. Although there is no unanimity of opinion, counts greater than 20–25 cells per mm[3] during the first week of life and equal to or greater than 10 to 25 cells per mm[3] beyond this period should cause suspicion of infection (Boyer et al., 1975; Nelson and Haltalin, 1971). Glitter cells are felt by many to be diagnostic of urinary tract infection. The single best source of urine for cultures is suprapubic bladder aspiration. Although theoretically any bacteria in urine obtained by this method is abnormal, virtually all infected infants will have counts equal to or greater than 10,000 to 100,000 colonies per mm[3]. On the other hand, colony counts of 100,000 colonies per mm[3] or greater must be present if urine is obtained by mid-stream collection or in a plastic receptacle applied to the perineum. If urine cultures yield counts less than 100,000 colonies per mm[3] or contain mixed bacterial populations, a repeat culture should be obtained by suprapubic aspiration.

A useful test to aid in differentiating upper from lower urinary tract disease in adults is examination of the urinary sediment for antibody-coated bacteria (Jones et al., 1974). When fluorescein-tagged anti-human globulin is utilized, antibody-coated bacteria causing renal parenchymal disease will be detected under the fluorescent microscope. This technique has been used in adult patients only; its application to urinary tract disease of infancy and childhood remains to be established. Preliminary evidence suggests that this test is not as helpful in differentiating upper versus lower tract disease as is elevation of the serum C-reactive protein value.

THERAPY. All infants with suspected or proved urinary tract infections should have blood and urine cultures obtained prior to initiating therapy. In general, antimicrobial agents should initially be administered parenterally because septicemia may occur in association with urinary tract infection, and antibiotic absorption after oral administration may be erratic in some neonates. Ampicillin plus kanamycin or gentamicin should be administered to symptomatic infants with bacteriuria prior to results of cultures and susceptibility studies. Final antibiotic selection is based upon these studies. In general, kanamycin or gentamicin is effective against the commonly encountered coliform bacteria. Because urinary concentrations of these drugs are high, the usual dosages may be reduced after septicemia has been ruled out.

A repeat urine culture taken 48 to 72 hours after initiation of appropriate therapy should be sterile or show a substantial reduction in the bacterial count. Infants with persistent bacteriuria should be evaluated for inappropriate therapy, obstruction or possible abscess formation. In the uncomplicated patient, therapy is usually continued for a period of approximately 10 days. Blood urea nitrogen and serum creatinine levels should be determined at initiation and completion of therapy. If there is evidence of renal failure, dosage and frequency of administration of these drugs, particularly the aminoglycosides, may need to be altered. Approximately 1 week after discontinuing therapy, a repeat urine culture is obtained. If the culture is positive, therapy is reinstituted and a thorough investigation of the urinary tract is made in order to rule out obstruction or abscess formation. In patients with recurrence of disease, it must be established whether the second episode represents relapse with the same organism or reinfection with a different pathogen.

All infants with documented urinary tract infections should have radiologic evaluation of the urinary tract. An intravenous pyelogram is obtained at the outset of therapy to rule out the possibility of gross congenital abnormalities of the urinary system. If obstruction is demonstrated, urologic procedures to insure proper drainage are mandatory if therapy is to be successful. Because of the possibility of ureteral reflux associated with bladder inflammation, many urologists prefer to obtain the voiding cystourethrogram several weeks after therapy has been completed.

**PROGNOSIS.** It is the physician's responsibility to be certain that neonates with documented urinary tract infections do not have congenital abnormalities of the urinary system. In such patients, recurrent urinary tract infections are common and physical growth may be retarded until definitive surgery has been performed. Every patient must have careful, long-term follow-up studies in order to detect recurrent infections, many of which will be asymptomatic.

# SEPTIC ARTHRITIS AND OSTEOMYELITIS

During the neonatal and infancy period the epiphysial plate is traversed by multiple small transepiphysial vessels that provide a direct communication between the articular space and the metaphysis of the long bones (Ogden and Lister, 1975). Thus, infection of a metaphysial site can spread across the growth plate to penetrate the epiphysis. Because these perforating vessels disappear at approximately 1 year of age, osteomyelitis is usually not associated with septic arthritis in older infants and children. There are two possible exceptions to this rule: osteomyelitis of the proximal femur and of the proximal humerus. The capsules of the hip and shoulder attach below the metaphysis of the femur and humerus, respectively. Infection of the epiphysial cartilage may rupture through the periosteum and enter the joint space, producing purulent arthritis. Because the capsular articulation of the hip and shoulder are permanent, osteomyelitis and septic arthritis may coexist, making the origin of infection difficult to establish. Because the inflammatory process of osteomyelitis or of septic arthritis can occupy the epiphysial and metaphysial sides of the growth plate, ischemia and necrosis of the plate may occur, resulting in permanent damage.

**ETIOLOGY.** *Staphylococcus aureus* is the most common etiologic agent of neonatal musculoskeletal infections. Group B streptococci are less commonly encountered and coliform organisms and Pseudomonas are infrequent pathogens (Weissberg et al., 1972, Dich et al., 1975, and Nelson, 1972). Antecedent trauma, umbilical vessel catheterization, respiratory tract disease and femoral venipunctures have been implicated in the pathogenesis of these infections in some infants.

**CLINICAL MANIFESTATIONS.** Initial signs and symptoms are usually nonspecific. Most infants are not brought to medical attention until local signs such as swelling, irritability and decreased motion of an extremity become apparent. Physical examination reveals swelling, localized pain on palpation and resistance to movement of the affected extremity. Localized heat and fluctuance are late findings. Occasionally, the diagnosis is made unsuspectingly when purulent material is obtained on attempted aspiration of the femoral vein. In this instance, the needle enters the swollen hip capsule.

Although blood cultures are frequently positive, clinically the infants usually do not appear septic. An exception is Group A beta-hemolytic streptococcal infection, in which the infant appears gravely ill.

**DIAGNOSIS.** Blood cultures should be obtained from all infants with suspected osteomyelitis or septic arthritis. In infants with septic arthritis a percutaneous needle aspiration of intraarticular pus should be performed; whereas in osteomyelitis direct needle aspiration of the affected periosteum and bone is attempted. If pus is obtained, the material should be Gram stained and cultured. Preliminary identification of the pathogen from stained smears is helpful in selecting initial antimicrobial therapy.

In patients with suspected septic arthritis, x-rays may be normal or show widening of the articular space and capsular swelling. Later in the course of disease, subluxation and destruction of the joint are common. In early osteomyelitis the normal roentgenographic water markings of the deep tissues adjacent to the affected bone are obliterated, indicating inflammation. Lifting of the periosteum from the bone may also be observed, but cortical destruction is unusual before the second week of illness, and new bone formation is a late finding. Resolution of bone changes is considerably slower than clinical improvement. (Weissberg et al., 1974). There is very little experience to date with scanning techniques of bone in newborn and young infants. This procedure offers the advantage of earlier diagnosis than can be achieved with ordinary roentgenograms.

**THERAPY.** Selection of initial antimicrobial therapy is based on results of examination of stained smears of aspirated purulent material and on the presence of associated clinical findings such as furuncles or cellulitis. If gram-positive cocci are observed, methicillin should be started. Either kanamycin or gentamicin is indicated if gram-negative organisms are noted. If no organisms are seen or if doubt exists regarding their identification, methicillin plus gentamicin or kanamycin should be used until results of the cultures are available. Direct instillation of an antibiotic into the joint space is unnecessary because most drugs will penetrate the inflamed synovium, and adequate concentrations are achieved in purulent material (Nelson, 1971). This also applies to treatment of osteomyelitis; direct instillation of antibiotics into acutely inflamed bone is unwarranted.

As a general rule, infection of the joint space and bone should be drained either by repeated aspiration or by surgery. Septic arthritis of the hip and shoulder is best treated with incision and drainage in order to prevent vascular compromise or extension of infection into the metaphysis. Orthopedic consultation should be obtained for all patients.

Antimicrobial therapy of neonatal musculoskeletal infections caused by staphylococci or coliform organisms is continued for a minimum of 3 weeks. Group B streptococcal infection is treated with penicillin G for approximately 2 weeks. The use of oral antibiotics as a substitute for parenteral therapy during the second and third weeks of therapy is unwise because of the difficulty in assuring complete compliance on the part of the parents and the lack of experience with this route of administration in neonates. In general, systemic symptoms disappear within several days of initiating therapy, although local signs such as heat, erythema and swelling may persist for 4 to 7 days. Full range of motion may not return to the involved limb for several months. Because of this, physical therapy should be instituted early in illness to prevent contractures. Complete resolution of the roentgenographic changes may take several months.

**PROGNOSIS.** Mortality from these diseases is rare. However, morbidity may be considerable, particularly when a weight-bearing joint such as the hip or knee is involved. Contractures and muscle damage may be permanent.

## OPHTHALMIA NEONATORUM

Paralleling the increased incidence of venereal disease in the general population, ophthalmia neonatorum is again being observed in some areas of the country (Snowe and Wilfert, 1973). *Neisseria gonorrhoeae* are acquired during passage through the infected birth canal when the mucous membranes come in contact with infected secretions. Infection usually becomes apparent within the first 5 days of life and is initially characterized by a clear, watery discharge, which rapidly becomes purulent. This is associated with marked conjunctival hyperemia and chemosis. Both eyes are usually involved, but not necessarily to the same degree. Untreated gonococcal ophthalmia may extend to involve the cornea (keratitis) and the anterior chamber of the eye. This may eventuate in corneal perforation and blindness. Until the introduction of adequate prophylactic measures, ophthalmia neonatorum was the most frequent cause of acquired blindness in the United States. Any infant presenting with a conjunctival discharge should have the material stained and cultured for gonococcus and other bacterial agents. Demonstration of gram-negative intracellular diplococci on stained smear is an indication for immediate penicillin therapy prior to definitive laboratory diagnosis.

**DIFFERENTIAL DIAGNOSIS.** Conjunctivitis occurring in the first days of life can be either chemical or bacterial in nature. Chemical irritants such as silver nitrate cause transient conjunctival hyperemia and a watery discharge, but this is not associated with a purulent discharge. Common bacterial agents associated with conjunctivitis in neonates are *S. aureus*, *N. gonorrhoeae* and *P. aeruginosa*. It is important to determine the specific etiology in order to select appropriate therapy and to prevent permanent sequelae to the eye. Viral conjunctivitis in a single nursery infant is unusual.

Conjunctivitis during the second or third week of life may be caused by viral, bacterial or chlamydial agents. Viral conjunctivitis is frequently associated with other symptoms of respiratory tract disease, such as rhinorrhea, cough and sore throat, and several individuals in the family unit may have simultaneous disease. In general, the discharge in viral conjunctivitis is watery or mucopurulent, but rarely purulent. Preauricular adenopathy is common. Staphylococci, streptococci and occasionally gonococci cause conjunctivitis in this age group. A smear of the purulent material is helpful in differentiating these etiologic agents. However, the presence of bacteria on a Gram-stained smear of material is not necessarily related etiologically to the conjunctivitis. Normal inhabitants of the skin and mucous membranes, such as staphylococci, diphtheroids and *Neisseria catarrhalis* may be observed.

Conjunctivitis caused by chlamydia (inclusion blennorrhea) is a venereally transmitted disease that is observed in infants 5 to 14 days of age (Goscienski, 1970). Clinical manifestations vary from mild conjunctivitis to intense inflammation and swelling of the lids associated with copious purulent discharge. Pseudomembrane formation and a diffuse "matte" injection of the tarsal conjunctiva are common. The cornea is rarely affected, and preauricular adenopathy is unusual. In the early stages of disease, one eye may appear more swollen and infected than the other, but both eyes are almost invariably involved. Diagnosis is made by scraping the tarsal conjunctiva and looking for typical cytoplasmic inclusions within epithelial cells, using Giemsa stain. These inclusions will not be seen on smears of purulent discharge, and cultures of the discharge yield various bacteria that are not related etiologically to the clinical disease. A simplified technique to cultivate chlamydia has been recently described, but is not generally available in most hospitals. Without treatment the acute inflammation continues for several weeks, merging into a subacute phase of slight conjunctival injection with scant purulent material. Occasionally chronicity develops, some cases persisting for over a year.

**THERAPY.** Ophthalmia neonatorum due to *N. gonorrhoeae* should be treated with parenteral and topical antimicrobial therapy. Crystalline penicillin G should be administered intravenously or intramuscularly in a dosage of 50,000 to 75,000 units per kg per day in two divided doses for infants under 1 week and in three divided doses for infants over 1 week of age. Duration of parenteral therapy is 7 to 10 days. In addition to systemic antibiotic treatment, the eyes should be washed with saline solution followed by topical administration of chloramphenicol or tetracycline. Initially, local therapy is given every 1 or 2 hours, and gradually the interval is increased to every 6 to 12 hours as clinical improvement is noted. Patients with ophthalmia neonatorum should be isolated, and strict handwashing techniques should be employed because of the highly contagious nature of the exudate. Conjunctivitis caused by other bacterial agents should be treated parenterally with the single most appropriate agent as judged by susceptibility testing of the organism.

Inclusion blennorrhea is treated by topical administration of 10 per cent sulfacetamide or 1 per cent tetracycline ointment applied every 3 to 4 hours for approximately 14 days. Marked reduction in swelling and discharge is observed within 24 hours of therapy. Antigonococcal prophylaxis at birth has little, if any, effect on chlamydial infection. Even with appropriate therapy, a small percentage of patients will have demonstrable scarring of the corneal limbus on follow-up examination. This finding is not usually associated with disturbed vision.

Ophthalmia neonatorum is a preventable disease. One per cent silver nitrate instilled in both eyes in the immediate neonatal period is 90 to 95 per cent effective in preventing gonococcal ophthalmia. Silver nitrate should not be irrigated with saline, as this may reduce efficacy. Ophthalmic ointments containing tetracycline or chloramphenicol are also effective prophylactic agents. Bacitracin ophthalmic ointment is not effective, and penicillin drops should not be used routinely because of the possible risk of sensitization.

## CUTANEOUS INFECTIONS

The most common bacteria causing skin infections during the neonatal period are *Staphylococcus aureus* and groups A and B streptococci. Disease caused by *S. aureus* can assume several clinical forms, the most common being pustular lesions. These tend to concentrate in the periumbilical and diaper areas, and rarely become invasive except when extensive areas are involved or when monitoring devices, catheters or other invasive procedures are necessary in gravely ill infants. A stained smear and a culture of an intact lesion are usually helpful in identifying the pathogen. The organisms should be phage typed (they usually belong to group I) so that if additional cases are encountered from the same nursery, these infants and others in the unit can be evaluated for the possibility of a nosocomial staphylococcal outbreak. If these infections are caused by the same phage type of staphylococcus, prompt measures should be instituted to determine

the source of infection and to prevent further colonization and disease.

Therapy of cutaneous staphylococcal disease depends on the extent of the lesions and the general clinical condition of the infant. Small, isolated pustules can be managed by local care using a mild cleansing agent or an antiseptic such as hexachlorophene or povidone iodine. Infants with more extensive cutaneous involvement or systemic signs of infection, or both, should be treated with parenteral antimicrobial agents. A penicillinase-resistant penicillin should be used initially; continuation of this drug will depend on the results of susceptibility testing.

The second form of neonatal staphylococcal disease has been previously described (see Septicemia) and is referred to as the expanded scalded-skin syndrome.

Group A beta-hemolytic streptococci occasionally cause disease in the nursery (Dillon, 1966). The most common manifestation is a low grade omphalitis characterized by a wet, malodorous umbilical stump with minimal inflammation. Disseminated disease occurs secondary to blood stream invasion or by direct extension to the peritoneal cavity by way of the umbilical vessels. Identification of one infant with group A streptococcal disease in a nursery necessitates cultural surveillance of the other infants and of the personnel in the unit. The organism is usually introduced into the nursery by asymptomatic nasopharyngeal infection of personnel or parents. When a nursery outbreak is suspected, specific M and T typing of the organism is useful in defining the source and spread of infection. Group B streptococci have been associated with cellulitis, impetiginous lesions and small abscesses in a few neonates. Penicillin is the drug of choice for streptococcal infections.

Necrotizing fasciitis is an unusual disease of newborn infants. This disease is frequently associated with surgical procedures, birth trauma or cutaneous infection (Wilson and Haltalin, 1973). Staphylococci, either alone or associated with streptococci, are usually causative. In this condition, subcutaneous tissues, including muscle layers, are invaded and the organism spreads along the fascial planes. Overlying skin may appear violaceous and is edematous, which imparts a thick "woody" sensation on palpation. The borders of the lesion are usually indistinct when compared to erysipelas, in which the borders are raised and easily palpated. Extensive surgery involving resection of destroyed tissue is imperative in treating necrotizing fasciitis. Blood and tissue cultures should be obtained, and methicillin is the drug of choice for initial therapy. Necrotic, fatty tissue may combine with calcium, resulting in tetany and convulsions.

BREAST ABSCESS. Although breast abscess is fairly common in neonates, there is very little written about this entity in current pediatric texts. Breast abscesses are most frequently encountered during the second or third weeks of life and occur more commonly in females, particularly those over 2 weeks of age. The disease does not occur in premature infants, presumably because of underdevelopment of the mammary gland in these infants. Bilateral disease is rare.

The major presentation of neonatal breast abscess is localized swelling with or without accompanying erythema and warmth. Systemic manifestations are uncommon, and only 25 per cent of these infants will have low-grade fever. *Staphylococcus aureus* is the major pathogen; coliforms and group B streptococci are encountered in a few infants. The diagnosis of breast abscess is best made by needle aspiration of the affected site. The single most important aspect of management is prompt incision and drainage by a skilled surgeon. Methicillin should be administered for approximately 5 days during the period of drainage. Experience with this condition in Dallas indicates that antimicrobial therapy plays a secondary role to adequate drainage (Rudoy and Nelson, 1975). Long-term follow-up studies suggest that some girls will have diminished breast tissue on the affected side.

## NOSOCOMIAL BACTERIAL INFECTIONS

Hospital-acquired (nosocomial) infections have become a significant problem in most hospitals and may affect 5 to 10 per cent of all hospitalized patients. The American Hospital Association (see References) strongly urges every hospital to establish an Infection Control Committee, the functions of which are principally two-fold: 1) prevention of nosocomial infection by education of all personnel and by routine surveillance procedures, and 2) prompt recognition and control of a nosocomial infection when it occurs. All hospitals should hire an infection control nurse to supervise and coordinate the infection control and surveillance programs.

When an infectious disease caused by the same organism appears in several infants from the same nursery over a short period of time, nosocomial infection should be suspected. The sick infants must be isolated and cultured in order to identify the pathogen. If a specific, single pathogen is responsible for the outbreak, epidemiologic investigations to determine the source and mode of transmission of infection are greatly facilitated. Specific identification by phage typing of staphylococci or pyocin typing of Pseudomonas can usually be performed by county or state laboratories. It is sometimes helpful to examine the antibiotic susceptibilities of the organism because a unique pattern may exist which can be used to identify carriers or inanimate objects harboring the microbe. The infection control nurse and physician must determine the extent and possible sources of nursery infection, and what measures should be taken to prevent further colonization and disease.

The following discussions of specific bacterial infections are intended to familiarize the reader with some of the more common nosocomial infectious problems encountered in nurseries. This section is not designed to be an exhaustive review of each or all nosocomial bacterial infections.

STAPHYLOCOCCAL INFECTION. Phage group I *Staphylococcus aureus* (phage types 29, 52, 52A, 79 and 80) caused significant hospital disease in the late 1950's and early 1960's. Disease ranging from pustules and omphalitis to pneumonia, septicemia and meningitis occurred in neonates during this period. Although the majority of infants are colonized with the epidemic strain during a staphylococcal outbreak, disease occurs in only a small percentage of these infants. Epidemic disease caused by phage group I organisms is relatively uncommon today, although it is reported that limited outbreaks of cutaneous staphylococcal disease occurred in some nurseries following discontinuation of routine 3 per cent hexachlorophene bathing. This does not appear to be a significant problem in most areas of the United States.

Disease caused by phage group II *Staphylococcus aureus* (phage types 3A, 3B, 3C, 55 and 71) in newborn and young infants has recently been encountered with increased frequency. Clinical manifestations caused by this organism have been broadly classified into the expanded scalded skin syndrome (Melish and Glasgow, 1971). Nursery epidemics of bullous impetigo caused by group II staphylococci have been reported (Anthony et al., 1972). The source of one outbreak was a member of the nursery staff, who was a carrier of the organism, while an infant reservoir of infection and a change in bathing technique may have contributed to the other outbreaks.

When staphylococcal disease occurs in a nursery, the extent of infection must first be determined. All infants and personnel associated with the index patient are cultured, and a random sampling is taken of the other infants. The nares and umbilicus of the infant, and the anterior nares and skin of personnel should be cultured. Active skin lesions are cultured also. All staphylococcal isolates are tested for coagulase production and phage type. A change in the percentage of infants colonized with *S. aureus* and an increase in the carriage of the specific virulent strain (phage type) are usually observed during nursery staphylococcal epidemics. As a general rule, fomites play a relatively minor role in nosocomial staphylococcal disease. Organisms carried on the hands of personnel have been implicated in outbreaks in several nursery epidemics.

It is often necessary for the physician to take certain precautionary measures before the results of the cultures and phage typing are available. Selection of the one or several measures necessary to control a nursery epidemic must be individualized (Sutherland, 1973). The measures commonly employed are as follows:

1. Isolation of all infants colonized with the virulent staphylococcus. It is advisable to form a cohort system in the nursery for exposed, but as yet non colonized, infants and for all new admissions to the nursery. These separate cohorts are maintained until discharge of the infants. Infected infants are removed from the cohort and placed in isolation.
2. Enforcement of infection control techniques such as gowning, limited access to the unit and thorough hand washing before and after handling each patient.
3. Use of antimicrobial agents. Topical antimicrobial therapy may be used for minor skin infections (pustules); parenteral antistaphylococcal therapy should be used for systemic staphylococcal diseases.
4. Initiation of routine bathing with antistaphylococcal cleansing agents such as 3 per cent hexachlorophene or application of triple dye to the umbilicus of all new admissions to the nursery.
5. Artificial colonization of infants with a less virulent staphylococcus such as the 502A strain (bacterial interference) (Shinefield et al., 1963).
6. Closing of the nursery.

ENTEROPATHOGENIC E. COLI. The infection control nurse and physician should be aware of the limitation of designating *E. coli* strains as enteropathogenic on the basis of serotyping only. As pointed out in the section on diarrheal diseases, non–enteropathogenic *E. coli* may cause serious disease in nurseries. If, however, an enteropathogenic strain is identified in a nursery infant, proper measures should be taken to prevent spread of this agent to other babies. Because diarrhea caused by enteropathogenic strains of *E. coli* occurs infrequently in the first week of life, nosocomial disease is usually confined to premature nurseries. The mother is frequently the source of infection for the index case; subsequent cases are usually transmitted from infant to infant by nursery personnel.

Any nursery infant with diarrhea should be suspected of having a potentially communicable disease and be treated accordingly. All neonates in proximity to the index case should be cultured immediately for potential bacterial pathogens and isolated from other infants in the nursery. The index case and each of the cohorts should have two stool cultures taken 24 hours apart. If there are no further symptomatic cases during the next 72 hours, and if the cultures are negative for pathogens, nothing further need be done, and the affected nursery can be opened to new admissions. If a bacterial pathogen is isolated from the index infant, this baby is isolated from all other infants and treated with appropriate therapy. If other infants develop watery stools or if asymptomatic carriers of the pathogen are detected, they should be placed in the same isolation room as the index infant and appropriately treated. If new cases continue to occur, personnel should be cultured to identify asymptomatic carriers.

GROUP A STREPTOCOCCAL INFECTION. Group A beta-hemolytic streptococcus was a common cause of puerperal and neonatal sepsis in the 1930's and early 1940's. With the advent of penicillin and its frequent use in maternity and nursery units, neonatal infections caused by this organism have become relatively uncommon. The primary source of group A streptococci in nursery outbreaks is either an attendant (nurse or physician) working in the unit or the mother. Once group A streptococci are introduced into a nursery, many infants become colonized but few develop clinical disease. The most common clinical manifestation is a low-grade, granulating omphalitis that fails to heal despite local measures. However, more significant disease may occur, including extensive cellulitis, septicemia, and meningitis.

Identification of one neonate with group A streptococcal infection is enough to warrant epidemiological investigations of the nursery. All infants in close contact with the index case, a random sampling of other infants, and all nursery personnel should be cultured. Nasopharyngeal and umbilical cultures from infants, and nasopharyngeal and rectal cultures from personnel should be obtained. Because nursery and maternity, personnel are frequently interchangeable, the epidemiological work-up should be coordinated with the obstetrical service of the hospital.

Infants with streptococcal disease should be treated with aqueous or procaine penicillin G. During nosocomial outbreaks, all asymptomatic infants colonized with group A streptococci should receive penicillin. The prophylactic use of penicillin for all new admissions to the nursery may also be indicated. Benzathine penicillin G has been used effectively as prophylaxis against group A streptococcal infection in several nursery outbreaks.

GRAM-NEGATIVE INFECTIONS. Routine nasopharyngeal and rectal cultures from normal newborn infants usually reveal one or more different coliform organisms. These bacteria and others represent the normal flora of the neonate's gastrointestinal tract. The intestine is frequently the source of systemic neonatal infections caused by coliform bacteria, particularly *E. coli* K1.

Over the past decade a number of nursery outbreaks caused by specific gram-negative bacteria have been described. Among the organisms incriminated were *Klebsiella pneumoniae, Flavobacterium meningosepticum, Pseudomonas aeruginosa, Proteus mirabilis, Serratia marcescens* and *Escherichia coli.* A common feature of these outbreaks is that the majority of colonized infants are asymptomatic; those who develop disease usually have pneumonia, septicemia or meningitis.

Infected fomites represent the single most common source of nursery outbreaks caused by gram-negative bacteria. Contaminated faucet aerators, sink traps and drains, suction equipment, bottled distilled water, cleansing solutions, humidification apparatus and incubators have been incriminated (Javett et al., 1956). In addition, healthy colonized infants or nursery personnel may act as a source of infection, the organism being transmitted among infants by way of hands or gowns of personnel. During epidemics, asymptomatic colonization of infants with the specific pathogen is variable and ranges from 0 to 90 per cent.

The general approach to nursery outbreaks caused by gram-negative organisms is similar to that caused by *Staphylococcus aureus.* Identification in a nursery or intensive care unit of an infant who harbors a potentially virulent pathogen such as *Pseudomonas aeruginosa* should serve as a warning. This infant should be isolated (preferably outside of the nursery) from the other infants and managed appropriately. All infants in the same unit should be cultured. If other infants are discovered to be asymptomatic carriers of the organism, they should be removed from the nursery and an epidemiological investigation initiated. Resuscitation and inhalation equipment, cleansing solution, washing facilities and other objects in the patient's environment should be cultured in order to identify the source of nosocomial infection. As a last resort, it may become necessary to close the nursery to new admissions until the source of infection is identified and appropriate measures have been taken to prevent new cases.

## NOSOCOMIAL VIRAL INFECTIONS

A number of viral agents have been incriminated in nursery outbreaks of infection (Eichenwald et al., 1967, and Overall and Glasgow, 1970). The original source of infection in these outbreaks is frequently the mother, who transmits the viral agent either transplacentally or by direct contact postnatally. A second common source of nosocomial viral disease is nursery personnel, particularly nurses and aides who have intimate contact with infants, and resident physicians who are assigned to nurseries for extended periods of time. Although the mechanisms accounting for spread of virus from infant to infant are not well defined, it appears likely that respiratory viruses are spread by the airborne route. In contrast, viruses causing diarrhea may be transferred from infant to infant by way of the hand-oral route, with the intermediary being nursery personnel. Viruses excreted in the urine in high concentrations may be aerosolized when diapers or sheets are changed. It should be pointed out that infected infants placed in closed incubators are not isolated from other infants in open bassinets within the same unit. This is because filtered air is brought into the

closed isolettes under slight positive pressure, thus causing leakage of potentially contaminated air back into the environment. Resuscitation and respiratory equipment, cleansing solutions and other objects in the infant's environment have not been shown to play a significant role in transmission of viral agents during nosocomial outbreaks.

During a nursery outbreak of viral infection, most infected infants are asymptomatic and serve as reservoirs for perpetuation of infection. More importantly, infants with minimal symptoms and signs of disease, such as sneezing, stuffy nose or several loose stools, may contribute significantly to transmission of the virus through the airborne or fecal-oral routes.

COXSACKIE VIRUSES.    There have been a number of well-documented nursery outbreaks of the encephalomyocarditis syndrome associated with Coxsackie B viruses (Javett et al., 1956). The $B_1$ through $B_5$ Coxsackie virus groups have been etiologically associated with this illness, and virus has been isolated from multiple organs, including the myocardium, brain, blood, kidney and liver. The clinical picture is of abrupt onset of fever, listlessness and feeding difficulty. Respiratory distress and cyanosis are noted frequently, and cardiac signs such as tachycardia, cardiomegaly, murmurs and gallop rhythm are present in most patients. Hepatosplenomegaly is common, and signs and symptoms referable to central nervous system involvement are present in one third of the patients. The newborn can apparently acquire his Coxsackie infection either in utero or after birth. The postnatally acquired disease has been traced to direct contact with either the mother or an attendant suffering from an illness that was clinically compatible with or proved to be caused by the Coxsackie agent.

ECHOVIRUSES.    Occasionally, a number of echovirus types have been found to cause illness in premature and newborn infants. However, considering the frequency with which infection occurs in the older infant and child, the newborn would generally appear to be extraordinarily resistant.

The clinical manifestations of echovirus infection are varied and range from mild diarrhea to overwhelming hepatic necrosis. Separate nursery outbreaks caused by the same echovirus type may produce different clinical diseases. For example, echovirus type 19 produced respiratory illness in a premature nursery outbreak associated with x-ray findings of cystic emphysema (Butterfield et al., 1963). In a separate outbreak of echovirus type 19, the initial clinical picture was strikingly similar to that of sepsis neonatorum and was characterized by overwhelming infection and hepatic necrosis (Philip and Larson, 1973). This disparity in the clinical diseases that characterize separate nosocomial outbreaks has been observed also for echovirus type 11.

ADENOVIRUS INFECTION. Infections with this group of agents appear to occur relatively rarely, except during sharply defined epidemics. Nursery outbreaks have been caused by adenovirus types 1, 2 and 3 (Eichenwald and Kotsevalov, 1960). Illness caused by these viruses varied from "snuffy nose syndrome," caused by the type 1 virus, to mild diarrhea, caused by adenovirus type 3. In one nursery outbreak, maternal antibodies acquired transplacentally did not completely protect against clinical disease. Adenovirus type 7 has been associated with fatal interstitial pneumonitis in one neonate.

RESPIRATORY SYNCYTIAL VIRUS INFECTION. This virus has caused two separate nursery outbreaks of bronchiolitis and pneumonia (Berkovich and Taranko, 1964). The patients initially demonstrated coryza and cough lasting several days, followed by the acute onset of dyspnea associated with roentgenographic evidence of pneumonia in the majority of infants. Bronchiolitis was diagnosed clinically in those not demonstrating x-ray findings. Several epidemics of respiratory illness due to influenza viruses have been described in newborn infants. It appears that the influenza virus may be acquired either congenitally or during the postnatal period.

When viruses are suspected as the cause of a nursery outbreak of illness, the affected infants should be isolated. Infants in close association with the index cases should be carefully observed and kept as a cohort separate from other infants in the nursery. All new admissions to the nursery should be isolated from infected infants and their cohorts. If virus isolation cannot be obtained within the institution, specimens should be sent to the county or state laboratory. It may become necessary to close the nursery to admissions if new cases of disease continue to occur despite isolation and cohort measures.

## REFERENCES

Adler, S. M., and Denton, R. L.: The erythrocyte sedimentation rate in the newborn period. J. Pediatr. *86*:942, 1975.

Albritton, W. L., Wiggins, G. L., and Feeley, J. C.: Neonatal listeriosis: distribution of serotypes in relation to age at onset of disease. J. Pediatr. *88*:481, 1976.

Al-Salihi, F. L., Curran, J. P., and Wang, J.: Neonatal trichomonas vaginalis. Pediatrics *53*:196, 1974.

Anthony, B., Giuliano, D., and Oh, W.: Nursery outbreak of staphylococcal scalded skin syndrome. Am. J. Dis. Child. *124*:41, 1972.

Baker, C. J., and Barrett, F. F.: Transmission of group B streptococci among parturient women and their neonates. J. Pediatr. *83*:919, 1973.

Baker, C. J., and Kasper, D. L.: Correlation of maternal antibody deficiency with susceptibility to neonatal group B streptococcal infection. N. Engl. J. Med. *294*:753, 1976.

Berkovich, G., and Taranko, L.: Acute respiratory illness in the premature nursery associated with respiratory syncytial virus infections. Pediatrics *34*:753, 1964.

Bland, R. D.: Otitis media in the first six weeks of life: Diagnosis, bacteriology and management. Pediatrics *49*:187, 1972.

Boyer, K. M., Peterson, N. J., Farzaneh, I., Patterson, C. P., Hart, M. C., and Maynard, J. E.: An outbreak of gastroenteritis due to *E. coli* 0142 in a neonatal nursery. J. Pediatr. *86*:919, 1975.

Brightman, V., Scott, T., Westphal, M., and Boggs, T.: An outbreak of Coxsackie B-5 virus infection in a newborn nursery. J. Pediatr. *69*:179, 1966.

Butterfield, J., Moscovici, C., Berry, C., and Kempe, C. H.: Cystic emphysema in premature infants. N. Engl. J. Med. *268*:18, 1963.

Ceruti, E., Contreras, J., and Neira, M.: Staphylococcal pneumonia in childhood. Am. J. Dis. Child. *122*:386, 1971.

Chanock, R., Zapikian, A., Mills, J., Kim, H., and Porrott, R.: Influence of immunologic factors in respiratory syncytial virus disease of the lower respiratory tract. Arch. Environ. Health *21*:347, 1970.

Chow, A. W., Leake, R. D., Yamauchi, T., Anthony, B. F., and Guze, L. B.: The significance of anaerobes in neonatal bacteremia: Analysis of 23 cases and review of the literature. Pediatrics *54*:736, 1974.

Dich, V. Q., Nelson, J. D., and Haltalin, K. C.: Osteomyelitis in infants and children. A review of 163 cases. Am. J. Dis. Child. *129*:1273, 1975.

Dillon, H. C.: Group A streptococcal infection in a newborn nursery. Am. J. Dis. Child. *112*:177, 1966.

DuPont, H. L., and Hornick, R. B.: Clinical approach to infectious diarrheas. Medicine *52*:265, 1973.

Edelman, C. M., Ogwo, J. E., Fine, B. P., and Martinez, A. B.: The prevalence of bacteriuria in fullterm and premature newborn infants. J. Pediatr. 82:125, 1973.

Eichenwald, H. F., and Kotsevalov, O.: Immunologic responses of premature and full-term infants to infection with certain viruses. Pediatrics 25:829, 1960.

Eichenwald, H. F., McCracken, G. H., and Kindberg, S.: Virus infections of the newborn. Progr. Med. Virol. 9:35, 1967.

Franciosi, R., Khostman, J., and Zimmerman, R.: Group B streptococcal neonatal and infant infections. J. Pediatr. 82:707, 1973.

Gorbach, S., and Khurana, C.: Toxigenic *Escherichia coli*. N. Engl. J. Med. 287:791, 1972.

Goscienski, P.: Inclusion conjunctivitis in the newborn infant. J. Pediatr. 77:19, 1970.

Howard, J. B., and McCracken, G. H.: The spectrum of group B streptococcal infections in infancy. Am. J. Dis. Child. 128:815, 1974.

Howard, J. B., and McCracken, G. H.: Reappraisal of kanamycin usage in neonates. J. Pediatr. 86:949, 1975.

Infection Control in the Hospital. 3rd Ed. Chicago, American Hospital Association, 1974.

Javett, S. N., Heymann, S., Mundel, B., et al.: Myocarditis in the newborn infant. J. Pediatr. 48:1, 1956.

Jones, S. R., Smith, J. W., and Sanford, J. P.: Localization of urinary-tract infections by detection of antibody-coated bacteria in urine sediment. N. Engl. J. Med. 290:591, 1974.

Kaijser, B.: *E. coli* O and K antigens and protective antibodies in relation to urinary tract infection. Goteborg, Sweden, University of Goteborg Press, 1972.

Kozinn, P. J., Taschdjian, C. L., Wiener, H., Dragutsky, D., and Minsky, A.: Neonatal candidiasis. Pediat. Clin. North Am. 5:803, 1958.

Lawson, J. S., and Hewstone, A. S.: Microscopic appearance of urine in the neonatal period. Arch. Dis. Child. 39:287, 1964.

Lincoln, K., and Winberg, J.: Studies of urinary tract infection in infancy and childhood. III. Quantitative estimation of cellular excretion in unselected neonates. Acta Paediat. 53:447, 1964.

McCracken, G. H.: Evaluation of intrathecal therapy for meningitis due to gram-negative enteric bacteria. Presented to the American Pediatric Society, Denver, 1975.

McCracken, G. H.: Group B streptococci: The new challenge in neonatal infections. J. Pediatr. 82:703, 1973.

McCracken, G. H.: Pharmacologic basis for antimicrobial therapy. Am. J. Dis. Child. 128:407, 1974.

McCracken, G. H., and Kaplan, J. M.: Penicillin treatment for congenital syphilis. A critical reappraisal. J.A.M.A. 228:855, 1974.

McCracken, G. H., and Mize, S. G.: A controlled study of intrathecal antibiotic therapy in gram negative enteric meningitis of infancy. Report of the Neonatal Meningitis Cooperative Study Group. J. Pediatr. 89:66, 1976.

McCracken, G. H., and Sarff, L. D.: Current status and therapy of neonatal *E. coli* meningitis. Hosp. Pract. October, 1974, p. 57.

McCracken, G. H., Sarff, L. D., Glode, M. P., Mize, S. G., Schiffer, M. S., Robbins, J. B., Gotschlich, E. C., Orskov, I., and Orskov, F.: Relation between *Escherichia coli* K1 capsular polysaccharide antigen

and clinical outcome of neonatal meningitis. Lancet 2:246, 1974.

Melish, M., and Glasgow, L.: Staphylococcal scalded skin syndrome: The expanded clinical syndrome. J. Pediatr. 78:958, 1971.

Melish, M., Glasgow, L., and Turner, M.: The staphylococcal scalded-skin syndrome: Isolation and partial characterization of the exfoliatin toxin. J. Infect. Dis. 125:129, 1972.

Miller, D., Gabrielson, M., Bart, K., Opton, E., and Horstmann, D.: An epidemic of aseptic meningitis primarily among infants caused by echovirus II-prime. Pediatrics 41:77, 1968.

Morehead, C. D., and Houck, P.: Epidemiology of pseudomonas infections in a pediatric intensive care unit. Am. J. Dis. Child. 124:564, 1972.

Nachum, R., Lipsey, A., and Siegel, S. E.: Rapid detection of gram-negative bacterial meningitis by the limulus lysate test. N. Engl. J. Med. 289:931, 1973.

Naidoo, B. T.: The cerebrospinal fluid in the healthy newborn infant. S. Afr. Med. J. 42:933, 1968.

Nelson, J.: Antibiotic concentrations in septic joint effusions. N. Engl. J. Med. 284:349, 1971.

Nelson, J. D.: Duration of neomycin therapy for enteropathogenic *Escherichia coli* diarrheal disease. Pediatrics 48:248, 1971.

Nelson, J. D.: Listeriosis. *In* Tice's *Practice of Medicine*, Vol. III. New York, Harper and Row, 1970, Chapter 40.

Nelson, J.: The bacterial etiology and antibiotic management of septic arthritis in infants and children. Pediatrics 40:437, 1972.

Nelson, J. D., and Haltalin, K.: Accuracy of diagnosis of bacterial diarrheal disease by clinical features. J. Pediatr. 78:519, 1971.

Ogden, J. A., and Lister, G.: The pathology of neonatal osteomyelitis. Pediatrics 55:474, 1975.

Overall, J., and Glasgow, L.: Virus infections of the fetus and newborn infant. J. Pediatr. 77:315, 1970.

Philip, A., and Larson, E.: Overwhelming neonatal infection with echo 19 virus. J. Pediatr. 82:391, 1973.

Platou, R.: Treatment of congenital syphilis with penicillin. Adv. Pediatr. 4:39, 1949.

Pryles, C. V.: Staphylococcal pneumonia in infancy and childhood. Pediatrics 21:609, 1958.

Robbins, J. B., McCracken, G. H., Gotschlich, E. C., Orskov, F., Orskov, I., and Hanson, L. A.: *Escherichia coli* K1 capsular polysaccharide associated with neonatal meningitis. N. Engl. J. Med. 290:1216, 1974.

Rudoy, R., and Nelson, J. D.: Enteroinvasive and enterotoxigenic *Escherichia coli*. Am. J. Dis. Child. 129:668, 1975.

Rudoy, R. C., and Nelson, J. D.: Breast abscess during the neonatal period: A review. Am. J. Dis. Child. 129:1031, 1975.

Sarff, L. D., McCracken, G. H., Schiffer, M. S., Glode, M. P., Robbins, J. B., Orskov, I., and Orskov, F.: Epidemiology of *Escherichia coli* K1 in healthy and diseased newborns. Lancet 1:1099, 1975.

Sarff, L. D., Platt, L. H., and McCracken, G. H.: Cerebrospinal fluid evaluation in neonates: Comparison of high-risk infants with and without meningitis. J. Pediatr. 88:473, 1976.

Shackelford, P. G., Campbell, J., and Feigin, R. D.: Countercurrent immunoelectrophoresis in the evaluation of childhood infections. J. Pediatr. 85:478, 1974.

Shinefield, H. R., Ribble, J. C., Boris, M., and Eichenwald, H. F.: Bacterial interference: Its effect on nursery-acquired infection with *Staphylococcus aureus*. I. Preliminary observations on artificial colonization of newborns. Am. J. Dis. Child. *105*:646, 1963.

Shurin, P. A., Alpert, S., Rosner, B., Driscoll, S. G., Lee, Y., McCormack, W. M., Santamarina, B. A., and Kass, E. M.: Chorioamnionitis and infant colonization with genital mycoplasmas. N. Engl. J. Med. *293*:5, 1975.

Snowe, R., and Wilfert, C.: Epidemic reappearance of gonococcal ophthalmia neonatorum. Pediatrics *51*:110, 1973.

Sutherland, J.: Comment. Pediatrics (Suppl.) *51*:351, 1973.

Thorley, J. D., Holmes, R. K., Kaplan, J. M., McCracken, G. H., and Sanford, J. P.: Passive transfer of antibodies of maternal origin from blood to cerebrospinal fluid in infants. Lancet *1*:651, 1975.

Warren, W. S., and Stool, S. E.: Otitis media in low-birth-weight infants. J. Pediatr. *79*:740, 1971.

Weissberg, E. D., Smith, A. L., and Smith, D. H.: Clinical features of neonatal osteomyelitis. Pediatrics *53*:505, 1974.

Wilson, H. D., and Haltalin, K.: Acute necrotizing fasciitis in childhood. Am. J. Dis. Child. *125*:591, 1973.

Wise, M. B., Beaudry, P. H., and Bates, D. V.: Long-term follow-up of staphylococcal pneumonia. Pediatrics *38*:398, 1966.

# 86    OTHER SPECIFIC BACTERIAL INFECTIONS

Only a few bacterial infections will be discussed in this chapter. They have been chosen chiefly because their manifestations in the neonatal period differ in some respects from those of later life.

## TUBERCULOSIS

Debré and LeLong demonstrated convincingly that tuberculosis is, in most instances at least, not inherited, but acquired by contact. They separated newborns from their tuberculous mothers immediately and in a large series found that none of the offspring had been infected. Similarly Ratner et al., reviewing carefully 260 infants born to mothers with tuberculosis at Sea View Hospital, found not one case of congenital tuberculosis, even though 39 of the mothers died of the disease shortly after delivery. There are nevertheless scattered throughout the literature examples of newborns dying of tuberculosis so early that prenatal infection must be accepted as the only possible mode of origin. In others, in whom evidence of illness became manifest somewhat later,

even though mother and child had been separated promptly after delivery, it appears likely that infection was acquired during birth by inhalation of infected amniotic fluid or vaginal secretions.

**INCIDENCE.** Beitzke laid down certain criteria which he believes indicate that tuberculous infection is truly congenital. *Mycobacterium tuberculosis* must be grown from the infant's tissues. A primary complex must be demonstrated in the liver indicating that bacilli were carried to it by the umbilical vein, or tuberculous lesions must be discovered at birth or within a few days thereafter. On the basis of these criteria Horley found in the literature 83 acceptable cases of congenital tuberculosis plus 41 of bacillemia without visible lesions. Considering the great frequency of the disease among young adults within the past century, prenatal hematogenous transmission must be exceedingly rare. Now that maternal tuberculosis can be successfully treated with a variety of chemical agents, transmission to the fetus ought to be, and almost surely is, even rarer.

**PATHOLOGY.** Hematogenous infection is manifested by enlargement and caseation of the glands at the porta hepatis plus disseminated tubercles throughout the liver, comprising the primary complex. In addition, tubercles are scattered through the lungs and spleen and other viscera, and the serous surfaces often are studded with them, while their cavities contain clear yellow fluid. Brain and meninges may be similarly involved. When lesions are most prominent in the lungs and a primary complex cannot be found in and about the liver, it is possible that the disease originated from inhalation of infected amniotic or vaginal contents at or shortly before delivery. The tubercles belong to Rich's category of soft tubercles showing local necrosis with little cellular reaction, indicating overwhelming infection with little host resistance.

**DIAGNOSIS.** Infants with truly congenital tuberculosis may give no indication of illness before their sudden death. Thus Horley's full-term female baby was born of a mother who had had pleural effusion in the fifth month and had miliary dissemination 2 months post partum. The infant seemed normal until the eighth day, when she died in the last of several attacks of cyanosis. Autopsy showed a primary hepatic complex and advanced miliary tuberculosis.

When infection has been acquired at birth, the onset of obvious illness has usually been delayed until 6 to 8 weeks. Premonitory signs were discovered retrospectively in many of these infants, the temperature curve showing unexplained spikes above normal and troughs of subnormality, as well as mild respiratory symptoms and unusual degrees of anemia. Attention has been called to the infant by the development of nasal discharge, cough, dyspnea, lethargy, anorexia, failure to gain, or by the passage of bloody stools indicating intestinal ulceration. By the time disease is suspected the lungs ordinarily show advanced, widespread areas of consolidation and hilar gland enlargement, with or without cavitation and miliary spread. Emphysema becomes more and more prominent as time passes. The course is long, and even in the face of vigorous therapy progression is the rule.

The tuberculin test is extremely unrelia-

ble. It remained negative through the entire course of one of Grady and Zuelzer's five reported infants who survived to 5 months, and only became positive in another at 8 months of age.

**MANAGEMENT. CONGENITAL TUBERCULOSIS.** If the mother has *miliary disease,* untreated in the last part of pregnancy, the infant is at greatest risk of having congenital tuberculosis. Such an infant deserves careful clinical evaluation, including a chest film, smear and culture of gastric washings and urine, examination and culture of the spinal fluid, and drug sensitivities determined on any organism recovered. The tuberculin test may not become positive for approximately 3 to 5 weeks or longer in such an infant, so reliance on a negative test is unwarranted. Separation of the infant from the mother, who would be hospitalized, is self-evident, and institution of INH, 10 mg per kilogram per day, is appropriate in the absence of manifest disease. If the infant has manifest disease, INH, 10 to 20 mg per kilogram per day, should be given for at least a year because of the serious nature of disseminated disease in infancy. Differences of opinion exist about the advisability of streptomycin in addition to INH. If the response is poor to INH, or drug sensitivity tests indicate resistance, streptomycin in the dose of 40 mg per kilogram every other day for some months would be indicated.

If the infant has tuberculous meningitis, triple drug therapy is indicated: streptomycin 40 to 50 mg per kilogram per day, INH 20 mg per kilogram per day and PAS 200 mg per kilogram per day. A recent study by Escobar and associates from Cali, Columbia, demonstrates the efficacy of prednisone at 1 mg per kilogram per day for the first 30 days of illness. Prednisone therapy should not be initiated until adequate blood levels of antituberculous drugs are achieved, presumably after about 48 hours of initiating treatment.

**INFANT OF A MOTHER ON THERAPY FOR PULMONARY TUBERCULOSIS.** A more frequent event is pregnancy in a mother with pulmonary tuberculosis on therapy. If the mother is sputum positive, the risk to the infant is of course greater than it is if she has been on treatment some months and is sputum negative. It would seem reasonable to separate the infant from the mother as long as she remains sputum positive. Once her sputum has converted to negative, and she is known to be taking her medication regularly, separation of the infant is not necessary. Such an infant remains at greater risk than normal, in part because of the likelihood of other unidentified cases of tuberculosis in the environment. It seems appropriate to consider such an infant a candidate for BCG or INH prophylaxis, whether or not separation from the mother occurs.

INFANT OF A MOTHER WITH TREATED TUBERCULOSIS. Finally, and perhaps most frequently, an infant may be born to a mother with a history of treated tuberculosis, off therapy for some years before pregnancy. The possibility of relapse in the mother would be greatest if her disease were arrested for less than 5 years. Since the risk to the infant of a mother with inactive tuberculosis depends on her likelihood of reactivation, careful and frequent examinations of the mother are essential. Indeed, a tuberculin test in all women during pregnancy and at the time of delivery would be desirable. A postpartum chest film and one 3 months and another 6 months later are indicated in tuberculin-positive mothers. The management of the infant is less clear under these circumstances. A minimal requirement would be a tuberculin test with 5 T.U. (0.1 ml intermediate PPD or 0.0001 mg) at three monthly intervals during the first year of life if BCG is withheld.

ROLE OF BCG. The arguments for BCG are based in part on the experience gained from its wide use in many countries with a very low incidence of subsequent tuberculosis and minimal complications. One study relevant to its role in newborn infants in tuberculosis households included 231 vaccinated by multiple puncture techniques and 220 control infants studied over a period of 19 years (Rosenthal et al.). The infants were returned to their respective homes only if the source case were "closed." Even so, the infectivity rate in the nonvaccinated controls was 36.5 per cent at one year, suggesting that the state of infectiousness of an adult cannot always be ascertained with accuracy. The results of

the Rosenthal study showed that there were three cases of tuberculosis among the 231 vaccinated infants, and eleven cases among the 220 controls. The controls included four deaths and four cases of miliary disease or meningitis; no deaths or disseminated disease occurred among the vaccinated. The strongest argument for BCG is the advantage gained from protection given at one time instead of daily, as with chemoprophylaxis. Kendig advocates the two-site method of BCG immunization, giving the material in two sites of the deltoid at the same time.

The arguments against BCG are that it is not always effective as shown in Rosenthal's study and in a large number of epidemiological studies. The efficacy varies in part because of different potencies of the antigen and variations in the physiological state of the host. During recent years the problem of differing reactions to the vaccine has been lessened by the availability of a freeze-dried preparation,* found to be comparable to the liquid Danish vaccine in testing on newborn infants (Griffiths and Gaisford). The immunizing dose is 0.1 ml by intradermal injection. A small red papule appears at the site of injection within 7 to 10 days, and may increase in size over the next few weeks. It leaves a smooth or pitted white scar in approximately 6 months. A tuberculin test should be performed in 2 or 3 months, and the immunization repeated if it is negative. Occasionally local granulomas and regional adenitis ensue. Another problem is the possibility that use of BCG could negate the value of subsequent tuberculin testing in a vaccinated individual. In general, the tuberculin reaction becomes small one year after BCG, and thus an increase in reactivity or a large reaction indicates human mycobacterial infection. Individual differences in tuberculin sensitivity, however, make the distinction often unreliable.

A special consideration with respect to INH prophylaxis in infants in the first days of life concerns the possible long-term pharmacologic agents, with respect to ab-

---

*Manufactured by Glaxo Laboratories, Ltd., Middlesex, England, and distributed by Eli Lilly and Co., Indianapolis, Indiana.

sorption and excretion, that have necessitated great care in matters of dosage and indications in infancy. Studies on INH blood levels in newborn infants and long-term follow-up of treated infants are not available. However, no adverse effects have been noted among infants treated with INH. Neurotoxicity in particular seems less common in children than adults. Some further reassurance comes from a study of the outcome of pregnancy in mothers on INH, including 50 on therapy at the time of conception. There was no increase in fetal loss or neonatal death, and no cancer detected among the 644 children followed up to 13 years (Hammond et al.).

### Nursery Exposure to Tuberculosis

Experiences in control of possible spread of infection from nursery personnel to infants has led Light et al. to propose 3 months of oral INH prophylaxis for all exposed infants. The arguments are that acquisition of fulminant disease may occur rapidly and in the absence of a tuberculin conversion. The time lag before effective immunity can be achieved with BCG makes this form of protection less desirable.

### Multiple Pseudocystic Tuberculosis of Bones

A case described by de Pape is mentioned briefly at this point because it appears to be an instance of congenital tuberculosis of bone.

An American Indian infant was born of parents who, unfortunately for themselves as well as for the certainty of the diagnosis in this case, both had strongly positive Wassermann results. The infant was normal at birth except for a notably swollen right fifth metacarpal. He soon became pale, weak and irritable, and at 10 weeks chronic purulent nasal discharge began. Cough and cervical node enlargement followed, then swellings over the skull and many of the long bones and fusiform enlargement of some digits. Hepatosplenomegaly developed. His own Wassermann test result was negative, but his Kahn test was weakly positive. The Mantoux test result was strongly positive, and x-ray films

of the lungs were suggestive of tuberculosis. Acid-fast bacilli were found in the aspirate from a fluctuant swelling over the forehead. In spite of treatment with streptomycin he died at 10 months. Autopsy showed widespread tuberculosis of the viscera and multiple loci of osseous tuberculosis.

Had the parents not had syphilis, one could be certain that this infant had acquired tuberculosis transplacentally. As it is, one cannot be sure that the original metacarpal lesion was not syphilitic and that the ultimate acid-fast infection was not a later superimposition. This reconstruction seems to be unlikely.

## DIPHTHERIA

The virtual disappearance of diphtheria from the scene in many metropolitan areas — in Baltimore only an occasional sporadic case has been reported since 1950 — inevitably decreases the consideration this disease receives in differential diagnosis. In view of the recent resurgence of other presumed eliminated infections, we must be careful lest a new generation of physicians who have had no experience with it forget its characteristics and its hazards.

**INCIDENCE.** In Baltimore the incidence for all age groups diminished from 260 per 100,000 in 1900 to 0 in 1957. Not all communities in the United States can boast such an enviable record, but all show tremendous declines. Diphtheria was never common in the neonatal period and is now almost non-existent in that age group. Yet occasional outbreaks are still encountered in nurseries, and the odd case still crops up.

A 1970 outbreak in Austin, Texas, resulted in 88 cases; three of the patients died. The authors came to the conclusion that to forestall an epidemic in a community, an immunization level of more than 80 per cent is required, not 70 per cent as usually taught. Twenty-five per cent of the affected children were under 4 years of age, but no mention was made of the incidence, if any, among newborns. This does not guarantee that you will never encounter one.

ETIOLOGY AND EPIDEMIOLOGY. *Corynebacterium diphtheriae,* generally of the gravis type, is the responsible organism. Its soluble toxin produces antitoxin in the host during the course of natural infection and may be used, modified to toxoid, as a potent antigen to stimulate the formation of antitoxin in inoculated persons. The antitoxic titer from either source persists for a variable number of years and is capable of being boosted by reinfection or by subsequent doses of toxoid. Many newborns receive no antitoxin from a mother whose natural or artificial antitoxin titer had diminished to the vanishing point over the course of years devoid of re-exposure either to *C. diphtheriae* to to stimulating injections. These infants are susceptible to diphtheria, and contact with an infected person or a healthy carrier may cause the disease.

Such was the situation in Curtin's case reported in 1953. The mother's level of antitoxin was less than 0.001 unit per cubic centimeter. A level of 0.005 unit is generally considered protective. A brother was found to be harboring *C. diphtheriae* in his pharynx, and his antitoxin concentration was 10 units per cubic centimeter; hence he was a healthy carrier. The infant became ill on the twentieth day of life.

DIAGNOSIS. We shall not go into the matter of diagnosis in detail. It differs in no respects from that in the older chiild. *Faucial* diphtheria is recognized by the characteristic membrane, *nasal* diphtheria by persistent discharge, often sanguineous, and the *laryngeal* form by slowly progressive hoarseness and aphonia and laryngotracheal obstruction. All are without sharp constitutional reaction. In all forms diagnosis is dependent upon bacteriologic identification of *C. diphtheriae.* Complications, chiefly myocarditis and postdiphtheritic paralysis, have been similarly encountered in the newborn.

TREATMENT. Diphtheria antitoxin must be given, intravenously when the condition appears serious, intramuscularly if the situation is not urgent. Doses of 20,000 to 50,000 units on 2 or 3 successive days will be more than sufficient. Preliminary testing for sensitivity must be carried out. Since penicillin has bactericidal effect upon *C.*

*diphtheriae,* it should be given in doses approximating 300,000 units every 8 to 12 hours. Erythromycin is effective in the event of penicillin sensitivity. Treatment of complications will be carried out as for older infants.

## TETANUS NEONATORUM

As knowledge of hygiene penetrates deeper and deeper into the more primitive corners of the world, tetanus of the newborn approaches ever more nearly its vanishing point. A disease with which many of us had to contend not at all infrequently 35 years ago has become a rarity in metropolitan areas. It remains an infrequent but still serious problem in less sophisticated rural communities in the United States and is still not uncommon in the hinterlands of Africa and Asia. La Force et al. found that there had been 507 cases of tetanus in the United States in 1965 and 1966. Of these, 54 patients were newborns. Marshall reviewed the experience with 2198 cases seen at the Hôpital Albert Schweitzer in Haiti between September 1957 and May 1966, with an overall mortality of 43 per cent from the disease.

ETIOLOGY AND PATHOGENESIS. The causative agent is the bacterium *Clostridium tetani.* This gram-positive, anaerobic spore-bearer produces a soluble toxin with a special affinity for nervous tissue. It is susceptible to penicillin and the tetracyclines. It gains entrance into the newborn's body by way of the stump of the umbilical cord which had been cut by an unsterile instrument or covered with an unclean dressing. Rarely a vaccination wound produced by an unclean instrument or upon contaminated skin imperfectly cleansed constitutes a portal of entry. The organism is long-lived by virtue of its spore-formation, is a normal inhabitant of the intestinal tract of many domestic animals, and hence abounds in the soil of many localities.

No natural immunity to tetanus exists. The blood of the newborn, however, contains roughly that amount of tetanus antitoxin which is present in his mother's blood, or a bit more. This content may be considerable if the mother has been actively immunized with tetanus toxoid. Peterson, Christie and Williams believe that concentrations as low as 0.01 antitoxin unit per milliliter may be protective against the disease, and levels higher than this may persist for years in actively immunized persons. Of La Force's 54 mothers, only three were sure they had received any form of tetanus toxoid immunization.

**DIAGNOSIS.** Signs appear between the sixth and fourteenth days after birth, most often at the beginning of the second week. Restlessness, irritability, and difficulty in sucking are followed within a day or two by fever, muscle stiffness and finally by convulsions. The temperature often rises to 104° and 106° F. Physical examination at this stage shows the characteristic trismus and risus sardonicus, and tenseness and rigidity of all muscles, including those of the abdomen. The fists are held tightly clenched and the toes rigidly fanned. Characteristic are the opisthotonic spasms plus clonic jerkings which follow sudden stimulation by touch or by loud noise.

Laboratory investigations are best held to a minimum, since any manipulation produces painful spasm. Diagnosis is clear from the clinical evidence alone, and studies of blood, urine and cerebrospinal fluid, in all respects normal, add nothing of value. Attempts should be made to cultivate the organism from the presumed portal of entry.

Tetany of the newborn should never be confused with tetanus. Infants with tetany appear well between their convulsive episodes. The infant who is generally rigid from birth trauma has shown evidences of brain injury from birth, before the first sign of tetanus could possibly appear. Extraocular palsies commonly are present and abdominal rigidity absent. Response to stimulation is depressed rather than increased.

**COURSE.** The infant may die within the week after onset from respiratory arrest during a convulsive episode. If he does not die, improvement will become manifest within 3 to 7 days by gradual decline of temperature, decrease in the number of episodes of spasm, and slow resolution of rigidity. Complete disappearance of all signs of illness may take as long as six weeks.

**TREATMENT.** The first requirement is for tetanus antitoxin to neutralize the circulating toxin not already bound to nerve tissue. Where tetanus immune globulin (human) is available, it should be given intramuscularly, in a dose of 1000 to 3000 units. If this is not available, equine or bovine tetanus antitoxin should be given intramuscularly, 10,000 units, on 2 successive days.

Penicillin should be given in a dose of 300,000 units every 12 hours. Oxytetracycline is bactericidal against vegetative forms, and should be given in its stead or in addition. The consensus appears to be that wide excision of the umbilicus is hazardous and does not appreciably improve chances for recovery.

Every known sedative has been used to control spasm, and there is no general agreement as to which one or ones should be chosen. Magnesium sulfate receives a high mark from many experienced observers. Its dose is approximately 1 ml of a 50 per cent solution intramuscularly every 6 hours. Avertin has been utilized with success in doses of 5 mg per pound repeated at six- to twelve-hour intervals, depending upon severity of spasm. Phenobarbital ($\frac{1}{8}$ to $\frac{1}{4}$ grain, or 8 to 16 mg, every 4 hours by mouth or one half this amount intramuscularly or intravenously) and chloral hydrate (5 grains, or 0.3 gm, every 3 to 6 hours by rectum) have been added, singly or in combinations, to the magnesium sulfate therapy. Diazepam (Valium) may be useful. It is difficult to assess their relative values. One aims at the ideal result of controlling spasm without depressing respiration, and one must feel one's way in each case. Curare appears to be too dangerous for routine use in the newborn, but may have to be resorted to if other drugs are ineffective. Howard and deVere have used intramuscular administration of meprobamate with no diminution of mortality, but with significant reduction in the number of days of spasms and of hospitalization.

Death may result from respiratory embarrassment due to severe laryngospasm. If this symptom is distressing, tracheotomy may have to be performed. Artificial respiration has been used with success by groups in South Africa with a significant reduction in mortality. Fluids are best given through an indwelling intravenous catheter at first, later through an indwelling gastric tube. The infant should be under close observation in a darkened room, and disturbed and stimulated as infrequently as possible. Active immunization with alum-precipitated or fluid toxoid should be begun as soon as the infant improves.

## TYPHOID FEVER

J. P. Crozer Griffith, one-time Professor of Diseases of Children at the University of Pennsylvania, and one of the early great pediatric clinicians, wrote his first treatise on typhoid fever in young infants before the turn of the twentieth century. He recognized not only that they could acquire the disease after birth, but also that babies born of mothers suffering from typhoid might acquire the infection in utero.

**INCIDENCE.** Typhoid fever attained epidemic proportions in the summer and fall of every year throughout most of the United States until the end of the first two decades of the 1900's. By 1902 Griffith was able to report in some detail on 18 patients below the age of 2½ years whom he had observed personally and upon 325 certain cases plus 92 somewhat doubtful ones which he had collected from the literature. Typhoid fever was still occurring with sufficient frequency in the early 1920's. Since that time it has declined in frequency until now we rarely encounter more than one or two cases a year among the infants and children of Baltimore. In 1902 Griffith and Ostheimer found 23 examples of congenital typhoid fever among their collected cases. We have not seen one in a pediatric experience which dates from 1923.

**DIAGNOSIS.** Weech and Chen described the course of a 3-week-old premature infant who was born after an uncomplicated pregnancy.

Five days *post partum* his mother had fever which proved later to be severe typhoid. The infant became febrile at the age of 26 days, but fever dropped to normal by crisis after 24 hours. The spleen was enlarged. White blood cell count was 11,000 per cubic millimeter. Culture of the blood revealed *B. typhosus* (*Salmonella typhi* in modern terminology). The next day a bright red papular eruption appeared over the entire body and lasted 2 days. The white cell count was now 17,000, of which 37 per cent were polymorphonuclears. He had no more fever for 3 weeks, and then low-grade elevation reappeared for a few days. Blood culture was still positive. Two weeks later it was negative. The only other symptom or sign was failure to gain. All other cultures, from stool and urine, remained consistently negative. Eleven Widal tests were performed throughout the course, and none was positive.

The authors comment upon the extreme youth of their patient, upon the mildness of the disease and the lack of gastrointestinal symptoms, upon the generalized exanthem which bore no resemblance to rose spots, upon the leukocytosis so unlike the leukopenic response of older persons, and upon the total failure to develop agglutinins.

**TREATMENT.** First chloramphenicol, then ampicillin were found to be highly effective against *S. typhi*. In the very young newborn, the well-known hazard of chloromycetin would make ampicillin the preferable antibiotic.

As an aside, we might mention that we observed an epidemic of typhoid in northern Mexico in the early 70's which was caused by a strain of *S. typhi* that was refractory to both chloromycetin and ampicillin. It was widely assumed that this strain developed because of the great overuse of these antibiotics.

**PROGNOSIS.** Nineteen of the 23 infants with congenital cases collected by Griffith died, three recovered, while the fate of one was not stated. This very grave outlook for the congenital form of typhoid fever did not apply to the postnatally acquired examples, as evidenced by the mildness of Weech's case. Yet only 23 of the infants below 1 year of age in Griffith's series survived, while 77 died. One would suppose that many milder cases with recovery were not diagnosed and placed upon record.

We can find no reports on series of cases of newborns treated with chloramphenicol or ampicillin.

## LISTERIOSIS (LISTERIA MONOCYTOGENES INFECTION)

**INCIDENCE.** Hood, looking particularly for this organism, found it 29 times in the

Charity Hospital of New Orleans in a 5-year period. Nineteen of these were in children. Nichols and Woolley, reviewing the cases of neonatal meningitis at The Children's Hospital of Michigan over an 8-year period, grew Listeria eight times, while finding gram-negative bacilli 15 times in a series comprising 46 examples. The Center for Disease Control in Atlanta received 40 isolates from newborn infants from state health departments in the 20 months from July 1973 to March 1975. It is, therefore, far from uncommon.

In 1965 Delta summed up all the cases in newborns reported to that date and discovered that they numbered 78.

**ETIOLOGY.** Listeriosis, due to *Listeria monocytogenes,* is an infection which is practically limited to persons debilitated by other disease and to pregnant women, from whom it may be transmitted to their newborn infants. Its unusual affinity for the pregnant animal, including the human, is remarkable.

The organism is a small, motile, gram-positive pleomorphic bacillus which is often mistaken for a diphtheroid. Although it is commonly found in many birds, rodents and cattle, no epidemiologic association with infected human beings has been discovered. Several recent communications have suggested strongly that there may be an occasional newborn-to-newborn spread of *L. monocytogenes* (Florman and Sundararajan).

**DIAGNOSIS.** As is the case with hemolytic streptococcus Group B neonatal infections, listeriosis appears to strike as an early form or a later onset form. The early form appears to be largely septicemic and to be associated with "prematurity, a history of obstetrical complications (perinatal fever, pyelitis or 'flulike' syndrome), a higher frequency of maternal isolates and an increased neonatal mortality" and "a late onset, predominantly meningitic form, characterized by normal birth weight, lower mortality, and the absence of obstetrical complications" (Albritton et al.).

**TREATMENT.** Since the organism is usually sensitive to penicillin, tetracyclines or ampicillin in vitro, treatment with penicillin and one or both of these other antibiotics is indicated. Gordon et al. have presented data more recently which indicate that "combinations of penicillin or ampicillin and kanamycin or gentamicin produce earlier and more complete in vitro killing of *Listeria monocytogenes* than any of the antibiotics used alone."

**PROGNOSIS.** Nichols and Woolley were able to save 12 of 13 patients. Not all series manifest such a high percentage of favorable outcomes, possibly because no premature infants were among their patients. This in itself is unusual.

## REFERENCES

Albritton, W. L., Wiggins, G. L., and Feeley, J. C.: Neonatal listeriosis: Distribution of serotypes in relation to age at onset of disease. J. Pediatr. 88:481, 1976.

Avery, M. E., and Wolfsdorf, J.: Diagnosis and treatment: Approaches to newborn infants of tuberculous mothers. Pediatrics 42:519, 1968.

Beitzke, H., cited by E. A. Harris, G. C. McCullough, J. J. Stone, and W. M. Brock (see below).

Curtin, M.: Neonatal diphtheria. Arch. Dis. Child. 28:127, 1953.

Debré, R., and LeLong, M.: The infant born of tuberculous parents, separated before contamination: Its growth and resistance to disease. Ann. Med. 18:317, 1925.

Delta, B. G.: Neonatal listerosis and the problem of retrieving medical information. Pediatrics 35:358, 1965.

de Pape, A. J.: Multiple pseudocystic tuberculosis of bone. J. Bone & Joint Surg. 36-B:637, 1954.

Escobar, J. A., Belsey, M. A., Duenas, A., and Medina, P.: Mortality from tuberculous meningitis reduced by steroid therapy. Pediatrics 56:1050, 1975.

Florman, A. L., and Sundararajan, V.: Listeriosis among nursery mates. Pediatrics 41:784, 1968.

Gordon, R. C., Barrett, F. F., and Clark, D. J.: Influence of several antibiotics, singly and in combination, on the growth of *Listeria monocytogenes*. J. Pediatr. 80:667, 1972.

Grady, R. C., and Zuelzer, W. W.: Neonatal tuberculosis. A.M.A. J. Dis. Child. 90:381, 1955.

Griffith, J. P. C., and Ostheimer, M.: Typhoid fever in children under two and a half years of age. Am. J. Med. Sci. 124:868, 1902.

Griffiths, M. I., and Gaisford, W.: Freeze-dried BCG. Vaccination of newborn infants with a British vaccine. Br. Med. J 2:565, 1956.

Hammond, E. C., Selikoff, I. J., and Robitzek, E. H.: Isoniazid therapy in relation to later occurrence of cancer in adults and in infants. Br. Med. J. 2:792, 1967.

Harris, E. A., McCullough, G. C., Stone, J. J., and Brock, W. M.: Congenital tuberculosis: A review of the disease with report of a case. J. Pediatr. 32:311, 1948.

Harvin, J. R., Hastings, W. D., Jr., and Baker, C. R. F.: Tetanus neonatorum. J. Pediatr. 32:561, 1948.

Hinds, M. W.: Pregnancy and tuberculosis. Am. Rev. Resp. Dis. *106*:785, 1972.

Horley, J. F.: Congenital tuberculosis. Arch. Dis. Child. *27*:167, 1952.

Howard, F. H., and de Vere, W.: Intramuscular Meprobamate in the treatment of tetanus in infants and children. J. Pediatr. *60*:421, 1962.

Hudson, F. P.: Clinical aspects of congenital tuberculosis. Arch. Dis. Child. *31*:136, 1956.

Kass, E. H.: Clinicopathological Conference, Children's Hospital Medical Center, Boston, Mass. A case of neonatal tuberculosis. J. Pediatr. *60*:145, 53, 1962.

Kendig, E.: *Disorders of the Respiratory Tract in Children.* Philadelphia, W. B. Saunders Co., 1967, p. 699.

La Force, F. M., Young, L. S., and Bennett, J. V.: Tetanus in the United States (1965–1966). N. Engl. J. Med. *280*:569, 1969.

Lawler, H. J.: Treatment of tetanus of the newborn. A.M.A. J. Dis. Child. *90*:701, 1955.

Light, I. J., Saideman, M., and Sutherland, J. M.: Management of newborns after nursery exposure to tuberculosis. Am. Rev. Resp. Dis. *109*:415, 1974.

Marshall, F. N.: Tetanus of the newborn. In *Advances in Pediatrics*, XV, S. Z. Levine (ed.): Chicago, Year Book Medical Publishers, 1968.

Merritt, K.: Tuberculosis in infants under one year of age. Am. J. Dis. Child. *38*:526, 1929.

Nichols, W., and Woolley, P. V.: Listeria monocytogenes meningitis. J. Pediatr. *61*:337, 1962.

Peterson, J. C., Christie, A., and Williams, W. C.: Tetanus immunization. XI. Study of the duration of primary immunity and the response to late stimulating doses of tetanus toxoid. A.M.A. J. Dis. Child. *89*:295, 1955.

Ratner, B., Rostler, A. E., and Salgado, P. S.: Care, feeding and fate of premature and full-term infants born of tuberculosis mothers. Am. J. Dis. Child. *81*:471, 1951.

Rosenthal, S. R., and others: BCG vaccination against tuberculosis in Chicago. Pediatrics *28*:622, 1961.

Weech, A. A., and Chen, K. T.: Typhoid fever: Report of a case in an infant less than one month of age. Am. J. Dis. Child. *38*:1044, 1929.

Weinstein, L.: Current Concepts: Tetanus. N. Engl. J. Med. *289*:1293, 1973.

Weinstein, L., and Murphy, T.: The management of tuberculosis during pregnancy. Clinics in Perinatology. Symposium on Management of the High Risk Pregnancy. W. B. Saunders Co., Philadelphia, 1974.

Zalma, V. M., Older, J. J., and Brooks, G. F.: The Austin, Texas, diphtheria outbreak: Clinical and epidemiological aspects. J.A.M.A. *211*:2125, 1970.

# 87

# VIRAL INFECTIONS OF THE FETUS

## RUBELLA

Since 1941, when Gregg first made the association of maternal rubella and cataracts in infants, physicians have been aware of the teratogenicity of the rubella virus. Not until the epidemic of 1964–65 in North America, however, were the multiple manifestations of the rubella syndrome fully appreciated, and the later consequences well delineated. Now, with an effective vaccine available, we hope that these few remarks about the disease in infants will become of historic interest only.

**ETIOLOGY.** Maternal rubella infection within a month before conception and through the second trimester may be associated with disease in the infant. The tera-

togenic effects predominate when the infection occurs within the first eight weeks; systemic disease, including encephalitis, may occur in the infant infected after the first trimester. The infant may excrete the virus for many months after birth despite the pressure of neutralizing antibody, and thus pose a hazard to susceptible individuals in its environment. Only rarely can the virus be recovered by one year of age. An exception is the cataract, which has harbored virus for as long as three years (Menser et al.).

**DIAGNOSIS.** The infected infants are usually born at term, but of low weight. They may show only a few manifestations of the disease such as glaucoma or cataracts, or may have a systemic illness characterized by purpuric lesions, hepatosplenomegaly, cardiac defects, pneumonia and meningoencephalitis. Table 87–1, from the study of Rudolph et al. in Houston, shows the distribution of findings in their extensive series. The skin lesions, which have been described as resembling a "blueberry muffin," are shown in Figure 87–1. Thrombocytopenia is commonly seen. Osseous lesions include a large anterior fontanel and striking lesions in the long bones. Linear areas of radiolucency and increased density are found in the metaphyses (Fig. 87–1 *D*). The provisional zones of calcification are also irregular. The changes in rubella are not pathognomonic of the disease, but resemble those of other viral diseases, such as cytomegalic inclusion disease.

The cardiac lesions include patent ductus arteriosus, septal defects and stenosis of the peripheral pulmonary arteries. Myocardial necrosis has been observed.

Among the manifestations that may occur after the newborn period ("late onset disease") are a generalized rash with seborrheic features that may persist for weeks, chronic lung disease such as described by

Phelan and Campbell, defective hearing from involvement of the organ of Corti or central auditory imperception, or even complete autism.

A few longitudinal studies of somatic growth reveal that most infants remain smaller than average through infancy, but grow at a normal rate. Stunting of growth was more common after rubella in the first 8 weeks of pregnancy than after later infection. A higher than expected incidence of diabetes mellitus has been reported after congenital rubella.

**LABORATORY.** The virus may be isolated from throat, spinal fluid, and occasionally urine. Serial antibody titers will distinguish between passively transferred antibodies from the mother and those produced by the infant. Elevated levels of IgM may be present, but need not be found in all infected infants (Overall and Glasgow).

**TREATMENT.** There is no specific therapy for the viremia. The infants may need blood transfusions, if bleeding, and general supportive measures.

The question of management of the pregnant woman who contracts the disease should be answered after weighing the known risks. A careful history of contacts, and evaluation of the mother's immune status are essential. If she has a high antibody titer the infant is protected. After exposure, 0.30 to 0.40 ml per kilogram of gamma globulin is advised. Once the disease is manifest, gamma globulin is of no help.

Then the question of interruption of pregnancy arises. Rubella acquired in the first 8 weeks carries the greatest risk, estimated to be a 10 to 20 per cent likelihood of fetal infection.

**PROGNOSIS.** The consequences of fetal rubella may not be evident at birth, but become apparent in subsequent months. Hardy et al. followed 123 infants with documented congenital rubella, and found that 85 per cent of them were not clinically suspect until after discharge from the nursery. Communication disorders, hearing defects, some mental or motor retardation, and small heads by one to three years of age were among the major problems to present after the newborn period. A predisposition to inguinal hernias was also noted.

**TABLE 87–1.** *Clinical Findings in 81 Infants With Congenital Rubella Syndrome* [*]

| | Group 1: Expanded Rubella Syndrome | Group 2: Classic Rubella Syndrome | Group 3: History of Maternal Rubella, Presumably Normal Baby |
|---|---|---|---|
| Number of Infants | 34 | 37 | 10 |
| Sex { Male | 26 | 23 | 7 |
| { Female | 8 | 14 | 3 |
| Mean gestational age (weeks) | 40.1 | 39.8 | 39.8 |
| Mean birth weight (gm.) | 2178 | 2533 | 3327 |
| Purpura | 78% | 0 | 0 |
| Thrombocytopenia (<140,000) | 100% | 0 | 0 |
| Hepatomegaly | 85% | 81% | 20% |
| Splenomegaly | 76% | 62% | 10% |
| Cardiac defects | 78% | 86% | 0 |
| Eye defects | 41% | 54% | 0 |
| Full fontanel | 69% | 43% | 0 |
| Positive viral isolation | 66% | 25% | 50% |
| Mortality | 32% | 8% | 0 |

[*] Rudolph, A. J., et al.: Am. J. Dis. Child., *110*:416, 1965.

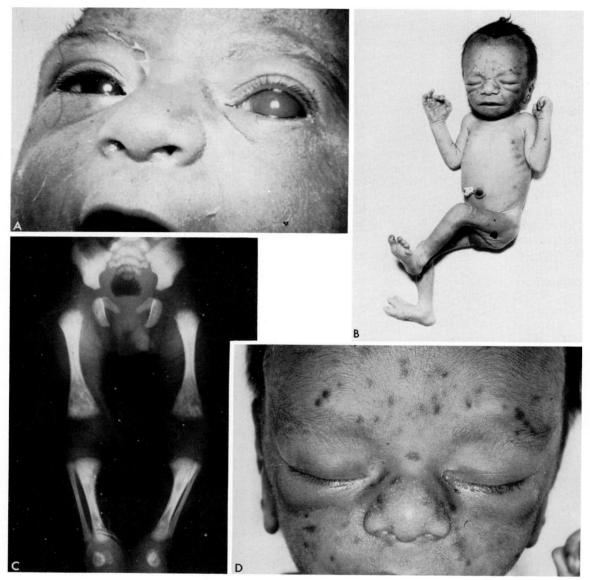

*Figure 87–1.* *A*, Note the prominence of the eyes and the clouding of the left eye typical of advanced congenital glaucoma. *B*, Term infant, underweight, with "blueberry muffin" rash over the face. *C*, Bone lesions in congenital rubella. The provisional zones of calcification are poorly defined. Multiple radiolucent defects are apparent. *D*, Closeup of rash shown in *B*. (Figure courtesy of Dr. A. J. Rudolph.)

An alarming ·report of chronic progressive panencephalitis with onset at age 11 years, after congenital rubella, appeared in 1975 by Weil et al. The patient was small for age, with sensorineural hearing loss of 60 decibels at age 4 years. At age 11 years he had the insidious onset of motor incoordination, ataxia and myoclonic jerks, with progressive deterioration. Although this complication of congenital rubella must be rare, it emphasizes that subacute sclerosing panencephalitis need not be restricted to the measles virus.

**PREVENTION.** Live attenuated rubella virus vaccine is now available, safe and effective (Lepow et al.), although the duration of immunity is uncertain. Given as a single subcutaneous injection, it is recommended for girls between ages 1 year and puberty, and for women of childbearing age with a negative hemaglutination inhibition antibody test. It should be given only if there is assurance that there is no likelihood of pregnancy for the next 2 months, because of a small potential hazard to the fetus. Administration in the immediate postpartum period is advisable. A mild rubella-like illness is sometimes seen after immunization, with arthralgia occasionally present 10 days to 2 weeks after injection.

## CYTOMEGALIC INCLUSION DISEASE

This disease has been recognized for a few decades as a serious, often fatal, infection of the newborn. Its pathologic manifestations in adults had been noted for many years as an incidental finding in a substantial number of routine autopsies performed upon adults in many geographic areas. Its etiologic agent has been sucessfully cultivated since 1955. Synonyms include generalized salivary gland virus infection, inclusion body disease and giant-cell inclusion disease, among others.

**INCIDENCE.** Salivary gland involvement has been reported in 10 to 30 per cent of consecutive autopsies on adults in different parts of the world, but in only 1 to 2 per cent of infants and children. In all the adults and the majority of the children it appeared to bear no relation to the illness which caused death in these series. The number of cases of the neonatal form now on record is quite large. From the most recent reports it would appear that large newborn services can expect to uncover two to five examples each year (Weller et al.; Hanshaw et al.; Medearis; etc.).

Serologic studies in Boston and Philadelphia showed that 30 to 60 per cent of pregnant women had detectable complement-fixing antibody. Virus can be isolated from 3 to 4 per cent of women; only rarely is the infant of a woman with viruria infected.

A prospective study by Reynolds et al. revealed cytomegalovirus excretion from urine or cervix in 12 per cent of pregnant women in Birmingham, Alabama. Infection present at birth was not documented in any of the infants, but 40 per cent of infants born to mothers excreting the virus ultimately became infected between the third and twelfth week after delivery. None of the infected infants manifested clinically recognizable illness, but most continued to excrete virus for many months.

**ETIOLOGY.** Long considered by many to be a protozoal infection, cytomegalic inclusion disease has been proved to be caused by a filtrable virus. Virus has been cultivated from the viscera of infants after death and also from the urine of affected babies during life. Viable virus is excreted into the urine for many months or years by most infected children (Emanuel and Kenny).

It is now evident that infection is transmitted from the mother, herself not ill, but harboring the virus, across the placenta to the fetus late in gestation. But it is also becoming clear that postnatal acquisition of the infection from close contacts is far from uncommon (Hanshaw et al.). Recurrence in subsequent pregnancies is rare, but has been reported by Embil et al. in Halifax.

**PATHOLOGY.** Characteristic multinuclear giant cells with both cytoplasmic and intranuclear inclusion bodies are found in many organs. Liver, lungs, brain, pancreas and kidneys contain them in large numbers. Mononuclear cell infiltration and diffuse fibrosis may be intense. In the brain are areas of necrosis, often subependymal and periventricular, and glial overgrowth, containing heavy deposits of calcium. Petechiae and larger hemorrhages involve skin and serous surfaces.

**DIAGNOSIS.** Infants infected with the virus are often prematurely delivered. In its classic form newborn infants have an acute progressive disseminating disease. They show petechiae and ecchymoses and are jaundiced at birth, or jaundice appears within a few hours and becomes intense. The liver and spleen are enlarged and firm from the start and may increase in size for a number of days. Fever to 102° and 103° may be found. Tachypnea and moderate dyspnea suggesting pulmonary involvement may appear. Pallor may or may not be striking. Puncture wounds bleed for many minutes, and hemorrhage from internal organs may cause death.

It is now apparent that a minority of infected newborn infants suffer from the so-called classic form. Elliott and Elliott were impressed by a "cerebral" form in which the principal pathologic findings were in the brain. Two of their three patients had purpura shortly after birth; the third did not. All three had elevated serum bilirubin concentrations, but only one of them had hepatosplenomegaly. Two died, but one survived.

Weller and Hanshaw were able to grow the virus from the urines of 17 nonfatal cases, repeatedly from 13 of them, in one for as long as 52 months. In 10 they felt sure that the infection was congenital, but in the other seven onsets were late (12 days to 7 weeks), so that they were not certain that their diseases had not been acquired postnatally. In many the clinical histories resembled those of neonatal hepatitis, and virus could be grown from liver biopsy tissue in five of these. In only two of the five, however, were typical inclusion bodies demonstrable in the liver. They speculated upon the possibility that the cytomegalic inclusion virus might be a common cause of neonatal hepatitis, even when the typical morphologic changes could not be found. Fourteen of these 17 either were microcephalic at birth or became so later. Of Emanuel and Kenny's seven examples only one, perhaps two, showed the fulminant disseminated symptom complex. The rest had early and prolonged jaundice, except for one, and enlargement of the liver or spleen or both. Hemorrhagic phenomena were noted in only three, only one or possibly three became mentally retarded, and none showed chorioretinitis.

An example of one nonclassic form was described by a group from the Babies' Hospital of New York.

A premature infant was quite well at birth, showing only a slightly enlarged liver and spleen. At the age of $5\frac{1}{2}$ weeks, after having gained from 1570 gm to 2200 gm, and after having behaved quite well in all respects, abdominal distention was noted. The liver and spleen were now very large. Blood was normal, platelets were not diminished, but cerebrospinal fluid was xanthochromic and contained an excess of red blood cells and protein. X-ray film of the skull revealed microcephaly and calcifications which appeared to outline dilated lateral ventricles. At $6\frac{1}{2}$ weeks chorioretinitis was noted in one eyeground. He improved for a

while, but had to be readmitted to hospital at 3 months because of vomiting, fever and the appearance of a petechial rash. Now his platelet count had fallen to 60,000 per cubic millimeter, and his liver and spleen had become huge. Inclusion bodies were found in the urine sediment, and the typical virus was grown from a specimen of urine. He was still alive at 1 year of age, retarded physically and mentally, and hydrocephalic. The Sabin dye tests and complement fixation tests for toxoplasmosis were negative in both mother and patient.

It is obvious that this form of cytomegalic inclusion disease is difficult to differentiate from congenital toxoplasmosis and that great reliance will have to be placed upon laboratory studies. It is also clear that the salivary gland virus may give rise to a number of dissimilar clinical syndromes.

**LABORATORY INVESTIGATIONS.** In the acute neonatal form the hemoglobin content at birth is normal or as low as 6 to 8 gm per 100 ml. If normal, it usually falls rapidly within the first few days in association with hemolysis. The white cell count is normal or elevated, but large numbers of nucleated red blood cells make the uncorrected count appear unusually high. Platelets are diminished in the stained smear, and counts as low as 5000 and as high as 50,000 per cubic millimeter are not at all infrequent. Prothrombin time is usually normal for the age, but may be lengthened.

The urine usually contains bile, but no urobilin. Albumin is commonly present, as are some red and white blood cells. Sediment which has been dried, cleared and stained with hematoxylin and eosin often demonstrates the characteristic inclusion bodies within desquamated renal epithelial cells (Fig. 87–2), so-called "owl's eye cells." Virus may be cultivated from the urine for an extraordinary length of time.

McCracken and Shinefield studied the immunoglobulins of eight newborn infants with cytomegalovirus disease. All had normal IgG levels, but *all had significantly increased levels of both IgM and IgA.* Hanshaw and his co-workers found an indirect fluorescent-antibody test for cytomegalovirus macroglobulin to be a convenient and sensitive diagnostic method.

The blood chemical findings are normal

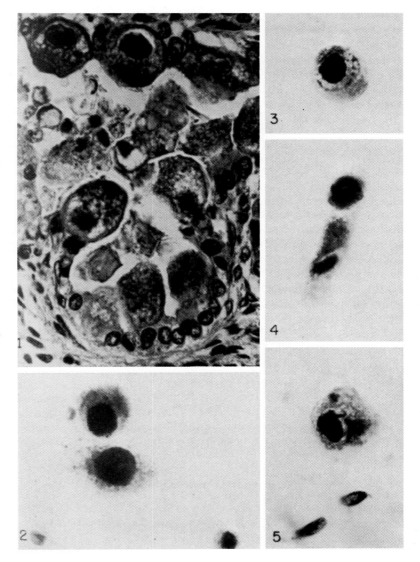

*Figure 87–2.* *1,* Renal tubule from a patient who died with cytomegalic inclusion disease. Note the intranuclear and intra-cytoplasmic inclusion bodies, with associated degeneration and desquamation of cells. Some of the necrotic cells appear as large masses of cytoplasm. *2, 3, 4,* Various types of cytomegalic cells observed in the urinary sediment from this infant. The shape of the cell in *3* suggests that it originated in the lower part of the collecting tubules or in the pelvis. In *4* note the two small desquamated cells that correspond in size to that of normal tubular cells. *5,* Cytomegalic cell and two normal cells from the gastric mucosa, observed in the sediment from a gastric washing. Hematoxylin and eosin, × 782. (Blanc, W. A.: Am. J. Clin. Path., 28:46, 1957.)

except for moderate to extreme hyperbilirubinemia. As much as 50 per cent of the bilirubin is direct-reacting, or conjugated.

**TREATMENT.** Antibacterial and antibiotic drugs have no effect upon the disease. Corticosteroids and cytotoxic agents have been used but without success. Transfusion is indicated for anemia. Exchange transfusion should be performed if the indirect-reacting bilirubin concentration approaches 20 mg per 100 ml.

**PROGNOSIS.** The majority of these infants who are symptomatic at birth die within the first week or two. A few survive and develop normally. Chorioretinitis, mi-

crocephaly or hydrocephalus with intracerebral calcifications, exactly like those which complicate toxoplasmosis and generalized herpes simplex, is to be expected in some of the survivors.

The possibility of asymptomatic infection in the newborn was noted by Starr and Gold in Cleveland. They found positive urine cultures in 1.57 per cent of 507 liveborn infants. Cytomegalovirus was recovered from the urine of all mothers of infected infants. Careful neurologic follow-up of infected infants is indicated, since some infected infants may have later developmental problems and microcephaly.

# COXSACKIE VIRUS DISEASE

Coxsackie group B viruses are enteroviruses capable of causing periodic outbreaks of illness with a wide spectrum of clinical manifestations. The infection is usually disseminated in the newborn infant.

**INCIDENCE.** The disease is surely rare, but the more general utilization of techniques for identification of viruses has already brought to light several series of 20 to 40 patients from single centers. We have encountered two within 1 year. These were reported by Robino et al. in 1962. Several outbreaks have by now been observed in newborn nurseries (Farmer and Patten).

**ETIOLOGY.** The two patients of Kibrick and Benirschke were infected with the group B-4 strain. Our two cases were caused by group B-2. Rawls et al. isolated an Echo 9 (Coxsackie A-23) from the tissues of one fatal neonatal example. Many are undoubtedly acquired by transplacental transmission, but the majority appear to be postnatally acquired group B viruses.

**PATHOLOGY.** Characteristic of many is diffuse myocardial inflammation, degeneration and necrosis. Inflammatory cells are mostly large mononuclears and lymphocytes. Liver, lungs, meninges, brain and adrenals may take part in similar pathologic alterations.

**DIAGNOSIS.** Fever, anorexia and vomiting initiate the illness. Often signs of heart failure, with rapidly enlarging heart and liver, diminishing strength of heart sounds and electrocardiographic changes of myocardial damage follow. In some infants the most prominent signs are the vomiting, lethargy and convulsions of meningoencephalitis. But the meningitis caused by this organism is more often signaled simply by unexplained fever and irritability. Signs of meningeal irritation are lacking more often than not (Nogen and Lepow). Pneumonitis is marked by dyspnea, cyanosis, rales and patchy infiltrations on the x-ray film. Hepatomegaly, mild to moderate jaundice, elevated bilirubin in the blood, a fair proportion of which is conjugated, and a lengthened prothrombin time with evidences of bleeding into skin and elsewhere indicate widespread involvement of the liver by the same inflammatory process.

In sum, the Coxsackie virus manifests a stronger affiliation for the myocardium than do any of the other infective agents which strike the newborn. Twelve of 23 of Kibrick and Benirschke's tabulated cases showed some signs of cardiac involvement. *The combination of myocarditis and meningoencephalitis strongly suggests Coxsackie infection.* The virus also produces pneumonitis and hepatitis. Rapid heart failure from myocarditis in the course of a generalized infection is the usual presenting sign. If the mother or some other member of the family had, within a week of the onset of the infant's illness, suffered from an influenza-like infection, the suspicion is strengthened, especially if pleurodynia had been part of the adult's symptomatology. Toxoplasmosis probably deserves second position among the diseases which cause simultaneous myocarditis and meningoencephalitis in a newborn infant, but the combination is a rarity in toxoplasmosis, a commonplace in Coxsackie infection. Sabin's dye test differentiates these two conditions.

**TREATMENT.** The myocarditis and heart failure must be treated by digitalization and the other measures detailed in the section devoted to disorders of the heart (p. 309). For the other manifestations therapy is directed toward individual symptoms.

**PROGNOSIS.** Nineteen of the 25 patients referred to above died within 1 to 14 days. Our two infants with proved cases also died. The outlook therefore is very grave.

## CASE 87–1

A white male infant was born to a 35-year-old multipara after a difficult breech delivery, but suffered no ill consequences. He breathed and cried spontaneously and seemed quite well. On the fourth postnatal day his mother became febrile, a few rales were heard in her chest, and her white blood cell count was low. On the fifth day the infant's temperature rose to 101.8° F, and later that day tachypnea with cyanosis and grunting expiration were noted. Pulse rate was 198 per minute. Physical examination was unrewarding. Hemoglobin was 14.7 gm, white blood cells numbered 4700 per cubic millimeter, urine showed albumin, 1+, blood culture proved to be sterile, and nasopharyngeal culture revealed no pathogens. He was given chloramphenicol, 100 mg every 8 hours by mouth, and penicillin, 300,000 units every 8 hours intramuscularly. On the sixth day the temperature rose to 103° F, respiratory rate was 80, pulse rate 220, the color was grayish blue, and the liver edge had descended 1.5 cm below the right costal margin. He was digitalized with Cedilanid. Lumbar puncture produced fluid containing protein in excess (2+ Pandy), 2500 red blood cells and 1200 white blood cells per cubic millimeter. Over the next few days his general condition improved slightly, but diarrhea developed with numerous blood-tinged, liquid, green stools. Stool cultures showed no pathogens. On the thirteenth day he went into severe shock, the temperature falling to 95.6°, the extremities becoming cold and mottled blue. A few clicking rales were heard throughout the lungs. The liver was down 3 cm and was firm. He died soon thereafter.

Antemortem diagnosis leaned strongly toward a disseminated viral infection, with myocarditis, pneumonitis and encephalomyelitis among its manifestations. Virus studies were made at the University Hospital of Baltimore (courtesy of Dr. Theodore Woodward) and were confirmed at the National Institutes of Health in Washington, D.C. Coxsackie virus B-2 was grown from cerebrospinal fluid, blood, throat washings and brain.

**COMMENT.** The onset of a febrile illness in this 5-day-old infant coincided with a similar illness in his mother. Tachycardia and heart failure developing in a previously normal heart suggested primary myocarditis, and cerebrospinal fluid alterations suggested encephalomyelitis. The combination of these two indicated generalized infection, with either a virus or toxoplasma the most likely pathogen. The former appeared the more probable cause in view of the simultaneous maternal illness and the absence of jaundice, hepatosplenomegaly and thrombocytopenia. (Since the appearance of this abstract in the first edition of this book this case and one other have been reported in detail by Robino, Perlman, Togo and Reback.)

## GENERALIZED HERPES SIMPLEX
### (Herpes hominis)

The virus of herpes simplex commonly produces in man a benign but protracted vesicular infection of skin and mucous membranes. Only rarely has it been known to invade the central nervous system of adults, and equally rarely its entrance into the blood stream has caused Kaposi's dermatitis herpetiformis (varicelliform eruption, eczema herpeticum). In 1952 Zuelzer and Stulberg reported generalized infection due to this virus, and their eight cases included six neonates and two infants between 1 and 2 years of age. Florman and Mindlin's carefully studied case appeared in the literature about the same time. Two distinct antigenic types of herpes simplex were described by Plummer et al. in 1968. One is associated with genital and neonatal infections, the other with oral infections. Infection in the infant is usually caused by Type II or genital type herpes virus.

**INCIDENCE.** To 1960 about 20 cases had been reported. With wider recognition, the next decade was marked by numerous reports of neonatal herpes. By 1968 Hovig et al. were able to find 68 cases in the literature.

**ETIOLOGY AND PATHOGENESIS.** The causative agent is the virus of herpes simplex. Transmission from mother to infant is not often transplacental, most infants apparently acquiring their infections during passage through the birth canal or by contact after birth. The mother may or may not show active herpetic lesions of the genitalia at the time of delivery.

**PATHOLOGY.** Macroscopically, many viscera, but chiefly liver, lungs and adrenals, are riddled with pale yellow, firm, necrotic nodules, measuring 1 to 6 mm in diameter. Under the microscope massive coagulation necrosis is seen to involve the parenchyma, stroma and vessels in these areas. Necrotizing, calcifying lesions of the brain may also be found.

**DIAGNOSIS.** The affected infants are usually premature or small and subpar full-term babies. They become ill between the fourth and eighth days of life or later. The first sign may be the appearance of groups of vesicles somewhere on the body. Two infants who developed vesicular lesions a few days after birth had been noted to have erythematous patches while they were still in the delivery room. Diagnosis is simplified by this sign, but unfortunately it has been present in less than half the reported cases. Conjunctivitis or keratoconjunctivitis is the presenting sign in many. There follow lethargy, anorexia, fever or fluctuating temperature, jaundice, usually not severe, enlargement of the liver and later of the spleen, at times dyspnea and cyanosis. Often a serious bleeding tendency develops, associated with profound thrombocytopenia. Exitus may be associated with bleeding, with apneic episodes or with convulsions and meningitis.

A few infants recover after long, stormy courses, but their ultimate prognosis is not good. Epstein and Crouch's infant showed psychomotor retardation at 6 months of age. One of the triplets reported by Florman and Mindlin had chorioretinitis at 3½ months, with resultant blindness, and severe mental retardation and spasticity. A second triplet, who had never had a neonatal illness, showed only chorioretinitis at 5 weeks of age.

Blood is not remarkable except for the late development of thrombocytopenia. Urine is normal except that albumin may be increased and bile may be present. Cultures from vesicles and blood are sterile for bacteria, a negative finding of considerable importance.

Material from vesicles or from the eye with conjunctivitis, or from organs *post mortem* inoculated into rabbit's cornea or chick embryo often yields the herpes simplex virus. The virus can be identified by cytopathic changes in tissue culture within 24 to 48 hours. More rapid diagnosis is sometimes possible by electron microscopy. The neutralization test is generally positive early, but weeks or months may elapse before it becomes positive. Fluorescent antibody against Type 2 virus can be demonstrated in the newborn's serum early.

**TREATMENT.** Prevention may be accomplished by recognition of maternal vulvar lesions on positive vaginal culture and delivery of the infant by cesarean section. Infants with the disease may be treated with 5-iodo-2-deoxyuridine, 50 to 100 mg per kilogram per day by continuous intravenous infusion. Since the drug may be toxic to bent marrow, its use should be restricted to infants in whom the diagnosis is established. It is not always effective. Other agents are under investigation.

CASE 87–2

A 5-day-old female infant was admitted to the Sinai Hospital of Baltimore because of fever, anorexia and lethargy. The mother had herpetic lesions about the genitalia at the time of delivery. After normal pregnancy and labor and spontaneous delivery the infant appeared quite well for the first four days, when a temperature of 102° F and anorexia were noted. On admission she was well developed, but a bit dehydrated, alert, with good cry. Temperature was 100.8° F, pulse rate 150 and respirations 40 to 50 per minute. A large pustular lesion was noted on the left cheek. The liver was felt 1.5 cm below the right costal mragin; the spleen was not palpable. White blood cells numbered 5600 per cubic millimeter; 73 per cent were polymorphonuclear. Hemoglobin was 16.9 gm per 100 ml. Blood cultures were negative, and cultures of the skin lesions were sterile.

In spite of chloramphenicol and penicillin the temperature remained elevated from 98 to 102° F. A few scattered skin lesions appeared during the fifth day, more on the seventh day, and these latter ones appeared vesicular. On this day a venipuncture wound bled for more than an hour, and platelets numbered 42,000 per cubic millimeter. She was given a transfusion. The liver and spleen gradually enlarged. The temperature became subnormal. She was given 100 ml of her mother's plasma in the hope that it might contain specific antibodies. Attacks of apnea and generalized convulsions followed. Death followed one of the apneic spells on the seventh hospital day, the twelfth day of life.

Autopsy showed extensive necrobiotic lesions characteristic of generalized herpes simplex in the liver, lungs and adrenals. There was hemorrhagic infiltration of the lesions, and many inclusion bodies were clearly visible within the cells. The brain was similarly involved. Hemorrhagic esophagitis was intense. Virus of herpes simplex was isolated from vesicles, blood, adrenals, lung and liver. Neutralization tests of the mother's blood were negative, those of the infant's blood were weakly positive and inconclusive.

**COMMENT.** This infant was undoubtedly infected during parturition by contact with the mother's herpes progenitalis. Skin lesions appeared on the fourth day, and new vesicles developed during the course. Unlike most instances of the disease, jaundice was never prominent. The liver and spleen enlarged, and thrombocytopenia with bleeding, and evidences of brain damage appeared. The virus was identified. Neutralizing bodies were not found in appreciable quantities in the mother or child.

In contrast to this infant is a baby who also was born to a mother with herpes progenitalis, but was sick at birth and had obviously been infected early in fetal life. The head was microcephalic, the eyes microphthalmic, and at birth the fingers and soles of the feet were covered with vesicles containing yellow purulent material. Cerebrospinal fluid was xanthochromic and contained an excess of protein, 160 red and 10 white blood cells per cubic millimeter. The liver and spleen were not large, and there was no thrombocytopenia. X-ray film of the skull showed dense periventricular calcification (Fig. 87–3). Herpes simplex virus was grown from both mother's and infant's skin lesions. We cite this example to point out that infection can take place transplacentally and very early in gestation, as well as at the moment of delivery, and also to demonstrate that periventricular calcification is not pathognomonic of toxoplasmosis or cytomegalic inclusion disease. It is possible that this represented a double

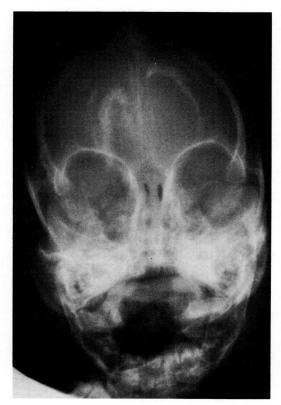

*Figure 87–3.* Herpes simplex disseminata; periventricular calcification.

infection, but no evidence supporting a second fetal pathogen has been discovered.

South et al. saw a case strikingly similar to this one. It seems clear now that herpesvirus type 2 may be transmitted across the placenta early, and may be teratogenic.

## POLIOMYELITIS

Prior to the 1950's acute infantile paralysis was largely a disease of early childhood. In epidemics in the 1950's its distribution pattern seemed to have changed so that many more adults and many more infants below 1 year of age were stricken. Part of this apparent shift may have been the result of greater awareness, but a genuinely higher attack rate for young babies seems to have been substantiated. Now that immunization is widely used, poliomyelitis is rarely seen in North America.

**INCIDENCE.** From 1947 to 1951, 29,656 cases of poliomyelitis were diagnosed in England; 1147 of these patients were less than 1 year old, 23 were less than 3 months old. Bates collected from the world literature 58 cases of neonatal disease, less than 1 month of age, of whom two were ill at birth, one sickened at 40 hours and five others before the fifth day of life.

**ETIOLOGY AND PATHOGENESIS.** Since the incubation period is approximately 10 days, those instances whose onsets antedate the tenth day must be transplacentally acquired. That pregnant women are somewhat more susceptible to the disease than other adults of the same age group is generally accepted. Fetal wastage is high among affected women, and both viremia (Bodian) and virus infection of the fetus and placenta (Schaeffer) have been demonstrated. Neonatal poliomyelitis manifesting itself after the tenth day is probably acquired, either during delivery from contamination with feces harboring the virus or by accidental contact after birth.

By far the great majority of newborn infants in countries where poliomyelitis is endemic are born with protective titers of antibody against the three main types. This was true of 86 per cent of the infants in the Philadelphia study of Pagano et al., while in Israel titers exceeded 1:4 in 87 to 94 per cent for the three types (Spigland and Goldblum). Passive immunity was gradually lost (about 50 per cent positive at three months, about 15 per cent at 6 months).

**PATHOLOGY.** In the newborn pathologic alterations are similar to those seen in older persons, but are apt to be extremely severe and widespread. Large necrotic areas with much hemorrhage and broadly cuffed vessels may be found throughout the spinal cord, medulla, basal ganglia and pons with less intense involvement of the motor and premotor cortical areas. Severe myocarditis is usually found, manifest by widespread focal necrosis and cellular infiltration.

**DIAGNOSIS.** Encephalomyelitic signs dominate the neonatal clinical picture, while those indicating meningeal irritation are virtually absent. Irritability, anorexia, vomiting and diarrhea may inaugurate the illness. Irritative phenomena such as localized twitching or muscle spasms or generalized convulsions may or may not precede paralyses. Flaccid palsy of one or several extremities may progress to involve all skeletal muscles and those of respiration. Rarely progression ceases and recovery takes place with or without permanent paralysis.

**TREATMENT.** There is no effective treatment.

**PREVENTION.** By now many series of newborn infants have been given poliomyelitis vaccine either by inoculation (Salk vaccine) or by mouth (Sabin vaccine). The oral Sabin vaccine is the best. Breast feeding should be discontinued for a few days after the infant is given the vaccine, since IgA antibodies in breast milk can inactivate the virus. Fewer newborns respond with a significant elevation of titer than do 3- to 6-month-old infants, approximately 50 per cent of the former versus 85 to 95 per cent of the latter. Antibody response to type 3 is much poorer than to types 1 and 2. Booster doses 4 to 12 months after the original challenge almost always induce a good antibody response whether or not there had been a good response to the first challenge. Failure to achieve a rise in titer after the original inoculation or ingestion probably is related to concentration of maternal antibody in the serum of the newborn.

By 1975 the number of children who had

not received their poliomyelitis prophylaxis has risen in many cities to an alarming height. If this persists we shall almost surely experience further epidemics of this frightening disease.

## VARICELLA

Congenital chickenpox is encountered infrequently. It is usually mild, but generalization of the infection may take place and cause death.

**INCIDENCE.** We have been able to discover about 40 certain case reports of congenital varicella in the literature. In two of these instances twins were affected. Since the incubation period is usually 14 days, and seldom as short as 10 days, an upper limit of 8 days for the appearance of the rash in the infant has been accepted as a sure indication that the disease was acquired transplacentally. The disease may also develop in the last 3 weeks of the first month of life as a postnatally acquired infection. This too is rare.

**ETIOLOGY.** The virus of varicella has been grown in suitable living media and has been seen under the electron microscope. Its characteristics are well known. Some difference of opinion still exists about the degree of immunity the newborn acquires from his mother. Our observation of family contacts leads us to the conclusion that many infants are indeed immune or partially so for the first 3 months of life, intimate exposure resulting in no disease or in a very mild attack. The only two instances we have seen of a second attack of varicella affected children whose first attacks had been exceedingly mild ones within the first few months of life.

Varicella has been shown to be caused by the same virus as herpes zoster. The lesions of zoster, along the distribution of peripheral nerves, have been seen very rarely in newborns, mainly in regions exposed to trauma. The mother of Feldman's infant had had herpes zoster at the onset of pregnancy, and the obstetrician and bacteriologist acquired the disease 10 to 15 days respectively after its appearance in the infant. The vesicular lesion occurs about the fourth to eighth day of life.

Rinvik describes the infant of a mother

who contracted varicella in the fourth month of her pregnancy. The 41-week baby was small and had congenital defects, pox-like scars and zigzag linear herpes zoster-like scars. He developed encephalomyelitis and chorioretinitis, and an elevated titer in his blood of varicella-zoster antibody. It seems not unlikely that this virus, like that of herpes simplex, may on rare occasions cross the placenta early enough to be teratogenic.

**DIAGNOSIS.** The manifestations of varicella in the newborn are often the same as those in the older child. Skin lesions may be present at birth or may crop out any day up to the eighth or tenth. Occasionally new lesions continue to appear for 7 or 8 days, a period of spread which would be highly unusual, but not unheard of, in later life. At times, too, the disease becomes generalized, producing meningoencephalitis, hepatitis and other visceral lesions, and causing death. Four of the reported patients succumbed in this fashion.

**TREATMENT.** Gamma globulin has not proved to be effective in the prevention of varicella in the same dosages which are effective against measles, hepatitis and poliomyelitis. Since the disease in a newborn may be fatal, it is important to give zoster immune globulin or plasma to the mother before delivery and to the infant at birth. Brunell et al. have demonstrated its protective effect in children, and presumably it will be useful in the neonate.

# WESTERN EQUINE ENCEPHALITIS

As far as we can determine, only one instance in which the virus of Western equine encephalitis may have been transmitted from mother to fetus has been reported.

Shinefield and Townsend cite the case of a mother who became ill 9 days after sleeping on an unscreened porch where she was repeatedly bitten by mosquitoes. The porch was contiguous to a yard in which there were forty chickens, a known reservoir host to the Western equine encephalitis virus. She had fever, lethargy and severe headache. Her antibodies to this organism rose to 1:128. Three days after the onset of her illness she delivered twins, one of whom became ill on the fifth day, the other 12 hours later. They had high fever, twitching, stiff neck,

bulging fontanels, cerebrospinal fluid pleiocytosis of 700 cells, of which 58 per cent were polymorphonuclear, and protein of 240 mg. per 100 ml. Cerebrospinal fluid sugar was not reduced. The fluid was sterile. Courses were stormy for 1 week, after which both recovered. Antibodies rose from 0 to 1:16 in one, from 0 to 1:128 in the other twin.

Since the incubation period of Western equine encephalitis is usually said to last from 4 to 21 days, and since the mother's own incubation period was clearly 9 days, the authors feel that the disease was almost surely acquired *ante partum* rather than at the moment of delivery. We cannot quarrel with this conclusion.

# REFERENCES

*Rubella*

Cooper, L. Z., Green, R. H., et al.: Neonatal thrombocytopenic purpura and other manifestations of rubella contracted in utero. Am. J. Dis. Child. *110*:416, 1965.

Cooper, L. Z., Ziring, P. R., Ockerse, A. R., et al.: Rubella: Clinical manifestations and management. Am. J. Dis. Child. *118*:18, 1969.

Desmond, M. M., et al.: Congenital rubella encephalitis: Effects on growth and early development. Am. J. Dis. Child. *118*:30, 1969.

Dudgeon, J. A.: Maternal rubella and its effect on the fetus. Arch. Dis. Child. *42*:110, 1967.

Gregg, N. M.: Congenital cataract following german measles in the mother. Tr. Ophthal. Soc. Austr. *3*:35, 1941.

Hardy, J. B., Monif, G. R. G., and Sever, J. L.: Studies in congenital rubella. Baltimore 1964–65. II. Clinical and virologic. Bull. Johns Hopkins Hosp. *118*:97, 1966.

Lepow, M. L., Veronelli, J. A., Hostetler, D. D. et al.: A trial with live attenuated rubella vaccine. Am. J. Dis. Child. *115*:639, 1968.

McCracken, G. H., Hardy, J. B., Chen, T. C., Hoffman, L. S., Gilkeson, M. R., and Sever, J. L.: Serum immunoglobulin levels in newborn infants. II. Survey of cord and follow up sera from 123 infants with congenital rubella. J. Pediatr. *74*:383, 1969.

Marshal, W. C.: The clinical impact of intrauterine rubella in intrauterine infections. *In* Elliott, K., and Knight, J. (Eds.): Ciba Foundation Symposium 10 (New series). Amsterdam, North Holland Publishers, 1973.

Michels, R. H., and Kenny, F. M.: Postnatal growth retardation in congenital rubella. Pediatrics *43*:251, 1969.

Overall, J. C., and Glasgow, L. A.: Virus infections of the fetus and newborn infant. J. Pediatr., *77*:315, 1970.

Phelan, P., and Campbell, P.: Pulmonary complications of rubella embryopathy. J. Pediatr. *75*:202, 1969.

Rowe, R. D.: Maternal rubella and pulmonary artery stenosis. Pediatrics *32*:180, 1963.

Rudolph, A. J., Singleton, E. B., et al.: Osseous manifestations of the congenital rubella syndrome. Am. J. Dis. Child. *110*:428, 1965.

Sever, J. L., Huebner, R. J., et al.: Serological diagnosis "en masse" with multiple antigens. Am. Rev. Resp. Dis. 88:Supp. 342, 354, 1963.

Weil, M. L., et al.: Chronic progressive panencephalitis due to rubella virus simulating subacute sclerosing panencephalitis. N. Engl. J. Med. *292*:994, 1975.

*Cytomegalic Inclusion Disease*

Alford, C. A., and Stagno, S.: Diagnosis of chronic perinatal infections. Am. J. Dis. Child. *129*:455, 1975.

Berenberg, W., and Nankervis, G.: Long-term follow-up of cytomegalic inclusion disease of infancy. Pediatrics *46*:403, 1970.

Blanc, W. A.: Cytologic diagnosis of cytomegalic inclusion disease in gastric washings. Am. J. Clin. Path. *28*:46, 1957.

Emanuel, I., and Kenny, G. E.: Cytomegalic inclusion disease of infancy. Pediatrics 38:957, 1966.

Embil, J. A., Ozere, R. L., and Haldane, E. V.: Congenital cytomegalovirus infection in two siblings from consecutive pregnancies. J. Pediatr. *77*:417, 1970.

Feldman, K. A.: Cytomegalovirus infection during pregnancy. Am. J. Dis. Child. *117*:517, 1969.

Fetterman, G. H.: A new laboratory aid in the clinical diagnosis of inclusion disease of infancy. Am. J. Clin. Path. *22*:424, 1952.

Guyton, P. B., Ehrlich, F., et al.: New observations in generalized cytomegalic-inclusion disease of the newborn: Report of a case with chorioretinitis. N. Engl. J. Med. *257*:803, 1957.

Hanshaw, J. B.: Congenital and acquired cytomegalovirus infection. Pediat. Clin. N. Amer. *13*:279, 1966.

Hanshaw, J. B., Betts, R. F., et al.: Acquired cytomegalovirus infection: Association with hepatomegaly and abnormal liver function tests. N. Engl. J. Med. *272*:602, 1965.

Hanshaw, J. B., Steinfeld, H. J., and White, C. J.: Fluorescent antibody test for cytomegalovirus macroglobulin. N. Engl. J. Med. *279*:566, 1968.

Hanshaw, J. B.: Congenital cytomegalovirus infection: A 15 year perspective. J. Infect. Dis., *123*:555, 1971.

McCracken, G. H., and Shinefield, H. R.: Immunoglobulin concentrations in newborn infants with congenital cytomegalic inclusion disease. Pediatrics *36*:933, 1965.

Medearis, D. N., Jr.: Observations concerning human cytomegalovirus infection and disease. Bull. Johns Hopkins Hosp. *114*:181, 1964.

Mercer, R. D., Luse, S., and Guyton, D. H.: Clinical diagnosis of generalized cytomegalic inclusion disease. Pediatrics *11*:502, 1953.

Reynolds, D. W., Stagno, S., Hosty, T. S., Tiller, M., and Alford, C. A.: Maternal cytomegalovirus excretion and perinatal infection. N. Engl. J. Med. *289*:1, 1973.

Silverman, W. A.: Clinical conference: Cytomegalic inclusion disease. Pediatrics *21*:682, 1958.

Smith, M. G., and Vellios, F.: Inclusion disease or generalized salivary gland virus infection. Arch. Path. *50*:852, 1950.

Stagno, S., Reynolds, D. W., and Alford, C. A.: Congenital cytomegalovirus (CMV) infection in two consecutive pregnancies. Clin. Res. *2*:124, 1973.

Starr, J. G., Bart, R. D., and Gold, E.: Inapparent congenital cytomegalovirus infection: Clinical and epidemiological characteristics in early infancy. N. Engl. J. Med. *282*:1075, 1970.

Starr, J. G., and Gold, E.: Screening of newborn infants for cytomegalovirus infection. J. Pediatr. *73*:820, 1968.

Weller, T. H.: The cytomegaloviruses: Ubiquitous agents with protein clinical manifestations. Part I, N. Engl. J. Med. *285*:203; Part II, *285*:267, 1971.

Weller, T. H., Macauley, J. C., et al.: Isolation of intranuclear inclusion producing agents from infants with illnesses resembling cytomegalic inclusion disease. Proc. Soc. Exp. Biol. & Med. *94*:4, 1957.

*Coxsackie Virus Disease*

Farmer, K., and Patten, P. T.: An outbreak of coxsackie B5 Infection in a Special Care Unit for Newborn Infants. New Zealand Med. J. *68*:86, 1968.

Kibrick, S., and Benirschke, K.: Severe generalized disease (encephalohepatomyocarditis) occurring in the newborn period due to infection with coxsackie virus, Group B. Pediatrics *22*:857, 1958.

Nogen, A. G., and Lepow, M. L.: Enteroviral meningitis in very young infants. Pediatrics *40*:617, 1967.

Overall, J. C., and Glasgow, L. A.: Virus infections of the fetus and newborn infant. J. Pediatr. *77*:315, 1970.

Rawls, W. E., Shorter, R. G., and Herrmann, E. C.: Fatal neonatal illness associated with echo 9 (coxsackie A-23) virus. Pediatrics *33*:278, 1964.

Robino, G., Perlman, A., et al.: Fatal neonatal infection due to coxsackie B2 virus. J. Pediatr. *61*:911, 1962.

*Generalized Herpes Simplex*

Charnock, E. L., and Cramblett, H. G.: 5-Iodo-2-deoxyuridine in neonatal herpesvirus hominis encephalitis. J. Pediatr. *76*:459, 1970.

Corbett, M. B., Sidell, C. M., and Zimmerman, M.: Idoxuridine in the treatment of cutaneous herpes simplex. J.A.M.A. *196*:441, 1966.

Epstein, H. C., and Crouch, W. L.: Herpes simplex of the newborn infant. Pediatrics *13*:553, 1954.

Florman, A. L., and Mindlin, R. L.: Generalized herpes simplex in an eleven-day-old premature infant. Am. J. Dis. Child. *83*:481, 1952.

Hovig, D. E., Hodgman, J. E., et al.: Herpes hominis (simplex) infection with recurrences during infancy. Am. J. Dis. Child. *115*:438, 1968.

Miller, D. R., Hanshaw, J. B., et al.: Fatal disseminated herpes simplex virus infection and hemorrhage in the neonate. J. Pediatr. *76*:409, 1970.

Nahmias, A. J., Josey, W. E., and Naib, Z. M.: Neonatal herpes simplex infection: Role of genital infection in mother as the source of virus in the newborn. J.A.M.A. *199*:164, 1967.

Nahmias, A. J., Josey, W. E., Naib, Z. M., et al.: Perinatal risk associated with maternal genital herpes simplex virus infection. Am. J. Obstet. Gynecol. *110*:825, 1971.

Nogen, A. G., and Lepow, M. L.: Enteroviral meningitis in very young infants. Pediatrics *40*:617, 1967.

Plummer, G., Waner, J. L., and Bowling, C. P.: Comparative studies of type 1 and type 2 herpes simplex viruses. Brit. J. Exp. Path., 49:202, 1968.

South, M. A., Tompkins, W. A. F., et al.: Congenital malformation of the central nervous system associated with genital type (type 2) herpesvirus. J. Pediatr. 75:13, 1969.

Torphy, D. E., Ray, C. G., et al.: Herpes simplex virus infection in infants: A spectrum of disease. J. Pediatr. 76:405, 1970.

Tuffli, G. A., and Nahmias, A. J.: Neonatal herpetic infection: Report of two premature infants treated with systemic use of idoxuridine. Am. J. Dis. Child. 118:909, 1969.

Zuelzer, W. W., and Stulberg, C. S.: Herpes simplex virus as the cause of fulminating visceral disease and hepatitis in infancy. Am. J. Dis. Child. 83:421, 1952.

*Poliomyelitis*

Bates, T.: Poliomyelitis in pregnancy, fetus and newborn. A.M.A. J. Dis. Child. 90:189, 1955.

Bodian, cited by T. Bates.

Katz, M., and Plotkin, S. A.: Oral polio immunization of the newborn infant, a possible method for overcoming interference by ingested antibodies. J. Pediatr. 73:267, 1968.

Lepow, M. L., Warren, R. J., Gray, N., Ingram, V. G., and Robbins, F. C.: Effect of Sabin Type I poliomyelitis vaccine administered by mouth to newborn infant. N. Engl. J. Med. 264:1071, 1961.

McConnell, A. A.: Poliomyelitis in infants under the age of six months. Arch. Dis. Child. 27:121, 1952.

Pagano, J. M., Plotkin, S. A., et al.: The response of premature infants to infection with attenuated poliovirus. Pediatrics 29:794, 1962.

Plotkin, S. A., Katz, M., et al.: Oral poliovirus vaccination in newborn African infants: The inhibitory effect of breast feeding. Am. J. Dis. Child. 111:27, 1966.

Pugh, R. C. B., and Dudgeon, J. A.: Fetal neonatal poliomyelitis. Arch. Dis. Child. 29:381, 1954.

Schaeffer, cited by T. Bates.

Siegel, M., and Greenberg, M.: Poliomyelitis in pregnancy: Effect on fetus and newborn infant. J. Pediatr. 49:280, 1956.

Spigland, I., and Goldblum, N.: Immunization of infants with formalinized poliomyelitis vaccine (Salk type). Pediatrics 25:812, 1960.

*Varicella-Zoster*

Brunell, P. A., Ross, A., et al.: Prevention of varicella by zoster immune globulin. N. Engl. J. Med. 280:1191, 1969.

Counter, C. E., and Korn, B. J.: Herpes zoster in the newborn associated with congenital blindness. Arch. Pediatr. 67:397, 1950.

Feldman, G. V.: Herpes zoster neonatorum. Arch. Dis. Child. 27:126, 1952.

Gaehde, cited by G. V. Feldman.

Meyers, J. D.: Congenital varicella in term infants: Risk reconsidered. J. Infect. Dis. 129:215, 1974.

Middlekamp, J. N.: Varicella in newborn twins. J. Pediatr. 43:573, 1953.

Rinvik, R.: Congenital varicella encephalomyelitis in surviving newborn. Am. J. Dis. Child. 117:231, 1969.

Shuman, H. H.: Varicella in the newborn. Am. J. Dis. Child. 58:564, 1939.

Waddington, H. K.: Congenital chickenpox: Report of a case in twins. Obstet. Gynecol. 7:319, 1956.

*Western Equine Encephalitis*

Medovy, H.: Western equine encephalomyelitis in infants. J. Pediatr. 22:308, 1943.

Shinefield, H. R., and Townsend, T. E.: Transplacental transmission of western equine encephalomyelitis in twins. J. Pediatr. 43:21, 1953.

# FUNGUS INFECTIONS

# 88

*Revised by Arnold Smith*

## COCCIDIOIDOMYCOSIS

Only two cases of coccidioidomycosis had been reported in infants less than 1 month of age by 1963. In both, the disease appeared to have been acquired from a parent postnatally. In 1964 Ziering and Rockas added another, listed as a 3-month-old, but whose first symptoms appeared within the first month. In addition to the rare human-to-infant transmission of coccidioidomycosis, it also appears that infants can be infected by porous fomites brought from an endemic area to one in which the disease is rare (Rothman et al.). This brief summary of the example described by

Townsend and McKey will serve to illustrate the problems of diagnosis and treatment.

### CASE 88–1

A 3-week-old white female infant had been well until 2 days before admission. The only pertinent fact in the family history was that the father had lived in the San Joaquin Valley for 12 years. The infant exhibited high fever, irritability and anorexia. She was acutely ill, with a temperature of 104° F, respirations 132 per minute. She was pale, and her neck was slightly stiff, her fontanel full, but not tense. Hemoglobin was 12.3 gm and fell to 8.2 gm after 1 week. White blood cells numbered 71,800, and fell gradually to 19,800, with normal differential counts. Cerebrospinal fluid showed 700 cells, 80 per cent polymorphonuclears, 195 mg of protein and 15 mg of sugar on admission. Cell count within the next month varied from 5 to 98, protein from 46 to 64 mg, sugar from 34 to 49 mg. Cerebrospinal fluid cultures were negative on four occasions, finally became positive for *C. immitis* one month after admission. The organism could never be grown from urine, blood, bone marrow or gastric washings. Complement fixation was positive for *C. immitis*, 4+, in the first dilution.

She seemed better 5 days after multiple antibiotic therapy had been started, but then the temperature began to spike. X-ray examination showed patchy infiltration of both lungs. The spleen became gradually larger; infiltration of lungs spread. Rimifon, streptomycin and para-aminosalicylic acid were given. In spite of this, cervical nodes and spleen grew larger, a papular rash appeared over the trunk, and she grew steadily weaker and died 2 months after admission. Autopsy showed disseminated coccidioidomycosis.

Interesting and disturbing is the fact that repeated coccidioidin skin test results were never positive.

**COMMENT.** This 3-week-old infant did not live in, but was exposed to a father who had lived in, the circumscribed desert region in our Southwest where coccidioidomycosis is endemic. The infection manifested itself first as a meningoencephalitis, followed by progressing pneumonitis and disseminated lesions, producing splenomegaly, glandular enlargement and an exanthem. No thrombocytopenia or purpura ever appeared. The skin test result never became positive. Cerebrospinal fluid cultures only became positive for the fungus 1 month after the onset. The complement fixation test gave the earliest confirmation of the diagnosis.

Ziering and Rockas achieved a notable success in treatment of their very ill baby, who had extensive pulmonary lesions, plus subcutaneous abscesses, osteitis and periostitis and iridocyclitis. He was given courses of amphotericin B over a period of 18 months without toxic effects. His complement fixation titer diminished and his skin test became positive, indications of marked improvement.

## CRYPTOCOCCOSIS

Cryptococcosis is caused by infection with *Torula histolytica* (*Cryptococcus neoformans*). It is important in the newborn, since it invades the central nervous system, where it sets up a meningoencephalitis which closely resembles that produced by toxoplasma and cytomegalic inclusion disease. Some of the earliest examples were reported by Neuhauser and Tucker. Emanuel et al. were able to find 23 affected children reported in the literature to 1961. Three definite and three almost certain cases showed illness within the first month of life.

**PATHOGENESIS.** Cryptococcus is an occasional inhabitant of the female genital tract, and it is believed that the infant acquires infection during passage through the birth canal. Symptoms begin so promptly after birth in some cases that one is forced to think seriously that infection may be transmitted transplacentally. It is, however, of interest that strains of *C. neoformans* pathogenic for man have been isolated from cow's milk, with or without concomitant bovine mastitis (Emmons, C. W.; Paunder et al.).

**DIAGNOSIS.** Neuhauser and Tucker's case I was a male infant 7 weeks old when admitted to hospital. He had been born after a precipitous delivery and was cyanotic after birth, requiring resuscitation. Twitchings and rigidity followed on the second day and did not entirely disappear for several weeks. He never ate well, was tube-fed, and in spite of this did not gain weight. Upon admission he was emaciated and chronically ill. The head was a bit large, there were cataracts in both eyes, and the spleen and liver were large. Opisthotonos, ankle clonus and positive Babinski reflex marked his neurologic examination. Cerebrospinal and subdural fluid contained an excess of protein and many red blood cells. Blood cell count was unremarkable, but no mention was made of platelets. He died suddenly after having been in hospital for 3 weeks. In this case it is difficult to date the onset, since many of the early symptoms might easily have stemmed from intracranial damage sustained at the time of birth.

Their case II began quite differently, the reason for admission on the nineteenth day of life being persistent, severe jaundice from birth. Abdominal enlargement was noted at 1 week; the urine was dark, and the stools were light. The spleen and liver were huge. Temperature never exceeded 100° F. He died 4 days after admission. No cause other than the patient's torula infection was found for the jaundice. Platelets were not mentioned.

In this example one wonders whether infection may not have begun before birth.

Case III of Neuhauser and Tucker again differed from the other two in mode of onset. The infant began to have convulsions and incessant crying at 2 weeks of age and was admitted to hospital 4 days later. He was well at birth and until he was 2 weeks old. The head, heart and lungs seemed normal on examination. The liver and spleen were very large. Neurologic examination showed only hyperactive reflexes. The platelets numbered only 66,000 per cubic millimeter. Otherwise the blood was normal, as was the urine. On the ninth hospital day he had gross hematuria. Death occurred on the following day.

X-ray films of the skulls of all three cases showed spotty calcifications within the substance of the brain. In case III interstitial pneumonitis, focal atelectasis and a large granulomatous lesion in the right upper lobe were noted in the chest x-ray. Two infants showed chorioretinitis, and two showed physical signs of central nervous system involvement. All had hepatosplenomegaly. Fever was almost nonexistent in all. All showed hydrocephalus and diffuse areas of focal degeneration throughout their brains.

It is clear that cases I and III are virtually indistinguishable from toxoplasmosis of early life on the basis of history and physical findings alone, while the story in case II, with the principal involvement centering in the liver, is highly suggestive of either cytomegalic inclusion disease or viral hepatitis. Diagnosis will have to depend upon exclusion of toxoplasmosis by Sabin's dye test and complement fixation studies, and exclusion of cytomegalic inclusion disease by inability to demonstrate inclusion bodies in the cells or urinary sediment or of gastric washings, and by virus culture. Cryptococcus has been seen in and cultivated from the cerebrospinal fluid of newborn infants five times, twice ante mortem and three times post mortem.

**TREATMENT.** Amphotericin B in a total intravenous dose of 30 mg per kilogram, administered in increasing increments beginning with 0.3 mg per kilogram over a 3 week period may be adequate therapy for disseminated disease with meningoencephalitis. In cases that progressively deteriorate or relapse, intrathecal therapy, in addition to the intravenous route, often produces a cure, particularly in the absence of underlying disease (Edwards et al.; Sarosi et al.). Since intrathecal therapy is often necessary over a protracted course, an intraventricular reservoir can facilitate this route if used with knowledge of the potential hazards (Diamond and Bennett). 5-Fluorocytosine (5-FC) should not be used alone, as the emergence of 5-FC resistant strains has been a major cause of treatment failure with this drug (Block et al.). This drug may have a role when used with amphotericin B, because the combination is synergistic in vitro and in vivo (Medoff et al.). Clinical trials with this combination are not available in adults or in children.

## DISSEMINATED HISTOPLASMOSIS

No very young infant has been observed who has suffered from the primary pulmonary form of histoplasmosis or from the localized granulomatous variety which involves skin, oropharynx, larynx or other viscera. This brief discussion will be limited therefore to the general disseminated form.

**INCIDENCE.** The disease is widespread in the United States and elsewhere, but certain areas seem to be heavily contaminated and their populations infected in large numbers. Cases are by no means confined to the broad central belt of high infection rate of which Tennessee appears to be the center. In our own section of the country the eastern shore counties of Maryland are the source of an appreciable number of histoplasma infections. Children below 2 years seem to be highly susceptible, and when they become infected, they almost always have the disseminated form. Cases developing within the first month of life are extremely uncommon, but many examples have been reported in the third month and later.

**ETIOLOGY.** The invading organism is a fungus, *Histoplasma capsulatum*. Depending upon environmental conditions, the fungus may grow in a yeast-like phase or in a mycelial phase. It is found in the soil in the mycelial phase, and it is from the soil that most human infection appears to be derived.

**DIAGNOSIS.** Infected infants become ill with fever, often spiking to high levels once a day, with rapid enlargement of the spleen and liver, bronchopneumonic pulmonary infiltrations of nonspecific nature, progressive anemia and thrombocytopenia. The disease resembles disseminated tuberculosis in some respects, but differs from it in the greater degree of hepatosplenomegaly, in the absence of miliary pulmonary involvement and in its failure to invade the meninges. Its later appearance, the usual but not invariable absence of jaundice and again its aversion to the central nervous system distinguish it from cytomegalic inclusion disease and toxoplasmosis. Differentiation from coccidioidomycosis and torulosis, which also make their appearance toward the end of the first month or later, may be impossible on clinical grounds alone. One will be influenced somewhat by geographic and epidemiologic considerations, but the final diagnosis will depend upon laboratory investigations.

A positive histoplasmin skin test is of use, but the result may be negative in as many as half of the early acute cases as well as in those patients who are severely ill with the disease. Histoplasmin reactions are not infrequently positive when other fungi are the responsible etiologic agents. By far the most reliable laboratory indication of the disease is growth of *Histoplasma capsulatum* from peripheral blood, liver biopsy or bone marrow samples, especially

the latter. The chief objection to this test is the length of time one must wait for the answer. Quickest and quite reliable confirmation can be obtained from demonstration of "specific histoplasmosis (H) and mycelia (M) precipitin bands by the micro-Ouchterlony technique" (Holland and Holland).

**TREATMENT.** Ethyl vanillate, Atabrine and hydroxystilbamidine have been used with some success. Amphotericin B appears to be far more effective than any of these. Little et al. reported four cures in children, three of whom were 3, 5 and 8 months of age at the time treatment was begun. The drug is given intravenously, in a daily dosage of 0.25 to 1.0 mg per kilogram, dissolved in 5 per cent dextrose to a concentration not exceeding 1.0 mg per 10 ml. The infusion must be given slowly over a period of 6 hours or more. Infusions are continued for 4 to 8 weeks, daily at first, later every alternate day. Headache, nausea and vomiting, and in some babies anaphylactoid-like reactions, are not uncommon side effects, but need not contraindicate continuation of therapy. We achieved a notable success by this method in a nearly moribund 4-month-old baby.

# CANDIDIASIS (MONILIASIS)

In the chapter on Infections of the Skin oral and cutaneous candidiasis are discussed (p. 952). We shall not go over this ground here, but shall confine ourselves to a brief résumé of several of the complications of thrush of interest to the neonatologist.

Attention should be called to the demonstration that gentian violet in the 1 per cent aqueous solution commonly used to treat oral thrush can cause mucous membrane lesions (Slotkowsky).

## DISSEMINATED CANDIDIASIS

This once rare disease is now becoming epidemic in many nurseries. This is probably the result of the intensive use of broad spectrum antibiotics in premature (and more vulnerable) infants and developmental, suboptimal leukocytic phagocytosis and killing of *Candida albicans* (Xanthou et al.); but the most important factor is the use of central venous hyperalimentation. *Candida albicans* grows in all alimentation solutions in use, but the rate is dependent on composition and temperature (Goldman and Maki). The organisms can reach densities of approximately 100,000 per ml and yet the solution appears clear to the eye; further infection due to contaminated intravenous fluids produced an insidious infection. A typical case has been reported by Hill et al.

The patient was a 1928 gm infant born to a 33-year-old primigravida at approximately 32 weeks' gestation. The infant, who was delivered by cesarean section because of placenta previa, required intubation and resuscitation in the delivery room. Because of persistent respiratory distress and periods of apnea, the patient was transferred to the University of Minnesota Neonatal Intensive Care Unit at approximately 12 hours of age. Severe hyaline membrane disease necessitated the use of respiratory therapy, and an umbilical artery catheter was inserted to monitor blood gases.

On the fifth hospital day, apnea, acidosis and questionable pneumatosis intestinalis observed on an abdominal x-ray prompted the institution and continuance of penicillin and kanamycin therapy, although blood, urine and cerebro-. spinal fluid cultures remained sterile. Hyperalimentation through the umbilical arterial catheter was started on the sixth hospital day. On the ninth hospital day a recurrence of apnea and acidosis prompted repeat cultures, and the antibiotic therapy was changed to ampicillin and gentamicin. The patient improved clinically, but after 4 days *Candida albicans* grew out in the blood culture drawn on the ninth day. The catheter in the umbilical artery was removed and replaced 12 hours later with an internal jugular venous catheter, and amphotericin B therapy was initiated. Four days later, after three negative blood cultures and a negative cerebrospinal fluid culture were obtained, the amphotericin B was discontinued. Urine cultures continued to yield 7000 to 50,000 colonies of *C. albicans* per milliliter. On the twenty-sixth hospital day, 17 days after the initial positive blood cultures, edema of feet, ankles and knees was observed. This was considered to have a vascular etiology and the extremities were elevated.

On the twenty-ninth hospital day, bilateral knee and ankle effusions developed and were accompanied by warmth and erythema. Synovial fluid contained numerous polymorphonuclear leukocytes (PMNs) but no organisms were seen on direct examination. *Candida albicans* subsequently grew from fluid obtained from both knees and the left ankle. Repeat urine cultures yielded 100,000 colonies of *C. albicans* per milliliter, although blood cultures remained sterile. A cerebrospinal fluid specimen obtained on the twenty-ninth hospital day contained six PMNs and 22 monocytes with a glucose of 29 mg per 100 ml and protein of 84 mg per 100 ml. This specimen also yielded *C. albicans* on culture.

This case illustrates several important principles in the diagnosis of disseminated candidiasis; the infection is septicemic, with blood cultures yielding the organism and the urine containing the organisms cleared by the kidney. Blood cultures obtained through the hyperalimentation catheter do sample infected thrombi adjacent to the tip, but do not aid in differentiating between disease that will resolve with catheter removal (Ellis and Spivack) and life-threatening illness. Peripheral blood cultures obtained by venipuncture are a more reliable indicator of ongoing candidemia. In overwhelming infections the organisms can be seen in stained smears of buffy coat preparations (Silverman et al.). Skin lesions can be seen (Bodey and Luna) and yield the organism on aspiration. Candida ophthalmitis is a frequent complication of candidemia (Fishman), and can serve as a focus for continued candidemia (Haring). Every infant in whom the diagnosis of candidal sepsis is suspected should have indirect funduscopic exam at regular intervals. Other manifestations of candidal sepsis in newborns are osteomyelitis (Freeman et al., Adler et al., Klein et al.), meningitis, endocarditis (Joshi and Wang, Shapira et al.) and arthritis.

Because of the importance of host factors, the course of disseminated candidiasis is unpredictable, making therapeutic generalizations impossible. If the infection is catheter related, the catheter should be removed. In most instances amphotericin B is administered until it is clear that there are no occult foci. In patients with meningitis, or when progressive clinical deterioration is present, 5-fluorocytosine is used in combination with amphotericin B.

## CONGENITAL CANDIDIASIS

Many examples of candidal infection acquired in utero have been reported by now. Dvorak and Gavaller's baby had a diffuse macular rash and respiratory distress at birth, and died at 34 hours of age. Autopsy showed extensive bronchopneumonia, the sections filled with hyphae and spores. The placenta was also heavily infected with the fungus.

In these instances, ascending infection produces chorioamnionitis with dissemination to the fetus, which can lead to spontaneous abortion (Ho and Aterman). In most instances, the severity of disseminated candidiasis acquired in utero is such that the infant expires before therapy can be considered (Schirar et al.).

It is also clear that the infant can be delivered with cutaneous candidiasis without systemic involvement (Rhatigan; Aterman). The lesions in Rhatigan's infant were yellow vesicles with a narrow red border. This infant's mother had had vaginal moniliasis for months prior to delivery, but no placental infection was found.

It thus appears that Candida, like bacteria, may infect the fetus by hematogenous dissemination from the umbilical vessels, leading to systemic infection, or be limited to cutaneous candidiasis.

## PNEUMONIA COMPLICATING ORAL THRUSH

Adams reported that five of eight infants who had oral thrush showed respiratory distress, cyanosis and leukocytosis. They all had signs of pneumonitis. In one who died Monilia were found invading the pulmonary parenchyma, and the author believed this to have been an example of true thrush pneumonitis. Winter cannot accept Adams' autopsied case as one of mycotic pneumonia, but believes that this complication has been demonstrated beyond doubt in a 1-year-old and in a number of older persons.

More recently it has become an unexpected finding at autopsies of newborn infants (Koenig). The course was not always fulminant and there is little specificity to the roentgenographic picture. Infants with thrush and pneumonia should be suspected of having Candida as the infecting agent, particularly if they have been pre-

treated with broad spectrum antibiotics. Isolation of *Candida albicans* from the blood of such infants is strongly suggestive of bronchopulmonary candidiasis, but demonstration of hyphae in tracheal aspirates or pulmonary tissue is the best evidence of infection. This is often difficult and hazardous because of the concomitant thrush and problems of bronchoscopy in sick infants.

Beckmann and Navarro recorded the following case history.

A 4 pound 11 ounce (2125 gm) infant was discharged from the nursery on the tenth day of life, well except for thick deposits of thrush upon the tongue. Gentian violet and 2 per cent ferric chloride solution were used locally, but the lesion became ulcerative and spread to involve all the oral and buccal mucous membranes. Cyanosis during feeding appeared, and rales were heard throughout both lungs. At 3 months of age he was admitted to hospital, weighing 5 pounds 6 ounces (2435 gm). His temperature was 98.6° F, and never rose during his stay. He was malnourished, cyanotic, critically ill. There were mucopurulent nasal and oral discharges. X-ray film showed patches of pneumonia, atelectasis and emphysema. Attempted feeding caused choking and cyanosis. Intravenous fluid therapy, transfusion, penicillin and Gantrisin failed to improve his condition. Mycostatin, 175,000 units by mouth every 6 hours, was begun. Within 48 hours his mouth was practically healed! The respiratory difficulty improved more slowly and was not gone until the second week.

The authors admit that the diagnosis of *C. albicans* pneumonitis was far from proved, but believe that the response to the fungicidal antibiotic was striking enough to be highly suggestive.

## THRUSH ESOPHAGITIS

A not inconsiderable number of cases have been reported in which oral thrush has advanced to involve the nasopharynx and the esophagus. When this occurs, swallowing becomes almost impossible, and during the attempts to swallow, much liquid appears to be aspirated into the tracheobronchial tree. Choking spells with cyanosis result.

Wolff et al. reported two examples from Birmingham, England.

The first concerned a female infant who weighed 6 pounds (2720 gm) at birth and seemed well until her sixteenth day, when anorexia and vomiting began. When she was admitted the next day, her general condition seemed good, but the tongue and buccal mucous membranes were covered with a white membrane from which *C. albicans* was identified by smear. After three days of treatment with 1 per cent gentian violet locally and 0.01 per cent solution, 4 cc three times a day by mouth, there had been no improvement. The following day pneumonia developed, which did not respond to a sulfonamide, later to penicillin. Profuse viscid discharge from the mouth and nose appeared. At this stage the infant could not swallow, and attempts led to repeated bouts of cyanosis. On the eighth day hydroxystilbamidine was begun, 15 mg (5 mg per kilogram) in 0.75 cc of water injected slowly into the intravenous infusion tubing. This was repeated every 12 hours. A staphylococcus, coagulase-positive, was grown from the blood. Streptomycin was given in addition to the other drug. Improvement began while she was on hydroxystilbamidine alone. After 6 days the intravenous drip was removed, and oral feedings were started. On the eighteenth day barium swallow showed that incoordination of swallowing was still present, much iodized oil entering the trachea during the act of deglutition. Gavage feedings were begun again and were able to be discontinued 1 week later.

Such contiguous spread should be suspected in infants with thrush when swallowing becomes difficult and aspiration seems to be taking place. Not surprisingly, the contiguous spread can be more anterior, and produce signs and symptoms of congenital stridor (Perrone).

## ENTERIC CANDIDIASIS

Kozinn and Taschdjian deplore the tendency to forget the possibility of enteric candidiasis in the differential diagnosis of diarrhea in the young infant. They stress that it is a not uncommon complication of thrush and that it may lead to systemic invasion and death.

The diagnosis should be suspected whenever diarrhea complicates thrush or cutaneous candidiasis, especially if the infant has been on antimicrobial therapy. Direct examination of stools reveals in many cases the mycelial form of the fungus, a finding which is much more significant than visualization of yeast forms.

Good clinical response and disappearance of the organisms can be attained with nystatin in 80 per cent of the cases. Amphotericin B may be helpful in severe cases.

## REFERENCES

Adams, J. M.: A reevaluation of the pneumonias of infancy. J. Pediatr. 25:369, 85, 1944.

Adler, S., Randall, J., and Plotkin, S. A.: Candidal osteomyelitis and arthritis in a neonate. Am. J. Dis. Child. 123:595, 1972.

Ashcraft, K. W., and Leape, L. L.: Candida sepsis complicating parenteral feeding. J.A.M.A. 212:454, 1970.

Aterman, K.: Pathology of candida infection of the umbilical cord. Am. J. Clin. Path. 49:798, 1968.

Beckmann, A. J., and Navarro, J. E.: Pneumonia complicating oral thrush treated with mycostatin, a new antifungal antibiotic. J. Pediatr. 46:587, 1955.

Block, E. R., Jennings, A. E., and Bennett, J. E.: 5-Fluorocytosine resistance in Cryptococcus neoformans. Antimicrob. Agents Chemotherap. 3:649, 1973.

Bodey, G. P., and Luna, M.: Skin lesions associated with disseminated candidiasis. J.A.M.A. 229:1466, 1974.

Burry, A. F.: Hydrocephalus after intra-uterine fungal infection. Arch. Dis. Child. 32:161, 1957.

Diamond, R. D., and Bennett, J. E.: A subcutaneous reservoir for intrathecal therapy of fungal meningitis. N. Engl. J. Med. 288:186, 1973.

Dvorak, A. M., and Gavaller, B.: Congenital systemic candidiasis: Report of a case. N. Engl. J. Med. 274:540, 1966.

Edwards, V. E., Sutherland, J. M., and Tyner, J. H.: Cryptococcosis of the central nervous system. J. Neurol. Neurosurg. Psych. 33:415, 1970.

Ellis, C. A., and Spivack, M. L.: The significance of candidemia. Ann. Intern. Med. 67:511, 1967.

Emanuel, B., Ching, E., Lieberman, A. D., and Golden, M.: Cryptococcus meningitis in a child successfully treated with amphotericin B, with a review of the literature. J. Pediatr. 59:577, 1961.

Emmons, C. W.: Cryptococcus neoformans, strains from an outbreak of bovine mastitis. Mycopath. Mycol. Appl. 6:231, 1953.

Fishman, L. S., Griffin, J. R., and Sapico, F. L.: Hematogenous candida endophthalmitis: A complication of candidemia. N. Engl. J. Med. 286:675, 1972.

Freeman, J. B., Wienke, J. W., and Soper, R. T.: Candida osteomyelitis associated with intravenous alimentation. J. Pediat. Surg. 9:783, 1974.

Goldman, D. A., and Maki, D. G.: Infection control in total parenteral nutrition. J.A.M.A. 223:1360, 1973.

Haring, H., Johnston, R., and Touloukian, R.: Successfully treated candida endophthalmitis. Pediatrics 51:1027, 1973.

Heiner, D. C.: Diagnosis of histoplasmosis. Pediatrics 22:616, 1958.

Henderson, J. L.: Infection in the newborn. Edinburgh Med. J. 50:535, 1943.

Hill, H. R., Mitchell, T. G., Matsen, J. M., et al.: Recovery from disseminated candidiasis in a premature neonate. Pediatrics 53:748, 1974.

Ho, C. Y., and Aterman, K.: Infection of the fetus by candida in a spontaneous abortion. Am. J. Obstet. Gynecol. 106:705, 1970.

Holland, P., and Holland, N. H.: Histoplasmosis in early infancy: Hematologic, histochemical and immunologic observations. Am. J. Dis. Child. 112:412, 1966.

Joshi, W., and Wang, N. S.: Repeated pulmonary embolism in an infant with subacute candida endocarditis of the right side of the heart. Am. J. Dis. Child. 125:257, 1973.

Klein, J. D., Yamauchi, T., and Horlick, S. P.: Neonatal candidiasis meningitis and arthritis: Observations and review of literature. J. Pediatr. 81:31, 1972.

Koenig, N. D.: Candida pneumonia in newborn infants. Deut. Med. Wchnschr. 96:818, 1971.

Kozinn, P., and Taschdjian, C. L.: Enteric candidiasis: Diagnosis and clinical considerations. Pediatrics 30:71, 1962.

Little, J., Bruce, J., Andrews, H., Crawford, K., and McKinley, G.: Treatment of disseminated infantile histoplasmosis with amphotericin B. Pediatrics 24:1, 1959.

Medoff, G., Comfort, M., and Kobayoshi, G. S.: Synergistic action of amphotericin B and 5-fluorocytosine against yeast-like organisms. Proc. Soc. Exp. Biol. Med. 138:571, 1971.

Neuhauser, E. B. D., and Tucker, A.: The roentgen changes produced by diffuse torulosis in the newborn. Am. J. Roentgenol. 59:805, 1948.

Perrone, J. A.: Laryngeal obstruction due to Monilia albicans in a newborn. Laryngoscope 80:288, 1970.

Peterson, J. C., and Christie, A.: Histoplasmosis. Pediat. Clin. N. Amer. 2:127, 1955.

Pounder, W. D., Amberson, J. M., and Jaeger, R. F.: A severe mastitis problem associated with *Crypto-coccus neoformans* in a large dairy herd. Am. J. Vet. Res. 13:121, 1952.

Rhatigan, R. M.: Congenital cutaneous candidiasis. Am. J. Dis. Child. 116:545, 1968.

Rothwamov, P. E., Graw, R. G., and Harria, J. C.: Coccidioidomycosis—possible fomite transmission. Am. J. Dis. Child. 118:792, 1968.

Sarosi, G. A., Parker, J. D., Doto, I. L., and Tosh, F. E.: Amphotericin B in cryptococcal meningitis. Ann. Intern. Med. 71:1079, 1969.

Schirar, A., Rendu, C., Vielk, J. P., et al.: Congenital mycosis (Candida albicans) Biol. Neonate 24:273, 1974.

Shapira, Y., Drucker, M., Russell, A., et al.: Candida endocarditis and encephalitis in an infant. Clin. Pediat. 13:542, 1974.

Silverman, E. M., Norman, L. F., and Goldman, R. T.: Diagnosis of systemic candidiasis in smears of venous blood stained with Wright's stain. Am. J. Clin. Pathol. 60:473, 1973.

Slotkowsky, E. L.: Formation of mucous membrane lesions secondary to prolonged use of one percent aqueous gentian violet. J. Pediatr. 51:652, 1957.

Townsend, T. E., and McKey, R. W.: Coccidioidomycosis in infants. Am. J. Dis. Child. 86:51, 1953.

Winter, W. G., Jr.: Candida (monilia) infections in children. Pediat. Clin. N. Amer. 2:151, 1955.

Wolff, O. H., Petty, B. W., Astley, R., and Smellie, J. M.: Thrush oesophagitis with pharyngeal incoordination treated with hydroxystilbamidine. Lancet 1:991, 1955.

Xanthou, M., Valassi-Adawn, E., Kintzonidou, E., et al.: Phagocytosis and killing ability of Candida albicans by blood leukocytes of healthy term and preterm babies. Arch. Dis. Child. 50:72, 1975.

Ziering, W. H., and Rockas, H. R.: Coccidioidomycosis: Long-term treatment with amphotericin B of disseminated disease in a three-month-old baby. Am. J. Dis. Child. 108:454, 1964.

# 89 PROTOZOAL INFECTIONS: CONGENITAL TOXOPLASMOSIS

The continuing researches of Sabin, Feldman and others within the past few decades have added immeasurably to our understanding of disease states caused by toxoplasma. The congenital form should now be recognized by competent pediatricians, and the laboratory tests required to ascertain the diagnosis should be made available in all medical centers.

**INCIDENCE.** Inapparent infection with the protozoon is widespread throughout the world. Population samples indicate that the percentage of adults with antibody is increased at lower geographical latitudes. Feldman found approximately 10 per cent positives, by complement fixation tests, in Iceland, 30 per cent in New Orleans and 65 per cent in Tahiti. But latitude is by no means the only determining factor. The number of positive reactors in Paris, for instance, is unusually high, and has been attributed to Parisians' fondness for raw or undercooked meat. As regards congenital toxoplasmosis, Eichenwald was able to comment upon the clinical findings in 75 infants and children, Feldman in 103, indicating that the disease cannot be termed rare. Nevertheless most of the observations were made upon children showing the end-results of their congenital disease, the figures therefore being retrospective and cumulative.

Serum specimens from 23,000 pregnant women in a collaborative project* were studied by Sever et al. for evidence of infection with toxoplasmosis. Thirty-eight per cent of the women had evidence of infection with toxoplasma at some time, but only 2.3 per cent had markedly elevated titers. The outcome of pregnancy was poorer in women with high titers. Only five infants among the entire group had definite congenital toxoplasmosis. The most recent estimates of frequency of congenital infection in the United States range from 1 to 4 in 1000 live births.

Desmonts and Couvreur, in Paris, reported that of 378 pregnant women with high initial toxoplasma antibody titers or seroconversion during pregnancy, 183 acquired the infection during pregnancy, a rate of 6.3 per 100 pregnancies. There were 11 abortions, seven stillbirths, and 59 cases of congenital toxoplasmosis. Of these, two died, seven had severe disease, 11 had mild disease and 39 had no symptoms or signs. Severe disease in the infant was noted only when maternal infections were acquired in the first two trimesters. Toxoplasma was isolated from the placentas of 25 per cent of those who acquired the infection during pregnancy.

**ETIOLOGY.** The disease is caused by infestation with *Toxoplasma gondii*, so named because it was first isolated in 1909 from a North African rodent called the gondi. The organism is generally classified as a protozoon. In addition to the large number of human beings who are infected,

---

*Collaborative Perinatal Research Study, National Institute of Neurological Diseases and Blindness, National Institutes of Health, Bethesda, Md.

if one may judge by positive skin test and antibody titer, many domestic and wild animals appear to harbor the organism. The domestic cat seems to be the main reservoir of the infective oocysts that are passed in the feces. Congenital toxoplasmosis is caused by invasion of the fetal blood stream by parasites during a stage of maternal parasitemia. It is likely that the parasitemia occurs only with initial infection, and in the absence of any maternal symptoms. This is important because it means that mothers whose infections become chronic and inapparent do not transmit the disease to subsequent fetuses. Infections acquired by the mother in the early trimesters of pregnancy are much more likely to be transmitted to the fetus than are those contracted later.

Postnatal infections also occur in children, but the youngest case we are aware of is that of a 7-month infant who became ill with diarrhea at 3 months of age. This was 1 month after the institution of unpasteurized goat's milk feeding, and was almost surely the result of that form of alimentation (Riemann et al.).

**PATHOLOGY.** The toxoplasma is a crescentic oval organism, 4 to 7 microns long, with a single eccentric nucleus. In tissues it is intracellular, and small or large agglomerates are often seen. In later stages the organism is often seen lying within a cystic space especially in the brain. This is termed a pseudocyst, since the wall is believed to represent the membrane of the cell which has been totally destroyed.

In the newborn the principal locus of infection is the central nervous system. Lesions consist of areas of necrosis in which calcium is ultimately deposited and throughout which pseudocysts or the naked parasite may be sparsely scattered. Similar lesions are less abundant in liver, lungs, myocardium, skeletal muscle, spleen and other tissues. There is little cellular inflammatory reaction, consisting mostly of lymphocytes, monocytes and plasma cells. The pathologic picture is not specific unless organisms or pseudocysts can be demonstrated.

**DIAGNOSIS.** The clinical picture in the minority of cases resembles that of cytomegalic inclusion disease in all respects. The tetrad of chorioretinitis, hydrocephalus or microcephalus, cerebral calcifications and mental retardation is highly suggestive in older infants and children. In newborns, skin hemorrhages and hepatosplenomegaly may be present at birth, and jaundice may be noted immediately or within a few hours. Platelets are reduced in number. More usual is a less explosive clinical pattern in which symptoms referable to the central nervous system overshadow those of the liver and spleen, lungs or bone marrow.

Thus Beckett and Flynn's case I was an infant born at term who seemed normal until the fifth day, when ptosis of one lid was noted. In the fourth week vomiting and pallor developed, while in the fifth week high-pitched cry, enlargement of the head and opisthotonos were noted. Examination at 6 weeks showed dehydration, pallor, sluggishness, hydrocephalus, bulging fontanel, separated sutures and right facial nerve palsy. The liver and spleen were not large, purpura was absent, platelets normal. Cerebrospinal fluid was grossly abnormal and xanthochromic, containing 200 red blood cells per cubic millimeter and 2900 mg of protein per 100 ml. X-ray film of the skull showed fine scattered calcifications.

The epidemiology in this example was noteworthy. The antibody titer of the mother against toxoplasma registered 1:4906, while that of a pet dachshund which had had "brain fever" with residual paralysis of one leg at the time of the infant's conception was 1:256!

Other more bizarre forms of the disease have been described. Silver and Dixon's case is one of the more remarkable ones, demonstrating how protean the manifestations of congenital toxoplasmosis can be.

This infant's course was one of increasing lethargy, poor appetite and bleeding manifestations until admission in his sixth week. Facial nerve palsy, hepatosplenomegaly, lethargy, pupillary membranes and cataracts were found. Cerebrospinal fluid was xanthochromic and contained a few white and red blood cells and 1000 mg of protein per 100 ml. X-ray film of the skull showed flaky calcific densities. His course in hospital was characterized by hypothermia, persistent hypernatremia and inability to concentrate urine except when treated with posterior pituitary extract. He also showed eosinophilia of the peripheral blood (30 per cent) and of the bone marrow.

**LABORATORY FINDINGS.** In the blood the hemoglobin content and red cell count may be normal or moderately to greatly reduced. Platelets are diminished in the visceral form, not in the encephalitic form. White blood cells are normal or somewhat elevated. Nucleated erythrocytes may be greatly increased. Direct bilirubin level is elevated in cases which go on to jaundice. Urine is usually normal with respect to albumin, sugar and sediment. Bile may be present in cases showing jaundice. The cerebrospinal fluid may have an increase in protein.

Sabin's dye test for antibodies is positive in high dilutions within the first two weeks of the acute phase and remains so, in slowly diminishing titer, for many years, perhaps for life. Mother's dye test is also strongly positive. Complement fixation test is negative at first, but rises with the passage of several weeks. This test remains positive for a limited time, perhaps 2 to 4 years.

Since IgG antibody possessed by the newborn may merely represent transplacentally transmitted maternal gamma globulin, a positive dye test at birth by no means indicates the disease; if it persists beyond 3 or 4 months, it probably does. More useful for quick diagnosis is the presence of specific IgM antibody, as demonstrated by a fluorescent-antibody test. Even this may give falsely positive results because of leakage of maternal blood into the fetal circulation (Remington et al.).

Isolation of toxoplasma may be accomplished by intracerebral or intraperitoneal inoculation of test material into mice.

**TREATMENT.** Sulfadiazine and its close relatives may have some effect in retarding multiplication of the protozoa. Pyrimethamine (Daraprim) has shown promise in treatment of the disease and should be tried in conjunction with sulfadiazine or trisulfapyrimidines, with which it may act synergistically. Langer has been impressed with the effectiveness of supronal (1-sulfanilyl-2 thiourea salt of 4-homosulfanilamide) combined with sulfamerazine.

**PROGNOSIS.** The outlook for survival is poor when the disease is manifest at birth and when it involves the liver and bone marrow predominantly. Those infants who become symptomatic after a few weeks and whose signs point almost entirely to central nervous system involvement often survive. Their ultimate prognosis is poor. Many suffer chorioretinitis in the acute phase or as late as the second or third month, with subsequent blindness. Many become microcephalic or hydrocephalic, and in most of these, scattered calcifications within the brain become demonstrable by x-ray examination. Psychomotor development is retarded, and they may be expected to end as severe mental defectives.

## REFERENCES

Beckett, R. S., and Flynn, F. J., Jr.: Toxoplasmosis: Report of two new cases with a classification and with a demonstration of the organisms in the human placenta. N. Engl. J. Med. 249:345, 1953.

Blattner, R. J.: Repeated congenital infection with Toxoplasma gondii: Comments on current literature. J. Pediatr. 64:452, 1964.

Ciba Foundation Symposium 10 (New Series). Intrauterine Infections. Elliott, K. and Knight, J., Eds. Amsterdam, Holland, Associated Scientific Publishers, 1973.

Desmonts, G., and Couvreur, J.: Cerebral toxoplasmosis, a prospective study of 378 pregnancies. N. Engl. J. Med. 270:1110, 1974.

Eichenwald, H.: Congenital toxoplasmosis. A study of one hundred fifty cases. Am. J. Dis. Child. 94:411, 1957.

Feldman, H. A.: The clinical manifestations and laboratory diagnosis of toxoplasmosis. Am. J. Trop. Med. 2:420, 1953.

Feldman, H. A.: Toxoplasmosis. N. Engl. J. Med. 279:1370, 1431, 1968.

Jacobs, L.: The biology of toxoplasma. Am. J. Trop. Med. 2:365, 1953.

Langer, H.: Repeated congenital infection with toxoplasma gondii. Obstet. Gynecol. 21:318, 1963.

Remington, J. S., and Desmonts, G.: Congenital toxoplasmosis: Variability in the IgM-fluorescent antibody response and some pitfalls in diagnosis. J. Pediatr. 83:27, 1973.

Remington, J. S., Miller, M. J., and Brownlee, I.: IgM antibodies in acute toxoplasmosis: I. Diagnostic significance in congenital cases and method for their rapid demonstration. Pediatrics 41:1082, 1968.

Riemann, H. P., Meyer, M. E. et al.: Toxoplasmosis in an infant fed unpasteurized goat milk. J. Pediatr. 87:537, 1975.

Sabin, A. B.: Toxoplasmosis: Current Status and Unsolved Problems. Am. J. Trop. Med. 2:360, 1953.

Schwartzberg, J. E., and Remington, J. S.: Transmission of toxoplasma. Am. J. Dis. Child. 129:777, 1975.

Sever, J. L.: Perinatal infections affecting the developing fetus and newborn. In The Prevention of Mental Retardation Through Control of Infectious Disease. Proceedings of a Conference, June 9–11, 1966. U.S. Department of Health, Education and Welfare, Public Health Service Publication No. 1692.

Silver, H. K., and Dixon, M. S., Jr.: Congenital toxoplasmosis: Report of case with cataract, "atypical" vasopressin-sensitive diabetes insipidus, and marked eosinophilia. A.M.A. J. Dis. Child. 88:84, 1954.

Tilden, I. L.: Congenital toxoplasmosis: Report of a fatal case in Hawaii. Hawaii Med. J. 12:355, 1953.

# INFECTIONS WITH SPIRAL ORGANISMS

# 90

## CONGENITAL SYPHILIS

Prior to 1945 the chapter on congenital syphilis in a textbook devoted to diseases of the newborn would have had to be the most important one in the section concerned with infections, by virtue of the great number of newborns affected and of the broad variety of clinical syndromes produced. If this chapter had been omitted in the 1950's and 1960's it would scarcely have been missed. In many parts of the United States a young pediatrician might have completed 3 years of residency in a large urban hospital without ever having encountered one case. Now the situation has changed. The disease is staging a modest comeback.

**INCIDENCE.** Thirty to 40 years ago, when we supervised the congenital syphilis clinic of the Harriet Lane Home, 60 to 80 infants and children showed up each week for arsenical therapy. A great many more were lost to view before completing their 2- to 3-year course of treatment. It was an unusual week if we did not discover three or four new examples in the general outpatient department. Then for several decades, a year or more might pass without our seeing one. The curve of incidence has shown a rise in the past few years, however.

ETIOLOGY AND PATHOGENESIS. The organism responsible for syphilis is the *Treponema pallidum.* This delicate, corkscrew-shaped, flagellated, highly motile spirochete is almost identical in appearance to *T. pertenue,* which causes yaws. These two diseases, like smallpox and cowpox, produce a cross-immunity for one another. This fact was driven home to us when, after having spent 2 years on yaws-infested Fiji and not having encountered one case of syphilis, we were transferred to yaws-free India, where syphilis became one of our main medical preoccupations.

Syphilis can be acquired by introduction of the treponema through an abrasion in the skin or mucous membrane or by transplacental transmission. Adults and some children become infected percutaneously, while young infants almost invariably receive their organisms from their mothers via the placenta and the umbilical vein. This crossing over may take place at any time beyond the fourth month of gestation, but ordinarily occurs in its later stages. Fetuses infected early may die in utero, but the usual outcome is the birth of an apparently normal infant who becomes ill within the first few weeks of life.

PATHOLOGY. Since treponemata irrupt into the fetal blood stream directly, the primary stage of infection is completely bypassed. There is no chancre and no local lymphadenopathy. Instead, the liver, the immediate target of the invasion, is flooded with organisms, which then penetrate all the other organs and tissues of the body to a lesser degree. Exactly where they take root and arouse local pathologic response, which in turn produces the presenting signs and symptoms, is unpredictable. Principal sites of predilection are the liver, skin, mucous membranes of the lips and anus, bones and the central nervous system. If fetal invasion has taken place early, the lungs may be heavily involved in a characteristic *pneumonia alba,* but this

condition is seldom compatible with life. Treponemata may be found in almost any other organ or tissue of the body, but they seldom set up inflammatory and destructive changes in loci other than the ones named above.

Under the microscope the tissue alterations consist of nonspecific interstitial fibrosis with or without evidences of low-grade inflammatory response in the form of round cell inflammation. Necrosis follows fairly regularly in bone, but only rarely in other tissues. Localization and gumma formation are not common in the neonate. Noteworthy is extensive extramedullary hematopoiesis in liver, spleen, kidneys and other organs.

DIAGNOSIS. The earliest sign of congenital syphilis is apt to be snuffles. The nose becomes obstructed and begins to discharge, at first clear fluid, later purulent or even sanguineous material.

Cutaneous lesions appear at any time from the second week on. They are sparse or numerous and are copper-colored, round, oval, iris-shaped, circinate or desquamative. Even more characteristic than their appearance is their distribution. Their favorite sites include perioral, perinasal and diaper regions. Palms and soles are involved also, but there the rash is soon replaced by diffuse reddening, thickening and wrinkling. In heavily infected infants the rash may become generalized. Mucocutaneous junctions become involved in typical fashion. The lips become thickened and roughened and tend to weep. Radial cracks appear which traverse the vermilion zone up to and a bit beyond the mucocutaneous margins of the lips. These are the beginnings of the radiating scars which may persist for many years as rhagades. Similar mucocutaneous lesions involve the anus and vulva, but in these locations one also encounters, though less frequently, the white, flat, moist, raised plaques known as condylomata.

X-rays films of the bones reveal characteristic osteochondritis and periostitis in more than 90 per cent of infants with congenital syphilis. In most the bone lesions are asymptomatic, but in a few, severe enough to lead to subepiphysial fracture and epiphysial dislocation, extremely painful pseudoparalysis of one or more extremities may supervene. X-ray alterations include an unusually dense band at the epiphysial ends below which is a band of translucency whose margins are at first sharp, but later become serrated, jagged and irregular. The shafts become generally more opaque, but spotty areas of translucency throughout them may given them a moth-eaten look. The periosteum of the long bones becomes more and more thickened. Epiphyses separate because the dense end plate breaks away from the shaft by fracture through the subepiphysial zone of decalcification. This is exactly what happens in the pseudoparalysis of scurvy, although the reason for the weakening of the subepiphysial bone is quite different. In syphilis pseudoparalysis appears within the first 3 months, in scurvy seldom before 5 months.

Signs of visceral involvement include hepatomegaly, splenomegaly and general glandular enlargement. Palpable epitrochlear nodes are not pathognomonic but are highly suggestive of congenital syphilis. The liver may be greatly enlarged, firm and nontender. Associated with this may be jaundice, which appears in the second or third week, is seldom intense and does not persist for many days. Anemia, probably indicative of bone marrow infection and hematopoietic suppression, may become severe. Lesions in the gastrointestinal tract and pancreas may occur, and produce distention and delay in passage of meconium.

A small number of the cases of congenital nephrosis are caused by *T. pallidum.*

Clinical signs of central nervous system involvement seldom appear in the newborn, even though one third to one half of those infected suffer such involvement. This is demonstrated by CSF changes of increased protein content, a mononuclear pleocytosis of up to 200 or 300 cells per cubic milliliter or by positive VDRL test.

Diagnosis is confirmed by dark-field visualization of treponemata in scrapings from any lesion or from any body fluid, by characteristic bone changes on x-ray and by positive serological tests for syphilis.

But these tests must be interpreted with caution. Since the IgG portion of reagin is transmitted across the placenta, its finding in the baby's serum means no more than that the mother has or has had syphilis. She may have been cured during pregnancy and yet still have quantities of reagin in her blood, or she may not have been treated at all and still not have passed the disease on to her fetus. A higher titer in the infant's blood than in the mother's is thought by many to be acceptable evidence of fetal infection, although we ourselves are not certain of this. Evaluation of IgM levels in fetal serum likewise indicates that the fetus has been infected, but it cannot be assumed that this infection is syphilis.

The only true specific test is a positive finding in the newborn's blood of IgM antibody against *T. pallidum,* IgM-FTA-ABS. This is fluorescent treponema antibody from which antibodies from treponemes other than pallidum have been removed by absorption. If positive, this finding is a true indicator of syphilis. But it is not always positive at first, even when infection is present in the infant, possibly because the infection had been acquired so late in pregnancy that specific antibodies had not had time to form.

Thus, when an infant's blood VDRL is positive at birth, one is not justified in making the diagnosis of congenital syphilis unless pathognomonic signs are also present. If they are not, serial determinations of reagin titer must be performed. If passively acquired, the titer will fall to zero within 4 to 12 weeks; it will slowly rise if the disease is actually present. If the IgM-FTA-ABS test is also positive at birth, treatment may be begun. If the test is negative, however, it should be repeated several times at 3 or 4 week intervals.

**TREATMENT.** McCracken's studies have convinced him that we must treat infants with central nervous system involvement somewhat differently from those without this localization. One reason for this is that he was unable to find adequate levels of penicillin in the cerebrospinal fluid of infants given the drug in the form of benzathine penicillin. His recommendations follow verbatim.

1. *Infants without central nervous system involvement.* Procaine penicillin G in a

single daily dose of 50,000 units per kilogram for 10 days, or benzathine penicillin G, 50,000 units per kilogram as a single dose intramuscularly are satisfactory for therapy of congenital syphilis without central nervous system involvement. The serum VDRL titer falls slowly after adequate microbial therapy; approximately 10 per cent have reactive tests at 2 years of age.

2. *Infants with central nervous system involvement.* Crystalline penicillin G, 30,000 to 50,000 units per kilogram in two or three doses or procaine penicillin G, 50,000 units per kilogram in one daily dose, is recommended for all infants with central nervous system syphilis. . . . Therapy should be continued for a minimum of 2 weeks and preferably for a total of 3 weeks. The spinal fluid cell count and protein content decrease slowly over a period of several months in the successfully treated patient.

Hardy et al. have reported a case, unique in their and our experience, of an infant who died of congenital syphilis, whose mother had received penicillin G 10 days before delivery, and who was given massive doses himself for 17 days after birth. In spite of all this, *T. pallidum* was recovered from the infant's eyes after his death. More recently, South reported a similar example of a baby born to a mother who had received presumably adequate treatment for syphilis.

## LEPTOSPIROSIS (WEIL'S DISEASE)

Lindsay and Luke reported the only case of congenital leptospirosis on record. It is briefly abstracted here because of its similarity to several of the other transplacentally transmitted infections.

CASE 90–1

An infant's mother had been a waitress in a restaurant known to be infested with rats, but she had never become ill. The infant was born at term, weighing 7 pounds 13 ounces (3540 gm); vernix and amniotic fluid were brown, but the infant seemed well. Icterus appeared at 34 hours, and listlessness, cyanosis, dyspnea and convulsions followed rapidly. The liver enlarged slightly. The blood was essentially normal, although platelets were not counted or

mentioned. The urine contained bile. Cerebrospinal fluid was normal. He died at 48 hours.

Autopsy revealed heavy lungs with bloody, frothy fluid in the trachea and bronchi. There were numerous subpleural hemorrhages, and the parenchyma was congested, edematous and hemorrhagic, but there was no inflammatory reaction. The enlarged liver showed extensive degenerative and necrotic changes with no evidence of bile stasis or regeneration. There were equally striking degenerative alterations of renal tubular epithelium, with protein and cellular casts within the tubules. Rare leptospirae were seen scattered throughout the liver sections stained by Dieterle and Levaditi stains. The mother's blood showed a high titer of agglutinins to *L. icterohaemorrhagiae* and *L. canicola*, which disappeared after a few months.

COMMENT. Weil's disease is contracted through contact with feces of infected rats. One cannot doubt that in this instance the mother acquired infection in this way, but that it remained asymptomatic. Leptospirae crossed the placenta and produced disease of the fetus which became apparent on the second day of extrauterine life and quickly caused death. Such transplacental transmission has been observed in animals.

## VIBRIO FETUS INFECTION

*Vibrio fetus* is a small, thin, gram-negative, polar flagellated spirillum. It is a common cause of abortion in sheep, cattle, goats and pigs. It is transmitted by the male venereally, the male not being rendered ill by it, to the female, in whom it causes inflammation of the fetal membranes.

By 1966, 34 cases of human infection had been reported, of whom four were newborns. No characteristic clinical pattern can be deduced from these few cases, but in all the organism could be grown from the spinal fluid. In one the presentation was that of meningitis, which was followed by subdural effusions and cystic cavitation of the cerebral hemispheres. This illness did not respond favorably to penicillin and chloramphenicol.

## NEONATAL HELMINTHIASIS

It is worthy of passing mention, at least, that a few newborn infants with neonatal infestations of a variety of worms have been reported. Chu et al. encountered an infant of 8 months' gestational age, delivered by cesarean section because of prolonged labor and fetal distress, whose mother passed a mature worm per vaginam. The infant was well on the second day but passed per rectum a 30 cm mature *Ascaris lumbricoides*, and another on the sixth day. The worm almost surely had penetrated the fetus's intestinal tract after migration into the uterus and across the placenta.

The authors point out that similar migrations have been reported for bilharzia, taenia and enterobius helminths.

### REFERENCES

Alford, C. A., Polt, S. S., et al.: Gamma-M-fluorescent treponemal antibody in the diagnosis of congenital syphilis. New Engl. J. Med. *280*:1086, 1969.

Chu, W-G., Chen, P-M., et al.: Neonatal ascariasis. J. Pediatr. *81*:783, 1972.

Eden, A. N.: *Vibrio fetus* meningitis in a newborn infant. J. Pediatr. *61*:33, 1962.

Hardy, J. B., Hardy, P. H., et al.: Failure of penicillin in a newborn with congenital syphilis. J.A.M.A. *212*:1345, 1970.

Lindsay, S., and Luke, J. W.: Fatal leptospirosis (Weil's disease) in a newborn infant. J. Pediatr. *34*:90, 1949.

McCracken, G. H., and Kaplan, M.: Penicillin treatment for congenital syphilis: A critical reappraisal. J.A.M.A. *228*:855, 1974.

Nelson, N. A., and Struve, V. R.: Prevention of congenital syphilis by treatment of syphilis in pregnancy. J.A.M.A. *161*:869, 1956.

Oppenheimer, E. H., and Hardy, J. B. H.: Congenital syphilis in the newborn: Clinical and pathological observations in recent cases. Johns Hopkins Med. J. *129*:63, 1971.

Rosen, E. U., and Richardson, N. J.: A reappraisal of the value of the IgM fluorescent treponemal antibody absorption test in the diagnosis of congenital syphilis. J. Pediatr. *87*:38, 1975.

Scotti, A. T., and Logan, L.: A specific IgM antibody test in neonatal congenital syphilis. J. Pediatr. *73*:242, 1968.

Wilkinson, R. H., and Heller, R. H.: Congenital syphilis: Resurgence of an old problem. Pediatrics *47*:27, 1971.

Willis, M. D., and Austin, W. J.: Human *Vibrio fetus* infection: Report of two dissimilar cases. Am. J. Dis. Child. *112*:459, 1966.

# DISORDERS OF UNCERTAIN ORIGIN

# 91

## LETTERER-SIWE DISEASE (ACUTE DISSEMINATED HISTIOCYTOSIS X)

The eponymic title seems preferable to the awkward descriptive name "acute nonlipid disseminated reticuloendotheliosis." This disease demonstrates many similarities to eosinophilic granuloma and Hand-Schüller-Christian disease, and the three are usually classified as reticuloendothelioses or histiocytoses. In the full-blown case of Letterer-Siwe's disease the patient develops fever, hepatosplenomegaly, lymphadenopathy, skin rash, destructive bone lesions, anemia, thrombocytopenia and recurring secondary infections.

**INCIDENCE.** Until 1955 only 41 cases had been reported, but in that year Batson et al. reported 15 additional ones for the Vanderbilt Clinic. We are inclined to the view that this remarkable incidence indicates unevenness in geographic distribution, since no other medical center to our knowledge has encountered so many cases. Their series astonished us in another regard in that four of the 15 had their onset within the first month of life, and in two infants skin rashes were noted at birth. Prior to this publication we had never thought of Letterer-Siwe disease as a neonatal affliction. By 1970 there had been four cases actually diagnosed within the first few days of life.

**ETIOLOGY AND PATHOLOGY.** Theories as to etiology range from those of specific infection, nonspecific tissue response to a variety of infective agents, tissue reaction as an abnormal immunologic response, through tumor, to some kind of hereditary defect. There have by now been reported one case in both members of an identical twinship, 16 families with two affected siblings, three with three and one with five siblings so affected (Miller).

The pathognomonic lesions are microscopic aggregations of large, pleomorphic mononuclear cells with contain no lipoid material. An admixture of plasma cells, lymphocytes, a few eosinophils and neutrophils is usually present. At times focal necrosis, at times proliferative fibrous tissue changes are present. These lesions may be found in skin, liver, spleen, lungs, lymph nodes and other organs and tissues.

**DIAGNOSIS.** The onset may be noted as early as the first day of life or at any time during the first year. In the Vanderbilt series two infants had skin manifestations at birth, and one was lethargic from birth. In one, abdominal enlargement due to enlargement of the liver and spleen was seen at 3 weeks. Onset in the 11 other cases was noted after the neonatal period. The authors made the point that evidences of infection were more prominent in infants with early onset than in those whose first manifestations appeared later. In some infants infection, chiefly respiratory and often complicated by discharging otitis media, preceded for some weeks the signs suggesting reticuloendotheliosis; in others the infections were clearly secondary.

Hepatosplenomegaly appears early in virtually all cases. General glandular enlargement of moderate degree is usual, but is not universal. Rash may herald the disease or may develop later. This ordinarily resembles and is mistaken for seborrheic dermatitis, since it appears first in the scalp and hairline, is more pronounced in the skin folds before becoming generalized, and the individual maculopapules composing it have greasy, scaly surfaces. Bone lesions are not encountered in all cases. When present, they are often overlaid by visible and palpable fluctuant swellings. These lesions in the skull and long bones are the sharply defined destructive ones characteristic of eosinophilic granuloma and generalized xanthomatosis. Pulmonary infiltration, found post mortem in all cases in the form of interstitial pneumonitis with infiltration of large mononuclear cells, may in a few infants become obvious clinically and be visualized in x-ray films. One infant

who failed to thrive from birth was found to have pulmonary infiltrates throughout both lungs, with diffuse histiocytic infiltration, and no other signs whatsoever (Aftimos et al.). This isolated pulmonary histiocytosis had been encountered before in a few adults, but never in an infant.

The course is rapidly or slowly progressive, in general more rapid in those whose onsets are earlier. It is marked by fever, anorexia, failure to gain and grow, and gradual fall of hemoglobin content and platelet count. Hemorrhagic manifestations may appear.

Batson et al. point out that differentiation may be difficult from acute histoplasmosis, which is also endemic in the region of Vanderbilt Hospital. When bone and skin lesions are present, one can be certain that the disease is reticuloendotheliosis. In their absence one has to rely upon biopsy appearance and ability or inability to culture *Histoplasma capsulatum* from lesions.

**TREATMENT AND PROGNOSIS.** Letterer-Siwe disease was at one time generally believed to be invariably fatal. However, two of Batson's infants survived. Remarkably enough, both of them were symptomatic from birth, one with skin rash, the other with persistent lethargy. Both were given Aureomycin for many months. Bierman, in 1966, was able to list eight cases of infants who improved after, and almost surely because of, antibiotic therapy.

More recent therapeutic efforts have bypassed antibiotics, utilizing instead vinblastine or 6-mercaptopurine, with or without prednisone. Lahey reviewed the outcomes in 83 patients, of whom 65 were less than 2 years old. Their diagnoses included the three varieties of histiocytosis, Letterer-Siwe, Hand-Schuller-Christian and eosinophilic granuloma. Of these 65 infants, treated with either vinblastine, vinblastine and prednisone or 6-mercaptopurine and prednisone, between 44 and 64 per cent achieved either good or complete remission.

# FAMILIAL ERYTHROPHAGOCYTIC LYMPHOHISTIOCYTOSIS

MacMahon et al. warn us not to confuse this entity with Letterer-Siwe disease.

These infants also become ill within the first few months of life, with fever, anorexia and wasting. The liver and spleen become very large, pallor progresses, and the blood shows increasing anemia, granulopenia and thrombocytopenia. Bone marrow reveals erythroid and myeloid hyperplasia and paucity of polymorphonuclear leukocytes. Some infants have nuchal rigidity, and their spinal fluids show a number of lymphocytes and histiocytes. Their downhill course may be temporarily halted by splenectomy.

The liver, spleen and at times the central nervous system reveal at biopsy or autopsy striking infiltration of lymphocytes and histiocytes which phagocytose erythrocytes greedily.

Several of the reported cases have involved two members of the same sibship. MacMahon believes that the disease resembles a primary proliferative state of the reticuloendothelial system more than a proliferative response to some antigenic stimulus.

## INFANTILE CORTICAL HYPEROSTOSIS

This unusual disorder had never been described by clinician or pathologist before 1930. It appears to represent a newly arrived entity upon the medical scene. Our inclusion of it among infections is unwarranted in the present state of knowledge of its etiology. Certain of its manifestations seem to fit an infective basis more closely than any other, and we literally know no better position in which to place it.

**INCIDENCE.** Since Caffey and Silverman's preliminary report in 1945 and Smyth's in 1946, many cases have been recorded in the literature. Staheli et al. were able to find more than 100 reports up to 1968. It can no longer be considered rare. The Sidburys saw 10 cases in their own private practice in the short period of 4 years.

**ETIOLOGY AND PATHOLOGY.** No infective agent, bacterial, viral, protozoal or other, has ever been implicated in the causation of the disease. Gene defect, allergy, and some form of vascular or collagen disturbance have been mentioned as possible causes; no sound evidence has come

forth in their favor. Gerrard et al. have tracked down three generations of one family to which their proband belonged and were able to find three almost certain cases in the first generation, four or five in the second, and six (out of 20 grandchildren) in the third generation. Transmission in this family strongly suggested that of an autosomal dominant. In other families the disorder appears to be transmitted as an autosomal recessive.

Pathologic study has shown the involved bones to be thickened by new deposition of immature lamellar bone. In some, but not all, cellular infiltration suggests that an inflammatory process is in progress. Eversole found intense inflammation in a biopsy specimen of an early case. Caffey states that "in the acute disease the periosteum is loose and thickened and has a gelatinous character with many mitotic figures in the cells. . . . The mucinous thickening in the periosteum usually extends directly into the neighboring tendons, fascias and intermuscular septa. In specimens taken several weeks after the onset, extensive muscular necrosis with fibrous replacement has been demonstrated."

**DIAGNOSIS.** The time of onset is an important diagnostic point. Onset is always before the age of 5 or 6 months. Changes which developed in utero and are present at birth indicate that prenatal onset is not too uncommon. The postnatal onset is usually sudden in an infant who had previously been well and whose nutrition is good. The first sign is swelling, commonly of the jaw or cheek on one or both sides, but not infrequently over a clavicle, ribs, scapula or any of the long tubular bones. Along with swelling come fever, irritability, loss of appetite, and pallor. The swellings are firm, tender and very poorly demarcated, seeming to be fixed and immobile and to taper off into the surrounding tissues. Mandibular hyperostosis imparts a moon-shaped appearance to the face, although the lower portion looks more swollen than the upper. Swellings over the extremities are fusiform, tender, fixed and nonfluctuant, and the overlying skin, although taut and shiny, does not seem very reddened, nor does it feel hot. Swelling over the scapula may induce an Erb's-like brachial palsy (Holtzman).

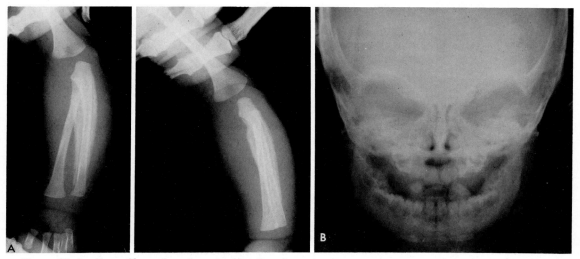

*Figure 91–1.* X-ray films of an 8-week-old infant from the Harriet Lane Home files whose case is not abstracted in the text. Swelling of the right forearm appeared by about 4 weeks of age. Aside from unwillingness to move the right arm, there were no symptoms. There was no fever. Biopsy of ulna showed dense scar tissue beneath the periosteum. A few lymphocytes and macrophages were seen and there was much osteoid and uncalcified bone in the sections.

*A,* Two views of the right arm show the broad, fusiform cortical thickening of the ulna. The humerus, radius and the metacarpals are not similarly involved. *B,* X-ray view of the skull and face shows unquestioned thickening of the mandible through its entire length. (The jaw, cheeks and face did not appear swollen to the clinician.)

The white blood cell count is elevated, with some polymorphonuclear increase, and the sedimentation rate is high. Alkaline phosphatase is generally elevated. Otherwise laboratory investigations contribute nothing.

X-ray films of the involved areas show subperiosteal deposition of new bone of little or great thickness (Fig. 91–1). If clinically uninvolved bones are also x-rayed, one is apt to find that others are involved in the same process. Brooksaler and Miller found 36 loci of hyperostosis in 11 cases. The mandible took part in the process in eight of the 11.

**COURSE.** The course is unpredictably variable. In some cases swelling disappears in a few weeks, in most within a few months, while in a few it persists for years. The courses in some infants are intermittent, swelling disappearing and fever subsiding for a time, then reappearing at the same or a different site; subsidence and exacerbation succeed one another a number of times.

**TREATMENT.** Antibiotics are of little or no help. ACTH and cortisone have been successful in reducing systemic manifestations, but apparently do not hasten the resolution of the osseous lesions. An initial dose of 5 to 10 mg per kilogram of cortisone, divided into four daily doses, or the equivalent dosage of one of the cortisone relatives, should be continued for several weeks and gradually tapered off over a period of months.

**PROGNOSIS.** The prognosis for life and for ultimate subsidence of the disease is good. Just how long the disease will last in an individual case cannot be foretold. Blank has reported a boy who had his initial attack at 4 months, which subsided but was followed by recurrences at 4, 6, 8, 10 and 11 years.

Of the eight patients whom Staheli et al. were able to follow for 6 or more years, all appeared well but two showed persistent asymmetry of the jaw, and one has synostoses between two ribs and between the tibia and fibula.

Barba, W. P., II, and Freriks, D. J.: The familial occurrence of infantile cortical hyperostosis in utero. J. Pediatr. *42*:141, 1953.

Batson, R., Shapiro, J. L., Christie, A., and Riley, H. D., Jr.: Acute nonlipid disseminated reticuloendotheliosis. A.M.A. J. Dis. Child. *90*:323, 1955.

Bierman, H. R.: Apparent cure of Letterer-Siwe disease. Seventeen-year survival of identical twins with nonlipoid reticuloendotheliosis. J.A.M.A. *196*:368, 1966.

Blank, E.: Recurrent Caffey's cortical hyperostosis and persistent deformity. Pediatrics 55:856, 1975.

Brooksaler, F., and Miller, J. E.: Infantile cortical hyperostosis. J. Pediat. *48*:739, 1956.

Caffey, J.: Infantile cortical hyperostosis: A review of the clinical and radiographic features. Proc. Roy. Soc. Med. 50:347, 1957.

Caffey, J., and Silverman, W. A.: Infantile cortical hyperostosis. J. Pediatr. 29:541, 559, 1946.

Cederbaum, S. D., Niwayama, G., et al.: Combined immunodeficiency presenting as the Letterer-Siwe syndrome. J. Pediatr. 85:466, 1974.

Eversole, cited by F. Brooksaler, and J. E. Miller.

Gerrard, J. W., Holman, G. H., Gorman, A. A., and Morrow, J. H.: Familial infantile cortical hyperostosis. J. Pediatr. 59:543, 1961.

Gotoff, J. P., and Esterly, N. B.: Editorial: Histiocytosis. J. Pediatr. 85:592, 1974.

Hertz, C. G., and Hambrick, G. W.: Congenital Letterer-Siwe disease: A case treated with vincristine and corticosteroids. Am. J. Dis. Child. *116*:553, 1968.

Holtzman, D.: Infantile cortical hyperostosis of the scapula presenting as an ipsilateral Erb's palsy. J. Pediatr. *81*:785, 1972.

Lahey, M. E.: Histiocytosis X: Comparison of three treatment regimens. J. Pediatr. 87:179, 1975.

MacMahon, H. E., Bedizel, M., and Ellis, C. A.: Familial erythrophagocytic lymphohistiocytosis. Pediatrics *32*:868, 1963.

McClure, P. D., Strachan, P., and Saunders, E. F.: Hypofibrinogenemia and thrombocytopenia in familial hemophagocytic reticulosis. J. Pediatr. 85:67, 1974.

Miller, D. R.: Familial reticuloendotheliosis: Concurrence of disease in five siblings. Pediatrics *38*:986, 1966.

Schoeck, V. W., Peterson, R. D. A., and Good, R. A.: Familial occurrence of Letterer-Siwe disease. Pediatrics *32*:1055, 1963.

Sidbury, J. B., and Sidbury, J. B.: Infantile cortical hyperostosis: An inquiry into the etiology and pathogenesis. New Engl. J. Med. 250:309, 1954.

Smyth, F. S., Potter, A., and Silverman, W.: Periosteal reaction, fever and irritability in young infants. A new syndrome? Am. J. Dis. Child. *71*:333, 1946.

Staheli, L. T., Church, C. C., and Ward, B. H.: Infantile cortical hyperostosis (Caffey's disease): Sixteen cases with a late follow-up of eight. J.A.M.A. *203*:384, 1968.

# XII

## Disorders of Nutrition

# 92

# FEEDING THE NORMAL NEWBORN

*By John R. Raye*

Although the American pediatrician cannot take much pride in his success in encouraging the use of human breast milk for infant feeding, pediatric research in this country has played a major role in the development of "humanized" proprietary formula. The broad use of these prepared formulas is perhaps the most significant change in infant feeding since the last edition of this book. Although, even today, prepared formula is clearly still not the ideal food, many of the lessons learned in its development have provided sound nutritional principles which are of value in understanding the growth requirements of all infants. In this chapter, we will review pertinent fundamentals of neonatal nutrition as they apply to the normal term infant (see also pages 60 and 61).

## FUNDAMENTALS

The basic purpose of all infant feeding is to provide appropriate nutrients in a manner which allows each individual to reach his or her full potential for cellular growth. Protein, fat, carbohydrate, minerals and vitamins are required to meet these needs. Within each broad nutrient category specific requirements also exist. Thus, the quality of each nutrient may be of equal importance to the total quantity. Too little of a required nutrient may result in growth restriction, while excess amounts of a specific nutrient may result in an inadequate or abnormal growth pattern.

Under normal circumstances, infants appear to regulate their daily volume intake on the basis of caloric intake. Fomon and co-workers have shown that as the caloric density of a formula is increased, ad lib intake decreases proportionally. For this reason, very high caloric density feedings may

result in inadequate daily fluid intakes. Best estimates suggest that the normal term infant needs approximately 120 kcal per kilogram per day to achieve full growth potential during the first month of life. Water requirements necessitated by this caloric load are in the range of 150 ml per kcal or 180 ml per kilogram per day. In general, most infant formulas contain 67 kcal per 100 ml, and this caloric density (20 kcal per ounce) meets both fluid and caloric requirements. Provision of adequate calories does not necessarily result in adequate growth, however. A specific distribution of calories among nutrient subgroups is necessary as well. Table 92–1 outlines the desirable percentage of calories to be provided daily from protein, fat and carbohydrate. It should be clear from this table, for example, why whole cow's milk is not ideal for infant feeding. It is apparent, however, that human breast milk and proprietary formula are similar both in caloric density and caloric distribution. Certain differences do exist, nevertheless, in the composition of the caloric sources.

## BREAST MILK AND FORMULA

NUTRITIONAL DIFFERENCES. A great deal has been written comparing the relative advantages of breast and formula feedings. Often, little objective data accompany the more fervent pleas for use of breast milk, and little impact seems to have been made on the public. Present estimates suggest that less than 15 per cent of the infants in this country are breast fed for 3 months or more. Many of the well known disadvantages of cow's milk feedings have been ameliorated by the development of proprietary "humanized" formula. Nevertheless, we still favor the use of human

TABLE 92–1.  *Percentage of Calories Obtained from Constituents of Feedings*

| | Desirable Range | Human | Type of Milk Prepared Formula | Cows (Whole) |
|---|---|---|---|---|
| Protein | 6–12 | 7 | 9 | 20 |
| Fat | 30–55 | 55 | 48 | 50 |
| Carbohydrate | 35–55 | 37 | 42 | 29 |

breast milk and we shall review those qualitative differences which seem pertinent in the comparison of breast milk and commercial formula. The composition of these milks is shown in Table 92–2.

It is clear that human milk has the lowest protein level of the milks. In spite of this, growth rates of infants fed breast milk are very similar to those fed the same volume of standard formula with similar caloric sup-

plies but higher protein content. One major qualitative difference between these proteins is the lactalbumin:casein ratio. High casein levels appear to result in firmer curd formation in the stomach, whereas whey proteins result in a softer, more flocculent curd. Animal experiments have suggested that whey protein is more efficiently utilized than casein, although this has not been confirmed in infant feeding studies.

TABLE 92–2.  *Comparison of Human and Cow's Milk with Proprietary Formula*

| | Human Milk | Cow's Milk | Proprietary Formula* |
|---|---|---|---|
| Water (ml per 100 ml) | 87 | 87 | 87–90 |
| Protein (gm per 100 ml) | 1.1 | 3.5 | 1.5 |
| Lactalbumen:casein ratio | 60:40 | 18:82 | 20:80 |
| Lactose (gm per 100 ml) | 6.8 | 4.9 | 7.0–7.2 |
| Fat (gm per 100 ml) | 4.5 | 3.7 | 3.6 |
| Linoleic (per cent of fat) | 7 | 1 | 21–41 |
| Calories (kcal per 100 ml) | 67–75 | 67 | 67 |
| Minerals | | | |
| Sodium (mEq per liter) | 7 | 22 | 9–11 |
| Potassium (mEq per liter) | 13 | 35 | 19–20 |
| Chloride (mEq per liter) | 11 | 29 | 11–16 |
| Calcium (mg per 100 ml) | 34 | 117 | 55–58 |
| Phosphorus (mg per 100 ml) | 14 | 92 | 43–46 |
| Magnesium (mg per 100 ml) | 4 | 12 | 4–5 |
| Iron (mg per 100 ml) | .05 | .05 | Trace–.15** |
| Copper (mg per 100 ml) | .04 | .03 | 0.4–0.6 |
| Total ash (gm per 100 ml) | 0.2 | 0.7 | 0.3–0.4 |
| Vitamins | | | |
| Vitamin A (I.U. per liter) | 1898 | 1025 | 1700–2500 |
| Thiamine ($\mu$g per liter) | 160 | 440 | 400–710 |
| Riboflavin ($\mu$g per liter) | 360 | 1750 | 630 |
| Niacin (mg per liter) | 1.5 | 0.9 | 4–8 |
| Pyridoxine ($\mu$g per liter) | 100 | 640 | 260–420 |
| Pantothenate (mg per liter) | 1.8 | 3.5 | 2–3.1 |
| Folacin ($\mu$g per liter) | 52 | 55 | 32–100 |
| B$_{12}$ ($\mu$g per liter) | 0.3 | 4 | 1–2 |
| Vitamin C (mg per liter) | 43 | 11 | 36–53 |
| Vitamin D (I.U. per liter) | 22 | 14 | 400–422 |
| Vitamin E (I.U. per liter) | 1.8 | 0.4 | 10–13 |
| Vitamin K ($\mu$g per liter) | 15 | 60 | 19–69 |

(Adapted from data assembled by Fomon, S. J.: Infant Nutrition, 2nd ed., Philadelphia, W. B. Saunders Co., 1974.)

*Range of composition of commonly used proprietary formula, Enfamil, Similac.

**Iron supplemented formula contains 12 mg per liter.

Raiha and colleagues, in comparing utilization of formula with whey to casein ratios of 60:40 and 18:82, did note increased renal losses of amino acids in the high casein group.

It has also been noted that human milk contains substantially more cystine than cow's milk. Although cystine is technically not an essential amino acid, the newborn infant has a relative deficiency in the ability to convert methionine to cystine. This results in a relative increase in the cystine requirement, which is more adequately met by breast milk.

Analysis of the qualitative differences in fat between breast and other milks again reveals significant differences. Although slightly higher in total fat content, the fatty acid composition of breast milk is such that fat absorption is superior to that of synthetic formula (Barnes et al.). This is a result of increased concentrations of medium chain triglycerides and monounsaturated fatty acids in human milk. Manufacturers of prepared formula have attempted to improve fatty acid absorption from their products by the addition of polyunsaturated fatty acids, such as linoleic, to the saturated fatty acids of cow's milk. Although fat absorption has been improved, vitamin E absorption has been decreased. György has also called attention to the lipase content of human milk, which results in the liberation of well absorbed free fatty acids.

Calcium absorption is superior with human milk feedings, and seems to parallel fat absorption. The hypocalcemia seen after several days of cow's milk feedings is due to both decreased calcium absorption and the high phosphate load of cow's milk. This "nutritional disease" is not seen in newborn infants fed breast milk. As noted in Table 92–2, little improvement has been made in altering the calcium to phosphorus ratio or total phosphate content of standard proprietary formula. Specific low solute formulas, however, are commercially available with improved calcium to phosphate ratios.

The carbohydrate of human milk as well as that of standard commercially available formula is exclusively lactose. On hydrolysis lactose yields a molecule of glucose and a molecule of galactose. Galactose is an important component of central nervous system lipids. Cow's milk contains only one half the human milk concentration of lactose, whereas commercial formulas have been supplemented with this sugar.

As noted in Table 92–2, the ash content of commercial formula is significantly higher than that of breast milk. This additional solute load must result in either increased water requirements, hyperosmolarity or edema. Davies has documented an increase in serum osmolarity in formula-fed infants. She has suggested that this hyperosmolarity may be aggravated by improper dilution of formula. The effects of this chronic, mild hyperosmolarity are not known. Taitz has speculated on the possibility of an increased risk of hyperosmolar dehydration, with its central nervous system sequelae, following episodes of diarrhea and vomiting. Similarly, high neonatal solute intakes in some animal models have been associated with the development of hypertension in the adult.

All proprietary formulas are supplemented with adequate amounts of appropriate vitamins for the term infant; however, these supplements may not be adequate for the premature infant (see Chapter 94). Breast milk, on the other hand, is low in some vitamins, particularly vitamins D and K. Following universal parenteral vitamin K supplementation at birth, adequate amounts of the vitamin are supplied to the growing infant by intestinal bacteria. Vitamin D supplementation is suggested for breast fed infants. The iron content of all natural milks is low (0.5 mg per liter). Although proprietary formulas that are not iron fortified contain no additional iron, those formulas that are iron fortified contain 12 to 13 mg per L. Following the study of Andelman and Sered in 1966, which documented early storage and subsequent utilization of dietary iron, the American Academy of Pediatrics Committee on Nutrition has recommended supplementary iron for all infants. This universal form of supplementation, although somewhat controversial, has received much support for two reasons: first, it is clear that iron deficiency during infancy is still widespread (Owens et al.), and second, that infant's intake of non-milk iron containing foods is not reliable (Dallman and Rios, et al.).

Fomon has recently commented on the

fluoride content of various milks. Human milk contains adequate amounts of fluoride when the drinking water contains more than 1 part per million of fluoride. In areas where the water content is less, breast-fed infants should receive supplemental fluoride to insure the intake of 0.5 mg of fluoride daily. Infants fed concentrated liquid or powdered formulas which are diluted with water should also receive fluoride supplementation when local water contains less than 0.3 parts per million. In this situation, 0.5 mg of additional fluoride daily is adequate.

This brief comparison of the composition of human milk and proprietary formula should suggest that while total calories and caloric distribution are similar some fundamental qualitative nutritional differences do exist. Certain non-nutritional differences also exist.

**NON-NUTRITIONAL DIFFERENCES.** The major non-nutritional advantages of breast feeding fall into three areas, increased resistance to infection, development of mothering and convenience.

Evaluation of the literature which suggests that breast feeding is superior to formula in protecting the infant from various forms of infection is hazardous at best. An early study by Mellander et al. clearly suggested that infants who were fed entirely on breast milk for the first 3 months of life had significantly fewer respiratory and diarrheal infections when compared to infants fed evaporated milk formula. In the only similar study using proprietary formula, Abebonojo observed no differences in the formula and breast milk fed groups. There are, however, objective reasons why such differences might exist. Colostrum and, to a larger extent, transitional milk are both high in secretory IgA. This antibody is thought to be surface active in the gastrointestinal tract and critical to the development of local gastrointestinal immunity. This IgA has been found unchanged in the stools of breast fed infants and thus appears to be resistant to digestion and capable of local activity. Warren and others, for example, have documented that the presence of polio antibodies in breast milk may prevent infection by vaccine virus in the infant.

In breast milk, factors other than immunoglobulins have been thought to play some role in protecting the infant from enteric infections. Breast milk contains large amounts of lysosome, which may have a direct bacteriocidal effect. Interesting work by Pitt et al. has demonstrated high concentrations of macrophages in fresh breast milk. These macrophages appeared to be capable of killing bacteria in vitro. In their rat model of necrotizing enterocolitis, these macrophages appeared to prevent development of disease. It is important to note that the antibacterial activity of these macrophages was diminished by either freezing or sterilizing the fresh breast milk but persisted with refrigeration up to 24 hours.

The presence in human milk of a factor that promotes growth of the bacterium *Lactobacillus bifidus* has also been noted. These bacteria are capable of producing lactic and acetic acids, resulting in an increased acidity of the stools of breast fed infants when compared to those who are formula fed. The combination of a lower pH and overgrowth by *L. bifidus* appears to result in diminished enteric colonization by *E. coli* and perhaps other invasive bacteria.

It has been suggested that other bacterial "resistance" factors are also present in human milk, but the roles of these in the prevention of infection are even less clear. For example, human milk is rich in lactoferin, an iron-binding protein which Bullen and co-workers have shown to inactivate *E. coli* both in vitro and in vivo. The addition of iron to this protein blocked this bacteriocidal ability. This latter finding has been suggested as an argument against routine iron supplementation of formula.

Thus, it appears that fresh human milk may play a direct role in protecting the gastrointestinal surface of the neonate. Many of these properties appear to be lost in processing or are completely lacking in proprietary formula. Excellent reviews of this material have been provided by Goldman and Smith and by Gerrard.

Breast-feeding has always been a unique form of mothering. In no other circumstance is there such physical closeness and emotional interdependence between mother and infant. Nevertheless, since the early 1900's, there has been a dramatic reduction in the number of women who breast-feed their infants. Estimates now would suggest that less than 15 per cent of women in the United States continue to breast-feed for 3 months or more. Over the past 10 years or so, however, this fraction has been fairly constant. It is not clear whether the reason for this relative disinterest in breast-feeding is economic, social, sexual, narcissistic or a combination thereof. It is of interest, however, that the majority of breast-feeders are of upper educational and social groups.

The close relationship fostered by the physical intimacy of breast-feedings has always been considered a positive stimulus for developing a secure and happy child. There is, however, little proof of this. In animal work, particularly with primates, in-

fants deprived of mothering appear to be less inquisitive and less secure, and have difficulty developing sexual and family behavior as adults. Klaus and co-workers have attempted to gather objective data regarding the development of this mothering behavior. Extended physical contact between mother and infant in the first 4 days of life significantly increased certain measures of mothering behavior. These measures included questions to evaluate closeness of mother-child contact and observations of soothing and touching behavior. Duration of en face positioning was also evaluated (Fig. 92–1). Differences in mother-child interaction between the routine and extended contact groups persisted up to 11

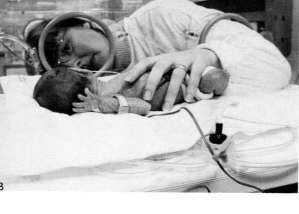

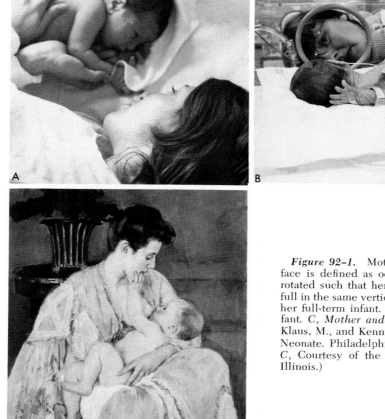

*Figure 92–1.* Mothers in the "en face" position. En face is defined as occurring when the mother's face is rotated such that her eyes and those of the infant meet full in the same vertical plane of rotation. *A,* A mother and her full-term infant. *B,* A mother and her premature infant. *C, Mother and Child,* by Mary Cassatt. (*A* and *B,* Klaus, M., and Kennell, J.: *In* The Care of the High-risk Neonate. Philadelphia, W. B. Saunders Company, 1973. *C,* Courtesy of the Art Institute of Chicago, Chicago, Illinois.)

months later. While bottle feeding clearly does not preclude extended physical contact, breast-feeding seems to almost guarantee it and, in addition, supplies both physiologic and sensory feedback to the mother. There would be no disagreement, however, that the quality of the experience may be of as much importance as the quantity.

Other objective evidence of the psychological advantages of breast-feeding is not available. As Newton has pointed out, well controlled studies are almost impossible because women who choose to breast-feed are different from those who do not: they may be less rigid and more physical. He has also suggested that the suppression of cyclic hormonal changes for the first several months of breast-feeding, which also result in amenorrhea, may influence the consistency of mother-child interaction.

The speculative nature of some of the above data cannot be denied. It is clear, however, that breast feeding is more economical than formula feeding. This is true even when the cost of the additional maternal food intake is considered (McKigney). Breast-feeding is also more convenient—no bottles to wash, no formula to mix and warm, no opportunity to overconcentrate or dilute the milk. The risk of contamination of the milk by enteric pathogens is very low. This fact has been of major importance in certain underdeveloped portions of the world. In these areas, attempts to improve infant nutrition by provision of milk supplements resulted in increased mortality rates because of formula contamination by impure water supplies.

Although bacterial contamination of breast milk does not occur, contamination of human milk by maternally ingested drugs does. In certain circumstances, this fact provides a clear contraindication to breast-feeding. The extensive review by Knowles in 1965, and a more recent review by O'Brien, should be in the files of every pediatrician. It is important to differentiate between the excretion of a particular drug and the significance of the intake of that drug by the infant. It is not often necessary to curtail breast-feeding for this reason, particularly when alternative forms of maternal medication are available.

Concern has also arisen over the effect of breast-feeding on neonatal jaundice. As a general rule, breast-fed infants do not appear to become more icteric than infants fed commercial formula (Dahms et al.). There does exist, however, a small group of infants who develop significant and prolonged hyperbilirubinemia in association with breast-feeding. In these infants, jaundice subsides rapidly on elimination of breast milk and returns on its reintroduction. It is thought that the presence of high concentrations of a steroid (3 alpha 20 beta pregnanediol) in the milk of these mothers may be responsible for this clinical observation. This steroid appears to inhibit bilirubin conjugation in vitro in certain animal species. There appears to be some doubt, however, whether this observation is true using human liver slices (Adlard and Lathe). Furthermore, when Ramos and his co-workers fed this steroid to infants, no significant increase in hyperbilirubinemia was noted. Regardless of the etiology, the clinical observation certainly is true. It is unlikely that this form of hyperbilirubinemia is responsible for clinical sequelae, and modest or prolonged icterus of this etiology is not a reason to terminate breast feeding.

I presume my prejudices are clear. The advantages of fresh, human breast milk, to me, certainly seem to outweigh those of either proprietary formula or evaporated milk formula. At present, however, it is not possible to distinguish objectively between the end products of different feeding regimes. It is also true that breast-feeding is not for everyone. The working mother may find breast-feeding impossible and should not be made to feel guilt. The mother who is uncomfortable with the degree of physical intimacy involved in breast-feeding is unlikely to succeed. The same is true of those who resent the social intrusion. One should never force a mother to breast-feed her infant, for little but frustration can be gained for mother, infant and physician. For those who are undecided, however, we must enthusiastically lay out the facts and develop their interest and confidence.

Unfortunately, the pediatrician usually sees the "maybe's" too late; that is, after delivery and after the administration of drugs to suppress lactation. At this point, in the midst of the turmoil of hospital routines, it is a rare woman who, without adequate preparation or inordinate desire, can suddenly make a go of it. Similarly, it is unusual to convince a woman to breast-feed an infant after previous children have been bottle raised. It seems that the conversion must take place in prenatal classes for primigravidas. Or perhaps we should accept the fact that although breast milk appears to be an ideal food, only those who have an "ideal" temperament will share it!

## BASICS OF BREAST-FEEDING

Perhaps the most important basis for breast-feeding, besides temperament, is a sound understanding of milk production. From this understanding comes the confidence to progress from a frustrating if not ticklish experience to successful and pleasureful feeding. Successful feeding requires two distinct physiologic processes on the mother's part. The first is milk production, which is mediated by prolactin, an anterior pituitary hormone. Milk production is stimulated by sucking and emptying the breast. The importance of emptying the breast in maintaining adequate milk production cannot be overemphasized. Little milk will be available to the infant, however, without adequate milk "let down." This second process, mediated by oxytocin secreted by the posterior pituitary, results in contraction of myoepithelial cells, rupture of holocrine secretory cells and transport of milk to the nipple area. The "let down" process releases the "hind milk," which is higher in fat content (4 to 7 per cent) than that which is first available within the ductile system ("fore milk"). The importance of confidence and relaxation in stimulating milk "let down" and milk production makes it crucial that the hospital environment is conducive to breast feeding. The initial appearance of colostrum, followed by transitional milk, and finally the appearance of real milk at 3 to 7 days should be anticipated landmarks. Manual expression or the use of the breast pump should be explained as useful techniques. The importance of emptying the breast as well as the significance of ductile plugging ("caking") and breast abscesses should be carefully explained, along with other aspects of breast and nipple care. Applebaum and Woody and Woody have provided some excellent guidelines for support of the "lost art" of counseling mothers in these regards.

Breast-feeding should begin when both mother and infant are alert and ready. Normally, this would be at 4 to 8 hours of age. Intiial feeds should be limited to 5 minutes per breast in order to stimulate but not irritate the nipples. The mother must be content with the dual role of this early nursing as stimulation for the initiation of milk production as well as a learning experience for both her and the infant rather than a nutritional "happening." Both must learn to relax and interact in a productive manner during these early sessions.

In the hospital, feedings should take place every 3 to 4 hours. They should be continued through the night in order to facilitate milk production and to avoid the discomfort of initial breast engorgement. As milk production increases, and nipples become less irritated, the period of nursing is extended to 10 minutes on each breast. By the end of the first week, nursing should be well established, with the infant sucking on one breast for 15 minutes and finishing for 10 to 15 minutes on the second breast. At the next feeding, the pattern is reversed. Supplemental bottles are to be avoided until milk production and mother-infant interaction are well established. After that period supplemental bottles may still result in decreased milk production, and their regular use should be discouraged.

## BASICS OF FORMULA FEEDING

Prior to the mid-1960's, feedings for term infants were often delayed for 18 to 24 hours after birth. The theoretical purpose of this delay was to allow the infant to excrete his "extra" water load. On closer examination of this practice, it became clear that this period was in fact a period of relative starvation and was associated with low blood sugars, acetonuria, elevated serum bilirubins and signs of poor hydration. On the basis of these data, there has been wide acceptance of the concept of early feeding. Following a period of relative inactivity after delivery, Desmond noted that by 3 to 6 hours the infant again becomes alert and active. At this time feedings should commence.

The first attempt at feeding should be distilled water. This food does not stimulate as vigorous sucking as sugar or milk solutions; however, Olson has demonstrated its relative lack of toxicity if aspirated directly into the lungs. She reported that in rabbits 5 per cent dextrose solution or milk when instilled directly into the trachea resulted in the clinical and pathological findings of aspiration pneumonia. Thus, if the first feeding is a trial of the sucking and swallowing mechanism, it seems reasonable to use a liquid that has little potential of causing pathology. On the other hand, Gresham has found that once these fluids have become mixed with gastric contents and then are aspirated into the lungs, the toxic effects of each are similar.

Following the initial test feeding, regular feedings of 20 calories per ounce of formula should be started on a 4-hour schedule. As soon as possible, the mother should be allowed to feed the infant in order to stimulate the development of mothering behavior, as noted previously. The artificial constraints imposed by taking the infant to the mother at a standard "feeding" time are most undesirable. In this respect, rooming in is to be strongly encouraged. In this situation, the mother and infant can begin to develop their own schedule of interaction, with the pleasure of feeding occurring when both are ready for it.

The pendulum of infant feeding programs varying from very rigid to completely unstructured now seems to lie halfway between those alternatives. A feeding schedule that results in the infant being fed every 3 to 5 hours upon waking and suggesting hunger seems sensible. A longer period between feedings is to be encouraged at night, again delaying until some interest is demonstrated by the infant. Feedings should take place in a comfortable, relaxed atmosphere, where the attentions of both mother and infant can focus on each other. Attentiveness and physical closeness are essential. Over the first few weeks, a productive routine will be established consisting of 5 or 6 feedings a day.

Some attention should be paid to the present vogue of infant overfeeding. As noted previously, a total intake of 180 ml per kilogram of standard formula provides adequate intake of all nutrients for the normal infant. Fomon has noted that mean intakes are in considerable excess of this amount. Significantly larger amounts given as a show of love or in competition to raise the "All American Baby" lead to high caloric and solute loads. Storage of these additional calories as fat may stimulate the multiplication of adipocytes. Hirsch has speculated that this increase in the number of fat cells may increase the risk of obesity in adult life. Similarly, high solute loads in infancy may be associated with an additional risk of hypertension in subsequent years (American Academy of Pediatrics, Committee on Nutrition).

## INTRODUCTION OF SOLID FOODS

An increasing tendency toward the early introduction of solid foods has accompanied the transition from breast- to bottle-feeding. At the present time, many mothers introduce cereals as early as 2 to 3 weeks of age, followed shortly by fruits, vegetables and finally meats. Although this practice is not clearly harmful, it does appear to increase the cost of infant feeding without any demonstrated advantage. Adequate nutrients in appropriate distribution are provided by either breast milk or cow's milk formula for the first 6 months of life. The high calorie and ash content of these supplemental foods again raises the question of long term effects noted previously for overfed infants. Davies has documented significantly elevated serum osmolarities in infants fed milk plus supplemental foods when compared to breast or formula fed infants. For these reasons, it seems proper to discourage the introduction of solids prior to 4 to 6 months of age.

## REFERENCES

Adebonojo, F. O.: Artificial vs. breast feeding. Clin. Pediatr. *11*:25, 1972.

Adlard, B. P. F., and Lathe, G. H.: Breast milk jaundice: Effect of $3_\alpha 20_\beta$-pregnanediol on bilirubin conjugation by human liver. Arch. Dis. Child. *45*:186, 1970.

American Academy of Pediatrics, Committee on Nutrition: Iron-fortified formulas. Pediatrics *47*:786, 1971.

American Academy of Pediatrics, Committee on Nutrition: Salt intake and eating patterns of infants and children in relation to blood pressure. Pediatrics 53:115, 1974.

Andelman, M. B., and Sered, B. R.: Utilization of dietary iron by term infants. Am. J. Dis. Child. *111*:45, 1966.

Applebaum, R. M.: The modern management of successful breast feeding. Pediat. Clin. North Am. *17*:203, 1970.

Barnes, L. A., Morrow, G., III, et al.: Calcium and fat absorption from infant formulas with different fat blends. Pediatrics *54*:217, 1974.

Bullen, J. J., Rogers, H. J., and Leigh, L.: Iron-binding proteins in milk and resistance to *Escherichia coli* infection in infants. Brit. Med. J. *1*:69, 1972.

Dahms, B. B., Krauss, A. N., et al.: Breast feeding and serum bilirubin values during the first 4 days of life. J. Pediatr. *83*:1049, 1973.

Dallman, P. R.: Iron, vitamin E and folate in the preterm. J. Pediatr. *85*:742, 1974.

Davies, D. P.: Plasma osmolarity and feeding practices in healthy infants in first 3 months of life. Br. Med. J. *2*:340, 1973.

Fomon, S J.: Infant Nutrition. 2nd ed., Philadelphia, W. B. Saunders Co., 1974.

Fomon, S. J.: What are infants fed in the United States? Pediatrics *56*:350, 1975.

Fomon, S. J., Filer, L. J., Jr., et al.: Influence of formula concentration on caloric intake and growth of normal infants. Acta Pediat. Scand. *64*:172, 1975.

Gerrard, J. W.: Breast-feeding: Second thoughts. Pediatrics *54*:757, 1974.

Goldman, A. S., and Smith, C. W.: Host resistant factors in human milk. J. Pediatr. *82*:1082, 1973.

Gresham, E. L.: Unpublished data.

György, P.: The uniqueness of human milk: Biochemical aspects. Am. J. Clin. Nutr. *24*:970, 1971.

Hirsch, J.: Adipose cellularity in relation to human obesity. Adv. Intern. Med. *17*:289, 1971.

Klaus, M., Jerauld, R., and Kreger, N.: Maternal attachment: Importance of the first postpartum days. N. Engl. J. Med. *286*:460, 1972.

Klaus, M., and Kennell, J.: Care of the mother. *In* Klaus, M., and Fanaroff, A. (Eds.): Care of the High-risk Neonate. Philadelphia, W. B. Saunders Co., 1973, pp. 98–118.

Knowles, J. A.: Excretion of drugs in milk — a review. J. Pediatr. *66*:1068, 1965.

McKigney, J.: The uniqueness of human milk: Economic aspects. Am. J. Clin. Nutr. *24*:1005, 1971.

Mellander, O., et al.: Breast feeding and artificial feeding; a clinical, serological and biochemical study of 402 infants, with a survey of the literature. The Norbotten Study. Acta Paediat. Scand. *48*(Suppl 116) 1959.

Newton, N.: The uniqueness of human milk: Psychologic differences between breast and bottle feeding. Am. J. Clin. Nutr. *24*:993, 1971.

O'Brien, J. E.: Excretion of drugs in human milk. Am. J. Hosp. Pharm. *844*, 1974.

Olson, M.: The benign effects on rabbits' lungs of the aspiration of water compared with 5 per cent glucose or milk. Pediatrics *46*:538, 1970.

Owen, G. M., Kram, K. M., et al.: A study of nutritional status of preschool children in the United States, 1968–1970. Pediatrics *53*:597, 1974.

Pitt, J., Barlow, B., et al.: Macrophages and the protective action of breast milk in necrotizing enterocolitis. Pediat. Res. *8*:384, 1974.

Raiha, N., Rassin, D., et al.: Milk protein quality and quantity. Pediat. Res. *4*:370, 1975.

Ramos, A., Silverberg, M., and Stern, L.: Pregnanediols and neonatal hyperbilirubinemia. Am. J. Dis. Child. *111*:353, 1966.

Rios, E., Hunter, R. E., et al.: The absorption of iron as supplements in infant cereal and infant milk. Pediatrics *55*:687, 1975.

Taitz, L. S.: Overfeeding in infancy. Proc. Nutr. Soc. *33*:113, 1974.

Warren, R. L., Lepow, M. L., et al.: The relationship of maternal antibody, breast feeding and age to the susceptibility of newborn infants to infection with attenuated poliovirus. Pediatrics *34*:4, 1964.

Woody, N. C., and Woody, H. B.: Management of breast feeding. J. Pediatr. *68*:344, 1966.

# 93

# FEEDING THE LOW BIRTH WEIGHT INFANT

*By John R. Raye*

The logarithmic expansion of knowledge regarding the care of low birth weight infants, both true prematures and infants who are small for gestational age, may deter even the most interested practitioner from actively participating in the care of these high risk infants. Although many of these infants should, in fact, receive specialized attention, the primary care physician ideally should remain involved in the care of most, either as a care coordinator or as a liaison with the family. For this reason, we will briefly review the basic principles of nutrition in the low birth weight infant and comment on some recently developed nutritional techniques.

## FUNDAMENTALS

A clearer understanding of the relation between nutrition and cellular growth has been brought about by the elegant animal studies of Winick, Dobbins, Cheek and others, and the clinical correlations in humans. These investigators have suggested that growth occurs in two phases (see Fig. 93–1). Intrauterine growth occurs primarily by cell division (hyperplasia), resulting in an increase in the total number of cells in each organ system. Growth in late infancy and beyond occurs by an increase in the size of the cells already present (hypertrophy). Growth in the neonatal period and for the first few months of life appears to result from a mixture of both processes. Each organ seems to have its own specific temporal pattern in this regard.

In animals, inadequate nutrition (generally a decrease in protein intake) throughout the period of cellular multiplication results in an irreversible diminution in the number of cells within specific organ systems, including the brain. This cell deficit leads to a limitation in potential organ growth and, in some cases, to a limitation in organ function as well. Evaluation of in-

fants who are born following a period of nutritional deprivation in utero has raised the possibility of similar findings in humans; that is, long term restrictions in organ growth and function as a result of irreversible cellular deficits (Fitzhardinge, Naeye, Drillien). Similar findings following severe postnatal malnutrition have been suggested by Lloyd-Still and co-workers.

On the basis of these data, the subject of neonatal nutrition in the premature and in the small-for-gestational-age infant has assumed a new focus, on nutrient supply for the maintenance of the full potential for cellular multiplication rather than simply for growth. Two additional points should be made: Although inadequate nutrition may cause a limitation of cellular multiplication, the human brain seems to be relatively spared. This may be because of its extended potential for cellular division, lasting for as long as 6 to 8 months after birth. Later restrictions in nutrition during periods of growth by increase in cell size (hypertrophy) are rapidly reversible and result in no long term residua. An example of this form of restriction would be the "catch up" growth seen following periods of nutritional deprivation in late infancy.

The body composition of the premature infant differs from that of the term infant in a number of ways. Although these differences have been detailed previously (Chapter 1), certain of them have important nutritional implications and will be mentioned here briefly. Total body water is significantly increased in premature infants. This appears to be due mainly to an increase in the extracellular fluid space, and results in an increased risk of water imbalance. Energy stores in the form of glycogen and particularly fat are markedly reduced in the preterm infant. Fat, for example, is virtually absent in infants under 1500 grams. Similarly, transplacental transport and storage of specific minerals such as calcium and iron occurs in late pregnancy, so that infants born prior to 34 to 36 weeks of gestation may lack the stores of these elements necessary for postnatal metabolic needs. In addition to these energy and mineral deficits, the high relative surface area increases heat and water losses. Initial oxygen consumption, although slightly below that of the term infant on a

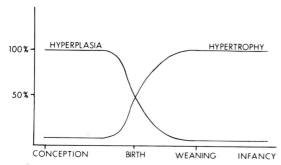

*Figure 93–1.* Approximate proportion of total growth occurring by each cellular process at various ages.

per kilogram basis, rises gradually over the next several weeks, finally exceeding that of the term infant by 20 per cent (Sinclair).

The small-for-gestational-age infant suffers from similar nutritional handicaps. Because of a relative decrease in transplacental transport of nutrients, energy stores are low. Cassidy has noted that as a manifestation of this intrauterine "starvation" the extracellular fluid space is large. Oxygen consumption, initially similar to that of the term infant, rises over the first 5 days of life and significantly exceeds that of the term infant over the next several weeks (Hill and Robinson).

Both types of low birth weight infants, then, suffer from low energy stores and high water turnover at a time when demands caused by rapid cellular multiplication are high. These facts, coupled with poor fat absorption and a gastrointestinal tract which may poorly tolerate the volume loads required to meet these metabolic demands, place the low birth weight infant in a precarious nutritional position.

### REQUIREMENTS

On the basis of the data noted above, it is clear that one must be vigorous in supplying the low birth weight infant a source of appropriate nutrition. The general caloric requirements for low birth weight infants are detailed in Table 93–1. For technical reasons, on the first day of life one often must be satisfied in supplying somewhat fewer than optimal calories. The initial aim is to supply at least 60 calories per kilogram per day to meet basic metabolic needs. An optimal caloric supply to meet general needs as well as to provide for growth requirements should be achieved as soon as possible. This should be a realistic goal by the fourth or fifth day. Methods to achieve these aims will be discussed subsequently; these have been recently reviewed by Heird and Driscoll and by Dweck.

The work of Davidson et al., and Omans et al. has established a general range of protein requirements for growth in low birth weight infants. Their infants grew well on 3 to 4 grams of protein per kilogram per day. Weight and length growth on lower protein intakes were significantly reduced. This was most apparent in the lowest weight groups, whose protein requirements on a per kilogram basis are highest. On protein intakes over 5 gm per kg per day, evidence of protein intoxication in the form of persistently elevated blood urea nitrogen was seen. Peripheral edema was seen to be associated with both higher and lower than optimal protein intakes. This was, on the one hand, a result of hypoproteinemia, and on the other, secondary to the high renal solute loads.

Formulas with appropriate protein but high mineral content have also resulted in the appearance of edema in low birth weight infants. Babson and Bramhall noted that when ash content of formula was high (0.87 gm per 100 ml) the additional weight gain noted was not accompanied by a similar increase in linear growth.

Total fluid requirements for the low birth weight infant are generally in the range of 80 to 150 ml per kg per day, depending on age (Table 93–2). These are basic requirements and must be increased appropriately in a number of situations. Phototherapy, for example, has been shown by Wu and Hodgman to increase insensible water losses by more than 100 per cent. This may result in an increase in daily water requirements in the range of 15 to 20 ml per kg per day. Even greater increases in daily water requirements are found in infants nursed under open radiant heat warmers (Williams and Oh). It is an interesting fact that, on a per kilogram basis, these additional losses increase as weight of the infant decreases. This is in part due to the higher relative surface area in proportion to the

*TABLE 93–1.  Estimated Requirements for Calories in the Low Birth Weight Infant*

| Item | Kcal per Kg per Day |
|---|---|
| Resting caloric expenditure | 50 |
| Intermittent activity | 15 |
| Occasional cold stress | 10 |
| Specific dynamic action | 8 |
| Fecal loss of calories | 12 |
| Growth allowance | 25 |
| Total | 120 |

(Data from Sinclair, J. C., et al.: Pediat. Clin. North Am., *17*:863, 1970.)

**TABLE 93–2.**

| Day | Fluid Requirements (ml per kg per day) |
|---|---|
| 1 | 80–100 |
| 2 | 100–120 |
| 3 | 120–140 |
| >3 | 150–180 |

total weight of the smaller infants. Roy and Sinclair have recently published an excellent review of this material. The range of water requirements reported by them somewhat exceeds those suggested here.

As mentioned previously, gastrointestinal fat absorption is impaired in the preterm infant. To some extent this is true in the small-for-gestational-age infant as well. Prepared formulas that are high in saturated and polyunsaturated fats, especially linoleic, are particularly poorly absorbed. The addition of linoleic acid to the saturated fat of cow's milk in an attempt to improve total fat absorption may result in clinically significant vitamin E deficiency (see p. 94). Tantibhedhyangkul and Hashim, and Roy et al. have recently documented improved fat absorption in the preterm infant with medium-chain triglycerides. Nitrogen absorption was significantly enhanced as well under these conditions.

As previously noted, a large fraction of transplacental mineral transport takes place in the last few weeks of gestation. The preterm infant who is born prior to this period has significantly decreased total body content of most minerals, most importantly of calcium and iron. Impaired transplacental transport may result in similar deficits, particularly of calcium, in the small-for-gestational-age infant. Hypocalcemia may be seen in the neonatal period, while the effects of iron deficiency are not evident for 8 to 10 weeks. Thus, calcium should be supplied to the low birth weight infant in a utilizable form; that is, not in formulas high in phosphate and unsaturated fatty acids. Some low birth weight infants may require additional oral or parenteral calcium supplementation. Iron, on the other hand, is generally supplied after the first week of life as oral supplements that achieve ade-

quate iron balance by the time additional iron utilization takes place (see pp. 25 to 27).

### TIMING

Calorie, protein and water intake by the low birth weight infant should begin as soon as possible following birth. Both the true premature and particularly the small-for-gestational-age infant are at risk for developing significant hypoglycemia, as meager energy stores are depleted if a reliable ongoing source of calories is not available. In general, the more severe the growth limitation the higher the risk of hypoglycemia, so that premature infants under 1500 grams and those with birth weights under the third weight percentile for gestational age should receive parenteral calories until an adequate gastrointestinal supply is achieved. Larger preterm infants benefit from early feedings as do term infants; these feedings result in significant elevations of mean blood sugar, less neonatal weight loss, improved intestinal motility and less subsequent hyperbilirubinemia (Wu et al., Rabor et al.).

### METHODS OF NUTRIENT SUPPLY

**MAJOR DECISIONS.** Prior to supplying nutrients to the low birth weight infant, certain procedural decisions must be made before the appropriate feeding technique can be selected. One must first decide whether or not the gastrointestinal tract can tolerate the introduction of nutrient materials. This decision should be based on an assessment of the adequacy of intestinal motility judged by bowel sounds, normal stooling patterns and lack of abdominal distention. Anatomic obstruction or decreases in motility can result from congenital malformations of the intestinal tract, hypoxia, hypokalemia or gastrointestinal disease processes such as meconium ileus, meconium plugging, Hirschsprung's disease or necrotizing enterocolitis. Increased intestinal transit times have been noted in very small infants without other obvious pathology. In the presence of signs of functional or anatomic intestinal obstruction, nutrients must be provided by the parenteral route.

If intestinal motility appears adequate, a second decision must be made regarding the level at which nutrients can be most safely delivered into the gut. Should one introduce feedings by mouth, directly into the stomach or beyond the pylorus? This decision must involve an evaluation of the adequacy and coordination of the sucking and swallowing mechanisms. Gryboski has demonstrated that these processes are not well developed until 34 to 36 weeks of gestational age. She has also noted that their coordination and efficiency tend to improve with postnatal age. Thus, it does not appear logical to attempt initial nipple feedings of infants who are less than 34 weeks of gestational age or who exhibit depression of these reflexes for other reasons.

The adequacy of gastric emptying must also be considered prior to nipple or direct intragastric feedings. The best way to do this is by evaluation of gastric residuals after a trial feeding. Silvero and Yu have each noted that hypoxia and respiratory distress markedly delay gastric emptying. They noted no differences, however, in the rate of gastric emptying between term, premature and small-for-gestational-age infants. They also found that gastric emptying is significantly more rapid when the infant is placed in the right-lateral or prone position, and that these positions should be used to facilitate emptying in most low birth weight infants.

It is also necessary to decide whether the infant can tolerate relatively low volume, intermittent feedings as its only caloric supply. Appropriately grown infants, who are greater than 34 weeks of gestational age, usually have energy stores which, although meager, will suffice for the delay between 3-hour feedings. Severely small-for-gestational-age infants, on the other hand, although physically able to ingest larger volumes of formula, may not have adequate energy stores to tolerate the period between feedings. These infants will require either parenteral caloric supplementation in addition to oral feedings or one of the continuous non-parenteral feeding techniques discussed below. This is also true, in general, for infants of less than 34 weeks of gestational age.

Infants who are tachypneic, with respiratory rates over 60 to 70, are also poor candidates for oral feedings. It is important to realize that the introduction of oral feedings introduces a second peak of morbidity and mortality (the first peak being birth itself). For this reason, it is important that risks other than those associated with feedings be minimal or at least well defined before oral feedings are instituted.

**NON-PARENTERAL METHODS OF NUTRIENT SUPPLY. ORAL.** If, in the larger low birth weight infant, oral feedings seem to be the technique of choice, as in the term infant, distilled water seems a reasonable fluid for the first feeding. This is followed by proprietary formula at a concentration of 20 to 24 calories per ounce. No advantage of either more dilute or more concentrated formula has been demonstrated. In fact, certain "elemental" high solute formulas have been associated with an increased incidence of necrotizing enterocolitis (Book et al.). An initial volume of 5 to 7 ml per kg per feeding is appropriate on a 3-hour basis, with increases, as tolerated, to 10–15 ml per kg per feeding by the third day. Subsequently, intakes are increased until requirements are adequately met.

**INTERMITTENT GAVAGE.** For infants who are not able to tolerate nipple feeding but who have adequate gastrointestinal function, gavage feedings may be instituted. A feeding catheter is passed either orally or nasally into the stomach. The position is confirmed by injection of a small bolus of air while listening over the stomach. Residual gastric fluid is measured, and formula is allowed to flow in by gravity. Forcing formula in under pressure increases the likelihood of gastric distention, regurgitation and aspiration. There seems no advantage to giving water or glucose water for the first gavage feeding, since once mixed with gastric fluid all materials appear to have the same potential pulmonary toxicity.

Volumes are as noted above for oral feedings. In gavage feeding, however, a more rational approach can be used in assessing gastric emptying and in determining the volume of subsequent feedings. Prior to each feeding, the residual volume from the previous feeding is aspirated and measured. When the amount of residual exceeds 4 ml per kg, feedings should be decreased in volume or the time interval between feedings increased. (Increasing gastric residuals may also be a helpful early diagnostic sign of infection, necrotizing enterocolitis, hypoglycemia or other problem interfering with gastric emptying.) Rates of gastric emptying are similar in term premature or small-for-gestational-age infants (Yu). In the infant under 1200 to 1500 gm, however, small gastric volumes may result in inadequate water and caloric supplies. In these circumstances supplemental parenteral fluid and calories may be essential to provide for the infant's nutritional requirements. In fact, in the very small infant, 24 to 48 hours of parenteral fluids may be required prior to the institution of gavage feedings.

The major problem with gavage feedings is the occasional appearance of bradycardia noted on tube passage. This bradycardia may be associated with apnea and cyanosis. This problem has been detailed by Hasselmeyer and Hon, who found that most reflex bradycardia occurred when the tip of the tube was 5 cm from the anterior nares, and occurred immediately on introduction of the tube. In some small infants, this vagal response may cause nurses considerable consternation. Generally, once the tube is in place the bradycardia is not persistent. In these sensitive infants, it may be advisable to leave the gavage tube in place between feedings. In most circumstances, however, feeding tubes should be removed between feedings to prevent partial withdrawal of the catheter into the esophagus, nasal ulcerations, gastric irritation and increased nasal airway resistance. If the tube is to be left in between feedings, the proximal end should be left open to allow for gastric decompression and to prevent regurgitation of gastric contents into the esophagus.

Recently, Wilkinson and Yu demonstrated a significant fall in arterial oxygen tension following intermittent gavage feedings as small as 6 ml per kg. This occurred 10 minutes post-feeding, with a mean decrease in oxygen tension of 13 mm of mercury and was accompanied with a rise in respiratory rate. Oxygen levels returned to prefeeding levels by 30 minutes. This brief period of hypoxia may have serious consequences in some infants.

CONTINUOUS GAVAGE. An alternate method for supplying fluids by gavage is by continuous infusion. This method has been presented by Landwirth and by Valmen et al., and utilizes an infusion pump to supply formula at an initial rate of 1–2 ml per hour, with increments until required volumes are achieved. Gastric residuals are checked periodically. This technique may result in higher daily feeding volumes than achieved by intermittent gavage feedings, particularly in the first few days of life. Post-feeding hypoxia may also be minimized by this technique. It does not eliminate the risks of development of significant gastric residuals or catheter dislodgment, however, and requires constant observation of the infant.

TRANSPYLORIC. Another constant infusion technique has received considerable attention over the past few years, that of infusion of formula beyond the pylorus, or continuous nasojejunal (or nasoduodenal) feeding. This technique, originally reported by Rhea and Kilby, has gained wide acceptance following subsequent reports by Rhea and co-workers and by Cheek and Staub. Following placement of the catheter in the stomach, the infant is placed on his right side, and the catheter is allowed to pass through the pylorus to the distal duodenum or jejunum. Transpyloric positioning of the catheter can be documented by aspiration of bile or alkaline material or by x-ray (see Fig. 93–2). If distal duodenal or jejunal positioning is achieved, isosmolar formula is infused at a rate of 60–80 ml per kilogram the first day with gradual increases each subsequent day to meet all daily fluid and caloric requirements. Initially, the tube is aspirated every hour to confirm placement and the adequacy of gastrointestinal motility.

The major advantages of transpyloric feeding is the low risk of gastric pooling of formula, leading to regurgitation and aspiration. Even with more proximal duodenal placement, significant gastric reflux of formula occurs in less than 15 per cent of patients. Thus, this technique can even be used on very sick infants with poor gastric emptying; for example, very adequate fluid and caloric intakes can be rapidly achieved in infants on respirators.

As with many other new techniques, however, significant complications are encountered as experience in the use of transpyloric feeding accumulates. The most

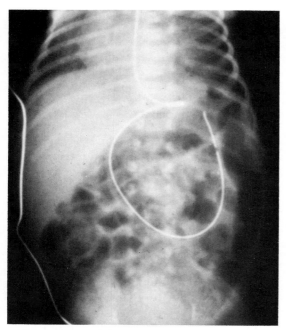

*Figure 93–2.* Abdominal film showing transpyloric feeding catheter in distal duodenum. Note marked displacement of duodenal loop secondary to catheter presence. (Case of Dr. Edwin L. Gresham. Printed with his kind permission).

clearly defined complication has been duodenal perforation. This was initially reported by Boros and Reynolds and subsequently by Sun et al. It has been suggested that this is a result of the use of polyvinyl chloride catheters, which seem to harden on prolonged intraintestinal exposure. For this reason, Rhea and colleagues have emphasized the advantage of use of barium-impregnated silicone catheters, which remain soft indefinitely. In their experience with almost 500 patients, use of these catheters has not been associated with a single perforation.

The possible relationship between the presence of a jejunal catheter and jejunojejunal intussusception has been reported by Chen and Wong, who also reported the appearance of necrotizing enterocolitis in an infant fed by this technique. Although this latter association may be purely coincidental, Challacombe has reported alterations in local intestinal flora following the introduction of jejunal tubes. Theoretically, an en-vironment favoring certain gas-forming bacteria associated with the infusion of hyperosmolar formula might well provide the triggering mechanism for development of this feared disease.

The gravity of the complications associated with this feeding technique requires that transpyloric feedings not be used routinely or without meticulous attention to technical details. When other oral feeding methods do not place an infant at jeopardy, they should be used initially. Nevertheless, the value of nasojejunal feeding cannot be underestimated in certain well defined clinical situations. Among these situations one might include infants on ventilators, infants with intermittent apnea requiring bag and mask ventilation and other circumstances where delays in gastric emptying preclude adequate gastric caloric intake. Wells and Zachman have recently demonstrated significant increases in rates of weight gain when nasojejunal feeding was compared to intermittent gavage feedings.

GASTROSTOMY. Brief mention should be made here about the use of gastrostomy as a method of feeding small infants. Although some controversy raged during the early 1960's regarding the role of this technique in our nutritional armamentarium, a controlled study published by Vengusamy and co-workers in 1969 clearly demonstrated that the routine use of gastrostomy for feeding low birth weight infants was associated with increased morbidity and mortality. At the present time, gastrostomy should be used only prior to or following gastrointestinal surgery, where it plays an important role in preventing subsequent gastric distention as well as in providing a route for feeding.

The techniques of nipple, gavage, continuous intragastric and transpyloric feedings provide the basis for the great majority of nutrient supply to the low birth weight infant. Parenteral feeding techniques, however, should be considered in situations in which adequate nutrition cannot be provided by non-parenteral means.

PARENTERAL METHODS OF NUTRIENT SUPPLY. The initial use of 10 per cent dextrose solutions in many low birth weight infants has become routine. In the immature infant, glucose solutions will safely provide partial daily water and calorie needs until the time when adequate volume and calories can be provided non-parenterally. These requirements are outlined in Tables 93–1 and 93–2. It is recommended that all infants who weigh less than 1750 grams be maintained on these simple solutions, starting by 6 hours of age and continuing until adequate amounts of nutrients are provided by alternate means. As the volume of non-parenteral feedings is increased, one should concomitantly reduce the parenteral glucose solutions. In normal circumstances, maintenance sodium (2 to 4 mEq per kg per day) and potassium (2 to 3 mEq per kg per day) are added on the second day. This form of supplementation should not be required after the third or fourth day. It is important to note that in very small infants even this glucose load may be excessive and may result in significant hyperglycemia and glycosuria. For this reason frequent Dextrostix and urine sugar testing should be done with an eye to decreasing glucose input. In general, the infusion site should be a peripheral vein unless an umbilical arterial catheter is required for blood sampling or pressure monitoring. The use of umbilical venous catheters is to be discouraged because of the risk of infection and thrombosis.

PARTIAL PARENTERAL NUTRITION. When longer delays occur before achieving adequate volumes of non-parenteral feeding, Benda and Babson have encouraged the addition of a source of amino acids (2 gm per 100 ml) to the standard 10 per cent glucose solution. They advocated additional calories in the form of ethanol (7 calories per gram) as well. More recently, the use of ethanol has been discouraged following a report by Peden and co-workers of ethanol intoxication in a significant number of infants who were followed with plasma alcohol levels. Although the osmolality of these amino acid and glucose solutions is quite high (900–1200 mOsm per kg), some success has been achieved in maintaining peripheral venous infusion sites. Controlled studies by Pildes et al. and Brans et al. have demonstrated modest increases in rates of weight gain in infants whose oral feedings were supplemented with glucose and amino acid solutions compared to those supplemented with simple glucose solutions. Complications of hyperglycemia, hyperosmolarity, hyponatremia and metabolic acidosis were noted frequently in Brans' series.

TOTAL PARENTERAL NUTRITION. One of the most exciting advances of the late 1960's was the demonstration by Dudrick that the use of parenteral solutions containing an amino acid source, glucose, minerals and vitamins could by itself support adequate long term growth in both experimental animals and man. Since that time, many modifications have been made in the composition of the infusate. Heird and Winters have recently published an excellent review of "the state of the art," and the composition of their infusate is shown in Table 93–3. Originally the nitrogen source was a hydrolysate of either casein or fibrin, but a mixture of pure crystalline amino acids at present appears to offer certain advantages. It should be noted that the nitrogen source, although contributing only 10 per cent of the total calories, is an essential factor in providing substrate for continued cellular multiplication.

The osmolality of this mixture is exceedingly high, in the range of 1800 mOsm per kg water. (Normal serum osmolality is 300 mOsm per kg water). One of Dudrick's major contributions, in fact, was the demonstration that an infusate of this type could be tolerated without marked elevations in serum osmolality when infused slowly into a central vein. His technique of superior vena cava placement through the

**TABLE 93–3.** *Composition of Total Parenteral Nutrition Infusate*

| Constituent | Amount |
| --- | --- |
| Nitrogen source | 2.5 gm per kg per day |
| Glucose | 25 to 30 gm per kg per day |
| Sodium (NaCl) | 3 to 4 mEq per kg per day |
| Potassium | 2 to 3 mEq per kg per day |
| Calcium (Ca gluconate) | 0.5 mEq per kg per day |
| Magnesium ($MgSO_4$) | 0.25 mEq per kg per day |
| Vitamins | |
| MVI | 1 ml per day |
| Vitamin $B_{12}$ | 5 to 10 $\mu$g per day |
| Folic acid | 50 to 75 $\mu$g per day |
| Vitamin $K_1$ | 250 to 500 $\mu$g per day |
| Total volume | 130 ml per kg per day |

(From Heird, W. C., and Driscoll, J. M., Jr.: Clinics on Perinatology 2:309, 1975.)

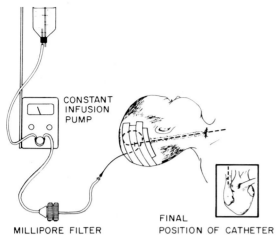

CONSTANT
INFUSION
PUMP

MILLIPORE FILTER

FINAL
POSITION OF CATHETER

**Figure 93–3.** Schematic depiction of the infusion technique for total parenteral nutrition. (From Heird, W. C., and Driscoll, J. M., Jr.: Clin. Perinatol. 2:309, 1975.)

jugular vein remains the most widely used technique of administration. The use of a distant cutaneous exit site (Fig. 93–3) seems to minimize the development of local thrombophlebitis with prolonged vessel catheterization.

The successful use of total parenteral nutrition depends in large part on meticulous attention to the technical details of infusate preparation and use. It should not be attempted where protocols for its preparation, administration and constant monitoring of its metabolic results have not been developed. It is beyond the scope of this work to detail the technical aspects of this form of parenteral nutrition. In general, the initial infusate contains significantly less glucose than noted in Table 93–3, and glucose concentrations are increased only in the absence of hyperglycemia. Thus, since most of the calories are in the form of glucose, initial caloric intakes may be low. Close attention must be paid to alterations in fluid and electrolyte balance of the patient, so that appropriate modifications may be made in the infusate composition. Because the infusate itself is an excellent culture media for both bacteria and yeasts, every precaution must be taken to prevent contamination of both infusate and infant. Use of the central venous line for the sam-

pling of blood or the injection of medication is to be avoided.

In spite of the most careful metabolic and microbiologic surveillance, the list of complications is long and the rate is moderately high. Generalized fungal infections due to *Candida* albicans have been a particular problem. Major common complications are listed in Table 93–4. In view of the seriousness of these problems, total parenteral alimentation should not be used when safer methods of nutrient supply are available. It is clear that this form of nutrition is essential in infants who have major abnormalities of the gastrointestinal tract; for example, major intestinal resection, short bowel syndromes, omphaloceles and gastroschisis or chronic diarrhea. Whether this technique has significant advantages in other situations is at present a matter of some controversy. Its use in very low birth weight infants has been advocated by some, although Driscoll and his co-workers in a careful analysis of their data have suggested that its routine use in this circumstance is not warranted.

*Intravenous Lipid.* Although intravenous lipid preparation has been used for some time in Europe, only recently have experimental trials been permitted in this country. This lipid is a soybean oil emulsion which provides 6 calories per gram and can be administered by peripheral vein. Cashore and colleagues have recently reported on the use of combined fat, glucose and protein hydrolysate supplements to oral feedings in a group of low birth weight infants. These supplements were administered peripherally and resulted in

**TABLE 93–4.** *Common Complications of Total Parenteral Nutrition*

*Metabolic*
  Hyperglycemia/hypoglycemia
  Azotemia
  Metabolic acidosis
  Hyperammonemia
  Abnormalities of liver function
  Abnormal serum amino acids

*Catheter related*
  Infection
  Dislodgment
  Erosion

rates of growth that exceeded those achieved by other previously discussed techniques. Complications, including hypernatremia, hyponatremia, hyperosmolality, azotemia and gross hyperlipemia were noted. A report by Andrew and co-workers has suggested that this lipid emulsion may displace bilirubin from its albumin binding sites. Thus, recommendations concerning the use of intravenous fat supplements must await further evaluation.

# REFERENCES

Andrew, G., et al.: In vivo effect of intralipid intravenous feeding on serum lipids and bilirubin in the neonate. Pediat. Res. 9:362, 1975.

Babson, S. G., and Bramhall, J. L.: Diet and growth in the premature infant. J. Pediatr. 74:890, 1969.

Benda, G. I., and Babson, S. G.: Peripheral intravenous alimentation of the small premature infant. J. Pediatr. 79:494, 1971.

Book, L. S., et al.: Necrotizing enterocolitis in infants fed on elemental formula. Pediat. Res. 8:379, 1974.

Boros, S. J., and Reynolds, J. W.: Duodenal perforation: Complication of neonatal nasojejunal feeding. J. Pediatr. 85:107, 1974.

Brans, Y. W., et al.: Feeding the low birth weight infant: Orally or parenterally? Preliminary results of a comparative study. Pediatrics 54:15, 1974.

Cashore, W. J., et al.: Nutritional supplements with intravenously administered lipid, protein hydrolysate and glucose in small premature infants. Pediatrics 56:8, 1975.

Cassady, G.: Body composition in intrauterine growth retardation. Pediat. Clin. North Am. 17:79, 1970.

Challacombe, D. N.: Bacterial microflora in infants receiving nasojejunal tube feeding. J. Pediatr., 85:113, 1974.

Cheek, D. B.: Maternal nutritional restriction and fetal brain growth. In Cheek, D. B. (Ed.): Fetal and Postnatal Cellular Growth. New York, J. Wiley and Sons, 1975, p. 111.

Cheek, J. A., and Staub, G. F.: Nasojejunal alimentation for premature and full-term newborn infants. J. Pediatr. 82:955, 1973.

Chen, J. W., and Wong, P. W. K.: Intestinal complications of nasojejunal feeding in low-birth-weight infants. J. Pediatr. 85:109, 1974.

Davidson, M., et al.: Feeding studies in low-birth-weight infants. J. Pediatr. 70:695, 1967.

Drillien, C. M.: The small-for-date infant: Etiology and prognosis. Pediat. Clin. North Am. 17:9, 1970.

Drillien, C. M.: Aetiology and outcome in low-birth weight infants. Develop. Med. Child. Neurol. 14:563, 1972.

Drillien, C. M.: Abnormal neurologic signs in the first year of life in low birth weight infants: Possible prognostic significance. Develop. Med. Child Neurol. 14:575, 1972.

Driscoll, J. M., Jr., et al.: Total intravenous alimentation in low-birth-weight infants: A preliminary report. J. Pediatr. 81:145, 1972.

Dudrick, S. J.: Long term total parenteral nutrition with growth, development and positive nitrogen balance. Surgery, 64:134, 1968.

Dweck, H. S.: Feeding the prematurely born infant. Clinic in Perinatology 2:183, 1975.

Fitzhardinge, P. M., and Steven, E. M.: The small-for-date infant, 1. Later growth patterns. Pediatrics 49:671, 1972.

Gryboski, J. D.: Suck and swallow in the premature infant. Pediatrics 43:96, 1969.

Hasselmeyer, E. G., and Hon E. H.: Effects of gavage feeding of premature infants on cardiorespiratory patterns. Military Med. 136:252, 1971.

Heird, W. C., and Driscoll, J. M., Jr.: Newer methods of feeding low birth weight infants. Clinics in Perinatology 2:309, 1975.

Heird, W. C., and Winters, R. W.: Total parenteral nutrition. The state of the art. J. Pediatr. 86:2, 1975.

Hill, J. R., and Robinson, D. C.: Oxygen consumption in normally grown, small-for-dates and large-for-dates new-born infants. J. Physiol. 199:685, 1968.

Landwirth, J.: Continuous nasogastric infusion feedings of infants of low birth weight. Clin. Pediatr. 13:603, 1974.

Lloyd-Still, J. D., et al.: Intellectual development after severe malnutrition in infancy. Pediatrics 54:306, 1974.

Naeye, R. L.: Structural correlates of fetal undernutrition. In Waisman, H. A., and Kerr, G. (Eds.): Fetal Growth and Development. New York, The McGraw-Hill Book Co., 1970, p. 241.

Omans, W. B., et al.: Prolonged feeding studies in premature infants. J. Pediatr. 59:951, 1961.

Peden, V. H., et al.: Intravenously induced infantile intoxication with ethanol. J. Pediatr. 83:490, 1973.

Pildes, R. S., et al.: Intravenous supplementation of L-amino acids and dextrose in low-birth-weight infants. J. Pediatr. 82:945, 1973.

Rabor, I. F., et al.: The effects of early and late feeding of intra-uterine fetally malnourished (IUM) infants. Pediatrics 42:261, 1968.

Rhea, J. W., and Kilby, J. O.: A nasojejunal tube for infant feeding. Pediatrics 46:36, 1970.

Rhea, J. W., et al.: Nasojejunal feeding: an improved device and intubation technique. J. Pediatr. 82:951, 1973.

Rhea, J. W., et al.: Nasojejunal (transpyloric) feeding: A commentary. J. Pediatr. 86:451, 1975.

Roy, C. C., et al.: Correction of the malabsorption of the preterm infant with a medium-chain triglyceride formula. J. Pediatr. 86:446, 1975.

Roy, R. N., and Sinclair, J. C.: Hydration of the low-birth-weight infant. Clinics in Perinatology 2:393, 1975.

Silverio, J.: Gastric emptying time in the newborn and nursling. Am. J. Med. Sci. 247:732, 1964.

Sinclair, J. C., and Silverman, W. H.: Intrauterine growth in active tissue mass of the human fetus, with particular reference to the undergrown baby. Pediatrics 38:48, 1966.

Sinclair, J. C., et al.: Supportive management of the sick neonate. Pediat. Clin. North Am. 17:863, 1970.

Sun, S. C., et al.: Duodenal perforation: A rare complication of neonatal nasojejunal tube feeding. Pediatrics 55:371, 1975.

Tantibhedhyangkul, P., and Hashim, S. A.: Medium-chain triglyceride feeding in premature infants: Effects on fat and nitrogen absorption. Pediatrics 55:359, 1975.

Valman, H. B., et al.: Continuous intragastric milk feeds in infants of low birth weight. Br. Med. J. 3:547, 1972.

Vengusamy, S., et al.: A controlled study of feeding gastrostomy in low birth weight infants. Pediatrics 43:815, 1969.

Wells, D. H., and Zachman, R. D.: Nasojejunal feedings in low-birth-weight infants. J. Pediatr. 87:276, 1975.

Wilkinson, A., and Yu, V. Y. H.: Immediate effects of feeding on blood-gases and some cardiorespiratory functions in ill newborn infants. Lancet 1:1083, 1974.

Williams, P. R., and Oh, W.: Effects of radiant warmer on insensible water loss in newborn infants. Am. J. Dis. Child. 128:511, 1974.

Winick, M.: Cellular growth in intrauterine malnutrition. Pediat. Clin. North Am. 17:69, 1970.

Winick, M., and Rosso, P.: Effects of severe, early malnutrition on cellular growth of brain. Pediatr. Res. 3:181, 1969.

Winick, M., et al.: Effects of early nutrition on growth of the central nervous system. Birth defects 10:29, 1974.

Wu, P. Y. K., and Hodgman, J. E.: Insensible water loss in preterm infants: Changes with postnatal development and nonionizing radiant energy. Pediatrics 54:704, 1974.

Wu, P. Y. K., et al.: "Early" versus "late" feeding of low birth weight neonates. Pediatrics 39:733, 1967.

Yu, V. Y. H.: Effect of body position on gastric emptying in the neonate. Arch. Dis. Child. 50:500, 1975.

# 94 DISORDERS OF VITAMINS AND TRACE MINERALS

*Revised by John R. Raye*

## GENERAL CONSIDERATIONS

In the United States of the mid-1970's vitamin deficiency states are rarely seen or even considered in a general pediatric practice. These deficiency syndromes are even more rare in the neonatal period. Several vitamins, the B group and C for example, appear to be actively transported across the placenta, so that extreme deficiency states in the mother are required for reduction of neonatal stores. Those vitamins that act as if passively transported to the fetus, although perhaps present in somewhat reduced concentrations in the newborn, appear to be adequate for the period prior to dietary accumulation in the term infant. However, the striking progress in increasing survival of the very small premature infant has brought with it a reassessment of "adequacy" of vitamin stores. Clinical and laboratory evidence of both vitamin and mineral deficiency states indica-tive of the pre-term infant's reduced stores and/or increased requirements have now been documented.

New methods of prolonged parenteral nutrition that require consideration of specific vitamin and mineral needs have reminded us of the many lessons learned during the formulation of our present proprietary formulas. The 1950's and 1960's abounded with examples of new formulas and new processing techniques, each of which reduced concentrations of vitamins previously found adequate in breast or condensed cow's milk. For the first time, in many instances, neonatal vitamin deficiency syndromes were recognized in the absence of severe maternal deficiency states. We must continually be chagrined at these iatrogenic diseases caused by "advances" in neonatal care.

Faddism, too, must bear its responsibility for iatrogenic disease. The use of high doses of vitamin A ("if a little is good...")

has merited as many case reports as deficiency of the vitamin. New dietary fads such as the severely deficient Zen macrobiotic diet must be watched with caution as they pass through their era of popularity. Similarly, one must continue to be aware that certain ethnic groups, by reason of dietary customs or availability, are at risk for specific vitamin deficiency syndromes.

Vitamin dependency syndromes representing alterations in vitamin requirements of specific individuals have assumed great practical and theoretical importance. In general, these are hereditary diseases involving specific biochemical abnormalities. Symptoms develop in the face of a normal body pool of the vitamin but are ameliorated when increased concentrations of the vitamin are present.

It is clear, therefore, that neither our increasing knowledge of neonatal medicine nor the wide use of proprietary formula, with its "full" complement of vitamin and mineral supplements has yet made this chapter superfluous.

## VITAMIN A DEFICIENCY

**INCIDENCE.** Outspoken vitamin A deficiency, as evidenced by its pathognomonic corneal signs, Bitot's spots and xerophthalmia, has not been reported within the first month of life. Chemical findings compatible with subclinical deficiency, however, are present in some mature and many premature infants. Prolonged intake of inadequate amounts of vitamin A may result in chemical evidence of deficiency appearing by 4 months of age. For these reasons a brief discussion of the syndrome will be presented. Infants with problems in dietary fat absorption, such as those with cystic fibrosis described by Keating and Fergin, are also at increased risk.

**ETIOLOGY.** One of the fat soluble vitamins, dietary vitamin A is obtained both as carotenoids and as vitamin A. Ingested vitamin A goes through a series of interconversions in the gut mucosa and liver. Carotenes are converted to a form of vitamin A in the intestinal mucosa during absorption. Increases in dietary fat and protein may increase daily vitamin requirements.

The mechanism of action of vitamin A,

other than in retinal pigment formation, is unknown. It has been suggested that the vitamin is important for cell growth and membrane stability. Certainly, the major pathological finding in vitamin A deficiency is squamous metaplasia of epithelial surfaces, with accumulation of keratinized cells.

In early pregnancy maternal vitamin A levels are low. At 16 weeks, levels begin to rise gradually, according to Gal and Parkinson, achieving values 1.5 times normal by term. Cord blood levels of vitamin A at term are not significantly different from maternal levels, although fetal carotenoid levels are significantly lower than the mother's. Mean cord levels were 23.6 $\mu$g per 100 ml of vitamin A and 12.5 $\mu$g per 100 ml of carotenoids. In general, serum vitamin A levels less than 20 mg per 100 ml have been accepted as evidence of low body stores. In term infants, levels then rise gradually over the first months of life.

Premature infants, on the other hand, may be handicapped with respect to vitamin A acquisition for a number of reasons. Henley and co-workers found low liver stores of vitamin A in infants who weighed less than 2500 grams who died on the first day of life. With respect to absorption of a test dose of the vitamin, premature infants again fared less well than term infants. Decreased absorption of the vitamin seemed to correlate with the decreased ability of the small premature infant to absorb dietary fat. At 3 weeks of age, one fourth of the preterm infants in their study who were not on vitamin A supplements had serum vitamin A levels below 20 $\mu$g per 100 ml. No infant on vitamin supplements fell below that level. Thus, adequate dietary vitamin supplementation is required to allow development of adequate body stores in the preterm infant.

**DIAGNOSIS.** Although clinical vitamin A deficiency has not been clearly identified in the first month of life, by 3 months of age the full-blown deficiency syndrome may be seen in infants on inadequate vitamin intake.

The case of Bass and Fisch is an excellent example of this course, which is marked by growth failure, anemia, epithelial metaplasia and increased intracranial pressure.

CASE 94–1

A female infant was born at term by spontaneous delivery. Birth weight was 7 pounds (3175 gm). Because of a history of milk allergy in siblings, the infant was immediately put on a soy milk diet without vitamin supplement. At the age of 3 1/2 months, the infant was brought to the physician's office because of marked enlargement of the breasts. No diagnosis was made. In 2 weeks, the infant had become extremely irritable and had a temperature of 100.5° F. The child appeared pale and extremely restless but did not look acutely ill. The breasts were still enlarged. There was marked bulging of the fontanel. The child had received no drugs. Lumbar puncture revealed bloody fluid under high pressure. Culture of the fluid showed no growth. Vitamin A deficiency was suspected. Urine could not be examined because the urethral opening could not be located, owing to excessive cornified epithelium. Penicillin was administered without improvement. Vitamin A was then given daily. In one day, the child's disposition had improved and the fontanel was softer. The next day the child was well. During the next few weeks, the gynecomastia gradually improved.

May et al. have suggested in a less well documented case the evidence of vitamin A deficiency in the premature may consist of failure to gain weight, hypoproteinemia and peripheral edema.

The clinical diagnosis of vitamin A deficiency can be confirmed by the finding of low serum vitamin levels and by clinical response to vitamin supplementation.

**TREATMENT.** Fomon has estimated the daily vitamin A requirement as 250 I.U. per day and suggested an advisable intake of 500 I.U. per day (Tables 94–1 and 94–2). Breast milk and standard formula contain approximately three times this amount per liter. Treatment of the deficiency state should be achieved by 5000 I.U. over a period of several days followed by maintenance therapy of 1500 per day. It should be remembered that vitamin A overdosage is in itself harmful and to be avoided.

## VITAMIN A EXCESS

Excessive vitamin A intake is capable of causing both an acute and a chronic form of toxicity. The chronic form, presenting with

**TABLE 94–1. Advisable Intakes of Vitamins**

| Vitamin | Daily Intake |
|---|---|
| A | 500 I.U. |
| D | 400 I.U. |
| E | 4 I.U.° |
| K | 15 μg |
| C | 20 mg |
| Thiamin | 0.2 mg |
| Riboflavin | 0.4 mg |
| Niacin°° | 5 mg |
| B$_6$ | 0.4 mg |
| Folacin | 50 μg |

°Greater intakes may be desirable for infants receiving formulas supplying more than 15 per cent of calories from polyunsaturated fatty acids (e.g., formulas in which approximately one half of the fat is supplied from corn oil or soy oil).

°°Including nicotinamide equivalents (60 mg tryptophan = 1 mg niacin).

(From Fomon, Samuel J., *Infant Nutrition*, 2nd ed., Philadelphia, W. B. Saunders Company, 1974.)

growth failure, hyperostosis and craniotabes, manifests itself only after months of overdosage and shall not be considered further here. The acute form, however, may be seen following a single massive dose of the vitamin and will be considered briefly. Also of interest is a recent report by Bernhardt and Dorsey that suggested the possible teratogenic effects of large doses of vitamin A in early pregnancy. Similar findings have been observed in animal studies.

**INCIDENCE.** No case of vitamin A tox-

**TABLE 94–2. Estimated Requirements for Vitamins**

| Vitamin | Requirement |
|---|---|
| A | 250 I.U./day |
| D | 100–200 I.U./day |
| E | 0.4 mg/gm PUFA° |
| K | 5 μg/day |
| C | 10 mg/day |
| Thiamin | 0.2 mg/1000 kcal |
| Riboflavin | <0.5 mg/1000 kcal |
| Niacin°° | 4.4 mg/1000 kcal |
| B$_6$ | 9 μg/gm protein |
| Folacin | <50 μg/day |

°Polyunsaturated fatty acid.

°°Including nicotinamide equivalents (60 mg tryptophan = 1 mg niacin).

(From Fomon, Samuel J., *Infant Nutrition*, 2nd edition, Philadelphia, W. B. Saunders Company, 1974.)

icity has been reported in the first month of life. Marie and See reported one infant at 8 weeks of age, and Knudson and Rothman another at 7 weeks. Since symptoms have been noted following a single dose of the vitamin, it is probable that instances will be observed within the neonatal period. Of some interest is the exceedingly high vitamin A content of polar bear liver (18,000 I.U. per gm). Arctic explorers who have ignored eskimo taboos and sampled it have developed severe symptoms of acutely increased intracranial pressure.

**ETIOLOGY.** The mechanism by which vitamin A causes its toxic effects is not known. It is interesting that toxicity is noted only following ingestion of vitamin A, not of carotenes. Ingestion of the latter substances results only in benign carotenemia.

**DIAGNOSIS.** The major symptoms following the ingestion of high doses of vitamin A appear to be related to an acute increase in intracranial pressure. Vomiting, irritability or lethargy and a bulging fontanel are seen.

CASE 94–2

Knudson and Rothman's case was a premature infant weighing 4 pounds 15 ounces (2240 gm). He was fed with Olac, which contains an adequate quantity of halibut liver oil, but was given by error an additional 10 drops of percomorph oil five times daily from the fourth to the seventh week. At this time his mother noted a bulging fontanel, and the baby was admitted to hospital. Here, aside from the tense fontanel, which was elevated to a height of 2 cm, a slightly enlarged liver, bilateral ankle clonus and mild tremors were noted. The cerebrospinal fluid spurted forth under greatly increased pressure, contained 30 cells, almost all mononuclears, and a faint trace of protein by the Pandy test. Improvement after lumbar puncture was rapid. Five days later, fine desquamation of the skin of the trunk and extremities was seen.

**TREATMENT.** Treatment consists of withholding further vitamin A intake until body stores return to normal.

## VITAMIN B₁ DEFICIENCY, BERIBERI

Deficiency of vitamin B₁ affects infants in two age groups. A congenital form develops within the first few days of life, and an infantile form is seen from 2 to 3 months after birth.

**INCIDENCE.** Although beriberi is common in Asian countries, where polished rice is the main dietary staple, both forms are exceedingly rare in this country. The congenital form, not reported in the United States since 1944, occurs only in infants born to mothers who are $B_1$ deficient. The infantile form has been reported at 2 to 7 months of age, following prolonged breast feeding by mothers who suffer from malnutrition. It has also been seen following feedings of improperly supplemented prepared formula, particularly some early soybean products.

**ETIOLOGY.** Thiamine, vitamin $B_1$, is indispensable in the human economy. It acts as a coenzyme in the conversion of pyruvic acid to acetaldehyde, one of the intermediate steps in the metabolism of carbohydrates. In the adult, withdrawal of thiamine from the diet produces symptoms within a week. $B_1$, however, seems to be actively transported across the placenta, and Slobody has reported that mean cord levels are twice maternal levels. This fact well may explain the rarity of congenital beriberi except in circumstances of extreme maternal deprivation.

Foman has recently suggested that the daily requirement of thiamine for infants is 0.2 mg per 1000 kcal per day. This amount is adequately supplied in cow's milk and in human milk as well. Human milk, however, is not rich in thiamine. In thiamine-deficient breast-feeding mothers, the relatively low margin of safety of $B_1$ supply to the infant may be inadequate over a period of months and may result in the appearance of infantile beriberi. Fehily has called attention to another possible form of vitamin $B_1$ deficiency in the breast-fed infant associated with the rapid onset of central nervous system depression, progressing to coma and death. She has suggested that this disease may be due to both inadequate intake of thiamine and to the accumulation of toxic by-products in the milk of deficient women.

**DIAGNOSIS.** Congenital beriberi presents within the first 3–4 days of life, usually within hours of birth. Rapid progression with congestive heart failure, convulsions and coma may be seen.

CASE 94–3

Van Gelder and Darby's case is one of the best-documented examples of neonatal beriberi. A mother had only mild edema and numbness and tingling of the hands and feet to show for her deficiency state. A 7 pound 5 ounce (3300 gm) infant was born after normal labor and delivery, but was cyanotic and needed resuscitation. For 3 hours he appeared well, but then again became blue. Examination revealed cyanosis, a few crackling rales at both bases behind, extreme tachycardia and an increased area of cardiac dullness. The liver edge was just palpable. X-ray study showed the heart to be very large (Fig. 94–1). Cyanotic spells recurred throughout the first day and were more frequent on the second. On this day the cry became feeble and hoarse. At 30 hours head retraction appeared, followed by convulsions and rigidity of the extremities. Without further diagnostic efforts, 50 mg of thiamine hydrochloride was given subcutaneously at 42 hours, and repeated at 50 hours. Convulsions and rigidity disappeared at 46 hours, but cyanosis persisted. By 62 hours improvement was dramatic. Thiamine was kept up, 50 mg every 8 hours, for 11 days. Heart rate and size steadily diminished. An electrocardiogram on the fourth day showed evidences of myocardial disease, but was normal after seven weeks.

Infantile beriberi, on the other hand, has an insidious onset. Symptoms of anorexia and lethargy are first noted at 2 to 3 months of age. Vomiting develops, and the infant may then rapidly deteriorate with congestive heart failure (misnamed the "pneumonic" phase). This is followed by a meningeal phase, with bulging fontanel, opisthotonos, coma and death. Cochrane has suggested that autopsy findings of degeneration of nerve cells and increased gliosis in pons, midbrain and medulla, with striking endothelial hyperplasia, may strongly support this diagnosis in the undernourished infant.

TREATMENT. As has been indicated, thiamine administration is the only therapeutic agent required. A dose of 10 mg every 6 to 8 hours should be sufficient. Supportive measures for the congestive heart failure should be provided. Seizures

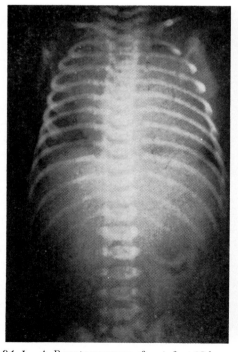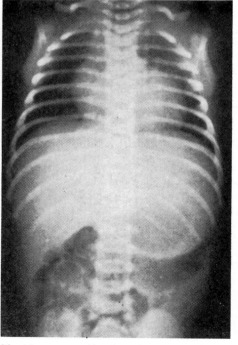

*Figure 94–1.* *A,* Roentgenogram of an infant 18 hours old with congenital beriberi, before thiamine therapy was instituted, showing an enlarged cardiac shadow. *B,* Roentgenogram of the child 11 days after administration of the first dose of thiamine, showing reduction in size of the cardiac shadow. (Van Gelder, D. W., and Darby, F. U.: J. Pediat. 25:226, 1944.)

in general respond promptly to thiamine administration without need of other anticonvulsant therapy. Clearly, the mother of the infant with either congenital beriberi or the infantile form secondary to breast feeding requires vitamin $B_1$ therapy as well.

## PYRIDOXINE DEFICIENCY AND DEPENDENCY

The active form of vitamin $B_6$ plays an important role as a coenzyme for a broad variety of reactions in amino acid, glycogen and short chain fatty acid metabolism. Clinical manifestations of body pool depletion of the coenzyme result in a clinically defined deficiency syndrome. Another form of $B_6$ "insufficiency" known as pyridoxine dependency is, however, of more immediate interest. In this form, the apoenzyme with which $B_6$ combines in its coenzyme function is modified so that unusually high concentrations of the coenzyme must be present to facilitate the enzymatic reaction and prevent either accumulations of substrate or deficiency of products of the reaction. As noted previously, $B_6$ acts broadly as a coenzyme and hence there are several forms of $B_6$ dependency.

**INCIDENCE.** True pyridoxine deficiency is extremely rare. It does not occur at birth but is a result of inadequate $B_6$ intake over the first months of life. In the early 1950's a modification in the processing of a particular prepared formula led to inactivation of the vitamin. This $B_6$ deficient formula resulted in an epidemic of seizures, which occurred at 6 weeks to 4 months of age in infants fed exclusively on this formula. The "epidemic" was elegantly reported by May. In general, and under normal conditions, both unprocessed cow's and human milk contain adequate amounts of the vitamin. It has been suggested, however, that breast-feeding by severely malnourished $B_6$ deficient mothers may result in a deficiency state in the infant. Both malabsorption and vitamin inhibition by drugs such as isoniazid and penicillamine have resulted in deficiency states in older children, but similar neonatal effects have not been noted.

The most common form of pyridoxine dependency in the neonatal period also presents with seizures, not unlike the deficiency syndrome. This form of vitamin dependency, however, is not due to a diminished transplacental or neonatal supply of the vitamin but rather to an increased vitamin requirement by specific individuals. More than 50 documented cases of pyridoxine dependent neonatal seizures have been reported from many parts of the world. As noted by Hunt in 1954, this abnormality of pyridoxine metabolism appears to be genetically determined and is inherited as an autosomal recessive. Other forms of $B_6$ dependency are associated with cystathioninuria, xanthurenicaciduria, homocystinuria and hyperoxaluria. All are hereditary. These forms have recently been reviewed by Scriver and Rosenberg and will not be discussed further.

**ETIOLOGY.** The naturally occurring forms of pyridoxine are widely distributed in nature in grains, meat and dairy products. These forms are converted in the body to pyridoxal-5'-phosphate, which, as noted previously, acts as a coenzyme for a broad variety of enzymatic reactions, particularly in amino acid metabolism. Heller and associates have noted the common occurrence of low pyridoxine levels in pregnant women. No abnormalities of maternal or fetal outcome, however, were found to correlate with low maternal $B_6$ levels. Brophy and Sriteri, however, reported low levels of pyridoxal phosphate in preeclamptic mothers, as well as evidence of decreased placenta transfer of the vitamin in these women. Contractor and Shane, and Brophy and Sriteri confirmed the low vitamin levels in pregnant women but noted that fetal cord blood levels at term were several times greater than maternal levels. These latter observations suggest active transport of the vitamin across the placenta and provide an explanation for absence of symptoms of the deficiency state in the immediate neonatal period. A group of premature infants studied by Reinken and Mangold, however, had low cord levels of pyridoxal-5'-phosphate at birth. These data may suggest that active transport of the vitamin occurs primarily late in pregnancy and that the premature infant may be at higher risk for development of the deficiency state.

In animals pyridoxine deficiency leads to

severe growth limitations, anemia, changes in skin and hair and seizures. In the infant, the major expression of either the deficiency or dependency state is seizures. It is felt that this manifestation is a result of decreased production of gamma-aminobutyric acid (GABA), a central nervous system inhibitory neurotransmitter. The active form of the vitamin appears to cocatalyze the conversion of glutamic acid to GABA with the apoenzyme glutamic acid decarboxylase. As noted by Schriver, deficiency of GABA predisposes the brain by hyperirritability and seizures. In the deficiency state, reduced amounts of the coenzyme pyridoxal-5′-phosphate are present. In the dependency state, the apoenzyme glutamic acid decarboxylase is altered so that markedly increased amounts of the coenzyme are required for the normal production of GABA. It is important to reemphasize that in the dependency state tissue vitamin levels are normal in the face of clinical symptoms. Why this particular enzyme system of all those affected by the vitamin seems to dominate the neonatal presentation of vitamin insufficiency is not known.

**DIAGNOSIS.** In May's original report of the 1953 deficiency "epidemic," extreme central nervous system irritability was the only early symptom of B₆ deficiency. As the degree of deficiency progressed, owing to lack of adequate vitamin intake, the onset of brief tonic-clonic seizures was noted at 1 to 4 months of age. Anemia and growth failure were not observed, although an earlier report by Snyderman et al. found both in retarded infants subjected to experimental vitamin deficiency. Rare subsequent reports of true deficiency states confirm seizures as the predominant clinical symptom.

In pyridoxine dependency, irritability and seizures are the sole symptoms. In the dependency state, however, seizures may start in utero, as reported by Bejsovec. In his report, 3 siblings appeared to have a severe form of the disease and all had intrauterine seizures beginning between the fifth and seventh month of gestation. It is interesting that in the third infant, seizures were controlled by high maternal doses of B₆.

In the majority of cases, however, seizures are noted in the first hours after delivery. The following case, described by Swaiman and Milstein, is typical.

CASE 94–4

The patient, a girl, was born at term and weighed 6 pounds, 10 ounces (3260 gm). The delivery was uncomplicated. There was no family history of seizures or neurologic disease. During her pregnancy, the mother did not receive supplemental pyridoxine.

The child appeared healthy until 3 hours of age, when she began having generalized major motor clonic seizures. The blood calcium was 8.5 mg per 100 ml, and blood sugar was 73 mg per 100 ml. The subdural space did not contain fluid, and the results of a spinal fluid examination were normal. Although the patient received phenobarbital, she had intermittent generalized seizures throughout the first day. The seizures gradually decreased in frequency during phenobarbital therapy, and by the seventh day of life, she no longer needed the drug. She was fed a commercial milk formula containing 0.3 mg pyridoxine per quart. No other vitamins were given.

At 17 days of age, the patient had another seizure, and daily phenobarbital therapy was resumed. She appeared overly sensitive to noise but otherwise was normal.

Subsequently, the patient had three generalized tonic major motor seizures. Administration of anticonvulsants, calcium and glucose failed to control the seizures, which continued intermittently for the next few days, until she received 100 mg of pyridoxine intramuscularly. The seizures stopped within an hour. Twitching began again 6 days later and was controlled with 10 mg of pyridoxine. She then remained seizure free on 25 mg of pyridoxine a day.

Occasionally, as in a case reported by Gentz, seizures may begin as late as 3 weeks of age, although some increase in muscle tone was noted earlier. In most cases, seizures have been brief and tonic-clonic in nature. An interesting feature is the inability of anticonvulsants to control this seizure disorder in contrast to the rapid control achieved by a single dose of 50 mg of pyridoxine. This feature has been considered of some diagnostic use. Frequently a single dose of pyridoxine is given to the neonate while in seizure in an early effort to rule out this diagnostic possibility. It has been widely suggested that this therapeutic trial is even more elegant when performed with EEG running. Control of seizures and reversion of EEG to normal within minutes after receiving the vitamin have been considered the ultimate in diagnostic orchestration. Iinuma and coworkers have tempered this approach slightly by suggesting that, although seizure control may be achieved rapidly, it may require up to 24 hours before the EEG returns to full normality.

Long-term followup of $B_6$ dependent children with seizures suggests normal development in those treated early and aggressively. Children whose diagnosis is delayed, with seizures persisting for weeks, or children who periodically experience inadequate $B_6$ supplements do not seem to fare as well.

The early onset and high continuing vitamin requirements should allow for clear differentiation of deficiency and dependency states. The tryptophan loading test, while normal in dependency states, results in an increase in xanthenurenic acid in true deficiency states. This is a result of the importance of $B_6$ as a coenzyme in the further breakdown of tryptophan and has been used to confirm the differentiation of these clinical entities.

**TREATMENT.** Prevention of the deficiency state requires only adequate vitamin $B_6$ supplementation. In general, 0.03 mg of pyridoxine a day is thought adequate for the neonate, and this amount is provided by proprietary formulas. Treatment of deficiency would simply require replenishment of the body pool and could be accomplished by daily 50 to 100 mg doses for several days.

Dependency states vary in vitamin $B_6$ requirements. In general, 25 to 100 mg of the vitamin are required daily to prevent irritability and seizures. This requirement apparently continues for life, although no long-term followup studies are available at present.

## VITAMIN C DEFICIENCY

Scurvy affects the newborn so rarely that a detailed discussion of the effects of vitamin C deficiency is not warranted. Of some interest, however, is the role of vitamin C in a form of transient tyrosinemia seen in premature infants.

**INCIDENCE.** Following the reports of Jackson and Park in 1935 and Ingalls in 1938 no subsequent cases of scurvy in the immediate neonatal period have been detailed. The first case, presented by Jackson and Park, was that of an infant born to a woman who in all probability also had the disease. This fact is of some interest following the report of Sherlock and Rothschild of scurvy appearing in a woman on a Zen macrobiotic diet. This diet has gained some popularity in certain health food circles and well may contribute subsequent neonatal cases to the literature.

**ETIOLOGY.** It appears that neonatal scurvy must be associated with maternal vitamin C deficiency. Vitamin C normally is transplacentally acquired by active transport, with fetal levels exceeding those of the mother. Whether preterm infants are more susceptible because of decreased transplacental acquisition of the vitamin is not known. Ingalls' three patients were all premature, but no concomitant description is given of maternal health. These infants were fed pooled breast milk, which is thought to contain enough ascorbic acid to prevent development of disease (43 mg per liter). It is interesting that cow's milk contains very little ascorbic acid and that the calf, unlike the human, can synthesize the vitamin. Man, apparently along with the Indian fruit bat and the guinea pig, has lost this ability. Although in this country all formula is now adequately supplemented with vitamin C, Grewar has had considerable experience with infants as young as 5 months who developed scurvy on diets made up exclusively of unfortified formula.

Ascorbic acid is essential for normal collagen synthesis by hydroxylation of proline as well as for normal function of osteoblasts and fibroblasts. In the preterm infant, interaction between ascorbic acid, protein intake and the enzymatic conversion of tyrosine to parahydroxyphenylpyruvic acid is of some importance. High protein intakes, over 5 gm per kilogram per day, lead to an accumulation of tyrosine which tends to inhibit its own enzymatic conversion. Ascorbic acid tends to reverse this inhibition and decrease serum and urine levels of tyrosine. This "neonatal tyrosinemia," as it was termed by Avery, appears to be a relatively common occurrence in premature infants

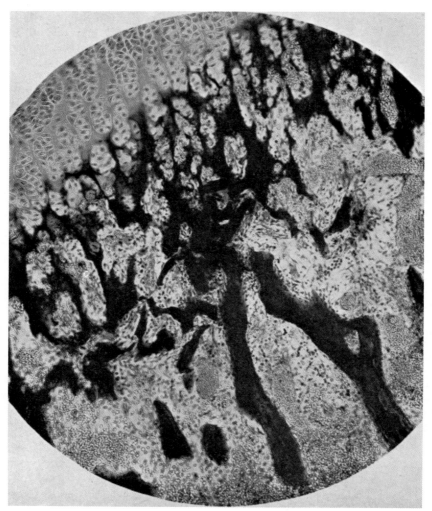

***Figure 94–2.***   Photomicrograph of histologic section from upper end of humerus to show typical scorbutic lesion. Above is the proliferative cartilage. The black network is the scorbutic lattice. Note how it is fractured. In the center the fragments are driven together into an impacted mass; to the left and right they lie crosswise, but appear to be free. To the histologist it is at once evident that the lattice is bare; i.e., no bone has formed on its surface. The supporting connective tissue of the marrow (*Gerüstmark*) is beautifully shown. Around the fragments of the lattice are osteoblasts. They surround the fragments loosely as swarms of bees surround the head of the person whom they are attacking. Under normal conditions they lie in orderly rows against the surfaces of the trabeculae. The blood vessels are full of red blood cells, but no hemorrhages are visible. (Jackson, D., and Park, E. A.: J. Pediatr., 7:741, 1935.)

and occurs occasionally in term infants fed high protein diets. The significance of the transient elevation of blood tyrosine and transient tyrosinuria, which tends to peak at the end of the first week of life, is not clear. In general, this form of vitamin C dependence is thought to be a transient developmental defect and of no long term

significance. Menkes and colleagues, however, have suggested that severe transient tyrosinemia may have some long term central nervous system residua. This subject and the differentiation of this entity from hereditary tyrosinemia have recently been reviewed by Scriver and Rosenberg.

**DIAGNOSIS.**   Because of its rarity, few

conclusions can be drawn regarding the clinical presentation of neonatal scurvy. Jackson and Park's infant presented only with weight loss and extreme irritability. Ingalls' patients were symptomatic. The classic signs of infantile scurvy, detailed by Grewar, of irritability, tenderness of lower limbs and weakness, as well as fever and gingival hemorrhages would be expected. Swelling of costochondral cartilages was prominent in his series. X-rays of the long bones show the characteristic findings of generalized osteoporosis, with thickening of the zone of provisional calcification, spur formation at the cartilage-shaft junction and subperiosteal hemorrhages. Caffey has noted the occasional difficulty in differentiating the radiographic picture of early scurvy from that seen in congenital syphilis. Neonatal copper deficiency may present a somewhat similar radiologic appearance (see p. 871).

**TREATMENT.** The recommended daily intake of ascorbic acid for neonates is 35 to 50 mg. In infants on high protein diets, as much as 100 mg per day may be required to cause reduction of elevated blood tyrosine levels. For the treatment of scurvy in infants, Grewar has recommended doses of vitamin C up to 1000 mg per day. By 5 days, improvement is seen and the dose may be reduced.

## VITAMIN D DEFICIENCY

The full spectrum of sequelae of fetal and neonatal vitamin D deficiency is still not clear. In 1930, Maxwell described classic rickets present at birth. Several recent reports have emphasized the appearance of rickets in small premature infants on inadequate vitamin D supplementation. Other reports have suggested that neonatal hypocalcemia with or without associated convulsions and late dental hypoplasia may as well be results of inadequate maternal or fetal vitamin D metabolism.

**INCIDENCE.** Certainly, florid rickets presenting in the neonatal period is extremely rare. Few cases have been added to Maxwell's original reports. Recently, however, Ford and co-workers, and Moncrieff and Fadahunsi have described congenital rickets in infants born of Asian immigrants with osteomalacia, and have suggested careful observation of this population. Interestingly enough, Maxwell's original cases were also infants of Asian mothers with a form of osteoporosis thought to represent nutritional rickets. Of perhaps more immediate interest is the report of Lewin and colleagues, who noted that almost all of their surviving infants who weighed less than 1000 grams at birth developed radiologic evidence of rickets at 2 to 3 months of life. These infants were not given supplemental vitamin D in addition to that supplied by commercial formula.

**ETIOLOGY.** Present knowledge suggests that vitamin D undergoes conversion to 25-hydroxyvitamin D in the liver, and a second subsequent hydroxylation to 1,25-hydroxyvitamin D in the kidney. This later metabolite appears to be the active form of the vitamin which is responsible for absorption of calcium from the gut and remodeling of bone. Vitamin D and 25-hydroxyvitamin D appear to cross the placenta by diffusion or facilitated diffusion according to Hillman and Haddad. Fetal and cord levels, therefore, reflect maternal serum levels. In the term infant following birth, levels are well maintained, whereas levels are low at birth and may fall over several weeks in premature infants with or without additional vitamin D supplementation (Hillman and Haddad). In the absence of adequate amounts of the active form of the vitamin, decreased calcium availability may occur. This may result in neonatal hypocalcemia, as noted by Rosen and co-workers, but certainly is not the only etiologic factor in this common disorder. Decreased calcium availability also leads to ineffective calcification of bone and teeth as a manifestation of vitamin D deficiency (Fig. 94–3).

**DIAGNOSIS.** At the present time, neonatal rickets is most often a purely radiologic diagnosis. Typical rarefaction and irregular fraying of the zone of provisional calcification of the radius and ulna, with some splaying of the metaphyses, is noted. Thickening of the costochondral junctions resulting in the "rachitic rosary" may be seen. Clinically, softening of cranial bones, craniotabes and fractures occur. Hypoplasia of dental enamel, particularly of incisors, may appear much later (Purvis and co-workers).

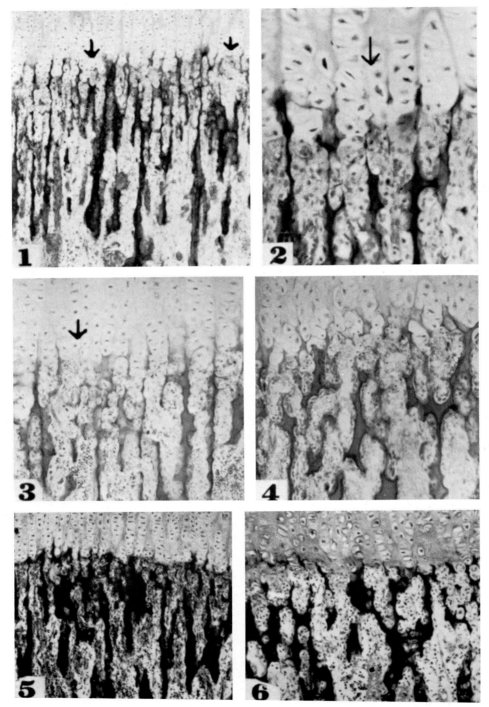

*Figure 94–3.    See legend on the opposite page.*

Biochemical alterations consist of low or normal serum calcium and phosphorus levels and high alkaline phosphatase levels. Vitamin D levels can be obtained. The association of some neonatal hypocalcemic seizures with vitamin D deficiency has been suggested by Roberts and colleagues. Whether or not this is a common event is unknown.

One of the cases summarized by Lewin and co-workers led to an unusual clinical presentation.

CASE 94–5

A girl born at 28 weeks' gestation and weighing 935 gm had moderate respiratory distress during the first 4 days of life. Recovery was uneventful. At the age of 2 months, she sustained a fracture of the shaft of the right radius; roentgenograms of knees and wrists showed moderately severe rickets. The serum calcium concentration was 9.8 mg per 100 ml and the phosphorus concentration was 4.6 mg per 100 ml. The alkaline phosphatase activity was 90 K.A. units per 100 ml. The intake of vitamin D during the first month of life had been 50 I.U. daily and was gradually increased to 200 I.U. daily by the end of the second month. Thus the average daily intake of vitamin D over the 2 month period was 103 I.U. Two weeks after starting vitamin D supplements, healing of bone lesions was observed.

**TREATMENT.** Vitamin D supplementation of infant formula is clearly the basis of both prevention and treatment. 400 I.U., the recommended daily requirement, appears to be adequate for both. In general, milk supplementation in the United States is based on the addition of 400 I.U. per quart. A small premature who may need less than 180 ml a day of formula to meet nutritional requirements will receive less than 80 I.U. of vitamin D a day. As detailed

by Lewin and co-workers and by Tulloch, this degree of supplementation may lead to the development of bony changes by 2 months of age. Thus, it is recommended that the preterm infant receive a full 400 I.U. of vitamin D daily regardless of size. It is interesting that Tulloch has suggested that the smallest infants may have increased daily requirements (800 I.U.), perhaps based on liver or renal enzymatic immaturity with regard to conversion of vitamin D to its active forms. Wolf et al. have made similar recommendations based on a comparison of alkaline phosphatase levels in premature infants given 500 or 1000 I.U. daily for the first 50 days of life. As yet this increased requirement has not been documented, although Hillman and Haddad noted little or no increase in the low serum levels of vitamin D in some premature infants given 400 I.U. daily either orally or intravenously over the first 5 to 6 weeks of life.

## VITAMIN E DEFICIENCY

The syndrome in the premature infant that we now recognize as Vitamin E deficiency was delineated as recently as the mid 1960's by Hassan, Oski, Ritchie and their respective co-workers. Prior to that time biochemical vitamin E deficiency, recognized for many years, was an interesting biochemical finding in search of a "disease" (see pp. 621 to 623).

**INCIDENCE.** Another disease of progress, clinical vitamin E deficiency probably does not occur in breast-fed infants. This is exclusively a disease of the small premature infant, and both the processing of cow's milk to create our current proprietary formula and the supplementation of this formula with iron have increased the risk of

---

*Figure 94–3. 1,* Rickets, acute, slight. Arrows indicate several areas in cartilaginous matrix between hypertrophic cells where disposition of inorganic materials is lacking (as indicated by failure to stain with hematoxylin). *2,* Rickets, acute, slight. Higher power to show area in matrix between several rows of hypertrophic cells where deposition of inorganic materials is faulty. *3,* Rickets, acute, slight. Focus of defective calcification in cartilage. *4,* Rickets, acute, moderate. Large focus of defective calcification in cartilage. *5,* Rickets, acute, severe. Except for a few areas there is virtual cessation of lime salt deposition in provisional zone of calcification. *6,* Rickets, acute, severe. Sudden and complete cessation of deposition of inorganic materials in areas of hypertrophic cells. The suddenness is evidenced by the adequacy (dark staining materials) beneath. (Follis, R. H., Park, E. A., and Jackson, D.: Bull. Johns Hopkins Hosp., *91:*480, 1952.)

clinical sequelae. In fact, in 1968 Ritchie's group noted some evidence of vitamin E responsive clinical or biochemical abnormalities in two thirds of the infants under 1500 grams that they investigated. This figure is undoubtedly high and perhaps has been reduced by alterations in infant formula since that time. Nevertheless, in dealing with small prematures one must continuously keep this clinical entity in mind.

**ETIOLOGY.** Vitamin E, a fat soluble vitamin (alpha tocopherol), crosses the placenta, but fetal serum levels are less than one fourth of those of the mother (Leonard et al., Mino et al.). Leonard has suggested that fetal levels change little during the course of pregnancy, although earlier studies by Dju and co-workers reported sharply reduced serum levels in the premature infant. After birth, vitamin E must be absorbed from the gastrointestinal tract. Term infants absorb the vitamin well, but premature infants have a marked reduction in absorption ability. Melhorn and Gross have demonstrated the postnatal maturation of E absorption, which in preterm infants tends to reach normal levels at about 40 post-conceptual weeks. Two other aspects of vitamin E absorption are of critical importance. Linoleic and other polyunsaturated fatty acids (PUFA) common in the vegetable oils, which are used to supplement many commercial formulas, decrease vitamin E absorption. Thus, as the amount of PUFA in the diet increases, the amount of vitamin E required to maintain an adequate serum level also increases. This has recently been documented by Williams et al. Breast milk, which is low in PUFA, has a high E/PUFA ratio and hence is ideal to promote vitamin E absorption. E/PUFA ratios greater than 0.6 are thought adequate for vitamin E absorption. In this regard, the advantages of breast milk have been clearly demonstrated by Lo and colleagues.

Melhorn and Gross have documented the ability of dietary iron supplements to block vitamin E absorption and increase hemolysis. The mechanism of this iron effect is not clear but is thought to be associated with the ability of iron to catalyze the non-enzymatic auto-oxidation of unsaturated fatty acids. Gross and Melhorn have recently suggested that this iron effect may not be a problem when using new water soluble vitamin E preparations.

The small premature infant then, in whom poor vitamin E absorption is aggravated by a diet high in PUFA and by the presence of supplemental iron, is at high risk for subsequent vitamin E deficiency. Cord levels of vitamin E tend to be in the range of 0.2 to 0.3 mg per 100 ml, a level below the 0.5 mg per 100 ml thought to be associated with metabolic defects. Normal levels are achieved in the term infant within 2 weeks but in the premature without appropriate E supplementation, levels may continue to fall over the first 6 to 8 weeks.

Although muscle necrosis and sterility may be seen in vitamin E deficient experimental animals and in severe vitamin E deficiency associated with prolonged steatorrhea outside of the neonatal period, the major effect of vitamin E deficiency in the neonate seems to be on red cell membrane stability. It is well known that the tocopherols are antioxidants, and it has been assumed that vitamin E contributes to stability of RBC membrane by preventing oxidation of lipids and sulfhydryl groups (Jacobs and Lux).

More recent work has suggested that vitamin E-selenium complexing may be an important step in stabilizing the red cell membrane. Regardless of mechanism, the vitamin E deficient red cell is subject to in vivo hemolysis and to hydrogen peroxide stimulated hemolysis in vitro.

**DIAGNOSIS.** The classic work of Oski and Barnes established the association of vitamin E deficiency and hemolytic anemia in the premature infant. In their cases the diagnosis was made between 6 and 8 weeks of age. Anemia accompanied by a mild reticulocytosis and pyknocytosis was found to correlate with low serum tocopheral levels. Red cell survival was significantly shortened to a half life of 11 to 15 days. No other clinical signs were observed, and the anemia responded promptly to vitamin E administration. Ritchie and co-workers, following the earlier work of Hassan's group, noted similar hematologic findings. In addition, they observed thrombocytosis with platelet counts as high as 600,000 per cubic milliliter. They also found that the patients often had subcutaneous edema of the legs and genitalia with puffiness of the eyelids. Serum proteins and electrolytes were normal. Occasionally, a papular erythematous rash was present. All findings disappeared within 2 to 3 weeks following vitamin E administration.

A major problem is the differentiation of this mild hemolytic anemia from the physiologic anemia of prematurity. The mild elevation of the reticulocyte count (5 to 8 per cent) in the face of a continuing fall in hemoglobin has been suggested by Dallman to be a helpful differentiating feature. The appearance of pyknocytes and thrombocytosis may also be useful. Vitamin E levels may be obtained, and serum levels less than 0.5 mg per 100 ml are considered low. The peroxide hemolysis test after the first 2 weeks of life is helpful. The increase in hemolysis seems to correlate well with the degree of E deficiency, although the test is not entirely specific for this vitamin effect. A normal peroxide hemolysis test, however, would make vitamin E deficiency very unlikely.

**TREATMENT.** When vitamin E deficiency has been demonstrated, treatment with 75 to 100 I.U. of alpha-tocopherol daily should be instituted. A response is seen within 2 weeks in the hematologic indices. Improved RBC survival and a decrease in peroxide hemolysis are seen within a few days. After a week the dose of alpha-tocopherol may be reduced to maintenance levels.

Most standard formulas contain 10 to 13 I.U. per Liter of alpha-tocopherol and have an adequate E/PUFA ratio. This appears to be adequate supplementation for prevention of E deficiency in most infants over 2000 grams. Smaller infants, especially those on iron supplementation, require higher doses of vitamin E, in the range of 15 to 25 I.U. daily. Recently Gross and Melhorn have presented data showing more effective absorption of a water soluble form of the vitamin, which at 25 I.U. daily achieved "sufficient" serum levels and prevented clinical evidence of deficiency in all infants studied.

## VITAMIN K DEFICIENCY

Without parenteral vitamin K supplementation to the newborn or parturient mother, vitamin K deficiency would rank as the most common deficiency syndrome of all. This disorder and its pathogenesis have been discussed in an earlier section and will not be reconsidered here (pp. 573 to 574).

## TRACE MINERAL DEFICIENCIES

A great deal of new information on the metabolic role of trace minerals has become available in the last few years. Particular attention has been focused on copper, zinc and chromium and their relationship to human disease. At the present time only copper deficiency has been recognized in the neonatal period.

## COPPER DEFICIENCY

Following reports of metabolic sequelae in copper deficient animals, a clinical syndrome associated with low serum levels of copper has been recognized in infants.

**INCIDENCE.** This entity seems to occur particularly in the small premature infant. It is interesting that two of the three cases of copper deficiency reported by Griscom and co-workers occurred in severely undergrown members of premature twin pregnancies. Small prematures maintained for prolonged periods on parenteral alimentation following bowel surgery also appear to be at risk. Clinical findings have not been reported prior to 2 months of age.

Danks and co-workers have suggested that Menkes' kinky hair syndrome, a sex linked metabolic disease, may also be a manifestation of copper deficiency secondary to a defect in intestinal copper absorption. In this form, deficiency symptoms have been noted in the first month of life.

**ETIOLOGY.** Copper is an essential nutrient combining with a number of proteins in the body. Copper-containing enzymes such as cytochrome oxidase are required for cellular respiration. The precise mechanism by which copper deficiency results in its characteristic symptoms, however, is unknown.

During fetal life, copper seems to be concentrated in the fetal liver. Levels are very high, exceeding those of the adult after 20 weeks' gestation (Widdowson et al.). Deficiency after birth appears to be the result of very low postnatal copper intake coupled with prematurity. In the premature, although hepatic copper concentrations may be high initially, the total amount of the element available during the period of rapid neonatal growth may be inadequate.

**DIAGNOSIS.** A sideroblastic anemia, neutropenia and bone abnormalities are among the most commonly reported findings in neonatal copper deficiency. This patient reported by Griscom and coworkers is typical.

**CASE 94–6**

This infant was a 680 gram member of a twin pair, born at 31 weeks gestation. Initial hospital course was uneventful without any respiratory distress. At 66 days of age, irritability and a low grade fever developed. A chest film showed irregularity of aeration with a distribution suggestive of aspiration. Healing fractures of the anterolateral portions of many ribs were evident; this led to a skeletal survey which showed separation of the left proximal humeral epiphyseal cartilage, severe systemic osteoporosis, poorly mineralized subperiosteal new bone along the shafts of the long bones, enlargement of the costochondral cartilages and metaphyseal cupping. The hematocrit was 17 per cent with a 1.3 per cent reticulocyte count. Neutropenia was noted. Vitamin intake, particularly of vitamins C and D, was adequate. At 71 days of age, the infant suffered a cardiorespiratory arrest. Pathological examination of the bones was compatible with copper deficiency, and a measurement of liver copper content was very low.

Bone lesions, as noted above, may include rib fractures and beading of costochondral cartilages. Osteoporosis, metaphyseal cupping and irregularities, epiphyseal separations and periosteal new bone formation may be seen. At times these findings may mimic those seen in scurvy.

Diagnosis is based on finding low serum copper levels and low serum ceruloplasmin. The reticulocyte response to copper administration should be rapid. Disappearance of the bone lesions and neutropenia should follow within 2 weeks. Serum, calcium, phosphorous and alkaline phosphatase levels should be normal.

**TREATMENT.** Ashkenazi and associates have recommended a dietary intake of copper between 100 and 500 $\mu$g per day. Their

treatment program for older infants with full blown deficiency states consisted of 1 to 3 mg of oral copper sulfate for several days, followed by maintenance dietary copper. In Menkes' syndrome, because of the defect in copper absorption, high daily oral doses of copper must be used.

## REFERENCES

Ashkenazi, A., Levin, S., et al.: The syndrome of neonatal copper deficiency. Pediatrics 52:525, 1973.
Avery, M. E., Clow, C. L., et al.: Transient tyrosinemia of the newborn: Dietary and clinical aspects. Pediatrics 39:378, 1967.
Bass, M. H., and Fisch, G. R.: Increased intracranial pressure with bulging fontanel. Neurology 11:1091, 1961.
Bejsovec, M., Kulenda, Z., and Ponca, E.: Familial intrauterine convulsions in pyridoxine dependency. Arch. Dis. Child. 42:201, 1967.
Bernhardt, I. B., and Dorsey, D. J.: Hypervitaminosis A and congenital renal anomalies in a human infant. Obstet. Gynecol. 43:750, 1974.
Brophy, M. H., and Siiteri, P. K.: Pyridoxal phosphate and hypertensive disorders of pregnancy. Am. J. Obstet. Gynecol. 121:1075, 1975.
Caffey, J.: Pediatric X-ray Diagnosis. 6th ed., Chicago, Year Book Medical Publishers, 1972, pp. 1237–1243.
Cochrane, W. A., Collins-Williams, C., and Donohue, W. L.: Superior hemorrhagic polioencephalitis occurring in an infant—probably due to thiamine deficiency from use of a soybean product. Pediatrics 28:771, 1961.
Contractor, S. F., and Shane, B.: Blood and urine levels of vitamin B$_6$ in the mother and fetus before and after loading of the mother with vitamin B$_6$. Am. J. Obstet. Gynecol. 107:635, 1970.
Dallman, P. R.: Iron, vitamin E and folate in the preterm infant. Pediatrics 85:742, 1974.
Danks, D. M., Campbell, P. E., et al.: Menkes' kinky hair syndrome. Pediatrics 50:188, 1972.
Dju, M. Y. et al.: Vitamin E (tocopherol) in human fetuses and placentae. Etud. Neonat. 1:1, 1952.
Fehily, L.: Human milk intoxication due to B$_1$ avitaminosis. Br. Med. J. 2:590, 1944.
Fomon, S. J.: Infant Nutrition. 2nd ed. Philadelphia, W. B. Saunders Company, 1974.
Ford, J. A., Davidson, D. C., et al.: Neonatal rickets in Asian immigrant population. Br. Med. J. 3:211, 1973.
Gal, I., and Parkinson, C. E.: Variations in the pattern of maternal serum vitamin A and carotenoids during human reproduction. Int. J. Vitamin Nutr. Res. 42:565, 1972.
Gentz, J., Hemfelt, S., et al.: Vitamin B metabolism in pyridoxine dependency with seizures. Acta Pediat. Scand. 56:17, 1967.
Grewar, D.: Infantile scurvy. Clin. Pediatr. 4:82, 1965.
Griscom, N. T., Craig, J. N., and Neuhauser, E. B. D.: Systemic bone disease developing in small premature infants. Pediatrics 48:883, 1971.
Gross, S., and Melhorn, D. K.: Vitamin E-dependent

anemia in the premature infant. III. Comparative hemoglobin, vitamin E and erythrocyte phospholipid responses following absorption of either water-soluble or fat-soluble d-alpha tocopheryl. J. Pediatr. 85:753, 1974.

Hassan, H., Hashim, S. A., et al.: Syndrome in premature infants associated with low plasma vitamin E levels and high polyunsaturated fatty acid diet. Am. J. Clin. Nutr. 19:147, 1966.

Heller, S., Salkeld, R. M., and Körner, W. F.: Vitamin $B_6$ status in pregnancy. Am. J. Clin. Nutr. 26:1339, 1973.

Henley, T. H., Dann, M., and Golden, W. R. C.: Reserves, absorption and plasma levels of vitamin A in premature infants. Am. J. Dis. Child. 68:257, 1944.

Hillman, L. S., and Haddad, J. G.: Human perinatal vitamin D metabolism. I.: 25-hydroxyvitamin D in maternal and cord blood. J. Pediatr. 84:742, 1974.

Hillman, L. S., and Haddad, J. G.: Perinatal vitamin D metabolism. J. Pediatr. 86:928, 1975.

Hunt, A. D., Stokes, J., Jr., et al.: Pyridoxine dependency: Report of a case of intractable convulsions in an infant controlled by pyridoxine. Pediatrics 13:140, 1954.

Iinuma, K., Narisawa, K., et al.: Pyridoxine dependent convulsion: Effect of pyridoxine therapy on electroencephalograms. Tohoku J. Exp. Med. 105:19, 1971.

Ingalls, T. H.: Ascorbic acid requirements in early infancy. N. Engl. J. Med. 218:872, 1938.

Jackson, D., and Park, E. A.: Congenital scurvy: A case report. J. Pediatr. 7:741, 1935.

Jacob, H. S., and Lux, S. E.: Degradation of membrane phospholipids and thiols in peroxide hemolysis: Studies in vitamin E deficiency. Blood 32:549, 1968.

Keating, J. P., and Fergin, R. D.: Increased intracranial pressure associated with probable vitamin A deficiency in cystic fibrosis. Pediatrics 46:41, 1970.

Knudson, A. G., Jr., and Rothman, P. E.: Hypervitaminosis A. Am. J. Dis. Child. 85:316, 1953.

Leonard, P. J., Doyle, E., and Harrington, W.: Levels of vitamin E in the plasma of newborn infants and of the mothers. Am. J. Clin. Nutr. 25:480, 1972.

Lewin, P. K., Reid, M., et al.: Iatrogenic rickets in low birth weight infants. J. Pediatr. 78:207, 1971.

Lo, S. S., Frank, D., and Hitzig, W. H.: Vitamin E and haemolytic anaemia in premature infants. Arch. Dis. Child. 48:360, 1973.

Marie, J. and Sée, G.: Hydrocephalic aigüe bénigne de nourisson après ingestion d'une dose massive unique, de vitamines A et D. Sem. Hôp. Paris 27:1744, 1951.

Maxwell, J. P., Hu, C. H., and Turnbull, H. M.: Foetal rickets. J. Path. Bacteriol. 35:419, 1932.

Maxwell, J. P.: Two cases of foetal rickets. J. Path. Bacteriol. 33:327, 1930.

May, C. D., et al.: Clinical studies of vitamin A in infants and in children. Am. J. Dis. Child. 59:1167, 1940.

May, C. D.: Vitamin $B_6$ in human nutrition: A critique and an object lesson. Pediatrics 14:269, 1954.

Melhorn, D. K., and Gross, S.: Vitamin E-dependent anemia in the premature infant. I. Effects of large doses of medicinal iron. J. Pediatr. 79:569, 1971.

Melhorn, D. K., and Gross, S.: Vitamin E-dependent anemia in the premature infant. II. Relationships between gestational age and absorption of vitamin E. J. Pediatr. 79:581, 1971.

Menkes, J. H., Welcher, D. W., et al.: Relationship of elevated blood tyrosine to ultimate intellectual performance of premature infants. Pediatrics 49:218, 1972.

Mino, M., and Nishino, H.: Fetal and maternal relationship in serum vitamin E level. J. Nutr. Sci. Vitaminol. 19:475, 1973.

Moncrieff, M., and Fadahunsi, T. O.: Congenital rickets due to maternal vitamin D deficiency. Arch. Dis. Child. 49:810, 1974.

Oski, F. A., and Barness, L. A.: Vitamin E deficiency: A previously unrecognized cause of hemolytic anemia in the premature infant. J. Pediatr. 70:211, 1967.

Purvis, R. J., Barrie, W. J., et al.: Enamel hypoplasia of the teeth associated with neonatal tetany: A manifestation of maternal vitamin D deficiency. Lancet 2:811, 1973.

Reinken, L., and Mangold, B.: Pyridoxal phosphate values in premature infants. Int. J. Vitam. Nutr. Res. 43:472, 1973.

Ritchie, J. H., Fish, M. B., et al.: Edema and hemolytic anemia in premature infants. N. Engl. J. Med. 279:1185, 1968.

Roberts, S. A., Cohen, M. D., and Forfar, J. O.: Antenatal factors associated with neonatal hypocalcaemic convulsions. Lancet 2:809, 1973.

Rosen, J. F., Roginsky, M., et al.: 25-Hydroxyvitamin D plasma levels in mothers and their premature infants with neonatal hypocalcemia. Am. J. Dis. Child. 127:220, 1974.

Scriver, C. R.: Vitamin $B_6$ deficiency and dependency in man. Am. J. Dis. Child. 113:109, 1967.

Scriver, C. R., and Rosenburg, L. E.: Amino Acid Metabolism and Its Disorders. Philadelphia, W. B. Saunders Co., 1973.

Sherlock, P., and Rothschild, O.: Scurvy produced by a Zen macrobiotic diet. J.A.M.A. 199:130, 1967.

Slobody, L. B., Willner, M. M., and Mestern, J.: Comparison of vitamin B levels in mothers and their newborn infants. Am. J. Dis. Child. 77:736, 1949.

Snyderman, S. W., Carretero, R., and Holt, E., Jr.: Pyridoxine deficiency in the human being. Fed. Proceed. 9:371, 1950.

Swaiman, K., and Milstein, J.: Pyridoxine dependency and penicillamine. Neurology 20:78, 1970.

Tulloch, A. L.: Rickets in the premature. Med. J. Australia 1:137, 1974.

Van Gelder, D. W., and Darby, F. U.: Congenital and infantile beriberi. J. Pediatr. 25:226, 1944.

Widdowson, E. M., Chan, H., et al.: Accumulation of Cu, Zn, Mn, Cr, and Co in the human liver before birth. Biol. Neonate 20:360, 1972.

Williams, M. L., Shott, R. J., et al.: Role of dietary iron and fat on vitamin E deficiency anemia of infancy. N. Engl. J. Med. 292:887, 1975.

Wolf, H., et al.: Der Bedarf an Vitamin D und an 25-Hydroxycholecalciferol bei frühgeborenen Kindern während der ersten Lebenszeit. Klinische Pädiatrie 187:331, 1975.

# XIII

# Disorders of the Skeletal System

We have discussed in prior sections some of the disorders of the skeletal system. Craniostenosis, microcephaly, encephalocele, myelocele and others will be found among disorders of the head and spine (p. 683 ff.), while osteomyelitis appears under infections (p. 788). Infantile cortical hyperostosis has been relegated to a subgroup entitled Disorders of Uncertain Origin (p. 835). Rickets and scurvy are to be found among the vitamin deficiency diseases (pp. 867, 865). There remains a miscellaneous group of disorders some of which involve bone alone, some joints alone, while in the remainder bone and other tissues are affected.

# 95

# THE FIRST ARCH SYNDROME, CLEFT LIP AND CLEFT PALATE

*Revised by F. Clarke Fraser*

Cleft palate and harelip have been recognized from earliest historic times. The clinical features of mandibulofacial dysostosis were first described by Treacher Collins in 1900. Pierre Robin later lumped together hypoplasia of the mandible, glossoptosis and cleft palate into a syndrome which bears his name. Modern students of these defects in the development of facial bones have become more and more inclined to consider them variable manifestations of one basic developmental error. McKenzie groups them all under the all-inclusive title of "the first arch syndrome," although the second branchial arch and temporal bone primordia are also involved in the developmental disturbance.

**INCIDENCE.** Although each member of the group is comparatively rare, their sum total is not inconsiderable.

**ETIOLOGY AND PATHOGENESIS.** Earlier observers recognized that the defects in this disorder were the results of "an inhibitory process occurring toward the seventh week of embryonic life and affecting the facial bones derived from the first visceral arch" (Mann and Kilner). Hövels graded the cases recorded up to 1953 and found a serial progression of involvement, from simple obliquity of the ocular fissures up to the most extensive facial hypoplasias, including complete agnathia. McKenzie believes that the origin of these defects can be ascribed to faulty vascularization, primarily of the first branchial arch, and to a lesser degree of the second arch. His view is supported by the experimental and clinical evidence of Poswillo and others that the basic defect can be hematoma formation during the anastomosis which precedes the formation of the stapedial arterial stem.

The first and second branchial arch syndromes involve an array of defects that are usually unilateral and include underde-velopment of the external ear, the middle ear ossicles, the condyle and ramus of the mandible, the zygomatic arch, the malar bone and often the temporal bone except for the petrous portion housing the inner ear. A group of syndromes share these features. Some are sufficiently different in the spectrum of defects displayed and in their genetic pattern to be considered separate entities; these include the Goldenhar, Treacher Collins and Hallermann-Streiff syndromes. The term "first (and second) arch syndrome" is best reserved for cases that are non-familial, usually unilateral and confined to the aural, oral and mandibular defects mentioned above.

## MANDIBULOFACIAL DYSOSTOSIS (TREACHER COLLINS SYNDROME)

**ETIOLOGY.** The basic developmental defect is unknown, but seems unlikely to result from post-hemorrhagic necrosis, as in the first arch syndrome. The inheritance is autosomal dominant, but with reduced penetrance and variable expressivity. About 60 per cent of cases are sporadic, and presumably fresh mutations, but near relatives should be examined carefully for minor signs of the syndrome before assuming that a patient is a sporadic case.

**DIAGNOSIS.** A fully developed mandibulofacial dysostosis includes defective eyes, ears and mandible. The ocular fissures are slanted downward from within out. There is a notch at the junction of the outer and middle thirds of the lower eyelid, and from this point the lid angles sharply upward toward the outer canthus. Eyelashes are absent or sparse in the outer two thirds of the lower lids. The mandible is small, the chin receding, the degree of overbite considerable. There is great variability in the amount of micrognathia. The zygomatic bones are often hypoplastic. The ears may be malformed in a number of different ways: the auricles either hypoplastic or large, floppy and low-set (Fig. 95–1), the external meatus stenotic or atretic, with skin tags, fistulas or flame-shaped areas of hypertrichosis between the tragus and the corner of the mouth. Associated defects such as high-arched palate, choanal atresia and others are occasionally present. Mental deficiency is not a feature of the syndrome.

Diagnosis may be obvious at a glance, or attention may be called to the infant by the nurse's report that it has considerable difficulty in sucking and swallowing. She may also note that there appears to be excessive mucus in the mouth and pharynx. Intermittent spells of cyanosis, as in the Pierre Robin syndrome, are not infrequent.

The differential diagnosis includes Goldenhar syndrome (oculo-auriculovertebral dysplasia), which is rarely familial, almost always unilateral, has notching of the upper rather than the lower lid, and epibulbar dermoids. Hemifacial microsomia (unilateral microtia, macrostomia and failure of the mandibular ramus and condyles to form) may be a variant of this, although it is more characteristic of the first arch syndrome.

**TREATMENT.** The first problems may be those concerned with feeding difficulties and the intermittent cyanosis and respiratory distress associated with micrognathia and glossoptosis. When this is overcome, one should look carefully into the matter of hearing disability. If any is present, the appropriate steps should be taken early. These may involve surgical correction of an atretic or stenotic external auditory meatus or the use of a hearing aid, and will surely call for special education. Finally, plastic surgery may be indicated to improve the child's appearance.

## MICROGNATHIA AND THE PIERRE ROBIN SYNDROME

Hypoplasia of the mandible, micrognathus, or micrognathia, is encountered in a few infants as a solitary defect. More often it is part of a group of signs which, described first by Robin as a clinical entity, has since borne his name. The Robin triad of micrognathia, cleft palate and glossoptosis leads to retraction of the sternum, cyanosis and malnutrition.

Micrognathia is also one of the numerous congenital anomalies that combine to make up the trisomy 18 (E, 16–18) syndrome (see p. 917).

**ETIOLOGY.** As mentioned above, some students of the problem believe the Robin

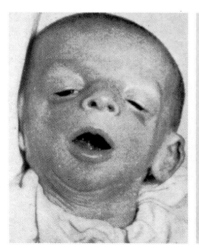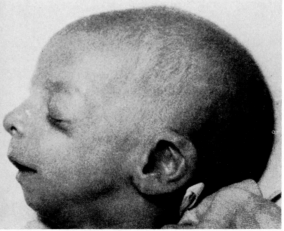

*Figure 95–1.* Typical Treacher Collins syndrome, or mandibulofacial dysostosis. *A,* Anterior view of the face shows the characteristic slanting, downward from within outward, of the lid slits. Also characteristic is the notching at the junction of the middle and outer thirds of the lower eyelid and the sharp angulation of the lid at that point. *B,* Lateral view, showing the receding jaw and the low-set, soft, slightly deformed external ear. (This example is one of those reported by McKenzie and Craig: Arch. Dis. Child., *30:*391, 1955. Photograph reproduced with the permission of the senior author.)

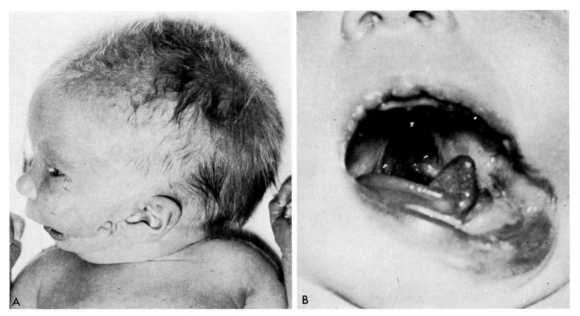

***Figure 95–2.*** *A*, Lateral view of face shows low-set malpositioned ear and extreme degree of micrognathia. In addition, a linear skin defect including several accessory skin tags runs from the ear to the corner of the mouth. *B*, With the mouth open one can see a large midline cleft in the posterior half of the palate. This combination of defects is more than is to be expected in the Treacher Collins syndrome or the Pierre Robin syndrome. It represents a more complicated error in development of the first visceral arch. This example was culled from the files of the Harriet Lane Home.

syndrome to be one manifestation of faulty development of the first branchial arch. Pruzansky and Richmond call attention to an older theory, which points out that mandibular micrognathia is a physiologic phenomenon in early intrauterine life and that at this time the tongue blocks the pharyngeal spaces and occupies part of the nasal cavity. If for some reason micrognathia persists, the tongue cannot fall out of the nasal cavity. Its presence there may prevent the palate from fusing, and cleft palate results.

Most cases are sporadic. Most of the reported familial cases appear to represent cases of the Stickler syndrome, which may also account for the reported association with eye problems (severe myopia, retinal detachment). Thus the family history, in cases of the Robin syndrome, should include inquiry into the presence in near relatives of joint problems, eye problems and deafness.

**DIAGNOSIS.** The pediatrician has not the equipment needed to make precise anthropometric measurements, nor are these necessary in order to arrive at a diagnosis of isolated micrognathia. A mandible which is so small that it imparts to its owner a "bird face" or, as Dennison prefers to call it, a "shrew face" cannot be overlooked. Lesser degrees of micrognathia need not cause concern unless bouts of cyanosis, due to glossoptosis, occur. In this event lateral x-ray films of the skull should suffice to show whether the tongue is displaced posteriorly and upward enough to encroach upon the airway. The severer grades lead to noisy, difficult breathing, and may indeed cause death. If not, it is apt to produce sternal cupping (pectus excavatum) and the Harrison's groove deformity of the lower ribs. There may also be such difficulty in swallowing that high degrees of malnutrition ensue, which may also be responsible for death. If cleft palate is associated, the Robin syndrome is complete. Associated congenital heart disease is not uncommon. Indeed heart failure without congenital defect has also been reported

(Jeresaty et al.). In this case failure, with cor pulmonale and pulmonary edema, resulted from the severe respiratory obstruction, similar in all respects to that which follows the hypoxia caused by hypertrophied tonsils and adenoids.

TREATMENT. Robin himself thought that postural treatment, so-called orthostatic nursing, sufficed in most cases. The infant was to be fed while lying on his abdomen with his chest elevated by a small pillow. The upward and outward reaching for the bottle which this position entailed would hasten the mandible's forward growth. At the outset, if respiratory distress is severe, tube feeding is useful and may have to be continued for several weeks. Some babies do not tolerate this well, and for them gastrostomy may be indicated.

Headgears have been devised which grasp the rami and exert a steady forward pull upon the lower jaw. Other traction devices have been advocated, one going so far as to thread a wire through the chin and attach it to pulley and weights.

The most widely accepted approach now concentrates upon the problem of preventing the tongue from falling backward to the point where it impedes respiration, by stitching its raw undersurface to the raw inner surface of the lower jaw. If cyanotic spells can be forestalled in this manner, and nutrition maintained, the mandible will in a few months grow sufficiently to accommodate the tongue in its proper position. The studies of Pruzansky and Richmond have made this fact clear. They have also emphasized the point that in severe cases in which cyanosis is persistent or in which severe cyanotic spells occur frequently one should not wait too long before resorting to tracheotomy.

Goldberg and Eckblom raise valid objections to the procedure of stitching the tongue to the lower lip and advocate a new and interesting therapeutic approach. They recommend placing a suture in the tongue, tying its ends to a rubber band, carrying this forward over a dowel over the end of the bassinet and fastening a weight to its end to supply gentle traction. During this first phase, feedings are carried out by gavage. At the end of 1 or 2 weeks the suture may be removed, and the tongue will remain forward. Then the infant may be fed by bottle with the aid of a palatine obturator; that is, a false palate, made of acrylic. This is continued as long as necessary.

## HARELIP

Harelip or cleft lip represents a failure of proper merging and fusion of the facial swellings that form the upper lip. The cleft may be no larger than a barely perceptible dent in the vermilion border or it may extend into the nostril; it may be unilateral or bilateral or midline. Most often it is unilateral and left-sided. It may or may not be associated with cleft palate; if it is, the palate defect appears to be a secondary consequence of the developmental disturbance resulting from the failure of lip closure. Other congenital defects may coexist. Additional congenital deformities need not, however, be confined to this area.

ETIOLOGY. Harelip, with or without cleft palate, occurs 40 times as often in siblings and children of the affected individual as in the general population; that is, in about 4 per cent. Its incidence is seven times the expected in aunts, uncles, nieces and nephews, and about three times the expected in first cousins (Carter). The risk for other malformations is not increased unless a genetic syndrome is involved.

It occurs in about 0.1 per cent of all births, and nearly twice as often in males as in females.

There are now over 50 recognized syndromes that include harelip or cleft palate, or both. Approximately 60 per cent are manifestations of mutant genes and the remainder do not seem to be familial. Although the deformity can be produced experimentally in animals by maternal dietary deficiencies, as well as by teratogens, only a few instances in humans can be related to agents such as thalidomide or rubella. Others in the non-familial groups are associated with chromosomal aberrations, notably D trisomy. The majority of cases of cleft lip or palate can be attributed to the interaction of several genes and several environmental factors.

DIAGNOSIS. This presents no difficulty.

TREATMENT. Cleft lips may be operatively repaired as soon as the surgeon desires. One need wait only until the initial weight loss has been regained and the nutritional state is satisfactory. Seldom does uncomplicated cleft lip, even if bilateral, cause any difficulty in feeding, except possibly in the immediate postoperative period.

## CLEFT PALATE

Imperfect closure of the palate, as of the lip, may vary from simple cleavage of the uvula and soft palate up to the most grotesque and serious malformations. Palatal clefts may be single and midline and unassociated with harelip. At their worst they are double clefts running from the soft palate forward to either side of the nose, continuous with widely spread cleft lip on each side, leaving the isolated intermaxillary process and the nose projecting upward between gaping slits in the face. As with cleft lip, other congenital defects often coexist.

**ETIOLOGY.** As with cleft lip, some cases are associated with syndromes that may result from mutant genes or chromosomal aberrations; a minority are caused by environmental insults, and most have a multifactorial basis. However, the genetic basis for isolated cleft palate appears to be different from that for cleft lip. Thus the sibs of a child with cleft palate have an increased risk of having a cleft palate (but not a cleft lip), whereas the sibs of a child with cleft lip have an increased risk of having a cleft lip (with or without cleft palate), but not of having an isolated cleft palate.

**TREATMENT.** The pediatrician's most important task when confronted with a newborn with a severe form of this disorder is to comfort the parents and relatives and to reassure them, no matter how dreadful the situation seems to be at that moment, that with clever plastic surgery a fairly good result can be anticipated. They must be told, not all at once, that a number of operations will have to be done, that feeding will present some difficulties, that speech training will be required and that excellent dentistry and orthodontia will be needed. In most medical centers teams of specialists in these various fields collaborate in supervising the child's progress; the final, and a very important, member of the team is a child psychiatrist. Through his efforts not only the child, but also the parents, will be assisted in surmounting

the distressing years of reconstruction. In smaller communities — and often in large cities — the pediatrician has to undertake this function.

Whenever we are confronted with this situation, we think, with intense satisfaction, of a 23-year-old young lady, formerly in our practice. She was a dreadful looking newborn who had, in addition to complete double cleft lip and palate, a tetralogy of Fallot. Now, after a Blalock-Taussig bypass operation and a second shunting procedure, and eight or 10 lip and palate repairs, she is pretty, animated, bright and well adjusted. Her lip scars are visible, but not deforming; her speech, which was imperfect and nasal a few years ago, is now almost perfect. Her surgeons deserve much credit, but her mother and grandmother deserve the lioness' share.

When the palatal malformation is severe, orthodontic appliances may be helpful in promoting improved alignment. They may be inserted during the first days of life (Oliver). Feeding has in our experience not been too difficult. In spite of their inability to create suction, these infants feed sufficiently well from a dropper or syringe. There is often some regurgitation through the nose, but this too is not excessive. For a time they may require a liquid concentrated feeding until they learn to manage solid foods. The palate will be repaired at 18 months or later.

## REFERENCES

Carter, C. O.: Genetics of common disorders Brit. Med. Bull. 25:52, 1969.

Davies, P.: Management of the Pierre Robin syndrome. Devel. Med. Child. Neurol. 15:359, 1973.

Dennison, W. M.: The Pierre Robin syndrome. Pediatrics 36:336, 1965.

Douglas, B.: A further report on the treatment of micrognathia with obstruction by a plastic procedure; results based on reports from 21 cities, 1948–1949. Plast. Reconstruct. Surg. 5:113, 1950.

Edgerton, M. T., Jr.: Plastic surgery for mandibular retrusion. Plast. Reconstruct. Surg. 6:450, 1950.

Fazen, L. E., Elmore, J., and Nadler, H. L.: Mandibulo-facial dysostosis (Treacher Collins syndrome). Am. J. Dis. Child. 117:700, 1969.

Fonkalsrud, E. W., and Jones, M.: Pierre Robin syndrome in infancy. Nasoesophageal intubation. Am. J. Dis. Child. 124:79, 1972.

Fraser, F. C.: The genetics of cleft lip and cleft palate. Am. J. Hum. Genet. 22:336, 1970.

Goldberg, M. H., and Eckblom, R. H.: The treatment of the Pierre Robin syndrome. Pediatrics 30:450, 1962.

Hövels, O., cited by J. McKenzie.

Jeresaty, R. M., Huszar, R. V., and Basu, S.: Pierre Robin syndrome: Cause of respiratory obstruction, cor pulmonale, and pulmonary edema. Am. J. Dis. Child. *117*:710, 1969.

Mann, I., and Kilner, T. P.: Deficiency of malar bones with defect of lower lids. Brit. J. Ophthalmol. 27:13, 1943.

McKenzie, J.: The first arch syndrome. Arch. Dis. Child. *33*:477, 1958.

Nisenson, A.: Receding chin and glossoptosis; a cause of respiratory difficulty in the infant. J. Pediatr. *32*:397, 1948.

Oliver, H. T.: Orthodontic treatment of the newborn

with clefts of the lip and palate. J. Canad. Dent. Assoc. *34*:196, 1968.

Oliver, H. T.: Construction of orthodontic appliances for the treatment of newborn infants with clefts of the lip and palate. Am. J. Orthodont. *56*:468, 1969.

Poswillo, D.: The pathogenesis of the first and second branchial arch syndrome. Oral Surg., Oral Med., Oral Path. *35*:302, 1973.

Pruzansky, S., and Richmond, J. B.: Growth of mandible in infants with micrognathia; clinical implications. A.M.A. J. Dis. Child. *88*:29, 1954.

# THE CHONDRODYSTROPHIES

## 96

*By F. Clarke Fraser*

The chondrodystrophies, or more properly the osteochondrodysplasias, are a heterogeneous group of disorders of cartilage and bone growth resulting in disproportionate short stature. In the past 15 years a bewildering array of distinct entities has been recognized. A recent proposed international nomenclature lists 44 entities, and the list continues to grow. Rimoin has recently published a useful review. This chapter will limit itself to those that present problems in infancy.

It is particularly important to obtain a precise diagnosis in those forms leading to prenatal or neonatal death, and every effort should be made to obtain photographs, measurements, roentgenograms and material for histological examination in such cases. Formerly these were usually categorized as "achondroplasia," but forms with other modes of inheritance occur, and proper genetic counseling depends on precise diagnosis.

### ACHONDROPLASIA

Achondroplasia is the most common the chondrodystrophies. It shows autosomal dominant inheritance, but about 80 per cent of these infants are born of normal parents and presumably represent fresh

mutations. Thus the recurrence risks for sibs of these sporadic cases is low, but the offspring each have a 50:50 chance of being affected.

The classical phenotype includes short limbs, rhizomelic (affecting the proximal segment most severely) dwarfism, a normally proportioned trunk and a large head with bulging forehead, depressed nose bridge and relatively prominent mandible. Mild ventricular dilatation is common, and internal hydrocephalus develops occasionally. The infant's limbs are covered with fatty folds of skin, and the hands extend only to about the hip joint. The hands are short and broad, with "trident" fingers, and there is limited extension and pronation of the elbows. Infants may be hypotonic and slow in motor development but are usually normal by the age of 2 years. X-ray films show the characteristic short, broad long bones, with flaring metaphyses, short, broad pelvis with horizontal acetabular roofs, and narrow, deep sacrosciatic notches, vertebral interpediculate distances decreasing from L1 to L5, narrow spinal canal and short skull base. Histologically (contrary to older reports) endochondral ossification is regular and well organized. Periosteal ossification is relatively increased, and it may be that the basic defect is a decrease in rate of endochondral

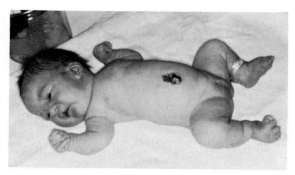

***Figure 96–1.*** Newborn infant with classic achondroplasia. Note the relatively long trunk and very short extremities.

ossification, with normal rate of membranous ossification, resulting in short, squat bones with cupped ends.

Treatment is of no avail. The psychological aspects of the unhappy situation must be handled with delicacy and care. No benefit is gained by withholding the details of diagnosis and prognosis from the parents.

## ACHONDROGENESIS

The term "achondrogenesis" has been used inconsistently in the literature; Rimoin suggests the following classification:

PARENTI-FRACCARO TYPE. This recessively inherited severe form of chondrodystrophy causes stillbirth or death early in life. The babies are small (25 to 29 cm, 900 to 1800 gm), the neck is very short, the arms are extremely short and stubby, the thoracic cavity is small and barrel-shaped. The membranous bones of the skull are variably ossified, rendering the skull soft; the vertebral column shows total lack of ossification of the vertebral bodies, but os-

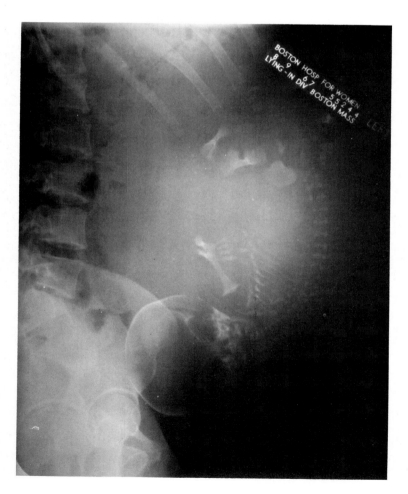

***Figure 96–2.*** A, Achondroplastic fetus in the uterus of a normal woman.

A

sification centers for the pedicles and arches are present. The ribs are short, narrow and expanded at the costochondral junction. There are no ossification centers in the sternum and the pelvis is poorly ossified. The long bones are extremely short and bowed, and are expanded at the metaphyses, with longitudinally projecting spurs.

Histologically, there is orderly cellular maturation until the hypertrophic zone, but calcification and ossification is disorderly, with haphazard capillary penetration.

LANGER-SALDINO TYPE. This form of achondrogenesis is also recessively inherited and results in severe dwarfism, and in stillbirth or early neonatal death. The head is very large in relation to the body, the neck is short and hidden in skin folds,

the trunk is short and squared, with distended abdomen and the limbs are very short. Ossification is much reduced in the lumbar vertebrae, sacrum, pubis and ischium, and the sacrum and pubic bones are not seen. The long bones are short, but usually not bowed, and the metaphyseal margins are irregular, with bony spurs. Histologically the epiphyseal cartilage appears lobulated and mushroomed, with increased vascularity. Resting cartilage is markedly hypercellular, with little matrix. Cellular column formation is absent at the growth plate and there is complete disorganization of endochondral ossification. The primary defect may affect matrix synthesis, with secondary disorganization of ossification.

The recurrence risk for sibs in both these types of achondrogenesis is 1 in 4, making

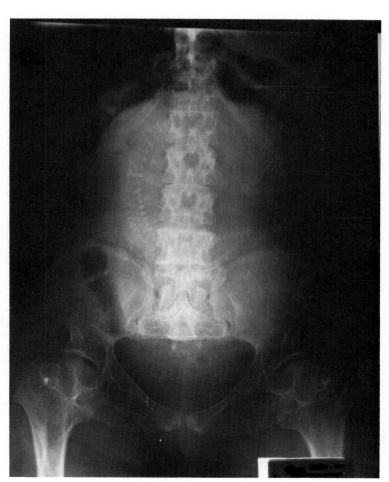

*Figure 96–2. Continued. B,* Achondroplastic mother with a normal fetus in uterus. (Courtesy of Dr. R. Wilkinson and N. T. Griscom, Boston Hospital for Women.)

B

it very important not to confuse them with achondroplasia or thanatophoric dwarfism.

The term achondrogenesis has also been applied (inappropriately) by Grebe to a non-lethal form of short-limb dwarfism, in which the limbs and hands are extremely short, the effect increasing distally so that the fingers are so short they may be functionless. About half of these cases have polydactyly. There are varying degrees of aplasia or hypoplasia of the bones of the limbs. Until the pathogenesis of this disorder is known, Rimoin suggests that the condition be known as Grebe disease.

## THANATOPHORIC DWARFISM

This lethal form of dwarfism is characterized by markedly shortened extremities, more rhizomelic than that of achondroplasia, a narrow thorax and a relatively large head, with bulging forehead, prominent eyes and depressed nose bridge. The thorax is very narrow in all dimensions, and is pear-shaped, with very short ribs; respiratory distress contributes to early death. The short extremities, which are covered by numerous skin folds, are held extended from the body. Hydrocephalus may be severe. X-ray examination reveals short long bones with marked bowing and irregular metaphyseal flaring and spicule-like cupping. The pelvis is small, with flat acetabulae, and with bony spicules projecting upward and downward from the medial surfaces of the ischium. Vertebral bodies are poorly developed and decreased in height; there is a lumbar stenosis and on frontal projection the lumbar vertebrae have an inverted-U appearance. Histologically there is generalized disruption of endochondral ossification.

There is no well-documented familial case, according to Rimoin, and the most likely cause seems to be a dominant mutation.

## DIASTROPHIC DWARFISM

Diastrophic dwarfism was formerly classified as achondroplasia, but shows autosomal recessive, rather than dominant, inheritance. It is a rhizomelic, short-limb dwarfism associated with club feet (meta-

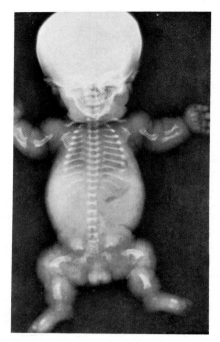

*Figure 96–3.* X-ray view of entire skeleton of newborn infant showing great shortening of all the extremities, great distortion in size and shape and irregularities of the epiphysial ends of the long bones. The head appears somewhat large in contrast to the face. (Aegerter, E., and Kirkpatrick, J. A., Jr.: *Orthopedic Diseases.* 3rd ed. Philadelphia, W. B. Saunders Company, 1968.)

tarsus varus and equinus, very resistant to therapy), ulnar deviation of broad, short hands with limitation of finger flexion, and a proximally inserted, hypermobile thumb held in abduction—a "hitchhiker thumb"—and cleft palate in about 25 per cent of cases. In the first few weeks of life most cases develop an acute inflammation of the ear pinnae that subsides, leaving a thick, firm ear with patches of calcification or even ossification eventually. Joint contractures and progressive scoliosis can be a problem.

The basic defect seems to be a generalized disease of cartilage, perhaps in the metabolism of the chondrocyte, leading to early cell death.

## CHONDRODYSPLASIA PUNCTATA

This heterogeneous group of disorders, is known also by several other names, two of which are chondrodystrophia calcificans congenita and congenital stippled epiphyses. The condition is characterized by radiographic stippling of the epiphyses and extraepiphysial cartilage. Stippling of the epiphyses can also be found in several other diseases, including the cerebrohepatorenal syndrome, multiple epiphysial dysplasia, GM₁ gangliosidosis, Smith-Lemli-Opitz syndrome, trisomies 18 and 21, and cretinism.

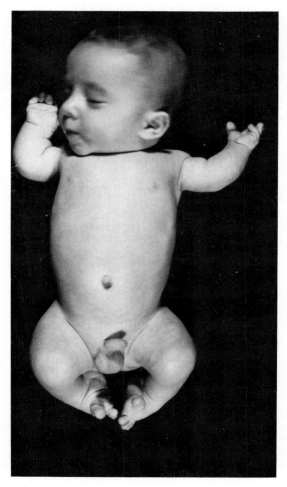

**Figure 96–4.** Diastrophic dwarfism. Note the normal head and face except for low-set ears with thickened pinnae, modest shortening of the trunk, and severe limb shortening. The club feet are resistant to treatment. The "hitch-hiker thumb" can be seen on the left hand. The great toe has a similar configuration. (Courtesy of Dr. Robert Wilkinson, Children's Hospital, Boston.)

The *rhizomelic* type of chondrodysplasia punctata is probably recessively inherited, and shows severe rhizomelic shortening of the limbs, joint contractures, cataracts (about 75 per cent), ichthyosiform erythroderma with alopecia, and a peculiar facies with depressed nose bridge. Many die in infancy, and those who survive are at risk for mental retardation, microcephaly and spastic paresis.

The *Conradi-Hunerman* type is less severe than the rhizomelic type, and many show autosomal dominant inheritance, though there may be heterogeneity. The dwarfing is not rhizomelic, and may be asymmetrical. Cataracts are less frequent (18 per cent), and intelligence is not impaired. The epiphysial calcifications may disappear.

## METATROPIC DWARFISM

This autosomal recessive disorder has frequently been confused with Morquio's disease. Affected infants have short limbs and normal body length, but kyphoscoliosis develops, resulting in short-trunk dwarfism. Although death may occur in infancy, survival to adulthood is common. X-ray films demonstrate marked platyspondyly, short long bones with irregular expanded metaphyses and flattened irregular epiphyses.

The Kniest syndrome, another form of short-trunk dwarfism, although radiologically similar to metatropic dwarfism, appears to be a separate entity, according to Rimoin. The condition may be associated cleft palate, hearing loss, myopia and limited joint movement. The genetics is unclear.

## CHONDROECTODERMAL DYSPLASIA

Otherwise known as the Ellis-van Creveld syndrome, this recessively inherited short-limb dwarfism is characterized by associated post-axial polydactyly, dystrophic nails and teeth, congenital heart disease in about 50 per cent of patients (usually atrial septal defect), varying degrees of fusion of the inner surface of the upper lip to the gingival margin and, occasionally, epispa-

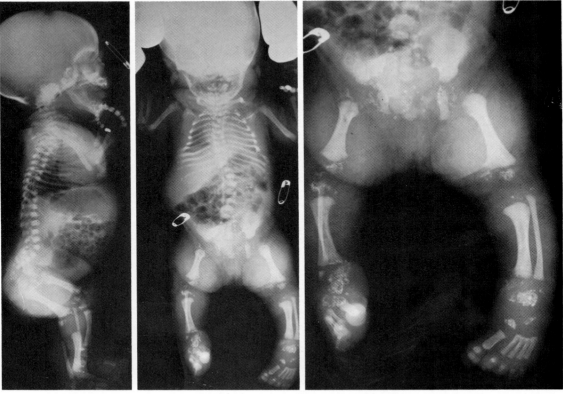

***Figure 96–5.*** Roentgenograms of skeletal system of an example of chrondrodysplasia punctata, rhizomelic, reported by Savignac. Note the short, broad bones, especially evident in the femora and tibiae. The ends of the long bones are somewhat distorted, but less so than is usual in classic achondroplasia. Most striking of all is the irregular, stippled calcification of the carpal and tarsal regions and in the neighborhood of all the joints. (Reproduced with the kind permission of the author, Dr. E. M. Savignac.)

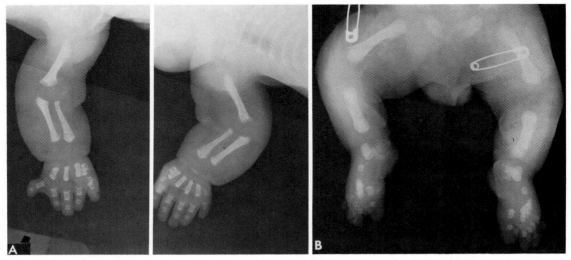

***Figure 96–6.*** Roentgenograms of upper extremities (*A*) and lower extremities (*B*) show shortening and broadening of the long bones, rounding and blunting of the ends of most, and wedging and irregularities of the ends of the humeri and of the upper ends of the ulnae.

This dwarfed, 1-month-old infant showed, in addition to the dyschondroplasia, polydactylism, syndactylism and absence of fingernails and toenails. This combination of defects comprises the Ellis–van Creveld syndrome. This case is not abstracted in the text. The films were discovered in the x-ray files of the Harriet Lane Home.

dias or hypospadias. The shortening of the limbs is mesomelic, with short, squat bones having expanded metaphyses. The phalanges are short and have cone-shaped epiphyses. The acetabular roof of the pelvis has a trident configuration. The mutant gene has a high frequency in certain Amish groups, but occurs also in other populations.

## ASPHYXIATING THORACIC DYSPLASIA

Somewhat similar to chondroectodermal dysplasia is asphyxiating thoracic dysplasia, or Jeune syndrome. It too is a recessively inherited short-limbed dwarfism, with similar radiological findings in the pelvis and the short tubular bones of the hand. Polydactyly occurs only occasionally, however, and ectodermal defects are rare. The thorax is extremely small, with shortened ribs, and respiratory death in infancy is common. Those who survive may have only a mild reduction in height as adults. (See also pages 193 and 194).

## SPONDYLOEPIPHYSIAL DYSPLASIA CONGENITA

This autosomal dominant form of spondyloepiphysial dysplasia can be distinguished at birth as a short-trunk dwarfism in which the child has a dysplastic spine and epiphyses, an unusual round face and extremely short neck. With time, dorsal kyphosis and lumbar lordosis exaggerate the disproportion. The limbs show some rhizomelic shortening. Cleft palate and clubfoot may occur, and over 50 per cent of patients have severe myopia or retinal detachment, or both. In the newborn there is retarded ossification of the epiphysial centers, especially of hips, knees and ankles. Further genetic heterogeneity probably remains to be sorted out.

## REFERENCES

Curran, J. P., Sigmon, B. A., and Opitz, J.: Lethal forms of chondrodysplastic dwarfism. Pediatrics 53:76–85, 1974.

Gefferth, K.: Metatropic dwarfism. *In* Intrinsic Diseases of Bone (H. J. Kaufman, ed.). Prog. Pediatr. Radiol. 4:137–151, 1973.

Jequier, S., and Dunbar, J. S.: The Ellis-van Creveld syndrome. *In* Intrinsic Diseases of Bone (H. J. Kaufman, ed.). Prog. Pediatr. Radiol. 4:167–187, 1973.

Kozlowski, K., Maroteaux, P., Silverman, F., Kaufmann, H., and Spranger, J.: Classification des dysplasies osseuses. Ann. Radiol. 12:965, 1969.

Langer, L. O.: Thoracic-pelvic-phalangeal dystrophy: Asphyxiating thoracic dystrophy of the newborn, infantile thoracic dystrophy. Radiology 91:447, 1968.

Murdoch, J. L., Walker, B. A., and Hall, J. G.: Achondroplasia—a genetic and statistical survey. Ann. Hum. Genet. 33:227, 1970.

Rimoin, David L.: *In* Harris, H., and K. Hirschhorn (eds.): Advances in Human Genetics, Vol. 5, Chap. 1, New York, Plenum Press, 1975.

Saldino, R. M.: Lethal short-limbed dwarfism: Achondrogenesis and thanatophoric dwarfism. Am. J. Roentgenol. 112:185, 1971.

Silverman, F. N.: Achondroplasia. *In* Intrinsic Diseases of Bone. Prog. Pediatr. Radiol. 4:94–124, 1973.

Spranger, J. W., and Langer, L. O., Jr.: Spondyloepiphyseal dysplasia congenita. Radiology 94:313, 1970.

Spranger, J. W., Langer, L. O., and Wiedemann, H. R.: Bone Dysplasias; An Atlas of Constitutional Disorders of Skeletal Development. Philadelphia, W. B. Saunders Co., 1974.

Spranger, J. W., Opitz, J. M., and Bidder, U.: Heterogeneity of chondrodysplasia punctata. Humangenetik 11:190–212, 1971.

Walker, B. A., Scott, C. J., Hall, J. G., Murdoch, J. L., and McKusick, V. A.: Diastrophic dwarfism. Medicine 51:1, 1972.

Wiedemann, H. R., Remagen, W., Heinz, H. A., Gorlin, R. J., and Maroteaux, P.: Achondrogenesis within the scope of connately manifested generalized skeletal dysplasia. Z. Kinderheilkd. 116:223, 1974.

# 97

# OTHER CONGENITAL DEFECTS INVOLVING BONES

*Revised by F. Clarke Fraser*

## MARFAN SYNDROME

Marfan syndrome is a hereditary disorder of connective tissue with many somatic manifestations including very long fingers, and was therefore also called "arachnodactyly" (spider fingers). Since several other syndromes show arachnodactyly, the term should not be used as a synonym for Marfan syndrome.

Inheritance is autosomal dominant, but those who carry the gene show much variation in the severity and variety of features expressed (variable expressivity) and occasionally fail to show any manifestations of the mutant gene (reduced penetrance), making counseling difficult. About 15 per cent or less do not have an affected relative and presumably represent fresh mutations. Since many of the features are not present at birth the condition is often difficult to diagnose at this stage unless there is an affected near relative.

**PATHOGENESIS.** Many of the pathologic alterations in Marfan syndrome can be attributed to an abiotrophy of connective tissue; i.e., to its imperfect structure leading to precocious weakening under stress. In the eye this leads to subluxation of the lens, in the musculoskeletal system to hyperextensibility of joints, kyphoscoliosis and inguinal hernia, in the great vessels to cystic medial necrosis which often terminates in dissecting aneurysm, and in the lungs to emphysema (Bolande and Tucker).

**DIAGNOSIS.** The sine qua non of the disorder is long, thin, tapering fingers and toes. From this sign the name "arachnodactyly" (literally, spider fingers) is derived. In addition, other skeletal deviations from the normal may be seen: long, slender arms and legs, dolichocephaly (long, narrow head), high-arched palate, joint laxity, kyphoscoliosis and pectus excavatum or carinatum. The upper to lower segment ratio is decreased, arm span is greater than height, the hand to height ratio is greater than 11 per cent, the foot to height ratio is greater than 15 per cent and the metacarpal index (length to width) is increased. Over the course of months or years abnormalities of other organs and systems may appear (or they may not, since formes frustes are common). These include muscle flabbiness and weakness and loss of deep reflexes, suggestive of Oppenheim's or Werdnig-Hoffmann's disease, eye defects, of which myopia and dislocation of the lens (usually upward) are the ones most frequently met, and cardiac disorders. These last are often mistaken for rheumatic heart disease, since the valves and chordae tendineae are involved in a fibrous thickening which produces murmurs similar to those of rheumatic endocarditis. The terminal event in many of these patients, rarely in infancy (one aged 9 months has been reported), more often in late childhood or early adulthood, is the growth and rupture of an aortic aneurysm. Pathologically, the great vessels will be seen to have undergone a gradual but relentless progression of cystic medial necrosis.

The disorder will be looked for carefully in infants in a family in which the diagnosis of Marfan syndrome has been made in a parent or other near relative. Indeed, Heldrich and Wright reported one case in which the diagnosis was made shortly after birth, largely because the patient's sister had been adjudged to have the disease. The presenting sign in both babies was dislocation of the hip. It may be suspected if the newborn has inordinately long, thin, tapering fingers and toes, especially if these are accompanied by dolichocephaly, joint laxity, myopia and the skeletal disproportions referred to above. One does not expect to find the cardiac and severe ocular abnormalities to be fully developed within the first months of life, but they have been seen this early.

The differential diagnosis includes *homocystinuria* (autosomal recessive) which can be ruled out by the absence of excess homocystine in the urine, and *congenital contractural arachnodactyly*, also dominantly inherited, in which the arachnodactyly is accompanied by multiple joint contractures and large, floppy ears. The distinction is important, as these patients do not develop the severe ocular and cardiac complications of Marfan syndrome, and the contractures improve with age.

**TREATMENT.** Treatment is symptomatic. The use of propranolol to reduce the probability of aortic aneuryism is under investigation. Preliminary results are discouraging.

**PROGNOSIS.** Prognosis is variable, depending upon whether cardiac and vascular complications supervene or not. In some they will, in others they will not, and there is no way of predicting which children will ultimately show these manifestations. Murdoch has calculated the life expectancy of persons with Marfan syndrome. The average age at death was 32 years. This rather dismal outlook may improve with increased awareness of the condition and continuing progress in management of the cardiovascular complications.

CASE 97–1

(This is Case J. G. of Bolande and Tucker, abstracted and reprinted here with the permission of the senior author.)

This 1-month-old white male infant was admitted with a diagnosis of congenital Marfan's syndrome. During breech extraction of the 7 pound 5 ounce (3510 gm) baby the left femur was fractured. Both mother and father are unusually tall and slender. On examination he measured 23½ inches (58 cm) and weighed 7 pounds 3 ounces (3450 gm). The head was narrow and long, the ears were soft and floppy, and there was an entropion of the right eye. A grade I systolic murmur was heard in the third left intercostal space. The extremities were long and thin, with extremely long hands, fingers, feet and toes, and a flail wrist on the left. Bilateral inguinal hernias were visible. Deep tendon reflexes were absent (Fig. 97–1).

Fluoroscopy revealed cardiac enlargement and pulmonary vascular congestion.

The murmur became louder and harsher, cardiac failure ensued, dislocation of the right lens

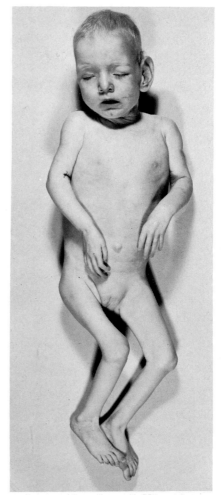

*Figure 97–1.* Photograph of infant with Marfan's syndrome. Note the extremely long arms and hands, legs and feet, the long, narrow skull, the very large ears and the dropped left wrist.

became obvious, the lungs became emphysematous, and the infant died after about five weeks in hospital.

**COMMENT.** This is an example of Marfan syndrome which was diagnosable shortly after birth, with many of the associated visceral lesions by the time of death, before the infant was 3 months of age.

## OSTEOGENESIS IMPERFECTA

The terminology and genetics of this group of diseases are confused. There is clearly a form showing autosomal dominant inheritance in which the carriers of the mutant gene usually have blue sclerae, and may also have bone fragility of varying degrees of severity (about 60 per cent), and otosclerotic deafness later in life (about 60 per cent). This condition is known as osteogenesis imperfecta tarda or osteopsathyrosis tarda. A variant without blue sclerae has been called Lobstein disease; it may represent another mutation at the same locus. The bone fragility may occasionally be so severe as to cause an occasional prenatal fracture.

Contrasted to this is osteogenesis imperfecta congenita (lethalis, gravis), in which the bone fragility is much more severe, leading to multiple intrauterine fractures and frequently stillbirth or neonatal death. Most cases are sporadic and may represent new mutations, but a minority show evidence of autosomal recessive inheritance. Thus parents of a sporadic case of the congenita type can be advised that (unless they are related) the risk of recurrence is probably very small, but that there is some chance that it is 1 in 4. The average risk may be roughly around 1 per cent. Unfortunately there is no way of distinguishing the two possibilities in an isolated case.

**INCIDENCE.** The intrauterine variety has an incidence of about 2.6 per 100,000 births and the tarda type about twice this.

**ETIOLOGY AND PATHOLOGY.** Dr. E. A. Park observed that osteocytes in the bones lie closely approximated in these infants, as though some substance which normally separates them were deficient. This fits in well with Follis's observations. He demonstrated clearly that the basic defect lies in the development of connective tissue. Histochemical studies showed that the infants are born with reticulum characteristic of early embryonic life which has failed in many places to mature into collagen fibers of the adult type (Fig. 97–2). Fractures then occur throughout the length of the bones exactly as they do at the epiphyses in scurvy where the collagen matrix is deficient.

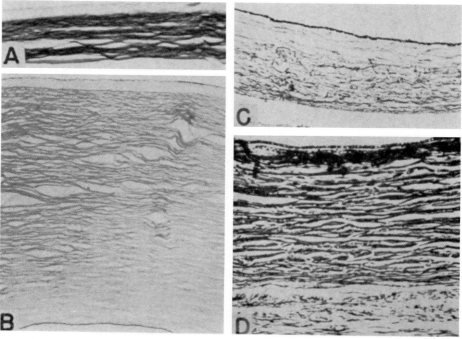

*Figure 97–2.* (*A* and *C* are from the patient; *B* and *D* are controls.) *A* and *B*, Corneas from infant being described and from control stained with periodic acid–Schiff technique. In addition to great difference in width the former stains red, while the latter is almost colorless. *C* and *D*, Scleras from infant with osteogenesis imperfecta and from normal infant. These exemplify difference in thickness and thin reticulum found in former (silver stain). (Follis, R. H., Jr.: J. Pediat. *41*:713, 1952.)

In the congenita type, shortening of all extremities from a multiplicity of fractures leads to an appearance resembling micromelia. The skull is soft, "like a membranous bag of bones" (Kraggs), because so little bone has been laid down. Subdural and subarachnoid hemorrhages often result from the trauma of delivery to this highly compressible skull and seem to be the immediate cause of death in many. Under the microscope no or little osteoid and no or few osteoblasts are found on the framework of the calcified cartilage matrix. The skin, corneas and sclerae are thin and demonstrate the immature reticulum mentioned earlier.

Remigio and Grinvalsky observed two newborn infants in whom there was, in addition to multiple fractures, immaturity of the cardiac and aortic connective tissue which actually was the cause of death of an older sister. This infant had other signs which also suggested Marfan's disease, and the question arose as to whether she had two coincident diseases or whether these two connective tissue disorders may be in some way related. The question was left unanswered.

**DIAGNOSIS.** The disorder has been recognized in utero when multiple fractures have been visualized by x-ray. After birth the stunted extremities, tapering at their ends, and the soft skull are the outstanding signs. By x-ray film the long bones are seen to be the sites of numerous fractures, as are the ribs.

The same soft, mushy skull is encountered in cleidocranial dystrophy, in congenital hypophosphatasia and in chondrodystrophia calcificans. Differentiation is simple, since in the first the clavicles are completely or partially missing, and in the second the epiphysial alterations resemble those of florid rickets, whereas in the last, stippled epiphyses are seen in the x-ray films (Fig. 97–3).

**PROGNOSIS.** Most infants with osteogenesis imperfecta congenita die in utero or during delivery. The few remaining liveborns seldom survive more than a few hours or at the most a few days. Infants with the less serious form who do survive

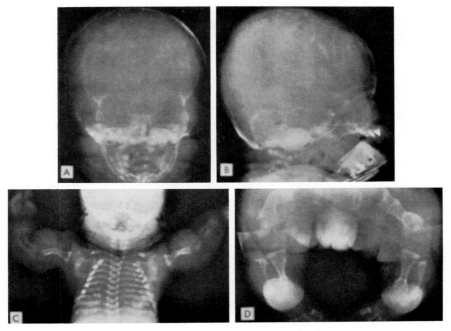

*Figure 97–3.* Osteogenesis imperfecta. A newborn with the severe form of the disease. In *A* and *B* note the inadequate mineralization of the cranial bones, the wide sutures and multiple centers of ossification. Multiple fractures of the extremities and rib cage are evident in *C* and *D*. The cortices are thin, and the spongiosa is deficient. (Aegerter, E., and Kirkpatrick, J. A., Jr.: Orthopedic Diseases. 3rd ed. Philadelphia, W. B. Saunders Company, 1968.)

grow up with varying degrees of deformity, or perhaps with only a few fractures that may not even lead to recognition of the disease until they themselves have an affected child.

**TREATMENT.** No treatment is effective.

## CLEIDOCRANIAL DYSOSTOSIS

Cleidocranial dysostosis is a developmental disorder in which multiple malformations of the skeleton are transmitted from generation to generation in an autosomal dominant pattern. It received its name from the fact that deformity of the skull and absence of clavicles are manifest in most cases, but either or both of these defects may be absent.

**INCIDENCE.** The disorder is rare, even though over 500 cases have been reported in the world literature. This apparent discrepancy is explainable by the fact that large aggregations of examples can be collected from the forebears, collaterals and progeny of almost every diagnosed patient.

**DIAGNOSIS.** The defect most often noted first is extreme softness of the skull. The fontanels are huge, the major sutures widely patent and the metopic suture widely separated. Very little membranous calvarial bone has been laid down before birth. There are other defects of facial bones of great variety. The clavicles are at times completely absent, while at other times one or two of the thirds may be missing or not joined. When both are absent, extraordinary mobility of the shoulders is possible to the point of approximating the acromial processes beneath the chin. Deformities, nonjunction and underdevelopment of the bones of the pelvis and of almost any other of the skeletal parts may coexist. The characteristic defects from which the disorder derives its name are shown in Figure 97–4. The soft skull of the newborn may be confused with that of osteogenesis imperfecta, hypophosphatasia or chondrodystrophia calcificans.

**PROGNOSIS.** The cranium completes its ossification slowly, the fontanels and metopic sutures often remaining open until adult life. The sutures generally remain depressed, leaving the frontal and parietal areas prominently bossed in "hot-cross bun" fashion. The permanent teeth may be late in erupting, and may have enamel hypoplasia, retention cysts and malformed roots. Morbidity and mortality are not increased by cleidocranial dystrophy.

**TREATMENT.** There is none available.

## HEMIHYPERTROPHY

This disorder is rare, and its etiology is unknown. There is little evidence that it is genetically transmitted, since, in the 135 cases reported up to 1961, it had recurred in two generations only a few times, in three generations only once. Some deviation from the normal process of twinning has been suggested as its cause.

Since about 1950 a large body of information has accrued concerning the association of congenital defects with malignancies of early life. Hemihypertrophy stands high on the list of those found with unusual frequency in the presence of Wilms' tumor and adrenal carcinoma. This matter is discussed more fully in Chapter 111 (p. 1013).

**DIAGNOSIS.** Some or all of the structures on one side of the body are noted to be larger than the corresponding ones on the other side. The time at which this inequality becomes apparent depends upon the degree of hemihypertrophy, which may vary within wide limits. Thus, in the case which we observed most recently, the only abnormality noted in the newborn nursery was that the tongue was too large to be contained within the mouth. Macroglossia was suspected. Shortly after returning home the mother suddenly made the observation that the right leg and arm seemed bigger and longer than those on the left. The pediatrician, and later an orthopedist, confirmed this finding, and then it became apparent that the hypertrophy of the tongue was limited to its right half. The face was similarly asymmetrical. The leg and arm of the affected side are larger in both length and girth, and measurements of the long bones by x-ray study show them to be longer than the contralateral ones. Growth continues for several years, making the discrepancy more noticeable, but toward puberty excessive growth ceases. By

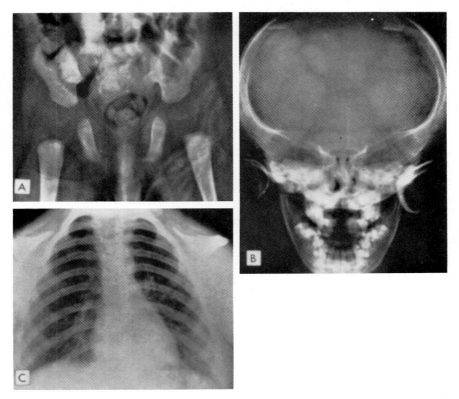

*Figure 97–4.* Cleidocranial dysostosis. *A* and *B*, Radiographs of the pelvis and skull of a male infant age 6 months. The pubic bones are underdeveloped; only a small portion of the body of each is evident. The epiphysial centers for the heads of the femora are tiny. The radiograph of the skull (*B*) shows widely patent sutures and fontanels, numerous centers of ossification in the cranial bones and an increase in the biparietal diameter. The facial bones are small. This child has no clavicles, and the radiograph of his mother's chest (*C*) reveals absence of clavicles. (Aegerter, E., and Kirkpatrick, J. A., Jr.: Orthopedic Diseases. 3rd ed. Philadelphia, W. B. Saunders Company, 1968.)

then one leg may be an inch or two longer than the other.

**TREATMENT.** Several methods have been used in the attempt to slow down excessive growth of the leg, in order to minimize both the limp and the scoliosis which result from discrepancy in leg length. Stapling a growing end is probably the most satisfactory method.

## SYNDROME OF CONGENITAL HEMIHYPERTROPHY, INTRAUTERINE DWARFISM AND ELEVATED URINARY GONADOTROPINS

Tanner's excellent study has shown that there is no justification for separating cases of this nature with hemihypertrophy (Silver syndrome) from those without it (Russell syndrome). The asymmetry is usually present in infancy, and may involve one side, or only the face, trunk or limbs. The face is triangular and small, with a broad forehead and small chin. The head thus may appear large but in fact tends to have a circumference somewhat below average. The mouth is often thin-lipped, with down-turned corners. Clinodactyly is frequent, and syndactyly, café au lait spots, muscle weakness and cryptorchidism may be present. Elevation of urinary gonadotropins may sometimes occur in both males and females but, contrary to previous claims, puberty is usually normal. Familial occurrence has been reported occasionally but most cases are sporadic.

# DEFECTS OF RADIUS AND THUMB

The skeletal dysplasias are so numerous and varied that their description is beyond the scope of this book. Bergsma's Atlas and Compendium is a useful source reference. However, defects of the radius are part of so many syndromes that their presence in the infant should lead the physician to look for associated abnormalities, since identifying the syndrome is important for both prognosis and genetic counseling. Radial dysplasias may range from complete absence of the radial ray to minimal hypoplasia of a low-set thumb. They may be sporadic or may be a feature of the following syndromes.

## GENETIC SYNDROMES

HOLT-ORAM SYNDROME. Varying degrees of radial dysplasia occur in association with congenital heart malformations, usually atrial septal defect but sometimes ventricular septal defect, transposition of the great vessels or single coronary artery. Some cases also manifest the Duane syndrome (a defect of ocular adduction). The inheritance is autosomal dominant.

FANCONI'S ANEMIA. Various combinations of anomalies including microcephaly, kidney malformations and skeletal defects, often including radial dysplasias, are present at birth, and a pancytopenic anemia develops later. The diagnosis can be confirmed by the presence of an excessive number of chromosome breaks in peripheral lymphocyte cultures. The inheritance is autosomal recessive.

THROMBOCYTOPENIA—ABSENT RADIUS SYNDROME. Also showing autosomal recessive inheritance, this syndrome is distinguished by the fact that the thumb is present, contrary to Fanconi's anemia. There is amegakaryocytosis, but this may be transient; if the infant survives the first year the prognosis is relatively good.

## "SPORADIC" SYNDROMES

THE VATER, OR VACTEL SYNDROME. This is a syndrome of unidentified etiology (although maternal ingestion of certain drugs is suspected) in which radial dyspla-

sia is associated with vertebral anomalies, anal atresia, tracheoesophageal fistula and cardiac defects.

THE THALIDOMIDE SYNDROME. This is really a series of syndromes, depending on the time of ingestion of the drug, and may "copy" several of the genetic syndromes described above. One hopes that this syndrome will not be seen again by neonatologists.

AFROFACIAL DYSOSTOSIS (NAGER). This syndrome includes, besides absence of thumbs and/or radii, cleft palate, micrognathia, gastroschisis and a rudimentary phallus.

## CHROMOSOMAL SYNDROMES

Radial dysplasia occurs occasionally in the trisomy 18 syndrome, with a low-set, retroflexible thumb being a more frequent feature. Absence or hypoplasia of the thumb may occur in patients with a deletion of chromosome 13 long arm.

## REFERENCES

Aegerter, E., and Kirkpatrick J. A.: Orthopedic Diseases: Physiology—Pathology—Radiology, 3rd ed. Philadelphia, W. B. Saunders Company, 1968.

Bergsma, D. (Ed.): Birth Defects Atlas and Compendium. National Foundation March of Dimes. Baltimore, Williams & Wilkins Co., 1973.

Bolande, R. P., and Tucker, A. S.: Pulmonary emphysema and other cardiorespiratory lesions as part of the Marfan abiotrophy. Pediatrics 33:356, 1964.

Carson, N. A. J., et al.: Homocystinuria: Clinical and pathological review of ten cases. J. Pediatr. 66:565, 1965.

Follis, R. H., Jr.: Osteogenesis imperfecta congenita: A connective tissue diathesis. J. Pediatr. 41:713, 1952.

Gellis, S. S., and Feingold, M.: Picture of the month: Congenital hemihypertrophy and adrenal carcinoma. Am. J. Dis. Child. 115:445, 1968.

Gordon, R. J., and Meskin, L. H.: Congenital hemihypertrophy: A review of literature and report of a case, with special emphasis on oral manifestations. J. Pediatr. 61:870, 1961.

Heldrich, F. J., Jr., and Wright, C. W.: Marfan's syndrome: Diagnosis in the neonate. Am. J. Dis. Child. 114:419, 1967.

Holmes, L. B., Moser, H. W., Halldorsen, S., Mack, C., Pant, S. S., and Matzilevich, B.: Mental Retardation. An Atlas of Diseases with Associated Physical Abnormalities. New York, Macmillan, 1972.

McKusick, V. A.: Heritable Disorders of Connective Tissue. St. Louis, 4th ed. C. V. Mosby Co., 1972.

Murdoch, J. L., Walker, B. A., Halpern, B. L., Kuzma,

J. W., and McKusick, V. A.: Life expectancy and causes of death associated in the Marfan syndrome. N. Engl. J. Med. *286*:804, 1972.

Remigio, P. A., and Grinvalsky, H. T.: Osteogenesis imperfecta congenita associated with conspicuous extraskeletal connective tissue dysplasias. Am. J. Dis. Child. *119*:524, 1970.

Tanner, J. M., Lejarraga, H., and Cameron, N.: The natural history of the Silver-Russell syndrome: A longitudinal study of thirty-nine cases. Pediat. Res. *9*:611–623, 1975.

Warkany, J.: Congenital malformations. Notes and Comments. Chicago, Year Book Medical Publishers, 1971.

# CONGENITAL DEFECTS INVOLVING JOINTS

# 98

*Revised by F. Clarke Fraser*

## CONGENITAL DISLOCATION OF THE HIP

The hip joint is only rarely completely dislocated at birth or within the first month of life. The more common lesion is subluxation; that is, a dislocatable hip with nearly stable reductions and an Ortolani click.

**INCIDENCE.** Estimates of frequency vary with the nature of the population and the intensity of screening. Surveys of infants in the first few days of life have provided figures ranging from 4 to 7 per 1000 live births. The likelihood of recurrence in sibs varies with sex of both proband and sib, ranging from roughly 5 per cent for the brothers of an affected female to about 20 per cent for the sisters of an affected male. These figures are for neonatal diagnosis; the proportion that would progress to overt dislocation is considerably less.

**ETIOLOGY.** Females are affected much more often than males, the overall reported ratio being eight females to one male. Whites outnumber blacks by 50 to 1. Noteworthy is the disproportion of breech positions among the affected babies. One out of about five of them has presented by the breech, whereas overall only one of about 40 fetuses is a breech presentation. In order to explain the disproportion of females over males, Andren and others

have looked for an endocrine factor in addition to the mechanical one of breech presentation. It is possible that maternal progesterone, acting upon the fetal uterus, produces relaxin, which affects the tensile strength of the ligaments about the hip adversely. Formerly most workers placed dysplasia of the joint in the primary role, subluxation and dislocation resulting from muscular pull and, eventually, weight bearing. The dysplastic joint is an imperfectly ossified one with a shallow acetabulum and a capsule which is soft and less elastic and strong than is normal. There appear to be genetic predisposing factors including a polygenic system influencing acetabular conformation and a major locus influencing joint laxity.

**DIAGNOSIS.** The diagnosis of actual dislocation of the femoral head out of the acetabular cavity is not difficult. But this is only rarely present at birth and may not become obvious for several months after birth. When present, at any age, it produces apparent shortening of the dislocated limb. One can discern shortening by pressing the knees flatly and firmly against the table top while holding the pelvis rigidly straight; that is, not tilted to one side or the other. The position of the soles should match perfectly. An additional sign of shortening is asymmetry of the creases of the thigh. In some infants all the creases of one thigh will appear to be higher than those of the other. In many one will see not only this, but also an extra crease or two in the seemingly shortened side. But an extra crease or two on one side is seen frequently in infants who have no other signs of dislocation of the hip and who grow up without ever exhibiting them.

The cardinal sign of subluxation, with or without actual dislocation, is inability to abduct the affected thigh. This can be demonstrated by flexing the thighs to a right angle, the infant lying supine, and attempting to bring them, outward and downward, one at a time, until they lie upon the table top. When a sharp click can be felt and heard consistently on one side (Ortolani's sign) and when the difference in ease of abduction between the two thighs is striking, one can be fairly certain that subluxation is present (Fig. 98–1). Minor differences or inconstant ones may not be considered diagnostic. This is especially true in the first week or two of life, when the newborn prefers to maintain vigorously his fetal "position of comfort." The leg on the affected side often is kicked less freely than the other. It may be held constantly in a position of slight internal rotation and flexion.

X-ray films of the dislocated hip show upward and outward malposition of the femoral head. The acetabular angle is generally greater than 30 degrees, whereas that of normals is generally below 30 degrees. There is unfortunately a fair amount of overlap. In the newborn, delay in ossification of the epiphysis of the femoral head is of no help, since this does not ordinarily occur until 6 weeks of age in the normal. But notable may be absence of any acetabular cupping, widening of the space between femur and pelvis and lateral displacement of the projected line of the long axis of the femur. This points, in normal hips, directly toward the position of the acetabulum, while in the dysplastic ones it misses the lateral margin of the ilium.

**TREATMENT.** Treatment is successful and simple in inverse proportion to the age at which it is begun. When diagnosed early, many subluxated hips can be prevented from ever dislocating by some simple device which holds the affected leg abducted and laterally rotated. Generally, splinting can be discontinued before the end of the third month. Cases diagnosed later may require longer splinting, and at times more drastic forms of intervention. The pediatrician in any case will not take it upon himself to detail the therapeutic measures needed.

## GENU RECURVATUM

This is a comparatively rare deformity, characterized by abnormal hyperextensibility of the knee joint.

**ETIOLOGY.** Many more females are affected than males. Many more babies with genu recurvatum present by the breech than is to be expected. Both of these statistical observations have been documented for congenital dislocation of the hip. They lend weight to the hormonal-postural theory of pathogenesis of both these disorders; that is, that maternal progesterone induces, via the fetal uterus, the production of relaxin, and that the abnormal stresses of the breech position distort one or both of the abnormally relaxed joints. The disorder may also occur as a feature in a number of syndromes, such as the Ehlers-Danlos, Marfan, Klinefelter and Turner syndromes.

**DIAGNOSIS.** The extended leg or both legs describe a concave arc when hyperextended at the knee (Fig. 98–3). Hyperextensibility is mild or severe; that is, the arc is shallow or deep. In severe cases there may be actual posterior dislocation of the knee.

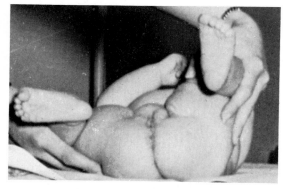

*Figure 98–1.* Infant with subluxation of left hip. The nurse is able to abduct the right thigh down to the level of the table, but not the left. (Pray, L. G.: Pediatrics, 9:94, 1952.)

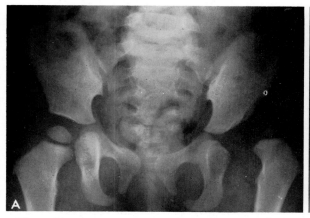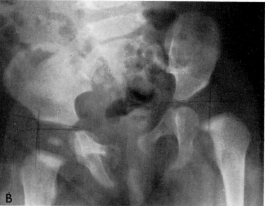

*Figure 98–2.* A, X-ray view of hips shows the right femoral head to be in its proper position with respect to its acetabulum. The left femur is placed considerably farther from the pelvis than is the right, its epiphysial center and its acetabulum are less well developed, and its long axis projected runs lateral to the edge of the ilium. B, The left femoral head is displaced slightly upward and outward, the acetabulum is shallow, and the epiphysial center is poorly developed. (Pray, L. G.: Pediatrics, 9:94, 1952.)

**PROGNOSIS.** Spontaneous improvement is the rule.

**TREATMENT.** Nothing need be done for cases of mild or moderate severity. Posterior splinting or, rarely, casting for 2 to 4 weeks is indicated for the most severe forms.

## ARTHROGRYPOSIS

Arthrogryposis multiplex congenita is an extraordinary condition in which the joints appear to be frozen, some in extension, some in flexion.

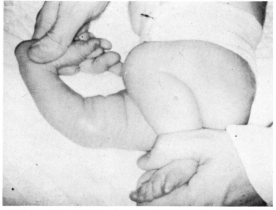

*Figure 98–3.* Genu recurvatum, right. The condition is unusually severe, with actual posterior dislocation of the knee.

**INCIDENCE.** It is a rare entity, although probably more common than one would think from the paucity of case reports.

**ETIOLOGY AND PATHOGENESIS.** Males are affected five times as often as females. Most cases are sporadic, but a number of familial occurrences have been reported, showing both autosomal dominant and autosomal recessive patterns of inheritance. It may also appear as a feature in a number of syndromes, including the COFS syndrome, congenital contractural arachnodactyly, congenital muscular dystrophy, diastrophic dwarfism, D and E trisomy, the Marden-Walker syndrome, the Potter syndrome and the Schwartz syndrome. It is important to identify such cases, for the recurrence risks vary widely from one to another.

Thus the etiology is undoubtedly heterogeneous, with both genetic and non-genetic types. The common factor may be restriction of joint movement in utero. It can be produced experimentally in chicks by infusion of curare. Therefore, the basic defect may be neurogenic, or myogenic or even mechanical, from oligohydramnios, for instance.

**PATHOLOGY.** Examination of the tissues shows striated muscle everywhere atrophied, with fatty replacement and some round cell infiltration. The articular capsules are thickened and inelastic.

It has thus become evident that arthrogryposis is a symptom-complex rather than

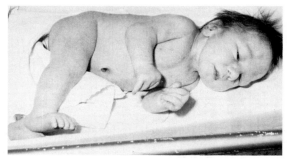

*Figure 98–4.*   Arthrogryposis congenita. One can see clearly the rigid extremities, the lower ones in extension, the upper ones in flexion, and the tightly balled fists.

a disease. It can be caused by cerebral or spinal cord lesions of various types or by primary muscle or connective tissue disorders. In the neuronal type, cell diminution or degeneration is generally demonstrable in the spinal cord.

**DIAGNOSIS.** At birth the infants are rigid. Their muscles are small, their joints thickened and inflexible. Commonly the large joints of the arms and legs are ankylosed in extension, the arms rotated inward, the thighs rotated outward. The hands and wrists are sharply flexed. The feet are often clubbed.

**TREATMENT.** Treatment includes physiotherapy and hydrotherapy directed toward increasing flexibility. Surgical intervention may be necessary to correct deformities. Slow improvement without

perfect restoration of function is to be expected.

**PROGNOSIS.** The oldest child we knew with this disorder was an 8-year-old boy. He had had the best possible orthopedic care, yet his disability was still great. He could walk, stiff-kneed, with the aid of a walker. His arms were still extended rigidly. He could use his hands and fingers fairly well. He was quite intelligent.

## GOUT

Gout strikes children rarely, young infants even more infrequently. It has, however, been described in a 5-week-old, and again in an infant in whom the onset was at or before 3 weeks of age.

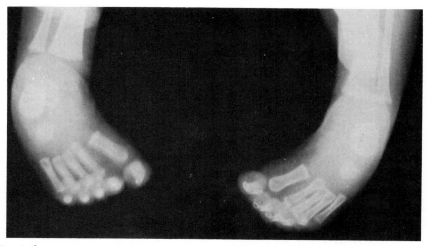

*Figure 98–5.*   Arthrogryposis in twins. Roentgenograms show the bones to be normal, but the soft tissues of the joint regions appear to be thickened and opacified. (Lipton, E. L., and Morgenstern, S. H.: A.M.A. J. Dis. Child. 89:233, 1955.)

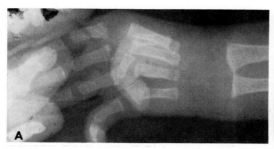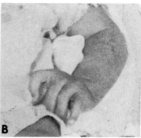

*Figure 98–6.* Arthrogryposis in twins. *A*, Roentgenogram of wrist of second twin. *B*, Photograph of arm shows the wrist fixed in dorsiflexion and the fingers tightly flexed. (Lipton, E. L., and Morgenstern, S. H.: A.M.A. J. Dis. Child. 89:233, 1955.)

This case, reported by Rosenthal, Gaballah and Rafelson, deserves brief summarization. It concerns a white male infant, born after normal pregnancy, labor and delivery, who weighed 8 pounds, 12 ounces (4205 gm) at birth. At 3 weeks his mother noted red-brown solid material on the diaper. At 7 weeks weight gain had been poor, and projectile vomiting began. Reddish-brown material increased in quantity in the diapers and accumulated on the penis.

At three months he was hospitalized for continued vomiting and dehydration. Weight was now ½ ounce above birth weight. He was pale and undernourished, but the rest of the examination revealed nothing abnormal. Urine pH was 4.5, specific gravity 1.008, albumin and sugar negative. Hemoglobin was 10.0 gm; white blood cells numbered 12,250 per cubic millimeter, with a normal differential. The blood nonprotein nitrogen level was 60 mg per 100 ml.

The red-brown material in the urine was identified as uric acid. Serum uric acid concentration was 18.6, urea nitrogen 67 and creatinine 2.3 mg per 100 ml.

The diagnosis of gout plus secondary renal insufficiency seemed justified.

Fluids were forced, and 1.0 gm of sodium citrate was given by mouth every 4 hours. As the pH of the urine rose, the precipitate disappeared. The blood uric acid level fell to 8.0 mg per 100 ml, where it remained. At 18 months the baby seemed well and weighed 11.82 kg, his urine was alkaline (he was still taking sodium citrate, 1.0 gm 4 times a day), and his serum urea nitrogen was 21 mg, his uric acid 8.3 mg per 100 ml.

There was a strongly positive family history for gouty diathesis in the family. A 15-year-old half-brother had urinary calculi, joint pains and a high uric acid level. He was improved by probenecid. The father also had renal calculi and an elevated blood uric acid level. The ma-ternal grandmother had a high blood uric acid level.

## DISORDERS OF THE FEET

It is impossible to treat the problem of congenital malformation of the feet with any degree of thoroughness because of limitations of space. We shall compromise by describing briefly three conditions which demand vigorous treatment soon after birth.

### PES CALCANEOVALGUS

This is the absolutely flat, at times slightly convex foot which often lies at rest dorsiflexed at an acute angle to the foreleg. When gentle pressure is applied to the sole of the foot, dorsiflexion increases easily until its dorsal surface lies in contact with the shin (Fig. 98–7).

These feet should be casted in the equinovarus position for 4 to 6 weeks, repeated several times if necessary. Continued treatment with tarsosupinator shoes, and perhaps with the Denis Browne bar, will probably be needed for several years.

### PES METATARSOVARUS

In this condition the heel and posterior half of the foot appear normal, but the forefoot angulates sharply inward. Thus the outer border of the foot is convex, while its inner border is concave (Fig. 98–8).

If the foot can be straightened by gentle traction, with the thumb held firmly over the apex of the convexity, no immediate

A

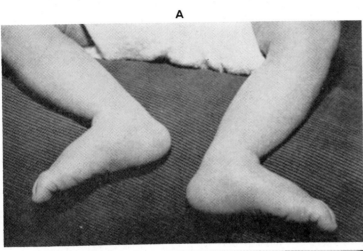

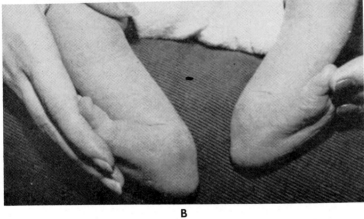

B

*Figure 98–7.* Calcaneovalgus deformity. *A*, Feet at rest; *B*, same feet under test. (Miller, W. R.: J. Pediatr. *51*:527, 1957.)

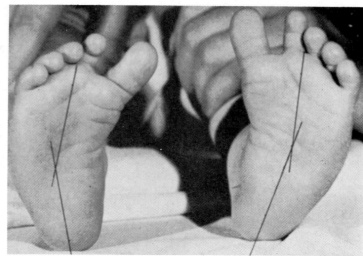

**Figure 98-8.** Metatarsus varus. (Miller, W. R.: J. Pediatr. *51*:527, 1957.)

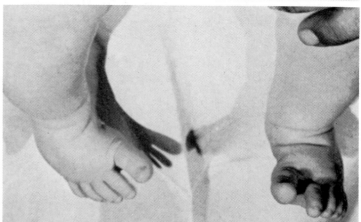

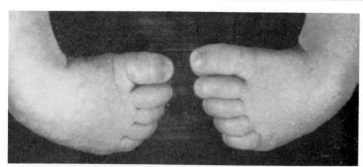

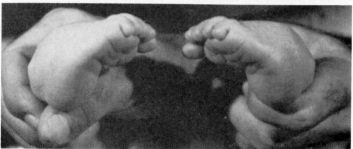

**Figure 98-9.** Congenital clubfeet. (Miller, W. R.: J. Pediatr. *51*:527, 1957.)

treatment is needed. If, on the other hand, the angulation is difficult or impossible to overcome, casting is probably indicated. Later use of corrective shoes may or may not be necessary.

### PES EQUINOVARUS

This is the classic clubfoot with sharp and tight hyperextension and incurving of the entire foot (Fig. 98–9). It is often a solitary defect, but not infrequently it is associated with congenital dislocation of the hip, myelomeningocele, arthrogryposis or other defects.

It requires immediate and long-continued orthopedic care. Most can be corrected by casting and subsequent shoe corrections. A few will require open operation.

### REFERENCES

Andren, L., and Borglin, N. E.: Disturbed urinary excretion pattern of oestrogens in newborns with congenital dislocation of the hip. Acta Endocrinol. 37:423, 1961.

Browne, D.: Congenital deformities of mechanical origin. Arch. Dis. Child. 30:37, 1955.

Charif, P., and Reichelderfer, T. E.: Genu recurvatum congenitum. Exhibit at A.M.A. Meeting, Atlantic City, June, 1963.

Dickerson, R. C.: Congenital dislocation of the hip. Pediatrics 41:977, 1968.

Fitti, R. M., and D'Auria, T. M.: Arthrogryposis multiplex congenita; case report. J. Pediatr. 48:797, 1956.

Miller, W. R.: Observations on the examination of children's feet. J. Pediatr., 51:527, 1957.

Rosenmann, A., and Arad, I.: Arthrogryposis multiplex congenita: Neurogenic type with autosomal recessive inheritance. J. Med. Genet., 11:91, 1974.

Rosenthal, J. M., Gaballah, S., and Rafelson, M. E.: Gout in infancy manifested by renal failure. Pediatrics 33:251, 1964.

von Rosen, S.: Diagnosis and treatment of congenital dislocation of the hip in the newborn. J. Bone Joint Surg., 44B:284, 1962.

Warkany, J.: Congenital Malformations. Notes and Comments. Year Book Medical Publishers, Chicago, 1971.

Wynne-Davies, R.: A family study of neonatal and late diagnosis, congenital dislocation of the hip. J. Med. Genet. 7:315, 1970.

# 99   MISCELLANEOUS DISORDERS OF THE SKELETAL SYSTEM

## CONGENITAL BOWING AND ANGULATION OF LONG BONES (CONGENITAL KYPHOSCOLIOTIC TIBIA, CONGENITAL PSEUDOARTHROSIS OF THE TIBIA)

As the name implies, this disorder consists in abnormal curvature of one or more bones which has developed in utero.

**INCIDENCE.**   The condition is rare.

**ETIOLOGY.**   No more than one case has ever been observed in a sibship, nor have successive generations been similarly affected. However, "many patients have been reported to have family histories of neurofibromatosis or stigmata of neurofibromatosis" (Gwinn and Barnes). The exact connection between the two, if there is any, is not known.

The cause is believed by some to lie in abnormal mechanical pressure upon the growing limb, although the not infrequent coexistence of other congenital malformations casts doubt upon this hypothesis. In Angle's case the "position of comfort" of the newborn infant seemed to consist in the soles of the feet being placed in the midportion of the convexity of the opposite femur. Angle inferred that the foot applied right angular pressure to the femur and acted as the fulcrum against which intrauterine forces acted.

**DIAGNOSIS.**   The tibia is by far the most frequently affected bone, some being angulated anteriorly, some posteriorly. Males are involved more often than females. Multiple osseous angulation is not too uncommon. Characteristically a deep dimple overlies the apex of the convexity. In the x-ray film the cortex is thickened on the con-

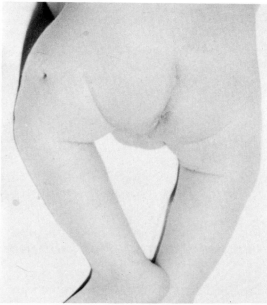

*Figure 99–1.* Photograph of lower limbs showing shortening and angulation of the femora. That of the left femur is seen clearly, and the characteristic dimple at the apex of the convexity is obvious. (Angle, C. R.: Pediatrics *13*:257, 1954.)

cave side, thinned on the convex side. Radiolucent cystic areas are not infrequently seen on x-ray within the mass of angulated bone. Actual fracture may take place at this point. When it does, nonunion, that is, pseudoarthrosis, often follows. This makes the prognosis for ultimate cure very gloomy.

TREATMENT. Treatment consists in orthopedic correction. This may necessitate operative fracture and casting.

## CONGENITAL LAXITY OF LIGAMENTS

This disorder derives its importance from the fact that it may easily be confused with more serious conditions. It is characterized by extreme laxity of ligaments and hypotonia of muscles. It is extremely rare.

ETIOLOGY. It is almost surely a hereditary defect, transmitted as a recessive trait. No pathologic structural alterations have been described.

DIAGNOSIS. Birth is without incident, and the newborn infant cries and breathes spontaneously. Thereafter he lies passively and moves very little, although he may suck well. The muscles feel extraordinarily flabby, as though they were composed of fat. All the joints show an abnormal range of movement. All sorts of acrobatic double-jointed positions can be attained without much effort and with no pain.

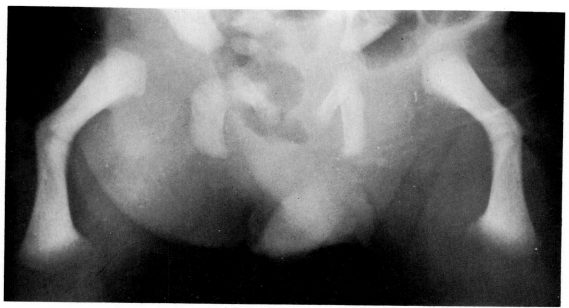

*Figure 99–2.* Roentgenogram of the femurs shows bilateral angulation and fracture. (Angle, C. R.: Pediatrics *13*:257, 1954.)

Differentiation must be made between congenital laxity of ligaments and all the other conditions in which hypermobility of the joints and muscular hypotonia are present. These include, in the neonatal period, mongolism, cutis laxa, the Ehlers-Danlos syndrome, atonic diplegia, amyotonia congenita (Oppenheim's disease), myasthenia gravis and glycogen storage disease of the cardiomuscular type, inter alia.

**PROGNOSIS.** This is excellent. The infant described by Catzel, from whose case report most of this summary was derived, was much improved by the end of his first year.

**TREATMENT.** None is indicated.

## CONGENITAL LUMBAR HERNIA

Lee and Mattheis recalled to attention this unusual malformation. We have encountered a case identical in all respects. As an acquired phenomenon, lumbar hernia, following accidental or surgical trauma, is not uncommon, but only a dozen of the congenital variety have been reported.

**ETIOLOGY.** This is plainly a developmental defect arising early in gestation. The lower ribs are distorted, hemivertebrae of the lower dorsal and upper lumbar region are usually found, and the fascial and muscle coats are thinned. Some muscles may indeed be missing. Its occurrence is inexplicable on embryologic grounds, since, as Nastin said, "Nothing in the development of the abdominal wall can account for the formation of a gap in the lumbar region."

**DIAGNOSIS.** At birth the entire lumbar area on one side is seen to protrude. The mass is soft and compressible, and within it no discrete tumor can be palpated. The only associated malformation in the above-mentioned authors' case was an undescended testis on the same side.

**TREATMENT.** Treatment is surgical. The defect is closed by imbrication of muscles, fasciae and aponeuroses.

## FRACTURES SUSTAINED DURING DELIVERY

Simple and depressed fractures of the skull have been discussed previously (p.

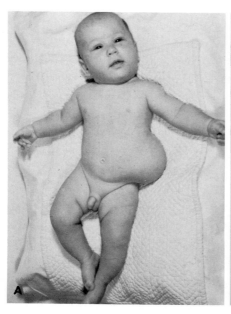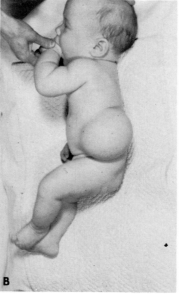

*Figure 99–3.* Photographs of an infant in the anteroposterior (*A*) and lateral (*B*) views show a grapefruit-sized mass projecting from the left flank. (Lee, C. M., Jr., and Mattheis, H.: Arch. Dis. Child. *32*:42, 1957.)

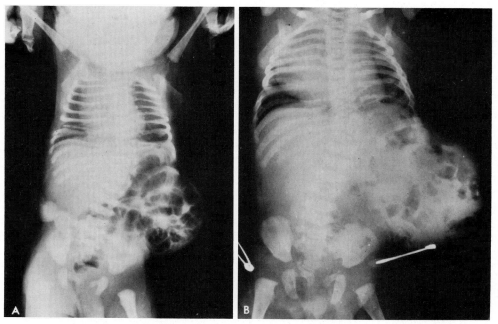

***Figure 99–4.*** Anteroposterior roentgenograms of the same infant show the mass to be filled with apparently normal bowel. Several of the lower thoracic vertebrae are deformed. (Lee, C. M., Jr., and Mattheis, H.: Arch. Dis. Child. *32*:42, 1957.)

696). Pathologic fractures sustained in utero are encountered in newborns with osteogenesis imperfecta (p. 890).

The clavicles are the bones most often fractured during delivery. Shoulder dystocia, probably the commonest cause of prolonged and difficult delivery, calls for vigorous, often violent, manipulation of the arm and shoulder. Resulting fracture of one clavicle may be incomplete, that is, greenstick, or complete. In the first instance no disability or pain need be present, and the first intimation that the accident occurred may be the discovery of a large callus in the second week of life. Complete fractures are manifest immediately after birth by the infant's refusal to move the affected arm, by crying as though in pain whenever the arm is moved, by tenderness and at times visible angulation or hematoma over the fracture site and by hypermobility of the bone. The Moro response is absent on that side. X-ray examination verifies the diagnosis.

Less often the humerus and even more rarely the femur can be fractured during delivery. Diagnosis of these conditions is not difficult and is made by eliciting their conventional signs, and verified by x-ray examination.

It must be remembered that the discovery of a fractured clavicle or humerus does not automatically rule out concomitant brachial plexus or peripheral nerve injury. Indeed, their presence augments the likelihood of the concomitance of one of these neurologic traumata. When a fracture is found, evidences of upper, lower or combined brachial palsy and of diaphragmatic paralysis will be sought out.

## EPIPHYSIAL INJURIES IN BREECH DELIVERY

Shulman and Terhune summarized knowledge of this disorder in 1951. That it is not excessively uncommon is indicated by the fact that they had observed four cases themselves.

**ETIOLOGY.** Firstborns are affected almost exclusively. The more rigid primiparous outlets call for greater force during extraction. Breech presentations requiring manual extraction or version and extraction are most liable to this type of injury, but it may occur in any delivery in which vigorous pulling is done. The upper epiphysis of the femur is the site most commonly involved, with the upper epiphysis of the humerus in the second numerical position. The usual traumatic result is separation of the epiphysis without dislocation.

**DIAGNOSIS.** Clinical signs do not become apparent until the second day. Then, if it is the upper femoral epiphysis that has been injured, the infant assumes the frog position, and the soft tissues over the upper thigh become full, tense and reddened. Pressure and passive motion cause pain. Low fever may be present, and also much irritability. All symptoms and signs clear within 1 to 2 weeks.

X-ray films show nothing until the end of the first week. At that time excessive subperiosteal calcification makes its appearance about the injured site. Dislocation of the epiphysis may be visualized.

Shulman's fourth case is of especial interest. On the tenth day of life this infant had great swelling and tenderness of the lower third of both thighs. X-ray film showed considerable subperiosteal calcification in these areas (Fig. 99–5), and his blood calcium level was 8.7 mg per 100 ml. Five days later he had three generalized convulsions, and his calcium level had fallen to 5.6 mg. The logical assumption was

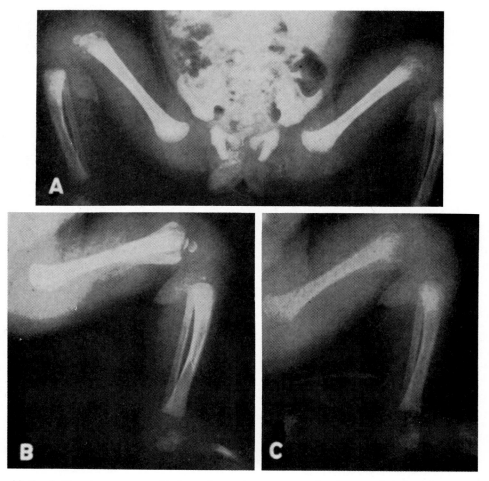

*Figure 99–5.* A, Roentgenogram at 11 days of age, showing osteochondritis and slight subperiosteal changes of lower third of both femora. B, Left, and C, right, on sixteenth day of life, showing definite subperiosteal calcification of both lower femora. (Shulman, B. H., and Terhune, C. B.: Pediatrics 8:693, 1951.)

that hypocalcemic tetany had followed withdrawal of calcium from the circulating blood during the phase of calcification of the callus.

**TREATMENT.** No treatment is needed unless there is dislocation. If there is dislocation, a cast may have to be applied.

## KLIPPEL-FEIL SYNDROME

The syndrome of short neck, associated usually with limitation of motion of the neck and low hairline, has been recognized in the newborn infant. Roentgenograms almost always show fusion of two or more of the bodies or arches of the cervical vertebrae, and not too infrequently the absence of one. Many of the affected infants have other congenital defects, some of them severe, but by no means all. These defects are apt to involve the nervous system.

Baird and his collaborators demonstrated that 12 of their 13 patients studied for inability to dissociate movements of their two hands showed these "mirror movements." Their significance is not known.

Most of these children grow quite slowly and end up short. Virtually no treatment is available for them.

## REFERENCES

Angle, C. R.: Congenital bowing and angulation of long bones. Pediatrics *13*:257, 1954.

Baird, P. A., Robinson, G. C., and Buckler, W. St. J.: Klippel-Feil syndrome: A study of mirror movement detected by electromyography. Am. J. Dis. Child. *113*:546, 1967.

Bound, J. P., Finlay, H. V. L., and Rose, F. C.: Congenital anterior angulation of the tibia. Arch. Dis. Child. *17*:179, 1952.

Catzel, P.: Congenital laxity of ligaments and hypotonia. Arch. Dis. Child. *30*:387, 1955.

Gwinn, J. L., and Barnes, G. R.: Congenital kyphoscoliotic tibia. Am. J. Dis. Child.

Lee, C. M., Jr., and Mattheis, H.: Congenital lumbar hernia. Arch. Dis. Child. *32*:42, 1957.

Nastin, cited by Lee and Mattheis.

Shulman, B. H., and Terhune, C. B.: Epiphyseal injuries in breech delivery. Pediatrics 8:693, 1951.

# XIV

# Constellations of Congenital Malformations (Odd-Looking Babies)

Repeatedly one sees babies born with various associated congenital malformations of such striking similarity of facies and other characteristics that one would expect a single teratogenic factor to be responsible for them all. In some such a factor can be assigned, but more often it cannot.

Described elsewhere in this volume are the visible features which stigmatize the following:

1. Hormonal deprivation or excess
   a. Cretinism
   b. Hypopituitarism
   d. Hyperadrenocorticism
   d. Infants of diabetic mothers
   e. Hypoparathyroidism
2. Errors of metabolism, for the most part inborn
   a. Phenylketonuria
   b. Homocystinuria

   c. Idiopathic hypercalcemia
3. Maternal drug ingestion
   a. Androgenic substances
   b. Thalidomide
   c. Fetal alcohol syndrome
   d. Dilantin syndrome
   e. Tridione syndrome
4. Exposure to radiant energy
   a. Microcephaly

Others are discussed in the sections devoted to disorders of the system which is most obviously involved in their deviation from the normal. Examples are the Pierre Robin syndrome, Treacher Collins syndrome, the dyschondroplasias, acrocephalo-syndactylism and others. There remain still others whose manifestations are so widespread that they cannot be classified by system. Some of these are included in the following pages.

**909**

# 100

## GROSS CHROMOSOMAL ABERRATIONS

*Revised by F. Clarke Fraser*

Only as recently as 1956 was it established that the modal number of chromosomes in the cells of man is 46. This diploid number represents 22 pairs of autosomes and two sex chromosomes, either two X's or an X and a Y. Spermatocytes and oocytes undergo meiosis in which the resulting cells (spermatids or oocytes) receive only one member of each pair. Thus the spermatozoon and the unfertilized ovum contain the haploid number of chromosomes, 22 autosomes and either an X or a Y. Fertilization means restoration of the chromosome number to 46 in the new individual so created.

It is not unexpected that mishaps befall during these complicated maneuvers. When errors in number, size or configuration result, visible under the microscope in properly prepared specimens, they are termed gross chromosomal aberrations, in contradistinction to the invisible alterations in single DNA nucleotides that result in the mutations underlying the inborn errors of metabolism.

A typical normal karyotype is shown in Figure 100–1. The 44 autosomes are divided into groups A (three pairs, 1, 2, 3), B (two pairs, 4, 5), C (seven pairs 6, 7, 8, 9, 10, 11, 12), D (three pairs, 13, 14, 15), E (three pairs, 16, 17, 18), F (two pairs, 19, 20) and G (two pairs, 21, 22). These are distinguished one from another by size, and by position of centromere which divides each chromosome into two arms (arms equal, metacentric; somewhat unequal, submedian; or with constriction almost at the end, acrocentric).

Furthermore, since 1973, innovations in staining techniques have revealed patterns of bands along the chromosomes so that each chromosome, and often specific regions of a chromosome, can be individually identified. Thus it is possible to detect much more subtle aberrations (deletions and rearrangements) than was previously possible. The illustration shows a karyotype prepared after G banding, using a modified Giemsa staining technique. These techniques have greatly increased the discrimination and precision of cytogenetic diagnosis, and the number of recognizable syndromes resulting from chromosomal aberrations is rapidly increasing. A convention has been adopted whereby the short arm of a chromosome is labelled p and the long arm q. Each band has a specific number. The relations between abnormalities in specific chromosomes and resultant alterations in phenotype are hardly understood at all.

Chromosomes may be abnormal in number, size or configuration. Such abnormalities are brought about by *nondisjunction* (failure of a pair of chromosomes to separate during meiosis), or breakage and subsequent rearrangements (*deletions, inversions, translocations* and others). A few individuals are *mosaics;* i.e. their body is made up of two or more cell lines, with different karyotypes.

From the data accumulated to the present time a few generalizations can be made.

1. Loss of any one entire autosome is almost always incompatible with life. At least four cases of complete monosomy, with survival for a number of years, have by now been described.

2. At least one X chromosome is requisite for life and development.

3. The Y chromosome is the male-determining chromosome. In its absence life and development may proceed, but in the female developmental pathway and, when there is only one X, far from perfectly.

4. Excesses of chromatin material, in the

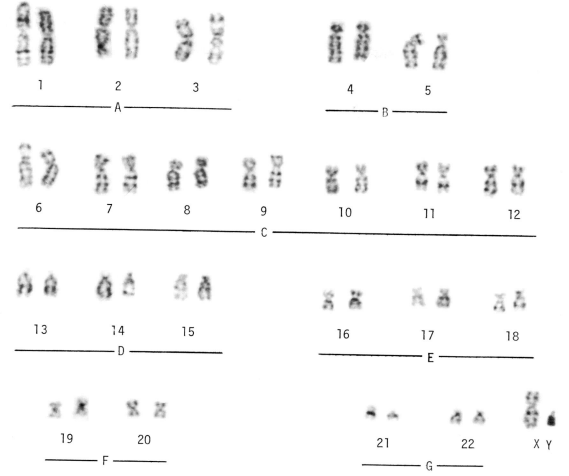

**Figure 100–1.**  Karyotype of normal male, showing banding produced by trypsin treatment of Seabright (1972). (Courtesy of Dr. Hope Punnett.)

form of extra entire chromosomes or of translocations or insertions of portions of chromosomes, are often compatible with continued life and development.

5. Gross chromosomal aberrations are *usually* associated with multiple congenital structural defects.

6. Mosaicism may exist in individuals who are phenotypically normal, or who have all the characteristics associated with their abnormal karyotype, or who show some but not all of the defects which usually result from that chromosomal aberration.

7. At least 10 well-defined clinical syndromes have been identified to date that correspond well with corresponding alterations in one autosome group (trisomies 13, 18, 21 and 22; deletion of the short arm of 4, 5 and 18; deletion of the short arm of 13, 18, 21 and 22). Other syndromes resulting from "partial trisomy" or deletion of specific segments of autosomes are gradually being delineated. Lewandowski and Yunis have prepared a useful list of the abnormal features occurring in the more recently recognized syndromes. Most of them are difficult to diagnose reliably by phenotype; if there is any suspicion of a chromosomal syndrome it is best to confirm it by karyotyping.

8. Two well defined clinical syndromes

result from specific aberrations of sex chromosomes (Turner's, XO, and Klinefelter's, XXY). A third is by no means uncommon (XYY), but at least one of the behavioral abnormalities ascribed to it has become the subject of heated controversy. A host of other aberrations of sex chromosomes have been encountered, but the constellations of congenital defects they produce are not so well defined.

The frequency of autosomal aberrations has been established as about 6 per 1000 births. However the use of modern banding techniques will undoubtedly increase this number considerably. Sex chromosome aberrations account for about one or two per thousand births. As many as 60 per cent of spontaneous abortions are associated with a chromosomal aberration according to the meticulous studies of the Boués.

The recent advances in cytogenetic techniques have also increased greatly the precision of prenatal diagnosis of chromosomal aberrations.

## DERMATOGLYPHICS

The study of ridge patterns on fingers and palms and of crease patterns on palms and digits dates back to the observations of Sir Francis Galton in 1892. The variations from the normal have been utilized more and more often in recent years for the diagnosis of syndromes, especially those associated with chromosomal aberrations.

These cannot be discussed in detail here, but have been reviewed recently by Preus. The most important patterns looked for are the following:

1. Fingerprints. These are conventionally classified as arches, loops or whorls, and loops are commonly designated as radial or ulnar, depending upon the orientation of their open end.

2. Transverse palmar lines. There should be two of these, and when there is only one, or the two are joined by a distinct bridge, this is classified as a simian crease. If the proximal transverse line extends to the ulnar border of the hand it is called a Sydney line.

3. Position of axial triradius. In normal individuals the axial triradius is found to lie near the proximal border of the palm. Displacement distally, that is, toward the center of the palm, occurs in normal individuals, but more frequently with a variety of syndromes. Its height can be measured as a percentage of the height from the distal wrist crease to the proximal crease at the base of the third digit. If this is greater than 40 per cent the axial triradius is referred to as t.' Bilateral t' occurs in 80 per cent of children with Down syndrome or trisomy 13, in roughly 20 per cent of children with trisomy 18, de Lange syndrome, and Rubinstein-Taybi syndrome, and in 3 per cent of normal children.

Baird has observed a family, thirteen of whose twenty-four members in three generations show complete absence of dermal ridges. This defect appeared to be transmitted as a dominant, nonsex-linked trait with variable penetrance.

## TRISOMY 21 (DOWN SYNDROME, MONGOLISM)

Trisomy 21 is an association of congenital anomalies which imparts to its subjects a characteristic facies. All of these children are by no means identical, but facies and body build are so similar that they bear a strong family resemblance. A common basic defect is reduced intellectual capacity, but even this is variable in degree and need not be present in all. Treatment is symptomatic, and prognosis is poor.

**INCIDENCE.** Among whites the incidence is between one and two per thousand live births, probably closer to one than to two. For many years it was alleged that Down syndrome did not occur in the Black and Asiatic races, but this is surely incorrect. Its incidence among them may be lower than it is in Caucasians.

**ETIOLOGY.** The frequency of Down syndrome is greatest in infants of mothers near the end of the child-bearing period, though this tendency appears to be decreasing.

In 1959 two teams of observers reported almost simultaneously the finding of an extra chromosome in the karyotypes of mongoloids. The forty-seventh chromosome seemed to fit into group G (21, 22);

hence the disorder was termed trisomy 21. The mechanism responsible for the extra chromosome was believed to be nondisjunction during meiosis, a "mistake" in the segregation of the chromosomes. This appeared to explain the observation that many of these infants were born to older mothers, since geneticists have long been aware that nondisjunction is a more frequent accident in their aging laboratory subjects than in the young. It also explains why the disorder is sporadic and not familial in most cases.

It soon became clear that not all Down syndrome children were trisomic for 21. A minority had the normal number of chromosomes, with two pairs of acrocentric autosomes in group G, but one atypical chromosome in another group. To take a frequent example, one of pair 13 may be missing, but replaced by a chromosome that appears to consist of the long arms of 13 and 21. These chromosomes arise by "robertsonian" translocation, in which the centromeres of 21 and 13 have fused; the short arms are lost, but their absence does not seem to have any effect. Hence these individuals possess a superabundance of 21 chromatin just as does the trisomy 21. These karyotypes are termed 46, translocation 15/21. Translocations of 21 to other chromosomes have been reported less commonly.

Translocations of this nature, unlike trisomies, are sometimes found in one parent and in other close relatives of the affected infant; hence this form of the disorder is familial and heritable, transmitted from one generation to others as an autosomal dominant. In these cases the association with increased maternal age does not appear. Such translocations need not produce abnormalities, if they are "balanced"—i.e. they have one 21, one 13 and the 13/15 translocation chromosome, so there is no excess chromosomal material. However, balanced carriers may produce unbalanced gametes, leading to abortion or chromosomal syndromes in the offspring. Fortunately such carriers may now take advantage of prenatal diagnosis (see Chapter 3).

The trisomic mongol, although himself or herself the result of a sporadic aberration, is capable of transmitting mongolism as a dominant. Fortunately few have produced offspring.

Finally, there have by now been reported a number of infants who are mosaics for trisomy 21 or translocations 15/21 or 21/22. Some have manifested all the defects of Down syndrome, some only a few of them. Some of this subgroup have attained an intellectual capacity within the range of normal. Mosaicism may explain the heretofore mystifying stories about children who had many of the stigmata of monogolism, but who were able nevertheless to keep up with and at times excel their peers in scholastic performance.

**DIAGNOIS.** Most infants with Down syndrome can be diagnosed at birth or at first glance. In a few the diagnosis may remain in doubt. Dermatoglyphic analysis can often establish or rule out the diagnosis with a high level of confidence. If there is a reasonable suspicion of Down syndrome a karyotype should be requested, to establish whether there is a regular trisomy or a translocation. If the latter, the parents should be karyotyped, and if they are translocation carriers other family members should be studied to identify those at increased risk. There are a number of characteristics which become manifest only later in life, but usually enough are sufficiently obvious from the moment of birth to make the diagnosis with assurance (Figs. 100–2 and 100–3). These may include (and it must be remembered that not all children with Down syndrome demonstrate *all* the anatomic defects of the syndrome) the following:

**SMALL SIZE.** Twenty per cent are prematurely born. Very few are as large as expected for their gestational ages.

**GLOBULAR BRACHYCEPHALIC SKULL.** The suboccipitobregmatic circumference is generally small; the skull is short and round.

**CHARACTERISTIC EYES.** The eyes slant upward from within outward. There is a prominent epicanthic fold involving the inner half of the upper eyelid. This is associated with a flat nose-bridge and tends to disappear as the child gets older. The eyeball is not recessed, giving rise to the flache Gesicht, the "flat face" noted by observers long ago. The iris may be speckled with Brushfield's spots, but this sign is rapidly obscured if the iris is darkly pigmented.

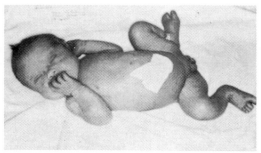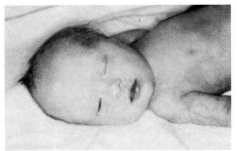

*Figure 100–2.* *A,* Overall view of Down syndrome infant made on the second day of life. General hypotonia is suggested by the relaxed appearance in what appears to be an awkward position. *B,* Head and face of the infant show the round, short skull, well developed epicanthus, slanting of lid slits upward from within outward, and shallow orbits.

RED CHEEKS. This sign may not be prominent immediately after birth, but it becomes increasingly so with the passage of months.

NARROW AND SHORT PALATE. (Shapiro et al.).

SHORT, FLAT-BRIDGED RETROUSSÉ NOSE.

PROTRUDING TONGUE. Later the dorsum of the tongue becomes dry, wrinkled and fissured, the so-called scrotal tongue.

LOOSE SKIN COVERING THE LATERAL AND DORSAL ASPECTS OF THE NECK.

CHARACTERISTIC HANDS. The fingers are short; the hands appear square. The thumb is low-set and separated a bit more than usual from the second finger. The fifth finger is apt to be short and incurved, to have but one transverse crease and to show absence or hypoplasia of its middle phalanx by x-ray study. The two usual transverse palmar creases are often replaced by a single deep one, the simian crease.

UMBILICAL HERNIA is often present.

CHARACTERISTIC FEET. The great toe is separated from the second toe. Between these toes a deep crease begins and continues in an arc around the thenar eminence to the medial edge of the sole.

MUSCULAR HYPOTONIA. This, associated with laxity of ligaments, permits extraordinary malleability. The great toe can easily be placed in the infant's mouth and the hand hyperextended until it lies flat against the dorsal aspect of the forearm.

NARROW ACETABULAR ANGLE, ILIAC INDEX (II) AND BROADENED ILIAL BONES, as determined by x-ray film.

RETARDED PSYCHOMOTOR DEVELOPMENT. This cannot be determined in the neonatal period, but will become manifest soon.

CONGENITAL HEART DEFECT. A common associated malformation is an interventricular septal defect, characteristically a persistent ostium primum.

DUODENAL ATRESIA. This congenital malformation is present in trisomy 21 children many times more often than it is in normals.

LEUKEMIA AND LEUKEMOID REACTIONS. A great many more trisomy 21 children

*Figure 100–3.* Photographs of two siblings with Down's syndrome caused by a translocation, not trisomy 21. (Warkany, J., et al.: Pediatrics 33:290, 1964.)

have these blood dyscrasias than do normal children, though the absolute frequency is fairly low.

**PROGNOSIS.** The hazards to life confronting children with Down syndrome are fairly numerous. They include, in chronologic order of appearance, coexisting severe congenital defects, to which they are inordinately liable. Among infants born with esophageal atresia, duodenal atresia and imperforate anus are included a large number of those with Down syndrome. Many of them have been reported among series of examples of annular pancreas. Congenital heart defects are common concomitants of the syndrome. Many of these turn out to be simple high interventricular septal defects, persistent ostium primum, which do little more than produce a loud murmur, but some are more complicated and more serious. Patients with Down syndrome are excessively liable to upper respiratory tract infections which, in preantibiotic days, often became lower respiratory tract infections and were responsible for many deaths. Few infants die for this reason nowadays.

The outlook for these children with respect to physical and mental development is discouraging. In a discussion limited to newborns this concerns us only because it has direct bearing upon the advice one has to give the parents. Almost all the signposts of development will appear late, in some moderately late, in some exceedingly so. In a study of the variability of trisomy 21, Levinson pointed out that whereas a few infants learned to sit alone between 6 and 8 months, most could not sit until they were over a year. A few learned connected speech, that is, sentence formation, by about 3 years of age, but most could not form sentences until they were more than 6 years old, some never learning how. The best equipped will fall into the classification of low grade morons, but most will have to be designated as imbeciles. Practically none are truly idiots. (However, these observations were based largely on children who were raised in institutions.) They are almost without exception pleasant, lovable, non-destructive children, who love music and are educable to a point far beyond that which we used to think possible. Smith and Wilson have prepared an inexpensive, well-illustrated book that provides useful information about the characteristics of children with Down syndrome, which parents of such children will find helpful.

**TREATMENT.** Once the diagnosis has been made with a fair degree of assurance, someone will almost surely suggest that the problem be solved by euthanasia. The suggestion may come from the obstetrician, from a nurse, from a member of the family who has been apprised of the situation, or it may occur to the pediatrician himself. Undeniably, euthanasia was resorted to, and not infrequently, in the past. It obviously presents an easy solution to what promises to be a long drawn-out, difficult situation. But the pediatrician must never allow himself to fall into this trap. Aside from the ethical considerations involved, euthanasia contravenes the laws of the state and makes the offending physician liable to severe penalties.

The next problem will inevitably concern itself with the disposition of the infant. Shall he be forthwith dispatched to a custodial home before the parents have the opportunity of becoming too attached to him, or shall he be taken home and reared as any other child would be? A generation ago the former decision was often taken, if the parents could afford the expense of custodial care. Now, under the benign influence of psychiatry, which has radically reoriented the thinking of pediatricians, the consensus appears to have swung in the other direction. The arguments are both positive and negative. On the positive side is the item that these children, in their own homes, receive the attention and affection to which every child is entitled. Under these circumstances their emotional life is not stunted, they respond to affection with affection, and their behavior patterns therefore approach more closely those of normal children. In addition, they are likely to develop intellectually to a point more nearly approximating their ultimate capacity, to become more amenable, to learn simple but important things such as toilet training, the ability to dress themselves and obedience to simple commands. Not only may they grow to the point at which they are no longer nuisances around the house but also they may develop skills which are quite useful. In this latter respect they can be helped considerably by attendance at special nursery schools, supervised by teachers trained in the education of the educable mentally retarded. In our own practice there are a number of trisomy 21 children who are the lights of their parents' lives. This is especially true if they are the only children of elderly parents, as they often are.

The prime argument against putting these infants away is that the children, if they survive institutional existence, grow up underdeveloped emotionally and intellectually, exactly as do many normals raised in institutions. Almost equally cogent is the effect of the decision to institutionalize upon some parents who, having consigned their child to the care of not-too-interested strangers, develop feelings of guilt which precipitate in them emotional disturbances of variable degree, some quite severe.

Many circumstances may have bearing upon the success or failure of home-rearing a retarded child. A child with Down syndrome who is, and who is apt to remain, an only child presents a considerably different problem from one who is the first of young parents who will, in all probability, have several other, normal children. This situation also differs a good deal from that in which the child is the last, as he often is, of a large family of normals. Another variable is the emotional makeup of the parents, particularly the mother. Is she calm, well balanced, on an even emotional keel herself? Or is she spoiled, self-indulgent, hypochondriacal, helpless in the face of even the minor problems incident to the rearing of a normal child? One wonders whether the discipline of rearing a defective child in her own home with all its implications of family and social stigma would be more likely to strengthen her or to break her completely. We cite these two examples as the two ends of a spectrum that contains innumerable personality makeups.

Indeed there are two spectra, for the father's pattern must be taken into account. In the case of one of our trisomy 21 girls, when last seen by us at 11 years of age,

home-rearing had been a complete failure because the father fits the description of the second hypothetical mother above. Now that there are two normal younger children, the presence in the household of a severely retarded, poorly trained, badly spoiled eldest child is making a shambles of the home, and it has become imperative that she be institutionalized. She has since been sterilized, with our full concurrence.

The decision as to whether to institutionalize will therefore be made after all the known facts have been taken into consideration. The young pediatrician would be well advised to call into consultation an older, more experienced one to aid him in arriving at the proper conclusion. Both the younger and the older pediatrician might well be helped by the advice of a psychiatrist.

## TRISOMY 22

This syndrome has been clearly defined only since the advent of modern banding techniques. The features include growth retardation, mental retardation, microcephaly, micrognathia, preauricular skin tags or sinuses, low-set, abnormal ears, cleft palate, congenital heart disease and digitalized or malopposed thumbs. The so-called "cat-eye" syndrome appears to result from partial trisomy 22. The main features are colobomas, hypertelorism, down-slanted (anti-mongoloid) palpebral fissures and anal atresia, as well as many features of full-blown trisomy 22, but without cleft palate.

## TRISOMY 18

After Down syndrome, the second gross autosomal aberration discovered capable of producing a fairly constant constellation of structural abnormalities was an extra chromosome in group E (16–18), now known to be trisomy 18.

**ETIOLOGY.** Nondisjunction appears to account for the majority of these cases. But, exactly as in trisomy 21, other defects in the karyotype were soon observed to be associated with the same clinical syndrome. Identical babies have been reported to have partial trisomy, translocations or mosaicisms. One has been recorded who had forty-eight chromosomes, an additional X (triple-X) as well as an extra group E autosome. In most instances mother and father had both passed their thirtieth year of age by the time the abnormal child had been conceived, but this is not invariably true. The same conditions of familial incidence and heredity apply to this syndrome as have been cited for Down syndrome.

**DIAGNOSIS.** The constellation of obstetrical and congenital abnormalities that earmarks these children includes the following (it must be remembered that, as in trisomy 21, not all the babies of this genre will manifest all the deviations from normal) (Fig. 100–4): 1) advanced parental age; 2) low birth weight after term gestation; 3) low-set, abnormal ears; 4) micrognathia (and microstomia); 5) mental retardation; 6) characteristically flexed fingers, with flexion contraction of the two middle digits, which are overlapped by the flexed thumb and index and little fingers; 7) congenital heart defect, almost always a ventricular septal defect, often coupled with

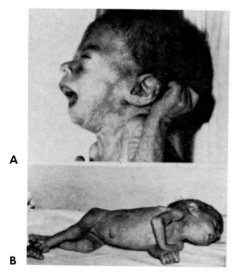

*Figure 100–4.* A, Photograph of head of newborn infant with trisomy E. This shows well low-set large ears and micrognathia. B, Demonstrates high degree of malnutrition, arthrogryposis and characteristic flexion deformities of the fingers. (Hecht, F., et al.: J. Pediatr. 63:605, 1963.)

patent ductus arteriosus; 8) rocker-bottom feet.

In addition to these almost universal abnormalities, many have ptosis of one or both eyelids, syndactyly, an abnormally jutting occiput, genitourinary defects, hernias and other scattered imperfections A few show the typical simian palmar crease, and dermatoglyphic studies reveal a preponderance of arch patterns. Arches on seven or more fingers occur in 80 per cent of cases, and less than six arches or more than two whorls is reason to be very skeptical of the diagnosis.

An observation of extraordinary interest was made by Alpert and his co-workers. Among 19 autopsied cases of the trisomy 18 syndrome, seven cases of neonatal hepatitis were discovered. Included in these seven were two of extrahepatic biliary atresia; in others, focal obliteration of bile ducts secondary to cholangitis was seen. This finding raises a number of intriguing questions. One has little to do with chromosomal aberrations but a great deal to do with the pathogenesis of congenital biliary atresia. Could these cases, or some of them, be due not to congenital defect, but to the consequences of fetal cholangitis? Such an idea has been suggested before, and this communication seems to offer strong supportive evidence to the hypothesis. Or—and more pertinent to our discussion—could the trisomic aberration itself, along with the hepatitis, be the result of early fetal infection? If so, one would expect mosaicism.

**PROGNOSIS.** Most of these babies die in early infancy, generally from heart failure. One, a partial trisomy, survived until 5½ years of age, while another of the same karyotype is still living at 7½ years. A third was living at 20 years at the time his report appeared. His karyotype was that of a translocation.

**TREATMENT.** Each defect must be treated on its own merits. Clearly, one can look forward to little benefit from therapy.

## TRISOMY 13

Trisomy of one of the group D autosomes, number 13, and mosaicisms of this aberration, are much less common than those of group E.

**DIAGNOSIS.** D trisomies have several defects in common with E trisomies. These are 1) psychomotor retardation, 2) malformed ears, 3) flexion deformities of wrist, hand and fingers, 4) congenital heart defects, 5) rocker-bottom feet, 6) simian creases.

In addition, they manifest abnormalities which are not characteristic of trisomy E. Such abnormalities are eye defects (microphthalmos, colobomata of iris and lids, cataracts); broad, flattened nose; failure of fusion of maxillary and palatal processes (harelip, cleft palate); umbilical defects (hernia, omphalocele); abnormalities of the genitals (in the female, bicornuate or septate uterus; in the male, cryptorchidism, small, anteriorly placed scrotum); cutaneous hemangiomas; gross defects of the brain (arhinencephaly and others); tendency to grand mal seizures, myoclonic jerks and severe breath-holding spells; skin defects of the scalp, and characteristic dermatoglyphics.

This group has assumed additional importance because of the finding in most of

them of several hematologic abnormalities. They have increased fetal hemoglobin (HbF), Bart's hemoglobin (gamma-4) and possibly embryonic hemoglobins (Gower 2). Walzer et al. added to these an abnormally low level of $HbA_2$. Their patient, a D-D translocation trisomy, had HbF levels consistently higher than expected and $HbA_2$ levels consistently lower from birth to 9 months of age, when he died. On the other hand, a patient of Wilson and Melnyk, with D-D translocation and *normal cell mosaicism*, did not show any hemoglobin abnormality.

**PROGNOSIS.** Death in early infancy is the rule. Some children survive for several years.

**TREATMENT.** Harelip and cleft palate may be repaired, and other defects amenable to surgical correction may be given appropriate therapy.

## LE CRI DU CHAT (CAT'S CRY) 5P SYNDROME

Lejeune observed three cases in which a deletion of the short arms of chromosome number 5 was associated with a consistent and characteristic constellation of malformations. This was the first autosomal deletion syndrome to be defined. As one would expect, the phenotypes described in these syndromes are quite variable, depending presumably on the extent and location of the deletion.

All his infants demonstrated microcephaly, micrognathia, epicanthus, oblique palpebral fissures, hypertelorism, low-set ears, severe mental retardation and *a peculiar cry resembling that of a cat*. However the facies is not as strikingly characteristic as it is in the trisomy syndromes.

The karyotype in all cases showed 46 chromosomes, but one autosome in the B group, number 5, was lacking part of the short arm.

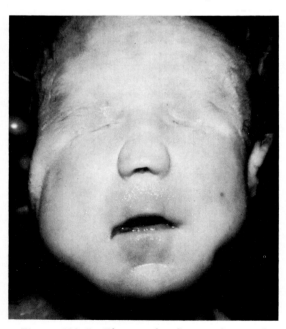

*Figure 100–5.* Photograph of a newborn infant with the trisomy D syndrome. Note microphthalmos and the bizarre nose with (in this case) a single centrally placed nostril. The ears are also low-set and malformed. (We are grateful to Dr. Barbara Migeon for this illustration.)

## THE 4P SYNDROME

A second deletion syndrome in the B group has been identified as involving the short arm of chromosome 4. The main features are low birth weight, profound psychomotor retardation, microcephaly, hypertelorism with a prominent glabella and broad nose, coloboma iridis, low-set, simple ears, a carplike mouth, cleft lip and palate, and hypospadias in males. The dermatoglyphic features include hypoplastic dermal ridges and, in 20 per cent, an increased frequency of bilateral simian creases.

## THE 18Q SYNDROME

Infants with deletions of the long arm of 18 are characterized by microcephaly, hypotonia, mental and physical retardation, mid-face hypoplasia, hypertelorism, retinal defects, large ears with a small canal, carplike mouth, long, tapering fingers, heart malformations (40 per cent), cryptorchidism, dimpled knuckles, elbows and knees, clubfoot and an excess of dermatoglyphic whorl patterns.

## THE 21Q SYNDROME

This syndrome which before "banding" was available was known as "G deletion syndrome I," is characterized by microcephaly, psychomotor retardation, downslanting (antimongoloid) palpebral fissures, a prominent nose bridge, large low-set ears, doliocephaly and hypertonia.

## THE 22Q SYNDROME

This syndrome, formerly called "G deletion syndrome II," is characterized by microcephaly, psychomotor retardation, low-set ears, epicanthal folds, flat nasal bridge, ptosis, bifid uvula, clinodactyly and syndactyly.

## GROSS ABERRATION OF SEX HORMONES

These are described in detail in the section devoted to Abnormalities of Sexual Differentiation (p. 509).

## REFERENCES

*General*

Baird, H. W., III: Kindred showing congenital absence of the dermal ridges (fingerprints) and associated anomalies. J. Pediatr. *64*:621, 1964.

Bergsma, D. (Ed.): Birth Defects Atlas and Compendium. Baltimore, Williams & Wilkins Company, 1973.

Boué, A., and Boué, J.: Chromosome abnormalities and abortion. *In* E. Coutinho and F. Fuchs (Eds.): Physiology and Genetics of Reproduction, Part B. New York, Plenum Press, 1974, pp. 317–339.

Forbes, A. P.: Fingerprints and palm prints (dermatoglyphics) and palmar flexion creases in gonadal dysgenesis, pseudoparathyroidism and Klinefelter's syndrome. N. Engl. J. Med. *270*:1268, 1964.

Hecht, F., Bryant, J. S., et al.: The nonrandomness of chromosomal abnormalities: Association of trisomy 18 and Down's syndrome. N. Engl. J. Med. *271*:1081, 1964.

Jacobs, P. A., Aitken J., Frackiewickz, A., Law, P., Newton, M. S., and Smith, P. G.: The inheritance of translocations in man. Ann. Hum. Genet. *34*:119–136, 1970.

Lewandowski, R. C., and Yunis, J. J.: New chromosomal syndromes. Am. J. Dis. Child. *129*:515, 1975.

Marden, P. J., Smith, D. W., and McDonald, M. J.: Congenital anomalies in the newborn infant including minor variations: A study of 4412 babies by surface examination for anomalies and buccal smear for sex chromatin. J. Pediatr. *64*:357, 1964.

Nitowsky, H., Sindhavananda, N., et al.: Partial 18 monosomy in the cyclops malformation. Pediatrics *37*:260, 1966.

Nora, J. J., and Fraser, F. C.: Medical Genetics: Principles and Practice. Philadelphia, Lea and Febiger, 1974.

Penrose, L. S., and Smith, G. F.: Down's Anomaly. Boston, Little, Brown and Company, 1966.

Preus, M., and Fraser, F. C.: Dermatoglyphics and syndromes. Am. J. Dis. Child. *124*:933, 1972.

Warkany, J., Weinstein, D., Soukup, S. W., Rubinstein, J. H., and Curless, M. C.: Chromosome analyses in a children's hospital. Selection of patients and results of studies. Pediatrics *33*:290, 454, 1964.

Waxman, S. H., Arakaki, D. F., and Smith, J. B.: Cytogenetics of fetal abortions. Pediatrics *39*:425, 1967.

*Down Syndrome*

Armendares, S., Urrusti-Sanz, J., and Diaz-del-Castillo, E.: Iliac index in newborns: Comparative values at term, in prematurity and in Down's syndrome. Am. J. Dis. Child. *113*:229, 1967.

Caffey, J., and Ross, S.: Pelvic bones in infantile mongolism. Am. J. Roentgenol. *80*:458, 1958.

Conen, P. E., and Erkman, B.: Combined mongolism and leukemia. Am. J. Dis. Child. *112*:429, 1966.

Friedman, A.: Radio-iodine uptake in children with mongolism. Pediatrics *16*:55, 1955.

Jacobs, P. A., Baikie, A. G., Brown, W. M. C., and Strong, J. A.: The somatic chromosomes in mongolism. Lancet *1*:710, 1959.

Levinson, A., Friedman, A., and Stamps, F.: Variability of mongolism. Pediatrics *16*:43, 1955.

Nichols, W. W., Coriell, L. L., Fabrizzio, D. A., Bishop, H. C., and Boggs, T. R.: Mongolism with mosaic chromosome pattern. J. Pediatr. *60*:69, 1962.

Nicolis, F. B., and Sacchetti, G.: Nomogram for the x-ray evaluation of some morphological anomalies of the pelvis in the diagnosis of mongolism. Pediatrics *32*:1074, 1963.

Shapiro, B. L., Gorlin, R. J., et al.: The palate and Down's syndrome. N. Engl. J. Med. *276*:1460, 1967.

Smith, D. W., and Wilson, A. A.: The Child with Down's Syndrome (Mongolism). Philadelphia, W. B. Saunders, 1973.

Weinstein, E. D., and Warkany, J.: Maternal mosaicism and Down's syndrome. J. Pediatr. *63*:599, 1963.

**E Trisomy**

Alpert, L. I., Strauss, L., and Hirschhorn, K.: Neonatal hepatitis and biliary atresia associated with trisomy 17–18 syndrome. N. Engl. J. Med. *280*:16, 1969.

Hecht, F., Bryant, J. S., Motulsky, A. G., and Giblett, E. R.: The no. 17–18 (E) trisomy syndrome. J. Pediatr. *63*:605, 1963.

Rohde, R. A., Hodgman, S. E., and Cleland, R. S.: Multiple congenital anomalies in the E trisomy (group 16–18) syndrome. Pediatrics *33*:258, 1964.

Uchida, J. A., Lewis, A. J., Bowman, J. M., and Wang, H. C.: A case of double trisomy no. 18 and triple-X. J. Pediatr. *60*:498, 1962.

Weber, F. M., and Sparks, R. S.: Trisomy E (18) syndrome: clinical spectrum in 12 new cases, including chromosome radioautography in 4. J. Med. Genet. *7*:363, 1970.

**D Trisomy**

Miller, J. Q., Picard, E. H., Alkan, M. K., Warner, S., and Gerald, P. S.: A specific congenital brain defect (arhinencephaly) in 13–15 trisomy. N. Engl. J. Med. *268*:120, 1963.

Smith, D. W., Patau, K., Therman, E., Inhorn, S. L., and DeMars, R. J.: The $D_1$ trisomy syndrome. J. Pediatr. *62*:326, 1963.

Walzer, S., Park, G. S., et al.: Hematologic changes in and $D_1$ trisomy syndrome. Pediatrics *38*:419, 1966.

Wilson, M. G., and Melnyk, J.: Translocation—normal mosaicism in $D_1$ trisomy. Pediatrics *40*:842, 1967.

**Cri du Chat Syndrome**

Dumars, K. W., Jr., Gaskill, C., and Kitzmiller, N.: Le cri du chat (crying cat) syndrome. Am. J. Dis. Child. *108*:533, 1964.

Hijmans, J. C., and Shearin, D. B.: Partial deletion of short arms of chromosome no. 5: Report of a case in a fraternal twin. Am. J. Dis. Child. *109*:85, 1965.

Lejeune, J., et al.: Deletion partielle du bras court du chromosome 5: Individualisation d'un nouvelle état morbide. Sem. hôp. Paris *25*:1069, 1964.

MacIntyre, M. N., Staples, W. I., LaPolla, J., and Hempel, J. M.: The "cat cry" syndrome. Am. J. Dis. Child. *108*:538, 1964.

# 101

# GENETIC COUNSELING

*By F. Clarke Fraser*

Genetic counseling deals with situations in which a person is concerned with the possibility that a disorder known or suspected to be genetic will occur in his or her family. In the present context the persons receiving counsel are usually the parents of a newborn child with a malformation, syndrome or disease who are concerned about the possibility of recurrence in a future child. The aim is to help the parents and family to comprehend the medical facts, to appreciate the way heredity contributes to the disorder, and the risk of recurrence, to understand the options for dealing with the risk of recurrence, to choose the course of action that seems appropriate to them and to act accordingly.

However, the genetic evaluation of the family begins well before the genetic counseling process. When prenatal diagnosis is involved, genetic evaluation may begin in early pregnancy (see Chapter 2). In the newborn nursery the genetic work-up is directed primarily toward diagnosis.

## GENETIC EVALUATION OF THE INFANT

The approach to genetic evaluation can be formulated as a series of questions:

1. Does the baby have a disease of clearly non-genetic origin, such as infection or birth trauma? Microcephaly, cata-

racts, retinopathy, heart defects and other abnormalities should raise the question of prenatal infection with rubella, toxoplasma, cytomegalic inclusion disease virus, herpes or other teratogenic organisms. A TORCH screening should be done in such cases—in 6 months it may be too late to verify the diagnosis. Did the mother take any drugs suspected of being teratogenic? It is useful to inquire about non-medical drugs such as LSD and marijuana at this point. With the exception of alcohol there is no evidence that these are teratogenic, but parents who have taken them may fear that this was the cause of the baby's disorder, and may need reassurance.

2. Does the baby have a disease of clearly genetic etiology, such as hemophilia, an inborn error of metabolism or a chondrodystrophy (see Table 100–1 for examples). The family history may be useful here, but the clinical and laboratory features will obviously provide the most important diagnostic information. Genetic heterogeneity should be kept in mind; that is, that conditions with similar clinical features may be genetically distinct. For instance, the Hurler form of mucopolysaccharidosis shows autosomal recessive inheritance whereas the Hunter form is X-linked, and achondroplasia has an autosomal dominant mode of inheritance, while achondrogenesis is autosomal recessive. If the disease does have a mendelian basis, a recurrence risk can be calculated according to the mode of inheritance of the disorder and the family history in the present case.

3. If the baby's disorder does not fall into either of the above categories, does the baby have features that suggest a syndrome? If so, the subsequent investigation and management will depend on the nature of the syndrome. Some syndromes are well known to pediatricians, others are so rare as to be "once-in-a-lifetime" events for the neonatologist and one must resort to appropriate compendia, atlases, and catalogues, or to consultation with a clinical geneticist experienced in syndromology, if available. It should be recognized, however, that many children with combinations of dysmorphic features so unusual, and a facies so striking, that one feels sure they have a syndrome nevertheless defy classifi-

cation by even the most experienced syndromologists. Furthermore, many dysmorphic features are age-dependent, and an infant who, as he grows older, will develop the facies associated in the physician's mind with a particular syndrome may have a quite different appearance at birth. Conversely, in some children, collections of minor anomalies that may lead one to suspect a syndrome may simply represent the "family facies," or be normal variants, or may even disappear in childhood.

4. When a syndrome cannot be identified, one must consider what further investigations are necessary. Is examination of the chromosomes indicated? The indications for karyotyping have continued to expand as improved methods of staining have allowed detection of progressively more subtle deletions, duplications and rearrangements of chromosomal material. Except where a specific, non-chromosomal syndrome has been identified, karyotyping should be considered in the baby who has multiple malformations, ambiguous genitalia or hypospadias of moderate or severe degree, or who exhibits unexplained small size or failure to thrive, especially when these are accompanied by dysmorphogenic features.

5. In any case, the family history should be screened for clues to the possible genetic basis for the baby's problem. Taking a detailed family history is usually neither feasible nor justified at the time of admission. On the other hand, following the time-honored practice of asking whether there are any relatives with "diseases of hereditary tendency," such as allergy, cancer, epilepsy, heart disease, insanity or tuberculosis, is not likely to be rewarding.

The most useful question to ask when taking the family history is whether problems similar to the present one have occurred in other members of the family. The answer will usually be negative, even when the disease is clearly genetic (since dominantly inherited diseases do not usually present in the newborn nursery, and recessive ones have only a one in four probability of recurrence), but when it is positive it can be very helpful. For example, a little girl was admitted in coma, following a measles infection. The fact that

**TABLE 101–1.**   *Selected List of Mendelian Disorders Presenting in the Newborn Period\**

Acrocephalosyndactyly (Apert). AD
Adrenogenital syndrome. AR
Albinism (several types). AR
Albinism, ocular. XR
Albinism, partial, with deafness. XR
Albinism with platelet defect (Hermansky-Pudlak). AR
Aniridia. AD
Anonychia with poly-, syn- or adactyly. AD
Arachnodactyly, Marfan. AD
Aortic stenosis, supravalvular. AD (few)
Asphyxiating thoracic dystrophy (Jeune). AR
Atrial septal defect. AD (few)
Cataract. AD, AR, XR
Cataract, acidosis, hypotonia, etc. (Lowe). XR
Cataract with microcornea. XR
Cerebrohepatorenal syndrome (Zellweger). AR
Chondrodystrophia calcificans congenita, Conradi type. AD
Chondrodystrophia calcificans congenita, rhizomelic type. AR
Cleft lip/palate with lip pits. AD
Cleft lip with lobster claw defect, etc. (EEC syndrome). AD
Cleft lip with popliteal web. AD
Cleft palate with face and digit anomalies—OFD I. XD
Cleft palate with face and digit anomalies—OFD II. AR
Cleft palate; deafness, characteristic facies, bone dysplasias (otopalatodigital). AR
Cleidocraniodysostosis. AD
Craniocarpal-tarsal dystrophy (whistling face). AD
Craniofacial dysostosis (Crouzon). AD
Cretinism, goitrous. AR
Cutis laxa. AR; less severe form. AD
Cutis, hyperelastosis (Ehlers-Danlos). AD
Cystic fibrosis of pancreas. AR
Deafness, congenital, severe. AD, AR, XR
Deafness with ECG conduction defects, freckles, etc. (Leopard). AD
Deafness, prolonged QT interval, cardiac arrhythmia (Jervell). AR
Deafness with preauricular pits or branchial sinus ± renal malformations. AD
Diabetes insipidus, ADH deficient. AD
Diabetes insipidus, nephrogenic. XR
Dislocations, multiple; flat facies, etc. (Larsen). AR
Dwarfism, achondrogenesis. AR
Dwarfism, achondroplasia. AD
Dwarfism, bird-headed (Seckel). AR
Dwarfism, diastrophic. AR
Dwarfism, mesomelic dyschondrosteosis (Leri). AD
Dwarfism, metatropic. AR
Dwarfism, pycnodysostosis. AR
Dwarfism, with cataracts, marble epiphyses, etc. (Cockayne). AR
Dwarfism, with fine, sparse hair (cartilage-hair hypoplasia). AR
Dwarfism, with polydactyly, tooth and nail defects (Ellis van Creveld). AR
Dwarfism, with spherophakia (Weil-Marchesani). AR
Dwarfism, with spondyloepiphysial dysplasia congenita. AD

\*A = autosomal; D = dominant; R = recessive; X = X-linked (inborn errors of metabolism are excluded).

**TABLE 101–1.** *Selected List of Mendelian Disorders Presenting in the Newborn Period*°
*(Continued)*

Dwarfism, with telangiectasias, chromosome breaks (Bloom). AR
Ectodermal dysplasia, anhidrotic. XR
Ectodermal dysplasia, hidrotic (Clouston). AD
Epidermolysis bullosa; simplex and dystrophic. AD
Epidermolysis bullosa lethalis. AR
Eyelids, displaced inner canthi, deafness, white forelock (Waardenburg). AD
Facial diplegia ± various anomalies (Möbius). Minority are AD or AR
Hemangiomatosis of von Hippel-Lindau. AD
Hydrocephalus with aqueductal stenosis. XL (some)
Ichthyosiform erythroderma. AR
Ichthyosis sauroderma. AR
Ichthyosis vulgaris. XR
Iridocorneal mesodermal dysgenesis, hypodontia (Rieger). AD
Iris hypoplasia with glaucoma. XR
Laurence-Moon-Biedl syndrome (post-axial polydactyly at birth). AR
Leprechaunism (AR)
Lymphedema (Milroy). AD (some)
Mandibulofacial dysostosis (Treacher-Collins). AD
Megalocornea, ± cataracts. XR, some AR or AD
Microphthalmia/anophthalmia. Usually sporadic, occasionally AD, AR, XR
Microphthalmia with digital anomalies. XR (some)
Muscular atrophy, progressive, spinal (Werdnig-Hoffman). AR
Myopathy, nemaline. AD (?)
Myopia, retinal detachment, joint degeneration (Stickler). AD
Nail-patella syndrome. AD
Nephrosis, congenital. AR (one type)
Neurofibromatosis. AD
Oculodentodigital dysplasia. AD
Optic atrophy, congenital (Behr). AR
Osteogenesis imperfecta lethalis. AR (few)
Osteogenesis imperfecta tarda. AD, occasionally AR
Osteomalacia from hypophosphatasemia. AR
Osteopetrosis, mild form. AD
Osteopetrosis, severe form. AR
Pachyonychia congenita. AD
Polcystic kidney disease, infantile. AR
Polycystic kidneys, microcephaly, polydactyly, cleft palate, etc. (Meckel). AR
Polydactyly, post-axial. AD (some)—also see various syndromes
Pseudoglioma retina (Norrie). XR
Ptosis, congenital. AD (reduced penetrance)
Ptosis, external ophthalmoplegia, myopia. XR
Radial absence with thrombocytopenia. AR
Radial defect with cardiac malformation (Holt-Oram). AD
Radial defect with other malformations, pancytopenia (Fanconi). AR
Radioulnar synostosis. AD
Retinal aplasia. AD or AR
Smith-Lemli-Opitz syndrome. AR
Spastic diplegia, ichthyosis, mental retardation (Sjögren-Larsson). AR
Syndactyly. AD (often)—see also various syndromes
Tibial absence, polydactyly. AD
Tuberous sclerosis. AD
Xanthomatosis, calcified adrenals, hepatosplenomegaly (Wolman). AR

°A = autosomal; D = dominant; R = recessive; X = X-linked (inborn errors of metabolism are excluded).

she had been acidotic was noted on the discharge summary, but its significance was not realized until review of the family history uncovered the fact that a sib had died in acidotic coma. The parents had been told (in another country) that this was caused by renal tubular acidosis, which was stated (incorrectly) to be non-genetic. Investigation of this clue led to the correct diagnosis, methylmalonic aciduria.

When surgery is contemplated it is also wise to inquire about relatives with bleeding tendencies or unusual reactions to anesthetics.

The patient's sibs should be listed by age and sex, and their state of health noted. The main reason for this is that parents sometimes do not recognize what constitutes a "similar problem," as the above example demonstrates. The causes of any deaths in sibs should be established. For example, the mother of a child admitted for "cerebral palsy" told me that a previous child had died of "pneumonia," but did not mention that the underlying cause was Tay-Sachs disease, which the second child also had.

If ancestors or collateral relatives are found to have diseases causing problems similar to that of the patient, a pedigree should be constructed so that the mode of inheritance can be evaluated.

Finally, one should ask about the possibility of parental consanguinity, since this can be a clue that the baby's problem may be caused by a recessively inherited disease and lead one to consider recessively inherited diseases that fit the clinical picture. If the baby's disease is unusual, the possibility of a hitherto unrecognized recessive disorder, with a one in four recurrence risk for sibs, should be kept in mind when there is parental consanguinity, even if no specific disease can be identified.

## COUNSELING THE FAMILY

It is difficult for anyone who has not had the experience to imagine the feeling of the parents of a baby who is born defective. They are shocked, bewildered, scared and often angered. Counseling at this point is directed largely to explaining the nature of the baby's disorder, and the short-term prognosis, and to providing as much emotional support as possible. This can, and probably should be, done by the family physician or pediatrician, who knows the parents, although it is sometimes left to the genetic counselor, particularly in cases of chromosomal problems and inborn errors of metabolism, in which the geneticist is involved in making the diagnosis. During this initial stage, the cause of the disorder is not one of the most important worries of the parents, except that they will often feel that the child's defect is a sign that they themselves are defective in some way, and may benefit by having these feelings aired. This is usually not the time to go deeply into the question of recurrence risks for future children, for in most cases the parents will not be listening. They should be made aware, however, that such information will be available later.

When the initial crisis is over and the parents become aware of the long-term significance of their baby's defect, they may begin to wonder more about the cause of the child's disease and, in particular, whether it might happen again. At this time the specifically *genetic* counseling should be done. If it is delayed too long, the parents may have already started another pregnancy, unaware of a high risk or burden, or have taken irreversible measures to prevent subsequent pregnancies, unaware that the risk and burden are low. To inform the parents that there is a risk of recurrence is particularly important if prenatal diagnosis is possible. Even if prenatal diagnosis is not necessary, parents still must be made aware of what the risks are so that they will neither be shocked by an unforeseen recurrence nor be deterred from having children when the risk is negligible, but be able to make an informed decision. It should not be assumed that they will actually do so; some parents are not helped by knowledge of the risk figures in choosing whether or not to have another baby and, in fact, enter a prolonged state of indecision in which they "let things take their course." Nevertheless, they should be given the information, since even these parents are usually able to recall the percentage risk quite accurately, and one cannot distinguish, in advance, those who will use the information in making their decision from those who will not.

## DETERMINING THE RECURRENCE RISK

In order to determine the recurrence risk it is useful to assign the disorder in question to one of four etiological categories: those due to an environmental agent, to a chromosomal aberration, to a multifactorial interaction, or to a mutant gene. To do this it is necessary, of course, to be certain that the diagnosis is correct, keeping in mind the possibility of genetic heterogeneity.

*Defects due to environmental agents* will recur in sibs only if the environmental agent recurs; therefore, we will not discuss this further.

### Defects Due to Chromosomal Aberrations

The recurrence risks here depend upon the nature of the aberration. For simple trisomies one can explain to the parents that the baby's extra chromosome arose as the result of a mistake in the pairing and separation of the chromosomes during formation of the sperm or egg, that it was an "accident" and is not likely to happen again, the risk being about 1 or 2 per cent for subsequent babies. This, however, is a high enough risk to justify the monitoring of subsequent pregnancies by amniocentesis (see Chapter 2).

When a translocation is involved, the risk cannot be estimated precisely, since it probably varies according to where the translocation segments are, and how they affect pairing and separation of the chromosomes. One can only say that the risk of a subsequent baby having a possibly harmful chromosomal aberration is higher than it is for a simple trisomy, but probably not as high as the theoretical expectation on the basis of random segregation; the important thing is to emphasize that the parents *can* have normal children, but that amniocentesis is necessary if they want to be certain that there will be no recurrence. The only exception is translocation of one chromosome to its homologue, in which case the outcome is certain to be an unbalanced complement for every offspring.

### Defects of Multifactorial Causation

In these conditions, which include most of the common malformations, the recurrence risks have been determined empirically, and can be provided by the counselor for the particular defect and family history. For normal parents with only one affected child the risk is usually of the order of 2 to 5%. For more complicated situations, one should consult the literature or a genetic counselor. It is important to inform parents of a child with anencephaly and/or spina bifida aperta of the recurrence risk, since subsequent pregnancies can be monitored by ultrasound and alphafetoprotein measurements.

### Defects Due to Mutant Genes

Here the recurrence risk depends on the mode of inheritance of the disorder and the family history. No doubt the reader will recall the principles of mendelian segregation, or will be able to find them in a good textbook of pediatrics or medical genetics. The following sections will serve as a brief refresher. There are three major patterns of mendelian inheritance.

AUTOSOMAL DOMINANT INHERITANCE. Autosomal simply means not sex-linked. Dominant mutant genes are those that manifest their presence even when the other gene of the pair is normal; that is, every carrier of a disease-causing mutant gene has the disease. Such diseases are rare, and an affected person almost always carries one mutant and one normal member of that pair; each offspring will receive either one or the other, and thus will have a 50:50 chance of being affected with the disease. Similarly, the affected person must have received the gene from somewhere, so that one parent should also be affected.

A certain amount of confusion can be caused by the fact that some individuals with dominantly inherited conditions represent fresh mutations, so that they do not have an affected parent. The family history is negative, thus the mutant individual is a "sporadic" case. The sibs of such a sporadic case will have a very low risk, but the offspring will have the usual 50:50 chance of being affected.

The more severe the effects of the mutant gene are, the greater will be the proportion of cases that are sporadic. To take an extreme example, a mutant gene that causes early death or sterility will always result in a sporadic case, since there will be no opportunity to transmit the gene. An example is the Apert type of acrocephalosyndactyly, in which few affected subjects have had offspring, so that almost all cases are sporadic. At the other extreme is the hydrotic type of ectodermal dysplasia, in which virtually all affected subjects have an affected parent. About 80 per cent of cases of achondroplasia are sporadic, indicating an intermediate degree of severity.

Another complication is the phenomenon of reduced penetrance. In certain conditions showing dominant inheritance, some carriers of the mutant gene do not show any manifestations of the disease. Various explanations can be advanced—examination has failed to detect subtle signs that are actually present, a developmental threshold has not been reached or (in diseases of variable age of onset) the signs of the disease have not yet appeared—and in some cases no explanation is known. The important thing is to recognize which diseases may do this (they include Marfan syndrome, neurofibromatosis and Treacher-Collins syndrome), since in a "sporadic" case a parent may actually carry the gene but not manifest it, and the risk for sibs will not be as low as it would for a new mutation. Thus the situation is complicated, and consultation with a genetic counselor may be useful.

AUTOSOMAL RECESSIVE INHERITANCE. In this condition the mutant gene does not produce disease when the other member of the pair is normal, but only when the other member (allele) is also mutant. The affected child must therefore inherit a mutant gene from each of the parents, who are themselves normal because they each carry a normal gene of that pair as well as the mutant allele. The child has one chance in two of getting the mutant gene from each parent, and therefore $1/2 \times 1/2 = 1/4$ chance of getting the mutant gene from both parents, and thus being affected. Similarly, any subsequent child of these parents will also have 1 chance in 4 of being affected.

If the parents are related, it is more likely that they will both carry the same mutant gene. This is why the frequency of cousin marriages is increased in the parents of children with rare, recessively inherited diseases.

These diseases are likely to result from enzyme deficiencies, and an increasing number are eligible for prenatal diagnosis (see Chapter 2).

X-LINKED RECESSIVE INHERITANCE. In females, recessive genes on the X chromosome behave as they do on the autosomes; there are two X chromosomes, and the mutant gene will usually, therefore, have a normal allele to mask its effect. (An exception resulting from X chromosome inactivation will be mentioned shortly.) In the male, however, there is only one X chromosome, so a "recessive" gene will be expressed. Thus a female carrier of one gene for, say, hemophilia A will not be a "bleeder." Each of her sons will receive either the X chromosome carrying the mutant gene or the one carrying the normal allele, and will thus have an equal chance of being affected or unaffected. Offspring of affected males will receive either the mutant-bearing X, and be carrier females, or the Y, and be unaffected sons.

The situation is complicated a little by the phenomenon of lyonization; that is, that in each cell of a female, one X chromosome is inactivated, so a female carrying a gene for, say, X-linked muscular dystrophy (Duchenne) is a mosaic (mixture) composed of cells in which the X carrying the mutant is active and cells in which the X carrying the normal allele is active. This is presumably why carrier females often show dystrophic patches in their muscles. Since inactivation occurs early in development, and is random with respect to which chromosome gets inactivated, occasionally in a great majority of the cells of a carrier female the X carrying the normal allele may be inactivated. This may account for the occasional carrier female who manifests the disease. It also explains why tests for carrier females usually do not detect all carriers—in the great majority of the cells of some carrier females the X carrying the mutant allele may be inactivated.

The most difficult situation to counsel for

X-linked recessive diseases is the "sporadic" case. When there are no affected relatives, one must decide whether the affected son represents a fresh mutation, in which case the mother is not a carrier, and the risk for future sons is low. Alternatively, the mutation may have occurred farther back in the family, but not have yet been transmitted to a male, in which case the mother will be a carrier and the risk for future sons will be 1/2. For some diseases, tests are available that will detect some carrier females, but usually not all, because of lyonization. Thus, for Duchenne muscular dystrophy, for example, an elevated creatine phosphokinase level is strong evidence that the mother is a carrier, but a normal level is not conclusive evidence that she is not.

The geneticist can estimate the probability that the mother of a sporadic case is a carrier on the basis of the available information. To begin with the simplest case, a first-born affected male with no maternal uncles, it can be calculated from the principles of population genetics that if the disease in question is lethal (as for Duchenne dystrophy) the probabilities are two out of three that the mother is a carrier to one out of three that she is not. The probability of not being a carrier increases with the number of unaffected sons born, with the number of unaffected brothers of the mother, although not so much, and with how far into the normal range the tests for carrier detection fall, so they must be calculated for each case. The important thing for the physician to realize is that even if there are no affected relatives one should not assume that the mother is not a carrier.

X-Linked Dominant Inheritance. This pattern of inheritance is relatively rare but examples do exist—for instance, hypophosphatemic rickets. The distinguishing feature is that men carrying the dominant mutant gene on the X chromosome will transmit it to all their daughters, who will be affected, but to none of their sons.

### Reaching a Decision

Now that the parents have some appreciation of the nature of their baby's disease and of the burden that it will impose upon the family, and have been informed of the risk of recurrence, it will be necessary for them to decide whether they want further children, and if not, what to do about it. Some geneticists maintain that the genetic counselor's role is simply to provide the facts in a non-directive way and let the parents decide what to do with them. Others feel that the parents will appreciate help in reaching a decision from someone they regard as having had experience in helping others to manage similar problems. It is difficult for the counselor to be completely non-directive in this situation. Certainly the counselor should never tell parents that they should or should not have children. Every case is unique and is influenced by a great many factors besides the scientific facts. The counselor may be able to provide helpful support while the parents talk through their problems. He should also be ready to refer them to appropriate sources, whether it be priest, social worker, psychiatrist, gynecologist or urologist, where indicated. Again, the pediatrician may be the best person to help the family at this stage, but the specialist in genetic counseling often seems to play the major role, perhaps by default. If so, he should take pains to inform the referring doctor of his findings and his evaluation of the family's response, especially where long-term follow up may seem desirable.

### REFERENCES

Bergsma, D. (Ed.): Birth Defects Atlas and Compendium. National Foundation March of Dimes. Baltimore, Williams & Wilkins Co., 1973.

Fraser, F. C.: Genetic counseling. Am. J. Hum. Genet. 26:636–659, 1974.

Holmes, L. B.: Current concepts in genetics. Congenital malformations. N. Engl. J. Med. 295:204, 1976.

Holmes, L. B., Moser, H. W., Halldorsen, S., Mack, C., Pant, S. S., and Matzilevich, B.: Mental Retardation. An Atlas of Diseases with Associated Physical Abnormalities. New York, The Macmillan Co., 1972.

Lewandowski, R. C., and Yunis, J. J.: New chromosomal syndromes. Am. J. Dis. Child. 129:515–529, 1975.

McKusick, V.: Mendelian Inheritance in Man. 4th edition. Baltimore, The Johns Hopkins Press, 1975.

Nora, J. J., and Fraser, F. C.: Medical Genetics: Principles and Practice. Philadelphia, Lea and Febiger, 1974.

Smith, D. W.: Recognizable Patterns of Human Malformation. 2nd edition. Philadelphia, W. B. Saunders Co., 1976.

Stevenson, A. C., and Davison, B. C. C.: Genetic Counselling. London, Heinemann, 1970.

# 102

The title of this chapter perhaps should read a bit differently, with the words "known to be" inserted before "caused by gross chromosomal aberrations." We say this because continuing improvements in cytogenetic techniques may eventually lead to the detection of small deletions, duplications or other aberrations consistently associated with some of these syndromes. In the meantime, their causes remain obscure.

As is true in all areas of neonatology, growth in this field has been extremely rapid. David W. Smith, in his monograph on this subject published in 1976, lists 221 recognizable patterns of human malformation. We do not propose to compete with him but shall limit our discussion to a few of the most common and the ones which, for historical and other reasons, interest us most. In our defense it should be pointed out that a not inconsiderable number of such constellations have been described in other sections, viz., cretinism, the first and second arch syndromes, the variety of dyschondroplasias, phocomelia, renal agenesis and a whole host of others.

## NUCLEAR AGENESIS (MOEBIUS SYNDROME)

Facial nerve palsy is most often unilateral and unassociated with other congenital palsies or defects. When it is bilateral, or when other congenital abnormalities of cranial nerves or of the osseous system of the face or extremities are present concomitantly, the syndrome may fall into the category of nuclear agenesis.

**INCIDENCE.** The condition is in-

frequent, but not extremely rare. Many instances have been misinterpreted as pseudobulbar palsies resulting from birth injury.

**ETIOLOGY AND PATHOLOGY.** The evidence in favor of genetic transmission is not strong. The pathologic evidence is difficult to interpret, but there seems to be aplasia of the nuclei of the facial nerves and of adjacent cranial nerve nuclei. This was considered to be the primary defect by Moebius, but some observers have felt that the failure of development of nuclei might be secondary to a primary defect of mesenchyma causing imperfect development of nerves. Evans, in his brilliant analysis of all possible etiologic factors, suggested that all the lesions found might be traced to leakage of cerebrospinal fluid down the branchial arches and limb buds shortly after the seventh week of gestation.

**DIAGNOSIS.** The sine qua non is facial nerve palsy. If it is bilateral, no other abnormalities must coexist to make Moebius syndrome a strong diagnostic possibility. If the palsy is unilateral, however, it is more likely to stem from an obstetric injury than from nuclear agenesis unless other congenital lesions coexist. These include one or more additional cranial nerve palsies, chiefly of extraocular movement, and of the palate, tongue and masseters. Micrognathia, high arched palate, syndactylism, Klippel-Feil deformity and club feet are some of the associated skeletal abnormalities.

The presenting sign is the extraordinary immobility of the face, as notable in the first few days of life as it is in later life. The facies mirrors no emotion, pleasant or unpleasant. This leads to the incorrect assumption of mental incompetence that will plague these afflicted children throughout life.

**TREATMENT.** Nothing can be done for the facial nerve palsy. Some of the associated defects are susceptible to treatment, and each of these deserves the best available therapy.

## LEPRECHAUNISM

The name for this complex and vaguely defined disorder was suggested by the elfin facies of the affected infants. They manifest also physiologic and pathologic deviations from the normal, pointing toward a complicated endocrine disturbance. It is exceedingly rare, probably recessively inherited.

**DIAGNOSIS.** The babies are small and develop slowly, both physically and mentally. Evans described his newborn infant as having sunken cheeks, a pointed chin, eyes set wide apart, with very dark irises, negroid nose and low-set ears. In Donohue's cases the ears were large and bat-like (Fig. 102–1). The hands and feet were large. Creases of the skin showed dark pigmentation. Nipples and areolae were large and protuberant. The clitoris was distinctly enlarged. Laparotomy revealed cystic ovaries.

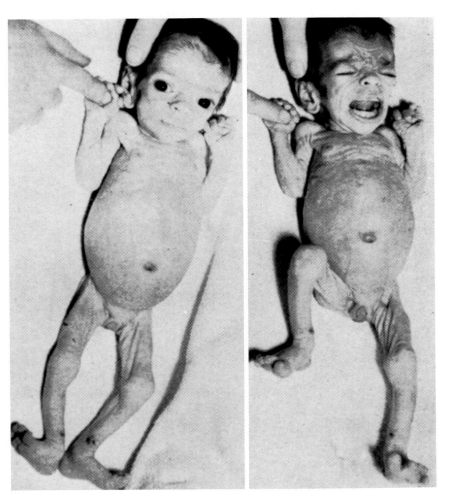

*Figure 102–1.* Note the extreme malnutrition, the huge ears, large eyes with black irises, the upturned nose, large mouth and pointed chin, and very large hands and feet.

Evans's careful studies revealed in his cases slightly elevated 17-ketosteroids and normal follicle-stimulating hormone (F.S.H.) excretion. Bone development was greatly retarded. Carbohydrate studies in his first example showed an excessive and unduly prolonged fall in response to insulin, but were essentially normal in all other respects. His second child showed, in addition, an unusually high and prolonged blood sugar response to epinephrine. The liver of this infant contained an excess of glycogen, as Donohue's had also shown.

Evans concluded that leprechaunism included two categories of endocrine disturbance: 1) an excess of estrogen causing enlarged cystic ovaries and mammary and clitoridean enlargement, and 2) pituitary deficiency giving rise to delay in growth, retardation of bone age, failure to respond to insulin-induced hypoglycemia, and wasting. He suggests that the primary defect may be overproduction of estrogens, which, in turn, may inhibit production of pituitary hormones, as they have been proved to do in the rat.

**TREATMENT.** If this hypothesis is correct, androgens might affect the condition favorably. Evans tried an 8-week course of methyltestosterone upon his second case with slight improvement in weight gain and in size of breasts. Length and bone age were not favorably influenced.

## THE ORAL-FACIAL-DIGITAL SYNDROME (OFD I SYNDROME)

As the name indicates, this constellation of multiple congenital defects involves structures within the oral cavity, of the face and of the extremities.

**ETIOLOGY.** In almost all cases the karyotypic pattern appears to be normal.

The disease is strongly familial and is almost entirely confined to females. Wahrman et al., themselves reporting a male with an XXY karyotype, cast doubt upon the correctness of the diagnosis in four of the five who had been reported up to 1966. Some of these, and the example described by Mandell and co-workers in 1967, about whose maleness there seems to be absolutely no question, are probably examples of the Mohr syndrome, sometimes called the OFD II syndrome. The consensus ap-

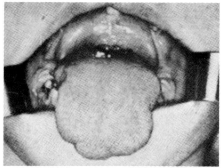

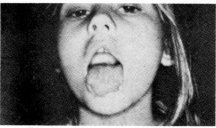

*Figure 102–2.* Photograph showing one of the characteristic tongue malformations in the oral-facial-digital syndrome. Note its irregular multifidity. (Ruess, A. L., et al.: Pediatrics *20*:985, 1962.)

pears to be that the OFD I syndrome is an X-linked dominant condition, almost always lethal in males.

**DIAGNOSIS.** The oral lesions include lobulations of the tongue, thick mucobuccal bands binding the tongue to the cheeks and gums, and palatal clefts and other anomalies of the palate. Facial deformities include shortness of alar cartilages and columella, median cleft of the lip and hypertelorism. At times there are alopecia and coarse hair and dry skin.

Brachydactyly, clinodactyly and syndactyly may involve the digits.

About half of the affected patients are mentally retarded.

**TREATMENT.** Plastic procedures are indicated for cleft lip and cleft palate and for freeing the tongue as much as is possible.

## OCULOAURICULOVERTEBRAL DYSPLASIA (GOLDENHAR SYNDROME)

In this constellation are to be found congenital defects of the eyes, ears, face, mandible and vertebral column. It resembles mandibulofacial dysostosis (Treacher Collins syndrome) in several ways, but differs from it in others.

**INCIDENCE.** The condition is very rare.

**ETIOLOGY.** The chromosomal pattern has been studied in a few examples, and no aberrations have been found. It is rarely a familial disease. The pathogenesis of the disorder therefore is not known.

**DIAGNOSIS.** Epibulbar dermoid cysts, colobomata of the upper lid, iris and choroid and at times microphthalmos characterize the eyes of these patients. The eyes do not commonly slant downward nor is the lower lid notched, as is the case in mandibulofacial dysostosis. The external and middle ear may be absent, displaced downward or malrotated, or there may be one or more ear tags. Asymmetrical facial and mandibular hypoplasia are typical. Hemivertebrae are common. Associated defects of heart, lungs (agenesis) and extremities are not infrequent. Mental deficiency occurs in only 10 to 15 per cent of cases.

**TREATMENT.** Conductive deafness is a major concern if both external auditory canals are incompletely developed, in which case a hearing aid should be used

from infancy. Plastic surgery is indicated for dermoids and ear tags; occasionally an external auditory canal can be created.

## CONGENITAL ECTODERMAL DYSPLASIA OF THE FACE

This is a unique combination of an extraordinary facial conformation with skin and hair abnormalities confined to the face.

**INCIDENCE.** Setleis et al. have encountered five such infants and children. They were unable to find any others reported.

**ETIOLOGY.** The five children were members of three families of Puerto Ricans. The authors concluded that the disorder was trasmitted as an autosomal recessive. No gross chromosomal aberrations were found in them.

**DIAGNOSIS.** The facies appears aged and leonine, the eyebrows sweep sharply upward and laterally, the nose is prominent with a rubbery, fleshy tip, and the mouth is large and arched downward. All these children had skin defects over the region of the temples, and one had a similar linear scar-like lesion on his lower lip and chin. The eyelashes were either missing on both lids,

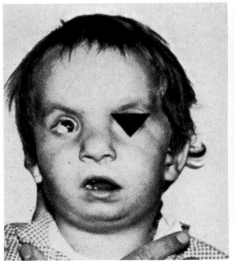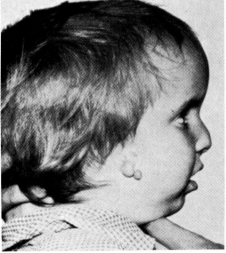

*Figure 102–3.* Note the epibulbar dermoid cyst of the right eye, and the virtually absent right external ear, its place taken by several rudimentary tags. This is typical oculoauriculovertebral dysplasia. (Gorlin, R. J., et al.: J. Pediatr. 63:991, 1963.)

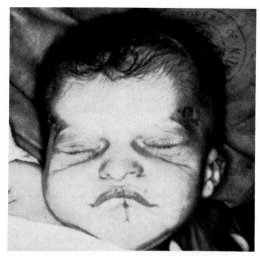

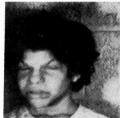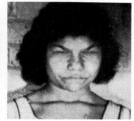

*Figure 102–4.* *A,* This newborn with congenital ectodermal dysplasia of the face shows two rows of eyelids on the upper lid, fleshy tip of nose and chin, symmetrical, round temporal skin defects, and a linear one involving the lower lip and chin. *B,* At a later age a heavy mop of scalp hair has developed, and the eyebrows have grown out in the characteristic upward and outward sweep. (Setleis, H., et al.: Pediatrics 32:540, 1963.)

or only on the lower lid, while there were multiple rows of lashes on the upper lids.

**TREATMENT.**   None is indicated.

## DE LANGE SYNDROME (TYPUS DEGENERATIVUS AMSTELODAMENSIS)

In 1933 de Lange described a group of infants whose resemblances were so marked that she thought they constituted a discrete entity.

**DIAGNOSIS.**   The infants and children are remarkable chiefly for their facial appearance and their unusual extremities. The facies is striking because of an unruly mop of coarse hair; a low irregular hairline making for a narrow forehead; thick eyebrows which meet in the midline; long eyelashes; flat nasal bridge and short up-turned nose with forward-tilting nostrils; a long upper lip; a crescentic mouth which curves downward, and a small mandible (see Fig. 102–5). The extremities are short and tapering, the digits particularly so, with incurved fifth finger.

In addition, these children are much smaller than average, both in height and weight, and their heads are small and brachycephalic. The ears are often low-set, and the neck is short and webbed. Simian creases are not uncommonly present. In the male the genitals are small, the testes hypoplastic. Ptacek et al. comment upon the fact that the nipples and umbilicus are tiny. Much lanugo hair grows over the shoulders, back and extremities of some of these infants. All are mentally retarded.

**PATHOLOGY AND PATHOLOGIC PHYSIOLOGY.**   Ptacek's   autopsied   17-month-old

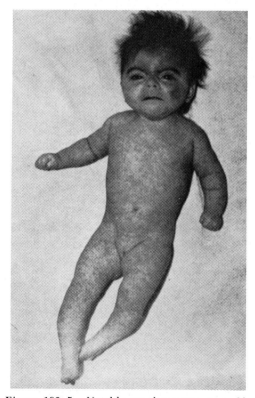

*Figure 102–5.*   Notable are the coarse mop of hair, growing low on the forehead, the eyebrows which cross the bridge of the nose to meet the midline, the short upward-tilted nose and the "carp mouth." The extremities are short and taper strikingly. (Ptacek, L. J., et al.: J. Pediatr. 63:1000, 1963.)

female showed extremely small, immature organs, a bicornuate uterus, virtual absence of germ cells in the ovaries and lack of myelinization of the brain. The thymus was tiny (0.8 gm). Two of Schlesinger's babies showed at postmortem examination microcephalic brains with grossly normal pituitary glands which, however, contained no basophilic cells. The thyroids revealed poor colloid formation in glands lined with low cuboidal epithelium. In one of his cases no lipoid could be demonstrated in the zona fasciculata of the adrenals.

In vivo studies of endocrine function have shown low protein-bound iodine and poor radioactive iodine uptake in some cases, but not all, persistently low blood sugar level after insulin sensitivity tests, and poor response of 17-hydroxysteroids after ACTH administration.

In sum, microcephaly, cortical atrophy and evidences of multiple endocrine defi-ciency, especially of trophic hormones of anterior pituitary origin, seem to be the main pathologic findings.

**ETIOLOGY.** Not many chromosome studies have been made, and most of the karyotypic patterns have been adjudged normal. Jervis and Stimson have seen an extra chromatin fragment, a bit smaller than the smallest chromosome, in some cells of four of their cases. Geudeke et al. saw what they interpreted as a deletion of the long arm of a B-group chromosome translocated to one of the G-group. Falek and his collaborators saw in the affected members of his unusual family a partial trisomy G, with the excess presumably derived from a deleted autosome 3. With findings so sparse and so different, one can do nothing except wait for further evidence.

Familial occurrence is the exception, and the risk of recurrence in a sib is probably considerably less than 5 per cent.

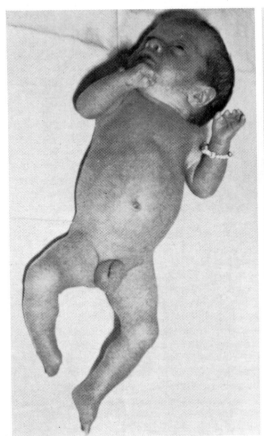

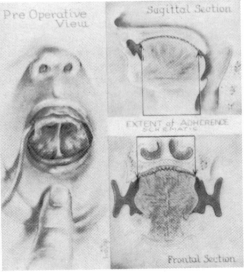

*Figure 102–6. A,* Photograph showing a well proportioned infant except for an extensive amputation of the right foot and more distal amputations of the toes of the left foot and the fingers of both hands. *B,* Diagrammatic sketch of the adhesion of almost the entire length of the dorsum of the tongue to the palate. (Wilson, R. A., et al.: Pediatrics *31:*1051, 1963.)

Virtually all the newborns are short and small at birth relative to their gestational age, possibly indicating placental insufficiency.

**PROGNOSIS.** Many feed poorly, gain slowly and die during infancy. Most of the survivors are institutionalized later because of severe mental defect.

**TREATMENT.** There is no effective therapy.

## ANKYLOGLOSSIA SUPERIOR

This is an unusual association of an oral lesion consisting of an extensive adhesion of the tongue to the palate with deformities of the extremities.

**INCIDENCE.** The disorder is rare.

**ETIOLOGY.** Buccal mucosal smears and chromosomal analyses have thus far revealed no aberrations. There is no increased familial incidence. No maternal drug ingestion has been implicated. The pathogenesis is unknown.

**DIAGNOSIS.** The tongue is firmly adherent to the palate, rendering sucking and swallowing impossible. The tongue may be hypoplastic, the palate highly arched, at times cleft. The most common malformations of the extremities are distal amputations of the digits or of the limbs a bit more proximally.

**TREATMENT.** Wilson et al. were able to free the tongue from the palate by blunt dissection. Little more can be done.

## SECKEL'S BIRD-HEADED DWARFISM

Seckel's name has become the eponym for a remarkable subgroup of microcephalic dwarfs. These infants are born small, with small heads in which sutures synostose prematurely. This, plus their large eyes, beaked noses, micrognathia and ears which are low-set and malformed, gives them an extraordinary and characteristic appearance. They are likely to have simian creases and clinodactyly. Associated congenital malformations often coexist.

The children grow very slowly and seldom attain an adult height of more than 3½ feet; mental development is equally slow. Their cerebrums are small, with a simple convolutional pattern resembling that of the chimpanzee.

The defect appears to be transmitted as an autosomal recessive.

## REFERENCES

Doege, T. C., Thuline, H. C., et al.: Studies of a family with the oral-facial-digital syndrome. N. Engl. J. Med. *271*:1073, 1964.

Donohue, W. L.: Clinicopathologic Conference at The Hospital for Sick Children. Dysendocrinism. J. Pediatr. *32*:739, 1948.

Donohue, W. L., and Uchida, I.: Leprechaunism: A euphemism for a rare familial disorder. J. Pediatr. *45*:505, 1954.

Evans, P. R.: Leprechaunism. Arch. Dis. Child. *30*:479, 1955.

Evans, P. R.: Nuclear agenesis: Möbius syndrome: The congenital facial diplegia syndrome. Arch. Dis. Child. *30*:237, 1955.

Gorlin, R. J., Jue, K. L., Jacobsen, U., and Goldschmidt, E.: Oculoauriculovertebral dysplasia. J. Pediatr. *63*:991, 1963.

Henderson, J. L.: The congenital facial diplegia syndrome: Clinical features, pathology and aetiology. A review of 61 cases. Brain *62*:381, 1939.

Jervis, G. A., and Stimson, C. W.: De Lange syndrome: The "Amsterdam type" of mental defect with congenital malformation. J. Pediatr. *63*:634, 1963.

Kushnick, T., Massa, T. P., and Bauksma, R.: Orofacialdigital syndrome in a male. J. Pediatr. *63*:1130, 1963.

Mandell, F., Ogra, P. L., et al.: Oral-facial-digital syndrome in a chromosomally normal male. Pediatrics *40*:63, 1967.

McKusick, V. A., Mahloudji, M., et al.: Seckel's bird-headed dwarfism. N. Engl. J. Med. *277*:279, 1967.

Nisenson, A., Isaacson, A., and Grant, S.: Mask-like facies with associated congenital anomalies (Möbius syndrome): Report of 3 cases. J. Pediatr. *46*:255, 1955.

Ptacek, L. J., Opitz, J. M., Smith, D. W., Gerritsen, T., and Waisman, H. A.: The Cornelia de Lange syndrome. J. Pediatr. *63*:1000, 1963.

Ruess, A. L., Pruzansky, S., Lis, E. F., and Patau, K.: The oral-facial-digital syndrome: A multiple congenital condition of females with associated chromosomal abnormalities. Pediatrics *20*:985, 1962.

Salmon, M. A., and Webb, J. N.: Dystrophic changes associated with leprechaunism in an infant. Arch. Dis. Child. *38*:530, 1963.

Schlesinger, B., Clayton, B., Bodian, M., and Jones, K. V.: Typus degenerativus amstelodamensis. Arch. Dis. Child. *38*:349, 1964.

Setleis, H., Kramer, B., Valcarcel, M., and Einhorn, A. H.: Congenital ectodermal dysplasia of the face. Pediatrics *32*:540, 1963.

Silver, H. K.: The de Lange syndrome. Am. J. Dis. Child. *108*:523, 1964.

Smith, D. W.: Recognizable Patterns of Human Malformation. 2nd ed., Philadelphia, W. B. Saunders Company, 1976.

Wahrman, J., Berant, M., et al.: The oral-facial-digital syndrome: A male-lethal condition in a boy with 47/XXY chromosomes. Pediatrics *37*:812, 1966.

Wilson, R. A., Kliman, M. R., and Hardyment, A. F.: Ankyloglossia superior (Palato-glossal adhesion in the newborn infant). Pediatrics *31*:105, 1963.

# XV

# Disorders of the Skin

No attempt has been made in this section to describe all the skin conditions which may be met in the neonatal period. We have perferred to limit consideration to those disorders which represent congenital defects, to infections which are unique to or have special characteristics in the neonatal period, to skin tumors which are encountered at birth or within the first month and to skin lesions which appear to result from toxic agents or hypersensitization in this age group.

# 103 CONGENITAL AND HEREDITARY DISORDERS OF THE SKIN

*By Nancy B. Esterly and Lawrence M. Solomon*

Numerous heritable disorders may be apparent in the newborn infant and may cause diverse aberrations of pigmentation, texture, elasticity and structural integrity of the integument. Some of these entities are confined to the skin, but others produce anomalies of several organ systems. Although, fortunately, most of these disorders are relatively uncommon, we have included the more frequently encountered, and particularly those that have a prominent cutaneous component.

## THE ICHTHYOSES

### HARLEQUIN FETUS

This severe type of congenital ichthyosis should not be confused with harlequin color change (see Chapter 106). This fortunately rare disorder is probably the extreme form of lamellar ichthyosis (non-bullous congenital ichthyosiform erythroderma) and is inherited as an autosomal recessive trait. Although the molecular defect is not known, x-ray diffraction analysis performed on the horny layer of one harlequin fetus demonstrated an abnormal cross-B fibrous protein as the major component (Craig, 1970).

The earliest known description in English was written by a clergyman, the Reverend Oliver Hart of Charleston, South Carolina, in 1750, and is as accurate as any in the medical literature:

The skin was dry and hard and seemed to be cracked in many places, somewhat resembling the scales of a fish. The mouth was large and round and wide open. It had no external nose, but two holes where the nose would have been. The eyes appeared to be lumps of coagulated blood, turned out, about the bigness of a plum, ghastly to behold. It had no external ears, but holes where the ears should be. The hands and feet appeared swoln, were crumpt up, and felt quite hard. The back part of its head was much open. It made a strange kind of noise, very low, which I cannot describe. It lived about eight and forty hours and was alive when I saw it.

The appearance and consistency of the skin of these infants has inspired innumerable metaphors. It has been likened to baked apple, tree bark, a loosely built wall, elephant or rhinoceros skin, a coat of mail

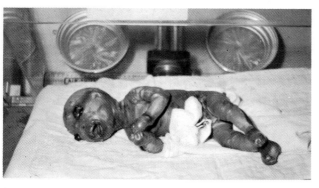

*Figure 103–1.* Harlequin fetus. (Photograph reproduced with the kind permission of Dr. Marvin Cornblath.)

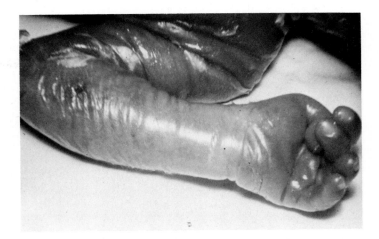

*Figure 103–2.* Shiny parchment-like membrane covering the arm and hand of a collodion baby.

and Moroccan leather. The skin is hard, brown, cracked and rigid, flattening the nose, ears and digits. Chemosis of the conjunctivae obscures the globes, the lips are gaping and the nails and hair are hypoplastic or absent. The viscera are usually normal. No treatment can be offered except humidity and lubrication, but these infants inevitably succumb to the disease because of inability to feed, maintain temperature and ventilate adequately. Survival beyond 6 weeks is unknown. Genetic counseling for the families of these infants is mandatory.

## COLLODION BABY

Collodion babies are also uncommon, although not as rare as the harlequin fetus. The infant is born tightly encased in a shiny membrane resembling parchment or oiled silk, which is perforated by scalp and lanugo hair. To some observers, the appearance suggests that the infant has been varnished or lacquered. The tautness of the membrane holds the face immobile and distorts the features. Motion of the limbs is also restricted. Within a day or two the membrane begins to fissure and peel, especially about the thorax and joints. In some instances, the skin beneath the membrane has a beefy-red color, and it may continue to scale or form a new membrane.

The collodion baby probably represents a phenotype for several genotypes. Many of these infants develop lamellar ichthyosis, but membranes have also been observed in patients with X-linked ichthyosis and, rarely, epidermolytic hyperkeratosis. Occasional infants subsequent to shedding of the membrane appear to have perfectly normal skin. No abnormality of the internal organs has been associated, and the mortality rate for these infants is low in contrast to that of the harlequin fetus (Esterly, 1968). A prolonged period of observation may be required to determine the outcome and prognosis. As soon as a reliable diagnosis is available, genetic counseling should be provided.

Treatment consists of humidity and lubrication with a bland ointment until the membrane has been desquamated.

## MAJOR TYPES OF ICHTHYOSIS

Six distinct types of ichthyosis have been delineated on the basis of their clinical and histologic features and their patterns of genetic transmission (Solomon and Esterly, 1973). Most of these disorders are apparent at birth. Briefly they can be outlined as follows:

1. ICHTHYOSIS VULGARIS. This is the most common form of ichthyosis and is inherited as an autosomal dominant trait. Onset is usually after the first 3 months of life. Scaling spares the flexural areas but affects the palms and soles.

2. X-LINKED ICHTHYOSIS. This variant affects males only and may be present at birth. The scales are large and dark, promi-

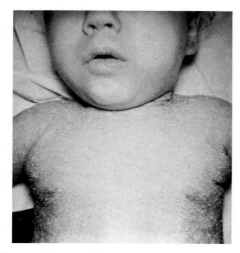

*Figure 103–3.* Infant with lamellar ichthyosis. Generalized scaling of the trunk with relative sparing of the face. The scales are finer and lighter in color than in older children with this disease.

nent on the neck and limbs with sparing of the palms and soles and variable sparing of the flexural areas. A deep corneal dystrophy may be detected by slit-lamp examination but usually is not apparent until late childhood or adolescence.

3. LAMELLAR ICHTHYOSIS (non-bullous congenital ichthyosiform erythroderma). Inherited as an autosomal recessive trait, this disorder is present at birth and is characterized by an erythroderma and large yellow-brown scales over the entire body, with involvement of all of the flexures as well as the palms and soles. Ectropion may be present and is progressive in severely affected individuals.

4. EPIDERMOLYTIC HYPERKERATOSIS (bullous congenital ichthyosiform erythroderma). Also affected at birth, these patients have a generalized erythroderma and small, thick, yellow, shotty scales. Scaling is accentuated in the flexural areas, and the palms and soles may be involved. The eruption of bullae, most frequently on the lower legs, is characteristic of the disease in infancy and childhood. Transmission is by an autosomal dominant gene.

5. ICHTHYOSIS LINEARIS CIRCUMFLEXA. This is a rare dermatosis, present at birth and transmitted as an autosomal recessive disorder. It is characterized by migratory, polycyclic lesions with a peripheral double-edged scale and hyperkeratosis of the flexural areas.

6. ERYTHROKERATODERMIA VARIABILIS. This type of ichthyosis is also very rare; it is inherited in an autosomal dominant fashion and can be detected in infancy. Affected individuals have transient migratory areas of discrete macular erythema as well as fixed hyperkeratotic plaques.

It is important to distinguish the various forms of ichthyosis so that the physician can offer a prognosis and appropriate genetic counseling to the family. Frequently the clinical picture and pedigree data provide sufficient information on which to base a diagnosis; however, at times a period of observation beyond the first 4 weeks of life is required to accurately assess the situation. A skin biopsy may help to solve a diagnostic dilemma, as all types of ichthyosis have a characteristic histologic pattern (Solomon and Esterly, 1973).

Therapy is restricted to topical preparations. Hydration of the stratum corneum is important and can be accomplished by bathing with a water dispersible bath oil. Lubrication with a bland adherent emollient such as petrolatum, Aquaphor or Eucerin should be provided immediately following the bath and whenever necessary throughout the day. Urea-containing emollients (10–20 per cent) are also effective preparations. Other available modalities such as vitamin A acid (0.1 per cent), lactic acid in petrolatum (5 per cent) and preparations containing propylene glycol (Keralyt) are not required in early infancy and should be reserved for older patients. Irritating soaps and detergents should be avoided. Extremes in temperature and excessively dry indoor heating also impose undue hardship on these individuals. The prognosis is related to the severity of the condition and the type of ichthyosis.

### SYNDROMES WITH ICHTHYOSIS AS A FEATURE

Several syndromes, identifiable in infants, have ichthyosis as a major feature (Solomon and Esterly, 1973). A few of these are listed below.

1. NETHERTON'S SYNDROME. Ichthyosis (lamellar or linearis circumflexa), hair shaft defects and atopic diathesis.
2. SJÖGREN-LARSSON SYNDROME. Lamellar ichthyosis, spastic diplegia and mental retardation.
3. RUD'S SYNDROME. Ichthyosis, epilepsy, mental retardation, sexual infantilism.
4. CONRADI'S SYNDROME. Patterned scaling, stippled epiphyses, cataract, bony anomalies. The scaling is transient in this disorder.

## ALBINISM

Oculocutaneous albinism is a congenital defect of pigmentation that is clinically manifest by hypopigmentation of the skin, hair and eyes, with associated photophobia and nystagmus. It is a disease that affects all races; estimates of gene frequency vary depending on the population under consideration. As with many genetic disorders, the incidence of affected individuals is increased in certain racial isolates, owing to the high percentage of consanguineous marriages.

Although all types of oculocutaneous albinism are inherited in an autosomal recessive fashion, genetic heterogeneity has been well established for this condition. The characteristic pigmentary changes are due to a defect in tyrosinase formation, which interferes with melanin synthesis. The three types of oculocutaneous albinism, 1) tyrosinase negative, 2) tyrosinase positive, and 3) yellow, can be distinguished on the basis of subtle clinical differences and by a hair bulb tyrosine test (Witkop, 1971).

Affected infants, whatever their race, have a marked decrease in skin pigment and yellow or white hair. The irides are blue-gray or pink in reflected light. Photophobia and nystagmus of variable degree are present, depending on the type of albinism. Visual acuity may be severely impaired. Associated abnormalities may include hemorrhagic diathesis (Hermansky-Pudlak syndrome), small stature and defective mentation. Deafness can occur in association with oculocutaneous albinism as well as with a number of other pigmentary disorders (Konigsmark, 1972).

In patients with the tyrosinase positive and yellow forms of albinism, some accumulation of pigment may accrue with increasing age. Concomitant with the development of pigment in the irides, visual acuity may improve significantly. There is no treatment for the albinism, but sun-screen preparations should be provided to protect against excessive exposure to sunlight.

## PARTIAL ALBINISM
## (PIEBALDISM)

Although the number of reported families with this disorder is low, the disease is believed to be more common than the literature would indicate. Partial albinism is a heritable disorder transmitted by an autosomal dominant gene. Ultrastructural studies show absence of melanocytes in the depigmented areas of skin and normal melanocytes in the uninvolved skin (Comings, 1966). A genetic defect in melanoblast differentiation has been proposed to account for these findings.

Partial albinism is present at birth but may be relatively inconspicuous if the infant is very fair-skinned. The amelanotic areas predominate on the ventral skin, with relative sparing of the dorsal surface. A favorite site of involvement is the central forehead, where a triangular or diamond-shaped defect extends to the scalp to produce a white forelock. Similar areas may be found on the eyebrows, chin, trunk, midarm and mid-leg. This disorder is readily differentiated from albinism, in which the absence of pigment is uniform. Vitiligo may have a similar appearance, but it is not congenital and usually does not remain fixed. Waardenburg's syndrome may also cause confusion. Occasional families may have associated defects such as sensorineural deafness and mental retardation (Telfer, 1971). The defects remain constant throughout life and are not amenable to treatment, although adequate cosmetic results may be achieved with the use of hair dyes and make-up (Covermark).

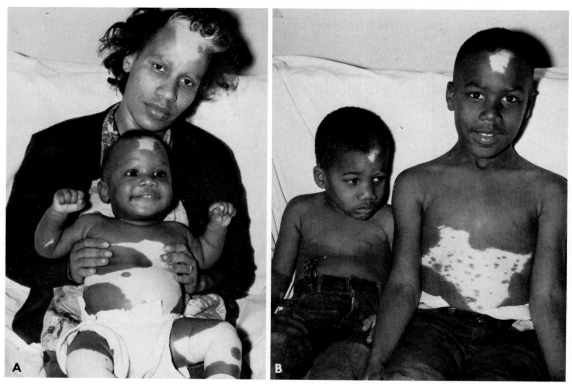

**Figure 103-4.** *A,* Mother and child with partial albinism. Both have patches on the forehead, although of different sizes and shapes. The areas of nonpigmentation on the infant's trunk and extremities are unusually extensive. *B,* Siblings with different degrees of partial albinism. (Jahn, H. M., and McIntire, M. S.: A.M.A. J. Dis. Child., 88:481, 1954.)

## APLASIA CUTIS CONGENITA (CONGENITAL ABSENCE OF SKIN)

Congenital absence of skin is a rare developmental anomaly which occurs most often on the scalp, but also may involve the skin of the trunk and extremities. The defects are usually along the midline of the scalp in the parietal or occipital areas, and may be solitary or multiple measuring up to several centimeters in diameter. Multiple defects, particularly those on the trunk and extremities, may be strikingly symmetrical in distribution. The lesion is sharply marginated, often oval or round, and can be ulcerated, bullous, cicatricial or covered with a tough membrane. The depth of the base can vary from the level of the dermis to that of the arachnoid, with defects in the calvarium and dura.

Histological examination of tissue from the defect demonstrates an absent epidermis and a diminished number of appendageal structures and dermal elastic fibers or, in deeper lesions, absence of all layers of the integument. No evidence of inflammation or pathogenic organisms is usually detectable.

Although most instances of aplasia cutis are sporadic, there are several well-documented pedigrees demonstrating autosomal dominant transmission of the defect (Fisher, 1973). Association with other developmental abnormalities, such as cleft lip and palate, syndactyly, clubbing of hands and feet, congenital heart disease, vascular lesions and malformations of the brain, also have been recorded in occasional patients (Fowler, 1973; Ruiz-Maldonado, 1974). In addition, scalp defects are frequently found in infants with trisomy D.

The cause of aplasia cutis congenita is

unknown. Incomplete closure of the neural tube has been suggested as an explanation for midline scalp lesions, but will not serve to explain defects elsewhere on the body surface. Healing of the lesions is usually uneventful, resulting in an atrophic or hypertrophic scar, which is always hairless. The repair process takes weeks to months, during which time little treatment is required. Secondary infections will respond to compresses and topical antibiotic ointment; if there is an associated bony defect, the patient must be observed for the possibility of a complicating meningitis. Those lesions, which fail to heal or produce cosmetically unacceptable scars, can be excised with primary closure (Kosnik, 1975). Punch-graft hair transplants may be attempted as an alternative procedure.

## INCONTINENTIA PIGMENTI

Also known as the Bloch-Sulzberger syndrome, incontinentia pigmenti is now widely recognized as a multi-system disease affecting structures of both ectodermal and mesodermal origin. The disorder is restricted almost exclusively to females, although a few affected males have been

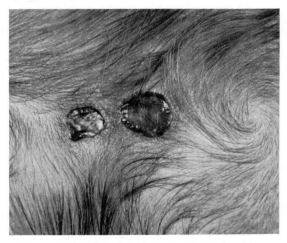

*Figure 103–5.* Two sharply punched-out ulcers on the scalp of a normal newborn male infant whose mother's labor and delivery were normal. The defects extended to the subcutaneous tissue and healed in three weeks with the formation of thin, white atrophic scars.

reported. The abnormal gene is believed to be transmitted on the X chromosome, with a dominant effect in females and a lethal effect in males. Several well-documented pedigrees demonstrating mother-daughter transmission have been recorded; an increased incidence of spontaneous abortions has been noted in these kindreds (Gordon, 1970).

The most striking feature of this disorder is the bizarre skin eruption which, in most patients, can be divided into three stages. The bullous phase, which generally lasts for the first 3 to 4 months, is characterized by widespread inflammatory vesicular lesions in a linear distribution on the scalp, trunk and extremities. The infant is otherwise well, although a peripheral eosinophilia as high as 50 per cent may be associated. The vesicular phase is superseded by the verrucous phase, in which warty lesions appear in roughly the same distribution as the blisters but are most pronounced on the hands and feet. The third stage, most familiar to pediatricians, consists of macular gray or brown pigmentation in whorls, stripes and feathered patterns that are independent of the sites of previous lesions. These pigmentary lesions may fade during the adolescent years or in adulthood. In an occasional infant the typical pigmentary changes are present at birth, and the first two stages are never evident (Lerer, 1973).

It is important to recognize the particular anomalies that accompany the skin changes in about 80 per cent of affected individuals. Central nervous system aberrations include seizures, microcephaly, retardation and spastic paralysis. Patchy alopecia, defective dentition, ocular abnormalities and, less commonly, cardiac and bony defects have all been documented repeatedly in affected children (Carney, 1976).

Differential diagnosis sometimes poses a serious problem during the neonatal period. Although the linear blisters are often so characteristic that they permit instant recognition of the disorder, at times certain procedures must be performed to exclude other bullous abnormalities (Solomon and Esterly, 1973). Skin biopsy during the bullous phase, although not pathognomonic, will show intraepidermal vesicles

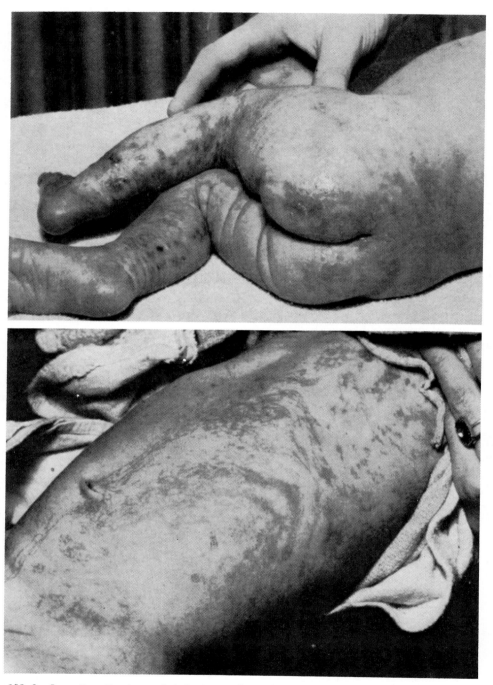

*Figure 103–6.* Incontinentia pigmenti. *A*, Lesions on buttocks and lower legs at age 1 month. *B*, Bizarre whorled pigmentation over left side of body at age 9 months. (Jackson, R., and Nigam, S.: Pediatrics, *30*:433, 1962.)

filled with eosinophils. Alterations in the epidermal melanocytes and dermal deposits of melanin are apparent in the later phases of the disease (Guerrier, 1974).

Treatment of the skin lesions is not necessary. Occasionally vesicular lesions become extremely inflamed or secondarily infected. In the latter instance, cool tap water compresses and antibiotic therapy may be required. If other anomalies are present, ongoing care should be provided by the appropriate specialists.

## CUTIS LAXA

Cutis laxa is a rare, genetically determined disorder in which the skin hangs in pendulous folds, producing a lugubrious facies and a grotesque, prematurely aged appearance. Both autosomal dominant and autosomal recessive forms have been described (Beighton, 1972). Males and females are affected equally. The disorder is distinct from Ehlers-Danlos syndrome, although the two conditions have, on occasion, been confused with one another.

The facies is characteristic, with a hooked nose, everted nostrils, a long upper lip and sagging cheeks. The infant may have a strikingly hoarse cry due to redundant laryngeal tissue. Individuals with the autosomal dominant form of cutis laxa suffer few ill effects, apart from their altered appearance, and enjoy good health and a normal life span. Pulmonary and cardiovascular manifestations are absent or minimal. In contrast, patients with the recessive form of the disorder are often seriously compromised and may die in childhood of pulmonary or cardiovascular complications. Systemic manifestations include diverticula of the gastrointestinal and urogenital tracts, rectal prolapse, multiple hernias, pulmonary emphysema and cardiac disease (Maxwell, 1969). A few infants have been reported who manifested additional defects, such as ambiguous genitalia, skeletal anomalies (Kaye, 1974), dislocation of the hips and intrauterine growth retardation.

Although the basic defect is unknown, all of the manifestations are attributable to abnormalities of the elastic tissue. Elastic fibers are diminished in the papillary and upper dermis, while those in the lower dermis undergo fragmentation and granular degeneration (Goltz, 1965). Similar changes occur in the elastic tissue of affected viscera. Plastic surgery can improve the physical appearance of these patients. The internal manifestations are not amenable to therapy.

## EHLERS-DANLOS SYNDROME

In contrast to cutis laxa, the skin of patients with Ehlers-Danlos syndrome is hyperextensible rather than loose-fitting and, when stretched, snaps back into place readily. Fragility of the skin is also characteristic, leading to easy bruising and bleeding; minor trauma may produce gaping wounds, which heal with cigarette-paper

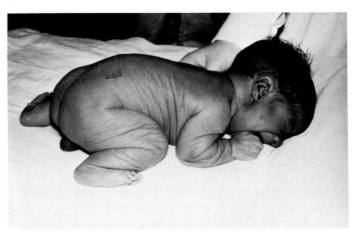

*Figure 103–7.* Newborn infant with dwarfism and cutis laxa.

**TABLE 103–1.    *Clinical Findings in Cutis Laxa and Ehlers-Danlos Syndrome***

|  | *Cutis Laxa* | *Ehlers-Danlos Syndrome* |
|---|---|---|
| Incidence | Approximately 30 reported cases | Cases number in hundreds |
| Inheritance | Autosomal recessive; autosomal dominant | Autosomal dominant; X-linked; autosomal recessive |
| Age of onset | Congenital; may be diagnosed in infancy; possibly an acquired form in adulthood | Congenital |
| Skin | Lax skin hangs in folds on body; does not stretch | Hyperelastic fragile skin is easily stretched, scarred and bruised; pseudotumors often present |
| Eye findings | Ectropion | Ectopic lens, blue sclerae |
| Defects in internal systems | Emphysema; hernias; rectal prolapse; intestinal and urogenital diverticula; cardiac anomalies | Emphysema uncommon; may have gastric atony and megacolon; urogenital involvement rare |
| Joints | Normal | Joints hyperextensible and unstable |
| Pathology | Elastic fibers may be fragmented and decreased in number | Elastic fibers appear normal, but increased in number |

scars that are often detectable over the forehead, knees, elbows and anterior lower legs. These patients tolerate surgical procedures poorly because of difficulty in healing and frequent dehiscence of surgical wounds. Other cutaneous findings include redundant skin on the palms and soles, molluscoid pseudotumors over pressure points and small, lipid-containing cysts which may calcify and which are identifiable radiologically as subcutaneous in location. Hypermobility of the joints with skeletal deformity and ocular manifestations such as epicanthal folds, blue sclerae, microcornea, retinal detachment and subluxation of the lens are frequently present. Although diverticula and hernias can occur, they are by no means as common as in cutis laxa (McKusick, 1972).

Genetic heterogeneity has been well established for Ehlers-Danlos syndrome; six forms have been delineated on the basis of differences in clinical findings (Beighton, 1970). It has been postulated that all forms of the Ehlers-Danlos syndrome are due to a defect in the collagen of the skin and other affected organs. A biochemical defect, deficiency of lysyl hydroxylase, has been demonstrated in type VI (Pinnell, 1972). Defective cross-linkage of the collagen is said to result from the deficiency of hydroxylysine and excess of lysine produced by the enzymatic aberration in type VI.

# EPIDERMOLYSIS BULLOSA

This group of diseases, all characterized by vesiculobullous lesions which arise in response to minimal trauma or shearing force to the skin, are most easily classified by the presence or absence of scarring (Esterly, 1974). Most authors recognize five distinct types of EB separable on the basis

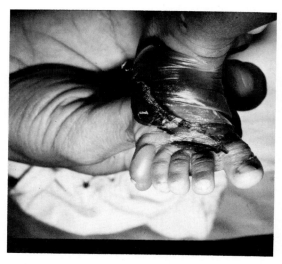

*Figure 103–8.*    Large hemorrhagic bulla on the dorsum of the foot and small tense clear blister on the fifth toe of an infant with a scarring form of epidermolysis bullosa.

of clinical and histologic features, although a few families have been described with variants of the well-known forms of this disorder. The five subgroups are as follows:

### EPIDERMOLYSIS BULLOSA SIMPLEX

The disorder, inherited as an autosomal dominant trait, is present at birth or early in infancy. Bullae arise most frequently over pressure points such as the elbows and knees, as well as on the legs, feet and hands. Mucous membrane involvement is minimal or absent. The extensive erosions that sometimes result from the trauma of birth may be mistaken for cutis aplasia. Nails may be lost but almost always regrow. The level of cleavage in the blister is in the basal layer of the epidermis and, for this reason, the disease does not cause scarring. The prognosis is relatively good and the propensity to blister may decrease with age.

### WEBER-COCKAYNE DISEASE

The blisters in this disease are usually limited to the hands and feet, although they occasionally occur elsewhere on the body. This type of EB, which is inherited in an autosomal dominant fashion, usually does not occur during the neonatal period. Cytolysis of the suprabasilar cells and marked dyskeratosis are the characteristic biopsy findings; healing proceeds without the formation of scars.

### EPIDERMOLYSIS BULLOSA LETALIS (HERLITZ TYPE)

Although the designation "letalis" implies an ominous prognosis, patients with this disorder exhibit varying degrees of severity as with other forms of EB, and not all patients die within the first year or two of life. The disorder is transmitted as an autosomal recessive trait. Bullae and moist erosions occur on the scalp, in the perioral area and over pressure points elsewhere on the body. Some of these erosions become the sites of vegetating granulomas. The hands and feet are relatively spared, and digital fusion, inevitable in the recessive dystrophic type of EB, does not occur.

Nails are affected and may be lost permanently. Mucous membrane erosions are inconspicuous and rarely cause distress of any significance; however, defective dentition is the rule. These patients grow poorly, appear malnourished and have a chronic recalcitrant anemia. The cleavage plane in the skin lesions occurs between the plasma membrane of the basal cell and the basement membrane. Since the separation does not involve the dermis, uncomplicated blisters heal without scarring.

### RECESSIVE DYSTROPHIC EPIDERMOLYSIS BULLOSA

This type of epidermolysis bullosa is inherited as an autosomal recessive trait and, as might be expected, consanguineous marriages are frequent in affected kindreds. These infants often have extensive denuded lesions at birth and during the neonatal period. Bullae may be hemorrhagic and occur on all surfaces, including the hands and feet; loss of nails is usual. Over subsequent years the mobility of the fingers and toes becomes severely restricted, as fusion of digits, bone resorption and the inevitable mitten-like deformity of the hands and feet ensue. Mucous membrane involvement may be severe, resulting in esophageal strictures and serious impairment of nutrition due to the restriction of oral intake. These bullae are subepidermal, and always eventuate in scarring.

### DOMINANT DYSTROPHIC EPIDERMOLYSIS BULLOSA

This variant of EB is less severe than the recessive dystrophic type. Although the bullae are subepidermal and heal with scarring, the disease may be relatively mild, involving mainly hands, feet and skin over bony protuberances. Nails may be lost. Milia are common and may appear in profusion in the soft, wrinkled scars; pigmentary changes are also usual. Mucous membrane lesions, if present, are mild, and general health may be unimpaired.

**DIAGNOSIS.** The diagnosis of infants with this group of diseases is not always easy. Bullous impetigo is probably the most commonly confused entity. A positive culture may indicate either secondary infection of epidermolysis bullosa or impetigo. Absence of organisms is suggestive of epidermolysis bullosa. The distribution of the lesions may be a diagnostic aid. Those of impetigo more often begin in the diaper region and spread peripherally whereas, in epidermolysis, the earliest lesions occur on extremities and those points that make closest contact with the crib sheets, such as the heels, wrists, knees and sacrum. The fluid within the bullae is more likely to be clear or hemorrhagic in epidermolysis, but turbid contents do not positively gainsay this diagnosis. A careful family history for blistering diseases should, of course, be taken. A biopsy of an induced blister also may help to confirm the diagnosis.

**TREATMENT.** There is no specific therapy for this group of disorders. Systemic corticosteroids have been ineffective except in the prevention of severe stricture formation in the esophagus from lesions of the recessive dystrophic type. Vitamin E orally, which has been advocated recently by some physicians, has been found by us to be ineffective in most cases. The infant should be protected from trauma as much as possible. Cribs, high chairs and infant seats should be well padded, and only soft toys offered for play. Clothing with metal closures should be avoided. If mucous membrane is involved soft nipples, bulb syringes and devices used for feeding infants with cleft palates should be employed. Bathing may have to be restricted to avoid excessive handling. Compresses with normal saline or 0.25 to 0.5 per cent silver nitrate for eroded areas may be helpful in some instances. Hot water should never be used, since warm temperatures are said to increase the tendency to blister. Petrolatum or non-sensitizing topical antibiotic ointments such as Polysporin should be applied to oozing or crusted areas to prevent adherence of the skin to clothing and sheets. Adhesive tape should never be applied, as large areas of epidermis may be torn off with its removal.

Every attempt should be made to ensure adequate nutrition, but growth may be impaired despite these efforts. Anemia should be anticipated in patients with severe disease, and high doses of supplemental iron

may be indicated from early infancy (Hruby, 1973).

## LUPUS ERYTHEMATOSUS

Infants born to mothers with acute and subacute systemic lupus erythematosus can manifest transient hematologic abnormalities as well as a positive LE cell test during the first few months of life. Occasionally, characteristic lesions of discoid lupus may be present in the newborn infant with no evidence of systemic disease (Jackson, 1964; Reed, 1967). The lesions are usually localized to the scalp, face and shoulders, and are erythematous, scaly, sharply demarcated, depressed areas with the characteristic carpet-tack scale. A skin biopsy from one of these lesions can be diagnostic; hyperkeratosis, follicular plugging, epidermal atrophy with degeneration of the basal cell layer and a periappendageal and perivascular lymphocytic infiltrate are present as typical histological features. Direct immunofluorescent studies on a snap-frozen biopsy specimen should demonstrate the deposition of immunoglobulin, most often

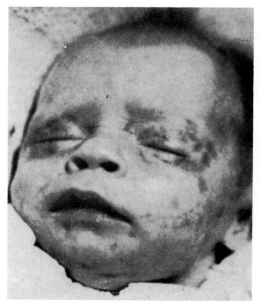

*Figure 103–9.* Newborn infant showing erythematous telangiectatic atrophic patches on eyelids, periorbital tissues and cheeks. (Jackson, R.: Pediatrics *33:*425, 1964.)

IgG, and complement at the dermal-epidermal junction. Appropriate tests for the collagen disorders should be performed on infant and mother (Vonderheid, 1976).

During the spring and summer months, affected infants should be protected from undue exposure to sunlight by application of one of the many available sun-screen preparations. The activity of the skin lesions may be controlled by local treatment with a fluorinated corticosteroid cream. The skin lesions are thought to be self-limited; however, good prognostic studies are not available, so that a predictable outcome cannot be assured.

## ECTODERMAL DYSPLASIAS

The term ectodermal dysplasia has been used traditionally to designate two particular disorders, hidrotic and anhidrotic ectodermal dysplasia. The term connotes abnormalities of the skin and its appendages, the sweat gland, the sebaceous gland and the hair follicle, but it has been applied to disease entities by many authors in instances in which abnormalities of nails, hair or teeth are a prominent feature of a particular syndrome. This practice has caused some confusion in the literature and, for this reason, we believe it is most helpful to define or qualify the type of ectodermal defect, if possible, when describing a particular entity. Although a number of entities might thus be included under this heading, we will confine our discussion to three: anhidrotic ectodermal dysplasia, hidrotic ectodermal dysplasia and the EEC syndrome.

### Hidrotic Ectodermal Dysplasia

Sweating response is normal in this form of ectodermal dysplasia. Hypoplasia, absence or dystrophy of the nails, sparse hair and hyperkeratosis of the palms and soles are characteristic. The teeth are usually normal but may be small and subject to decay. The disorder is inherited as a autosomal dominant trait.

### Anhidrotic Ectodermal Dysplasia

The anhidrotic form of this disorder is probably of greater interest to the neonatol-ogist and pediatrician, as it may cause difficulties during the first year of life. The most serious disturbance is the absence of sweating, due to rudimentary or absent eccrine sweat glands, which results in marked heat intolerance and episodes of hyperpyrexia during infancy (Richards, 1969). If the possibility of this disorder is not considered, such infants may undergo numerous hospitalizations and tests until the true nature of the problem is appreciated.

Patients with anhidrotic ectodermal dysplasia have several identifiable features which, although sometimes difficult to appreciate in a small infant, should permit the physician to make the diagnosis. The skin is pale, thin and dry, with a prominent venous pattern over most of the body, but hyperpigmented and wrinkled in the periorbital area. The facies is characteristic, with frontal bossing, depression of the central face, saddle nose, thick protruding lips and a prominent chin. The hair is sparse, is usually blond, and has an unruly appearance. The changes in dentition cannot, of course, be appreciated until late infancy. Hypodontia with conical, poorly formed teeth are the rule; these changes can be detected on x-rays of the jaws prior to eruption of the teeth. Atrophic rhinitis, diminished lacrimation, hoarseness, hypoplastic

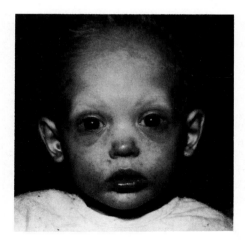

*Figure 103–10.* Female with fully expressed anhidrotic ectodermal dysplasia. Note sparse, wispy hair, hyperpigmentation around the eyes, depressed nasal bridge, protruding lips and ears.

or absent mucous glands in nasotracheo-bronchial passages are frequent findings in these patients (Reed, 1970). If the diagnosis is in doubt, a skin biopsy will demonstrate the absence of eccrine sweat glands. Techniques used to elicit sweating, such as pilocarpine iontophoresis or examination of the sweat pores on the palm with O-phthalaldehyde, can also be utilized to demonstrate the defect (Esterly, 1973). Atopic dermatitis occurs with increased frequency in these children (Reed, 1970).

In most families, the disorder is transmitted as an X-linked recessive, with the fully expressed disease appearing only in males. Carrier females may be detected by minor clinical stigmata or by decreased sweat pore counts and abnormal dermatoglyphic findings (Crump, 1971; Esterly, 1973). However, females with the complete syndrome have been carefully documented and, in these families, an autosomal recessive gene appears to be operating (Gorlin, 1970).

Once the diagnosis is made, it is important to educate parents so that these children are protected from overexertion and undue exposure to heat. Defective lacrimation can be palliated by the use of artificial tears. The nasal mucosa should be treated with saline irrigations to remove adherent crusts, followed by application of petrolatum. Regular dental evaluations should be started early in life and prostheses constructed, if necessary, to maintain good nutrition and to improve the appearance of the child prior to starting school. Some of these children also require a wig and reconstructive procedures later in life to improve facial configuration.

## EEC SYNDROME

The EEC syndrome, which has been defined relatively recently, consists of ectodermal dysplasia (E), ectrodactyly (E) and cleft lip and palate (C). This syndrome affects both ectodermal and mesodermal tissues and is probably an inherited disorder, although the genetic transmission is not well defined. The cutaneous and appendageal anomalies include diffuse hypopigmentation affecting both skin and hair, scanty scalp hair and eyebrows, dystrophic nails and small teeth with enamel hypoplasia. Sweating appears to be intact and sweat glands are present on skin biopsy. The clefting of the lip is usually complete and bilateral, and the palate has a median cleft. Dry granulomatous lesions in the corners of the mouth consistently yield *Candida albicans* on culture. Anomalies of the hands and feet include lobster claw deformity, syndactyly and clinodactyly. Other findings include scarred lacrimal ducts, blepharitis and conjunctivitis, xerostomia, conductive hearing loss and, occasionally, retardation. Although incomplete forms of this syndrome have been documented, the fully developed EEC syndrome should not be confused with other types of ectodermal dysplasia (Pries, 1974).

## REFERENCES

Beighton, P.: The dominant and recessive forms of cutis laxa. J. Med. Genet. 9:216, 1972.

Beighton, P.: The Ehlers-Danlos Syndrome. London, William Heinemann Medical Books Ltd., 1970.

Carney, R. G., Jr.: Incontinentia pigmenti. A world statistical analysis. Arch. Dermatol. 112:535, 1976.

Comings, D. E., and Odland, G. F.: Partial albinism. J.A.M.A. 195:519, 1966.

Craig, J. M., Goldsmith, L. A., and Baden, H. P.: An abnormality of keratin in the harlequin fetus. Pediatrics 46:437, 1970.

Crump, J. A., and Danks, D. M.: Hypohidrotic ectodermal dysplasia. J. Pediatr. 78:466, 1971.

Esterly, N. B.: The ichthyosiform dermatoses. Pediatrics 42:990, 1968.

Esterly, N. B., and Hruby, M. A.: Epidermolysis bullosa letalis in two brothers. Birth Defects: Original Article Series 10(10):154, 1974.

Esterly, N. B., Pashayan, H. M., and West, C. E.: Concurrent hypohidrotic ectodermal dysplasia and X-linked ichthyosis. Am. J. Dis. Child. 126:539, 1973.

Fisher, M., and Schneider, R.: Aplasia cutis congenita in three successive generations. Arch. Dermatol. 108:252, 1973.

Fowler, G. W., and Dumars, K. W.: Cutis aplasia and cerebral malformation. Pediatrics 52:861, 1973.

Goltz, R. W., Hult, A. M., Goldfarb, M., and Gorlin, R. J.: Cutis laxa. Arch. Dermatol. 92:373, 1965.

Gordon, H., and Gordon, W.: Incontinentia pigmenti: Clinical and genetical studies of two familial cases. Dermatologica 140:150, 1970.

Gorlin, R. J., Old, T., and Anderson, V. E.: Hypohidrotic ectodermal dysplasia in females. A critical analysis and argument for genetic heterogeneity. Z. Kinderheilkd. 108:1, 1970.

Guerrier, C. J. W., and Wong, C. K.: Ultrastructural evolution of the skin in incontinentia pigmenti (Bloch-Sulzberger). Dermatologica 149:10, 1974.

Hruby, M. A., and Esterly, N. B.: Anemia in epidermolysis bullosa letalis. Am. J. Dis. Child. *125*:696, 1973.

Jackson, R.: Discoid lupus in a newborn infant of a mother with lupus erythematosus. Pediatrics *33*:425, 1964.

Kaye, C. J., Fisher, D. E., and Esterly, N. B.: Cutis laxa, skeletal anomalies, and ambiguous genitalia. Am. J. Dis. Child. *127*:115, 1974.

Konigsmark, B.: Hereditary childhood hearing loss and integumentary system disease. J. Pediatr. *80*:909, 1972.

Kosnik, E. J., and Sayers, M. P.: Congenital scalp defects: Aplasia cutis congenita. J. Neurosurg. *42*:32, 1975.

Lerer, R. J., Ehrenhranz, R. A., and Campbell, A. G. M.: Pigmented lesions of incontinentia pigmenti in a neonate. J. Pediatr. *83*:503, 1973.

Maxwell, E., and Esterly, N. B.: Cutis laxa. Am. J. Dis. Child. *117*:479, 1969.

McKusick, V. A.: Heritable Disorders of Connective Tissue. Saint Louis, The C.V. Mosby Co., l972.

Morgan, J. D.: Incontinentia pigmenti (Bloch-Sulzberger syndrome). Am. J. Dis. Child. *122*:294, 1971.

Pinnell, S. R., Krane, S. M., Kenzora, J., and Glimcher, M. J.: A new heritable disorder of connective tissue with hydroxylysine-deficient collagen. N. Engl. J. Med. *286*:1013, 1972.

Pries, C., Mittleman, D., Miller, M., Solomon, L. M.,

Pashayan, H. M., and Pruzansky, S.: The EEC syndrome. Am. J. Dis. Child. *127*:840, 1974.

Reed, W. B., Lopez, D. A., and Landing, B.: Clinical spectrum of anhidrotic ectodermal dysplasia. Arch. Dermatol. *102*:134, 1970.

Reed, W. B., May, S. B., and Tuffanelli, D. L.: Discoid lupus erythematosus in a newborn. Arch. Dermatol. *96*:64, 1967.

Richards, W., and Kaplan, M.: Anhidrotic ectodermal dysplasia: An unusual cause of hyperpyrexia in the newborn. Am. J. Dis. Child. *117*:597, 1969.

Ruiz-Maldonado, R., and Tamayo, L.: Aplasia cutis congenita, spastic paralysis and mental retardation. Am. J. Dis. Child. *128*:699, 1974.

Solomon, L. M., and Esterly, N. B.: Neonatal Dermatology. Philadelphia, W. B. Saunders Co., 1973.

Telfer, M. A., Sugar, A., Jaeger, E. A., and Mulchay, J.: Dominant piebald trait (white forehead and leukoderma) with neurological impairment. Am. J. Hum. Genet. *23*:383, 1971.

Vonderheid, E. C., Koblenzer, P. J., Ming, P. M. L., and Burgoon, C. T., Jr.: Neonatal lupus erythematosus. Arch. Dermatol. *112*:698, 1976.

Witkop, C. J., Jr., White, J. G., Nance, W. E., Jackson, C. E., and Desnick, S.: Classification of albinism in man. Clinical Delineation of Birth Defects, Part XII, Skin, Hair and Nails. Baltimore, Williams & Wilkins, 1971, p. 13.

# INFECTIONS OF THE SKIN

## 104

*By Nancy B. Esterly and Lawrence M. Solomon*

The newborn skin may be the site of a variety of lesions of infectious origin. Some types represent localized disease, whereas others are a reflection of generalized disease. Although certain systemic infections, such as disseminated herpes simplex (p. 813), varicella-zoster (p. 816) and pseudomonas sepsis produce characteristic skin lesions, these lesions have been described in the appropriate chapter as a feature of the total clinical pictures. Other systemic infections, such as cytomegalic inclusion disease, toxoplasmosis and rubella, cause less distinctive lesions, which are not specific for the particular disease entity; these, also, are described else-

where. In this chapter, we will confine our discussion to those infections that are primarily cutaneous in nature.

## BULLOUS IMPETIGO

Impetigo is one of the most common infections that plague the infant and neonatologist. The disease may occur sporadically in an individual infant, or it may involve a number of infants simultaneously or sequentially in an epidemic form. Although usually not life threatening, the possibility of bacteremic spread to visceral organs should not be overlooked. Constant surveillance of nursing techniques in the nursery is mandatory to prevent the initiation of epidemics. The appearance of a single case demands immediate investigation and possible revision of these techniques.

The number of cases originating in a given nursery is related to the physical facilities and adequacy of care in handling the infants. Overcrowding, insufficient nursery personnel, carelessness in the simple matters of washing and gowning on the part of both nurses and physicians, and other infractions of elementary rules of hygiene may lead to an increased incidence of impetigo. This is particularly true now that hexachlorophene bathing has been abandoned as standard nursery procedure because of the potential neurotoxicity of the compound, if it is absorbed. If modern nursery procedures are fastidiously observed, however, the recommendations for skin care proposed by the Committee on the Fetus and Newborn (1974) should be adequate to prevent the occurrence of impetigo. Furthermore, it appears that enforced aseptic techniques actually may be more effective in preventing superficial skin infection than is the routine use of hexachlorophene bathing (Gehlbach, 1975).

Bullous impetigo is caused by a coagulase-positive hemolytic *Staphylococcus aureus.* Most often the organism can be classified as one of the group 2 phage types (Albert, 1970), although occasional infections can be attributed to organisms in other phage groups (Faden, 1974). In contrast to some of the congenital blistering diseases, the lesions of bullous impetigo usually appear during the latter part of the first week or as late as the second week of life. The diaper region is the one most frequently involved, but bullae may arise anywhere on the body surface. The blisters may vary considerably in size, and may spread to contiguous areas often forming arcs or circles, but usually do not exhibit the characteristic grouping in grape-like clusters seen in the cutaneous eruptions of herpes simplex infection. Staphylococcal bullae are flaccid, filled with straw-colored or turbid fluid, and rupture easily, leaving a red, moist, denuded base, which then becomes covered by a thin varnish-like crust. These lesions are very superficial, re-epithelialize rapidly and do not result in scars.

The diagnosis is suggested by the demonstration of gram-positive cocci on smears of the blister fluid and confirmed by identification of the organism on culture of material from the blister.

Treatment should be instituted promptly, and strict isolation maintained until the lesions have resolved. Compresses with sterile water, normal saline or 0.1 per cent silver nitrate solution applied every few hours will cause maceration, rupture and drying of blisters. Extremely limited infections may be treated with a topical antibiotic ointment, preferably Polysporin. More extensive lesions require a systemically administered antibiotic that will effectively eradicate a penicillinase-producing strain of staphylococcus. Ultimately, the sensitivities of the organism cultured should determine the choice of antibiotics.

## TOXIC EPIDERMAL NECROLYSIS (RITTER'S DISEASE; SCALDED SKIN SYNDROME)

Traditionally called Ritter's disease when it occurs in the newborn infant, this disorder is now included with nonstreptococcal scarlatiniform eruption and bullous impetigo under the heading of staphylococcal scalded skin syndrome (Melish, 1971). Although a similar cutaneous reaction pat-

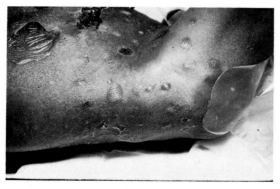

*Figure 104–1.* Bullous impetigo. Multiple intact and ruptured bullae on the abdomen, hip and thigh of a newborn infant. No underlying erythema is present.

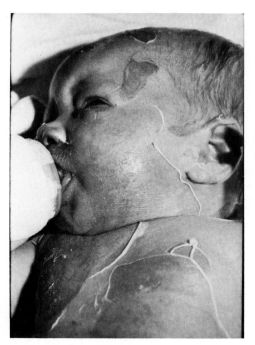

*Figure 104–2.* Toxic epidermal necrolysis (Ritter's disease, scalded skin syndrome). Intense erythema and peeling of large areas of epidermis.

The onset of toxic epidermal necrolysis is often abrupt, and the disease may progress with astonishing rapidity. Affected infants have an intense, generalized erythema, which most often starts on the face and spreads to the contiguous skin. Facial edema may be quite striking. Oozing from the conjunctival area and crusting around the nose and mouth give the infant a characteristic "sad mask" appearance. The reddened skin is exquisitely sensitive to touch and the formation of flaccid bullae may precede widespread exfoliation in which the skin peels in large sheets, leaving a moist, red, denuded surface. The denudation, which can be induced by light stroking with the examining finger, is called Nikolsky's sign, and can always be elicited in the exfoliative form of the disease. Separation usually occurs first on the face and in the flexural areas and may be incomplete, leaving a rolled edge of epidermis at the junction of the unpeeled and desquamated areas. The skin over the hands and feet may be shed in a glovelike fashion. Infants with scalded skin syndrome may be toxic or appear relatively well, but fluctuations in body temperature, poor feeding and irritability due to skin tenderness, are usual manifestations of the infection. With rapid, widespread denudation, fluid balance may become a serious problem. Conjunctivitis, omphalitis or other localized inflammatory lesions may be prominent, depending on the portal of entry of the organism.

Approximately 2 to 3 days after onset, the denuded areas become dry, and a flaky desquamation ensues. Resolution occurs in another 3 to 5 days, leaving no residual lesions. Since the intraepidermal cleavage plane is at the level of the granular layer, scarring occurs only in instances of secondary complications.

The infant with the less severe form of this disease, the scarlatiniform eruption, also exhibits a generalized erythema, but Nikolsky's sign is absent. The skin has a sandpaper-like texture similar to that of streptococcal scarlet fever; however, the palatal enanthem, strawberry tongue and perioral pallor are lacking. Instead, perioral erythema with subsequent fissuring and crusting result in the rather characteristic facial appearance. A dry, flaky desquama-

tern may result from drug hypersensitivity in the older child or adult, toxic epidermal necrolysis in the infant is virtually always a staphylococcal disease. As might be expected because of their common origin, all three forms of the scalded skin syndrome may be seen simultaneously in a nursery epidemic of staphylococcal disease.

Although initial reports suggested that all patients with Ritter's disease were infected with group 2 phage type staphylococci (Melish, 1971; Albert, 1970; Anthony, 1972), more recent evidence suggests that strains in other phage groups are also capable of causing scalded skin syndrome (Kondo, 1974; Faden, 1974). These organisms produce an erythrogenic exotoxin called exfoliatin, which causes the intraepidermal separation responsible for the clinical manifestations of blistering and exfoliation of large sheets of skin. The toxin has been isolated, purified, and partially characterized (Kondo, 1973, 1974), and has been studied extensively in the murine model (Melish, 1970; Elias, 1974).

tive phase also occurs at the end of the first week in this form of the disease.

The only helpful laboratory procedures are bacterial cultures. Blood cultures should be obtained, since sepsis, although uncommon, may supervene. In the exfoliative form, fluid from intact bullae is usually sterile; however, exudate from denuded or crusted areas may yield the organism. Purulent drainage from any area, such as the conjunctival sac, is also a good source of the staphylococcus, as are nasopharyngeal or throat cultures. Phage typing is of interest and should be obtained, if possible. Gram stains of material obtained for culture may be used to confirm the clinical diagnosis if clumps of gram-positive cocci can be demonstrated. Polymorphonuclear leukocytes may be sparse or absent on smear. The presence of a peripheral leukocytosis cannot be depended upon as a reliable indication of infection.

The differential diagnosis includes severe seborrheic dermatitis, $C_5$ dysfunction syndrome, epidermolytic hyperkeratosis (bullous congenital ichthyosiform erythroderma), epidermolysis bullosa, erythema multiforme and diffuse cutaneous mastocytosis. Further studies, including a skin biopsy, may be required in confusing situations, but the clinical picture of toxic epidermal necrolysis is usually sufficiently characteristic to make the diagnosis. Although extremely uncommon, it should be appreciated that boric acid poisoning in the young infant causes a clinical picture indistinguishable from that of toxic epidermal necrolysis. Appropriate toxicology studies must be performed to confirm this diagnosis (Rubenstein, 1970).

Since most of the staphylococcal strains which cause this syndrome are penicillinase-producing organisms, systemic administration of a penicillinase-resistant penicillin is the therapy of choice. Corticosteroids are not indicated in the staphylococcal form of toxic epidermal necrolysis. Fluid and electrolyte replacement and measures to maintain normal body temperature may be required. Crusted and denuded areas may be treated with compresses of normal saline solution; application of a bland emollient may accel-

erate the return to normal during the flaky desquamative phase.

## OTHER STAPHYLOCOCCAL SKIN LESIONS

Staphylococci may also cause superficial pustulosis, folliculitis or localized cutaneous abscesses. Superficial lesions, if limited, may respond to compresses and topical antibiotic therapy. Deeper lesions will require systemic antibiotic therapy and, occasionally, surgical intervention. Procedures such as fetal monitoring may induce abscess formation and associated osteomyelitis. Although usually not a pathogen, *Staphylococcus epidermidis* also has been implicated in this type of lesion (Overturf, 1975).

## CANDIDIASIS

Candidal infections during the neonatal period are most often manifest as mucosal lesions (thrush) or as localized or generalized dermatitis. Rarely, umbilical cord granulomas or a widespread systemic mycosis may occur. The relatively high incidence of localized mucosal or cutaneous lesions can be attributed to the acquisition of *Candida albicans* as normal flora in the oral cavity and gastrointestinal tract by a significant number of infants (Kozinn, 1957). One longitudinal study of infants from birth through 1 year of age demonstrated a maximal isolation peak in infants 4 weeks of age, when 82 per cent of infants were found to have candida in the mouth (Russell, 1973). *Candida albicans* is not a saprophyte of normal skin as is erroneously stated in many textbooks. In infants, the yeast is deposited on the surface of the integument via the saliva and feces. The original source of the yeast, in most instances, is the mother, who may be a vaginal or intestinal carrier of the organism or who may have had overt disease during her pregnancy.

The peak incidence of thrush occurs during the beginning of the second week of life. The lesions are readily recognized as plaques of white, friable, pseudomem-

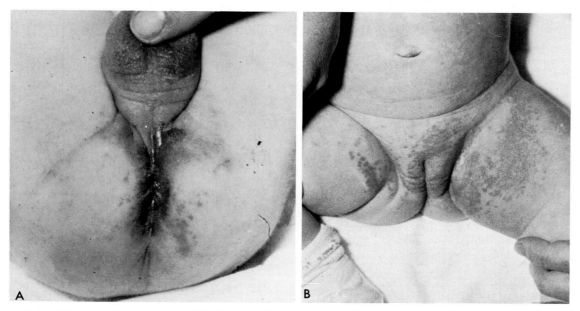

*Figure 104–3.* *A*, Cutaneous candidiasis in an infant 6 days of age. Note spreading of dermatitis from the anal region. *B*, Cutaneous candidiasis of 10 days' duration in an infant eight months of age. Note confluent plaques and satellite lesions (Kozinn, P. J., Taschdjian, C. L., Dragutsky, D., and Minsky, A.: Pediatrics *20*:827, 1957).

branous material on an erythematous base distributed over the tongue, palate, buccal mucosa and gingivae. Both yeast and mycelial fungal elements can be demonstrated on a potassium hydroxide preparation of material removed from a typical lesion. The diagnosis may be confirmed by identification of the organism on culture. Oral lesions usually respond promptly to a course of nystatin suspension 100,000 to 200,000 units P.O. four times daily for 10 to 14 days.

Localized candidal infections of skin are also common in infants. Intertriginous areas, particularly the diaper area, are most commonly affected, but even facial eruptions can occur, presumably by acquisition of the organism during passage through the vagina. Multiple tiny vesicopustules erode and merge, forming bright, erythematous, scaly plaques, often with a scalloped edge bordered by a fringe of epithelium. Scattered satellite vesicopustules develop beyond the margins of the plaque and are

one of the hallmarks of cutaneous candidiasis. Diaper area eruptions usually result from contamination of the perineal skin with feces containing *C. albicans;* therefore, it is usual to have involvement of perirectal skin. The moisture and maceration of the diaper and flexural areas encourage proliferation of the yeast; pruritus and burning associated with the dermatitis may cause extreme discomfort.

When involving the perineal skin, cutaneous candidiasis may be confused with superficial staphylococcal infection or with a primary irritant diaper dermatitis. Potassium hydroxide preparations of scrapings from involved skin will disclose budding yeasts and mycelia, confirmatory evidence of yeast infection. Localized cutaneous candidiasis should be treated with a specific candidicidal agent, nystatin, miconazole or amphotericin B in a cream, ointment, lotion or powder. Generally, ointments are the most soothing and best tolerated.

Occasionally a widespread cutaneous

dermatitis occurs either as a result of spread from an untreated localized plaque or by contamination of the entire integument during the process of birth. Superficial vesicopustules rupture, leaving a denuded surface with a ring of detached epidermis. The lesions spread peripherally, forming confluent plaques of dermatitis with generalized scaling. Mucous membrane involvement may be associated. Extensive cutaneous lesions may occur in normal newborns, in infants with an underlying dermatologic disease, such as acrodermatitis enteropathica or ichthyosis, in patients with immunodeficiency disease or in those with chronic mucocutaneous candidiasis and endocrinopathies. Confusion with other types of infection, including congenital syphilis and seborrheic dermatitis, is possible, and the presence of yeast should be confirmed by potassium hydroxide preparation and culture. Normal infants respond rapidly to application of anticandidal topical agents; patients with underlying disease may be refractory to therapy.

Intrauterine infection with *C. albicans* may result in lesions of the placenta and fetal membranes and characteristic granulomas of the umbilical cord (Schirar, 1974). The cord lesions are multiple yellow-white papules, usually measuring 1 to 3 millimeters in diameter. A mixed inflammatory cell infiltrate and fungal elements are demonstrable on histologic sections of the cord lesions prepared with the appropriate stains (Aterman, 1968). Although prolonged rupture of membranes occurred in some instances, in others the membranes remained intact until immediately prior to delivery (Lopez, 1968). In addition to cord lesions, some of these infants have had generalized cutaneous involvement, and candida has been recovered as well from the lungs and gastrointestinal tract (Lopez, 1968).

## STREPTOCOCCAL INFECTIONS

Cutaneous streptococcal infections occur in the newborn, but are less common than staphylococcal infections. *Group A streptococci* may cause disease of epidemic proportions (Dillon, 1966) following introduction of the organism into the nursery by maternal carriers or nursery personnel. The umbilicus is a frequent site of infection, which is manifested by seropurulent drainage from the umbilical stump and erythema and pustules on the contiguous abdominal skin. Conjunctivitis, paronychia, vaginitis and an erysipelas-like eruption have also been described (Geil, 1970; Dillon, 1966). Since sepsis and meningitis may result, infected infants should be treated promptly and strict isolation instituted. As with staphylococcal infection, serious efforts should be made to identify the source of the organism. These infections respond readily to penicillin, which should be administered for a 10-day course.

*Group B streptococci* are now one of the most frequently encountered pathogens in the newborn nursery. Early onset disease (first week of life), probably acquired in utero or during delivery, is most commonly manifested as septicemia with respiratory distress and shock. Late onset disease (after the first week of life) is acquired postpartum, and more often takes the form of meningitis. Patients with early onset disease may harbor the organism on the skin. A recent report suggests that the group B streptococcus should be included in the list of organisms capable of causing impetigo neonatorum. Belgaumkar (1975) has re-

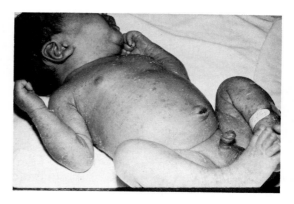

*Figure 104–4.* Infant of 10 days with generalized vesicopustular, scaly eruption sparing only the face and scalp. Oral mucosa was not involved. Hyphae and budding yeasts were seen on KOH preparation, and *Candida albicans* was cultured from the lesions. The infant's mother had a candidal vaginitis during the pregnancy.

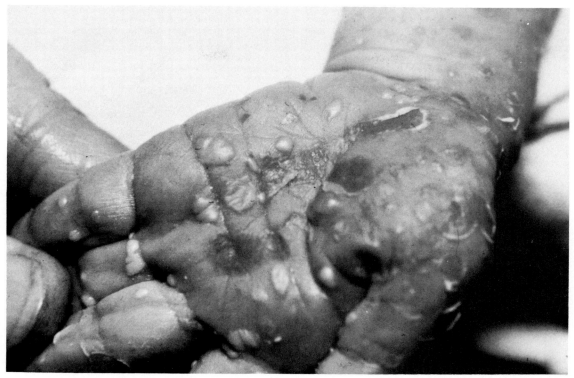

*Figure 104–5.*  Congenital cutaneous candidiasis—pustular stage—in a 6 day old infant. A maculopapular rash was present at birth. (Courtesy of P. J. Kozinn, N. Rudolf, A. A. Tariq, M. R. Reale, and P. K. Goldberg.)

ported a term infant with widespread superficial ulcerations and crusted lesions noted at birth. Membranes had ruptured 22 hours prior to delivery, but the lochia was negative for group B streptococci on culture. Rapid healing ensued following a course of parenteral penicillin. With the emergence of this organism as a primary pathogen in the newborn infant, it is possible that cutaneous disease due to group B streptococci will become a more common phenomenon in the nursery population.

## REFERENCES

Albert, S., Baldwin, R., Czekajewski, S., van Soestbergen, A., Nachman, R., and Robertson, A.: Bullous impetigo due to group II *Staphylococcus aureus.* Am. J. Dis. Child. *120*:10, 1970.

Anthony, B. F., Giuliano, D. M., and Oh, W.: Nursery outbreak of staphylococcal scalded skin syndrome. Am. J. Dis. Child. *124*:41, 1972.

Aterman, K.: Pathology of candida infections of the umbilical cord. Am. J. Clin. Pathol. *49*:798, 1968.

Belgaumkar, T. K.: Impetigo neonatorum congenita due to group B beta-hemolytic streptococcus infection. J. Pediatr. *86*:982, 1975.

Committee on Fetus and Newborn. Skin care of newborns. Pediatrics *54*:682, 1974.

Dillon, H. C., Jr.: Group A Type 12 streptococcal infection in a newborn nursery. Am. J. Dis. Child. *112*:177, 1966.

Elias, P. M., Mittermayer, H., Tappeiner, G., Fritsch, P., and Wolff, K.: Staphylococcal toxic epidermal necrolysis (TEN): The expanded mouse model. J. Invest. Dermatol. *63*:467, 1974.

Faden, H. S., Burke, J. P., Everett, J. R., and Glasgow, L. A.: Nursery outbreak of scalded skin syndrome due to group I *Staphylococcus aureus.* APS SPR Absts. May 1974, p. 424.

Gehlbach, S. H., Gutman, L. T., Wilfert, C. M., Brumley, G. W., and Katz, S. L.: Recurrence of skin disease in a nursery: Ineffectuality of hexachlorophene bathing. Pediatrics *55*:422, 1975.

Geil, C. C., Castle, W. K., and Mortimer, E. A., Jr.: Group A streptococcal infections in newborn nurseries. Pediatrics *46*:489, 1970.

Kondo, I., Sakurai, S., and Sarai, Y.: New type of exfoliatin obtained from staphylococcal stains, belonging to phage groups other than group II, isolated from patients with impetigo and Ritter's disease. Infect. Immun. *10*:851, 1974.

Kondo, I., Sakurai, S., and Sarai, Y.: Purification of exfoliatin produced by *Staphylococcus aureus* of bacteriophage group II and its physicochemical properties. Infect. Immun. 8:156, 1973.

Kozinn, P. J., Taschdjian, C. L., Dragutsky, D., and Minsky, A.: Cutaneous candidiasis in early infancy and childhood. Pediatrics *20*:827, 1957.

Lopez, E., and Aterman, K.: Intrauterine infection by *Candida*. Am. J. Dis. Child. *115*:663, 1968.

McCracken, G. H., Jr.: Group B streptococci: The new challenge in neonatal infections. J. Pediatr. 82:703, 1973.

Melish, M. E., and Glasgow, L. A.: Staphylococcal scalded skin syndrome: The expanded clinical syndrome. J. Pediatr. 78:958, 1971.

Melish, M. E., and Glasgow, L. A.: Staphylococcal

scalded skin syndrome—development of an experimental model. N. Engl. J. Med. *282*:1114, 1970.

Overturf, B. D., and Balfour, G.: Osteomyelitis and sepsis: Severe complications of fetal monitoring. Pediatrics 55:244, 1975.

Rubenstein, A. D., and Mesher, D. M.: Epidemic boric acid poisoning simulating staphylococcal toxic epidermal necrolysis of the newborn infant: Ritter's disease. J. Pediatr. 77:884, 1970.

Rudolph, R. I., Schwartz, W., and Leyden, J. J.: Treatment of staphylococcal toxic epidermal necrolysis. Arch. Dermatol. *110*:559, 1974.

Russell, C., and Lay, K. M.: Natural history of *Candida* species and yeasts in the oral cavities of infants. Arch. Oral Biol. *18*:957, 1973.

Schirar, A., Rendu, C., Vielh, J. P., and Gautray, J. P.: Congenital mycosis (*Candida albicans*). Biol. Neonate *24*:273, 1974.

# 105

# NEVI AND CUTANEOUS TUMORS

*By Lawrence M. Solomon and
Nancy B. Esterly*

There is no universally accurate or even satisfying definition of the word "nevus." By common usage, it has come to mean a cutaneous malformation represented by a localized collection of cells in a considerably advanced state of differentiation. The distinction between hamartoma and nevus is not clear. In a nevus, the aggregation of cells in the skin may originate from any tissue normally found in skin, and may attempt to become functional (i.e., produce pigment or keratin) or may form imperfect versions of their destined structures (i.e., abortive hair follicles, blood vessels, sebaceous glands).

Pinkus (1969) believes that nevi are derived from pluripotential epithelial germ buds in the basal layer of the epidermis that undergo aberrant development. It is possible that a disturbance in tissue growth factors may also play a significant role in their genesis.

The clinical forms of cutaneous nevi are extremely numerous, and a discussion of each would be beyond the scope of this chapter. For this reason, we have sum-

marized the spectrum of nevi to be found in Table 105–1. We will discuss the most common and important nevi in the following pages.

## VASCULAR NEVI (HEMANGIOMAS) AND OTHER MALFORMATIONS

Localized vascular malformations, nevi, or hemangiomas occur extremely frequently in the pediatric population. The incidence of all vascular nevi is probably about 6 to 25 per cent. We believe that for the numbers to be more accurately considered they should be separated into cavernous hemangiomas, about 5 to 10 per cent, and nevus flammeus, about 30 per cent (Harris, 1975). Hemangiomas may be superficial (about 65 per cent), subcutaneous (15 per cent), or mixed (20 per cent) (Rook, 1972). The clinical appearance of the lesion often does not correspond exactly to the histopathological classification. Two types of hemangiomas have been described: capillary and cavernous. Capillary

**TABLE 105–1.** *Spectrum of Nevi*

*Epidermal*
Keratinocytic (Epidermal) Nevi

Nevus unius lateris
Systematized verrucous nevi
Small verrucous nevi
Ichthyosis hystrix
Unilateral congenital ichthyosiform erythroderma
Epidermal nevus syndrome
Benign congenital acanthosis nigricans
Porokeratosis of Mibelli

Appendageal (Organoid) Nevi

Sebaceous nevi \
Hair follicle nevi / comedo nevi
Apocrine duct nevi
  (nevus syringocystadenoma papilliferus)

Melanocytic Nevi

*Dermal*
Melanocytic Nevi
Vascular Nevi
Connective Tissue Nevi

Collagen
Elastic tissue
Digital fibroma
Juvenile fibromatosis
Osteoma cutis

Nervous Tissue Nevi

Nasal glioma
Meningioma

*Subcutaneous Tissue*

Lipoma
Nevus lipomatosis superficialis
Michelin tire baby

*Mixed*
Benign teratomas (Dermoids)

(From Solomon, L. M., and Esterly, N. B.: Neonatal Dermatology. Philadelphia, W. B. Saunders Co., 1973.)

sideration is whether the lesions are strictly cutaneous or are associated with other abnormalities.

### TELANGIECTATIC NEVI

These lesions are among the most frequent abnormalities of the skin of the newborn infant. They are designated nevus flammeus as a group but may be subdivided into salmon patch, nuchal nevus, and port-wine stain. The typical lesion is flat, is bright to dark red and has a sharp border.

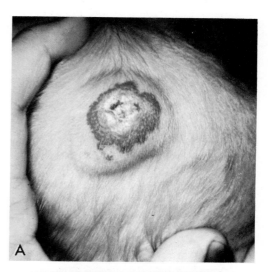

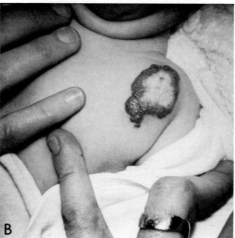

*Figure 105–1.* *A*, Mixed capillary and cavernous hemangioma with small central ulceration on the scalp of an infant. *B*, Involuting strawberry hemangioma with central gray fibrotic area.

hemangiomas consist of dilated vessels, often associated with endothelial proliferation, and develop fibrotic changes as they resolve. Cavernous hemangiomas have, in the lower dermis, large irregular spaces filled with blood, lined by a single layer of endothelial cells and by a fibrous wall of varying thickness. Both pathological changes may be found in different portions of many hemangiomas. Clinically, one can classify cutaneous hemangiomas in the neonatal period into two types: flat telangiectatic nevi (nevi flammeus, port-wine stain) and raised angiomas (capillary, cavernous or mixed). A second useful con-

Those found at the base of the skull tend to remain with increasing age. A paler variety of nevus flammeus may be found over the eyelids, between the eyes and on the mid-forehead (salmon patch). Hemangiomas in these sites tend to be less visible as the skin becomes less translucent, and may fade completely. However, in moments of

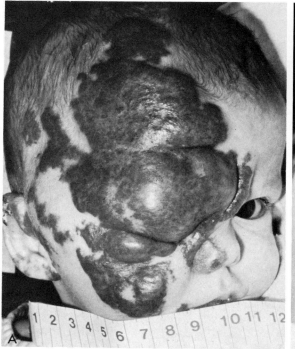

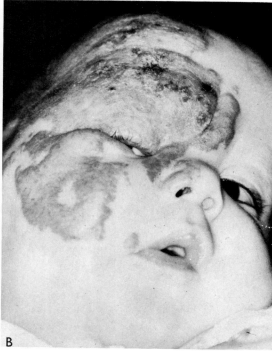

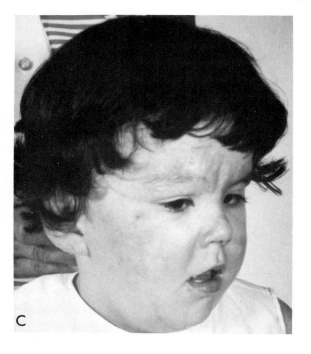

*Figure 105–2.*   *A,* A port wine stain was noted at birth, and by 3 weeks of age had expanded as shown in the figure. After 11 weeks of prednisone (20 mg per day) the lesion had regressed, as shown in *B. C,* Nearly complete regression is evident by age 4 years. She is a normally intelligent child whose only residual problem is strabismus.

anger, during intense exercise or flushing, the lesion may become visible. Telangiectatic nevi on other sites, such as the cheeks, usually do not fade but instead acquire a purplish hue, which suggests the term "port-wine stain." Nevus flammeus may, in fact, be found almost anywhere on the body or on any mucosal surface.

Macular telangiectatic nevi occur in the following conditions with varying frequency: Trisomy 13, Rubinstein-Taybi syndrome, Wiedemann-Beckwith syndrome, pseudothalidomide syndrome (SC syndrome), Wyburn-Mason syndrome and the epidermal nevus syndrome.

### STURGE-WEBER SYNDROME

A nevus flammeus affecting the skin innervated by the ophthalmic portion of the trigeminal nerve may be a sign of Sturge-Weber syndrome (Alexander and Norman, 1960). This syndrome represents a congenital malformation (not hereditarily transmitted) of the vessels of the skin, meninges and, frequently, the ocular orbit. The malformation is most often unilateral , but bilateral involvement is not rare (about one in 10 cases). The clinical features are port-wine nevus, perimeningovascular calcification, seizures, hemiparesis and mental retardation. Ocular complications include glaucoma, buphthalmos, choroidal angiomas and optic atrophy. The hemangioma may also involve the mouth, tongue and buccal mucosa.

Careful neurologic and ophthalmologic examinations and electroencephalographic studies should be performed during infancy as a basis for future evaluations. Periodic assessment of intelligence and behavior and radiographic examination of the skull not only may confirm the diagnosis but, more importantly, may indicate the degree of severity of the process. In some patients only minimal central nervous system involvement will occur, while in others the disorder may cause profound retardation and frequent seizures. Longitudinal observation of the patient is required before prognosis can be predicted. The radiographic finding of double-contoured ("tram-line") calcification in the cerebral cortex is not seen during infancy but develops during childhood. Unilateral depression of cortical activity and episodes of spike discharges are the most characteristic EEG changes.

Treatment measures include anticonvulsant drugs, management of glaucoma and a masking screen (Covermark) for the skin lesions. In severely affected infants neurosurgical procedures aimed at removal of abnormal meningeal and cortical tissue have been palliative (Peterman, 1958). Plastic repair of gingival overgrowth due to either hemangioma or anticonvulsant therapy also may be indicated.

### CAVERNOUS AND CAPILLARY (STRAWBERRY) HEMANGIOMAS

These hemangiomas may be single or multiple. The lesions are raised and may be felt as a mass in the skin or deeper tissues. The borders can be well or poorly defined. Superficial lesions are bright red, lobulated and somewhat compressible. Deeper lesions may have a bluish hue or be flesh-toned if the overlying skin is not significantly involved. Histologic examination of these lesions usually is not helpful, since they often have a mixed picture. About one fourth of the lesions are present at birth (Simpson, 1959; Rook, 1972) and approximately 10 per cent of newborn infants are affected (Holmdahl, 1955), with a somewhat higher incidence in preterm infants (Harris, 1975).

**EVOLUTION.** Most of these lesions increase in size during the first 3 to 6 months of life. A subsequent stationary interval is followed by involution, which may take a variable period of time. The vast majority of hemangiomas resolve by 7 to 9 years of age without treatment (Margileth, 1971). Involution of an individual strawberry hemangioma is heralded by the appearance of gray fibrotic plaques on the surface, a change in color to a darker hue and softening of the mass. As healing progresses, the skin may return to normal color or be streaked by a few telangiectatic vessels. The texture of the healing skin is flabby at first, but improves with time. Those patients we have followed whose hemangiomas have been allowed to involute spontaneously have achieved a more successful cosmetic result than those subjected to surgical or radiological intervention.

**COMPLICATIONS.** The following complications may occur in cavernous and capillary hemangiomas:

1. Local: Necrosis, ulceration, hemorrhage, and infection.
2. Those caused by impingement on particular structures: obstruction of vision, interference with respiration, hearing impairment and interference with nutrition.
3. Systemic: Hemangiomas in internal organs, congestive heart failure, thrombocytopenia (Kasabach-Merritt syndrome).
4. Those after treatment with radiation, surgery or injection of sclerosing agents: Scarring, ulceration, damage to internal organs, local impairment of growth.
5. Psychological and social problems.

**TREATMENT.** For uncomplicated hemangiomas, the treatment of choice is patient observation. The lesion should be measured regularly and its growth recorded and followed. In our experience, parents inevitably show signs of anxiety and a need for constant reassurance. Before-and-after photographs of involuted lesions in other children often alleviate parental concern. Local compression of accessible lesions has recently been advocated (Mangus, 1973).

1. Treatment of local complications: Massive hemorrhage is rare. Minor episodes of bleeding will respond to compression. Necrotic, ulcerated and infected areas should be cultured and treated with appropriate antibiotics, either topically or systemically. The ulcers will heal, but scarring may result.
2. When large hemangiomas interfere with vital functions or sight, surgical intervention or the use of systemically administered corticosteroids (prednisone, 2 mg per kg in a single daily morning dose or an alternate day regimen) for 6 to 12 weeks may initiate involution of the lesion (Fost, 1968; Brown, 1972).
3. Hemangiomatous involvement of internal organs such as the liver, gastrointestinal tract or bladder, high output congestive heart failure, or Kasabach-Merritt syndrome (see below) are life threatening conditions which require active intervention. Prednisone in large doses has been helpful in some infants, but unfortunately not all patients respond.
4. The prime complication of therapy is scarring. Regrowth after surgery is not uncommon. All one can do in such instances is to wait for involution and follow with plastic repair and cover-up cosmetic screens such as Covermark.
5. A small number of hemangiomas simply will not resolve in spite of all one may do. For this reason, an unequivocally certain prognosis of resolution may be premature. The subsequent psychological and social problems of these individuals require constant support from the physician and social agencies. We have found that if patients are willing to express their feelings openly, they seem to cope with the issue somewhat better. On rare occasions, psychiatric help should be sought.

### KLIPPEL-TRENAUNAY-WEBER SYNDROME

A vascular nevus may involve an entire limb or large area and cause hypertrophy of skin, subcutaneous tissue, muscle and bones. The cutaneous lesion, which is usually visible at birth, affects boys more often than girls (Mullins, 1962). Associated deformities include venous varicosities, capillary or cavernous hemangiomas and arteriovenous fistulas. Treatment is not very effective, and surgical repair and occasionally amputation may have to be considered, owing to severe deformity and functional loss of a limb.

**DIFFUSE NEONATAL HEMANGIOMATOSIS (DISSEMINATED HEMANGIOMATOSIS, VISCERAL HEMANGIOMATOSIS, MILIARY HEMANGIOMATOSIS).** Numerous cutaneous lesions may be present at birth or develop within the first few weeks of life. The most commonly involved organ systems are the central nervous system, liver, gastrointestinal tract and lungs, although any organ may be involved. Affected infants may develop high-output congestive failure, pulmonary obstruction, neurological deficit or gastrointestinal hemorrhage leading to early death (Holden, 1970; Burman, 1967).

The cutaneous lesions are small, dome-shaped and red or dark blue. The presence of a profusion of hemangiomas in the skin should alert the physician to search for internal involvement (rarely, visceral involvement is not found). Systemic corticosteroid therapy is the treatment of choice (Brown, 1972). The prognosis, though extremely grave, is not necessarily hopeless, since some infants with involvement of internal organs have survived.

### KASABACH-MERRITT SYNDROME

During the first few months of life (Shim, 1968) a rapidly expanding capillary or cavernous hemangioma may be complicated by the development of thrombocytopenia. A few infants have developed this complication with lesions as small as 5 or 6 centimeters in diameter. Thrombocytopenia is followed by bleeding, anemia and, occasionally, splenomegaly. Bleeding is believed to be caused by a trapping of platelets in the hemangioma and a depletion of circulating clotting factors (Konstras, 1963; Rodriguez-Erdmann, 1971). Hypofibrinogenemia and decreased factors II, V, VII and VIII may be found. Red blood cell and platelet survivals are also shortened. The prognosis of Kasabach-Merritt syndrome is serious, and the results of various forms of treatment are difficult to evaluate. Administration of systemic corticosteroids and surgical extirpation have been followed by improvement in thrombocytopenia. Radiation has also been advocated. Splenectomy is not indicated for this condition.

### CUTIS MARMORATA TELANGIECTATICA CONGENITA (CONGENITAL GENERALIZED PHLEBECTASIA)

Localized areas of vascular ectasia result in a bluish-red network of vessels which forms a reticulated pattern over portions of the trunk and extremities (Mizrahi, 1966; Way, 1974). Nodules resembling varicosities, superficial ulcerations and telangiectatic nevi or other defects may be associated (Petrozzi, 1970). Improvement in appearance is usual but does not always occur. If hypertrophy of a limb results, it is difficult to distinguish from Klippel-Trenaunay-Weber syndrome.

### CIRSOID ANEURYSM (ARTERIOVENOUS FISTULAR MALFORMATION)

This rare lesion may be found anywhere on the body but is usually located on the

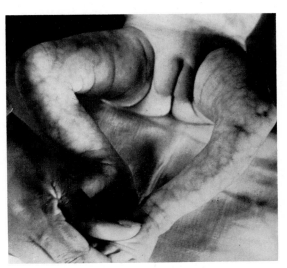

*Figure 105–3.* Cutis marmorata telangiectatica congenita. Note the striking network of dilated vessels most distinct over the extremities (Humphries, J. M. J. Pediatr. 40:486, 1952).

scalp. The lesion may be several centimeters in size, is elevated and warm, and often pulsates. A murmur may be auscultated in the area of involvement. Angiography may identify one or more central feeding vessels. These vessels should be tied or the lesion surgically extirpated at some time during early childhood. A fistulous aneurysm may complicate a cavernous hemangioma.

### BLUE RUBBER BLEB NEVUS SYNDROME

This interesting and exceedingly rare syndrome (Fretzin, 1965) consists of multiple cavernous hemangiomas of skin, mucous membrane, bowel and, less frequently, spleen, liver and central nervous system. Numerous lesions may be present at birth. They range in size from 1 millimeter to several centimeters, and have three peculiar characteristics: they look like blue ballooning rubber nodules, they are tender to palpation, and they are surmounted by droplets of sweat. Treatment is restricted to resection of involved areas of bowel. Blue rubber bleb hemangiomas do not resolve spontaneously.

### RARE VASCULAR NEVI

Other rare vascular tumors that may occur in the newborn include linear verrucous hemangioma, benign juvenile hemangioendothelioma, hemangiopericytoma, and multiple glomus tumors.

## LOCALIZED MALFORMATIONS OF THE LYMPHATIC VESSELS

Localized nevoid tumors of lympathic vessel origin (lymphangiomas) are less common than hemangiomas in infants. A mixed tumor consisting of lymphatics and blood vessels may also occur; however, at times it is difficult to distinguish the tissue of origin of a vascular tumor, especially if bleeding into a lymphatic bleb has occurred. Four morphologic forms of lymphangioma have been distinguished. The histological features of all are basically quite similar: They consist of dilated lymph channels forming cystic structures of varying size and lined by a simple endothelium, characteristic of a lymphatic vessel.

LYMPHANGIOMA CIRCUMSCRIPTUM. Lymphangioma circumscriptum is the most common variant of lymphangioma encountered in the infant (Peachy, 1970). It is usually located on the upper portion of the limbs, in the axillary or inguinal folds, and on the oral mucosa. The lesion consists of a grapelike cluster of very thin-walled translucent vesicles filled with a clear or somewhat bloody fluid. The surrounding skin may have a red to wine color and be somewhat verrucous. Although most of the lesions appear to be very superficial, there is most often an associated anomaly of the deeper vessels. Biopsy or incision of a group of vesicles may result in chronic drainage which may be repaired only by excision of the entire lesion and application of full thickness grafts. This form of lymphangioma may recur even after extensive surgery.

SIMPLE LYMPHANGIOMA. The simple lymphangioma is exceedingly rare and occurs as a simple skin-colored nodule on the head, thorax or oral mucosa. Chronic drainage and recurrence following surgical excision may complicate management.

DIFFUSE LYMPHANGIOMA. This lymphangioma, a more diffuse lesion, presents as a large, ill-defined, soft tissue mass involving skin, subcutaneous tissue and muscle on the trunk, extremities, face,

lips or tongue. Marked enlargement of the affected area may result from invasion by the cystic lymphatics complicated by stasis and infection. Surgical intervention is often impractical in these cases but may be the only alternative when oral lesions interfere with feeding.

CYSTIC HYGROMA (CAVERNOUS LYMPHANGIOMA). More localized, but in many ways similar to diffuse lymphangioma, the hygroma is a large, multiloculated, translucent lesion that may involve any part of the body but most frequently affects the face, trunk and shoulder girdle area. It expands rapidly. Surgery may not be curative, but an attempt at excision should be made before the lesion reaches unmanageable proportions.

LYMPHEDEMA. Lymphedema is swelling as a result of lymphatic stasis. A widespread defect (or aplasia) of lymphatic channels may result in the characteristic brawny edema. Females are affected more frequently than males. The lower limbs are the sites of predilection, but other sites may also be involved, and, rarely, chylothorax or ascites may be present. When the legs are involved and autosomal dominant transmission can be demonstrated, the eponym Milroy's disease may be applied. Patients with diffuse lymphatic malformations require extensive radiological contrast studies for adequate evaluation and lifetime vascular supportive treatment to the affected areas. It should be stressed that the underlying defect in many of the lymphedemas is unclear, and that arteriovenous dysfunction may also be involved in the pathogenesis of the swelling. Lymphedema of the legs occurs in the Turner syndrome.

## PIGMENTED NEVI

Pigmented lesions occur less frequently on the skin of the newborn than in the adult. Pigmented lesions may be caused by hyperactivity of the pigment-forming cells (melanocyte) in the epidermis, by collections of cells of melanocytic origin in the basal areas of the epidermis and high in the dermis (melanocytic nevus cells) or by collections of spindle-shaped melanocytic cells deep in the dermis (dermal melanocytes). The location of the melanocytic cells in the skin, the degree of melanin production, and the numbers of cells present are the variables that determine the size, shape, surface and color of the nevus.

Not all known types of melanocytic lesions occur in the newborn. Those that do are described in the following paragraphs.

### CAFÉ-AU-LAIT SPOTS

Café-au-lait spots are flat lesions of light brown color in whites and of darker brown color in blacks. They vary in size from a couple of centimeters in their largest diameter to much larger lesions that cover a significant portion of the surface anatomy. The surface is usually uniform in color, but minor variations may occur. Single small lesions (under 3 cm) are found in 19 per cent of normal newborn infants (Whitehouse, 1966). Much larger lesions or the presence of six or more café-au-lait spots (Crowe, 1956) connote an existing underlying pathological condition, usually neurofibromatosis or Albright's syndrome (McCune-Albright syndrome).

NEUROFIBROMATOSIS. Neurofibromatosis is an autosomal dominant disease that occurs about once in 3000 live births. The cutaneous manifestations in the newborn infant are limited to the presence of a few café-au-lait spots, which become more numerous as the child grows. Axillary freckling is an almost invariable feature of the syndrome as well. The protuberant cutaneous tumors, consisting of perineural elements, usually appear in late childhood and adolescence. Neurofibromatosis is a complex disease with multiorgan involvement, and these patients should be carefully observed for other manifestations of the disease (Crowe, 1956). Of interest to the physician faced with the need to discriminate between the café-au-lait spots of neurofibromatosis and those of other conditions are the studies of Johnson (1970) and Benedict (1968). On electron microscopic examination of the café-au-lait spot of neurofibromatosis, one may find giant melanosomes in the affected melanocytes and keratinocytes. The melanocytes are also large and produce abnormal pigment. These changes are found in most patients with neurofibromatosis, only rarely in Albright's syndrome and not at all in insignificant café-au-lait spots in normal infants.

ALBRIGHT'S SYNDROME (MCCUNE-ALBRIGHT SYNDROME). Albright's syndrome (Albright, 1937) consists of polyostotic fibrous dysplasia, endocrine dysfunction, sexual precocity (in females), and large café-au-lait spots. The café-au-lait lesions in this syndrome may be unilateral, have irregular borders, are elongated and very large, and usually contain melanocytes with normal-appearing melanosomes.

CAFÉ-AU-LAIT LESIONS IN OTHER SYNDROMES. Café-au-lait lesions are also found inconstantly in the epidermal nevus syndrome, ataxia-telangiectasia, and Bloom's syndrome. In Silver's syndrome, they are spike-shaped.

### FLAT MELANOCYTIC NEVI (JUNCTION NEVI)

Flat, dark-brown to black, sharply demarcated melanocytic nevi are found in about 3 per cent of newborn white infants (Pack, 1956) and in about 16 per cent of black infants. They vary in size and grow proportionately with the infant. Most frequently, one may find one or two lesions in normal infants, but more numerous melanocytic nevi are found in a number of syndromes, such as the epidermal nevus syndrome and

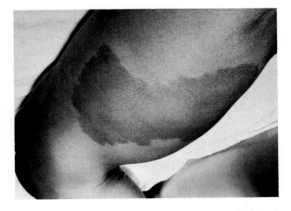

*Figure 105–4.* Large café-au-lait spot on the trunk of a newborn infant.

giant hairy nevus. The presence of these lesions in profusion, either at birth or within the first month of life, usually signifies a more widespread disorder. Flat nevi have a characteristic histological appearance. They consist of nests of cuboidal cells clustered at the base of the epidermis, at the junction with the dermis. For this reason flat melanocytic nevi are called junctional nevi.

The differential diagnosis of junctional nevi may include urticaria pigmentosa, postinflammatory hypopigmentation, and juvenile lentigines. Neither freckles nor ordinary lentigines are seen at birth or during the first few months of life. The lentiginous spots found in the leopard syndrome appear after the first year of life, and those in the Peutz-Jeghers syndrome appear at about puberty. In generalized hereditary lentiginosis, an autosomal disease with mental retardation and nystagmus, the numerous lentigines are present at birth.

The treatment of simple junctional nevi depends, in part, on their location. The most frequent concern of parents and pediatricians is the lesions' potential for malignant transformation. The risk for small lesions (1 to 2 cm) is minimal. Large or disfiguring melanocytic nevi may be surgically excised. There is no pressing concern for early surgery if the lesion is unchanging and excision may wait until the child will

best tolerate it physically and psychologically.

## MONGOLIAN SPOTS, BLUE NEVI, NEVI OF OTA AND ITO

More than 90 per cent of Black and Oriental infants but less than 5 per cent of white children (Pratt, 1953) are born with mongolian spots, deep-brown to slate-gray or blue-black, large macular areas of varying size located over the lumbosacral area. Although the buttocks area is the most frequent site, multiple lesions involving the lower limbs, back, flanks and shoulders are not uncommon.

Mongolian spots represent collections of spindle-shaped melanocytes located deep in the dermis. Most mongolian spots gradually fade during the first few years of life, but some may remain for a lifetime as a slate-gray discoloration.

Nevus of Ota is a blue or black discoloration involving the orbital and zygomatic area. The sclera and fundus on the affected side also may appear to be stained black. When the lesion is located in the deltotrapezius area, it is called nevus of Ito. A biopsy is not necessary, since the lesion is clinically quite characteristic. Treatment of nevus of Ota is only of concern after the child starts school and should include an adequate cosmetic cover (such as Covermark) for the affected area. Surgery should be avoided.

## RAISED MELANOCYTIC NEVI

BLUE NEVI. Blue nevi are so called because of their deep Prussian blue color and are, on occasion, found at birth (Lund, 1962) on the scalp, face, arms or buttocks. These are oval, dome-shaped tumors, which protrude above the skin surface, in contrast to the flat bluish nevi described in the preceding paragraphs. Two types of blue nevi have been histologically described: in one, the melanocytic component is similar to that found in mongolian spot, and in the second, the melanocytes take the form of cuboidal cells with a pale vacuolated cytoplasm.

GIANT HAIRY NEVI. Giant hairy nevi are, from the perspective of the neonatol-

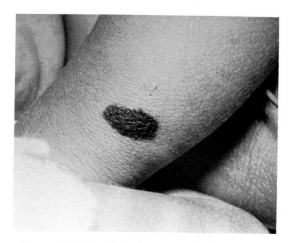

*Figure 105–5.* Dark brown irregular junctional nevus present at birth on the limb of an infant.

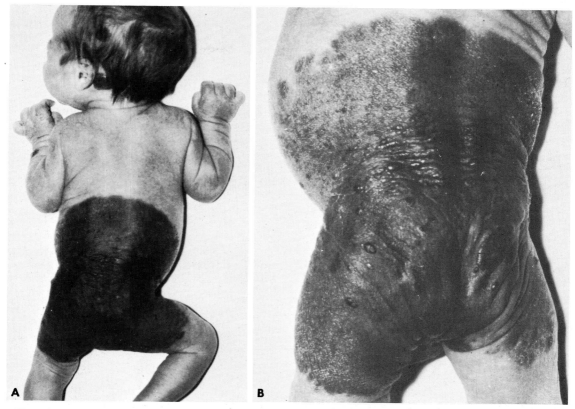

*Figure 105–6.* *A*, Newborn infant with large black nevus covering the "bathing trunk" area. The closer view (*B*) permits visualization of the nodular surface typical of giant hairy nevi.

ogist, the most important of the congenital pigmented nevi. This is true because of their more than occasional propensity toward malignant degeneration (Reed, 1965; Greeley, 1965). These nevi vary in size from lesions of several centimeters to massive deformities covering half the body, usually in the thoracic area. Extremely large lesions involving the back, thorax and abdomen are called bathing-trunk nevi. The lesion is invariably noticed at birth, is raised, fleshy, brown or black, has a leathery or cerebrate surface and the pigment may appear to spill over, staining the surrounding skin with a junctional halo. Coarse hair grows in the area but may not be apparent until childhood. Histologically the lesion consists of a plethora of melanocytic nevus cells. These cells may be pigment laden or clear, cuboidal or spindle shaped, and invade the entire cutis, subcu-

taneous tissue and even muscle, fascia and periosteum. In the area of the scalp and neck, the meninges may also be involved, resulting in central nervous system disorders and leptomeningeal melanosarcoma (Reed, 1965; Hoffman, 1967).

About 10 to 15 per cent of patients with giant pigmented hairy nevi of the bathing trunk type develop malignant melanoma. For this reason, it is desirable to remove these lesions surgically. The postoperative course in patients undergoing extensive procedures may be very difficult, but the dangers inherent in giant nevi warrant a drastic surgical approach.

## WHITE MACULES

Localized areas of hypopigmentation on the skin of the newborn infant are prognostically significant. A distinction must first be made between vitiligo (or complete depigmentation) and hypopigmentation. The vitiliginous lesion is dead white when fully developed, and may be seen in ordinary daylight, even in fair skinned infants. The hypopigmented lesion is slightly lighter in color than the surrounding skin and, in fair-skinned children, may require exposure of the skin to a Wood's light to be made apparent. Simple hypopigmented macular plaques may be seen as an innocent unchanging localized defect in melanocyte function (achromic nevus), in congenital giant halo nevi containing a flat junction nevus surrounded by an area of hypopigmentation (Berger, 1971), as a result of post-inflammatory hypopigmentation, as a pale vascular anomaly called nevus anemicus (Greaves, 1970) or as evidence of an incipient hemangioma.

Small oval areas of hypopigmentation, often in the shape of a European-mountain-ash leaflet, are found at birth on the thorax and limbs of 90 per cent of infants with tuberous sclerosis (Fitzpatrick, 1971). The number of white spots may be quite variable, but their presence should alert the pediatrician to the need for a careful genetic history and thorough examination (of the infant and all members of the family) for further evidence of tuberous sclerosis. When a question exists about the nature of a hypopigmented macule, a biopsy specimen taken from it and prepared for electron microscopic examination may help to resolve the issue. In vitiligo and partial albinism, a few or no melanocytes may be found. Melanocytes are present in the white macule of tuberous sclerosis, but the melanosomes are poorly pigmented.

Tuberous sclerosis is an autosomal dominant disease characterized by the development of multiple fibroangiomas, which ultimately may affect the skin (digital fibromas, adenoma sebaceum); the central nervous system (intercerebral tubers), leading to intracerebral calcification and seizure disorders; and the eye (retinal glial tumors). Moderate to severe mental retardation and seizures may be associated. The prognosis depends on the number of organs involved and the extent of fibroangiomatous involvement of individual organs. Serious complications of tuberous sclerosis include hamartomas of the lung and kidney and rhabdomyomas of the heart.

## EPIDERMAL NEVI

Epidermal (epithelial, verrucous) nevi represent congenital disturbance of keratinocytes, resulting in hyperkeratosis and hypertrophy of the epidermis. These lesions may be present at birth and continue to spread during the first decade of life. Less frequently, they appear after the neonatal period. A spectrum of epidermal lesions may be seen on different anatomic areas of the same patient. The lesions may be deeply or slightly pigmented, be well or poorly demarcated, and have either a unilateral or bilateral distribution. Affected skin varies from warty to scaly. Given the morphological variability of epidermal nevi, it is not surprising to find a host of Latin names describing them. Until evidence is accumulated to distinguish these lesions on other than strictly morphological grounds, we prefer to consider epidermal nevi as a group. A brief description of some of the common morphological variants follows:

1. *Nevus Unius Lateris:* A linear, highly verrucous lesion that streaks across a variable portion of the anatomy. The lesion may be strictly unilateral on one surface and cross the midline on another surface of the body. If the limbs are affected, nail deformity is frequent. When the scalp, face or neck are involved, the adnexal tissues, such as the sebaceous glands, may participate by becoming enlarged. If a large part of the body is affected, the process may be referred to as systematized epithelial nevus. When the sebaceous gland element on the scalp is very prominent, some authors prefer the term linear nevus sebaceous.

2. *Verrucous nevi:* A more localized form consists of a short (6 to 10 cm) warty streak across the thorax, arm or abdomen. Occasionally (in the neck or axilla) the warty element is so localized as to result in a narrow string of small, soft tumors resembling seborrheic keratoses, but

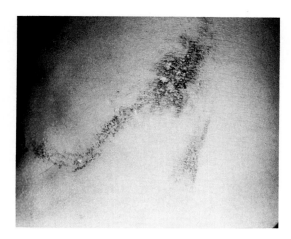

*Figure 105-7.* Linear hyperkeratotic epidermal nevus on the back and lateral thorax.

more fleshy in consistency. Smaller epidermal nevi may be represented by a 2 to 3 centimeter linear lesion on the scalp or face, frequently mistaken for a melanocytic nevus.

3. *Ichthyosis Hystrix:* This variant is a scaly eruption often involving both sides of the body, but in some areas stopping abruptly at the midline. The patterns formed result in an appearance of marbling, feathery streaks, sheets or whorls on the skin.

**HISTOPATHOLOGY.** Two distinctive forms of epidermal disorder may be seen:

1. Hyperkeratosis, papillomatosis and a decrease in the granular layer.
2. Hyperkeratosis and vacuolization (ballooning) of the cells, which may give rise to microvesicles in the epidermis.

The former description is more often seen in nevus unius lateris and the latter in ichthyosis hystrix; however, we have seen both histological pictures in biopsies taken from different areas in the same patient or in different stages of a single lesion.

**EPIDERMAL NEVUS SYNDROME.** The epidermal nevus syndrome (Solomon, 1975) consists of widespread epidermal nevi (any type mentioned above); bony abnormalities, including kyphoscoliosis, hemihypertrophy, discordance in limb length and vertebral anomalies; central nervous system disorders, including seizures, mental retardation and hemiplegia; and vascular disorders, primarily hemangiomas of skin and of the central nervous system. We have seen one case of Wilms' tumor with epidermal nevus but without hemihypertrophy. Other systemic malignancies also occur in this syndrome.

**TREATMENT.** The optimal treatment of epidermal nevi of small dimension is simple excision down to the subcutaneous tissue. Lesions recur if underlying dermis is not removed. Since malignant degeneration (usually basal cell epitheliomas) may occur at a later date (Swint, 1970), it is preferable to excise smaller lesions, but large lesions are difficult to treat surgically and it may be impractical to attempt surgery in all but exposed areas.

**PROGNOSIS.** Epidermal nevi in any other area except the scalp and face are unpredictable. Continued spread may persist until puberty. We have seen none resolve spontaneously. Affected infants should have a thorough physical examination and appropriate radiologic and electroencephalographic studies if defects in bony structure or neurologic function are detected.

### JUVENILE XANTHOGRANULOMA

About one fifth of infants with juvenile xanthogranuloma have visible lesions at birth (Helwig, 1954), and in two thirds they are present by 6 months of age (Nomland, 1959). Xanthogranulomas are benign tumors of fat-laden histiocytic cells and Touton giant cells associated with a

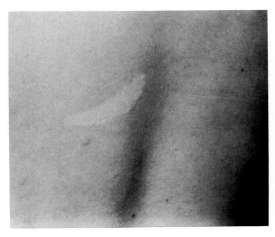

*Figure 105-8.* White leaf macule on the back of a patient with tuberous sclerosis.

chronic inflammatory process. In the majority of affected infants, the lesions are confined to the skin of the upper half of the body. Usually they are firm, red-yellow papules; macules, nodules or confluent lesions are rare (Esterly, 1972). Most of the lesions resolve spontaneously within 6 to 12 months of onset but may leave residual pigmentary or atrophic changes. The infants are otherwise healthy and have no abnormalities of serum lipids.

Ocular involvement is the only complication of concern. Cellular infiltrates may invade the iris, ciliary body, episclera or entire orbit. The ocular tumors may precede, coincide with or follow the onset of skin lesions, and may present as unilateral glaucoma, hyphema, uveitis, heterochromium iridis or proptosis (Zimmerman, 1965; Gaynes, 1967). Ocular lesions may require treatment by x-irradiation or systemically administered corticosteroids to avoid serious sequelae (Gaynes, 1967; Smith, 1968). Very rarely, lesions have developed in the lung, testis or pericardium. The cutaneous lesions do not require treatment.

## DERMOIDS

Dermoids are firm, egg-shaped tumors that occur along certain lines of embryonic

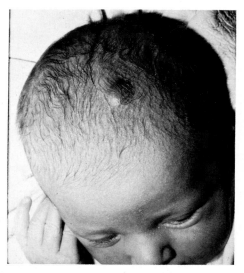

***Figure 105–9.*** Solitary juvenile xanthogranuloma on the scalp, a typical site for these lesions.

closure, particularly on the lateral forehead and around the external superior portion of the orbit. These encapsulated masses contain a mixture of epidermal components such as hair, keratin and sebaceous material. They are benign and need not cause concern. For cosmetic reasons they may be excised conservatively without complication.

## MASTOCYTOSIS (URTICARIA PIGMENTOSA)

Mastocytosis is a disease of undetermined origin. Although pedigrees of affected individuals have been carefully studied, the question of genetic transmission remains unresolved. Mast cells may infiltrate the skin and result in a variety of lesions of differing prognostic significance (Solomon and Esterly, 1973). Infants may have solitary lesions, a generalized maculopapular eruption or, rarely, diffuse thickening of the skin (Sagher, 1967).

The solitary tumor may be discovered at birth or may develop shortly thereafter. The lesion is often oval, pink, yellow or light brown, and measures under 6 centimeters in length. It is raised, has a pebbly surface and feels rubbery, and may appear anywhere on the body surface. If rubbed or traumatized, mastocytomas develop a wheal (Darier's sign), and in the newborn infant may blister or become hemorrhagic. On occasion, a blister may be the sole presenting sign of a localized mast cell infiltrate.

All forms of the disease are due to an infiltrate of mast cells in the dermis which may be demonstrated by Giemsa stain. Symptoms are due to release of histamine from the mast cells. Itching is usual and, with widespread lesions, and occasionally with solitary lesions, massive histamine release may result in episodes of flushing, irritability, tachycardia, respiratory distress and hypotension. Coagulopathy may occur rarely. In the systemic form of the disease, the liver, spleen, lymph nodes, bone marrow and gastrointestinal tract may show evidence of mast cell invasion (Sagher, 1967).

Solitary cutaneous lesions usually have no systemic component and may be treated

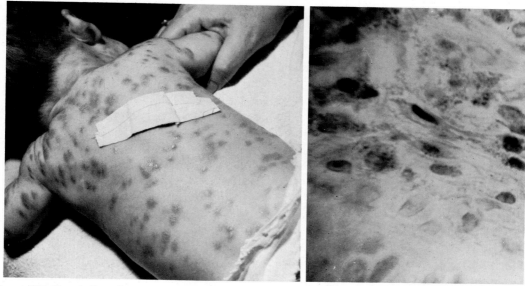

*Figure 105–10.* *A,* Deeply pigmented nodules and macules on the back of an infant with urticaria pigmentosa. A group of vesicles is visible just below the Band-aid which covers the biopsy site. *B,* Microscopic section from biopsy of patient stained with Giemsa stain. The mast cells can be identified as spindle-shaped cells containing granules which are located in the upper dermis.

conservatively without recourse to extensive studies and with every expectation that the lesion will resolve spontaneously within a few years. The maculopapular form also has a relatively good prognosis in childhood. Systemic involvement carries a poor prognosis.

In patients with any form of mastocytosis, the following should be avoided: trauma to the lesions, hot showers, excessive rubbing, aspirin, codeine, polymyxin B and procaine (all histamine releasers). Cyproheptadine hydrochloride in regular doses may offer some relief when symptoms become bothersome.

## REFERENCES

Albright, I., Butler, A. M., Hampton, A. O., and Smith, P.: Syndrome characterized by osteitis fibrosis disseminata, areas of pigmentation and endocrine dysfunction with precocious puberty in females. N. Engl. J. Med. *216*:727, 1937.

Alexander, G. L., and Norman, R. M.: The Sturge-Weber Syndrome. Bristol, John Wright and Sons, 1960.

Benedict, H. P., Szabo, G., Fitzpatrick, T. B., et al.: Melanotic macules in Albright's syndrome and in neurofibromatosis. J.A.M.A. *20*:618, 1968.

Berger, R. S., and Voorhees, J. J.: Multiple congenital giant nevocellular nevi with halos. Arch. Dermatol. *104*:515, 1971.

Brown, S. H., Jr., Neerhout, R. C., and Fonkalsrud, E. W.: Prednisone therapy in the management of large hemangiomas in infants and children. Surgery *71*:168, 1972.

Burman, D., Mansell, P. W. A., and Warin, R. P.: Miliary hemangiomata in the newborn. Arch. Dis. Child. *42*:193, 1967.

Crowe, F. W., Schull, W. J., and Neel, J. V.: A Clinical, Pathological and Genetic Study of Multiple Neurofibromatosis. Springfield, Charles C Thomas, 1956.

Esterly, N. B., Sahihi, T., and Medenica, M.: Juvenile xanthogranuloma: An atypical case with study of ultrastructure. Arch. Dermatol. *105*:99, 1972.

Fitzpatrick, T. B., and Mihm, M. C.: Abnormalities of the melanin pigmentary system. *In* Fitzpatrick, T. B., Arndt, K. A., Clark, W. H., Jr., Eisen, A. Z., Von Scott, E. J., and Vaughan, J. H. (eds.): Dermatology in General Medicine. New York, McGraw-Hill, 1971, p. 1591.

Fost, N. C., and Esterly, N. B.: Successful treatment of juvenile hemangiomas with prednisone. J. Pediatr. *72*:351, 1968.

Fretzin, D. F., and Potter, B.: Blue rubber bleb nevus. Arch. Intern. Med. *116*:924, 1965.

Gaynes, P. M., and Cohen, G. S.: Juvenile xanthogranuloma of the orbit. Am. J. Ophthalmol. *63*:755, 1967.

Greaves, M. W., Birckett, D., and Johnson, C.: Nevus anemicus: A unique catecholamine dependent nevus. Arch. Dermatol. *102*:172, 1970.

Greeley, P. W., Middleton, A. G., and Curtain, J. W.: Incidence of malignancy in giant pigmented nevi. Plast. Reconstr. Surg., 36:26, 1965.

Harris, L. E., Stayura, L. A., Ramirez-Talavera, P. F., and Annegers, J. F.: Congenital and acquired abnormalities observed in live born and stillborn neonates. Mayo Clin. Proc. 50:85, 1975.

Helwig, E., and Hackney, V. C.: Juvenile xanthogranuloma. Am. J. Pathol. 30:625, 1954.

Hoffman, H. J., and Freeman, A.: Primary leptomeningeal melanoma in association with giant hairy nevi. Report of two cases. J. Neurosurg. 26:62, 1967.

Holden, K. R., and Alexander, R.: Diffuse neonatal hemangiomatosis. Pediatrics 46:411, 1970.

Holmdahl, K.: Cutaneous hemangiomas in premature and mature infants. Acta Paediatr. 44:370, 1955.

Johnson, B. L., and Charneco, D. R.: The café-au-lait spot in neurofibromatosis and normal individuals. Arch. Dermatol. 102:442, 1970.

Kontras, S. G., Green, O. C., King, L., and Diran, R. J.: Giant hemangioma with thrombocytopenia. Am. J. Dis. Child. 105:188, 1963.

Lund, H. A., and Kraus, J. M.: Melanotic tumors of the skin. Fascicle 3, Atlas of Tumor Pathology. Armed Forces Institute of Pathology. Washington, D. C., 1962.

Mangus, D. J.: Continuous compression therapy of hemangiomas: Evaluation in two cases. Plast. Reconstr. Surg. 49:490, 1973.

Margileth, A. M.: Developmental vascular abnormalities. Med. Clin. North Am. 18:773, 1971.

Mizrahi, A. M., and Sachs, P. M.: Generalized congenital phlebectasia. Am. J. Dis. Child. 112:72, 1966.

Mullins, J. F., Naylor, D., and Pedetski, J.: The Klippel-Trenaunay-Weber syndrome (nevus vasculosus osteohypertrophicus) Arch. Dermatol. 86:202, 1962.

Nomland, R.: Nevoxanthogranuloma. J. Invest. Dermatol. 22:207, 1959.

Pack, G. T., and Davis, J.: Moles. N.Y. State. J. Med. 56:3998, 1956.

Peachy, R. D. G., Lim, C. C., and Whimster, J. W.: Lymphangioma of skin. A review of 65 cases. Br. J. Dermatol. 83:519, 1970.

Peterman, A. F., Hayles, A. B., Dockerty, M. B., and Love, J. G.: Encephalotrigeminal angiomatosis (Sturge-Weber disease): Clinical study of 35 cases. J.A.M.A. 167:2169, 1958.

Petrozzi, J., Rahn, E. K., Mofenson, H., and Greensher, J.: Cutis marmorata telangiectatica congenita. Arch. Dermatol. 101:74, 1970.

Pinkus, H., and Mehregan, A. H.: A Guide to Dermatohistopathology. New York, Appleton-Century-Crofts, Inc., 1969, pp. 352–354.

Pratt, A. G.: Birthmarks in infancy. Arch. Dermatol. 67:302, 1953.

Reed, W. B., Becker, S. W., Sr., Becker, S. W., Jr., and Nickel, W. R.: Giant pigmented nevi, melanoma and leptomeningeal melanocytosis. Arch. Dermatol. 91:100, 1965.

Rodriguez-Erdmann, F., Button, L., Murray, J. E., and Moloney. Kasabach-Merritt syndrome: Coaguloanalytical observations. Am. J. Med. Sci. 261:9, 1971.

Rook, A.: Angiomatous nevi. In Rook, A., Wilkinson, D. S., and Ebling, F. J. G. (eds.): Textbook of Dermatology. 2nd Ed. Blackwell Scientific Pub., London, 1972, p. 140.

Sagher, F. and Evan-Paz, Z.: Mastocytosis and the Mast Cell. Chicago, Year Book Medical Publishers, 1967.

Selmanowitz, V. J., Orentreich, N., Tiangco, C. C., and Demis, D. J.: Uniovular twins discordant for cutaneous mastocytosis. Arch. Dermatol. 102:34, 1970.

Shim, W. K. T.: Hemangiomas of infancy complicated by thrombocytopenia. Am. J. Surg. 116:896, 1968.

Simpson, J. R.: Natural history of cavernous hemangiomata. Lancet 2:1057, 1959.

Smith, J. L. S., and Ingram, R. M.: Juvenile oculodermal xanthogranuloma. Br. J. Ophthalmol. 52:696, 1968.

Solomon, L. M., and Esterly, N. B.: Neonatal Dermatology. Philadelphia, W. B. Saunders Co., 1973.

Solomon, L. M., and Esterly, N. B.: Epidermal and other congenital organoid nevi. Curr. Probl. Pediat. Nov. 1975.

Solomon, L. M., Fretzin, D. F., and De Wald, R. L.: The epidermal nevus syndrome. Arch. Dermatol. 97:273, 1968.

Swint, R. B., and Klaus, S. W.: Malignant degeneration of an epithelial nevus. Arch. Dermatol. 101:56, 1970.

Way, B. H., Herrmana, J., Gilbert, E. F., Johnson, S. A. M., and Opitz, J. M.: Cutis marmorata telangiectatica congenita. J. Cutan. Pathol. 1:10, 1974.

Whitehouse, D.: Diagnostic value of the Café-au-lait spot in children. Arch. Dis. Child. 41:316, 1966.

Zimmerman, L. C.: Ocular lesions of juvenile xanthogranuloma. Am. J. Ophthalmol. 60:1011, 1965.

# 106

# MISCELLANEOUS SKIN DISORDERS

*By Lawrence M. Solomon and
Nancy B. Esterly*

In this chapter, we will discuss a number of mysterious cutaneous disorders that cause concern to the physician or mother. Most of these disorders are self-limited, some are quite serious and the pathogenesis of only one of them (miliaria) is understood. They share one common characteristic: All may be diagnosed with certainty, and, for this reason, a clear concept of the clinical process and the requisites for establishing a diagnosis are essential for pediatricians.

## SEBORRHEIC ECZEMA

**DEFINITION.** Perhaps a word about terminology is appropriate because of the commonly expressed bewilderment about what the terms "eczema," "dermatitis," and "seborrhea" mean. Some authors consider the term "eczema" to be synonymous with "dermatitis." For the purposes of discussion, we would like to consider this term to represent a "family" of diseases, whereas "eczema" may be considered a genus (more specific) and "atopic eczema" as a species of cutaneous disorder. The qualifying adjective "seborrheic" describes a type of inflammatory skin disease that has a particular appearance and evolution and is therefore fairly specific (Rostenberg and Solomon, 1965).

**APPEARANCE.** Seborrheic eczema or dermatitis is a common disorder having two peaks of occurrence in early infancy. It appears during the first week or two of life as "cradle cap" or "milk crust" and then again from the end of the first month to the third month, this time as a more widespread process involving the scalp, ears, forehead and flexural areas, including the perineum (Beare, 1972).

The primary lesion of seborrheic eczema is a greasy, yellow, flaky scale on an erythematous base. The scales coalesce to form patches that may, in flexural areas such as the ear folds, erode and leave fissures which weep and become infected. Other areas that may become involved are the neck folds, arm and leg folds and the diaper area.

**ETIOLOGY.** The cause of seborrheic eczema is unknown, but it is one of the group of eczemas that appear to be endogenous in origin, as opposed to the exogenous eczemas caused by, for example, primary irritants, infections, or topical allergens. There has been considerable speculation as to the relationship of seborrheic eczema to atopic eczema, a disease that occurs in the older infant. Certainly, the cutaneous lesions and distribution in both conditions are often similar. Furthermore, occasional cases of seborrheic eczema diagnosed with assurance when first seen in the month-old infant may, on prolonged observation, evolve

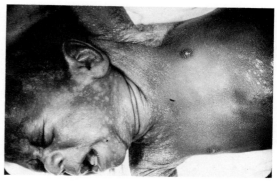

*Figure 106–1.* Infant with seborrheic eczema on the face and neck, and in the axillae. Note the scaling and hypopigmentation. Temporary hypopigmentation is common in black infants with this disorder.

into typical atopic eczema. It is almost impossible on strictly morphological grounds to say that any one child with seborrheic eczema will not develop atopic eczema. It may be reasonable to consider the greasy, scaling eruption of seborrhea as one of the morphological components of atopic eczema.

**EVALUATION.** Most infants with seborrheic eczema seem perfectly well except for the dermatitis.* The eruption may last 3 to 6 weeks or longer, heal and never reappear, or it may, as mentioned above, evolve into atopic dermatitis. In the rare infant, seborrheic eczema may become a generalized process with full-blown exfoliative erythroderma, or *Leiner's disease.* In Leiner's disease, severe diarrhea, gram-negative septicemia and wasting accompany the dermatitis. Familial cases of Leiner's disease have an ominous prognosis (Jacobs, 1972). It has recently become apparent that Leiner's disease may be a manifestation of a functional defect of the fifth component of complement (C5). The administration of plasma was life-saving for the infants studied (Jacobs, 1972).

**TREATMENT.** For cradle cap: Frequent shampooing is the secret to effective management of the condition. Sebulex shampoo or Fostex cream or (in the winter months) Zetar shampoo should control the problem and may be used daily or two or three times a week, depending on the severity of the scaling. When the scaling persists, 1 per cent salicylic acid *or* 3 per cent sulfur in cold cream may be applied to the scalp following the shampoo.

For seborrheic eczema in flexures or diaper area: Bathe the infant with *tepid* water containing a little Alpha Keri oil (advise the mother to expect a slippery infant). Any uncomplicated soap, such as Dove soap, will do. Dress in cotton clothing and avoid wool, nylon or abrasive synthetic fabrics. Absorbent, disposable diapers are acceptable, but should be changed frequent-

ly. The perineum may be protected with a simple zinc ozide paste.* The soiled paste can be removed with mineral oil at each diaper change, then fresh paste applied. One per cent hydrocortisone cream may be used up to four times a day for brief periods, periodically (8 to 14 days), to accelerate resolution. It is frequently wise to culture the perineal area, where pustules or ulceration may herald supervening infection with Candida or pathogenic bacteria. Appropriate treatment should be instituted, if pathogenic organisms are identified. The infant's room should be humidified in winter and air conditioned in summer, since infants with widespread dermatitis may have difficulty tolerating extremes of heat, dryness or humidity.

## HARLEQUIN COLOR CHANGE

This condition is not to be confused with an entirely different disorder called harlequin fetus. Harlequin color change is characterized by reddening of one half of the body and simultaneous blanching of the other half. A sharp line of demarcation runs from the center of the forehead, down the nose and chin and trunk, very nearly in the midline. Occasionally, the line of demarcation may be incomplete, sparing the face and genitalia. Harlequin color change occurs most frequently in low birth weight infants, but the color change may be seen in a few otherwise normal infants on the third and fourth days of life, and occasionally earlier or later. Apparently the color change is accentuated by the gravitational force, since turning the body from one side to the other induces blanching of the upper half and reddening of the lower side. The total duration of these episodes may vary from a few minutes to several hours. Harlequin color change occurs most often during the first 4 days of life (Mortensen, 1959), but some infants may still experience such episodes up to 3 weeks of age. There is no accompanying change in respiratory rate, pupillary reflexes, muscle tone,

---

*The presence of purpura and systemic manifestations, such as listlessness, poor feeding, failure to thrive, recurrent fever or hepatosplenomegaly, should alert the physician to the possibility that the eczematous process may be a manifestation of a serious underlying illness, such as Wiskott-Aldrich syndrome or histiocytosis (Solomon and Esterly, 1973).

---

*Zinc ozide 30 per cent, talc 30 per cent, petrolatum 40 per cent.

or response to external stimuli. Harlequin color change probably represents a state of vascular instability related to temporary inadequacy of the autonomic nervous system. It has no pathologic significance, requires no treatment and can be expected to disappear no later than the third week of life.

## ACNE NEONATORUM

Acne neonatorum is usually a self-limited process, but has most interesting physiologic, genetic and pathologic implications. The lesions can be found at birth or may not be noticed until several weeks postnatally. They appear in crops on the cheeks, nose, chin and, occasionally, forehead. Individually, each lesion may be an open comedo (a blackhead), a closed comedo (a granular, pale papule) or an inflammatory papule. Cystic lesions very rarely occur. The patients in this age group are almost always boys. In infantile acne, which occurs after 3 months of age, there is only a small preponderance of males over females.

Acne neonatorum is, surprisingly, sometimes difficult to distinguish at first examination from other common conditions found in the newborn. The differential diagnosis and discriminating features include the following:

1. Erythema toxicum—there are lesions on

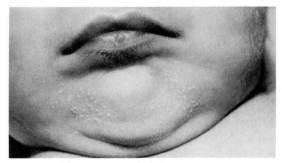

*Figure 106–3.* Numerous grouped milia on the chin of a newborn infant.

the trunk. The process usually resolves in 72 hours.
2. Milia*—the lesions are smaller, are uniform in appearance, and are all white. Comedones are absent.
3. Miliaria rubra—the lesions tend to be vesiculopustular and widespread, mostly involving intertriginous areas.

---

*A rare exception is the giant milia found on the face and ears in the orofacial–digital syndrome. These cystic lesions are usually very striking, and examination of the mouth, hair and hands should resolve the diagnostic dilemma.

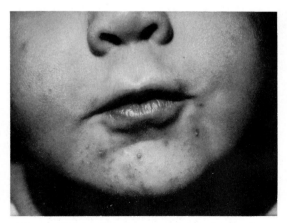

*Figure 106–2.* Papules, pustules and comedones (acne) on the chin and cheeks of an infant male.

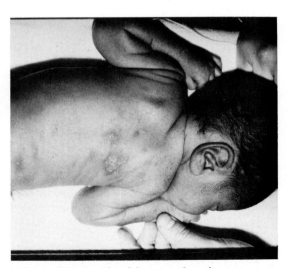

*Figure 106–4.* Florid lesions of erythema toxicum on the back of a newborn infant. The pustules are large and surrounded by an erythematous halo. Smears of the pustular contents showed only eosinophils.

4. Sebaceous gland hyperplasia—these are uniform, pinpoint, yellow, non-inflammatory papules without comedones.

5. Candidiasis—scrapings and culture from the lesions should resolve this possible source of confusion.

6. Follicular eczema in the older infant may closely mimic the changes seen in acne. The presence of eczema elsewhere on the body should alert the astute observer to the diagnosis.

7. An acneiform eruption of the forehead and face may be caused by excessive use of petrolatum, oils, or creams.

The cause of acne neonatorum has not been elucidated, but certain elements that may contribute to the process have been studied. In most instances, the infant does not suffer from an endocrine disturbance, since the urinary excretion of 17-ketosteroids is normal (Tromovitch, 1963). There is, however, a strong genetic component to the process, since a familial tendency for acne is frequently present (Hellier, 1954). The fact that infants with infantile acne tend to develop severe acne later in life (Hellier, 1954) suggests that the acnegenic process in the infant is related to a genetically determined end organ (pilosebaceous unit) hyperresponsiveness to maternal androgens that have crossed the placental barrier. The usually temporary nature of neonatal acne supports this view. It is also interesting to note that infants with the feminizing testis syndrome, who are unable to respond to testosterone, never develop infantile (or adolescent) acne.

In most instances, given the self-limited nature of the process, no special treatment of neonatal acne is required. In severe cases a mild salicylic acid or sulfur-containing lotion, such as lotio alba or Komed lotion, will suffice. Creams, ointments and topical steroids should be avoided. The face may be washed with plain soap and water or Fostex soap. Caution is necessary in using irritant scrubs or lotions (such as retinoic acid or benzoyl peroxide) on infants with very fair skin, since one may stimulate more of an inflammatory reaction than one bargained for. Similarly, irritants used on black skin may cause unwanted hyper- or hypopigmentation at the site of treatment.

## MILIA AND SEBACEOUS GLAND HYPERPLASIA

Milia are formed in about 40 per cent of full-term infants (Gordon, 1949). They are multiple (single lesions are called milium), 1-to-2 millimeter sized cystic white lesions that occur on the face of the newborn. The sites of predilection are the cheeks, nasolabial folds, forehead, nose, ears, chin and periorbital areas. Large milia (more than 2 millimeters) are found in the orofacial—digital syndrome (Solomon, 1970). Rarely milia may occur in unusual sites, such as on the arms and legs or the penis.

Histologically, a milium represents a defect in pilosebaceous formation in which an invagination of epidermal tissue forms a keratin-producing pocket which eventually may lose its canalicular attachment to the surface and, thereby, become a cyst lined by several layers of keratin-producing cells. The expressed contents of milial cysts resemble tiny white pearls.

The most frequent confusion in diagnosis stems from the resemblance of milia to the lesions of sebaceous gland hyperplasia, which occur in the same areas and are the result of maternal androgen on the infant's sebaceous glands. The papules of sebaceous gland hyperplasia are smaller (pinpoint) lesions, which are more yellow and from which sebaceous material can be expressed. Even if confusion exists, one is justified in a conservative, non-interventive approach to management, since both lesions tend to be self-limited. Milia usually exfoliate within a few weeks without scarring. Even the large milia of the OFD syndrome exfoliate in 3 to 4 months, but these lesions do leave pitted scars.

### Epstein's Pearls

These tiny cystic lesions occur in about 85 per cent of newborn infants and are the oral mucosal variant of cutaneous milia. The lesions are usually grouped , firm and movable, and are opaque white, in contrast to mucinous cysts, which are larger, translucent and somewhat firmly adherent to the alveolar tissue. Epstein's pearls are also self-limited, but take a longer time to disappear than do cutaneous milia (Solomon and Esterly, 1973).

## ERYTHEMA TOXICUM NEONATORUM

Erythema toxicum is an inflammatory cutaneous disease of unknown origin that affects about half of all full-term newborns. It occurs more frequently among term-weight infants (2 kg and more) and less frequently among preterm infants (Harris, 1956; Taylor, 1957; Carr, 1966). We have seen lesions present on the skin at birth. In the majority of infants, the lesions develop at between 24 and 48 hours but may occur as late as 2 weeks postpartum. No predilection of the disease for race, sex, season or geographic location has been noted.

The basic lesion in erythema toxicum is a small (1 to 3 mm) papule, which becomes a sterile vesicle, usually white and firm, and surrounded by a halo of erythema and some edema. An entire lesion may measure about 1 to 3 centimeters across. The number of lesions present may vary from a few to dozens. The areas most frequently involved are usually the chest and back, but the arms, legs, buttocks and face may not be spared. Individual lesions may last only a few hours, but the eruption usually lasts 3 to 6 days, disappearing spontaneously. Recurrence is rare. There is no evidence of systemic manifestations accompanying the process, other than a peripheral blood eosinophilia of varying degree.

On examination of histological secretions prepared from a lesion of erythema toxicum, one finds eosinophil-filled intraepidermal vesicles and an intradermal inflammatory component, also heavily infiltrated with eosinophils but containing other polymorphonuclear leucocytes and a few lymphocytes. These cells, usually accompanied by edema, tend to localize around superficial blood vessels, and especially around the superficial portion of the pilosebaceous organ. The eosinophilic infiltrate has suggested to some authors that erythema toxicum is a disease of hypersensitivity, but studies attempting to incriminate chemical or microbiological substances, either acquired transplacentally or vaginally

from the mother, drugs, topical irritants, sebum or milk, have failed to provide conclusive evidence for this hypothesis. At present, all that can be said with certainty is that erythema toxicum is a benign inflammatory disease of unknown cause.

The differential diagnosis of erythema toxicum may occasionally raise some troublesome doubts. Entities that may be considered as possible alternatives to the diagnosis include miliaria rubra, pyoderma and candidiasis. Miliaria rubra usually affects the flexures, face, arms and legs, and rarely disappears as rapidly without treatment as does erythema toxicum; nor do the vesicles contain eosinophils in abundance. Pyoderma and cutaneous candidiasis may be identified by Gram stain and KOH preparation and culture of the pustular contents. Furthermore, polymorphonuclear leucocytes predominate in the pustule of pyoderma. A useful diagnostic procedure when the diagnosis is in doubt consists of preparing a Wright- or Giemsa-stained smear from the intralesional contents. The presence of large numbers of eosinophils may be considered strong evidence to support a diagnosis of erythema toxicum.

Erythema toxicum requires no treatment, since it resolves spontaneously within a brief period. Not infrequently, however, a mother may worry about the eruption, and reassurance should be provided.

## MILIARIA

Miliaria is a cutaneous eruption caused by a functional or morphological disturbance in sweat secretion. In the days before air-conditioned nurseries were commonplace, miliaria was a frequent occurrence; however, with the advent of environmental humidity and temperature control, it has decreased sharply in frequency. Lately, with the use of phototherapy for hyperbilirubinuria, we are once more observing an increase in this minor cutaneous nuisance. This recrudescense is probably brought about by the heat generated by the lights placed over the incubators.

Miliaria takes two principal clinical forms, depending on the site of obstruction in the sweat duct. The less serious form, *miliaria crystallina,* consists of small, very superficial, clear, thin-walled, noninflammatory vesicles, resulting from sweat retention localized in the epidermis just below the stratum corneum. *Miliaria rubra* consists of small, erythematous, grouped papules, and results from rupture of the intraepidermal portion of the sweat duct. The resultant vesicle is found at the level of the basal layer of the epidermis and may be surrounded by many inflammatory cells. The papules may become pustular if the inflammatory component is prominent.

The distribution of miliaria is usually accentuated in the intertriginous areas, but it is not uncommon to find the face, scalp and shoulders also involved.

During the first few days of life, the differential diagnosis of miliaria includes erythema toxicum, candidal infection and early pyoderma. Culture, Gram stain and KOH preparation of vesicular contents should resolve the question regarding the presence of yeast or bacteria. The vesicles of erythema toxicum are usually full of eosinophils. Treatment of miliaria should be conservative. The infant may be placed in a cooler, less humid environment, and the application of calamine lotion to the body folds should result in resolution of the lesions in several days.

## SCLEREMA NEONATORUM

Sclerema neonatorum is a serious, uncommon disorder occurring in the first or, less commonly, second week of life in debilitated or preterm newborns, and results in widespread stone-hard, non-pitting induration of the skin. The affected infant is immobilized and feels cold to the touch. The face is fixed in a mask-like expression; the joints are stiff. Systemic manifestations are always present and may include sepsis, pneumonia, gastroenteritis and, occasionally, multiple congenital anomalies. Body temperature and blood pressure are unstable, feeding is poor and apneic spells are common. Complications such as central nervous system depression, cyanosis, respiratory distress and convulsions frequently supervene. Changes in blood urea nitrogen and potassium, and decrease in blood car-

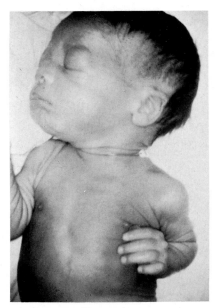

*Figure 106–5.* Sclerema neonatorum. Note the masklike expression on the face, "pseudotrismus" of the partially immobilized mouth, and thickening of the skin over the face, arms and hands. (From the Collection of the American Academy of Pediatrics. Reproduced with permission of the officers of the Academy).

bon dioxide (Levin, 1965) may reflect the severe constitutional stress.

The cause of sclerema neonatorum is unknown, but biochemical and crystalline changes in the subcutaneous fat of affected infants have suggested a shift in its composition toward an increase in triglycerides (Horsefield, 1965) and in the ratio of saturated to unsaturated fats (Kellum, 1965). Specifically, palmitin and stearin were found to be increased with abnormal excess formation of a large crystalline structure of these substances in the subcutaneous fat.

The histological changes in sclerema are not highly specific; surprisingly little inflammation is in evidence. On examination of sections from biopsies, one usually sees edema and thickening of the interlobular septae of the fat panniculus.

The treatment of sclerema neonatorum is essentially that of management of a very sick infant. Maintenance of normal body temperature, control of infection, adequate nutrition and balance of fluid and electrolyte are required. Corticosteroid therapy has been advocated for this disorder, but controlled studies have not shown steroids to be effective in altering the mortality rate (Levin, 1961), which approaches 50 per cent. If the infant can be maintained during the first month of life, resolution of the process may occur.

## SUBCUTANEOUS FAT NECROSIS

The lesions of subcutaneous fat necrosis are very similar to those of sclerema neonatorum, and the pathogenesis leading to the two diseases may be identical, but the former process is highly localized, whereas the latter is diffuse; the infant with sclerema is usually very sick, whereas subcutaneous fat necrosis may be a benign self-limited process. Subcutaneous fat necrosis is usually discovered within the first two weeks of life, most frequently between the fifth and tenth day, but may be found as early as the second or as late as the twenty-

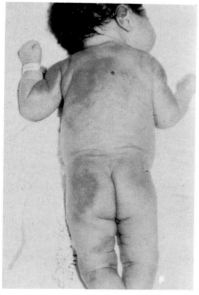

**Figure 106–6.** Rear view of newborn showing several large discolored and slightly swollen areas. They are irregular in size and shape and no doubt felt firm and were not hot or tender. They are large areas of subcutaneous fat necrosis.

fourth day. The lesions are sharply circumscribed nodules or plaques, hard and of a dusky red-purple hue. Most often they are found in areas where a fat pad is present: cheeks, buttocks, back, arms and thighs. The affected area may have an uneven surface and a sharp margin delineating it from surrounding normal skin. The lesions may become the site of dystrophic subcutaneous calcification, and in some infants hypercalcemia may accompany the process. When cutaneous calcification is present, radiographic examination of the skin may provide supportive evidence for the diagnosis. Heavy calcification may lead to extrusion and drainage of a liquefied material from the discharging lesion. The drainage site (usually sterile) often heals with scarring.

Although most infants appear to suffer few systemic complications of subcutaneous fat necrosis, some do refuse to feed, vomit, fail to thrive, become irritable and develop fever. Rarely, visceral calcification may supervene (Sharlin, 1970).

Numerous causes have been ascribed to subcutaneous fat necrosis. Most prominent among these are obstetrical trauma and hypothermia. Obstetrical trauma is commonly observed without the consequences of fat necrosis and the maintenance of normal body temperature is a common problem in healthy preterm infants, so that one must take a reserved attitude toward these suppositions. It is probable that if these factors contribute to fat necrosis they do so only in infants susceptible to the disease.

The management of subcutaneous fat necrosis depends on the severity of the process, on the presence of draining ulcerations and on systemic complications. In all cases *warm or hot packs to the lesions should be avoided.* In most infants, the process is self-limited and resolution occurs over a period of a few weeks to months without much residual atrophy or scarring. Where fluctuant areas are present, careful needle aspiration may reduce scarring. In infants with hypercalcemia or visceral calcification, restriction of oral calcium intake, decrease in vitamin D intake and administration of corticosteroids systemically may aid in resolution of the process.

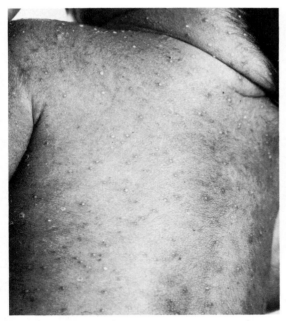

*Figure 106–7.* Numerous superficial pustules on the neck and back of a 1 day old infant. A few pustules have ruptured, leaving a collarette of scale.

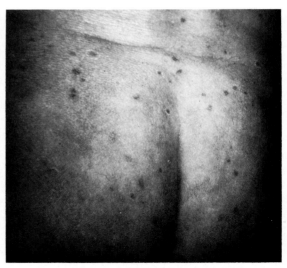

*Figure 106–8.* Transient neonatal pustular melanosis. Hyperpigmented macules on the lower back and buttocks, some of which are encircled by scale. (From Ramamurthy, R. S., Reveri, M., Esterly, N. B., Fretzin, D. F., Pyati, S. P., Sethupathy, R. and Pildes, R. S.: Transient neonatal pustular melanosis. J. Pediatr. [in press].)

## TRANSIENT NEONATAL PUSTULAR MELANOSIS

This benign disorder occurs relatively frequently in the newborn and is usually apparent at birth. Characteristic lesions consist of small, superficial pustules, which rupture easily, leaving a collarette of fine scale, and hyperpigmented macules, which are often discernible at the sites of unroofed pustules. The macules are seen more commonly at birth and may represent end-stage lesions of pustules that have ruptured in utero. The lesions may be profuse or sparse and can involve all body surfaces, including the palms, soles and scalp. Areas of predilection are the forehead, anterior neck and submental area, lower back and shins.

The cause of the eruption is unknown. Affected infants are otherwise well. Gram stains and bacterial cultures obtained from intact pustules are uniformly negative for organisms. Wright-stained smears of pustular fluid contain cellular debris, polymorphonuclear leukocytes and few or no eosinophils. The differential diagnosis includes erythema toxicum and staphylococcal pyoderma, which can usually be distinguished on the basis of the above studies. The pustules last about 48 hours, the macules may persist for up to 3 months. The disorder is transient and self-limited, and requires no therapy.

## REFERENCES

Beare, J. M., and Rook, A.: The newborn. *In* Rook, A., Wilkinson, D. S., and Ebling, F. J. G. (eds.): Textbook of Dermatology. 2nd Ed., Philadelphia, F. A. Davis Co., 1972, p. 168.

Carr, J. A., Hodgeman, J. E., Freedman, R. J., and Levan, N. E.: Relationship between toxic erythema and infant maturity. A.M.A. J. Dis. Child. *112*:129, 1966.

Harris, J. R., and Schick, B.: Erythema neonatorum. A.M.A. J. Dis. Child. 92:27, 1956.

Hellier, F. F.: Acneiform eruptions in infancy. Brit. J. Dermatol. 66:25, 1954.

Horsefield, G. J., and Yardley, H. J.: Sclerema neonatorum. J. Invest. Dermatol. 44:326, 1965.

Jacobs, J. C., and Miller, M. E.: Fatal familial Leiner's disease: A deficiency of the opsonic activity of serum complement. Pediatrics 49:225, 1972.

Kellum, R. E., Ray, T. L., and Szijarto, L.: Leprechaunism (Donohue's syndrome). Arch. Dermatol. 97:372, 1968.

Levin, S. E., Bakst, C. M. and Isserow, L.: Sclerema neonatorum treated with corticosteroids. Brit. Med. J. 2:1533, 1961.

Levin, S. E., and Milunsky, A.: Urea and electrolyte levels in the serum in sclerema neonatorum. J. Pediatr. 67:812, 1965.

Mortensen, O. and Stougard-Andresen, P.: Harlequin color change in the newborn. Acta Obstet. Gynec. Scand. 38:352, 1959.

Rostenberg, A., Jr., and Solomon, L. M.: Infantile eczema and systemic disease. Arch. Dermatol. 98:41, 1968.

Sharlin, D. N., and Koblenzer, P.: Necrosis of sub-cutaneous fat with hypercalcemia. A puzzling and multifaceted disease. Clin. Pediatr. 9:290, 1970.

Solomon, L. M., and Esterly, N. B.: Eczema in Neonatal Dermatology. Philadelphia, W. B. Saunders Co., 1973, p. 125.

Solomon, L. M., and Esterly, N. B.: Transient Cutaneous Lesions in Neonatal Dermatology. Philadelphia, W. B. Saunders Co., 1973, p. 43.

Solomon, L. M., Fretzin, D., and Pruzansky, S.: Pilosebaceous dysplasia in the oral-facial-digital syndrome. Arch. Dermatol. 102:596, 1970.

Taylor, W. B., and Bondurant, C. P.: Erythema neonatorum allergicum. Arch. Dermatol. 76:591, 1957.

Tromovitch, T. A., Abrams, A. A., and Jacobs, P. H.: Acne in infancy. A.M.A. J. Dis. Child. 106:230, 1963.

# XVI

## Disorders of the Eye

There are only a few ophthalmic disorders that demand immediate attention in the neonatal period. Even when one of these is present, it is the consulting ophthalmologist rather than the pediatrician who almost always will direct or carry out treatment. Nevertheless, it behooves the pediatrician to have sufficient knowledge in this field to know when it is safe and proper to mark time and when he must act with all possible speed in order to save vision, and possibly life. Opportunities to save life will be limited to early recognition of malignancy and the immediate institution of appropriate therapy. There are more chances to save sight. Most pressing, although also rare, is his need to suspect the presence of congenital glaucoma. In this situation a delay of days may mean the difference between good and bad vision for life. Early treatment of some cataracts is indicated in order to minimize the period of amblyopia, which, if too prolonged, leads to permanent impairment of sight. For the same reason definitive treatment of severe congenital squint should not be delayed.

Retrolental fibroplasia will be discussed in the following chapter (p. 985), while xerophthalmia appears among the vitamin deficiencies (p. 859).

## STRABISMUS

A great many infants and children manifest strabismus during attempts to accommodate their eyes for near or far gaze. Since newborns make little or no attempt to accommodate, one is not concerned with this variety in them. Attention in this age period is limited to the paralytic (incomitant) form, to congenital squint, usually convergent (congenital nonaccommodative esotropia), and to pseudostrabismus.

### INCOMITANT (PARALYTIC) STRABISMUS

When the stormy period of a severe episode of birth cerebral damage subsides, an extraocular palsy which appeared during its active stage may persist. Or if a newborn survives a bout of meningoencephalitis caused by toxoplasma, cytomegalic inclusion virus or other organism, the strabismus which accompanied it may not disappear. If it does not disappear after 1 or 2 months, the probability is that an extraocular muscle group has been paralyzed permanently. Differential diagnosis of this neurologic form from any other variety is simple.

Advice as to treatment is less simple, for two reasons. First, the amount of brain damage in other fields may be so great that repair of the relatively unimportant deviating eye seems unwarranted.

The second consideration is that surgery for paralytic strabismus is not too satisfactory. One cannot strengthen or cure a paralyzed muscle. The most one can do is to improve its position somewhat by recessing or weakening opposing muscles. A transplantation of the lateral portions of the vertical rectus muscles is occasionally used for a paralytic lateral rectus muscle but only slight improvement can be expected.

### CONGENITAL NONACCOMMODATIVE ESOTROPIA

This form of crossed eyes is considerably more frequent than is the incomitant form. Often one notes the squint at birth, but at times the pediatrician first becomes aware of it at the first or second monthly examination. Diagnosis in the neonatal period is not simplified by the fact that the baby does not yet follow light, an achievement

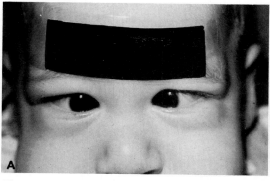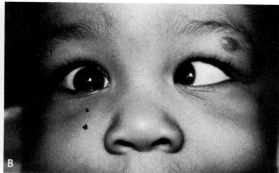

*Figure 107–1.* Strabismus. *A*, The internal strabismus is bilateral and symmetrical. *B*, Demonstrating the squint of congenital nonaccommodative esotropia of the left eye. There is also a hemangioma of the left upper eyelid. At operation both internal rectus muscles were found to be short, fibrous and ropelike in consistency. (From the collection of Dr. Arnall Patz.)

he ordinarily learns at the age of 3 months. Until that time one must rely upon eye movements made in response to noises or to rolling the head from side to side. The eyes in repose seek the midline, often symmetrically, but not too rarely with one eye more sharply deviated medially than the other. When lateral gaze is attempted, rotation cannot be accomplished all the way to the external canthus. In severe examples one or both eyes cannot rotate as far as the midline.

It has been our experience that many of the milder examples clear with the passing months and that no treatment is ever indicated. More severe ones should be referred promptly to the ophthalmologist. Competent pediatric ophthalmologists are beginning to attempt earlier surgical correction of those eyes which are firmly fixed in a distinctly abnormal position. An eye which gazes constantly at the bridge of the nose or upward and outward will frequently become amblyopic.

### PSEUDOSTRABISMUS

Most diagnostic errors relative to eye position of which parents and pediatricians alike are guilty have to do with confusing pseudostrabismus with true strabismus. An appearance of eye-crossing does not necessarily signify strabismus. Apparent squinting arises from the fact that in many infants' eyes the breadth of sclera visible medial to the iris is narrowed by the overhanging epicanthus. This is accentu-

ated when the space between the eyes is small. Because narrowing of the band of white in this location usually indicates deviation of the eye toward the midline, the observer subconsciously interprets such narrowing as being due to muscle imbalance. This superficial misinterpretation can be corrected by noting the excessive epicanthus and by careful attention to the position of the light reflexes in the eyes in various positions. The bright points of reflex will be seen to fall in corresponding locations in each eye no matter which way the gaze is directed if the condition is pseudostrabismus (Fig. 107–2). When true strabismus is present, the points of light will be asymmetrical in some or all positions. It goes without saying that nothing but parental reassurance is required for pseudostrabismus.

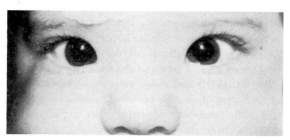

*Figure 107–2.* Child aged six months. Note wide bridge of nose and prominent epicanthus simulating strabismus. Flash bulb reflection is centered in each pupil, showing that eyes are straight. (Patz, A.: Maryland State M.J., 8:600, 1959.)

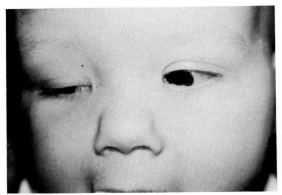

**Figure 107–3.** Unilateral congenital ptosis. (From the collection of Dr. Arnall Patz.)

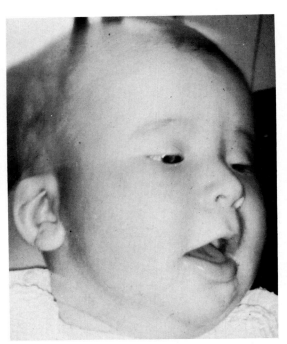

**Figure 107–4.** Bilateral congenital ptosis of the eyelids.

## CONGENITAL PTOSIS

Inability to raise one or both upper eyelids is encountered as a solitary congenital defect or in association with inability to move the eyeball upward. The combination stems from total failure of the superior rectus muscle to develop, and with it its offshoot, the levator palpebrae superioris. Isolated ptosis results when the superior rectus muscle forms and becomes functional, but its bud either fails to form entirely or produces a defective levator. It may be unilateral or bilateral (Figs. 107–3 and 107–4).

Congenital ptosis should not be confused with upper facial nerve palsy in which the main disability is that of closing the eye tightly rather than opening it widely. Drooping lids, common in myasthenia gravis of older patients, are not often a sign of myasthenia of the newborn.

Congenital ptosis is generally hereditary, and this isolated defect of the levator palpebrae superioris is usually transmitted as a dominant.

**TREATMENT.** Consists in a plastic surgical procedure well after the neonatal period has passed.

## NYSTAGMUS

True nystagmoid movements are seen rarely in the neonatal period. When they are present at birth or soon thereafter, the probability of subdural hematoma or some other form of intracranial damage comes to mind. Nystagmus is common in the pyridoxine dependency syndrome. These oscillating movements are often poorly sustained and may be apparent only when the eyes are deviated conjugately to one side or the other. Nystagmus which is constant, or present whenever the infant attempts to fix his gaze, suggests that central vision has been impaired. Such impairment may result from opacification in the lens (cataract) or in the vitreous (retrolental fibroplasia), from hazing of the cornea (glaucoma and others), from macular scarring due to chorioretinitis, from retinoblastoma or from a hereditary defect.

*Congenital idiopathic nystagmus,* in which no abnormality of cornea, lens, media or retina can be discovered, affects males more often than females. Its mode of genetic transmission has not been completely clarified. Head nodding, amblyopia, hypermetropia and deficiency of ocular pigment may be associated defects, and later on total color blindness and day blindness may become apparent. It can be expected to remain static for life, but many patients make a satisfactory adjustment to the visual difficulty it entails.

Nystagmus noted within the first week of life often disappears with subsidence of the underlying injury. If it persists, or if it is first recognized later on in the first few months of life, careful ophthalmologic examination is indicated. Remedial defects must receive prompt treatment.

## REFERENCES

Costenbader, F. D., and Albert, D. G.: The management of strabismus. Pediat. Clin. N. Amer. 5:153, 1958.

Harley, R. (Ed.): Pediatric Ophthalmology. Philadelphia, W. B. Saunders Co., 1975.

Ophthalmic Pathology: An Atlas and Textbook. American Academy of Ophthalmology and Otolaryngology and The Armed Forces Institute of Pathology.

Patz, A.: The management of some common pediatric eye problems. Maryland State Med. J., 8:600, 1959.

Von Noorden, G. K., and Maumenee, A. E.: Atlas of Strabismus. 2nd Ed., St. Louis, C. V. Mosby, 1974.

# OTHER NEONATAL DISORDERS OF THE EYES

# 108

*Revised by Arnall Patz*

## RETROLENTAL FIBROPLASIA

Retrolental fibroplasia (RLF) was virtually unheard of prior to 1942, when Terry first identified it as a specific disorder of prematurity. By 1950 this entity had become the largest cause of child blindness in the United States, greater than all other causes combined. After discovery of the etiological role of oxygen in the 1950's, the incidence of the disease decreased dramatically throughout the world. Yet, cases of RLF continue to occur even up to the present time, in spite of the most careful restriction of oxygen. Indeed, recent cases of RLF have been described in which no oxygen, or oxygen for only a few hours, was administered. Also, RLF has occasionally occurred where repeated arterial oxygen tension ($Pa_{O_2}$) values were under 100 mm Hg.

During the 1960's, when several investigators demonstrated severe oxygen deprivation in premature infants with the idiopathic respiratory distress syndrome (RDS), a change in treatment modality occurred, in which oxygen was used more liberally. Infants with RDS required high incubator concentrations of oxygen to raise the $Pa_{O_2}$ to levels compatible with survival and prevention of brain damage. The specter of increased mortality and brain damage resulting from restriction of oxygen to prevent blindness was brought up by several investigators.

Not until the late 1960's and early 1970's did the capability for monitoring arterial blood gases become more widespread. The most common practice has been to insert a catheter into the umbilical artery, localizing the catheter tip in the descending aorta. This has provided a source for monitoring arterial oxygen as well as other blood chemistries. An occasional infant who has right-to-left shunting may have a significantly greater $PO_2$ level reaching the brain than that measured in the descending aorta below the shunt. Temporal artery, right brachial or radial artery sampling circumvents this problem of shunting but these methods require a highly sophisticated team and can present problems in obtaining frequent blood samples. Some investigators utilize arterialized capillary blood from the fingers by heating the digits on the right hand. The validity of the "arterial" $PO_2$ taken in this manner is subject to question. Yet, in one large nursery where this method was used and careful eye examinations were performed, the incidence of RLF over a period of 5 years was as low as several centers using umbilical arterial samples.

At the present time there appears to be an irreducible minimum of RLF cases in spite of the most meticulous arterial $PO_2$ monitoring. For example, occasional babies who have had $Pa_{O_2}$ levels never exceeding 100 mm on repeated samplings have developed classic proliferative disease. Fortunately, the majority of these leave only minor cicatricial changes, but occasionally these will progress to significant permanent damage. Furthermore, there have been documented changes indistinguishable from retrolental fibroplasia in stillborn infants and those living for only a few hours after birth. The presence of these abnormal new vessels indicates that causes other than the excess use of oxygen in the nursery can produce the basic pathogenetic changes of RLF. Therefore, prematurity, per se, is fundamental to the development of the disease, and excess oxygen can be considered

the major precipitating or aggravating factor.

Earlier studies by Owens and Owens raised the possibility that vitamin E administration might have an effect on the disease. Subsequent studies in the 1950's by other investigators failed to confirm these original reports. More recent observations, however, by Boggs, Johnson and Schaeffer have again raised the possibility that Vitamin E supplements may have a protective effect upon RLF. It is possible that when modest amounts of oxygen are given, such as in current practice, Vitamin E supplements may have a protective effect. However, controlled studies are needed to document this concept.

### MECHANISM OF OXYGEN ACTION

The retina is unique in that prior to the fourth month of gestation it contains no blood vessels. The embryonic hyaloid system in the vitreous provides nourishment up to this period. Starting at 4 months' gestation, the hyaloid system regresses as the retina becomes vascularized, starting from the optic nerve. The nasal retina becomes fully vascularized by approximately 8

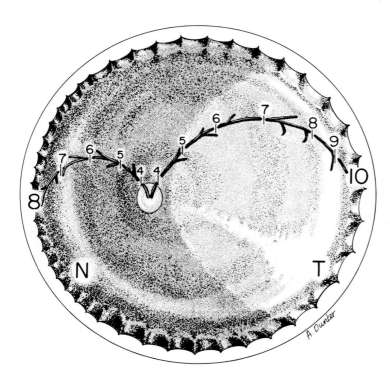

*Figure 108–1.* Schematic drawing of the posterior segment of the eye. The retina is avascular until 4 months' gestation, at which time vessels start from the optic nerve, reaching nasal periphery at 8 months' gestation. Temporal periphery is not vascularized until 1 month after birth of the *full-term* infant. This explains predilection of temporal periphery for RLF and occasional cases of RLF in full-term infants.

OXYGEN IN RLF

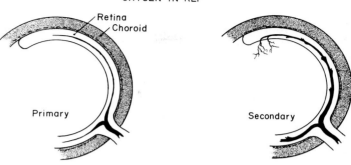

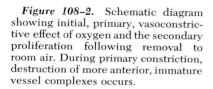

*Figure 108-2.* Schematic diagram showing initial, primary, vasoconstrictive effect of oxygen and the secondary proliferation following removal to room air. During primary constriction, destruction of more anterior, immature vessel complexes occurs.

months' gestation, but the temporal retinal periphery, which is farther away from the optic nerve, is not completely vascularized until approximately 1 month after birth of the full-term infant (Fig. 108–1). This pattern is significant, as the more immature portions of the retina have been shown in experimental studies to be more sensitive to oxygen. Experimental animals lose their sensitivity to retinal vessel damage when the retina is fully vascularized. Accordingly, the temporal periphery, which is less completely vascularized at any particular stage of gestation, is more vulnerable in humans and animals. A predilection for the temporal retina is well documented. With this in mind when examining young children, particularly where cooperation is limited, special attention should be given the temporal periphery. Chances are greater than 90 per cent that if no disease is present in the temporal periphery, the remainder of the retina will be normal. Since the temporal retina is farthest removed from the optic nerve and is not fully vascularized until 1 month after birth for the full-term infant, the occasional case of RLF reported in the full-term infant is explained.

The effects of oxygen on the infant or experimental animal with an incompletely vascularized retina can be conveniently divided into the initial response to oxygen and a secondary response after removal to room air (Figure 108–2). In the initial, or primary, response a severe vasoconstriction is present. During the exposure to oxygen, direct injury to the vessel endothelium occurs, and ultimate obliteration of the more immature vessel complexes results. After removal to air, new vessel formation occurs

at the area of retinal capillary damage and obliteration. These new vessels erupt through the surface of the retina to grow into the vitreous in the classical manner of proliferative retinopathy, very similar to that seen in diabetic and sickle cell disease. The changes after the intravitreal proliferation of new vessels are relatively nonspecific. These vessels invariably leak proteinaceous material, and in more advanced cases hemorrhages occur from these intravitreal new vessel formations. Traction produced by vitreoretinal adhesions detaches the retina (Fig. 108–3). Active RLF may regress at any stage of the proliferative disease, depending upon the amount of scar tissue in the temporal periphery, the amount of dragging of the retinal vessels across the disc and the temporal displacement of the macula (heterotopia). Many infants who have had active proliferative disease but who regress without further scar

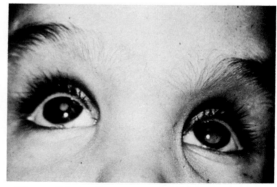

*Figure 108–3.* Stage V retrolental fibroplasia with total detachment of the retina, presenting as a white membrane in the pupil (leucocoria). The child is totally blind. One pupil does not dilate, owing to posterior adhesions of iris to lens.

tissue will develop a high degree of myopia. The mechanism for this refractive change is unknown.

It should be recognized by the pediatrician that the *early* active proliferative disease occurs in the mid-periphery of the retina at about the equator of the eye. The changes can usually be detected around the time of discharge from the nursery. The abnormal proliferating vessels are farther anterior than can be visualized with the routine hand-held ophthalmoscope used by most pediatricians. Only with the indirect ophthalmoscope can the mid-periphery be adequately visualized. If active disease is found, periodic ophthalmoscopic examination is recommended to determine if the disease is progressive. If it is progressive, treatment by photocoagulation may be considered, but this is still an experimental form of therapy and its use must be weighed against the possibility that spontaneous regression will occur. Examination for the primary or vasoconstrictive effect of oxygen has not proved feasible and is not recommended.

At the time of this writing the precise arterial $PO_2$ levels that can be sustained without having a significant risk to the retina are still undocumented. The general guideline of maintaining the arterial $PO_2$ at levels beneath 100 mm Hg seems reasonable for practical management of the infant requiring oxygen therapy in the premature nursery. It is possible, however, that in an occasional premature infant the $Pa_{O_2}$ levels achieved by breathing room air alone may be sufficient to damage the retinal vessels which, if developing in utero, would have sustained a lower $Pa_{O_2}$.

## CONGENITAL CATARACT

Congenital cataract, that is, cataract which is present at birth or which becomes apparent within the first few weeks, is rare.

**ETIOLOGY.** One of three etiologic factors underlies its development. In the majority the disorder is hereditary, usually transmitted as a dominant trait from an affected parent to half the offspring of either sex. The unaffected siblings are not carriers. In some the disorder results from

maternal rubella in the first trimester of pregnancy. Other toxic influences upon the fetus early in gestation lead to cataract formation in experimental animals and may well have the same effect in human beings. The third causative factor is the enzymatic deficiency of congenital galactosemia. In this category cataract is not present at birth, but may make its appearance as early as the second week of life. The finding of Richter and Duke, that rats exclusively on commercial yogurt develop cataracts, they attribute almost certainly to that product's high galactose content. One might add that cataracts are almost always present in babies with Lowe's syndrome and in several other constellations of congenital defects.

**DIAGNOSIS.** Diagnosis is made by careful inspection of the eyes at the original examination in the newborn nursery and at each subsequent monthly checkup. A bright light should be thrown not only directly toward the eye, but also tangentially across the cornea. Small opacities will be visible only in cross-illumination or in the light reflected from the eyegrounds. For this procedure one looks at the lens through the plus 8.00 lens of an ophthalmoscope from a distance of about 6 inches. The observation of nystagmus calls for the most scrupulous examination of the lenses, since nystagmus appears in all cases in which central vision has not become established.

**TREATMENT.** Treatment must be left in the hands of a competent ophthalmologist. Whether or not one should operate and, if so, what type of operation should be performed and when, are questions about which there is no unanimity of opinion. The pediatrician can be of little help in making these decisions.

CASE 108–1

The mother of a white female infant contracted German measles 2 weeks after the onset of gestation. The infant was born at term, weighed 7 pounds 5½ ounces (3320 gm) and was declared normal at the first examination. On the second day a heart murmur was noted, and this persisted. Spells soon began in which she turned white, then dusky. Her eyes seemed to "wander," and she clearly had not learned to recognize her mother by the age of 3 months, when we first saw her. At this time her eyes were making constant "searching movements," and bilateral central cataracts were visible (Fig.

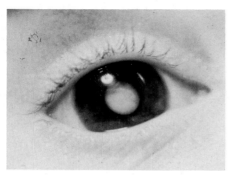

**Figure 108–4.** Congenital cataract. The opaque lens stands out sharply. (From the collection of Dr. Arnall Patz.)

108–4). The congenital heart lesion was ascertained to consist of an intraventricular septal defect and a patent ductus arteriosus. The right eye was operated upon at the age of 7 months, the ductus ligated 1 week later.

**COMMENT.** This mother had two normal children, aged 2½ and 1½ years, and contracted German measles very early in her third pregnancy. The infant was born with two of the principal defects that often characterize early fetal infection.

## CONGENITAL GLAUCOMA

No disease illustrates so well one facet of the importance of the pediatrician in the newborn nursery as does congenital glaucoma. Unprepared though he is to treat the disorder medically or surgically, the mere fact that he suspects its presence may mean the difference between good vision and blindness. For if one delays seeking expert advice until signs are outspoken, prognosis will probably have been gravely altered.

**ETIOLOGY.** Primary congenital glaucoma is an inborn defect transmitted genetically as an autosomal recessive. Intraocular tension rises as a result of an imbalance between production and outflow of aqueous humor. Obstruction to outflow depends upon some abnormality of development and insertion of the iris. The disorder is rare. Since the rubella epidemic of 1964 and thereafter, a great many cases of undoubted glaucoma have been reported by numerous observers. Some babies born after fetal rubella manifest cloudy corneas, which, however, clear after a period of from 1 week to several months. Without other confirmatory signs these should not

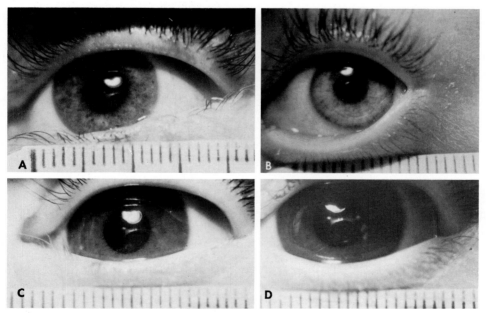

**Figure 108–5.** *A,* Normal eyeball with cornea of normal size. It measures 10 mm in diameter. *B,* Small eyeball with microcornea, measuring 6.5 mm across. This photograph is included for comparison and contrast. *C,* Early glaucoma, without hazing of cornea or tearing of Descemet's membrane. The cornea is 13.5 mm wide. *D,* Early glaucoma measuring 14.0 mm in diameter. (From the collection of Dr. Arnall Patz.)

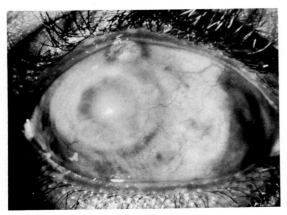

*Figure 108–6.* Late congenital glaucoma. Note the unusual breadth of the cornea and its diffuse haziness. Pericorneal vascular congestion is striking. (From the collection of Dr. Richard Hoover, Baltimore.)

be considered glaucoma. They may well represent viral keratitis. But some behave exactly as do primary glaucomas of genetic origin, and must be included in this category. Indeed, "all infants with congenital rubella should be studied for the possibility of congenital glaucoma" (Weiss et al.). Remarkably often a positive culture will still be found.

**DIAGNOSIS.** Unfortunately, most cases when first seen already show homogeneous opacification of both corneas, with broadening of their diameters and increased intraocular tension. Diagnosis should be suspected if the cornea is unusually large. Most of us are not in the habit of measuring the diameter of the cornea in newborns, and as a general rule this practice is hardly necessary. We should, however, strive to obtain a good look at every cornea as part of our original examination and to fix in our mind's eye its size relative to that of the eyeball. When in doubt, we should measure its breadth, and if this exceeds 11 mm we should call for help. Signs that may be present in addition to abnormal size or inequality are haziness or cloudiness of the corneas, and blepharospasm. Buphthalmos, or tremendous enlargement of the entire eyeball, is an end-stage of the disease for which little can be accomplished. The ophthalmologist will verify the suspected diagnosis by measuring intraocular tension and by examining the chamber angle under

a special microscope. Both tonometry and gonioscopy must be performed under anesthesia.

**TREATMENT.** Treatment will consist in immediate surgery, the details of which need not concern us here.

For emphasis we should like to quote a few lines from Barkan and Ferguson. "Damage done by glaucoma is permanent and irreparable, so that early diagnosis and surgical therapy are the only effective means of combating this disease. Half of the cases could be recognized at birth by a careful look at the eyes of newborns. The rest can be recognized if watched for in routine examinations during the first four to five months of life."

## CONGENITAL NONFAMILIAL MYOPIA

We were confronted once by an instructive newborn whose eyes appeared prominent. They seemed slightly proptosed, the corneas we judged to be a bit broader than usual, and the intraocular tension, to our not too discriminating palpation, appeared to be increased. We were certain this was an example of early glaucoma. Our ophthalmologic consultant, Dr. Richard Hoover, arrived at a different conclusion. The corneal breadth was indeed at the upper limit of normal, but intraocular tension was not elevated. Refraction revealed myopia in each eye measuring −9 diopters.

Congenital myopia differs from the usual form in that it is nonfamilial, is present at birth and does not progress. The familial form commonly does not become apparent for several years, after which it increases in degree for several more years before reaching a state of relative stability.

## EVERSION OF THE EYELIDS

The eyelids of the newborn may be everted at birth secondarily, that is, in the presence of microphthalmos, buphthalmos, lid defects or other abnormalities of the eyes. Primary eversion, without discoverable contributing cause, has been reported only a few times. Stillerman et al. added three examples, in two of whom all four

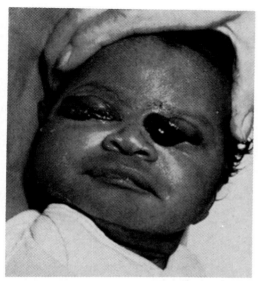

*Figure 108–7.* At 10 days of life, note the marked edema of both conjunctivae of the upper lids while the eversion of the lids has practically returned to normal. (Stillerman, M. L., Emanuel, B., and Padorr, M. P.: J. Pediatr. *69*:656, 1966.)

lids were everted at birth, in the other only the two upper ones. The bulbar conjunctivae, facing outward of course, were swollen and red, edematous, chemotic and hyperemic. In none had there been obstetrical difficulties and in none were there other ocular abnormalities. All returned to normal in a few weeks, following the application of an ophthalmic ointment and moist sterile gauze dressings.

## REFERENCES

Aranda, J. V., Saheb, N., Stern, L., and Avery, M. E.: Arterial oxygen tension and retinal vasoconstriction in newborn infants. Am. J. Dis. Child. *122*:189, 1971.

Avery, M. E., and Oppenheimer, E. H.: Recent increase in mortality from hyaline membrane disease. J. Pediatr. 57:553–558, 1960.

Barkan, O., and Ferguson, W. J.: Congenital glaucoma. Pediat. Clin. N. Amer. 5:225, 1958.

Chandler, P. A.: Congenital cataract. Pediat. Clin. N. Amer. 5:169, 1958.

Johnson, L., Schaffer, D., and Boggs, T. R., Jr.: The premature infant, vitamin E deficiency and retrolental fibroplasia. Am. J. Clin. 27:1158, 1974.

Kerr, J. D., and Scott, G. J.: The retinopathy of prematurity. Arch. Dis. Child. 29:543, 1954.

McDonald, A. D.: Cerebral palsy in children of very low birth weight. Arch. Dis. Child. 38:579–588, 1963.

Owens, W. C., and Owens, E. J.: Retrolental fibroplasia in premature infants. Am. J. Ophthalmol. 32:1, 1949.

Patz, A.: Oxygen studies in retrolental fibroplasia: Clinical and experimental observations. First Edward L. Holmes Memorial Lecture. Am. J. Ophthalmol. 38:291, 1954.

Patz, A.: Retrolental fibroplasia. Survey Ophthal. 14:1–29, 1969.

Patz, A.: The role of oxygen in retrolental fibroplasia. Trans. Amer. Ophth. Soc. 66:940–985, 1968.

Richter, C. P., and Duke, J. R.: Cataracts produced in rats by yogurt. Science, 168:1372, 1970.

Richter, C. P., and Duke, J. R.: Yogurt-induced cataracts: Comments on their significance in man. J.A.M.A. 214:1878, 1970.

Stillerman, M. L., Emanuel, B., and Padorr, M. P.: Eversion of the eyelids in the newborn without apparent cause. J. Pediatr. 69:656, 1966.

Weiss, D. I., Cooper, L. Z., and Green, R. H.: Infantile glaucoma: A manifestation of congenital rubella. J.A.M.A. 195:725, 1966.

Zimmerman, L. E., and Font, R. L.: Congenital malformations of the eyes: Some recent advances in knowledge of the pathogenesis and histopathological characteristics. J.A.M.A. 196:684, 1966.

# INFECTIONS WITHIN AND ABOUT THE EYE

# 109

*Revised by Arnall Patz*

The eye and its surrounding tissues are subject to a variety of infections in the neonate. They may be classified etiologically as bacterial, viral or protozoal, or anatomically as conjunctivitis, uveitis, chorioretinitis, dacryocystitis and herpes simplex ophthalmicus, inter alia. From the clinical standpoint it might be wiser to discuss them in this latter setting.

# CONJUNCTIVITIS

## CHEMICAL CONJUNCTIVITIS

Much of the conjunctivitis one formerly encountered in the first few days of life derived from chemical and mechanical irritation caused by the instillation of drops or ointment into the eye in order to prevent gonorrheal ophthalmia. Indeed, this chemical ophthalmia occurred so frequently after the use of silver nitrate solution that workers were stimulated to seek less irritating substitutes. Margileth found that severe inflammatory reactions followed the instillation of one drop of 1 per cent silver nitrate, washed out immediately with sterile normal saline solution, in more than 50 per cent of infants. Lloyd, quoted by Ormsby, observed similar reactions in 50 per cent of his cases. Reactions to the various substitutes used never approached this figure, ranging from 1 per cent when penicillin or bacitracin ointment or penicillin solution was used (Margileth), to slightly higher percentages, never more than 5 per cent, in a number of other studies.

It is significant that the Committee on Ophthalmia Neonatorum of the National Society for the Prevention of Blindness recommends the use of 1 per cent silver nitrate prophylaxis without adding distilled water or normal saline after instillation of the drops. At the present time prophylactic drops are required by 47 states. Silver nitrate is specified in 15 states. In 33 states, and the District of Columbia, silver nitrate or "other equally effective medication" must be used. In two states, no designation of medication is specified but prophylaxis is required.

Chemical conjunctivitis differs from infective forms in that it becomes apparent almost immediately after the instillation. By the time infants are transferred from delivery room to nursery the eyes are often puffy and reddened, the palpebral conjunctivae are red and thickened, and a small amount of mucopus is visible in the conjunctival sac. Smears show few or no organisms, and cultures reveal no pathogenic bacteria. Without treatment the eyes clear within 2 to 5 days. No complications or sequelae are to be anticipated, although Mallek, Spohn and Mallek believe the chemical irritation to be responsible for some cases of dacryostenosis.

## GONORRHEAL OPHTHALMIA

This serious disorder was commented upon early in the Christian era by Soranus. The association between maternal vaginal discharge and neonatal conjunctivitis was recognized in the mid-nineteenth century. Its etiologic agent was discovered in 1879, and successful prophylaxis was begun in 1881.

**INCIDENCE.** Prior to the institution of prophylactic therapy the frequency of the disease varied considerably from country to country and between groups of various economic levels, but an incidence of 10 per cent was not unusual in some urban communities. Since prophylaxis was begun this figure has fallen to 0.0 to 0.1 per cent. The percentage of children admitted to schools for the blind because of neonatal ophthalmia fell from 24 in 1906 through 1911 to 0.3 in 1958 and 1959 (Barsam).

**ETIOLOGY.** The responsible organism was isolated by Neisser in 1879 and was named *Neisseria gonorrhoeae*. The same organism can be discovered in the mother's vaginal flora.

**DIAGNOSIS.** Discharge from the eyes appears on the second or third day of life. If untreated, the infection progresses rap-

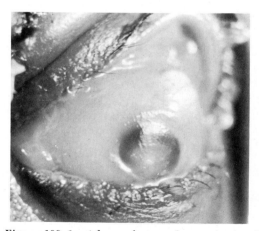

*Figure 109–1.* Advanced case of gonorrheal ophthalmia. Note the intense panophthalmitis with reddening and thickening of both the bulbar and the tarsal conjunctiva and ulceration of the cornea and sclera. (From the collection of Dr. Arnall Patz.)

idly until the eyes become puffy and the conjunctivae intensely red and thickened, while the conjunctival sac contains a few drops of green purulent material. The conjunctivae may become so edematous that they project out between the closed lids. Discharge may run in a constant stream down the cheeks. In the preantibiotic era corneal hazing and ulceration followed not infrequently, and opaque staphyloma or microphthalmos from rupture at the point of corneal ulceration used to be not uncommon outcomes in severe cases.

**PROPHYLAXIS.** Two years after Neisser had identified the responsible organism Credé began to instill one drop of 2 per cent silver nitrate solution into each eye of every one of his newborn babies. He promptly reduced the frequency of gonorrheal ophthalmia in his clinic from 10 to 0.5 per cent. Later the strength was reduced to 1 per cent, and this preventive method was made legally mandatory in most civilized countries. As a result, this dangerous disease almost vanished.

Recently physicians in widely scattered clinics concerned themselves with the fact that 50 per cent or more of the infants treated by the Credé method suffered chemical conjunctivitis. Various alternatives were proposed. The most radical recommended discontinuation of any prophylaxis, since gonorrhea had become so rare and was so readily curable by a short course of treatment with one of several antibacterial agents. Mellin and Kent put this approach to the test in the Babies Hospital of New York from April through October of 1957. During this no-prophylaxis period the incidence and severity of conjunctivitis diminished greatly. But four of those cases that did occur were sufficiently pronounced to be called ophthalmia neonatorum, and from three of these *N. gonorrhoeae* was cultivated. One more positive culture was obtained from a "sticky eye." After October 1957, prophylaxis was reinstituted.

Various kinds of preventive therapy in the way of instillation of drops or ointment into the eyes have been tried. Sulfacetamide solution and ointment were used by Ormsby, bacitracin ointment by Margileth, and penicillin in drops and ointments of several strengths and by intramuscular injection by many others. All gave satisfactory results. A carefully controlled study by Davidson, Hill and Eastman demonstrated beyond doubt that penicillin ointment containing 100,000 units per gram, later reduced to 50,000, instilled into each eye once, gave perfect protection against gonorrhea in a population of mothers from 2.7 per cent of whose cervices *N. gonorrhoeae* could be cultivated. Equally good results were obtained by the routine intramuscular injection of 50,000 units. Nevertheless penicillin is not completely without danger. It carries the hazard of Herxheimer reaction when given parenterally to an infected infant, and of the development of permanent ocular sensitivity when instilled into the eye. Barsam feels, and we find it hard to disagree, that 1 per cent silver nitrate is still the safest prophylactic agent if it can be properly packaged, handled and administered.

**TREATMENT.** If prophylaxis is unsuccessful, perhaps because the medicament had not been applied properly into the eye, and the disease develops, it is easy enough to cure. Penicillin intramuscularly, 100,000 units every 4 to 6 hours, and frequent topical applications of penicillin solution for several days should suffice. If sensitivity to penicillin develops, the sulfonamides and tetracyclines are almost equally efficacious.

## OPHTHALMIA DUE TO ORGANISMS OTHER THAN GONOCOCCUS

Cultures from discharging eyes of newborns reveal in descending order of frequency staphylococcus, pneumococcus, nonhemolytic or green-producing streptococcus, *Escherichia coli* or some other gram-negative bacillus. Many cultures are sterile or grow out one or more nonpathogenic bacteria. Conjunctival scrapings from these eyes, stained by the Giemsa technique, may show within the cytoplasm of epithelial cells characteristic blue-staining granules of inclusion blennorrhea.

Clinically, these various forms of conjunctivitis are almost impossible to distinguish. One may suspect that the virus causing inclusion blennorrhea is at fault rather than a bacterium if onset is delayed 10 to 12 days. Otherwise the differences are slight and far from pathognomonic. Rather than make a guess of little value, one should rely upon studies of stained smears, cultures and conjunctival scrapings.

The first principle of *treatment* consists in rigid isolation of newborns with conjunctivitis. Mild infections may be treated after culture solely with ointments containing bacitracin or neomycin, or both. Severer ones call for local and parenteral therapy with the antibacterial agent appropriate to the responsible organism. Penicillin is the drug of choice against pneumococcus, sulfadiazine against inclusion blennorrhea, ampicillin or kanamycin against *E. coli* and methicillin against staphylococcus. Sensitivity tests in vitro are recommended.

## DACRYOSTENOSIS

Only rarely does obstruction of a lacrimal duct become apparent within the neonatal period. Occasionally it does, toward the end of the first month, in an infant who secretes more tears than is usual at that early age. An eye remains constantly wet, and from time to time a clear drop wells up and courses down the cheek. Mild infection repeatedly involves these eyes, the secretion becoming turbid and yellow and the conjunctivae becoming infected.

Infections can be controlled readily by the use of an appropriate antibiotic solution into the eye two or three times a day. Nothing further need be done for at least 6 months, by which time the duct will almost always have become patent. If not, the passage of a probe to dilate the duct may then be contemplated.

## DACRYOCYSTITIS

When infection within the lumen of a stenosed lacrimal duct is neglected, the lacrimal sac may become deeply involved. The result is puffiness and redness of the skin in the corner between the inner angle of the eye and the bridge of the nose (Fig. 109–2). Pressure upon the cystic mass may force purulent material upward through the punctum on the lower lid margin near the external canthus, or downward into the nose.

It is advisable to treat dacryocystitis conservatively. An appropriate antibiotic should be given orally or parenterally, and instilled frequently into the eye and naris

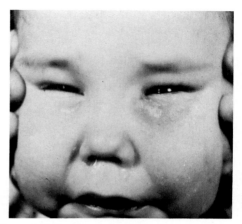

*Figure 109–2.* Acute dacryocystitis. Note the swollen, reddened lower lid and the cystic swelling in the angle between the eye and the bridge of the nose. (From the collection of Dr. Arnall Patz.)

on the affected side while hot wet compresses are applied externally. If improvement does not take place within a few days, one may have to resort to probing the duct. External incision should seldom be required.

## UVEITIS

The fetal eye manifests an extraordinary susceptibility to chorioretinitis. Many infections acquired transplacentally localize in this situation, as well as a few acquired postnatally. Toxoplasmosis, cytomegalic inclusion disease, disseminated herpes virus infection, rubella and syphilis are some of the diseases in which chorioretinitis may be one sign. But involvement of the iris and ciliary body, iridocyclitis, is extremely uncommon.

Figure 109–3 shows the eye of a newborn who probably suffered this complication. At birth the pupils were virtually occluded by a dense fibrous membrane, and at operation firm adhesions between the iris and lens (synechiae) were noted. This appeared to have resulted from uveitis suffered during gestation, which had healed completely by the time of birth. There was no hepatomegaly or splenomegaly, and no other signs indicating activity of infection were discovered. The Sabin dye tests for toxoplasmosis on both mother and child were strongly positive. No other proof was adduced, but it is assumed by the consulting ophthalmologist (Dr. A. Patz) that this represented a per-

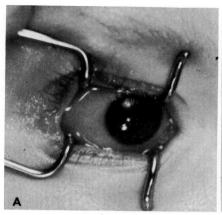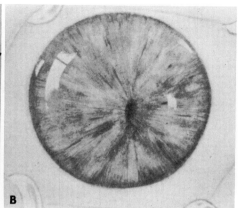

*Figure 109–3.* *A,* Photograph of eye of newborn described in the text. *B,* Artist's conception of the lesion. The pupil resembles a tightly closed camera shutter. This is the contracted fibrosed iris, firmly bound down to the lens and fixed. (From the collection of Dr. Arnall Patz.)

sistent pupillary membrane resulting from intrauterine toxoplasmosis.

## ORBITAL CELLULITIS

This fairly serious disorder is encountered in the newborn, but rarely. It usually follows conjunctivitis or ethmoid sinusitis but may appear without a discoverable portal of entry. It is characterized by chemosis, proptosis and impaired motility.

Treatment should consist of incision and drainage, perhaps after a brief period of antibiotic therapy.

## REFERENCES

Barsam, P. C.: Specific prophylaxis of gonorrheal ophthalmia neonatorum. N. Engl. J. Med. *274*:731, 1966.

Committee on Ophthalmia Neonatorum, National Society for the Prevention of Blindness. The Sight-Saving Review, *43*:11, 1973.

Davidson, H. H., Hill, J. H., and Eastman, N. J.: Penicillin in prophylaxis of ophthalmia neonatorum. J.A.M.A. *145*:1052, 1951.

Egan, J. A.: Localized sensitivity of eye to penicillin. Am. J. Ophthalmol. *34*:289, 1951.

Hepner, R., and Hagar, D.: Staphylococcal orbital sepsis in newborn infants. South. Med. J. *53*:922, 1960.

Kimura, S. J., and Hogan, M. J.: Uveitis in children. Pediat. Clin. N. Amer. 5:173, 1958.

Mallek, H., Spohn, P., and Mallek, J.: On the comparative use of silver nitrate and penicillin in the eyes of the newborn. Canad. Med. Assoc. J. *68*:117, 1953.

Margileth, A. M.: Comparison of ocular reactions using penicillin and bacitracin ointments in ophthalmia neonatorum prophylaxis. J. Pediatr. *51*:646, 1957.

Mellin, G. W., and Kent, M. P.: Ophthalmia neonatonum: Is prophylaxis necessary? Pediatrics *22*:1006, 1958.

Ormsby, H. L.: Ophthalmia neonatorum. Canad. Med. Assoc. J. *72*:576, 1955.

The over-all number of tumors of the eye that appear within the neonatal period is small. Most of them are hamartomas or choristomas and the most common of these are dermoids and hemangiomas. The one malignant neoplasm of utmost importance in this age period is retinoblastoma. It is imperative that this diagnosis by made promptly and therapy instituted without delay. An apparent neoplasm that must be differentiated from tumor in this location is encephalocele, presenting either in the orbit or in the angle between the eye and the bridge of the nose.

## HEMANGIOMA

As has been indicated earlier (p. 957), the upper lids are a common site for the port-wine stains of nevus flammeus. These may be faint or exceedingly prominent. When present, one or more of the same type can be expected to be located over the

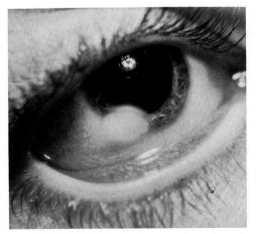

***Figure 110–1.*** Dermoid of the eye. There is a dead-white cyst arising at the limbus and overlying portions of both the cornea and the conjunctiva. (From the collection of Dr. Arnall Patz.)

nuchal region. The faint ones fade within a few months, the more deeply colored ones within a few years. They need no treatment.

Hemangiomas not infrequently involve the palpebral conjunctivae. These may take the form of nevus flammeus also, imparting a deeper purplish color to a portion of the conjunctiva and thickening it slightly. Or, as in the skin, the tumors may be more deeply seated cavernous hemangiomas producing visible bulges within the eyelid which protrude into the conjunctival sac (Fig. 110–1). Not infrequently hemangiomas of the conjunctiva are accompanied by similar nevi elsewhere. In one of our patients thick, deep angiomas covered the lower lid, conjunctiva, the pharyngeal wall and the tonsil on one side. Thin, superficial nevi in this location require no treatment. Deeper ones may have to be treated because of their sheer size and the irritation they may inflict upon the eyeball. We prefer surgical excision to x-irradiation. Prior to either, cortisone probably deserves a trial for 10 days to 2 weeks.

Hemangiomas may also be present within the orbit. These may be of sufficient size to produce proptosis and disturbances of extraocular movement. They almost invariably project out of the orbit into an eyelid, where they are visible beneath the tarsal conjunctiva. Like hemangioma everywhere, their natural tendency is toward ultimate shrinking and disappearance. One should allow them plenty of opportunity to subside. If either proptosis or fixation of the eyeball is serious, or if the tumor seems to be growing, some form of treatment is indicated. A course of prednisone should be tried first. A dose of 2 to 3 mg per kilogram per day for 10 to 14 days will allow assessment of its effect. If the hemangioma has regressed, the steroids can be tapered until the lowest dose needed to prevent growth is ascertained. We have maintained some infants on low doses of prednisone for many months, and then stopped medication with no recurrence. Occasionally steroids are ineffective, and careful x-irradiation in trustworthy hands is indicated.

## CHORISTOMAS

Epibulbar choristomas include dermoids, dermolipomas, complex choristomas, dermis-like choristomas, ectopic lacrimal gland tissue and osseous choristomas (Elsas and Green).

Dermoids are the most commonly encountered epibulbar lesions in the newborn and usually are located near or straddling the limbus temporally and slightly inferiorly (Fig. 110–1). Fine hairs emanate from the surface, and an arc of lipid may be present in the cornea after a clear zone. Surgery for such lesions is for cosmetic purposes only. Difficulties may be encountered at surgery for several reasons: no cleavage plane exists between the lesion and the eye; rare intraocular extension is observed; and, occasionally, a scleral staphyloma may be encountered in association with the dermoid.

Limbal dermoids occurring in association with aural fistulae or extra-auricular appendages may be features of the oculoauricular vertebral dysplasia syndrome of Goldenhar (see p. 930).

The cystic types of dermoids are congenital lesions encountered most frequently in the upper lid or in the orbit superotemporally, or in both areas. These cysts may be very small at birth, but continue to enlarge throughout life. Only 20 to 25 per cent are clinically evident at birth.

Histopathologically, the solid dermoid of the limbus consists of a dermis-like connective tissue in which pilosebaceous apparati are present. The dermoid cyst is filled with keratinous debris, contains a variable number of hair shafts and sebaceous material, is lined by keratinized stratified squamous epithelium and a dense corium-like connective tissue in which pilosebaceous apparati are present and have continuity with the cyst lumen.

Dermolipomas consist of a dermis-like connective tissue and adipose tissue, and are most frequently encountered superotemporally in the conjunctiva, giving the lid a fullness. Surgery for these lesions is strictly cosmetic; complications can be encountered, especially if overzealous excision is attempted. If removal is done, only the superficial portion or enough to correct the cosmetic defect should be excised. There is no clear cleavage plane between the lesion and subjacent tissue, and there may be deeper orbital extension and connections with the fascial sheaths of the superior and lateral rectus muscles. The lesion may also involve the five to seven orifices and ducts of the lacrimal gland.

## RETINOBLASTOMA

Once uniformly fatal, retinoblastoma, the most common intraocular malignancy of childhood, can now be detected and treated successfully enough to preserve both life and vision. Retinoblastoma occurs with a frequency of 1 case per 17,000 to 34,000 live births. The tumor may be present at birth; however, the diagnosis is most frequently made between the ages of 1½ and 2 years.

**PATHOLOGY.** The tumor arises in the retina and may extend in a mound-like fashion internal to the retina (endophytic) or external to the retina (exophytic). Multiple sites of origin in the same and fellow eye are common and do not necessarily arise simultaneously. The tumor tends to undergo necrosis, giving a characteristic pattern of collarettes of viable tumor around blood vessels, separated by necrotic areas, which often develop calcification (Fig. 110–2).

The tumor may extend into the vitreous as nonvascularized seedings. According to Ellsworth, such vitreous seeding of the tumor is a sign of poor prognosis. Extension of the tumor into the anterior chamber may produce signs of inflammation or glaucoma, or both, either of which may mask the underlying neoplasm and result in delays in diagnosis and therapy. The most common route of extraocular extension is along the optic nerve, by which the tumor gains access to the subarachnoid space and intracranial cavity.

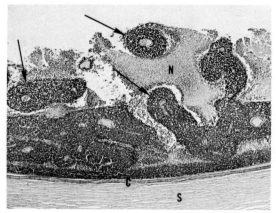

**Figure 110-2.** Characteristic pattern of retinoblastoma with extensive necrosis (N) and a collarette of viable tumor cells around blood vessels (arrows); (sclera, S), (choroid, C). Hematoxylin and eosin (× 45).

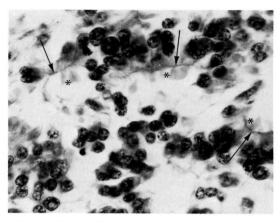

**Figure 110-4.** Fleurettes of retinoblastoma containing a structure analogous to the external limiting membrane of the retina (arrows) and rudimentary photoreceptors (asterisks). Hematoxylin and eosin (× 850).

Invasion of retinoblastoma into the vascular choroid is a potential source of hematogenous spread of the tumor. In advanced cases, direct extension through the sclera into the orbit may occur.

Three forms of cytodifferentiation have been recognized. The first is the Homer Wright rosette, which consists of a ring of tumor cells around a central area containing fibrillar material and no acid mucopolysaccharide. This pattern of tumor cells is seen also in neuroblastoma and medulloblastoma. Flexner-Wintersteiner rosettes (Fig. 110–3) are specific for retinoblastoma, and consist of a ring of low columnar cells

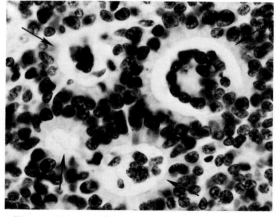

**Figure 110-3.** Flexner-Wintersteiner rosettes of retinoblastoma (arrows). Hematoxylin and eosin (×750).

with basally located nuclei around a lumen in which a hyaluronidase-resistant acid mucopolysaccharide is present. Filamentous cytoplasmic projections of the tumor cells extend into the lumen and have rudimentary photoreceptor differentiation. T'so et al. have described clusters of cells (fleurettes) (Fig. 110–4), which have more definite photoreceptor differentiation.

**HEREDITY.** Approximately 6 per cent of retinoblastoma cases are familial. The mode of transmission is autosomal dominant with penetrance varying between 20 and 95 per cent, but most frequently stated to be 80 per cent. Ellsworth (1969) considers both familial and sporadic retinoblastoma to be due to germinal mutations, but that penetrance is low in unilateral sporadic cases and high in bilateral sporadic cases. The probability of bilateral retinoblastoma in sporadic cases is from 18 to 31 per cent, whereas in hereditary cases it is 92 to 95 per cent if a parent is affected, 83 per cent if two or more siblings are affected, and 60 per cent if a distant relative is affected.

**GENETIC COUNSELING.** In cases of established hereditary retinoblastoma, the gene is generally transmitted to 50 per cent of offspring. Normal parents with one affected child and with no prior family history will have a 4 to 7 per cent probability of producing a second offspring with retinoblastoma. Normal parents with two or more affected children will have a 50 per cent probability of producing a genetically affected offspring, the incidence of retinoblastoma being dependent on penetrance. A survivor of bilateral sporadic retinoblastoma will produce clinically affected offspring in 50 per cent of cases, whereas a survivor of unilateral sporadic retinoblastoma will produce clinically affected children in 10 per cent of offspring.

**DIAGNOSIS.** The most frequent sign, observed in about 56 per cent of patients with retinoblastoma (Ellsworth, 1969), is leukocoria (white pupil). The white reflex in the pupil is frequently observed by the child's mother.

The presence or onset of strabismus is the second most common sign (20 per cent). This sign is particularly important, since the general physician may be the first to examine such a patient. We believe infants and children with strabismus should have an ophthalmoscopic examination to rule out the possibility of retinoblastoma. Often, this can be accomplished by wide dilation of the pupil, restraint of the child, and examination with an indirect ophthalmoscope. If such is not possible, examination should be performed under sedation or anesthesia.

Other, less-common, presenting signs and symptoms include: a red, painful eye with

glaucoma, 7 per cent; orbital cellulitis, 3 per cent; unilateral mydriasis, 2 per cent; heterochromia, 1 per cent; hyphema, 1 per cent. In 3 per cent of cases, the retinoblastoma was observed at the time of a routine examination.

Other conditions can be confused clinically with retinoblastoma. These conditions are listed in Table 110-1.

**PROGNOSIS.** Both clinical and histopathologic features have been found to be of some help in prognosticating the course of retinoblastoma. If distant metastases are demonstrated, the disease is invariably fatal, despite current modes of chemotherapy and radiation.

The size and extent of disease within the globe has been found useful in determining therapy and prognosis (Ellsworth, 1969). Table 110-2 lists these five clinical categories. Histopathologic criteria in estimating prognosis include optic nerve invasion, choroid invasion, scleral extension, epibulbar extension and degree of cytodifferentiation.

**TREATMENT.** Enucleation of the eye is the treatment of choice in patients who have large tumors in one eye and no family history of retinoblastoma (Groups IV and V; Table 110-2). Children with small,

**TABLE 110-1.** *Diagnosis in 265 Patients with Lesions Simulating Retinoblastoma (Howard and Ellsworth, 1965)*

| Diagnosis | Per Cent of Total |
|---|---|
| Persistent hyperplastic primary vitreous | 19.0 |
| Retrolental fibroplasia | 13.5 |
| Posterior cataract | 13.5 |
| Coloboma of choroid or disc | 11.5 |
| Uveitis | 10.0 |
| Nematode endophthalmitis | 6.5 |
| Congenital retinal fold | 5.0 |
| Coats' disease | 4.0 |
| Old vitreous hemorrhage | 3.5 |
| Retinal dysplasia | 2.5 |
| Tumor other than retinoblastoma | 1.5 |
| White-with-pressure sign | 1.0 |
| Juvenile xanthogranuloma | 1.0 |
| Retinoschisis | 1.0 |
| Tapetoretinal degeneration | 1.0 |
| Endophthalmitis | 1.0 |
| Persistent tunica vasculosa lentis | 1.0 |
| Miscellaneous | 3.5 |
| | 100.0 |

**TABLE 110-2.** *Prognosis Based on Size and Extent of Tumor (Ellsworth, 1969)*

Group I—very favorable, 95 per cent cure
   A. Solitary tumor, less than 4 disc diameters in size, at or behind the equator
   B. Multiple tumors, none over 4 disc diameters in size, all at or behind the equator
Group II—favorable, 87 per cent cure
   A. Solitary tumor, 4 to 10 disc diameters in size, at or behind the equator
   B. Multiple tumors, 4 to 10 disc diameters in size, behind the equator
Group III—doubtful, 67 per cent cure
   A. Any lesion anterior to the equator
   B. Solitary tumors larger than 10 disc diameters and behind the equator
Group IV—unfavorable, 69 per cent cure
   A. Multiple tumors, some larger than 10 disc diameters
   B. Any lesion extending anterior to the ora serrata
Group V—very unfavorable, 34 per cent cure
   A. Massive tumors involving over half of retina
   B. Vitreous seeding

unilateral tumors (Group I, II and III; Table 110–2) that are diagnosed early because of the onset of strabismus, or because of a family history, or detection at a routine ophthalmologic examination, are treated primarily with radiotherapy rather than enucleation. In bilateral cases, there is usually more-advanced tumor in one eye. Such patients are treated by enucleation of the more-advanced eye and by radiation therapy, with or without chemotherapy, for the second eye. Ellsworth (1969) generally restricts chemotherapy to those patients in Groups IV and V.

Bilateral advanced tumors in Groups IV and V are treated by irradiation and chemotherapy. Selected cases of small residual or new tumor growth can be treated by other techniques, such as cryotherapy, photocoagulation, radon-seed implantation and cobalt-60 application.

In more recent years, some authorities have been stressing focal techniques, such as localized betatron therapy from the side, cobalt plaques, photocoagulation and cryosurgery, in the treatment of single or multiple tumors of 10 mm or less (Bedford, 1975). Tumors larger than 10 mm would appear to be best treated by whole eye irradiation.

Some authors (Bedford, 1975) appear to be moving away from the opinion that the worst-affected eye, or the involved eye in unilateral cases, should be treated by enucleation. It would appear that the only indication for enucleation is the clinical suspicion that the optic nerve may be involved because of tumor at or adjacent to the disc.

## REFERENCES

Bedford, M. A.: Treatment of retinoblastoma. Adv. Ophthalmol. *31*:2–32, 1975.

Doxanas, M. T., Green, W. R., Arentsen, J. J., and Elsas, F. J.: Lid lesions of childhood: A histopathologic survey at the Wilmer Institute (1923–1974). J. Pediat. Ophthalmol. *13*:5, 1976.

Elsas, F. J., and Green, W. R.: Epibulbar tumors in childhood. Am. J. Ophthalmol. 79:1001, 1975.

Ellsworth, R. M.: The practical management of retinoblastoma. Trans. Am. Ophthalmol. Soc. 67:462, 1969.

Fost, N. C., and Esterly, N. B.: Successful treatment of juvenile hemangiomas with prednisone. J. Pediatr. 72:351, 1968.

Howard, G. M., and Ellsworth, R. M.: Differential diagnosis of retinoblastoma. A statistical survey of 500 children. I. Relative frequency of the lesions which simulate retinoblastoma. Am. J. Ophthalmol. 60:610, 1965.

Iliff, C. E., and Ossofsky, H. J.: Tumors of the Eye and Adnexa in Infancy and Childhood. Springfield, Ill., Charles C Thomas, 1962.

Nicholson, D. H., and Green, W. R.: Tumors of the eye, lids, and orbit in children. *In* Harley, R. D. (Ed.): Pediatric Ophthalmology. Philadelphia, W. B. Saunders Co., 1975.

T'so, M. O. M., Fine, B. S., and Zimmerman, L. E.: The Flexner-Wintersteiner rosettes in retinoblastoma. Arch. Pathol., 88:664, 1969.

T'so, M. O. M., Zimmerman, L. E., and Fine, B. S.: The nature of retinoblastoma. I. Photoreceptor differentiation: A clinical and histopathologic study; II. Photoreceptor differentiation: An electron microscopic study. Am. J. Ophthalmol. 69:339, 350, 1970.

# XVII

## Miscellaneous Disorders

# 111

# CONGENITAL MALIGNANT DISORDERS

*By Allen D. Schwartz*

Many tumors peculiar to individual organs and specific localities of the body have been discussed in their appropriate sections. Thus, retinoblastoma is discussed among the disorders of the eye (Chap. 110), and teratoma in the chapters devoted to the nasopharynx, abdomen and sacrococcygeal region. Here we will discuss the more common malignant disorders that may occur in the neonate without including an exhaustive list of case reports of every congenital tumor recorded in the literature.

A study of death certificates by Fraumeni and Miller during the 5 year period 1960 to 1964 revealed that the death rate from malignant diseases under 28 days of age was 6.24 per one million live births (Table 111–1). Over one half of cancer deaths in the neonatal period occurred in the first week of life and over one third occurred on the first day (Table 111–2). However, a study of mortality differs markedly from one of incidence since certain malignancies may be rapidly fatal, others may lead to death beyond the neonatal period, while a large number of others are curable or undergo spontaneous regression. Wells' classic review of 255 congenital malignant neoplasms (Table 111–3) is probably the most extensive recording of solid tumors diagnosed during the neonatal period. Retinoblastoma, which was omitted from Wells' series, is seldom discovered during the first month of life unless a careful ophthalmologic evaluation is performed in a child whose parent or sibling has the neoplasm. The average age of diagnosis of retinoblastoma is 18 months. The most common malignant disorders found in the newborn are retinoblastoma, neuroblastoma, congenital sarcoma, Wilms' tumor, primary hepatic tumors and leukemia. Teratomas are often present at birth; however, most are benign neoplasms.

## PATHOGENESIS

### Transplacental Tumor Passage

Malignant disease in the mother is very seldom transmitted across the placenta to

**TABLE 111–1.** *Mortality from Malignant Neoplasms in the United States Under 5 Years, as Compared with Under 28 Days of Age, 1960 to 1964*[*]

| Neoplasms | No. Deaths under 5 Years | No. | Deaths under 28 Days Rate Per $10^6$ Live Births | Per Cent[†] |
|---|---|---|---|---|
| Leukemia | 4592 | 44 | 2.11 | 1.0 |
| Neuroblastoma | 1049 | 27 | 1.30 | 2.6 |
| Brain tumor | 1035 | 7 | 0.34 | 0.7 |
| Wilms' tumor | 696 | 9 | 0.43 | 1.3 |
| Liver cancer, primary | 196 | 10 | 0.48 | 5.1 |
| Teratoma | 111 | 9 | 0.43 | 8.1 |
| Sarcoma, type specified | 1940 | 12 | 0.58 | 1.2 |
| Other | | 12 | 0.58 | |
| Total | 9619 | 130 | 6.24 | 1.4 |

*Fraumeni, J. F., and Miller, R. W.: Am. J. Dis. Child. 117:186, 1969.

†Percentage of neonatal deaths among type-specific cancers under 5 years of age, e.g. for leukemia = (44 × 100)/4592 = 1.0.

TABLE 111-2.    *Deaths from Neonatal Cancer According to Specific Diagnosis, Age and Sex*[*]

| Neoplasms | <24 hr | Age –6 days | 1–4 weeks | Sex Male | Female |
|---|---|---|---|---|---|
| Leukemia | 10 | 9 | 25 | 21 | 23 |
| Neuroblastoma | 13 | 2 | 12 | 15 | 12 |
| Sarcoma | 7 | 1 | 4 | 7 | 5 |
| Liver cancer, primary | 4 | 3 | 3 | 6 | 4 |
| Wilms' tumor | 1 | 6 | 2 | 6 | 3 |
| Teratoma | 7 | 1 | 1 | 4 | 5 |
| Brain tumor | 3 | 1 | 3 | 4 | 3 |
| Other | 6 | 5 | 1 | 4 | 8 |
| Total | 51 | 28 | 51 | 67 | 63 |

[*]Fraumeni, J. F., and Miller, R. W.: Am. J. Dis. Child. *117*:186, 1969.

the fetus. Wells accepted as certain only four examples of such occurrences. Two were melanosarcomas, which caused death of the children, in one instance at 8 months with metastasis to the liver, and in the other at 10 months with disseminated disease. In both instances the placenta had extensive metastases. A maternal lymphosarcoma was discovered in one infant's liver, and a bronchogenic carcinoma had metastasized to the skin of the knee of a fourth fetus.

A small number of cases of malignant melanomas of the mother with spread to the fetus have been reported since Wells' review in 1940 (Holland, 1949; Cavell, 1963; Brodsky et al., 1965). The infant reported by Cavell recovered from the metastatic disease. Kasdon has recorded two instances of Hodgkin's disease occurring in infants of mothers with the disorder. Multiple myeloma has been reported in a small number of pregnant women. In two instances no abnormal myeloma protein was found in the infants, but a transient abnormal protein thought to be passively transferred from the mother was demonstrated in two others. None of the infants had evidence of disease.

Leukemia has not been found to occur in newborn infants of women with this malignancy, although two children of affected mothers developed the disease at 5 and 9 months of age. In these instances, both mothers and children had acute lymphoblastic leukemia (Cramblett et al.; Bernard et al.). Although leukemia in mice can be transmitted to their offspring by viruses in

TABLE 111-3.    *Summary of Recorded Congenitally Malignant Tumors (Not Including Retinal Tumors)*[*]

| | Accepted | Probable | Possible | Total |
|---|---|---|---|---|
| Malignant renal tumors | 5 | 11 | ? | 16 |
| Malignant adrenal neuroblastoma | 17 | 15 | 21 | 53 |
| Malignant extra-adrenal neuroblastoma | 6 | 4 | ? | 10 |
| Congenital sarcoma | 33 | 29 | 53 | 115 |
| Teratoma: malignant at birth | 1 | 2 | ? | 3 |
| Tumors of undetermined nature | 3 | 1 | 7 | 11 |
| Carcinoma of liver | 0 | 1 | 9 | 10 |
| Malignant hemangioendothelioma of liver | ? | ? | 15 | 15 |
| Hepatic tumors of undetermined character | ? | ? | 4 | 4 |
| Carcinoma, excluding liver | 0 | 0 | 5 | 5 |
| Cerebral glioma | 1 | 1 | 2 | 4 |
| Malignant endothelioma, excluding liver | ? | ? | 5 | 5 |
| Melanoma malignum | 0 | 2 | 2 | 4 |
| | 66 | 66 | 123 | 255 |

[*]Wells, H. G.: Arch. Pathol. *30*:535, 1940.

breast milk, there is no evidence that leukemia is passed on to the human infant in this manner.

The development of choriocarcinoma in an infant as a complication of placental choriocarcinoma is rare. In at least four instances both mother and infant have been affected. This represents tumor transmission from the fetus to the mother because the trophoblast, the site of origin, is composed of fetal, not maternal tissue. In all of the recorded cases, summarized by Witzleben and Bruninga, there was either a recognized placental choriocarcinoma or absence of a primary site in the infants with disseminated malignancy. These authors stressed the characteristic presentation of hematemesis or hemoptysis, anemia, hepatomegaly and pulmonary metastasis in the infant. The diagnosis is established by the demonstration of elevated urinary or plasma gonadotropin levels.

## Environmental Factors

The review of Fraumeni and Miller showed no significant annual variation or aggregation of cases of neonatal cancers in the United States. Children exposed prenatally to the atomic bombs in Hiroshima and Nagasaki have no significant excess of mortality from leukemia or other cancers. In 1971 Herbst et al. reported that large doses of stilbesterol given to pregnant women were related to the development of adenocarcinoma of the vagina in their daughters of that pregnancy from 14 to 22 years later. A relationship between exposure in utero to stilbesterol and its close synthetic analogs during the first half of pregnancy with the later development of clear-cell adenocarcinoma of both vagina and cervix now appears to be well-established. There is also evidence that a number of carcinogens, when given to the experimental animal at a critical point in pregnancy can lead to cancers late in the life of the offspring. Thus although there are no data to suggest that environmental factors are responsible for the development of neonatal malignant disease, the relationship of prenatal exposure to various agents and carcinogenesis in later life remains to be determined.

## Host Factors

Certain host factors seem to predispose an individual to the development of neoplastic disease. There is an increased incidence of leukemia in persons with Down's syndrome, Fanconi's aplastic anemia and Bloom's syndrome and of leukemia and lymphoreticular malignancies in individuals born with immunodeficiency disorders such as ataxia-telangiectasia, Wiskott-Aldrich syndrome, and congenital thymic alymphoplasia. Miller found Down's syndrome to be more common than usual among siblings of children with leukemia. It is of interest that both Down's syndrome and leukemia occur more frequently among children of older mothers. Borges et al. found that four of 25 non-mongoloid children with acute leukemia had cytogenetic variants of prezygotic origin and suggested that the aneuploid cell might be more susceptible to malignant change.

Although the risk of developing leukemia is increased slightly in a dizygotic twin or other sibling of a child who has the disease, the chance of developing leukemia is greatest in a monozygotic twin. If one monozygotic twin has leukemia, the co-twin has approximately a 25 per cent chance of developing leukemia, usually within weeks or months of the diagnosis in the sibling.

A small number of well-defined hereditary disorders such as neurofibromatosis, tuberous sclerosis or basal-cell carcinoma syndrome are associated with an increased incidence of certain neoplasms. Also, kindreds have been reported in which multiple members developed the types of malignant diseases that usually occur in sporadic fashion. Although the number of such families is small, it is hard to escape the conclusion that, at least in some instances, heredity plays some role in the development of malignancy.

## Congenital Defects

An unexpectedly large number of tumors common to the infant occur in children who have certain congenital defects. Children with Wilms' tumor have an increased incidence of congenital aniridia and anomalies of the genitourinary tract. Congenital hemihypertrophy occurs excessively with Wilms' tumor, adrenocortical neoplasia and hepatoblastoma, and is also associated with hamartomas and with the visceral cytomegaly syndrome described by Beckwith. Hamartomas occur commonly in children with Wilms' tumor and adrenocortical neoplasia. One child has been reported with hepatoblastoma and Wilms' tumor; another, with congenital hemihypertrophy, had an adrenocortical adenoma and years later developed a Wilms' tumor. Of interest is the fact that Beckwith's visceral cytomegaly syndrome affects the kidney, adrenal cortex and liver, the three organs that develop the malignancies associated with hemihypertrophy. These relationships among hemihypertrophy, visceral cytomegaly syndrome, hamartomas and malignancy have been reviewed by Miller.

In certain experimental animals it has been shown that the same toxic agent is teratogenic to the fetus in the second quarter of pregnancy and carcinogenic in the latter half of pregnancy (Napalkov). This observation and the association of childhood neoplasias with congenital anomalies suggests that there is a close relationship between oncogenesis and teratogenesis.

## CONGENITAL LEUKEMIA

Leukemia rarely occurs during the first month of life. Approximately 90 per cent of the neonatal cases reported have been acute myelogenous leukemia, in contrast to the predominance of acute lymphoblastic leukemia found in later childhood. To date, no child born to a mother with leukemia has been found to have the disease during the neonatal period. Instances of familial neonatal leukemia must be extremely rare, as only one report of such a family has appeared in the literature. Campbell et al. (1962) described male and female siblings who died at 10 and 8 weeks of age of myelogenous leukemia, and a third female in the family who died at 4 weeks of age with a clinical course similar to her siblings, although a definite diagnosis was not made.

**DIAGNOSIS.** The clinical manifestations of leukemia may be evident at birth, with the presence of hepatosplenomegaly, petechiae and ecchymoses. Leukemic cell infiltration into the skin, leukemia cutis, results in nodular fibroma-like masses. These tumors are freely movable over the subcutaneous tissue and result in a blue or gray discoloration to the overlying skin (Fig. 111-1). Such cutaneous lesions are commonly found when the disease appears at birth and have been found in stillborn premature infants with leukemia. They may be the first clinical signs of the disease. At birth many of the infants have respiratory distress due to either leukemic infiltration in the lungs or atelectasis. The author has seen one infant who developed severe respiratory difficulty soon after birth from a fatal pulmonary hemorrhage, presumably secondary to thrombocytopenia.

In those infants who develop signs of the disease within the first month but in whom

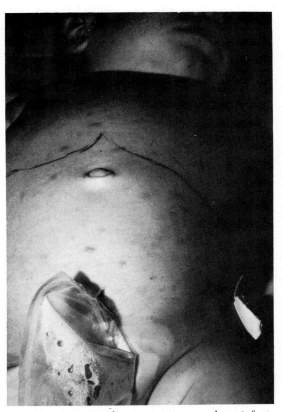

*Figure 111-1.* Leukemia cutis in a newborn infant.

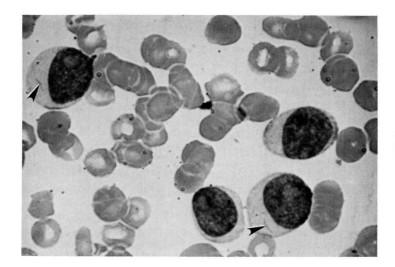

*Figure 111–2.* Malignant blast cells with Auer rods (arrows) present in cytoplasm diagnostic of acute myelogenous leukemia.

no detectable signs of leukemia were noted at birth, the symptoms are often ill defined, with low grade fever, diarrhea, hepatomegaly and failure to gain weight. Hemorrhagic manifestations are often the first sign of the disease and leukemia cutis is uncommon.

Hemoglobin levels are often normal at first, but soon fall to low levels. Total white blood cell counts may be within normal limits or diminished, but leukocytosis is usually present. White cell counts of 150,000 to 250,000 per mm³ or more are not unusual, and counts as high as 1,300,000 per mm³ have been recorded. Leukocyte counts often rise progressively before death. There is usually a predominance of blast cells and immature granulocytes. Auer rods may be present in the blast cells (Fig. 111–2). These intracellular inclusions are composed of lysosomes, and are considered to be pathognomonic of acute myelogenous leukemia.

**DIFFERENTIAL DIAGNOSIS.** A number of newborn infants reported in the older literature who were originally thought to have leukemia were later found to have other diseases. The predominance of myelogenous leukemia in this age group has contributed to the difficulty in differentiating the disorder from leukemoid reactions. Confusion with infections such as congenital syphilis, cytomegalovirus infection, toxoplasmosis and bacterial septicemia may occur because of the leukocytosis, organo-

megaly and thrombocytopenia that may accompany these diseases. The low platelet counts and leukemoid reactions reported in infants with congenital amegakaryocytic thrombocytopenia may also lead to an incorrect diagnosis of leukemia, but the absence of radii commonly seen in these children is a major clue to the correct diagnosis.

Several infants who were reported to have leukemia were later discovered to have severe erythroblastosis fetalis. Such infants usually have hepatosplenomegaly, large numbers of nucleated erythroblasts in the peripheral blood and, occasionally, thrombocytopenia. Small infiltrates of extramedullary erythropoiesis may appear in the skin and superficially resemble leukemia cutis.

Infants with neonatal neuroblastoma often have hepatomegaly, with discolored nodules in the subcutaneous tissue. Their blood counts are usually normal, and specimens of bone marrow, if involved, reveal small clusters of neuroblastoma cells which can be distinguished from the bone marrow replaced by leukemic cells.

**PATHOLOGY.** Biopsy or autopsy shows heavy infiltration of many immature leukocytes into extrahematopoietic tissues. The bone marrow is hypercellular, with a marked predominance of the immature cells of the series affected, either myeloid or lymphoid. Cirrhosis of the liver has been noted at autopsy in several infants.

**THERAPY AND PROGNOSIS.** The course of the disease is usually one of rapid deterioration and death from hemorrhage and infection. Although the length of survival has been significantly prolonged in children with leukemia, there has been little experience in treating the neonate. The author is aware of one newborn infant with acute lymphoblastic leukemia who experienced a remission for a year following the use of multiple chemotherapeutic agents. Drugs used in the treatment of myelogenous leukemia in older children and adults, such as cytosine arabinoside, 5-azacytidine, cyclophosphamide, and vincristine may be of value, but reports of the use of such agents in treating neonatal leukemia have been anecdotal, with the infant usually experiencing a poor or short response. Spontaneous remissions, which occur in Down's syndrome infants with leukemia, rarely are experienced by the normal child. One infant with a normal karyotype has been reported who had a transient spontaneous remission which lasted until the age of nine months, when the child finally had a relapse and died of acute myelogenous leukemia (van Eys and Flexner, 1969).

### LEUKEMIA WITH DOWN'S SYNDROME

An increased incidence of acute leukemia in children with Down's syndrome is now well recognized. A review of the world literature by Rosner and Lee revealed 227 children with both disorders; 31 per cent had acute myeloblastic leukemia and 69 per cent had acute lymphoblastic leukemia. Among 47 newborn mongoloids with leukemia, 58 per cent had myeloblastic leukemia and 42 per cent had lymphoblastic leukemia. Eighteen additional Down's syndrome infants who had a transient disorder initially indistinguishable from acute myelogenous leukemia experienced complete clinical and hematologic recovery. In those with "transient leukemia" who died of other causes no evidence of leukemia could be found at postmortem examination. It has been suggested by Ross and associates that this disorder is due to a defect in the regulation of granulocyte multiplication and maturation, possibly related to the chromosomal abnormality. The increased incidence of neonatal polycythemia in

Down's syndrome patients observed by Weinberger and Oleinick have led these investigators to propose that abnormality in the regulation of hematopoiesis is not limited to granulocyte production. However, a number of mongoloid infants with transient leukemia have had recurrence of their disease leading to death, indicating that the disorders of marrow dysfunction and neonatal leukemia may not be separate entities but intimately related.

The high incidence of spontaneous remission of leukemia in infants with Down's syndrome makes it difficult to interpret their response to antileukemic therapy. It may be most prudent to withhold the use of chemotherapeutic agents in this unusual group of neonates unless the clinical course is one of rapid deterioration.

### NEUROBLASTOMA

Neuroblastoma is the most common malignant tumor in infancy. The neoplasm originates from neural crest cells that normally give rise to the adrenal medulla and sympathetic ganglia. In infancy, the first clinical manifestations are usually due to the presence of metastatic disease rather than the primary tumor. Yet despite the occurrence of widespread disease, the prognosis in the neonate is remarkably good.

**CLINICAL MANIFESTATIONS.** Neuroblastoma may present as a tumor mass anywhere sympathetic neural tissue normally occurs. Over half of affected children have the primary tumor within the abdomen, arising in the adrenal medulla or a sympathetic ganglion. The tumor may arise in the posterior mediastinum, and because of bronchial obstruction the symptoms may be either increasing dyspnea or pulmonary infection. The neoplasm may also arise in the head, neck or pelvis. Involvement of the stellate ganglion may result in a Horner's syndrome, although in the author's experience this has more commonly been a complication of surgical removal of the tumor mass than a presenting symptom. The neoplasm arising from a sympathetic ganglion has an unusual tendency to grow into the intervertebral foramina, causing spinal cord compression and resultant paralysis. Careful periodic neurologic evaluation should be carried out on the child with a neuroblastoma arising from a sympathetic ganglion, since the onset of cord compression may necessitate emergency neurosurgical intervention. The late diagnosis of this complication has resulted in permanent paraplegia.

Metastatic lesions, especially of the skin and liver, are common presenting findings during the neonatal period. Often the primary site cannot be discovered at operation or autopsy. The skin nodules often have a bluish color. Hawthorne et al. found that the nodules first become erythematous for 2 or 3 minutes after palpation and then blanch, presumably owing to vasoconstriction from release of catecholamines from the tumor cells. They consider this to be a diagnostic sign of subcutaneous neuroblastoma.

The liver often bears the brunt of metastatic dissemination, becoming studded with innumerable foci of tumor growth. The tumor almost always presents in the newborn as a rapidly growing hepatic neoplasm. Hagstrom reported a fetus that could not be delivered intact because the abdomen contained a nodular 700 gm liver, resulting in dystocia. The abdomen had to be opened and much of the liver cut away piecemeal before delivery could be accomplished. The right adrenal gland was entirely replaced by a neuroblastoma. An infant reported by Larimer was delivered easily, but severe respiratory difficulty and cyanosis, apparently due to abdominal distention, were noted at birth. The child lived only 9 hours. Autopsy showed a huge 425 gm liver filled with bulging spherical nodules, a right adrenal gland weighing 83 gm and filled with neuroblastoma, and metastatic involvement of mesenteric lymph nodes and the left adrenal gland.

Neuroblastomas arising from sympathetic ganglia lower in the abdomen give rise to the clinical pictures consistent with their locations. Thus presacral neuroblastomas may simulate presacral teratomas and be distinguished from them only by biopsy. Hepler's case is an instructive example. A 3-week-old male infant had been unable to void from birth, and an indwelling catheter had been passed into his bladder. A tumor of the lower part of the abdomen could be felt. By rectum the mass was palpable, filling the hollow of the sacrum and extending forward to the symphysis. A cystogram showed the bladder to be displaced upward and to the left. A preoperative diagnosis of presacral teratoma was made. At operation, most of the tumor was removed and proved to be a neuroblastoma. Postoperatively 1260 roentgens of x-irradiation were given over a 2-month period. The remainder of the tumor disappeared, and the child was well four years later.

Several children with neuroblastoma have been reported whose sole presenting symptom was persistent, intractable diarrhea. Green et al. described two patients with chronic diarrhea who were discovered to have chest masses, and a third who had a mass in the region of the left adrenal gland that contained stippled calcifications. The children were thought to have had either cystic fibrosis or celiac syndrome before the roentgenographic discoveries were made. Their symptoms dramatically abated following surgical removal of their tumors. It is believed that such symptoms are due to excessive excretion by the tumor of one or more catecholamines or their metabolic end products.

The association of acute myoclonic encephalopathy and neuroblastoma has been described by numerous authors. This usually consists of rapid multidirectional eye movements (opsoclonus), myoclonus and truncal ataxia in the absence of increased intracranial pressure. In many instances neurological improvement occurred once the tumor had been removed. Despite the fact that it has been suggested that the encephalopathy is due to toxic neurological effects of catecholamine catabolites, at least one child has been described who developed neurologic symptoms 19 months following removal of the tumor and return to normal of the previously elevated levels of urinary catecholamines.

A report from the Netherlands suggests that there may be signs and symptoms in mothers whose fetuses have neuroblastoma. Voûte and co-workers have reported six women who had sweating, pallor, headaches, palpitations, hypertension and tingling in the feet and hands during the eighth and ninth months of pregnancy. All of the women delivered children who were diagnosed as having neuroblastoma shortly after birth or during the first few months of life. Because the mothers' symptoms disappeared postpartum, the authors proposed that they were caused by fetal catecholamines entering the maternal circulation. It is not known how commonly this syndrome occurs.

Occasionally a newborn infant with congenital neuroblastoma may be thought to have erythroblastosis. The infant reported by Falkinburg and Kay developed severe jaundice and, because of hepatosplenomegaly, was mistakenly thought for a time to have hemolytic disease of the newborn. An increase of nucleated red cells was noted in the child's blood. Anders et al. described two newborn infants with congenital neuroblastoma which had metastasized to the liver and placenta who were thought to have hydrops fetalis. In one the diagnosis was established by histologic examination of the placenta.

In summary, abdominal neuroblastoma of the newborn most commonly manifests itself by enlargement of the liver alone. An additional mass, the primary tumor, sometimes may be palpable beneath it. Otherwise unexplained persistent diarrhea may be the only sign. Metastases to lungs, bones, skull and orbit are rare in the neonate, although clumps of tumor cells are often found if one carefully examines bone marrow aspiration specimens (Fig. 111–3). In 1965 Schneider et al. reported on 56 cases of neonatal neuroblastoma recorded in the English literature since 1940. Fifty-two per cent had metastases at the time of the original diagnosis, but only 3

per cent had metastasized to bone. The liver was involved in 65 per cent, and subcutaneous metastases were seen in 32 per cent. These figures differ strikingly from those for older infants and children (Table 111–4).

**CATECHOLAMINES.** In 1957 Mason et al. reported an increased excretion of pressor amines in the urine of an infant with neuroblastoma. Subsequent studies in children with neuroblastoma have shown elevated levels of norepinephrine, its biochemical precursors and its metabolites in the urine, including dopa, dopamine, normetanephrine, homovanillic acid (HVA) and vanillylmandelic acid (VMA). According to Williams and Greer, 95 per cent of patients will have an elevated urinary excretion of VMA or HVA, or both. Occasional cases, however, have no elevation of catecholamines. It is therefore important to measure urinary catecholamines in a child prior to surgical removal of a neuroblastoma or initiation of therapy in order to determine whether or not it is a catecholamine-producing tumor. This unique property of the neoplasm not only can be used as an aid in diagnosis but also as a useful means of assessing the response to therapy or detecting the recurrence of tumor.

**PATHOLOGY.** The most primitive histologic subgroup of this tumor, the neuroblastoma, is very cellular and is composed of small round cells with scant cytoplasm. The ganglioneuroma, its more benign

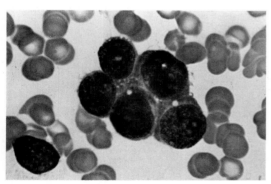

**Figure 111–3.** Clump of neuroblastoma cells found in bone marrow aspiration.

**TABLE 111–4.** *Incidence of Metastases in the Newborn with Neuroblastoma*°

|  | Number | Percentage | All Ages (per cent) |
|---|---|---|---|
| Liver | 20 | 64.6 | 24.3 |
| Subcutaneous | 10 | 32.3 | 2.6 |
| Marrow | 3 | 9.7 |  |
| Lung | 2 | 6.5 | 13.2 |
| Spleen | 2 | 6.5 | 2.0 |
| Kidney | 2 | 6.5 | 2.0 |
| Pancreas | 2 | 6.5 |  |
| Brain | 2 | 6.5 | 15.8 |
| Bone | 1 | 3.2 | 47.4 |
| Nodes | 1 | 3.2 | 32.2 |
| Pleura | 1 | 3.2 |  |
| Myocardium | 1 | 3.2 |  |
| Periadrenal | 1 | 3.2 |  |

°Schneider, K. M., Becker, J. M., and Krasna, I. H.: Pediatrics 36:359, 1965.

counterpart, is composed of large, mature ganglion cells with abundant cytoplasm, while the ganglioneuroblastoma is intermediate in the degree of cellular differentiation. However, the histologic appearance of an individual tumor may show various degrees of cellular maturation. Although attempts have been made to correlate prognosis with histologic grading, there appears to be a much better correlation between prognosis and both clinical staging of the disease and the patient's age at the time of diagnosis. Thus most oncologists have not found the finer points of histologic grading to be a major factor in influencing therapy or determining prognosis.

**PROGNOSIS.**  It has been known that the chance of survival of a patient with neuroblastoma is inversely correlated with the age of the child at the time of diagnosis. The infant who has widespread disease appears to have a better chance of survival than the older child with a lesser degree of tumor dissemination.

The site of origin also has been considered to be a factor influencing survival, and a more favorable prognosis has been observed in children with mediastinal neuroblastoma. An evaluation by Evans and co-workers of 100 cases confirmed this observation, but it was felt that the prognosis was good in such children only because they seldom had metastatic disease. Based upon their findings, these investigators proposed a clinical staging for children with neuroblastoma that appeared to be helpful in predicting the ultimate prognosis. Children with Stage I disease had tumor limited to the organ of origin; those with Stage II had regional tumor spread that did not cross the midline; Stage III tumors extended across the midline; and Stage IV disease included patients with distant metastases to lymph nodes, lung, brain or bone. Those with a greater degree of spread tended to have a poorer prognosis, and in those with Stage IV disease the malignancy was usually fatal.

One unique group of patients with disseminated disease had such a good prognosis, however, that a separate category called Stage IV–S was proposed to distinguish them from other patients with widespread involvement. This special group of children had remote spread of tumor involving the liver, skin, and/or bone marrow without roentgenographic evidence of skeletal metastases. This pattern seemed to occur most commonly in infancy. Eighteen of 20 infants under the age of 1 year with Stage IV–S disease reported by D'Angio and associates were cured of their disease. The 2 year survival of all of those with Stage IV–S disease was 84 per cent as compared to 5 per cent survival in those with Stage IV disease. This association between age at the time of diagnosis, clinical staging and survival is shown in Table 111–5.

A number of children have been reported to have experienced spontaneous tumor regression despite the presence of metastases. In other instances, malignant neuroblastomas have apparently undergone maturation into benign ganglioneuromas. The following example of a spontaneous regression was reported by Schwartz and associates.

CASE REPORT 111–1

A 2-month old Caucasian girl was referred to the Children's Memorial Hospital of Chicago with a chief complaint of "lumps in the skin" since birth. The lesions were purple, and blanched when pressure was applied. A biopsy of one of the skin lesions was diagnostic of neuroblastoma. Results of a bone marrow exam-

*TABLE 111–5.  Two Year Survival of 234 Children with Neuroblastoma**

| Age (months) | Stage | | | | | |
| --- | --- | --- | --- | --- | --- | --- |
| | I | II | III | IV | IV-S | Total |
| <12 | 10/11 | 14/15 | 2/4 | 4/17 | 18/20 | 48/67 |
| 12–23 | 4/5 | 5/8 | 3/7 | 0/26 | 1/1 | 13/47 |
| 24+ | 2/3 | 4/12 | 3/13 | 3/88 | 2/4 | 14/120 |
| Total | 16/19 | 23/35 | 8/24 | 7/131 | 21/25 | 75/234 |

*D'Angio et al.: Lancet *1*:1046, 1971.

ination, liver-spleen scan, and roentgenograms of the chest and skeleton were normal. An intravenous pyelogram revealed lateral displacement of the left ureter, suggesting a left paravertebral mass. Urinary VMA excretion was elevated to 90 $\mu$g per mg of creatinine (normal: 20 $\mu$g per mg of creatinine or less). A diagnosis of disseminated neuroblastoma was made, the primary tumor probably arising from a left paravertebral sympathetic ganglion in the abdomen. No therapy was administered. The skin lesions completely resolved by 4 months of age (Fig. 111–4), at which time a repeat intravenous pyelogram showed no evidence of the paravertebral mass. The urinary excretion of VMA decreased to 8 $\mu$g per mg of creatinine. At 2 years of age, the child was well and had no evidence of neuroblastoma.

The diagnosis of neuroblastoma was made before the age of 6 months in 21 of 29 cases collected by Everson and Cole in which spontaneous regression occurred. The remainder were diagnosed between 6 and 24 months of age. This relationship of

spontaneous regression to age has also been noted by Evans et al., who noted that the majority of those with tumor regression were under 6 months of age and were usually those with Stage II or Stage IV-S disease. Stage I patients, however, could not be evaluated because the tumor was usually completely resected.

The incidence of spontaneous regression of neuroblastoma may be more common than is clinically evident. Beckwith and Perrin detected the presence of microscopic clusters of neuroblastoma cells, termed neuroblastoma in situ, in the adrenal glands of a significant number of infants under the age of 3 months with no clinical evidence of tumor upon whom post mortem examinations were performed. They estimated the incidence of neuroblastoma in situ to be about 40 times greater than the number of cases of clinically diagnosed disease. Based upon their findings, they proposed that the great majority of

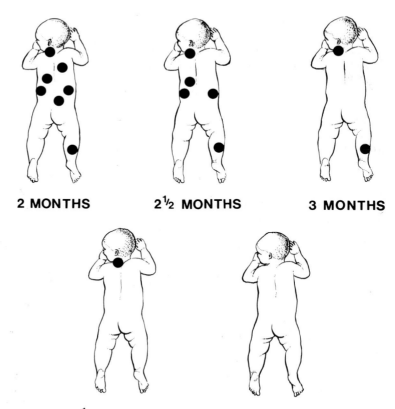

*Figure 111–4.* Spontaneous regression of skin lesions of disseminated neuroblastoma. (Schwartz, A. D., et al.: J. Pediatr. 85:760, 1974.)

**2 MONTHS**  **2½ MONTHS**  **3 MONTHS**

**3½ MONTHS**  **4 MONTHS**

these tumors either degenerated or underwent differentiation to normal tissue. Turkel and Itabashi, however, believe that such neuroblastic nodules represent normal changes in the developing adrenal gland, and noted their presence in 100 per cent of 169 fetal adrenal glands they examined. Whether or not neuroblastoma in situ is a true neoplasm, it completely disappears after 3 months of life under normal circumstances.

TREATMENT. The unpredictable course of neuroblastoma, with its occasional spontaneous maturation or regression, not only makes the tumor unusual but also causes difficulty in evaluating therapy. The impressive collection of cases reported by Bodian suggested that massive doses of vitamin $B_{12}$ led to cure, but subsequent evaluation of the collected experiences of others failed to confirm these observations. One likely explanation for Bodian's successful results was that his series was heavily weighted with young patients who experienced spontaneous remission. Reports that surgical assault on the primary tumor may influence regression of distant metastases must also be interpreted with caution in view of the natural history of the disease.

The response of neuroblastoma to chemotherapy is often dramatic, with the most impressive results occurring in children under the age of 1 year. The two most commonly employed drugs are vincristine sulfate and cyclophosphamide. Yet, despite well-documented initial regression of tumor, the use of these drugs has done little to improve survival in this disease, as shown by the data collected by Leikin and co-workers. The tumor is radio responsive and radiation therapy has been successfully used to shrink large tumor masses and relieve symptoms of pain and spinal cord compression. However, its routine use to eradicate residual tumor after surgery has not been conclusively demonstrated to affect ultimate survival.

The policy of most oncologists is to completely resect, if possible, the Stage I neuroblastoma. Available data can support no specific treatment regimen in view of the lack of influence of chemotherapy on the ultimate prognosis of those with Stage III or IV disease. There is some evidence that irradiation is of benefit in patients with Stage III disease, but it appears to be unrelated to survival in Stage I, II, and IV disease (Koop and Schnaufer). The extremely high fatality rate in older children with regional extension or disseminated disease warrants an aggressive approach with further evaluation of newer therapeutic agents. The observations by the Hellstroms that neuroblastoma is capable of evoking both cell mediated and humoral immune responses in the host may eventually lead to newer forms of immunotherapy. It has been suggested that the infant with the special pattern of metastases classed as Stage IV-S disease be observed for a period of time before the decision is made to initiate therapy, because the high cure rate in this group may be due to spontaneous tumor regression.

## WILMS' TUMOR

Wilms' tumor, or nephroblastoma, the most common intra-abdominal tumor of childhood, was first described as a clinical entity in 1899. In contrast to neuroblastoma, the increasing rate of cure of this neoplasm as a result of treatment has been one of the dramatic success stories in the field of cancer therapy. The establishment of a National Wilms' Tumor Study has helped to rapidly accumulate information regarding the prognosis and therapy of this tumor, which results in death if untreated.

CLINICAL MANIFESTATIONS. In the majority of children with Wilms' tumor either an abdominal mass or an increase in abdominal size is noted as the first clinical evidence of a disease which is often discovered by a parent and brought to the attention of the physician. The tumor lies deep in the flank, is attached to the kidney or is part of it, and is usually firm and smooth. It seldom extends beyond the midline, even though it may grow downward beyond the iliac crest. In about 10 per cent of all cases tumors involve both kidneys. Gross hematuria is a rare presenting symptom, but microscopic hematuria is found in approximately one fourth of the cases. According to Sullivan and co-workers, hematuria in Wilms' tumor is not a poor prognostic sign, as it is in adults with hypernephroma. Hypertension, noted in older infants and children upon occasion, has not been observed in the newborn.

Wilms' tumor is seldom diagnosed at birth or during the neonatal period, although several tumors have been so large as to have caused dystocia during delivery. Wells reported five certain cases and 11 probable ones in this age group. In addition to the infants reported by Wells, Hartenstein found seven more cases that were diagnosed in the neonatal period and added one of his own. Of the 77 children treated at the M. D. Anderson Hospital and Tumor Institute over a period of 18 years, only one was diagnosed during the first month of life (Sullivan et al.).

Rare cases of Wilms' tumor associated with polycythemia have been reported. This finding has apparently been secondary to an increased production of erythropoietin by the neoplasm. The demonstration of elevated plasma erythropoietin levels in five of eight non-polycythemic children with Wilms' tumor studied preoperatively by Murphy and colleagues led these investigators to suggest that this test may be useful in the diagnosis and evaluation of response to therapy.

**ASSOCIATED CONGENITAL ANOMALIES.** The association between Wilms' tumor, hemihypertrophy, congenital aniridia, hamartomas and genitourinary defects has been discussed earlier in this chapter. The finding at birth of hemihypertrophy should alert the physician to observe the child for the possible development of Wilms' tumor, adrenal cortical tumor or hepatoblastoma. A number of cases of pseudohermaphroditism, nephron disorders and Wilms' tumor have also been reported. Occasionally, certain members of a family may have the congenital anomaly and another have the neoplasm. Meadows et al. reported one family in which a mother had congenital hemihypertrophy, three of her children had Wilms' tumor, and a fourth had a urinary tract anomaly. Aniridia is usually inherited in an autosomal dominant pattern with high penetrance and little variability of phenotypic expression. The child with aniridia who has Wilms' tumor does not have this usual inheritance pattern but has sporadic congenital aniridia. Pilling reported 26 children with aniridia, 20 of whom had the sporadic type. Seven of the 20 developed

Wilms' tumor. It appears that the risk of developing Wilms' tumor is higher if the sporadic aniridia is accompanied by a major genitourinary tract anomaly or severe mental retardation, or both. There are two reports of aniridia in monozygous twins, but only one member of each pair developed Wilms' tumor (Miller, R. W.). This striking association of Wilms' tumor with a number of congenital abnormalities and disorders of growth control strongly suggests that common teratogenic and oncogenic factors may be at work. Reports of subtle chromosomal abnormalities in two newborn infants with Wilms' tumor (Giangiacomo et al.; Ladda et al.) and reports of tumors occurring in siblings and identical twins indicate that hereditary factors at times may play a major role in the development of this neoplasm.

**PROGNOSTIC FACTORS.** Three factors seem to influence the response to therapy and ultimate prognosis of the child with Wilms' tumor: the histologic pattern, the age of the patient at the time of diagnosis and the extent of disease. Tumors with better differentiation, showing glomeruloid and tubular formation, indicate a better chance for survival than those with more anaplastic and sarcomatous patterns. Younger patients have a more favorable prognosis, but this may be accounted for by the fact that the disease is usually less extensive in the younger child.

Several clinical staging systems have been proposed, the most common one now in use being that devised by the National Wilms' Tumor Study Group. This staging system is as follows:

Group   I: Tumor limited to the kidney and completely resected.
Group  II: Tumor extending beyond the kidney but completely resected.
Group III: Residual nonhematogenous tumor confined to the abdomen.
Group IV: Hematogenous metastases.
Group  V: Bilateral renal involvement either initially or subsequently.

The clinical staging appears to be the most important factor in predicting survival,

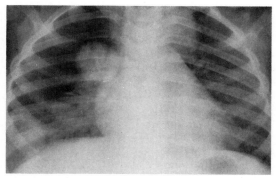

*Figure 111–5.* Pulmonary metastases of Wilms' tumor.

tine is more effective than using either drug alone. Clinical trials have demonstrated that Adriamycin is also active against Wilms' tumor and may further improve the response in patients with more advanced disease when used in conjunction with the other therapeutic modalities. Thus Wilms' tumor, a neoplasm which is fatal if untreated, presently has a cure rate of greater than 80 per cent and the use of newer therapeutic agents may continue to improve these remarkably successful results.

those with more extensive spread having the poorer prognosis. Therefore, adequate evaluation of the extent of tumor involvement is essential and should include at the minimum an intravenous pyelogram and a roentgenographic evaluation of the lungs, the most commonly involved area of hematogenous spread (Fig. 111–5). Other commonly involved sites of metastatic spread are the liver, retroperitoneum, peritoneum, mediastinum and pleurae.

**THERAPY AND PROGNOSIS.** Prior to 1950 the two major modalities of therapy for the treatment of Wilms' tumor, surgical removal and radiation therapy, resulted in cure rates approaching 50 per cent. The advantage of treatment with the chemotherapeutic agent actinomycin D was demonstrated in 1966 by Farber, who reported an 89 per cent survival rate in children who had no evidence of metastatic disease at the time of diagnosis and who were followed for at least 2 years, and a 53 per cent survival rate in those presenting with evidence of metastatic disease. The drug therapy appeared to prevent clinical hematogenous metastases following surgical removal and radiation to the tumor bed by presumably destroying nondetectable, microscopic tumor foci, especially in the lungs. Vincristine sulfate also has been shown to have striking activity against Wilms' tumor and appears to be as effective as actinomycin D.

Information accumulated by the National Wilms' Tumor Study indicates that multiple courses of actinomycin D are more effective than a single course in suppressing pulmonary metastases, and that using a combination of actinomycin D and vincris-

## CONGENITAL MESOBLASTIC NEPHROMA

A number of neonatal renal tumors have previously been confused with the typical nephroblastoma, and have been referred to as "congenital Wilms' tumors." These neoplasms are now considered to be a separate entity and are termed mesoblastic nephromas or fetal renal hamartomas. The congenital mesoblastic nephroma was clearly distinguished from Wilms' tumor in 1967 by Bolande and co-workers, who emphasized its benign nature. The involved kidney is usually greatly enlarged and distorted by the tumor, but, unlike Wilms' tumor, there is usually no lobulation, necrosis, hemorrhage or discrete capsule between neoplasm and compressed kidney (Fig. 111–6). The histologic picture is of a preponderance of interlacing bundles of

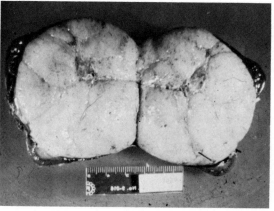

*Figure 111–6.* Congenital mesoblastic nephroma compressing and nearly totally replacing the kidney.

spindle-shaped cells within which dysplastic tubules and glomeruli are irregularly scattered. Extrarenal infiltration is common, especially into the perihilar connective tissues.

The vast majority of patients have been cured by nephrectomy alone. It has been suggested that the previous confusion with Wilms' tumor might account for the excellent survival rates reported in infants. There is good evidence that more patients with mesoblastic nephroma have died as a result of aggressive chemotherapy and irradiation than from the tumor itself. Nephrectomy is the treatment of choice; however, in very rare instances the tumor has been unusually aggressive. Because of the occasional case in which there is recurrence, it is now recommended that when the surgical margins are involved or uncertain, or the typical appearance of congenital mesoblastic nephroma is not present, additional therapy is indicated in addition to removal of the involved kidney.

## HEPATIC MALIGNANCIES

Primary malignant tumors of the liver are uncommon in infants and children; the two major histologic types are hepatoblastoma and hepatocellular carcinoma. Hepatoblastomas usually occur in infants and are rarely seen after 3 years of age. Of the 129 cases reported by Exelby and co workers, almost half were 18 months or younger, 11 were under 6 weeks of age, and 3 were newborns. Hepatocellular carcinomas, however, appear to have a bimodal age distribution, occurring either in the very young child below 4 years or between the ages of 12 and 15 years. Both types of tumors occur more commonly in males.

The most common presenting symptoms of hepatic tumors are an upper abdominal mass or an enlarging abdomen. Anorexia, weight loss and pain also frequently occur. Laboratory studies of liver function are rarely helpful in establishing a diagnosis and are usually normal. Alpha fetoprotein, an alpha-1 globulin that occurs normally in the fetus and disappears in the first few weeks of life, is often present in the serum of the child with hepatic malignancy. A number of children with hepatoblastoma have elevated levels of the amino acid cystathionine in their urine. If present, cystathioninuria may differentiate between hepatoblastoma and a number of benign and malignant disorders, but this finding also occurs in about 50 per cent of patients with neuroblastoma, a neoplasm which commonly spreads to the liver in the young child.

Hepatic calcification is demonstrated in 20 per cent of cases on the plain abdominal roentgenogram. Radioisotopic liver scanning usually demonstrates the presence of a neoplasm, and is useful in following regeneration of the liver after hepatic lobectomy and in diagnosing tumor recurrence. Angiography is useful in determining whether both lobes of the liver are involved. If one lobe is free of malignancy and there is no evidence of distant metastatic disease, a lobectomy of the involved portion of the liver should be performed despite the high operative mortality. At the present time surgery appears to be the only means for cure. In the large series cited above there was no evidence that radiation therapy or chemotherapy controlled disease which could not be totally resected. When incomplete excision was performed no patient survived, but 60 per cent of those with hepatoblastoma and 33 per cent with hepatocellular carcinoma were cured if the tumor could be completely excised.

## REFERENCES

Alpert, M. E., and Seeler, R. A.: Alpha fetoprotein in embryonal hepatoblastoma. J. Pediatr. 77:1058, 1970.

Anders, D., Kindermann, G., and Pfeifer, U.: Metastasizing fetal neuroblastoma with involvement of the placenta stimulating fetal erythroblastosis. J. Pediatr., 82:50, 1973.

Aron, B. S.: Wilms' tumor—a clinical study of eighty-one patients. Cancer 33:637, 1974.

Beckwith, J. B.: Mesenchymal renal neoplasms of infancy revisited. J. Pediat. Surg. 9:803, 1974.

Beckwith, J. B., and Perrin, E. V.: In situ neuroblastoma: A contribution to the natural history of neural crest tumors. Amer. J. Pathol. 43:1089, 1963.

Bernard, J., Jacquillat, C., Chavalet, F., Boiron, M., Stoitchkov, Y., and Tanzer, J.: Leucémie Aiguë d'une Enfant de 5 Mois Née d'une Mère Atteinte de Leucémie Aiguë au Moment de L'Accouchement. Nouv. Rev. Franc. Hémat. 4:140, 1964.

Bodian, M.: Neuroblastoma: An evaluation of its natural history and the effects of therapy, with particular reference to treatment by massive doses of vitamin $B_{12}$. Arch. Dis. Child. 38:606, 1963.

Bolande, R. P.: Congenital and infantile neoplasia of the kidney. Lancet 2:1497, 1974.

Bolande, R. P., Brough, A. J., and Izant, R. J.: Congenital mesoblastic nephroma of infancy: A report of eight cases and the relationship to Wilms' tumor. Pediatrics 40:272, 1967.

Borges, W. H., Nicklas, J. W., and Hamm, C. W.: Prezygotic determinants in acute leukemia. J. Pediatr. 70:180, 1967.

Brodsky, I., Baren, M., Kahn, S. B., Lewis, G., Jr., and Tellum, M.: Metastatic malignant melanoma from mother to fetus. Cancer 18:1048, 1965.

Campbell, W. A. B., Macafee, A. L., and Wade, W. G.: Familial neonatal leukaemia. Arch. Dis. Child. 37:93, 1962.

Cavell, B.: Transplacental metastasis of malignant melanoma. Acta Paediat. Suppl. 146:37, 1963.

Cramblett, H. G., Friedman, J. L., and Najjar, S.: Leukemia in an infant born of a mother with leukemia. N. Engl. J. Med. 259:727, 1958.

D'Angio, G. J., Evans, A. E., and Koop, C. E.: Special pattern of widespread neuroblastoma with a favorable prognosis. Lancet 1:1046, 1971.

Delalieux, C., Ebinger, G., Maurus, R., and Sliwowski, H.: Myoclonic encephalopathy and neuroblastoma. N. Engl. J. Med. 292:46, 1975.

Engel, R. R., Hammond, D., Eitzman, D. V., Pearson, H., and Krivit, W.: Transient congenital leukemia in 7 infants with mongolism. J. Pediatr. 65:303, 1964.

Evans, A. E., D'Angio, G. J., and Randolph, J.: A proposed staging for children with neuroblastoma. Cancer 27:374, 1971.

Evans, A. E., Gerson, J., and Schnaufer, L.: Spontaneous regression of neuroblastoma. J. Nat. Cancer Inst. (in press).

Everson, T. C., and Cole, W. H.: Spontaneous Regression of Cancer: A Study and Abstract of Reports in the World Medical Literature and of Personal Communications Concerning Spontaneous Regression of Malignant Disease. Philadelphia, W. B. Saunders Company, 1966, pp. 88–163.

Exelby, P. R., Filler, R. M., and Grosfeld, J. L.: Liver tumors in children in particular reference to hepatoblastoma and hepatocellular carcinoma: American Academy of Pediatrics Surgical Section Survey—1974.

Falkinburg, L. W., and Kay, M. N.: A case of congenital sympathogonioma (neuroblastoma) of the right adrenal simulating erythroblastosis fetalis. J. Pediatr. 42:462, 1953.

Farber, S.: Chemotherapy in the treatment of leukemia and Wilms' tumor. J.A.M.A. 108:826, 1966.

Fleming, I., and Pinkel, D.: Clinical staging of Wilms' tumor. J. Pediatr. 74:324, 1969.

Fraumeni, J. F., and Miller, R. W.: Cancer deaths in the newborn. Amer. J. Dis. Child. 117:186, 1969.

Geiser, C. F., Baez, A., Schindler, A. M., and Shih, V. E.: Epithelial hepatoblastoma associated with congenital hemihypertrophy and cystathioninuria: Presentation of a case. Pediatrics 46:66, 1970.

Giangiacomo, J., Penchansky, L., Monteleone, P. L., and Thompson, J.: Bilateral neonatal Wilms' tumor with B-C chromosomal translocation. J. Pediatr. 86:98, 1975.

Green, M., Cooke, R. E., and Lattanzi, W.: Occurrence of chronic diarrhea in three patients with ganglioneuromas. Pediatrics 23:951, 1959.

Gross, L.: Transmission of mouse leukemia virus through milk of virus-infected C3H female mice. Proc. Soc. Exp. Biol. Med., 109:830, 1962.

Hagstrom, H. T.: Fetal dystocia due to metastatic neuroblastoma of the liver. Am. J. Obst. Gynecol. 19:673, 1930.

Haicken, B. N., and Miller, D. R.: Simultaneous occurrence of congenital aniridia, hamartoma, and Wilms' tumor. J. Pediatr. 78:497, 1971.

Hartenstein, H.: Wilms' tumor in a newborn infant: Report of a case with autopsy studies. J. Pediatr. 35:381, 1949.

Hawthorne, H. C., Nelson, J. S., Witzleben, C. L., and Giangiacomo, J.: Blanching subcutaneous nodules in neonatal neuroblastoma. J. Pediatr. 77:297, 1970.

Hellstrom, K. E., and Hellstrom, I.: Immunity to neuroblastoma and melanomas. Ann. Rev. Med. 23:19, 1972.

Hepler, A. B.: Presacral sympathicoblastoma in an infant causing urinary obstruction. J. Urol. 49:777, 1943.

Herbst, A. L., Ulfelder, H., and Poskanzer, D. C.: Adenocarcinoma of the vagina: Association of maternal stilbesterol therapy with tumor appearance in young women. N. Engl. J. Med. 284:878, 1971.

Holland, E.: A case of transplacental metastases of malignant melanoma from mother to fetus. J. Obst. Gynaec. Brit. Emp. 56:529, 1949.

Jablon, S., and Kato, H.: Childhood cancer in relation to prenatal exposure to atomic-bomb radiation. Lancet 2:1000, 1970.

Joshi, V. V., Kay, S., Milstein, R., Koontz, W. W., and McWilliams, N. B.: Congenital mesoblastic nephroma of infancy: Report of a case with unusual clinical behavior. Am. J. Clin. Pathol. 60:811, 1973.

Kasdon, S. C.: Pregnancy and Hodgkin's disease. Am. J. Obst. Gynecol. 57:282, 1949.

Kersey, J. H., Spector, B. D., and Good, R. A.: Cancer in children with primary immunodeficiency diseases. J. Pediatr. 84:263, 1974.

Koop, C. E., and Schnaufer, L.: The management of abdominal neuroblastoma. Cancer 35:905, 1975.

Ladda, R., Atkins, L., Littlefield, J., Neurath, P., and Marimuthu, K. M.: Computer-assisted analysis of chromosomal abnormalities: Detection of a deletion in aniridia/Wilms' tumor syndrome. Science 185:784, 1974.

Larimer, R. C.: Neuroblastoma (sympathogonioma) of the adrenal in a newborn infant. J. Pediatr. 34:365, 1949.

Leikin, S., Evans, A., Heyn, R., and Newton, W.: The impact of chemotherapy on advanced neuroblastoma. Survival of patients diagnosed in 1956, 1962, and 1966–68 in Children's Cancer Study Group A. J. Pediatr. 84:131, 1974.

Lergier, J. E., Jiménez, E., Maldonado, N., and Veray, F.: Normal pregnancy in multiple myeloma treated with cyclophosphamide. Cancer 34:1018, 1974.

MacMahon, B., and Levy, M. A.: Prenatal origin of childhood leukemia—evidence from twins. N. Engl. J. Med. 270:1082, 1964.

Martin, E. S., and Griffith, J. F.: Myoclonic encephalopathy and neuroblastoma. Am. J. Dis. Child. 122:257, 1971.

Mason, G. A., Hart-Mercer, J., Millar, E. J., Strang, L. B., and Wynne, N. A.: Adrenaline-secreting neuroblastoma in an infant. Lancet 2:322, 1957.

Meadows, A. T., Lichtenfeld, J. L., and Koop, C. E.: Wilms' tumor in three children of a woman with congenital hemihypertrophy. N. Engl. J. Med., *291:* 23, 1974.

Miller, R. W.: Down's syndrome (mongolism), other congenital malformations and cancers among the sibs of leukemic children. N. Engl. J. Med. 268:393, 1963.

Miller, R. W.: Persons at exceptionally high risk of leukemia. Cancer Res. 27:2420, 1967.

Miller, R. W.: Relation between cancer and congenital defects: An epidemiologic evaluation. J. Nat. Cancer Inst. 40:1079, 1968.

Miller, R. W.: Wilms' tumor: Evidence against Knudson's hypothesis (?). Childhood Cancer Etiology Newsletter No. 15, 1975.

Moe, P. G., and Nellhaus, G.: Infantile polymyoclonia–opsoclonus syndrome and neural crest tumors. Neurology 20:756, 1970.

Murphy, G. P., Mirand, E. A., Johnston, G. S., Gibbons, R. P., Jones, R. L., and Scott, W. W.: Erythropoietin release associated with Wilms' tumor. Johns Hopkins Hosp. Bull. *120:*26, 1967.

Napalkov, N.: *In* Tomatis, Mohr, and Davis (eds.): Transplacental carcinogenesis. International Agency for Research on Cancer Scientific Publication No. 4, 1973.

Perez, C., Kaiman, H. A., Keith, J., Mill, W. B., Vietti, T. J., and Powers, W. E.: Treatment of Wilms' tumor and factors affecting prognosis. Cancer, *32:*609, 1973.

Pierce, M. I.: Leukemia in the newborn infant. J. Pediatr. 54:691, 1959.

Pilling, G. P.: Wilms' tumor in seven children with congenital aniridia. J. Pediat. Surg. 10:87, 1975.

Reimann, D. L., Clemmens, R. L., and Pillsbury, W. A.: Congenital acute leukemia: Skin nodules, a first sign. J. Pediatr. 46:415, 1955.

Rosner, F., and Lees, S. L.: Down's syndrome and acute leukemia: Myeloblastic or lymphoblastic? Report of forty-three cases and review of the literature. Am. J. Med., 53:203, 1972.

Ross, J. D., Moloney, W. C., and Desforges, J. F.: Ineffective regulation of granulopoiesis masquerading as congenital leukemia in a mongoloid child. J. Pediatr. 63:1, 1963.

Sawitsky, A., and Desposito, F.: A survey of American experience with vitamin $B_{12}$ therapy of neuroblastoma. J. Pediatr. 67:99, 1965.

Schneider, K. M., Becker, J. M., and Krasna, I. H.: Neonatal neuroblastoma. Pediatrics 36:359, 1965.

Schwartz, A. D., Dadash-Zadeh, M., Lee, H., and Swaney, J. J.: Spontaneous regression of disseminated neuroblastoma. J. Pediatr. 85:760, 1974.

Spear, G. S., Hyde, T. P., Gruppo, R. A., and Slusser, R.: Pseudohermaphroditism, glomerulonephritis with the nephrotic syndrome and Wilms' tumor in infancy. J. Pediatr. 79:677, 1971.

Stark, C. R., and Mantel, N.: Effects of maternal age and birth order on the risk of mongolism and leukemia. J. Nat. Cancer Inst. 37:687, 1966.

Sukarochana, K., and Kiesewetter, M. B.: Wilms' tumor: Factors influencing long-term survival. J. Pediatr. 69:747, 1966.

Sullivan, M. P., Hussey, D. H., and Ayala, A. G.: Wilms' tumor. *In* Sutow, W., Vietti, T., and Fernbach, D. (Eds.): Clinical Pediatric Oncology. St. Louis, The C. V. Mosby Co., 1973, p. 359.

Transplacental carcinogenesis (Editorial). Lancet *1:*1425, 1973.

Turkel, S. B., and Itabashi, H. H.: The natural history of neuroblastic cells in the fetal adrenal gland. Am. J. Pathol. 76:225, 1974.

Van Eys, J., and Flexner, J. M.: Transient spontaneous remission in a case of untreated congenital leukemia. Am. J. Dis. Child. *118:*507, 1969.

von Studnitz, W., Käser, H., and Sjoerdsma, A.: Spectrum of catechol amine biochemistry in patients with neuroblastoma. N. Engl. J. Med. 269:232, 1963.

Voorhess, M. L.: Neuroblastoma with normal urinary catecholamine excretion. J. Pediatr. 78:680, 1971.

Voûte, P. A., Jr., Wadman, S. K., and van Putten, W. J.: Congenital neuroblastoma: Symptoms in the mother during pregnancy. Clin. Pediat. 9:206, 1970.

Weinberger, M. M., and Oleinick, A.: Congenital marrow dysfunction in Down's syndrome. J. Pediatr. 77:273, 1970.

Wells, H. G.: Occurrence and significance of congenital malignant neoplasms. Arch. Pathol. 30:535, 1940.

Williams, C., and Greer, M.: Homovanillic acid and vanilmandelic acid in diagnosis of neuroblastoma. J.A.M.A. 183:836, 1963.

Witzleben, C. L., and Bruninga, G.: Infantile choriocarcinoma: A characteristic syndrome. J. Pediatr. 73:374, 1968.

Wolff, J. A.: Advances in the treatment of Wilms' tumor. Cancer 35:901, 1975.

Wolff, J. A., D'Angio, G., Hartmann, J., Krivit, W., and Newton, W. A.: Long-term evaluation of single versus multiple courses of actinomycin D therapy of Wilms' tumor. N. Engl. J. Med. *290:*84, 1974.

# XVIII

## Neonatal Pharmacology

# 112

# PRINCIPLES OF NEONATAL PHARMACOLOGY

*By Allen H. Neims, Jacob V. Aranda and Peter M. Loughnan* *

A 1500 gram premature infant born in North America is exposed to about 20 prescribed drugs between conception and discharge from the nursery. On the average, four to 10 medications are given to the mother and reach the fetus or infant transplacentally or through breast milk; after birth, the low-birth-weight infant is usually exposed to about seven agents by nursery routine (e.g., vitamin K, triple-dye, penicillin ophthalmic ointment and cyclopentolate) and seven drugs prescribed for specific indications. Total xenobiotic exposure is substantially greater since over-the-counter medications, alcohol, nicotine, caffeine, and environmental pollutants such as heavy metals and polycyclic hydrocarbons must be considered. The extent of exposure is emphasized by the presence of salicylate, hexachlorophene and caffeine in many random cord plasma samples. Common chemicals such as these can affect the developing mammal (Table 112–1).

The current trend of fetal and neonatal exposure to drugs is complex. Widespread knowledge of the tragic consequences of early exposure to thalidomide has prompted a cautious approach by physicians and patients. The tendency to limit exposure in the population at large, however, has been offset by the progressive regionalization of high-risk perinatal care and the coincident emergence of an attitude of aggressive diagnostic and therapeutic intervention. This attitude has added new dimensions to drug utilization, with respect to benefit and potential risk for the infant before, during, and after birth.

The scope of treatment before birth expands rapidly with reports of the use of propranolol, vitamin $B_{12}$, and, especially, agents such as glucocorticoids designed to accelerate the lung maturation. During birth, interpretation of sophisticated cardiopulmonary data gathered from the fetus during monitoring now requires an awareness of the modification of these functions by drugs. Finally, the breadth of current neonatal therapeutics is emphasized by a recent drug utilization survey conducted in the Neonatal Intensive Care Unit of the Montreal Children's Hospital, wherein it was found that more than 70 different drugs were prescribed for 320 infants (Table 112–2). Many specific medications have been discussed earlier; this chapter is designed to tabulate adverse effects and to stress certain general principles of perinatal therapeutics.

## ADVERSE DRUG REACTIONS: AN OVERVIEW

### THE FIRST TRIMESTER

The actions of drug on host and host on drug do not remain constant during development. Although it is pragmatic to distinguish between teratology and perinatal adverse drug reactions, any such classification remains arbitrary. Human development is a continuous process, with various tissues and functions maturing in distinctive, yet integrated, fashion from conception to puberty; even the tempo of maturation of a given tissue varies between individuals. Nonetheless, the earlier in gestation a harmful xenobiotic is encountered the more likely is the adverse effect to be unpredictable from an adult data

*The authors express appreciation to the MRC of Canada and Hoffmann-LaRoche, Basel, Switzerland, for support of studies used as examples in this chapter.

**TABLE 112–1.** *Possible Effects of Environmental Chemicals on the Fetus and Newborn*

*Ethanol:* Chronic maternal consumption is associated in human beings with the "fetal alcohol syndrome": high perinatal mortality, mental deficiency, retarded growth, and ocular, joint and cardiac malformations.[1] Withdrawal syndrome might occur after birth. Consumption just before birth might provoke hypoglycemia in premature infants; postnatal interaction with CNS depressant drugs remains possible.

*Caffeine:* Fetal breathing movements in sheep are stimulated by caffeine. Caffeine citrate has been utilized in treatment of apnea of prematurity.[2]

*Smoking:* Chronic cigarette smoking in mothers has been associated with fetuses of low weight; the possibility of increased perinatal mortality has been debated.[3-5] Smoking inhibits breathing movements in human beings and sheep,[6,7] probably through the hypoxia provoked by decreased uterine blood flow. Some women who smoke exhibit induced levels of placental aryl hydrocarbon hydroxylase activity.[8,9]

*Lead:* Exposure of rats during the suckling period causes hyperactive behavior at adulthood.[10]

*Organic Mercury:* Maternal poisoning is associated with an exaggerated fetal death rate and severe neurological defects, including seizures and movement disorders (Minamata disease).[11,12]

*Tetrachlorobiphenyl:* Maternal poisoning, Yusho disease, may be associated with an exaggerated fetal death rate; there is characteristic brown discoloration of the skin, as well as decreased birth weight and gingival hyperplasia.[13]

[1]Jones, K. L., et al.: Lancet *1*:1076, 1974. [2]Aranda, J. V., et al.: Clin. Res. *23*:611A, 1975. [3]Butler, N. R., et al.: Br. Med. J. *2*:127, 1972. [4]Meyer, M. B., and Comstock, G. W.: Am. J. Epidemiol. *96*:1, 1972. [5]Rush, D., and Kass, E. H.: Am. J. Epidemiol. *96*:183, 1972. [6]Gennser, G., et al.: Am. J. Obstet. Gynecol. *123*:861, 1975. [7]Manning, F. A., and Feyerabend, C.: Br. J. Obstet. Gynaecol. *83*:262–270, 1976. [8]Nebert, D. W., et al.: Cancer Res. *29*:1763, 1969. [9]Welch, R. M., et al.: Clin. Pharmacol. Ther. *10*:100, 1969. [10]Silbergeld, E. K., and Goldberg, A. M.: Exp. Neurol. *42*:146, 1974. [11]Tatetsu, S., and Harada, M.: Adv. Neurol. Sci. (Tokyo) *12*:181, 1968. [12]Snyder, R. D.: N. Engl. J. Med. *284*:1014, 1971. [13]Miller, R. W.: Teratology *4*:211, 1971.

**TABLE 112–2.** *Drugs Most Commonly Used in a Referral Neonatal Intensive Care Unit*[1]

| Drug | Per Cent Infants Exposed (n = 320) |
|---|---|
| Penicillin | 42.2 |
| Kanamycin | 41.6 |
| Gentamicin | 28.8 |
| Ampicillin | 27.5 |
| Calcium gluconate | 24.7 |
| Sodium bicarbonate | 22.5 |
| Furosemide | 10.6 |
| Chloramphenicol | 9.4[2] |
| Phenobarbital | 8.8 |
| Digoxin | 6.3 |
| Cloxacillin | 5.9 |
| Mycostatin | 4.7 |
| Methicillin | 4.7 |
| Diazepam | 3.8 |
| Multivitamin | 20.9 |
| Iron | 9.7 |

[1]Aranda, J. V., et al.: J. Pediatr. *89*:315–317 (1976).
[2]Usually ophthalmic solution.

base. The tragic and irreversible morphologic consequences of early exposure to thalidomide, androgenic steroids and folate antagonists are only too apparent (Table 112–3). But it would be foolish to conclude that all adverse drug-host interactions in the first trimester are associated with irreversible and obvious morphologic toxicity. A reversible effect may go unnoticed; a morphologically trivial, yet functionally important, toxic reaction may go unrecognized; and an effect with delayed expression may escape assignment of drug causality. The postpubertal vaginal adenocarcinoma associated with exposure in utero to diethylstilbestrol underscores our ignorance (Herbst et al.).

## THE PERINATAL PERIOD

By the perinatal period, *documented* adverse drug reactions have usually been the

**TABLE 112–3.   *Predictability of Adverse Drug Effects***

| Drug and Predictability[1] | Effect[2] |
|---|---|
| *Drug Exposure in Early Gestation* | |
| Thalidomide (−) | Amelia, phocomelia, CHD, acheiria, anomalies of eye, ear and intestinal tract |
| Narcotic Analgesics (−) | Associated with IUGR |
| Phenytoin (±Phenobarbital) (−) | Congenital anomalies (see text) |
| Amphetamine (−) | ?Biliary atresia, CHD |
| Salicylate (−) | ?Anomalies of nervous system, gastrointestinal tract and talipes |
| Trimethadione (−) | ?Fetal wastage, IUGR, CHD, cleft lip and palate |
| Progestins (−) | ?CHD and other anomalies |
| Oral anticoagulants (−) | ?Nasal anomalies, stippled epiphyses |
| Oral hypoglycemics (−) | ?Fetal wastage |
| Diethylstilbestrol (±) | Vaginal adenosis, adenocarcinoma |
| Sex steroids (±) | Masculinization of female fetus |
| Folate analogues (±) | Multiple anomalies; fetal wastage |
| Propylthiouracil, Iodine (+) | Goiter |
| *Drug Exposure in the Perinatal Period* | |
| Phenytoin/Phenobarbital (−) | Vitamin K-related coagulation defects |
| Oxygen (−) | Retrolental fibroplasia |
| Sulfonamides, benzoate, furosemide (±) | Displacement of bilirubin from albumin |
| Tetracycline (±) | Staining of teeth, retardation of bone growth |
| Phenobarbital (±, +) | Withdrawal syndrome, decreased hyperbilirubinemia, CNS depression |
| Short-acting barbiturates (+) | CNS depression |
| General anesthetics (+) | CNS depression |
| Regional anesthetics (+) | Bradycardia, seizures, acidosis, CNS depression |
| Lithium (+) | Hypotonia, CNS depression |
| Diazepam (+) | Hypotonia, CNS depression, hypothermia |
| Atropine (+) | Tachycardia |
| Hexamethonium bromide (+) | Paralytic ileus |
| Chlorpromazine (+) | Extrapyramidal dysfunction |
| Narcotic analgesics (+) | Respiratory depression, withdrawal syndrome |
| Acetylsalicylate (+) | Bleeding, platelet dysfunction, decreased factor XII |
| Reserpine (+) | Nasal stuffiness, lethargy, bradycardia, impaired temperature regulation |
| Oral hypoglycemics (+) | Thrombocytopenia, severe hypoglycemia |
| Diazoxide (+) | Hyperglycemia |
| Dicumarol (+) | Bleeding |
| Thiazide diuretics (+) | Thrombocytopenia, salt and water depletion |
| Magnesium sulfate (+) | Hypotension, CNS depression |
| Chloramphenicol (+) | Gray-baby syndrome |
| Hexachlorophene (+) | Status spongiosus |

[1]Predictability:

   +, drug action a known side effect in human beings beyond the neonatal period.

   −, not *now* predictable from an adult data base.

   ±, partially predictable *now* from adult data base by either (a) target organ or (b) mechanism of action.

[2]Original references contained in Pomerance and Yaffe, Smithells, Wilson, or Warkany.

result of pharmacologic or toxic actions of the agent that occur in adults as well. Inappropriate dosing and unexpected portals of entry have played important causative roles in perinatal toxicity. The application of relatively simple pharmacokinetic principles and an awareness of unusual modes of drug acquisition could have prevented many of these unfortunate accidents. Examples are tabulated in Table 112–3. In many cases, premature and/or low-birth-weight infants have proved most susceptible.

The foregoing considerations should not detract from the possibility of unpredicted, and perhaps subtle and permanent, toxicity from agents administered perinatally. Certain features of the neonate do predispose to unique adverse reactions. Rapid growth accentuates the discoloration of teeth and the suppression of bone elongation associated with exposure to tetracycline. Hematologic and hepatic circumstances predispose the infant to the hyperbilirubinemic effect of vitamin K analogues, and to the exaggerated kernicterus coincident with displacement of bilirubin from albumin by drugs such as sulfisoxazole. The association between retrolental fibroplasia and oxygen could not have been anticipated. Indeed, expensive and difficult follow-up studies will probably reveal other adverse effects of current therapeutic regimens, especially with respect to reproductive and neurological function (Chung et al.). This possibility makes formal governmental approval of agents such as theophylline (for apnea of the premature) and glucocorticoid (for prevention of respiratory distress syndrome) difficult.

Finally, the distinctions between permanent and transient, morphological and functional or harmless and harmful drug reactions are not always clear-cut. The depression of fetal and neonatal breathing movements in lambs and humans that is associated with therapeutic doses of barbiturates or diazepam serves to illustrate this situation. Without monitoring, transient depression of fetal breathing will go unrecognized. If labor is monitored, the suppression of breathing movements may alarm the unaware physician despite the normality of blood gas determinations; speculatively, such pharmacological action could

also modify the meaning of amniotic fluid tests for lung maturity. After birth, related respiratory depression predisposes to hypoxia and, at times, necessitates mechanical ventilation. Diazepam and the barbiturates probably inhibit fetal respiratory movements by a direct action on fetal brain. The suppression of fetal breathing movements caused by these depressants is probably less harmful than that caused by nicotine, the mechanism of action of which is likely to involve reduction of uterine blood flow and fetal hypoxia.

## DRUGS IN EARLY PREGNANCY

During early gestation, most toxicologic and pharmacologic attention has focused on the unpredictable adverse effects on fetus of drugs administered to the mother. Our ignorance relates to an inability to predict confidently the fetal pathological effects from chemical structure or from animal experiments, and to our inability to identify the individual fetuses at risk. More is known about the relationship between the timing of insult and the subsequent lesion. This discussion concentrates on three areas: 1) the extent and duration of fetal exposure to drugs taken by the mother; 2) the clinical quandary engendered by "suspected teratogens"; and 3) recent advances in fetal pharmacology that pertain to these problems.

### FETAL ACQUISITION OF DRUG

Most xenobiotics that reach the embryo and fetus are first encountered by the mother, and potential exposure includes metabolites generated by the maternal organism. The placenta can no longer be viewed as a barrier that prevents entry of these foreign compounds into the fetus. Although valuable information about placental transfer has been obtained from study of the chronic fetal sheep model, and from the human being at the time of therapeutic abortion and term, both sets of data must be applied cautiously. Interspecies differences can be substantial, and the placenta itself is not static during the course of gestation.

Only endogenous compounds, or drugs

that closely resemble them, are likely to be transported actively or by facilitative diffusion across the placenta. Most drugs traverse the placenta by simple passive diffusion, but rates of transfer vary appreciably between compounds. The rate of simple diffusion is governed by many factors, which include the gradient of free drug, its molecular weight, solubility in lipid, and degree of ionization. These criteria are similar to those described for diffusion through any biological membrane, but distinctive aspects of different membrane systems have been observed. Drugs of low molecular weight and substantial hydrophobicity, such as morphine, caffeine and diazepam, cross the placenta rapidly. Others that are more hydrophilic or larger, such as salicylate, succinylcholine, heparin and insulin, traverse the placenta more slowly. Since metabolism tends to impart hydrophilicity, metabolites are likely to enter the fetus more slowly than parent drugs. Affixation of drug to maternal plasma protein will decrease the rate of placental transfer because maternal concentrations of free drug will have been correspondingly decreased. Any differences between mother and fetus with respect to plasma protein binding of drug will be reflected by differences in plasma concentrations of total drug (not unbound drug) at equilibrium.

For drugs that equilibrate rapidly between mother and fetus (or better, between uterine vein and umbilical vein), the quantitative aspects of fetal exposure mimic closely those of the mother within certain constraints of maternal rates of absorption, elimination and uterine blood flow (Fig. 112–1). The quantitative significance of changes in uterine and umbilical blood flow on placental transfer rates depends on the rapidity of diffusion. Uterine blood flow is decreased by certain drugs including epinephrine, methoxamine and nicotine.

The kinetic situation is more complex when rates of diffusion across the placenta are lower. After a single dose of a drug that diffuses slowly and passively across the placenta, the fetal maternal plasma concentration ratio will vary from less than to greater than unity as a function of time (Fig. 112–1); cord plasma concentrations of free drug that surpass maternal values do

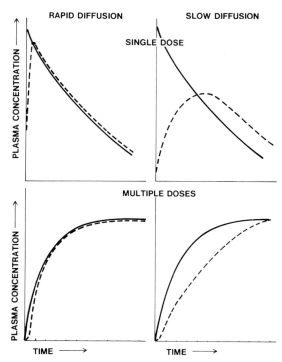

*Figure 112–1.* Schematic representation of maternal (———) and fetal (– – – –) plasma concentrations of drug with time after single intravenous or multiple doses. Simple transplacental diffusion rates that are rapid (left) or slow (right) are hypothesized.

not necessarily indicate active transport. Minuscule fetal accumulation after a single maternal dose does not imply low fetal concentration of drug at steady state. Slow transfer rates do not preclude the teratogenic potential for a drug administered chronically during pregnancy.

The placenta itself may not be inert with respect to the metabolism of drugs. The presence of oxytocinase and sulfatase activities might be important. The placenta can exhibit substantial amounts of at least one type of xenobiotic oxidative activity: aryl hydrocarbon hydroxylase. This placental activity, attributable to a subclass of the cytochrome P-450 mono-oxygenase system, is increased by maternal cigarette smoking in some individuals. Although a related hepatic mono-oxygenase system is involved in most drug oxidations, it seems that only a few foreign compounds serve as substrates for the human placental system. The most likely explanation relates "to the fact that human placental cytochrome P-450 exhibits a high specificity with respect to substrate binding as well as to the positional hydroxylation of steroid molecules" (Juchau). Further investigations of placental oxidative, conjugative and hydrolytic activities are needed.

The capacity of the maternal organism to dispose of drugs cannot be ignored in considerations of fetal exposure. The ultimate source of drug elimination is the mother, yet clinical pharmacologic studies in the gravid woman are scarce. Many maternal changes do occur as the result of pregnancy, and some will surely influence fetal exposure to xenobiotics. These include, in the third trimester, a substantial decrease in plasma albumin concentration (approximately 1 gm per 100 ml), an increase in glomerular filtration rate, and changes in blood flow and its distribution. There is some evidence to suggest deficient drug oxidation (meperidine) and glucuronidation (salicylamide). The effects of illnesses such as pre-eclampsia and toxemia of pregnancy on pharmacokinetic variables remain virtually unexplored.

## SUSPECTED TERATOGENS

The thalidomide disaster has dramatically alerted the community to the devastating potential teratogenic effects of a minor hypnotic agent. Anomalies are produced with high frequency upon exposure to thalidomide, and some of the abnormalities (phocomelia, major anomalies of the ears and auditory canal) are both very gross and very rare. These facts enabled astute observers to establish the cause-effect association rapidly.

Of deep concern in the present decade is the difficult problem posed by suspected teratogens. The establishment of a cause-effect relationship between the maternal ingestion of a drug and congenital anomalies is difficult when (a) the drug only rarely evokes the adverse effect, and (b) the abnormality itself is not uncommon (e.g., cleft lip and palate).

To illustrate the problems we will continue to face in this area, consider phenytoin. In 1968, Meadow reported a higher than expected incidence of cleft lip and palate in association with maternal anticonvulsant usage. Other congenital anomalies, including malformation of the heart, were also implicated. Subsequent reports, some anecdotal and all retrospective, described widely discrepant incidences of cleft palate in exposed infants. Between 1971 and 1975, a series of studies from different countries revealed that infants born to mothers receiving anticonvulsant drugs during early pregnancy had an overall malformation rate approximately two to four times greater than control groups. The fetuses of epileptic women not receiving anticonvulsants did not appear to be at increased risk. The number of patients in the latter category was small, and one could argue that the epilepsy itself in that group was likely to be less severe.

In addition to cleft palate, certain congenital heart defects, delayed psychomotor development and cerebral malformations, a few specific abnormalities have been attributed to phenytoin. These include unusual and characteristic facies and distal phalanges (Loughnan et al.; Hanson and Smith). One large study comprising about 50,000 pregnancies focused on certain abnormalities selected from the above list, and indicated a barely significant ($p \approx 0.03$) association between congenital malformations and the use of phenytoin in the first trimester. The association also approached statistical significance when phenytoin was utilized after 4 months of gestation only; similar findings apply to fetuses of women with convulsive disorders *not* treated with the hydantoin. The actual incidence rates for these three groups were 6 of 98, 4 of 78 and 3 of 101, respectively. These data are included not to minimize significance but rather to emphasize the difficulty in deriving unqualified conclusions even in comprehensive, expensive and time-consuming studies.

The fact that many investigators have independently reached the conclusion that overall malformation rates of epileptic women treated with anticonvulsants are two to four times higher than expected cannot be ignored. Nevertheless, it remains possible that the epilepsy itself, or some other, unrecognized, confounding factor may explain the association. It is our current opinion that the association of anomalies with a specific anticonvulsant is not yet known. Phenytoin and phenobarbital are the most commonly used anticonvulsants; it is not surprising that, rightly or wrongly, they are under most suspicion. However, there is no evidence to indicate that available alternative agents are any safer. If a mother's seizures are insignificant in type, or very infrequent, a trial without anticonvulsant therapy may be warranted. This may also apply if, for reasons of inadequate dose or compliance, plasma concentrations of drug are found to be minuscule. On the other hand, where anticonvulsant therapy is clearly indicated, it is our opinion that it should be continued. Although one would recommend the lowest dose consistent with seizure control, the dose-response aspects of human anticonvulsant teratogenicity are unknown.

Wilson has estimated that about 2 to 3 per cent of developmental defects in man can be attributed with confidence to specific drugs and environmental chemicals. The etiologies in about 70 per cent of defects are unknown, and interactions of xenobiotics with genetic factors, infections, and various disorders remain feasible. Wilson lists as "suspected of some teratogenic potential" phenytoin, phenobarbital, trimethadione, dextroamphetamine, phenmetrazine, tolbutamide and other sulfonureases, and alkylating agents. Alcohol and warfarin can be included. A second category of "drugs possibly teratogenic under some conditions" includes aspirin, some antibiotics, antituberculous agents, quinine, imipramine, insulin and female sex hormones. Each requires a risk to benefit analysis in individual patients, not unlike that advocated above for phenytoin. Certain drugs once suspect but now thought to "pose little or no risk at recommended usage levels" include bacteriostatic sulfonamides, meclizine and current "tranquilizers and antiemetics generally."

## TRENDS IN RESEARCH

Marketing approval for a new drug requires animal investigations for teratogenic potential. Unfortunately, screens with common laboratory mammals are not foolproof, even though attempts are made to employ animals whose route(s) of drug metabolism resemble those of man. The extensive utilization of primates would be expensive, and the benefits of such a maneuver are not yet clarified. Many reasons can be cited speculatively for the occasional inadequacies of animal models. It is almost too obvious to recall the numerous ways in which species differ at the genetic, cellular, tissue and functional levels. Moreover, the fact that many xenobiotics are likely to prove teratogenic in only a small fraction of exposed individuals in any given species limits confident extrapolation.

The recent demonstration of drug-oxidizing capacity in certain human fetal tissues as early as the sixth week of gestation bears significantly on these questions of species and individual variability. The oxidative process can generate electrophilic metabolites, such as epoxides and N-hydroxides, that are potentially teratogenic, mutagenic or carcinogenic (Fig. 112–2). Under most circumstances, analogous activity is virtually absent in non-primate mammalian fetal tissue. The implications for teratogenic screening are apparent.

Upon exposure to polycyclic hydrocarbons, aryl hydrocarbon hydroxylase activity is induced in mouse fetal liver in mid-gestation. Nebert and colleagues have found that the abilities of fetal and adult mice to respond to this induction are under the control of a small number of genes. Phenotypic responsiveness is associated with a predisposition to the teratogenic effects of aryl hydrocarbons, even when the fetuses are compared to non-responsive phenotypes within the same uterus. The sum of these findings, as well as studies of detoxification enzymes such as epoxide hydrase and glutathione-S-epoxide transferase (Fig. 112–2), promises to open new dimensions in our understanding of teratology.

## DRUGS IN THE PERINATAL PERIOD

Many aspects of perinatal therapeutics and toxicology can be approached through consideration of the dose-response relationship. Quantitative aspects of this relationship are based on the reversible interaction between drug and hypothetical tissue receptor, the occupancy of which generates unit biological response. Overall response is then a function of the concentration of unbound drug in the vicinity of

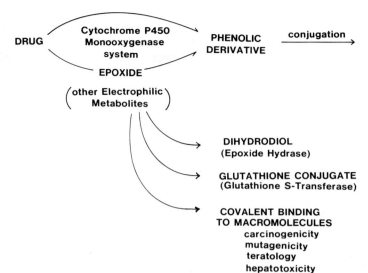

*Figure 112–2.* Toxification-detoxification potential of the cytochrome P-450 mono-oxygenase and related systems.

the receptor(s). In most cases, correlation of response with plasma concentration of drug (especially of unbound drug) represents a refinement of the classic dose-response relationship.

We must first ask whether or not the relationship between biological response and plasma concentration of unbound drug is identical in newborns and adults. On the one hand, many functions are intact at birth; on the other, brief observation of a 1000 gram premature infant convinces one that important pharmacodynamic differences must exist. Although these differences are likely to become the focus of perinatal pharmacology, especially with continued improvement of noninvasive technology, available information is sparse. Indeed, historical survey reveals that most pharmacologic mishaps that have occurred at the time of delivery or in the newborn nursery resemble adult drug overdose situations (Table 112–3). In those circumstances wherein plasma concentrations have been measured, the intoxicated neonate is found to exhibit drug concentrations that exceed the accepted adult therapeutic range. These high concentrations have usually been the result of unintentional portals of entry (placenta, inadvertent fetal injection, breast milk, skin, conjunctiva, and so forth), or of inappropriate dose schedules. The former problem can be ameliorated only by awareness and contin-

ued suspicion; recent tabulations of drug concentrations in breast milk are available (Ayd; Vorherr). The latter problem, that of neonatal dose schedules, occupies most of the remainder of this chapter.

We believe that the reliable achievement in newborns of plasma concentrations of unbound drug within the range defined as safe and efficacious in children and adults would in many cases afford substantial improvement in therapeutic result. The accomplishment of this objective is feasible but not simple. The difficulties are illustrated clearly by the two infants depicted in Figure 112–3. Each was full-term but

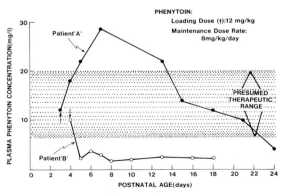

*Figure 112–3.* Plasma phenytoin concentration versus age curves in two infants (A and B) with asphyxic seizures. Each was treated with phenytoin, 8 mg per kg per 24 hours, after a loading dose of 12 mg per kg.

experienced asphyxic seizures soon after birth. There were no obvious clinical differences between the two at the time of initiation of anticonvulsant treatment with phenytoin. Each infant received an intravenous loading dose of 12 mg per kg of body weight and a maintenance dose rate of 8 mg per kg per day, a regimen designed to achieve and maintain a plasma concentration of about 15 mg per liter. The phenytoin concentrations observed after the loading dose conformed to predictions, and seizures ceased. Infant A, however, experienced a substantial increase in the plasma concentration of phenytoin over the next few days to the potentially toxic level of 28.6 mg per liter. Without alteration of the maintenance dose rate, concentrations of phenytoin decreased progressively over the next 2 to 3 weeks. Infant B experienced a sharp decrease in phenytoin concentration immediately after initiation of maintenance therapy. By the age of 3 to 4 weeks both infants were found to exhibit plasma concentrations of phenytoin of less than 5 mg per liter, and seizures recurred in one.

Complexity derives from the fact that most routes of drug elimination (Fig. 112–4) are more or less deficient in the newborn. The magnitude of the deficiency, as well as the rapidity and extent of functional maturation, is a function of 1) the pathway, 2) the drug, 3) postnatal age, 4) gestational age, and 5) individual factors presumably including genetic composition, general condition, specific illness, nutritional state, drug interactions, among others. We shall explore the implications of these pharmacokinetic characteristics (including defi-cient plasma protein binding), first with theophylline as an example of a drug, which like phenytoin, is dependent on oxidation for elimination. Discussion of theophylline in the context of treatment of apnea of the premature is not to be taken as an endorsement of the drug for this purpose.

## DEFICIENT PLASMA PROTEIN BINDING

The binding of many drugs, including theophylline, phenytoin, phenobarbital, salicylate and penicillins, to plasma protein is diminished in the newborn relative to the non-pregnant adult. Since unbound drug in plasma is considered to be the pharmacologically active fraction, a more intense response may be obtained in the newborn than in the adult at the same concentration of total drug in plasma. In adults with asthma, increasing bronchodilation is observed over the plasma concentration range of total theophylline, 5 to 20 mg per liter, but toxicity becomes more likely above 20 mg per liter. Let us assume tentatively the applicability to newborns with apnea of this upper limit of desired concentration, since it is set by toxicity, not efficacy. At the theophylline plasma concentration of 17 mg per liter, 56 per cent of the drug is affixed to protein in adult plasma. The therapeutic plasma concentration range in adults of 10 to 20 mg per liter, therefore, corresponds to 4.4 to 8.8 mg per liter of unbound theophylline. Only 36 per cent of theophylline is bound to protein in full-term newborn cord plasma. The concentration limits for unbound drug of 4.4 to

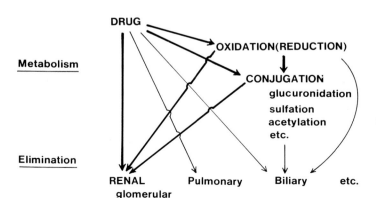

*Figure 112–4.* Schematic summary of major routes of drug elimination.

8.8 mg per liter would therefore correspond to a concentration range for total theophylline of 6.9 to 13.8 mg per liter. Binding may be even more deficient in plasma from premature infants, but data with theophylline are unavailable. This computed range for theophylline is remarkably similar to that (6.6 to 11.0 mg per liter) found appropriate by Shannon and colleagues during treatment of premature infants with apnea.

The postnatal age at which adult-like binding is attained is unknown, since most studies have been restricted to cord plasma samples. With phenytoin, most of the deficiency has disappeared before the age of 3 months. Hyperbilirubinemia accentuates the deficiency with the hydantoin, and probably other drugs as well (Rane et al.).

The cause (or causes) of the deficient plasma protein binding of drugs at birth is not yet defined. It is in part due to decreased plasma albumin concentrations (also applicable to the gravid woman at term), but competition by endogenous ligands or qualitative differences in neonatal plasma protein, or both, remain possible contributors. Decreased plasma protein binding need not affect dosage computations. It will, however, influence the translation of adult therapeutic plasma concentration ranges to the newborn. It will also affect calculations of volume of distribution based on plasma concentrations of total drug (see below). Finally, for an increasing list of drugs including phenytoin and theophylline, concentration within erythrocytes and saliva reflect the concentration of unbound drug in plasma.

## DECREASED RATES OF OXIDATIVE METABOLISM OF DRUGS

The patient's capacity to clear or eliminate a drug determines the rate at which it must be given to maintain a given plasma concentration. The disposition of the drug after a single intravenous dose and the steady-state concentration generated by a given maintenance dose rate are closely related. A two-year-old child with asthma (*C*) and a two-week-old premature infant with apnea (*D*) were treated with single intravenous doses of theophylline (4 mg per kg in 15 minutes). The log plasma concentration versus time curves are depicted in Figure 112–5. Plasma concentrations of total rather than unbound drug are presented because that is the usual manner in which such data are obtained. In both patients, the log of the plasma concentration (log $C_P$) of theophylline decreases linearly with time after a brief distributive phase. For the present purpose, we conclude from these data that the disappearance of drug from plasma is first-order, and that the entire body behaves kinetically as if it were a single compartment. In other words, over any given period of time, a certain percentage (not amount) of the theophylline remaining in the body is eliminated; and after the first few minutes, the plasma concentration reflects, or is proportional to, the concentration of drug in other portions of the body. These concepts apply with more or less accuracy to kinetic analyses of a wide variety of drugs. Some, such as diazepam and digoxin, require assumption of multicompartmental models for adequate interpretation; others, such as salicylate and ethanol, require analysis by saturation kinetics.

The time required for the plasma concentration of drug to decrease to one half its initial value is termed the half-life (t½). The apparent volume of distribution of the drug ($V_D$) can be computed from dose and

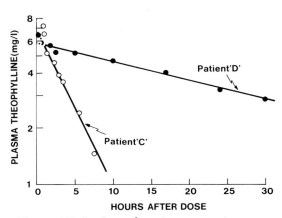

*Figure 112–5.* Log plasma concentration versus time curves for theophylline in a 2-year-old child with asthma (C) and a 2-week-old premature infant with apnea (D) after a single intravenous dose (4 mg per kg) administered in 15 minutes.

$C_P{}^o$, the hypothetical plasma concentration of drug at time zero (Fig. 112–5):

$$V_D(L/kg) = Dose\ (mg/kg)/C_P{}^o\ (mg/L).$$

It follows, of course, that the loading dose needed to generate a given plasma concentration is that concentration times $V_D$. $V_D$ is not meant to relate to a definable physiological or anatomical space. Body clearance rate ($Cl_B$) can be computed from $V_D$ and $t^{1/2}$:

$$Cl_B\ (L/hr/kg) = V_D[(L/kg) \times 0.693]/t^{1/2}\ (hr)$$

The values ($t^{1/2}$; $V_D$; $Cl_B$) for theophylline in 1 to 4 year old children with asthma ($n = 10$) and premature infants with apnea ($n = 6$) are presented in Table 112–4. Although $V_D$ in the newborn infants is somewhat increased, the predominant difference pertains to a diminished clearance rate, itself a reflection of a markedly prolonged $t^{1/2}$. Since the dose rate required to maintain a given steady-state concentration of theophylline ($C_P{}^{ss}$) is proportional to $Cl_B$ [$C_P{}^{ss}(mg/L) = $ Dose rate $(mg/kg/hr)/Cl_B$ $(L/hr/kg)$], the administration of maintenance doses designed to generate a plasma concentration of theophylline of 10 mg/L in 1 to 4 year old children would have generated concentrations greater than 50 mg/L (presumably toxic!) in the infants a few days after initiation of therapy. Since a greater fraction of total drug in plasma is unbound in the infants, the chances of toxicity would be even further enhanced.

**TABLE 112–4.** *Theophylline Elimination in Premature Newborns and Young Children*

| Age | Premature Infants[1] 3–15 days | Children[2] 1–4 yrs |
|---|---|---|
| $t^{1/2}$ (hr) | 30.2 (14.4–57.7) | 3.4 (1.9–5.5) |
| $Cl_B$ (ml/hr/kg) | 14 (10–21) | 100 (67–163) |
| $V_D$ (L/kg) | 0.62 (0.39–0.96) | 0.46 (0.29–0.67) |

[1]Aranda, J. V., et al.: N. Engl. J. Med. 295:413–416, 1976. Plasma values computed from blood values. Ranges in parentheses.
[2]Loughnan, P. M., et al.: J. Pediatr. 88:874 (1976).

Besides this effect on maintenance dose rate, these pharmacokinetic features of the neonate, drug oxidation, and elimination in general, have other implications:

1. The effects of a drug acquired transplacentally can be surprisingly prolonged.
2. The long $t^{1/2}$ allows recommendation that the daily maintenance dose be divided into fewer doses than would be necessary in young children.
3. This recommendation is strengthened by the observation that the absorption of many drugs administered orally to newborns is slow, albeit complete.
4. The prolonged $t^{1/2}$ implies that the need for a loading dose is greater in neonates than in young children, since four to five $t^{1/2}$'s are required to reach $C_P{}^{ss}$.
5. Since the $V_D$'s of many drugs are not grossly dissimilar in newborns and young children, loading dose (mg/kg) will vary less with age than does maintenance dose rate, especially if account is taken of decreased binding to plasma protein. Perinatal changes in extracellular water and fat contents are probably responsible for many of the small changes seen in $V_D$.

## VARIABILITY IN ELIMINATION BY OXIDATIVE METABOLISM

The relative deficiency in the capacity to oxidize a drug at birth, as well as the rate of maturation of that capacity, varies with the drug. Both characteristics, the deficiency at birth and the rate of maturation, also exhibit marked individual variability. Most drugs, including phenytoin, phenobarbital, diazepam, amobarbital, tolbutamide, nortriptylene, mepivacaine, theophylline and caffeine, exhibit prolonged $t^{1/2}$'s and/or low $Cl_B$'s shortly after birth (Neims et al.). Carbamazepine does not. Even among those drugs poorly disposed of, there are quantitative differences; for example, elimination of the methylxanthines is substantially slower than that of phenytoin, both relative to adult values. As the capacity to oxidize these drugs improves, there is a concomitant diminution in individual variation. The rate of maturation seems more rapid with phenytoin and phenobarbital than with the methylxanthines. $Cl_B$ for phenytoin surpasses relative adult values by age

2 weeks, whereas $Cl_B$ for theophylline is still deficient at age 2 months. There is little evidence to support the view that xenobiotic induction, midgestationally or perinatally, plays an important role in these processes.

The influences of gestational age and birth per se are not clearly defined. The capacities to oxidize antipyrine and diazepam are more deficient in premature infants than in their full-term counterparts. There is good evidence in guinea pigs and some evidence in human beings that birth per se does initiate maturation of drug oxidative function, although the rate of maturation may be slower in very-low-birth-weight infants. That aspect of birth which triggers maturation is undefined. The two- to fourfold deficiency in $Cl_B$ associated with most oxidized drugs at birth correlates well with fetal hepatic concentrations of cytochrome P-450 mono-oxygenase activity observed midgestationally. The dependence of deficiency and rate of maturation on drug per se can be attributed speculatively to differing maturational sequences for the different subclasses of cytochrome P-450, each of which likely possesses distinctive substrate specificity. The adrenal gland could play a role in these processes. The influences of specific illness, general condition, hypoxemia, nutritional state, drug interactions (e.g., prenatal treatment with glucocorticoid) and other factors on oxidative drug capacity remain virtually unexplored.

## DRUGS THAT UNDERGO CONJUGATION BEFORE ELIMINATION

Certain important conjugative processes, especially glucuronidation, are also deficient at birth. This deficiency has contributed to the chloramphenicol-induced "gray baby syndrome" (Burns et al.), and it may also play a role in the potential toxicity of hexachlorophene in low-birth-weight infants. Most of the comments made above in reference to oxidation apply as well to the processes of glucuronidation. One exception is the virtual absence of glucuronidative capacity in midgestational human fetal liver. Sulfation, as distinct from glucuronidation, is active in the neonate, as evidenced by metabolite patterns of acetaminophen. Acetylation, glutathione conjugation, mercapturic acid formation and conjugation with amino acids are processes likely to be somewhat deficient at birth. Maturational characteristics of hepatic blood flow, transport of drugs into hepatocytes, intracellular binding of drugs and biliary secretion, alone or in combination, are likely to influence the disposition of certain drugs.

## DRUGS ELIMINATED BY THE KIDNEY

The most important characteristics of the neonatal renal function relative to drug elimination include a low glomerular filtration rate, glomerular preponderance, nephron heterogeneity, low effective renal blood flow and low tubular function compared to the adult. Neonatal glomerular filtration rate is about 30 per cent of that of the adult expressed per unit surface area; adult values are reached at about one year of age (Weil). The renal clearance of inulin, a measure of GFR, is about 20 ml/min/1.73 $M^2$ during the first 12 hours (Oh). This increases to 35 to 45 ml/min/1.73 $M^2$ during the first week and progressively thereafter to the adult level of 125 ml/min/1.73 $M^2$ kg at 1 to 2 years of age. The plasma disappearance rates of aminoglycosides, kanamycin and gentamicin, which are eliminated mainly by glomerular filtration, reflect these changes in GFR. The dosage schedules recommended for these drugs have taken these variables into account.

Renal blood flow may influence the rate at which drugs are presented to and eliminated by the kidney. The average values for effective renal plasma flow, as measured by the para-aminohippurate clearance ($C_{PAH}$), is 90 ml/min/1.73 $M^2$ in the neonate less than 12 hours of age, assuming complete extraction of PAH). Rapid changes occur during the first week, and these values increase to 150 to 200 ml/min/1.73 $M^2$. Adult values of about 600 ml/min/1.73 $M^2$ are achieved by age 1 to 2 years. Even when these values are corrected (PAH extraction is 60 per cent in infants, compared to greater than 92 per cent in adults), the renal plasma flow is still low in the infants.

The most commonly used drugs in a newborn intensive care unit population are antibiotics, particularly the penicillins.

Since more than 90 per cent of administered penicillin in adults is eliminated by tubular secretion, low tubular function in the newborn infant results in decreased clearance rates, especially during the first few days of life. Progressive maturation in tubular function occurs and renal clearance of many antibiotics has been shown to depend on postnatal age (McCracken et al.). The inverse, of course, applies to t½. The mean t½ of penicillin G is 3.2 hours in full-term infants 0 to 6 days of age, 1.7 hours in infants 7 to 12 days of age, and 1.4 hours in infants 14 days of age or older. The serum t½ of ampicillin in full-term infants is 3.1 to 4.7 hours by 3 days of age, and 1.7 to 2.3 hours by 7 to 10 days of age (Kaplan et al.). Analogy with the kinetic discussion of oxidized drugs is obvious. Dose and frequency adjustments have been recommended for the most commonly used antibiotics in the newborn period (McCracken).

These functions are dependent upon the gestational age of the infant. The low-birth-weight neonate has the lowest capability to excrete drugs, but there are little data concerning drug elimination in very immature neonates. During the first 3 days of life, serum ampicillin t½'s are 4.7 to 6.3 hours in premature infants, compared to 3.1 to 4.7 hours in the full-term newborns (Kaplan et al.). Methicillin t½'s are 3 times longer in premature than in full-term neonates. The difference in renal drug elimination between the very small (<1000 gm) and the larger premature or full-term infant should be seriously considered with drugs that have a low therapeutic index. Serum digoxin concentrations of 6.1 ng/ml and 1.4 ng/ml are observed in <1000 gm and >2500 gm infants, respectively, on the same maintenance dose rate (Table 112–5). Serum digoxin levels above 2 ng/ml tend to be associated with toxicity in adults.

Renal elimination of drugs may be modified by preceding or intercurrent pathophysiologic states. Increasing evidence indicates that renal function in respiratory distress syndrome and following perinatal asphyxia is impaired (Guignard et al.; Dauber et al.). The mechanism (or mechanisms) responsible for these impaired renal functions is not clear. Hypoxia per se may decrease renal drug elimination in the

**TABLE 112–5.  Serum Digoxin Concentrations in Infants[1]**

| Birth Weight | Serum Concentration of Digoxin |
|---|---|
| (Grams) | Mean in ng/ml (Number of Patients) |
| < 1000 | 6.1 |
| 1000–1250 | 4.4    (4) |
| 1250–1500 | 3.5    (3) |
| 1500–2000 | 2.1    (2) |
| 2000–2500 | 2.0    (4) |
| 2500 | 1.4    (1) |

[1]From Pinsky, W. W. et al.: Ped. Res. 10:333, 1976. Serum concentrations were obtained following loading dose of 31 ± 4.2 µg/kg and maintenance dose rate of 8.2 ± 2.6 µg/kg/24 hours.

newborn, since a two-fold prolongation in amikacin serum t½'s has been noted in hypoxemic infants (Mirhij et al.).

## CLINICAL IMPLICATIONS OF THE PHARMACOKINETIC CHARACTERISTICS OF THE NEWBORN

The sum of these observations on neonatal drug elimination gives us some clinical therapeutic guidelines, but creates many uncertainties. If rapid drug effect is needed, a loading dose (mg/kg) similar to that used in children is likely to be appropriate. To prevent the slow accumulation of drug to toxic levels, initial maintenance dose rates (mg/kg/day) are likely to be substantially lower than those for older children. The maintenance dose rate will likely require gradual augmentation to values possibly higher than those applicable in young children. Finally, both the initial maintenance dose rate and its rate of postnatal increment are likely to exhibit a degree of individual variability that occasionally prohibits establishment of fixed dosage rules, especially in the few days after birth. The therapeutic index of the drug will influence clinical flexibility. Appropriate caution, clinical awareness and monitoring of drug concentrations provide the best solutions at this time.

## HYPERBILIRUBINEMIA, BILIRUBIN DISPLACEMENT AND DRUGS

One must first distinguish between drugs that increase bilirubin load, such as excessive doses of vitamin K analogues, and agents that displace bilirubin from albumin, such as sulfisoxazole, salicylate, benzoate and furosemide. Although both groups may increase the risk of kernicterus, the serum concentrations of bilirubin increase with the former but decrease with the latter. The potential for drugs to compete with bilirubin for binding to plasma protein is assessed in vitro by methods that depend on such processes as the adsorption of bilirubin to Sephadex or erythrocytes, peroxidation of free bilirubin and fluorescence quenching.

Since the affinity constant that describes the interaction between bilirubin and the first binding site on albumin is about 1 nM, it is unlikely that any of the drugs in common use will displace substantial amounts of bilirubin from that site. Bilirubin affixed to the second binding site is less tightly bound (association constant, approximately $1\mu M$), and displacement by certain drugs is feasible. At given concentrations of serum bilirubin and albumin, the competitive process would assume most clinical significance in those infants in whom, for unknown reasons, the first binding site on albumin is available for only 0.5 to 0.7 mole-equivalents of bilirubin (Kapitulnik et al.). In such infants, if the serum albumin concentration is 3 g per 100 ml, the second binding site is partially occupied by bilirubin when the serum concentration of the latter exceeds 12 mg per 100 ml. Prematurity, acidemia, and low serum albumin concentration, as well as hyperbilirubinemia, weigh against the use of drugs known to displace bilirubin from albumin. The extent of displacement is a function of the plasma concentration of displacing drug; in this clinical circumstance higher drug potency provides therapeutic advantage.

## REFERENCES

Aranda, J. V., Cohen, S., and Neims, A. H.: Drug utilization in a newborn intensive care unit. J. Pediatr. 89:315–317, 1976.

Aranda, J. V., Sitar, D., Parsons, W., Loughnan, P., and Neims, A. H.: Pharmacokinetic aspects of theophylline in premature newborns. N. Engl. J. Med. 295:413–416, 1976.

Avery, M. E.: Pharmacological approaches to the acceleration of fetal lung maturation. Br. Med. Bull. 31:13–17, 1975.

Ayd, F. J. (Ed.): Breast Milk. International Drug Therapy Newsletter, 8:33–39, 1973. (Ayd Medical Communications Ltd., Publ.)

Burns, L. E., Hodgman, J. E., and Cass, A. B.: Fatal circulatory collapse in premature infants receiving chloramphenicol. N. Engl. J. Med. 261 1318–1321, 1959.

Chung, L. W. K., Weimar, W. R. Jr., Hales, B., and Neims, A. H.: Perinatal toxicology: The question of delayed and residual effects. *In* Sellers, E. M. (Ed.): Clinical Pharmacology of Psychoactive Drugs. Toronto, Alcohol and Addiction Foundation, 1975, p. 15–33.

Dauber, I. M., Krauss, A. N., Synchyk, P. S., and Auld, P. A. M.: Renal failure following perinatal anoxia. J. Pediatr. 88:851–855, 1976.

Guignard, J. P., Torrado, A., Mazouni, S. M., and Gautier, E.: Renal function in respiratory distress syndrome. J. Pediatr. 88:845–850, 1976.

Hanson, J. W., and Smith, D. W.: The fetal hydantoin syndrome. J. Pediatr., 87:285–290, 1975.

Herbst, A. L., Ulfelder, H., and Poskanzer, D. C.: Adenocarcinoma of the vagina. Association of maternal stilbesterol therapy with tumor appearance in young women. N. Engl. J. Med. 284:878–881, 1971.

Juchau, M. R.: Mixed-function oxidation in the human placenta. *In* Morselli, P. L., Garattini, S., and Sereni, F. (Eds.): Basic and Therapeutic Aspects of Perinatal Pharmacology. New York, Raven Press, 1975, pp. 29–38.

Jusko, W. J.: Pharmacokinetic principles in pediatric pharmacology. Pediat. Clin. N. Amer. 19:81–100, 1972.

Kapitulnik, J., Horner-Mirashan, R., Blondheim, S. H., Kaufmann, N. A., and Russell, A.: Increase in bilirubin-binding affinity of serum with age of infant. J. Pediatr. 86:442–445, 1975.

Kaplan, J. M., McCracken, G. H., Horton, L. J. et al.: Pharmacologic studies in neonates given large dosages of ampicillin. J. Pediatr. 84:571–577, 1974.

Levy, G., Procknal, J. A., and Garrettson, L. K.: Distribution of salicylate between neonatal and maternal serum at diffusion equilibrium. Clin. Pharmacol. Ther. 18:210–214, 1975.

Loughnan, P. M., Gold, H., and Vance, J. C.: Phenytoin teratogenicity in man. Lancet 1:70–72, 1973.

Loughnan, P., Sitar, D., Ogilvie, R., Eisen, A., Fox, Z., and Neims, A. H.: Pharmacokinetic profile of theophylline in young children. J. Pediatr. 88:874–879, 1976.

McCracken, G. H.: Pharmacologic basis for antimicrobial therapy in newborn infants. Am. J. Dis. Child. 28:407–419, 1974.

McCracken, G. H., Ginsburg, C., Chrane, D. F. et al.: Clinical pharmacology of penicillin in newborn infants. J. Pediatr. 82:692–698, 1973.

Meadow, S. R.: Anticonvulsant drugs and congenital abnormalities. Lancet 2:1296, 1968 (Letter to the Editor).

Medical Letter. Drugs in breast milk. 16(6):25–28, 1974.

Mirhij, N., Reeves, M. D., and Roberts, R. J.: Effects of hypoxia on amikacin pharmacokinetics (abstract). Pediat. Res. 10:333, 1976.

Neims, A. H., Warner, M., Loughnan, P., and Aranda, J. V.: Developmental aspects of the hepatic cytochrome P-450 monooxygenase system. Ann. Rev. Pharmacol. *16*:427–445, 1976.

Odell, G. B.: The dissociation of bilirubin from albumin and its clinical implications. J. Pediatr. *55*:268–279, 1959.

Oh, W., Arulla, R. A., Oh, M. A., and Lind, J.: Renal and cardiovascular effects of body tilting in the newborn infant. A comparative study of infants born with early and late cord clamping. Biol. Neonate *10*:76–92, 1966.

Pinsky, W. W., Jacobsen, J. R., Gillette, P. C., Burdine, J. A., Adams, J. M., Rudolph, A. J., and McNamara, D. G.: Serum digoxin levels in premature infants. (Abstract) Ped. Res. *10*:333, 1976.

Pomerance, J. J., and Yaffe, S. J.: Maternal medication and its effect on the fetus. Curr. Probl. Pediat. *4*:1–60, 1973.

Rane, A., Lunde, P. K., Jalling, B., Yaffe, S. J., and Sjoqvist, F.: Plasma protein binding of diphenylhydantoin in normal and hyperbilirubinemic infants. J. Pediatr. *78*:877–882, 1971.

Robinson, J. R., Felton, J. S., Thorgeirsson, S. S., and Nebert, D. W.: Pharmacogenetic aspects of drug toxicity and teratogenesis in the newborn. *In* Morselli, P. L., Garattini, S., and Sereni, F. (Eds.): Basic and Therapeutic Aspects of Perinatal Pharmacology. New York, Raven Press, 1975, pp. 29–38.

Shannon, D. C., Gotay, F., Stein, I. M., Rogers, M. C., Todres, I. D., and Moylan, F. M. B.: Prevention of apnea and bradycardia in low-birth-weight infants. Pediatrics *55*:589–594, 1975.

Smithells, R. W.: Environmental teratogens of man. Br. Med. Bull. *32*:27–33, 1976.

Van Petten, G. R.: Fetal cardiovascular effects of maternally administered tricyclic antidepressants. *In* Morselli, P. L., Garattini, S., and Sereni, F. (Eds.): Basic and Therapeutic Aspects of Perinatal Pharmacology. New York, Raven Press, 1975, pp. 83–88.

Vorherr, H.: Drug excretion in breast milk. Postgrad. Med. *56*:97–104, 1974.

Warkany, J.: Congenital Malformations. Chicago: Year Book Medical Publishers, 1971, pp. 84–96.

Weil, W. B. Jr.: Evaluation of renal function in infancy and childhood. Am. J. Med. Sci. *229*:678, 1955.

Wilson, J. G.: Present status of drugs as teratogens in man. Teratology *7*:3–15, 1973.

Yaffe, S. J., and Juchau, M. R.: Perinatal pharmacology. Ann. Rev. Pharmacol. *14*:219–238, 1974.

# Appendices

# Appendix I

## PRINCIPLES OF FULL-TERM AND PREMATURE INFANT CARE IN NURSERIES*

Revised with assistance from Drs. Ronald Gutberlet and Elizabeth Brown

Ideally, most infants should be delivered in institutions capable of providing perinatal intensive care. Certain, "high risk," pregnancies should alert the medical staff to arrange delivery in a setting capable of prenatal monitoring and neonatal intensive care. Since about 40 per cent of neonatal problems are unpredictable, the need for transport of some infants to regional centers becomes apparent. A physician–nurse team from the center may go to the hospital of birth, stabilize the infant in a transport incubator, collect all pertinent facts about the pregnancy and delivery, see the parents and then accompany the infant in an ambulance or helicopter to the referral center.

I. *Medical Services and Policies*

A pediatrician, preferably board-certified, should be designated medical director of nurseries. He or she should be responsible for

1. Laying down written regulations with respect to all routines. These should cover in detail all aspects of the care and feeding of normal newborns, isolation of sick or suspect ones, nurses' notes, physicians' examination forms and notes, etc.
2. Daily rounds by himself (herself) or a qualified attending pediatrician.
3. Teaching conferences at regular stated intervals for obstetrical and pediatric house staff and attendants. A fetal mortality clinical-pathologic conference at least once a month is mandatory, and at least one neonatal morbidity conference each month is advisable.

II. *Nursing Service*

A. Supervisor
A registered nurse with special training in the care of newborns, and especially of premature infants.
B. Nurses and Nurses' Aides
1. Full-term nursery. One nurse or aide to 12 infants at all times of the day and night. One graduate nurse for no more than 24 full-term infants at all times.

---

*Adapted, in greatly modified form, from the pamphlet "Hospital Care of Newborn Infants," issued by the American Academy of Pediatrics.

2. Intermediate care nursery. A ratio of one nurse to four premature infants is recommended.
3. Neonatal intensive care nursery. A ratio of one nurse to one or two infants is desirable.

III. *Physical Care*

A. Regular Nurseries
(For babies weighing 5 pounds or more, or more than 36 weeks gestational age, delivered with sterile technique from uninfected mothers whose membranes had been ruptured less than 24 hours)
   1. Nursery units, as constructed in the following four paragraphs, should, if at all possible, be used intermittently. Newborns are assigned to units in such sequence that one unit is always empty. This should then be thoroughly cleaned and aired for a few days before babies are again assigned to it.
   2. Capacity: Eight to 12 bassinets per nursery unit, with one nurses' station and service unit for each two nursery units.
   3. Space: A minimum of 24 square feet per bassinet, preferably 30, with 2 feet between bassinets. Cubicles are not necessary or desirable.
   4. Environment: Temperature about 75° F, humidity about 50 per cent. Air-conditioning desirable if obstetrical suite is air-conditioned also.
   5. Equipment: Hot and cold running water and hexachlorophene dispensers with knee or foot control in each unit. Examining room adjacent to each unit, preferably with window through which babies are passed for examination.

B. Observation Unit
(For infants (1) whose mother's membranes had been ruptured 24 hours or more before delivery, (2) whose amniotic fluid had been discolored, viscid or foul-odored, (3) whose mothers have fever or obvious respiratory or skin infection and for babies delivered under unsterile conditions)
   1. Capacity: One bassinet per 10 to 15 regular nursery bassinets.
   2. Reversibility: Infants admitted to the observation unit may be transferred to the regular nursery if no infection becomes manifest in 24 to 48 hours, unless they had been exposed to an infected infant within that unit.

C. Neonatal Intensive Care Unit
The director of this unit should be full time with special training in neonatalogy.
   1. Capacity: From an obstetrical service which delivers 100 mothers a month one can expect five to ten low birth weight infants to be born each month. Three to six of these should weigh between 5 and 5½ pounds and can therefore be cared for in the regular nursery. Two to four will require premature nursery care. Since their average stay is about 30 days, facilities for four low birth weight infants per 100 deliveries to accommodate the maximum number anticipated each month ought to be sufficient. High risk and sick infants may also go to this facility, where nursing care, availability of house staff and special equipment should be optimal.

2. Nursing: One nurse for three infants is desirable; 1 nurse for each infant on a respirator is required.
3. Space: 30 to 50 square feet per bassinet.

IV. *Feeding*

A. Full-Term Infants
   1. Nothing by mouth until stable.
   2. Water every 4 hours for the next one or two feedings.
   3. Then milk feeding.
      a. Breast feeding every 3 or 4 hours thereafter, omitting the 2 A.M. feeding until the fourth night if desired.
         (1) Glucose water may be offered after each breast feeding until milk comes in.
         (2) Supplementary formula not to be offered without good reason.
      b. Bottle feeding at 8 or 12 hours and every 4 hours thereafter, unless demand feeding is specifically ordered by the attending pediatrician.
         (1) First day—usual house formula (20 calories per 30 ml).
         (2) Offer ½ ounce (15 ml) every 4 hours for 12 hours, then 1 ounce (30 ml) the next 24 hours, then increase ½ ounce every day as tolerated up to 3 ounces (90 ml).
         (3) Bottle-fed babies should be taken to their mothers at least twice a day for feedings, preferably for every feeding.
         (4) Offer water ad lib. if crying between feedings.
B. Premature Infants
   The feeding of premature infants must be individualized on the basis of the infant's vigor, the quality and quantity of nursing service available and generalizations about his nutritional requirements. During the first week of life the infant's minimal food requirements must be met without exceeding his ability to ingest and retain the food offered. The pediatrician after consultation with the nurse must prescribe in writing the detailed feeding orders:
   1. Technique of feeding; i.e., choice of nipple, indwelling catheter or gavage as indicated by the individual infant's sucking and swallowing ability. This decision is based on the nurse's and physician's estimate of the infant's status.
   2. Time of initiation of feedings: Vigorous infants may be given the first test feeding of water at 4 hours. The fluid requirement of 60 to 100 ml per kilogram per day may be given parenterally, using a mixture of one-third saline and two-thirds 5 or 10 per cent glucose in water during the first 24 to 48 hours in infants who are distended and in whom peristalsis cannot be demonstrated. Infants cared for in open warmers or low humidity environments may lose water through evaporation and require up to 200 ml per kg per day after the first week of age.
   3. The interval between feedings must be specified.
   4. The amount of each feeding and subsequent increases are ordered and are illustrated below. A SCHEDULE SUCH AS THIS MUST BE USED AS A BASE FROM WHICH ONE INDIVIDUALIZES THE FEEDING OF EACH INFANT ACCORDING TO HIS ABILITY TO INGEST AND RETAIN THE AMOUNT OFFERED.

### Guidelines for Feeding

| Weight | 1200 Gm° | 1200–1500 Gm° | 1500–2000 Gm° | |
|---|---|---|---|---|
| Feeding Interval: | q 2 hr | q 2–3 hr | q 3–4 hr | |
| Hours of Life | ml/feed | ml/feed | ml/feed | Type of Feeding # |
| 4–8 | 1–2 | 2–3 | 5–15 | sterile water × 1 |
| | 1–2 | 2–3 | 5–15 | D10W × 2°° |
| 8–12 | 1–2 | 2–3 | 5–15 | D10W : formula 1:1 |
| 12–24 | 2–4 | 4–6 | 5–15 | D10W : formula 1:1 |
| 24–48 | 3–6 | 6–9 | 10–25 | D10W : formula 1:1 |
| 48–72 | 4–8 | 8–12 | 15–35 | D10W : formula 1:1 |
| 72+ | 5–10 | 10–15 | 20–45 | full strength formula |
| Increment per feed per day after 72 hrs | 1–2 | 2–3 | 5–15 | formula |

°Infants less than 1200 grams, or larger infants in respiratory distress, may require IV feeding until they can tolerate sufficient enteral intake. If this period is prolonged, IV protein ± fat solutions should be considered.

#Feedings should be increased only if the preceding step is well tolerated as measured by gastric aspirates of less than 2 to 4 ml, no abdominal distention and no significant blood or sugar in stools.

°°D10W = 10 per cent dextrose in water.

5. The composition of the feeding mixture must be indicated. Premature infant formulas are available commercially. Widely advocated are those that have a low solute load, modified protein, and reduced fat. They are well tolerated in a concentration of .67 or .8 calorie per cubic centimeter, except in infants under 1200 grams, who may not tolerate more than 0.67 calories per cc.

6. No infants are to be fed by propping the bottles.

## V. Skin Care

Bathing upon transfer to the nursery. Some bathe daily thereafter, some do not.

## VI. Drugs and Vitamins

A. Indications for antibiotics *other than* overt infection
 1. Ruptured membranes with active labor over 12 hours and premature birth
 2. Foul-smelling, discolored or viscid amniotic fluid and premature birth
 3. Prolonged or complicated labor and premature birth
 4. Suspected infection in infant after nose, throat, urine, CSF and blood cultures have been performed
B. Dosages of antibacterial drugs (see Appendix IV)
 For gonorrheal ophthalmia prophylaxis:
  One drop of 2 per cent silver nitrate in each eye, or a 1 per cent solution in wax ampules.

    C. Vitamins
        1. Vitamin $K_1$: If mother has received none during labor, infant should be given one dose of 1.0 mg intramuscularly.
        2. Vitamin C
           a. In full-term infants 50 mg per day to be begun at 1 or 2 weeks of age.
           b. In premature infants 50 mg twice a day to be begun the day after oral feedings have been instituted, continued until an ACD mixture is started at one week of age.
        3. Vitamins A and D: One may safely wait until 1 or 2 weeks of age to add these.
        4. If a term infant is receiving a formula with vitamins in it, added vitamin drops would not be necessary.
        5. Vitamin E: If none in formula, give 15 to 25 I.U. daily (see page 870).

VII. *Humidity*

Fifty-five to 65 per cent; higher with increased concentrations of oxygen.

VIII. *Oxygen*

    A. All oxygen orders should be left by the pediatrician at concentration desired, not by flow as liters per minute. All nurseries for premature infants *must* be equipped with an oxygen analyzer in good working order, and should have facilities to measure arterial oxygen tensions.
    B. The oxygen concentrations in hoods and incubators should be determined hourly by a nurse on the nursery service and recorded on the infant's chart.

IX. *Nurse's special notes will be initiated promptly by the nursery nurse for all babies, and the physician should be notified for any of the following findings:*

a. Early jaundice
b. Labored breathing
c. Suspicion of any infection
d. Elevated or very low temperature
e. Cyanosis or pallor
f. Abdominal distention
g. Poor feeding or failure to eat
h. Vomiting
i. Loose stools
j. Excessive crying or hyperactivity
k. Twitching or convulsive movements
l. Excessive quietness or inactivity
m. "Baby doesn't look right"
n. No stools in twelve hours
o. No urine in twenty-four hours

All babies should have respirations and apical pulse recorded every four hours or more frequently as indicated.

Apical pulse is counted for 1 full minute, using a stethoscope. Respirations must be counted when the infant is asleep or quiet, preferably midway between feedings.

# Appendix II

## RESUSCITATION IN OBSTETRICAL DELIVERY ROOM

Revised with assistance of Dr. Ronald Gutberlet

*TIME* IS OF UTMOST IMPORTANCE. *DELAY* IS DAMAGING TO THE INFANT. *ACT* PROMPTLY, ACCURATELY AND *GENTLY*.

### Equipment

1. Infant warmer with heat on.
   The following are to be available and checked before each delivery.
   a. Full oxygen tanks and masks; one premature mask available in each resuscitator.
   b. Catheters: Numbers 8 and 10 polyethylene (sterile) (see p. 1044).
   c. Cole infant endotracheal tubes, sizes 10, 12, 14, dry, sterilized.
   d. DeLee suction trap with Rausch two-hole catheter (boiled), or wall suction.
   e. Plastic infant airway.
2. Infant laryngoscope with premature and newborn blade—available at all times.
3. Stethoscope—chained to each resuscitator.
4. Bulb syringe—(in obstetrical delivery setup).
5. Stopwatch.

### General Routine for All Babies

1. Suction the nose and oropharynx with the bulb syringe or catheter. This should be done as soon as possible after complete delivery. The baby should be kept below the level of the perineum to prevent loss of blood from the infant into the placenta. Then the cord should be clamped and cut and the infant placed at once in 15-degree Trendelenburg position in the warmed resuscitator. No attempt to tie the cord should be made at this time. The infant should be dried.
2. An evaluation should be made of the infant at 60 seconds and 5 minutes after birth, according to the criteria suggested by Apgar.

The following five objective signs are evaluated and each given a score of 0, 1 or 2. A score of 10 indicates an infant in the best possible condition.

| Score | Heart Rate | Respiratory Effort | Muscle Tone | Reflex Irritability (Response to Catheter in Nostril) | Color |
|---|---|---|---|---|---|
| 0 | Absent | Absent | Limp | No response | Blue, pale |
| 1 | Slow (below 100) | Slow Irregular | Some flexion of extremities | Grimace | Body pink Extremities blue |
| 2 | Over 100 | Good crying | Active motion | Cough or sneeze | Completely pink |

3. The baby must be kept *warm*, watched by a delivery room nurse. If further care is indicated, she should give the infant oxygen by mask at once, while notifying the anesthetist, obstetrician or pediatrician of the baby's condition.

*Clinical Classification of Infants*

*Usual Score*

  I. Apneic infants
    A. Moderately depressed, good heart beat                           4–7
    B. Severely depressed                                           0–3
 II. Infant breathing with poor air exchange, is cyanotic or pale, has gasping, shallow or intermittent respirations           4–7
III. Normal infant                                                8–10

*Group I.* Procedure for Severely Depressed Infant
    Direct laryngoscopy for diagnosis, aspiration of secretions, intubation and bag or mouth-to-endotracheal tube respiration should be done immediately.

Technique of laryngoscopy and bag ventilation
1. Place towel under infant's shoulders.
2. Laryngoscope is held in the left hand and introduced into the right side of the infant's mouth. Shift laryngoscope to center when the glottis is in view.
3. The laryngoscope should now be between the base of the tongue and the epiglottis. Now tilt the tip of the instrument upward to raise the epiglottis out of the way and thus expose the entrance to the trachea.
4. Introduce the endotracheal tube under direct vision from the right side of the infant's mouth and push tip into the tracheal orifice and advance it up to the flange.
5. Withdraw laryngoscope carefully so as not to displace tube, and then blow air or oxygen into tube.
6. The presence of the tube in the trachea can be proved by having air or oxygen cause the chest wall to rise.
7. Inflate the lungs with oxygen, delivered by bag or mouth applied to the tube, approximately 30 times a minute. Observe excursion of chest wall to judge appropriate volumes.
8. The endotracheal tube is removed when the infant is breathing spontaneously and the heart rate is maintained at 100 per minute or more.

External cardiac massage

If no heart beat is present, compression of the mid-sternum against the vertebral column at a rate of 100 to 120 per minute is indicated. During inflation of the lungs by artificial respiration, cardiac massage should be stopped, then resumed during expiration.

*Group II.* Infant breathing, but with poor air exchange, cyanotic or pale with gasping, shallow or intermittent respirations.
1. Give 100 per cent oxygen by mask.
2. Establish more adequate airway.
    a. Suction nose and oropharynx with catheter quickly and efficiently.
    b. Intubate trachea under direct vision at once for any of the following indications:
        i. Unequal respiratory movements or unequal expansion of lungs, when comparing both sides of the chest.
        ii. Retractions occurring immediately or soon after birth.
        iii. Inadequate air entry.
        iv. Any question of laryngeal anomalies which obstruct air exchange.
3. Stimulation of extremities with massage or a brisk slap on feet.
4. If the infant becomes apneic, oxygen by intermittent positive pressure is indicated.
5. Examination by pediatrician should be done as soon as possible, with particular attention to heart sounds, rate and rhythm, resonance and air exchange, retractions, muscle tone, Moro reflex and abdomen (liver size). Get an x-ray film of the chest if there is any reason to suspect diaphragmatic hernia or pneumothorax.

*Group III.* Normal Infants

Infants are vigorous and cough or cry within seconds. No further procedures are necessary.

ASPIRATION OF GASTRIC CONTENTS is indicated after the initiation of normal respiration if hydramnios was present, or if it is probable that the infant aspirated blood or meconium that he may subsequently vomit. Approximate measurement of fluid should be done and noted on infant's chart. (DeLee trap = 30 ml)

1. TECHNIQUE. A number 8–10 French suction catheter attached to a DeLee trap should be introduced into the esophagus through the mouth and with slow rotary movements advanced until it is 10 to 20 cm (5 inches) from the mouth. Then advance the catheter 2 to 3 cm (1 inch) more and aspirate, putting moderate pressure on the epigastrium.
2. If amount exceeds approximately 20 ml or if there is difficulty in passing tube, a pediatrician should be alerted and notified.

Anomalies such as atresias, tracheoesophageal fistula, and others, may first be suspected at this time.

*DRUGS*

Analeptics have no role in stimulating the first breath. The only drugs that are useful are the narcotic antagonists if maternal narcotics were excessive. Naloxone hydrochloride (Narcan) can be given in a dose of 0.01 mg/kg intravenously or intramuscularly.

### Correction of Acidosis

Severely asphyxiated infants may not respond to artificial respiration alone. Five to 10 ml of a solution of 25 mEq per 100 ml of $NaHCO_3$ in 10 per cent glucose by push into the umbilical vein is reasonable.

### *Maximum Catheter Measurements for Endotracheal Suction in Newborns*[*]

Weight of Baby

7.0 cm
☐ 500 gm

8.0 cm
☐ 600–1000 gm

9.0 cm
☐ 1100–1500 gm

10.0 cm
☐ 1600–2000 gm

11.0 cm
☐ 2100–2500 gm

12.0 cm
☐ 2600–3000 gm

13.0 cm
☐ 3100–3500 gm

14.0 cm
☐ 3600–4000 gm

[*]Measure catheter along appropriate line for weight. Add length of E-T tube which is sticking out of *mouth*. This is the *maximum* safe distance for insertion of suction catheter through E-T tube. (Courtesy of Kathryn D. Anderson, Children's Hospital-National Health Center, Washington, D.C.)

## REFERENCES

Apgar, V.: A proposal for a new method of evaluation of the newborn infant. Current Res. Anesth. 32:4, 1953.

Apgar, V.: Infant resuscitation. Postgrad. Med. 19:447, 1956.

Avery, M. E., and Fletcher, B. D.: The Lung and Its Disorders in the Newborn Infant. 3rd ed. Philadelphia, W. B. Saunders Company, 1974.

Day, R., Goodfellow, A. M., Apgar, V., and Beck, G. J.: Pressure time relations in the safe correction of atelectasis in animal lungs. Pediatrics 10:593, 1952.

James, L. S.: Onset of breathing and resuscitation. Pediat. Clin. N. Amer. 13:621, 1966.

Safar, P., and McMahon, M.: Mouth-to-airway emergency artificial respiration. J.A.M.A. 166:1459, 1958.

Silverman, W. A., and Anderson, D.: A controlled clinical trial of effects of water mist on obstructive respiratory signs, death rate and necropsy findings among premature infants. Pediatrics 17:1, 1956.

# Appendix III

## A PLAN FOR THE MANAGEMENT OF NEWBORN INFANTS WITH SUSPECTED ERYTHROBLASTOSIS

The instructions in force at the Sinai Hospital of Baltimore were composed by Dr. Eugene Kaplan and the full-time Pediatric Staff, with revisions by Dr. Ronald Gutberlet.

### OBSTETRIC RESPONSIBILITY

1. Early recognition of maternal isosensitization.
2. Follow-up of maternal titers and amniotic fluid pigment during pregnancy.
3. Notification of the responsible pediatrician before delivery of each sensitized mother. The maternal history with respect to previous immunization experience and fetal outcome, the estimated duration of this pregnancy and weight of this fetus are basic facts essential to the proper evaluation of the newborn infant and must be communicated to the pediatrician before actual delivery.
4. Elective section or medical induction should be performed for the indications listed in Chapter 71 at a time convenient to the pediatrician and the laboratory in order to ensure essential clinical and laboratory help for a severely affected infant.
5. Clamping the umbilical cord early to prevent unnecessary placental transfusion of sensitized fetal erythrocytes.
6. Assuring the collection of essential cord blood specimens.

### PEDIATRIC RESPONSIBILITY

1. The pediatrician is directly responsible for the care of each infant born to an immunized mother. Upon notification of an expected delivery he must initiate preparations by the blood bank, delivery room personnel, and laboratory. A supply of *fresh* group O Rh-negative blood must be assured before delivery.
2. He must attend the delivery, quickly evaluate the newborn's clinical status, collect cord blood specimens, and direct procedures and decisions relative to replacement transfusion.
3. Proper diagnosis of Rh erythroblastosis includes positive direct Coombs test on infant blood, and demonstrable maternal antibody.
4. He must complete and record a physical examination of the infant as noted at birth.

5. Infants of Rh-negative mothers said to be unsensitized must have a cord Coombs test, hemoglobin, and blood grouping. These infants must be watched particularly.
6. ABO erythroblastosis causes early icterus without severe anemia or visceromegaly. The direct Coombs test result is often negative, but striking spherocytosis is evident in blood smears, and free homologous antibody is commonly present in the infant's serum, if looked for early. The nursery personnel must be constantly alert for icterus in the first 12 hours and immediately notify the responsible resident.

## REPLACEMENT TRANSFUSION IN Rh ERYTHROBLASTOSIS

I. *Purpose*
   A. To prevent early death from anemic heart failure.
   B. To prevent later death or sequelae from kernicterus.
II. *Indications*
   A. At birth
      1. Immediate exchange is indicated for frank hydrops or anemic heart failure.
      2. Early exchange is indicated for cord hemoglobin less than 14 gm per 100 ml or cord bilirubin in excess of 4 mg per 100 ml.
   B. In first 24 hours
      1. Bilirubin rise of 0.5 mg per hr or more which threatens to exceed 20 mg per cent.
      2. Prematurity increases kernicterus risk. Exchange transfusion is indicated if anemia or icterus appears in first 12 to 18 hours.
      3. Lethargy, irritability, deviation from normal body tone or temperature may indicate early exchange.
      4. Albumin priming before replacement may be useful before the exchange transfusion, 1.0 gm per kg.
III. *Preparation of Blood*
   A. Type
      If selected before birth of infant:
      Group O, Rh negative, compatible with maternal serum, and of low titer.
      If selected after birth of infant:
      Rh negative blood of same major group as infant red cells.
   B. Freshness
      Coagulation factors and platelets decrease, and $K^+$ and contamination risks increase rapidly during storage. When possible, use blood less than 48 hours, certainly less than 96 hours old. Do not delay treatment in severe disease if fresh blood is not available.
   C. Anticoagulant
      Citrate-phosphate-dextrose is the preferable anticoagulant. Heparin advocates must use heparinized blood within 24 hours.
   D. Packed vs. whole blood
      Concentrated blood (by aspiration removal of excess plasma) is preferred when initial treatment is for real or threatened anemic heart failure.
      Whole blood is preferable when treatment is primarily for bilirubin withdrawal.

E. Temperature

Should approximate room temperature if time permits. Avoid rapid warming of refrigerated blood.

IV. *Procedure*

A. The infant

Pre-exchange — Aspirate stomach contents

Administer vitamin $K_1$, 1 mg

During exchange — Constant monitoring by senior assistant.

Airway, body temperature, safe venous pressure (6-12 cm blood), cardiovascular stress signals such as restlessness, salivation, rales, changes in cardiac rate, rhythm, sounds, or EKG patterns. (Continuous EKG monitoring is valuable.) Slow down or stop procedure temporarily for any stress signal.

After transfusion — Obtain preterminal blood specimen for Hgb or Hct, and bilirubin. Follow postexchange values every 6 to 12 hours p.r.n.

B. The replacement transfusion

1. Terminal hemoglobin should not be less than 12 gm per 100 ml before withdrawal of catheter.
2. Amount of replacement: 160 to 180 ml per kg; more if conditions are favorable; less if anemia is severe.
3. Rate of replacement, 2 to 4 ml per minute per kilogram. Sicker infants should receive slower replacement procedures.
4. Calcium administration: For each 100 ml citrate blood replacement, give 1 to 2 ml of 10 per cent Ca gluconate. If bradycardia is observed, omit the next dose or give ½ dose for each 50 ml replaced.

# Appendix IV

## PHARMACOPEIA FOR THE NEWBORN PERIOD

Compiled with the assistance of Dr. Russell Asnes

ABBREVIATIONS: P.o.—by mouth  
I.v.—intravenously  
P.r.—by rectum  

I.m.—intramuscularly  
S.c.—subcutaneously  
Top.—locally

| Drug | Route and Dose | Special Hazards |
|------|----------------|-----------------|
| Achromycin | *See* Tetracyclines | |
| ACTH | I.m.; 3–5 units/kg/day, in 4 divided doses | |
| Actinomycin D | I.v.; 75 mg/kg, divided into 5 daily doses. Into tubing of rapidly flowing infusion | |
| Adrenalin | *See* Epinephrine | |
| Albumin, salt-free | I.v.; 1.0 gm/kg slowly | Hypervolemia, heart failure |
| Amphotericin B | (1) I.v.; 0.25–1.0 mg/kg/day, diluted to at least 1.0 mg/10 ml, in slow drip<br>(2) Top.; as 2% ointment (in liquid petrolatum 95%, polyethylene 5%) | Nephrotoxic |
| Ampicillin | Infants less than 24 hours: 50 mg/kg q 12 hr I.m.<br>Over 24 hours: 50 mg/kg q 8 hr I.m. | |
| Ascorbic acid | *See* Vitamin C | |
| Atabrine | P.o.; approximately 5 mg/kg b.i.d. or t.i.d. | |
| Atropine | (1) S.c.; 0.01 mg/kg Repeat q 2 hr p.r.n. | Hyperthermia, especially in brain-damaged, mentally defective or Down syndrome infants |
| Avertin | P.r.; 10 mg/kg/day q 6–8 hr. | |
| Bacitracin | (1) I.m. or I.v.; 500 units/kg/day, divided into 4 equal doses<br>(2) Top.; as ointment (500 units/gm), q 4–8 hr | Nephrotoxic |
| Banthine | P.o.; 3–5 mg q 4 hr a.c., increasing cautiously | Hyperthermia |
| Belladonna tincture | P.o.; 0.1 ml (0.03 mg atropine) q 4 hr a.c., increasing cautiously to flushing | Hyperthermia |
| Benadryl | P.o.; 5 mg/kg/day, divided into 4–6 equal doses, a.c. | |

| *Drug* | *Route and Dose* | *Special Hazards* |
|---|---|---|
| Blood (packed cells) | I.v.; 5 ml/kg. Repeat p.r.n. | |
| Blood (whole) | I.v.; 10 ml/kg. Repeat p.r.n. | |
| Calcium gluconate (9% calcium) | (1) I.v.; 0.5–1.0 gm/kg/day, in 2 or 3 divided doses. Dilute to 10% solution<br>(2) P.o.; 0.5–1.0 gm per dose, 2–4 times daily, diluted to 5% solution in milk or other fluid | Bradycardia if injected too fast<br><br>Necrosis from extravascular leakage<br>Gastric necrosis and calcification if too concentrated |
| Calcium lactate (13% calcium) | P.o.; 0.5 gm/kg/day in divided doses | Same as above |
| Carbenicillin | I.v.; 100–200 mg/kg/day divided in 4 doses | |
| Chloral hydrate | Hypnotic, P.o. or P.r.; 50 mg/kg/day<br>Sedative, P.o. or P.r.; 25 mg/kg/day | |
| Chloramphenicol | Premature infants, 10–25 mg/kg/day<br>Full-term infants, 50 mg/kg/day<br>P.o.; in 6 divided doses<br>I.m. or I.v.; in 3–4 equal doses | Death due to hepatic immaturity<br>"Gray baby syndrome" |
| Chloromycetin | *See* Chloramphenicol | |
| Chlorpromazine (Thorazine) | P.o., i.m., i.v. 2.0–2.5 mg/kg/day divided in 4 doses. | |
| Chlortetracycline | *See* Tetracyclines | |
| Chlor-Trimeton | P.o.; 0.5 mg/kg/day, divided into 4–6 equal doses, a.c. | |
| Colistin | I.m.; 1.5–5.0 mg/kg/day in 2 divided doses<br>P.o.; 15 mg/kg/day in 3–4 divided doses | |
| Cortisone | P.o.; 0.5–2 mg/kg/day, in 4 equal doses, reducing slowly to minimal effective dose, withdrawing cautiously | Spread of infection |
| Daraprim (pyrimethamine) | I.v.; 0.05 mg/kg/day | For toxicity folic acid 10 mg. |
| Demerol (meperidine) | P.o.; or I.m.; 1.0–1.5 mg/kg/dose q 4 hr p.r.n. | |
| Desoxycorticosterone acetate (DOCA) | I.m.; 1–5 mg/day, as required | |
| Dexamethasone | I.m. or I.v.; 0.5–1.0 mg every 6–8 hours | |
| Diamox | I.v. or P.o.; 5 mg/kg/day, divided into 3 equal doses | |
| Diazepam (Valium) | P.o., i.m., i.v.; 0.1–0.8 mg/kg/24 hr | |
| Dicumarol | P.o.; 30 mg daily, more or less, titrated by clotting time | |
| Digalen | P.o.; total dose 0.025 gm/kg, in 3–6 divided doses, at 6 hr intervals<br>Maintenance dose, $\frac{1}{10}$ total dose per day | |
| Digitalis | P.o., I.m. or I.v., same as Digalen | |

| *Drug* | *Route and Dose* | *Special Hazards* |
|---|---|---|
| Digoxin | P.o., I.m., or I.v.; total digitalizing dose 0.050 mg/kg (50 micrograms), ½ total dose stat, remainder in 2 divided doses at 4–6 hr intervals. Maintenance dose, ¼ total dose, in 2 divided doses daily | |
| Diphenylhydantoin sodium (Dilantin) | An intravenous loading dose is 8 mg/kg P.o., I.m. or I.v.; 3–5 mg/kg/day divided into 3 doses. Increase cautiously after second week up to 10 mg/kg/day. Blood levels indicated at higher doses. | |
| Diphtheria antitoxin | I.m. or I.v. 20,000–50,000 units/day for 2 or 3 successive days | Hypersensitivity reaction |
| Diuril | P.o.; 20–40 mg/kg/day in 2 divided doses | |
| DOCA | *See* Desoxycorticosterone acetate | |
| Epinephrine | S.c.; 1:1000 aqueous solution, 0.01 ml/kg/dose Repeat q 2–4 hr p.r.n. | |
| Erythromycin | P.o.; 50 mg/kg/day, in 4 divided doses I.m. or I.v.; 30–50 mg/kg/day in 3–4 divided doses | |
| Ethacrynic acid | I.v.; 1.0 mg/kg. Dilute with 5% dextrose and water and give over a 5-minute period | |
| Fibrinogen | I.v.; 50 mg/kg. Repeat p.r.n. as determined by clotting time | |
| Fluorocortisone | Top.; as 0.2–0.25% ointment, 3–4 times daily | |
| Folic acid | I.m.; 5 mg. Repeat in 7–14 days | |
| Furosemide | P.o. or I.v.; 1.0 mg/kg/dose | |
| Gamma globulin | I.m.; preventive—0.22 ml/kg I.m.; attenuating—0.05 ml/kg I.m.; for agammaglobulinemia, 1 ml/kg, repeated every 2–4 weeks | |
| Gantrisin | P.o.; 100 mg/kg/day in 4 equal doses I.m., I.v.; 50–75 mg/kg/day in 4 equal doses | In prematures or in presence of jaundice may lead to kernicterus |
| Gentamicin | 1.5 mg/kg/dose q 8 to 12 hr I.m. | |
| Gentian violet | Top.; as 1–2% aqueous solution, b.i.d. (skin) Top.; as 1% aqueous solution, b.i.d. (mouth) | |
| Glucagon | I.m. or I.v.; 30–100 $\mu$g/kg. May repeat after 6–12 hr. | |
| Heparin | Initial dose: I.v.; 50 units/kg Maintenance dose: 100 units/kg q 4 hr I.v. Titrate dose to yield 20–30 minute clotting time or 2–3 times pre-heparin clotting time | Intractable bleeding |
| Hydrocortisone | P.o.; 3–10 mg/kg/day, in 4 equal doses I.m. or I.v.; 25–50 mg, repeat q 6 hr p.r.n. | Spread of infection |

| Drug | Route and Dose | Special Hazards |
|------|----------------|-----------------|
| Hydroxystilbamidine | I.v.; in slow drip, 5 mg/kg in 1.0 ml of water, q 12 hr | |
| Indomethacin | P.o.; 0.1 mg/kg | |
| Insulin | For diabetic acidosis, 1 unit/kg initially, then ½–1 unit/kg q 1–3 hr p.r.n. | |
| Iron | P.o.; 6 mg/kg/day elemental iron | |
| Isoniazid | P.o.; 10 mg/kg/day, single dose | |
| Isuprel (isoproterenol) | I.v.; 1 $\mu$g/ml 5% dextrose and water, given as a drip at a rate of 1.0 cc/minute until effect is obtained | |
| Kanamycin | I.m., I.v.; 15 mg/kg/day divided into 2–4 doses | Nephrotoxic, ototoxic |
| Magnesium sulfate | I.m.; 0.2 ml/kg/dose 50% sol. q 4–8 hr (For tetanus neonatorum or other repeated convulsions) | Hypotension |
| Mecholyl | S.c.; 0.2 mg/kg. Increase by 25% and repeat q 15 minutes until desired effect. For paroxysmal tachycardia | Cardiac arrest. Antidote: atropine |
| Meprobamate | P.o. or I.m.; 10–25 mg/kg/day, divided into 2–3 doses | |
| Mercuhydrin | I.m.; 0.25–0.5 ml q other day, increase if necessary | |
| Mestinon | I.m.; 0.1–0.4 mg q 4–8 hr P.o.; 1.0–2.0 mg q 4–12 hr | |
| Methicillin (Staphcillin) | If under 24 hours of age, 100 mg/kg q 12 hr I.m. Over 24 hours of age, 100–200 mg/kg divided q 8 hr I.m. | |
| Methylene blue | Top.; 1% or 2% sol. I.v. for methemoglobinemia, 1% sol. 0.1–0.2 ml/kg I.v. slowly | |
| Methyl scopolamine nitrate | *See* Skopyl | |
| Morphine sulfate | S.c.; 0.1–0.2 mg/kg/dose q 6 hr p.r.n. | |
| Mycostatin | P.o.; 100,000–200,000 units q 6 hr Top.; as 2% ointment (in liquid petrolatum 95%, polyethylene 5%) 3–4 times daily | |
| Nalline (nalorphine) | I.m. or I.v.; 0.1–0.2 mg/kg/dose | |
| Naloxone HCl (Narcan) | 0.01 mg/kg/dose. May repeat in 3–5 minutes. | |
| Neomycin | P.o.; 50–100 mg/day in 3–4 equal doses Top.; 0.5% ointment, 3–4 times daily | |
| Neostigmine | P.o.; 6–8 mg/day, divided into 4–8 doses | Cardiac arrhythmia |
| Nicotinic acid | 6 mg/day | |
| Nystatin | *See* Mycostatin | |
| Oxacillin (prostaphlin) | I.m., I.v.; 50–200 mg/kg/day, divided into 6 doses | |

| Drug | Route and Dose | Special Hazards |
|------|----------------|-----------------|
| Oxytetracycline | *See* Tetracyclines | |
| Pancreatin | P.o.; 0.3–0.5 gm with each feeding<br>P.r. and into colostomy; 0.3–0.5 gm in sufficient liquid (for meconium ileus) | |
| Papaverine | I.v., I.m.; 6 mg/kg/day, in 4 divided doses | |
| Para-amino salicylic acid | Not advised for newborns | |
| Paraldehyde | P.o., P.r., I.m.; 0.15 ml/kg. Repeat q 4–6 hr p.r.n. | |
| Paregoric | P.o. 3–6 drops every 3–4 hr | |
| Penicillin | I.m., I.v.; aqueous solution 20,000–50,000 units/kg/day. Increase to 2–3 million units/day for serious infections. Divide into 4–6 doses.<br>I.m.; 200,000 units/kg divided over 3–15 days (for treatment of congenital syphilis).<br>Locally, as ointment, 50,000 units/gm (for prevention of gonorrheal ophthalmia).<br>For treatment gonococcal ophthalmia 50,000 units/kg/day for 7 days, plus local drops | |
| Pentabarbital | Same as Phenobarbital | |
| Phenobarbital | P.o., I.m.; 8–12 mg/kg/day, divided into 4–6 doses | |
| Pitressin (aqueous) | S.c.; 1–3 ml/day, divided into 3 equal doses | |
| Plasma | I.v.; 20 ml/kg. Repeat p.r.n. | |
| Polymyxin B | I.m., I.v.; 2.5 mg/kg/day. Intrathecally, 1–2 mg qd for 3–5 days, then q.o.d. as long as needed. Solutions containing procaine should not be used for intrathecal administration | Nephrotoxic and neurotoxic |
| Prednisone | P.o.; 1–3 mg/kg/day, divided into 4 doses | |
| Priscoline | P.o.; 5–10 mg q 4–6 hr. | |
| Pro-Banthine | P.o., I.m.; 1–2 mg/kg/day, divided into 3 to 6 doses | |
| Prostigmin | I.m.; 0.5–1.0 mg q 4–6 hr<br>P.o.; 1.0–5.0 mg q 4–8 hr | |
| Protamine sulfate | I.v.; 1.0 mg for each 1.0 mg heparin in previous 4 hr | |
| Pyribenzamine | P.o.; 5–10 mg/kg/day, divided into 4–6 doses | |
| Pyridoxine | *See* Vitamin $B_6$ | |
| Quinidine | P.o., I.m., I.v.; 4 mg/kg/dose<br>Repeat q 2 hr until desired effect or toxicity | Check with electrocardiogram before each dose. Discontinue if QRS interval greater than 0.10 second |
| Silver nitrate | For gonorrheal ophthalmia prophylaxis, One drop 2% solution in each eye | |

| Drug | Route and Dose | Special Hazards |
|---|---|---|
| Sodium bicarbonate | For correction of acidosis: 5–15 mEq/100 ml – usually 60–80 cc/kg/day I.v. For resuscitation: 25 mEq/100 ml, 10 cc I.v. stat | |
| Sodium chloride | P.o.; 2–5 gm daily, added to total intake (for adrenocortical insufficiency) | |
| Solu-Cortef | I.m., I.v.; *see* Hydrocortisone | |
| Staphcillin | *See* Methicillin | |
| Streptomycin | I.m.; 40 mg/kg/day, divided into 2–4 doses | |
| Sulfadiazine | P.o.; 100 mg/kg/day, divided into 4–6 doses S.c., I.v.; 50–100 mg/kg/day, divided into 2–4 doses | Slow renal clearance may lead to excessively high blood levels. Contraindicated in presence of jaundice |
| TEM (triethylene melamine) | P.o.; 1–5 mg per day in courses of 4–5 days | Bone marrow depression |
| Tensilon | S.c., I.m.; 0.1 ml (as test for myasthenia gravis) | |
| Terramycin | *See* Tetracyclines | |
| Tetanus antitoxin | I.m., I.v.; 10,000–20,000 units on 2 successive days | |
| Tetracyclines | P.o., I.m., I.v.; 50 mg/kg/day in 4 divided doses orally; 2–3 divided doses by injection | May stain teeth |
| THAM (tris-hydroxymethylamino-methane) | 0.3 Molar solution in 10 gm per 100 ml glucose (pH 8.85). Dose: 1.0 ml/kg for each 0.1 pH unit below 7.4. Rate 1.0 ml/min by intravenous push. | |
| Thiamine | *See* Vitamin $B_1$ | |
| Thiomerin | I.m.; 0.1–0.25 ml/dose. May repeat every other day | Repeated urine examinations necessary |
| Thyroid extract | P.o.; 0.015 gm daily. Increase as indicated | |
| Tocopherol | *See* Vitamin E | |
| Valium (diazepam) | For convulsions: 0.2 mg I.v. up to 2.0 mg Tranquilizer: p.o., im., iv. 0.1–0.8 mg/kg/24 hrs. | |
| Vitamin A | P.o.; preventive, 600–1000 units/day | |
| Vitamin $B_1$ (thiamine) | P.o.; preventive, 0.5–1.0 mg q.d. I.m.; therapeutic, 10 mg q 6–8 hr | |
| Vitamin $B_6$ (pyridoxine) | P.o.; preventive, 100 $\mu$g/liter of ingested formula P.o.; therapeutic, 2–5 mg/day Test dose for dependency, 50 mg I.v. | |
| Vitamin C (ascorbic acid) | P.o.; preventive, 25–50 mg/day, 100 mg mg/day for premature infants. P.o. or I.m.; therapeutic, 100 mg q 4 hr | |

| Drug | Route and Dose | Special Hazards |
|------|----------------|-----------------|
| Vitamin D | P.o.; preventive, 400 units/day | |
| Vitamin E | None additional needed in newborn period | |
| Vitamin K₁ oxide | I.m.; preventive, 1.0 mg, one dose only<br>Im.; therapeutic, 2.5–5.0 mg q 6–12 hr, titrated by prothrombin time | |

### Placental Transfer of Antibiotics[*]

| Antibiotic | Route of Administration | Time Elapsed After Administration | Maternal-Fetal Ratio | Authors |
|------------|------------------------|-----------------------------------|----------------------|---------|
| Chloramphenicol | Oral | 1 hr | 1 | Scott et al., 1960 |
| Penicillin G | I.m. | 1 hr<br>2 hr<br>6 hr | 3<br>2<br>1.4 | Woltz et al., 1945 |
| Long-acting penicillin | I.m. | 1 hr<br>2 hr<br>6 hr | 2<br>2<br>0.8 | Woltz et al., 1945 |
| Dicloxacillin | I.v. | 1½ hr | 3.3 | MacAuley et al., 1968 |
| Cephalothin | I.v. | Immediately afterward | 2.5 | MacAuley et al., 1968 |
| Tetracyclines | I.m. | 1 hr<br>2 hr | 4<br>2 | Elliott et al., 1957 |
| Ampicillin | I.m. | ½ hr<br>1 hr<br>2 hr | 2<br>1<br>0.33 | Blecher et al., 1966 |
| Streptomycin | I.m. | 1 hr | 4 | Grasset et al., 1951 |
| Erythromycin | Oral | 1 hr | Not detectable in fetal blood | Kiefer et al., 1955 |
| Rifomycin | I.m. | 1 hr | 20 | Mainardi and Sacchetti, 1966 |

[*]Courtesy of Dr. F. Sereni, University of Milan, Italy.

### Correlations Between Gestation Length and Embryonic and Fetal Bodily Dimensions

| Week of Gestation | Crown-rump Length (cm) | Weight (G) | Biparietal Diameter (cm) |
|:---:|:---:|:---:|:---:|
| 6 | 0.5 | | |
| 7 | 0.8 | 0.07 | |
| 8 | 1.5 | 0.22 | |
| 9 | 2.5 | 0.88 | |
| 10 | 3.5 | 3.5 | |
| 11 | 4.6 | 6.0 | |
| 12 | 5.7 | 11.0 | |
| 13 | 6.8 | 19.0 | |
| 14 | 8.1 | 33.0 | |
| 15 | 9.4 | 55.0 | |
| 16 | 10.7 | 80.0 | |
| 17 | 12.1 | 120.0 | 3.7 |
| 18 | 13.6 | 170.0 | 4.0 |
| 19 | 15.3 | 253.0 | 4.4 |
| 20 | 16.4 | 316.0 | 4.8 |
| 21 | 17.5 | 385.0 | 5.2 |
| 22 | 18.6 | 460.0 | 5.5 |
| 23 | 19.7 | 542.0 | 5.75 |
| 24 | 20.8 | 630.0 | 5.95 |
| 25 | 21.8 | 723.0 | 6.1 |
| 26 | 22.8 | 823.0 | 6.2 |
| 27 | 23.8 | 930.0 | 6.35 |
| 28 | 24.7 | 1045.0 | 6.5 |
| 29 | 25.6 | 1174.0 | 6.65 |
| 30 | 26.5 | 1323.0 | 6.85 |
| 31 | 27.4 | 1492.0 | 7.1 |
| 32 | 28.3 | 1680.0 | 7.3 |
| 33 | 29.3 | 1876.0 | 7.6 |
| 34 | 30.2 | 2074.0 | 7.8 |
| 35 | 31.1 | 2274.0 | 8.1 |
| 36 | 32.1 | 2478.0 | 8.35 |
| 37 | 33.1 | 2690.0 | 8.6 |
| 38 | 34.1 | 2914.0 | 8.9 |
| 39 | 35.1 | 3150.0 | 9.2 |
| 40 | 36.2 | 3405.0 | 9.55 |
| 41 | | 3600.0 | 9.8 |
| 42 | | 3650.0 | 9.85 |
| | | 3750.0 | 10.0 |
| | | 3900.0 | 10.2 |
| | | 4000.0 | 10.3 |
| | | 4200.0 | 10.6 |

Data based on the study of Bartolucci: Amer. J. Obstet. Gynecol. *122*:439, 1975. Courtesy of Iffy, L., et al.: Pediatrics *56*:173, 1975.

### Thyroid Function Values

| Age | Protein Bound Iodine µg % | BEI or $T_4$ (µg %) | Free $T_4$ (µg %) | $T_3$ uptake % |
|:---:|:---:|:---:|:---:|:---:|
| Maternal | 7.4 ± 0.4 | 14.2 ± 2.6 | 3.37 ± 0.64 | |
| Cord | 6.8 ± 0.4 | 12.6 ± 4.0 | 3.57 ± 0.84 | 16.3 |
| 0–12 hours | 8.3 ± 2.4 | | 5.4 ± 0.3 | |
| 12–24 hours | 10.1 ± 1.4 | | | |
| 1–3 days | 12.0 ± 2.4 | | 8.6 ± 0.4 | |
| 3–7 days | 10.9 ± 1.8 | 9.9 ± 2.1 | | 19.8 |
| 1–5 weeks | 7.4 ± 1.8 | 4.6 ± 0.3 | | 17.5 |
| | (Mean ± S. E.) | | | |

Data of Fisher and Odell (1966); Oddie and Fisher (1967); Marks, Hamlin, and Zack (1966); Czerichow et al. (1970); and Marks et al. (1961).

## Body Composition of the Reference Fetus

| Gestational Age (weeks) | Body Weight (gm) | Water (gm) | Protein (gm) | Lipid (gm) | Other (gm) | Water (gm) | Protein (gm) | Ca (mg) | P (mg) | Mg (mg) | Na (meq) | K (meq) | Cl (meq) |
|---|---|---|---|---|---|---|---|---|---|---|---|---|---|
| | | *per 100 gm body weight* | | | | *per 100 gm fat-free weight* | | | | | | | |
| 24 | 690 | 88.6 | 8.8 | 0.1 | 2.5 | 88.6 | 8.8 | 621 | 387 | 17.8 | 9.9 | 4.0 | 7.0 |
| 25 | 770 | 87.8 | 9.0 | 0.7 | 2.5 | 88.4 | 9.1 | 615 | 385 | 17.6 | 9.8 | 4.0 | 7.0 |
| 26 | 880 | 86.8 | 9.2 | 1.5 | 2.5 | 88.1 | 9.4 | 611 | 384 | 17.5 | 9.7 | 4.1 | 7.0 |
| 27 | 1010 | 85.7 | 9.4 | 2.4 | 2.5 | 87.8 | 9.7 | 609 | 383 | 17.4 | 9.5 | 4.1 | 6.9 |
| 28 | 1160 | 84.6 | 9.6 | 3.3 | 2.4 | 87.5 | 10.0 | 610 | 385 | 17.4 | 9.4 | 4.2 | 6.9 |
| 29 | 1318 | 83.6 | 9.9 | 4.1 | 2.4 | 87.2 | 10.3 | 613 | 387 | 17.4 | 9.3 | 4.2 | 6.8 |
| 30 | 1480 | 82.6 | 10.1 | 4.9 | 2.4 | 86.8 | 10.6 | 619 | 392 | 17.4 | 9.2 | 4.3 | 6.8 |
| 31 | 1650 | 81.7 | 10.3 | 5.6 | 2.4 | 86.5 | 10.9 | 628 | 398 | 17.6 | 9.1 | 4.3 | 6.7 |
| 32 | 1830 | 80.7 | 10.6 | 6.3 | 2.4 | 86.1 | 11.3 | 640 | 406 | 17.8 | 9.1 | 4.3 | 6.6 |
| 33 | 2020 | 79.8 | 10.8 | 6.9 | 2.5 | 85.8 | 11.6 | 656 | 416 | 18.0 | 9.0 | 4.4 | 6.5 |
| 34 | 2230 | 79.0 | 11.0 | 7.5 | 2.5 | 85.4 | 11.9 | 675 | 428 | 18.3 | 8.9 | 4.4 | 6.4 |
| 35 | 2450 | 78.1 | 11.2 | 8.1 | 2.6 | 85.0 | 12.2 | 699 | 443 | 18.6 | 8.9 | 4.5 | 6.3 |
| 36 | 2690 | 77.3 | 11.4 | 8.7 | 2.6 | 84.6 | 12.5 | 726 | 460 | 19.0 | 8.8 | 4.5 | 6.1 |
| 37 | 2940 | 76.4 | 11.6 | 9.3 | 2.7 | 84.3 | 12.8 | 758 | 479 | 19.5 | 8.8 | 4.5 | 6.0 |
| 38 | 3160 | 75.6 | 11.8 | 9.9 | 2.7 | 83.9 | 13.1 | 795 | 501 | 20.0 | 8.8 | 4.5 | 5.9 |
| 39 | 3330 | 74.8 | 11.9 | 10.5 | 2.8 | 83.6 | 13.3 | 836 | 525 | 20.5 | 8.7 | 4.6 | 5.8 |
| 40 | 3450 | 74.0 | 12.0 | 11.2 | 2.8 | 83.3 | 13.5 | 882 | 551 | 21.1 | 8.7 | 4.6 | 5.7 |

Data of Ziegler, E. E., et al., University of Iowa, Iowa City, 1975.

## Estimated Daily Requirements of Premature Infants[*]

| | 750–1000 | 1000–1250 | 1250–1500 | 1500–1750 | 1750–2000 | 2000–2250 | 2250–2500 | 2500–2750 | 2750–3000 |
|---|---|---|---|---|---|---|---|---|---|
| **Growth and Non-Growth Body Weight Intervals (gm)** | | | | | | | | | |
| **Energy** | | | | | | | | | |
| Growth (kal) | 21 | 46 | 68 | 79 | 93 | 104 | 114 | 111 | 108 |
| Non-growth (kcal) | 71 | 94 | 117 | 133 | 156 | 180 | 204 | 215 | 239 |
| Total (kal/kg) | 105 | 124 | 127 | 130 | 133 | 133 | 134 | 124 | 121 |
| **Protein** | | | | | | | | | |
| Growth (g) | 1.78 | 3.45 | 4.44 | 4.79 | 4.85 | 4.90 | 4.68 | 4.27 | 3.77 |
| Non-growth (g) | 0.87 | 1.12 | 1.37 | 1.62 | 1.87 | 2.12 | 2.37 | 2.62 | 2.87 |
| Total (g/kg)[**] | 3.02 | 4.06 | 4.22 | 3.94 | 3.58 | 3.30 | 2.96 | 2.62 | 2.30 |
| **Sodium** | | | | | | | | | |
| Growth (mEq) | 0.95 | 1.68 | 2.10 | 2.21 | 2.21 | 2.21 | 2.10 | 1.89 | 1.57 |
| Non-growth (mEq) | 0.18 | 0.23 | 0.28 | 0.34 | 0.39 | 0.44 | 0.49 | 0.55 | 0.60 |
| Total (mEq/kg) | 1.29 | 1.69 | 1.73 | 1.56 | 1.38 | 1.24 | 1.09 | 0.92 | 0.75 |
| **Potassium** | | | | | | | | | |
| Growth (mEq) | 0.31 | 0.73 | 1.05 | 1.15 | 1.26 | 1.36 | 1.36 | 1.36 | 1.15 |
| Non-growth (mEq) | 0.20 | 0.26 | 0.32 | 0.38 | 0.43 | 0.49 | 0.55 | 0.61 | 0.66 |
| Total (mEq/kg) | 0.58 | 0.88 | 0.99 | 0.94 | 0.90 | 0.87 | 0.80 | 0.75 | 0.63 |
| **Calcium** | | | | | | | | | |
| Growth (mg) | 148 | 317 | 442 | 530 | 592 | 632 | 660 | 627 | 592 |
| Non-growth (mg) | — | — | — | — | — | — | — | — | — |
| Total (mg/kg) | 169 | 282 | 321 | 326 | 316 | 300 | 278 | 239 | 206 |
| **Phosphorus** | | | | | | | | | |
| Growth (mg) | 49 | 110 | 148 | 172 | 188 | 197 | 202 | 194 | 177 |
| Non-growth (mg) | 12 | 27 | 37 | 43 | 47 | 49 | 50 | 49 | 44 |
| Total (mg/kg) | 70 | 121 | 135 | 132 | 125 | 116 | 106 | 93 | 77 |
| **Magnesium** | | | | | | | | | |
| Growth (mg) | 9.0 | 18.5 | 25.5 | 30.0 | 33.5 | 35.5 | 37.0 | 35.5 | 32.5 |
| Non-growth (mg) | — | — | — | — | — | — | — | — | — |
| Total (mg/kg) | 10.3 | 16.4 | 18.6 | 18.5 | 17.8 | 16.7 | 15.6 | 13.5 | 11.3 |

[*]Assuming extent of intestinal absorption as follows: energy: 75 per cent absorption for infants weighing 750 to 1500 gm, 80 per cent for those weighing 1500–2500 gm and 85 per cent for those weighing more than 2500 gm; protein: 75 per cent absorption at 750–1250 gm, 77 per cent at 1250–1500 gm, 80 per cent at 1500–2250 gm, 83 per cent at 2250–2500 gm and 85 per cent above 2500 gm; sodium and potassium, 95 per cent absorption throughout; calcium, 40 per cent, phosphorus, 80 per cent and magnesium, 20 per cent throughout.

[**]Based on arithmetic mean weight for the weight interval. (Data of O'Donnell, A. M., Ziegler, E. E., and Fomon, S. J., reproduced with permission of Dr. Fomon.)

# Appendix V

## ILLUSTRATIVE FORMS AND NORMAL VALUES

*Premature Weight Chart*

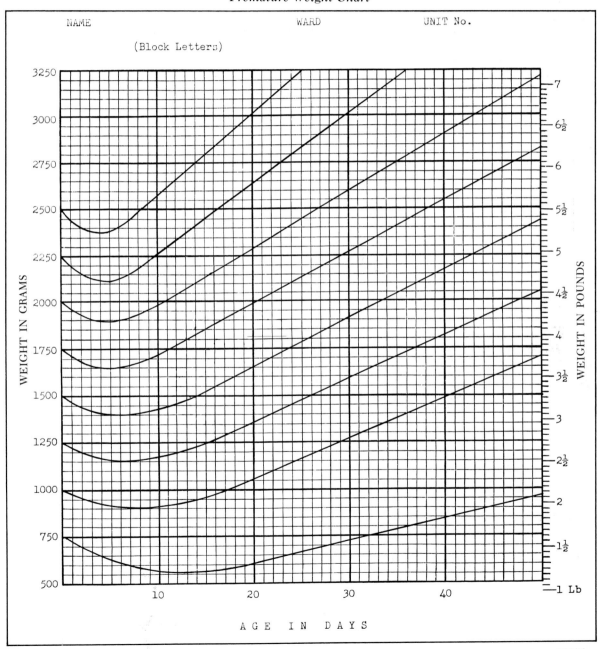

*Obstetrics Hospital Admission Form*

THE JOHNS HOPKINS HOSPITAL

**OBSTETRICS**

**HOSPITAL ADMISSION**

HISTORY NO.

PATIENT'S NAME

**BABY HISTORY NO.**

Admitted _____ M _____ 19____ (In Labor _____ Hrs.) By Dr. _____

Age _____ Parity _____ E.D.C. _____ S.T.S.: ☐ Pos. ☐ Neg.

Blood Type _____ Rh. ☐ Pos. ☐ Neg. Antibodies: ☐ Pos. ☐ Neg. Last Titre _____
DATE

Family & Past History (Describe Positive Information Rx-dates etc.) _____

Obstetric History Comments _____

   Complications prev. pregs. _____

   Complications this preg. _____

   Drugs this preg. _____

GENERAL CONDITION: ☐ Good ☐ Fair ☐ Critical ☐ Moribund ☐ Febrile ☐ Afebrile

HEART_____LUNGS_____

RUPTURE OF MEMBRANES (Time & Date)_____ M _____ 19_____ Cervix _____ cms

     ☐ Spontaneous ☐ Artificial ☐ Premature ☐ Early ☐ Late

PRESENTATION: Admission _____ Full dilatation _____ Delivery_____

LABOR: Onset ☐ Spontaneous ☐ Induced

   Onset _____ M _____ 19 _____ Full dilatation _____ M _____ 19 _____

   Child born _____ M _____ 19 _____ Placenta delivered _____ M _____ 19 _____

   Oxtoxic: (P.P.)_____ Blood Loss _____ c.c. ☐ measured ☐ estimated

   Duration of labor_____ hrs. 1st stage _____ hrs. 2nd stage _____ hrs. 3rd stage _____ hrs.

Analgesia:     Time Given     Drugs     Dose     Route

1.

2.

3.

Anesthesia: Time Started _____ Method & Agent _____

   Delivery: ☐ Spontaneous ☐ Operative

        INDICATION            OPERATION

_____

_____

_____

_____

_____ Epis: _____ Tear: _____ ☐ Repaired

NEWBORN INFORMATION: Sex _____ Apgar Score _____ At Three Min. _____

Immed. Condition: ☐ Good ☐ Fair ☐ Poor

RESUSC.: 02 MASK 02 IPP M-M IPP M-T IPP INTUB. #DRUGS Massage Other

Physical Examination (Comment if abnormal)

Cord:    No. of Vessels:

Placenta:    Wt.

Measurements:

| | | |
|---|---|---|
| Birth Weight | _____ | gms |
| Body Length | _____ | cms |
| C.R. Length | _____ | " |
| Shoulders | _____ | " |
| SOB (circ.) | _____ | " |
| BIP | _____ | " |

JHH FORM 3.069 (REVISED 5-66) REPLACING 8009 & 6

Physician in charge: Dr. _____ Delivered by: Dr. _____

### Normal Blood Chemistry Values, Term Infants

| Determination | Sample Source | Cord | 1–12 hr | 12–24 hr | 24–48 hr | 48–72 hr |
|---|---|---|---|---|---|---|
| Sodium, mEq/L[*] | Capillary | 147 (126–166) | 143 (124–156) | 145 (132–159) | 148 (134–160) | 149 (139–162) |
| Potassium, mEq/L | | 7.8 (5.6–12) | 6.4 (5.3–7.3) | 6.3 (5.3–8.9) | 6.0 (5.2–7.3) | 5.9 (5.0–7.7) |
| Chloride, mEq/L | | 103 (98–110) | 100.7 (90–111) | 103 (87–114) | 102 (92–114) | 103 (93–112) |
| Calcium, mg/100 ml | | 9.3 (8.2–11.1) | 8.4 (7.3–9.2) | 7.8 (6.9–9.4) | 8.0 (6.1–9.9) | 7.9 (5.9–9.7) |
| Phosphorus, mg/100 ml | | 5.6 (3.7–8.1) | 6.1 (3.5–8.6) | 5.7 (2.9–8.1) | 5.9 (3.0–8.7) | 5.8 (2.8–7.6) |
| Blood urea, mg/100 ml | | 29 (21–40) | 27 (8–34) | 33 (9–63) | 32 (13–77) | 31 (13–68) |
| Total protein, gm/100 ml | | 6.1 (4.8–7.3) | 6.6 (5.6–8.5) | 6.6 (5.8–8.2) | 6.9 (5.9–8.2) | 7.2 (6.0–8.5) |
| Blood sugar mg/100 ml | | 73 (45–96) | 63 (40–97) | 63 (42–104) | 56 (30–91) | 59 (40–90) |
| Lactic acid, mg/100 ml | | 19.5 (11–30) | 14.6 (11–24) | 14.0 (10–23) | 14.3 (9–22) | 13.5 (7–21) |
| Lactate, mm/L[†] | | 2.0–3.0 | 2.0 | | | |

[*]Acharya and Payne: Arch. Dis. Childhood *40*:430, 1965.
[†]Daniel, Adamsons, and James: Pediatrics 37:942, 1966.

### Normal Blood Chemistry Values, Low Birth Weight Infants, Capillary Blood, First Day[*]

| Determination | <1000 | 1001–1500 | 1501–2000 | 2001–2500 |
|---|---|---|---|---|
| Sodium, mEq/L | 138 | 133 | 135 | 134 |
| Potassium, mEq/L | 6.4 | 6.0 | 5.4 | 5.6 |
| Chloride, mEq/L | 100 | 101 | 105 | 104 |
| Total $CO_2$, mEq/L | 19 | 20 | 20 | 20 |
| Urea, mg/100 ml | 22 | 21 | 16 | 16 |
| TSP, gm/100 ml | 4.8 | 4.8 | 5.2 | 5.3 |

[*]Data from Pincus et al.: Pediatrics, *18*:39, 1956.

## Normal Values for Cerebrospinal Fluid*

|  | *Prematures* | *Term Babies* |
|---|---|---|
| Color | Xanthochromic mostly | Clear or xanthochromic |
| White cell count | 8–10 (range 0–44) | 6–8 (range 0–34) |
| Protein | 180 mg per 100 ml (range 40–180) | 45 mg per 100 ml (range 30–102) |

Protein content, highest on the first day, tends to be under 50 mg per 100 ml by 1 month.
Sugar and chlorides must be compared to values in blood.

*Data from Samson: Ergebn. d. inn. Med. u. Kinderh. *41*:553, 1931; Otilia: Acta Paed. *35*: Suppl. 8, 1948; Bauer et al.: J. Pediat. *66*:1017, 1965; Wolf and Hoepffuer: World Neurol. *2*:871, 1961; and Widell, Acta Paed. *47*: Suppl. *115*, 1958.

## Hematologic Values*

|  |  | *1–3 days* | *4–7 days* | *2 weeks* | *4 weeks* | *6 weeks* | *8 weeks* |
|---|---|---|---|---|---|---|---|
| <1200 gm birth weight | Hgb | 15.6 | 16.4 | 15.5 | 11.3 | 8.5 | 7.8 |
|  | Retic | 8.4 | 3.9 | 1.9 | 4.1 | 5.4 | 6.1 |
|  | Plat | 148,000 ±61,000 | 163,000 ±69,000 | 162,000 | 158,000 | 210,000 | 212,000 |
|  | Leuk | 14,800 ±10,200 | 12,200 ±7000 | 15,800 | 13,200 | 10,800 | 9900 |
|  | Seg | 46 | 32 | 41 | 28 | 23 | 23 |
|  | Band | 10.7 | 9.7 | 8.0 | 5.9 | 5.8 | 4.4 |
|  | Juv | 2.0 | 3.9 | 5.3 | 3.6 | 2.6 | 2.0 |
|  | Lymph | 32 | 43 | 39 | 55 | 61 | 65 |
|  | Monos | 5 | 7 | 5 | 4 | 6 | 3 |
|  | Eos | 0.4 | 6.2 | 1.0 | 3.7 | 2.0 | 3.8 |
|  | Nuc/RBC | 16.7 | 1.1 | 0.1 | 1.0 | 2.7 | 2.0 |
| >1200–<1500 gm birth weight | Hgb | 20.2 | 18.0 | 17.1 | 12.0 | 9.1 | 8.3 |
|  | Retic | 2.7 | 1.2 | 0.9 | 1.0 | 2.2 | 2.7 |
|  | Plat | 151,000 ±35,000 | 134,000 ±49,000 | 153,000 | 189,000 | 212,000 | 244,000 |
|  | Leuk | 10,800 ±4000 | 8900 ±2900 | 14,300 | 11,000 | 10,500 | 9100 |
|  | Seg | 47 | 31 | 33 | 26 | 20 | 25 |
|  | Band | 11.9 | 10.5 | 5.9 | 3.0 | 1.4 | 2.1 |
|  | Juv | 5.1 | 2.4 | 2.7 | 1.8 | 1.7 | 1.6 |
|  | Lymph | 34 | 48 | 52 | 59 | 69 | 64 |
|  | Monos | 3 | 6 | 3 | 4 | 5 | 5 |
|  | Eos | 1.3 | 2.2 | 2.5 | 5.1 | 2.6 | 2.3 |
|  | Nuc/RBC | 19.8 | 0.8 | 0 | 0.4 | 1.4 | 1.0 |

*Wolff and Goodfellow: Pediatrics *16*:753, 1955.

## TERM NEWBORN

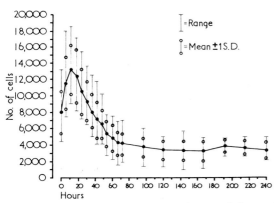

Means, ranges, and means ±1 SD of neutrophils on 15 full-term healthy babies during the first 10 days of life.

## PREMATURES

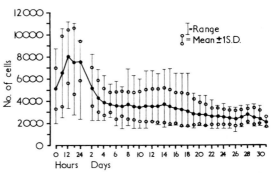

Means, ranges, and means ±1 SD of neutrophils of 14 healthy babies during the first month of life (13 premature +1 small for dates).

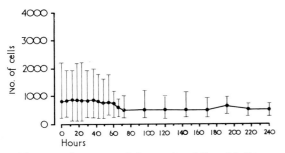

Means and ranges of the eosinophils of full-term babies during the first 10 days of life.

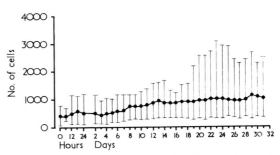

Means and ranges of eosinophils of low birth weight babies during the first month of life.

Data of M. Xanthou: Arch. Dis. Child. 45:242, 1970.

## TERM NEWBORN

## PREMATURES

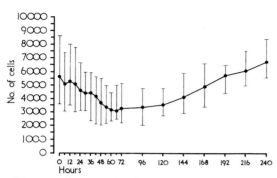

Means and ranges of lymphocytes of full-term babies during the first 10 days of life.

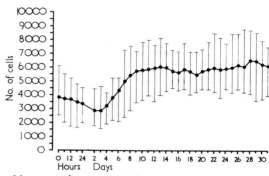

Means and ranges of lymphocytes of low birth weight babies during the first month of life.

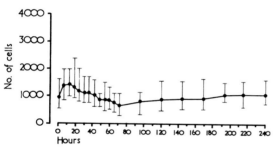

The mean and range of the monocytes healthy full-term babies during the first 10 days of life.

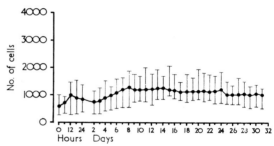

Means and ranges of monocytes of low birth weight babies during the first month of life.

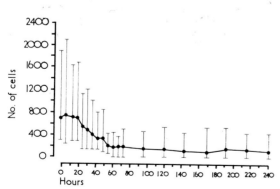

Means and ranges of metamyelocytes of full-term babies during the first 10 days of life.

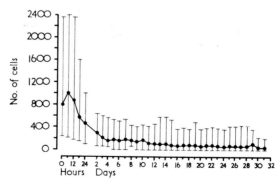

Means and ranges of metamyelocytes of 14 healthy babies during the first month of life.

### *Average Systolic, Diastolic and Mean Blood Pressures during the First 12 Hours of Life in Normal Newborn Infants Grouped According to Birth Weight**

| Birth Weight | Hour | 1 | 2 | 3 | 4 | 5 | 6 | 7 | 8 | 9 | 10 | 11 | 12 |
|---|---|---|---|---|---|---|---|---|---|---|---|---|---|
| 1001 to 2000 gm | Systolic | 49 | 49 | 51 | 52 | 53 | 52 | 52 | 52 | 51 | 51 | 49 | 50 |
| | Diastolic | 26 | 27 | 28 | 29 | 31 | 31 | 31 | 31 | 31 | 30 | 29 | 30 |
| | Mean | 35 | 36 | 37 | 39 | 40 | 40 | 39 | 39 | 38 | 37 | 37 | 38 |
| 2001 to 3000 gm | Systolic | 59 | 57 | 60 | 60 | 61 | 58 | 64 | 60 | 63 | 61 | 60 | 59 |
| | Diastolic | 32 | 32 | 32 | 32 | 33 | 34 | 37 | 34 | 38 | 35 | 35 | 35 |
| | Mean | 43 | 41 | 43 | 43 | 44 | 43 | 45 | 43 | 44 | 44 | 43 | 42 |
| Over 3000 gm | Systolic | 70 | 67 | 65 | 65 | 66 | 66 | 67 | 67 | 68 | 70 | 66 | 66 |
| | Diastolic | 44 | 41 | 39 | 41 | 40 | 41 | 41 | 41 | 44 | 43 | 41 | 41 |
| | Mean | 53 | 51 | 50 | 50 | 51 | 50 | 50 | 51 | 53 | 54 | 51 | 50 |

*Kitterman, J. A., Phibbs, R. H., and Tooley, W. H.: Pediatrics 44:959, 1969.

### *Representative Values in Normal Infants at Term**

| | Umbilical vein | 30 min | 1–4 hr | 12–24 hr | 24–48 hr | 96 hr | Reference |
|---|---|---|---|---|---|---|---|
| | | | | Arterial Blood | | | |
| pH | 7.33 | | 7.30 | 7.30 | 7.39 | 7.39 | Reardon et al. (1960) |
| PCO$_2$ mm Hg | 43 | | 39 | 33 | 34 | 36 | Oliver et al. (1961) |
| HCO$_3$ mEq/liter | 21.6 | | 18.8 | 19.5 | 20 | 21.4 | Nelson et al. (1962, |
| Po$_2$ mm Hg | 28 ± 8 | | 62 ± 13.8 | 68 | 63–87 | | 1963) |
| O$_2$ saturation | | | 95% | 94% | 94% | 96% | |
| Crying vital capacity ml (for 3 kg infant) | | 77 range (56–110) | | | 92 (69–128) | 100 | Sutherland and Ratcliff (1961) |
| Functional residual capacity, ml/kg | | 22 ± 8 | 25 ± 8 | 21 ± 1 | 28 ± 7 | 39 ± 9 | Klaus et al. (1962) |
| Lung compliance ml/cm H$_2$O/kg | | 1.5 ± 0.05 | | 2.0 ± 0.4 | | 1.7 | Cook et al. (1957) |
| Lung compliance/FRC ml/cm H$_2$O/ml | | | 0.04 ± 0.10 | .053 ± 0.009 | | 0.065 | Chu et al. (1964) Cook et al. (1957) |
| Right to left shunt as percentage cardiac output | | | 22% (range 11–29%) | 24% (17–32%) | | | Prod'hom et al. (1964) |

| | | Comment | Reference |
|---|---|---|---|
| Respiratory frequency | 34/min. range 20–60 | 1–2 days 1–11 days | Cook et al. (1955) Cross (1949) |
| Resistances cm H$_2$O/liter/sec | 29, 26 18 ± 6/3 | Total lung resistance Airway resistance | Cook et al. (1949), Swyer et al. (1960), Polgar (1962) |
| Flow rates ml/sec | 48–37 161–106 | Max. insp., max. exp. rest crying | Swyer et al. (1957), Long and Hull (1961) |
| Ventilation ml/kg/min | 200 | | Cook et al. (1955), Nelson et al. (1962) |
| Dead space ml | 4.4–9.2 | Term infants | Nelson et al. (1962), Cook et al. (1955), Strang (1961) |
| Alveolar ventilation ml/kg/min | 120–145 | First 3 days of life | Nelson et al. (1962) |
| O$_2$ consumption ml/kg/min | 6.2 | At neutral temperature | Oliver and Karlberg (1963) |
| CO$_2$ production ml/kg/min | 5.1 | At neutral temperature | Oliver and Karlberg (1963) |
| Alveolar-arterial O$_2$ differences mm Hg | 28 ± 10, room air 311 ± 70, 100% O$_2$ | Age 7 hr to 42 days Age 6 to 58 hr, 3 infants | Nelson et al. (1963) |
| Arterial-alveolar CO$_2$ differences mm Hg | 1.8 ± 3.8 | Age 3 to 74 hours | Nelson et al. (1962) |

*From Avery, M. E., and Normand, C.: Anesthesiology 26:510, 1965.

## Temperature Equivalents

| Celsius | Fahrenheit | Celsius | Fahrenheit |
|---------|-----------|---------|-----------|
| 34.0 | 93.2 | 38.6 | 101.4 |
| 34.2 | 93.6 | 38.8 | 101.8 |
| 34.4 | 93.9 | 39.0 | 102.2 |
| 34.6 | 94.3 | 39.2 | 102.5 |
| 34.8 | 94.6 | 39.4 | 102.9 |
| 35.0 | 95.0 | 39.6 | 103.2 |
| 35.2 | 95.4 | 39.8 | 103.6 |
| 35.4 | 95.7 | 40.0 | 104.0 |
| 35.6 | 96.1 | 40.2 | 104.3 |
| 35.8 | 96.4 | 40.4 | 104.7 |
| 36.0 | 96.8 | 40.6 | 105.1 |
| 36.2 | 97.1 | 40.8 | 105.4 |
| 36.4 | 97.5 | 41.0 | 105.8 |
| 36.6 | 97.8 | 41.2 | 106.1 |
| 36.8 | 98.2 | 41.4 | 106.5 |
| 37.0 | 98.6 | 41.6 | 106.8 |
| 37.2 | 98.9 | 41.8 | 107.2 |
| 37.4 | 99.3 | 42.0 | 107.6 |
| 37.6 | 99.6 | 42.2 | 108.0 |
| 37.8 | 100.0 | 42.4 | 108.3 |
| 38.0 | 100.4 | 42.6 | 108.7 |
| 38.2 | 100.7 | 42.8 | 109.0 |
| 38.4 | 101.1 | 43.0 | 109.4 |

To convert Celsius to Fahrenheit:

$$9/5 \times \text{Temperature} + 32$$

Example: To convert 40° Celsius to Fahrenheit
$$9/5 \times 40 = 72 + 32 = 104° \text{ Fahrenheit}$$

To convert Fahrenheit to Celsius

$$(\text{Temperature minus } 32) \times 5/9$$

Example: To convert 98.6° Fahrenheit to Celsius
$$98.6 - 32 = 66.6 \times 5/9 = 37° \text{ Celsius}$$

### Conversion of Pounds and Ounces to Grams

| Ounces | 1 lb | 2 lb | 3 lb | 4 lb | 5 lb | 6 lb | 7 lb | 8 lb |
|--------|------|------|------|------|------|------|------|------|
| | | | | Grams | | | | |
| 0 | 454 | 907 | 1361 | 1814 | 2268 | 2722 | 3175 | 3629 |
| 1 | 482 | 936 | 1389 | 1843 | 2296 | 2750 | 3204 | 3657 |
| 2 | 510 | 964 | 1418 | 1871 | 2325 | 2778 | 3232 | 3686 |
| 3 | 539 | 992 | 1446 | 1899 | 2353 | 2807 | 3260 | 3714 |
| 4 | 567 | 1021 | 1474 | 1928 | 2381 | 2835 | 3289 | 3742 |
| 5 | 595 | 1049 | 1503 | 1956 | 2410 | 2863 | 3317 | 3771 |
| 6 | 624 | 1077 | 1531 | 1985 | 2438 | 2892 | 3345 | 3799 |
| 7 | 652 | 1106 | 1559 | 2013 | 2466 | 2920 | 3374 | 3827 |
| 8 | 680 | 1134 | 1588 | 2041 | 2495 | 2948 | 3402 | 3856 |
| 9 | 709 | 1162 | 1616 | 2070 | 2523 | 2977 | 3430 | 3884 |
| 10 | 737 | 1191 | 1644 | 2098 | 2552 | 3005 | 3459 | 3912 |
| 11 | 765 | 1219 | 1673 | 2126 | 2580 | 3033 | 3487 | 3941 |
| 12 | 794 | 1247 | 1701 | 2155 | 2608 | 3062 | 3515 | 3969 |
| 13 | 822 | 1276 | 1729 | 2183 | 2637 | 3090 | 3544 | 3997 |
| 14 | 851 | 1304 | 1758 | 2211 | 2665 | 3119 | 3572 | 4026 |
| 15 | 879 | 1332 | 1786 | 2240 | 2693 | 3147 | 3600 | 4054 |

### Conversion of Inches to Centimeters

| Inches | cm | Inches | cm | Inches | cm |
|--------|------|--------|-------|--------|-------|
| 10 | 25.40 | 15 | 38.10 | 20 | 50.80 |
| 10½ | 26.67 | 15½ | 39.37 | 20½ | 52.07 |
| 11 | 27.94 | 16 | 40.64 | 21 | 53.34 |
| 11½ | 29.21 | 16½ | 41.91 | 21½ | 54.61 |
| 12 | 30.48 | 17 | 43.18 | 22 | 55.88 |
| 12½ | 31.75 | 17½ | 44.45 | 22½ | 57.15 |
| 13 | 33.02 | 18 | 45.72 | 23 | 58.42 |
| 13½ | 34.29 | 18½ | 46.99 | 23½ | 56.69 |
| 14 | 35.56 | 19 | 48.26 | 24 | 60.96 |
| 14½ | 36.83 | 19½ | 49.53 | | |

## Composition of Frequently Used Formulas

| Formula | Dilution | cal/cc or ml | Protein | Fat | CHO | Type of carbohydrate | Na | K | Ca | P° | Remarks |
|---|---|---|---|---|---|---|---|---|---|---|---|
| | | | Percentage composition | | | | mEq per L | | mg per L | | |
| Alacta | 15 gm/100 ml | 0.67 | 5.0 | 2.0 | 7.0 | Lactose | 32 | 45 | 1580 | 1200 | |
| Baker's | 1:1 | 0.67 | 2.2 | 3.3 | 7.0 | Lactose, dextrose, maltose, dextrins | 17 | 23 | 870 | 700 | Trace of iron |
| Beniflex | | 0.80 | 2.84 | 3.7 | 9.1 | Lactose, sucrose | 20 | 32.5 | 500 | 464 | |
| Breast | | 0.67 | 1.2 | 3.5 | 7.0 | Lactose | 7 | 14 | 340 | 155 | 133 mOsm/L |
| Bremil (liquid) | 1:1 | 0.67 | 1.5 | 3.5 | 7.0 | Lactose | 13 | 22 | 600 | 400 | Trace of iron |
| Bremil (powder) | 1 tbsp powder/2 fluid oz water | 0.67 | 1.5 | 3.5 | 7.0 | Lactose | 16 | 36 | 600 | 400 | Trace of iron |
| Cow's milk | 1:1 | 0.67 | 3.3 | 3.7 | 4.8 | Lactose | 25 | 35 | 1240 | 950 | 362 mOsm/L |
| Enfamil (liquid) | 1:1 | 0.67 | 1.5 | 3.7 | 7.0 | Lactose | 11 | 16 | 650 | 500 | 1 mg iron/L |
| Enfamil (powder) | | 0.67 | 1.5 | 3.7 | 7.0 | Lactose | 11 | 16 | 650 | 500 | |
| Enfamil with iron | 1:1 | 0.67 | 1.5 | 3.7 | 7.0 | Lactose | 11 | 16 | 650 | 500 | 8 mg iron/L |
| Goat's milk | | 0.67 | 3.3 | 4.1 | 4.7 | | | | | | |
| Isomil | 1:1 | 0.67 | 2.0 | 3.6 | 6.8 | Corn syrup, solids, sucrose | 13 | 18 | 700 | 500 | 12 mg iron/L |
| Lactum (liquid) | 1:1 | 0.67 | 2.7 | 2.8 | 7.8 | Lactose, dextrins, maltose | 17 | 28 | 1020 | 780 | |
| Lactum (powder) | 1 measuring cup powder/2 fluid oz | 0.67 | 2.7 | 2.8 | 7.8 | Lactose, dextrins, maltose | 21 | 29 | 1020 | 780 | |
| Lofenalac | 1 measuring cup/2 fluid oz. water | 0.67 | 2.2 | 2.7 | 8.5 | Maltose, dextrin, starch, sucrose, gluconic acid | 26 | 34 | 1000 | 700 | |
| Lonalac | 1 measuring cup/28 fluid oz water | 5 cal./gm. | 3.4 | 3.5 | 4.8 | Lactose | 1 | 34 | 1200 | 1150 | Low sodium |
| Modilac | 1:1 | 0.67 | 2.15 | 2.7 | 7.8 | Lactose, dextrose, maltose, dextrins | 17 | 21 | 800 | 605 | 10 mg iron/L |
| Mullsoy (liquid) | 1:1 | 0.67 | 3.1 | 3.6 | 5.2 | Sucrose, invert sugar | 16 | 40 | 1200 | 800 | Soybean protein |
| Mullsoy (powder) | 1 tbsp. powder/2 fluid oz water | 0.67 | 3.1 | 4.0 | 4.5 | Sucrose, dextrose | 26 | 35 | 1300 | 765 | |
| Nutramigen | 1 measuring cup powder/2 fluid oz water | 0.67 | 2.2 | 2.6 | 8.5 | Sucrose, starch | 17.4 | 25.6 | 1000 | 700 | Casein hydrolysate; 50 mOsm/L |
| Olac | 1 measuring cup/2 fluid oz water | 0.67 | 3.4 | 2.7 | 7.5 | Lactose, dextrins, maltose | 26 | 36 | 1280 | 986 | |
| Premature formula (Mead Johnson) | 1:1 | 0.8 | 2.8 | 3.7 | 9.1 | Lactose, sucrose | | | 900 | 750 | Trace iron |
| Probana | 1 measuring cup/2 fluid oz | 0.67 | 3.9 | 2.0 | 7.3 | Lactose, dextrose, fructose, sucrose, dextrins, starch | 26 | 31 | 1000 | 900 | |
| Prosobee | 1:1 | 0.67 | 2.5 | 3.4 | 6.8 | | | | 800 | 600 | |
| Similac (liquid) | 1:1 | 0.67 | 1.7 | 3.4 | 6.6 | Lactose | 11 | 28 | 670 | 517 | Trace of iron |
| Similac with iron (liquid and powder) | 1:1 | 0.67 | 1.7 | 3.4 | 6.6 | Lactose | 11 | 28 | 670 | 517 | 12 mg iron/L |
| Similac (powder) | | 0.67 | 1.7 | 3.4 | 6.6 | Lactose | 15 | 28 | 770 | 510 | Trace of iron |
| Similac PM 60/40 | 1 measuring cup/2 fluid oz | 0.67 | 1.5 | 3.4 | 7.2 | Lactose | 7 | 14 | 330 | 170 | 2 mg iron/L |
| SMA-14 | 1:1 | 0.67 | 1.1 | 3.7 | 7.2 | Lactose | 7.8 | 11.2 | 400 | 310 | 5.3 mg iron/L |
| SMA-26 | 1:1 | 0.67 | 1.5 | 3.6 | 7.2 | Lactose | 6.5 | 14 | 420 | 330 | 7.5 mg iron/L |
| SMA-29 | 14.2 gm powder and water to 100 ml | 0.67 | 1.65 | 2.2 | 9.8 | Lactose | 0.44 | 12.5 | 140 | 170 | Trace of iron |
| Sobee | 1:1 | 0.67 | 3.2 | 2.6 | 7.7 | Soya carbohydrate, sucrose, dextrins, maltose | 22 | 33 | 1000 | 544 | |

°Calculated for valance of 1.8.

### Examples of Commercially Prepared Formulas with Protein From Soy Isolate or Soy Flour

| | Soy isolate | Soy flour |
|---|---|---|
| **Components** | | |
| Protein | Soy isolate | Soy flour |
| Fat | Vegetable oils | Vegetable oils |
| Carbohydrate | Corn syrup solids and/or sucrose | Corn syrup solids and/or sucrose |
| **Examples** | | |
| | Isomil (Ross) | Sobee (Bristol Myers)[*] |
| | Neo-Mull-Soy (Syntex) | Mull-Soy (Syntex) |
| | Pro-Sobee (Mead Johnson) | |
| | Nursoy (Wyeth) | |
| **Major constituents (gm/100 ml)** | | |
| Protein | 1.8–2.5 | 3.1–3.2 |
| Fat | 3.0–3.6 | 2.6–3.6 |
| Carbohydrate | 6.4–6.8 | 5.2–7.7 |
| Minerals | 0.4–0.5 | 0.5–0.8 |
| **Caloric distribution (% of calories)** | | |
| Protein | 12–15 | 19 |
| Fat | 45–48 | 35–49 |
| Carbohydrate | 39–40 | 32–46 |
| **Minerals per liter** | | |
| Calcium (mg) | 700–950 | 1060–1200 |
| Phosphorus (mg) | 500–690 | 530–800 |
| Sodium (meq) | 9–24 | 16–22 |
| Potassium (meq) | 15–28 | 33–41 |
| Chloride (meq) | 7–15 | 14–16 |
| Magnesium (mg) | 50–80 | 75 |
| Copper (mg) | 0.4–0.6 | 0.4 |
| Zinc (mg) | 2.0–5.3 | 3.0 |
| Iodine ($\mu$g) | 70–160 | 70–160 |
| Iron (mg) | 8.5–12.7 | 5.0–8.5 |
| **Vitamins per liter** | | |
| Vitamin A (I.U.) | 2100–2500 | 1590–2110 |
| Thiamin ($\mu$g) | 400–700 | 530 |
| Riboflavin ($\mu$g) | 600–1060 | 850–1060 |
| Niacin (mg) | 5.0–8.4 | 7.4–9.5 |
| Pyridoxine ($\mu$g) | 400–530 | 420–430 |
| Pantothenate (mg) | 2.6–5.0 | 1.0–2.6 |
| Folacin ($\mu$g) | 50–100 | 70 |
| Vitamin $B_{12}$ ($\mu$g) | 2.0–3.0 | 2.1 |
| Vitamin C (mg) | 50–55 | 42–53 |
| Vitamin D (I.U.) | 400–423 | 423 |
| Vitamin E (I.U.) | 9–11 | 5–11 |
| Vitamin K (mg) | 0.09–0.15 | 0.09 |

[*]Not marketed in the United States.

From Fomon, S.: Infant Nutrition. 2nd ed. Philadelphia, W. B. Saunders Co., 1974. Reproduced by permission.

### Selected Special Formulas (Mead Johnson)

| | Nutramigen | Lofenalac | Portagen | Pregestimil |
|---|---|---|---|---|
| **Components** | | | | |
| Protein | Casein hydrolysate | Casein hydrolysate | Sodium caseinate | Casein hydrolysate |
| Fat | Corn oil | Corn oil | MCT and corn oil | MCT and corn oil |
| Carbohydrate | Sucrose and tapioca starch | Tapioca starch and corn syrup solids | Corn syrup solids and sucrose | Glucose and tapioca starch |
| **Major constituents (gm/100 ml)** | | | | |
| Protein | 2.2 | 2.2 | 2.3 | 2.2 |
| Fat | 2.6 | 2.7 | 3.2 | 2.8 |
| Carbohydrate | 8.6 | 8.7 | 7.7 | 8.8 |
| **Caloric distribution (% of calories)** | | | | |
| Protein | 13 | 13 | 14 | 13 |
| Fat | 35 | 35 | 42 | 36 |
| Carbohydrate | 52 | 52 | 44 | 51 |
| **Minerals per liter** | | | | |
| Calcium (mg) | 950 | 950 | 710 | 950 |
| Phosphorus (mg) | 660 | 660 | 560 | 740 |
| Sodium (meq) | 14 | 21 | 18 | 14 |
| Potassium (meq) | 27 | 27 | 27 | 24 |
| Chloride (meq) | 24 | 23 | 18 | 23 |
| Magnesium (mg) | 80 | 80 | 138 | 80 |
| Manganese (mg) | 2.1 | 2.1 | 2.1 | 2.1 |
| Copper (mg) | 0.64 | 0.64 | 1.06 | 0.64 |
| Zinc (mg) | 4.2 | 4.2 | 4.2 | 4.2 |
| Iodine ($\mu$g) | 70 | 69 | 106 | 69 |
| Iron (mg) | 12.7 | 12.7 | 12.7 | 12.7 |
| **Vitamins per liter** | | | | |
| Vitamin A (I.U.) | 2120 | 2120 | 2820 | 2120 |
| Thiamin ($\mu$g) | 635 | 635 | 1060 | 635 |
| Riboflavin ($\mu$g) | 1060 | 1060 | 1270 | 1060 |
| Niacin (mg) | 8.5 | 8.5 | 12.7 | 8.5 |
| Pyridoxine ($\mu$g) | 530 | 530 | 1370 | 530 |
| Pantothenate (mg) | 3.2 | 3.2 | 7.4 | 3.2 |
| Folacin ($\mu$g) | 50 | 50 | 70 | 50 |
| Vitamin $B_{12}$ ($\mu$g) | 2.6 | 2.6 | 3.5 | 2.6 |
| Vitamin C (mg) | 55 | 55 | 56 | 55 |
| Vitamin D (I.U.) | 423 | 423 | 282 | 423 |
| Vitamin E (I.U.) | 10.6 | 10.6 | 10.6 | 10.6 |
| Vitamin K (mg) | 0.11 | 0.11 | 0.04 | 0.11 |

*Examples of Commercially Prepared Milk-Based Formulas Marketed in the United States**

| Components | | | |
|---|---|---|---|
| Protein | Nonfat cow milk | Demineralized whey and nonfat cow milk | Nonfat cow milk and soy-protein isolate |
| Fat | Vegetable oils | Vegetable oils and oleo oil | Corn oil |
| Added carbohydrate | Lactose or corn syrup solids | Lactose | Sucrose |
| *Examples* | | | |
| | Enfamil† (Mead Johnson) Similac‡ (Ross) | SMA§ (Wyeth) | Similac Advance (Ross) |
| *Major constituents (gm/100 ml)* | | | |
| Protein | 1.5–1.6 | 1.5 | 3.6 |
| Fat | 3.6–3.7 | 3.6 | 1.6 |
| Carbohydrate | 7.0–7.1 | 7.2 | 6.6 |
| Minerals | 0.3–0.4 | 0.3 | 0.7 |
| *Caloric distribution (% of calories)* | | | |
| Protein | 9 | 9 | 26 |
| Fat | 48–50 | 48 | 27 |
| Carbohydrate | 41–43 | 43 | 47 |
| *Minerals per liter* | | | |
| Calcium (mg) | 550–600 | 445 | 1000 |
| Phosphorus (mg) | 440–455 | 330 | 800 |
| Sodium (meq) | 11–17 | 7 | 17 |
| Potassium (meq) | 16–28 | 14 | 32 |
| Chloride (meq) | 12–24 | 10 | 29 |
| Magnesium (mg) | 40–48 | 53 | 85 |
| Sulfur (mg) | 130–160 | 145 | 310 |
| Copper (mg) | 0.4–0.6 | 0.4 | 1 |
| Zinc (mg) | 2.0–4.2 | 3.2 | 4.0 |
| Iodine (µg) | 40–69 | 69 | 100 |
| Iron (mg) | trace–1.5‖ | 12.7 | 18 |
| *Vitamins per liter* | | | |
| Vitamin A (I.U.) | 1700–2500 | 2650 | 3000 |
| Thiamin (µg) | 400–650 | 710 | 750 |
| Riboflavin (µg) | 600–1000 | 1060 | 900 |
| Niacin (mg) | 7–8.5 | 7 | 10 |
| Pyridoxine (µg) | 320–400 | 423 | 700 |
| Pantothenate (mg) | 2.1–3.2 | 2.1 | 5 |
| Folacin (µg) | 50–100 | 32 | 100 |
| Vitamin $B_{12}$ (µg) | 1.5–2.0 | 1.1 | 2.5 |
| Vitamin C (mg) | 55 | 58 | 50 |
| Vitamin D (I.U.) | 400–423 | 423 | 400 |
| Vitamin E (I.U.) | 8.5–12.7 | 9.5 | 6.3 |

*Some are marketed in other countries as well.
†Enfalac in Canada.
‡Multival in some European countries.
§S-26 in other countries. Product marketed as SMA in other countries has different composition.
‖Products also available with 12 to 13 mg iron per liter.
(From Fomon, S.: Infant Nutrition. 2nd ed. Philadelphia, W. B. Saunders Co., 1974. Reproduced by permission.)

## DRUGS EXCRETED IN MILK (Courtesy of Dr. Peter Goldman)

When prescribing drugs to the nursing mother one must consider the added risk that these drugs may pass to the nursing infant. Most drugs get into the milk by passive diffusion; few, if any, are more concentrated to any significant extent in the mother's milk than in her plasma. Thus there is an inherent safety factor because the drug is transferred to the baby in discrete amounts only during the nursing period. The following table illustrates this dilution factor for some of the drugs that have been studied.

*Concentration of Various Drugs in Maternal Blood and Breast Milk Under Normal pH Conditions*

| Drug Administered (Therapeutic Dosage) | Drug Levels (unit/100 ml) Plasma or Serum (pH 7.4) | Milk (pH 7.0) | Administered Drug Appearing in Milk (%/day) |
|---|---|---|---|
| Aspirin | 1–5 mg | 1–3 mg | 0.5 |
| Bishydroxycoumarin | 11–16.5 mg | 0.2 mg | 0.5 |
| Chloral hydrate | 0–3 mg | 0–1.5 mg | 0.6 |
| Chloramphenicol | 2.5–5 mg | 1.5–2.5 mg | 1.3 |
| Chlorpromazine | 0.1 mg | 0.03 mg | 0.07 |
| Colistin sulfate | 0.3–0.5 mg | 0.05–0.09 mg | 0.07 |
| Cycloserine | 1.5–2 mg | 1–1.5 mg | 0.6 |
| Diphenylhydantoin | 0.3–4.5 mg | 0.6–1.8 mg | 1.4 |
| Erythromycin | 0.1–0.2 mg | 0.3–0.5 mg | 0.1 |
| Ethanol | 50–80 mg | 50–80 mg | 0.25 |
| Ethyl biscoumacetate | 2.7–14.5 mg | 0–0.17 mg | 0.1 |
| Folic acid | 3 $\mu$g | 0.07 $\mu$g | 0.1 |
| Imipramine hydrochloride | 0.2–1.3 mg | 0.1 mg | 0.1 |
| Iodine 131 | 0.002 $\mu$c | 0.13 $\mu$c | 2–5 |
| Isoniazid | 0.6–1.2 mg | 0.6–1.2 mg | 0.75 |
| Kanamycin sulfate | 0.5–3.5 mg | 0.2 mg | 0.05 |
| Lincomycin | 0.3–1.5 mg | 0.05–0.2 mg | 0.025 |
| Lithium carbonate | 0.2–1.1 mg | 0.07–0.4 mg | 0.12 |
| Meperidine hydrochloride | 0.07–0.1 mg | trace (<0.1 mg) | <0.1 |
| Methotrexate | 3 $\mu$g | 0.3 $\mu$g | 0.01 |
| Nalidixic acid | 3–5 mg | 0.4 mg | 0.05 |
| Novobiocin | 1.2–5.2 mg | 0.3–0.5 mg | 0.15 |
| Penicillin | 6–120 $\mu$g | 1.2–3.6 $\mu$g | 0.03 |
| Phenobarbital | 0.6–1.8 mg | 0.1–0.5 mg | 1.5 |
| Phenylbutazone | 2–5 mg | 0.2–0.6 mg | 0.4 |
| Pyrilamine maleate | – | 0.2 mg | 0.6 |
| Pyrimethamine | 0.7–1.5 mg | 0.3 mg | 0.3 |
| Quinine sulfate | 0.7 mg | 0.1 mg | 0.05 |
| Rifampin | 0.5 mg | 0.1–0.3 mg | 0.05 |
| Streptomycin sulfate | 2–3 mg | 1–3 mg | 0.5 |
| Sulfapyridine | 3–13 mg | 3–13 mg | 0.12 |
| Tetracycline hydrochloride | 80–320 $\mu$g | 50–260 $\mu$g | 0.03 |
| Thiouracil | 3–4 mg | 9–12 mg | 5 |

Modified from Vorherr, H.: The Breast: Morphology, Physiology, and Lactation. New York, Academic Press, Inc., 1974.

# INDEX

*Note:* Page numbers in *italics* refer to illustrations. Page numbers followed by (t) refer to tables.